Encyclopedia of Radiation Oncology

Luther W. Brady and Theodore E. Yaeger (Eds.)

Encyclopedia of Radiation Oncology

With 257 Figures and 156 Tables

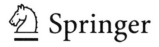 Springer

Editors
Luther W. Brady, MD
Distinguished University Professor
Hylda Cohn/American Cancer Professor Of
Clinical Oncology
Professor of Radiation Oncology
Drexel University College of Medicine
MS 200
216 North Broad St.
Philadelphia, PA 19102
USA

Theodore E. Yaeger, MD
Department of Radiation Oncology
Wake Forest University School of Medicine
Winston-Salem, NC 27157-0001
USA

ISBN 978-3-540-85513-2   ISBN 978-3-540-85516-3 (eBook)
ISBN 978-3-540-85517-0 (print and electronic bundle)
DOI 10.1007/978-3-540-85516-3
Springer Heidelberg Dordrecht London New York

Library of Congress Control Number: 2012936046

The Encyclopedia of Radiation Oncology is dedicated to all the families of the authors who allowed the editors work diligently and effectively in producing the Encyclopedia. It is also dedicated to the mentorship of the outstanding past leaders in radiation oncology; Simon Kramer, M.D., Gilbert Fletcher, M.D., and Henry Kaplan, M.D.

Luther W. Brady MD
Theodore E. Yaeger MD
Jay Reiff PhD
Reiner Class PhD
Stephan Mose MD

Preface

The Encyclopedia of Radiation Oncology represents a Herculean world-wide effort made on the part of many associate editors to develop basic statements relative to general oncology, radiation physics, radiation biology and clinical therapies. It is intended to serve as an informational document with cross references and references built on the style and construction of an encyclopedia. It is not a definitive text book in oncology but the groundwork for initial knowledge on a wide variety of topics that involve oncology, especially those related to modern radiotherapy.

The data has been put together in such a method to cover all of the important and newer oncologic viewpoints, including some controversies. It relates the many aspects of radiation therapy physics, the contemporary data with regard to radiation biology and, mostly, applied clinical oncology practice. As an encyclopedia, this represents a reference document serving as a springboard for the identification of substantial areas of noteworthy oncology subject matters. Topics needing further investigation should be found more fully developed in the suggested referenced journals and textbooks in oncology related to each chapter. Also, the cross references can identify related areas of interest within the encyclopedia leading to a variety of comparative subjects.

The authors are hopeful that this encyclopedia will serve as a useful strategic reference document for medical students, residents in oncology, non-oncologic medical practiioners as well as practicing radiation oncologists, medical oncologists, medical physicists, dosimetrists, biotherapists and the surgical aspects of oncology.

Acknowledgments

The editors would like to acknowledge the support of all the contributing authors to the preparation of this Encyclopedia. Without the ongoing continuing persistent input, the Encyclopedia could never have been finished. To all the families who suffered the indignities of the time committed by the authors and editors, you deserve our complete and everlasting praise and thanks.

About the Editors

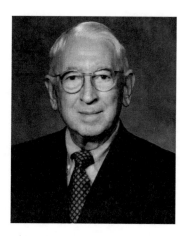

Luther W. Brady
Distinguished University Professor
Hylda Cohn/American Cancer Professor Of Clinical Oncology
Professor of Radiation Oncology
Drexel University College of Medicine
MS 200
216 North Broad St.
Philadelphia, PA. 19102
USA

Luther W. Brady, M.D., one of the world's foremost oncologists, is Hylda Cohn/American Cancer Society Professor of Clinical Oncology and Distinguished University Professor in the Department of Radiation Oncology at Drexel University College of Medicine, Philadelphia, Pennsylvania. Former Chairman of the Department of Radiation Oncology and Nuclear Medicine at Hahnemann University, Dr. Brady stepped down in 1996, having built during a distinguished tenure a department reputed for its teaching excellence and innovative approaches in the treatment of cancer. In June 1996, the University announced establishment of the Luther W. Brady, M.D. Professorship in Radiation Oncology in his honor. The following year, 1997, the Faculty Committee promoted Dr. Brady to the institution's highest academic rank of University Professor. In 1999, in recognition of exceptional contribution and accomplishment in the field of oncology, the American Medical Association presented Dr. Brady with the AMA Distinguished Service Award Gold Medal. Later that same year the Philadelphia County Medical Society granted him the 1999 Strittmatter Award, one of the most illustrious honors given for high achievement in the field of medicine. The Chairmanship in the Department of Radiation Oncology became open unexpectedly in January 2001, and Tenet Health System appointed Dr. Brady Interim-Chair of Radiation Oncology at Hahnemann University, Medical College of Pennsylvania (MCP), and Graduate Hospitals until a suitable candidate was located. He was appointed formally on January 26, 2001.

He has held the rank of Professor since 1963 and, in 1970, was appointed Chairman of the Department of Radiation Oncology and Nuclear Medicine. In 1975, he was named the Hylda Cohn/American Cancer Society Professor of Clinical Oncology. Hahnemann recognized Dr. Brady's enormous professional commitment and dedication by establishing the Luther W. Brady Pavilion in 1980. When Hahnemann University and Medical College of Pennsylvania merged in 1994 he was named Head of the combined MCP/Hahnemann University Department of Radiation Oncology and Nuclear Medicine.

Dr. Brady is a Fellow of the American College of Radiology and a Fellow of the American College of Radiation Oncology. He has been a member of the American College of Radiology Board of Chancellors, Chairman of the Commission on Radiation Oncology, and has served on numerous College committees. As well, he was Chairman of the Radiation Therapy Oncology Group, a nationwide consortium to evaluate forms of cancer treatment. From 1991 to 1993 he served as appointed Chairman of the Radiation Oncology Committee for ACGME (Accreditation Council for Graduate Medical Education).

Dr. Brady has received three medals honoring his outstanding contributions made in the arts and education:

- City of Philadelphia Distinguished Honoree Medal (1993) in appreciation for his many years of commitment to all of the cultural arts
- George Washington University Society Medal (1995) by the Trustees of the University
- James B. Colgate Society Medal (1995) by the Trustees of Colgate University in recognition and appreciation for his valuable contributions to Colgate University

His remarkable accomplishments during his career have been recognized in manifold ways. In 1990 Dr. Brady received the degree of Doctor of Science, Honoris Causa, from Lehigh University. That same year, George Washington University granted him the Distinguished Alumni Achievement Award. In 1995 he was elected to the University Board of Trustees of George Washington University, and in 1996 he was appointed to the Governing Board of the University's School of Medicine and Medical Center. In Japan in 1996 he received the honorary degree of Doctor of Medicine, Honoris Causa, from the Toyama Medical and Pharmaceutical University, and in 1997 the University of Heidelberg awarded him an honorary doctoral degree "doctoris medicinae honoris causa," a special and rare event in the oldest German university.

Honors have been numerous in Dr. Brady's career. Elected to Alpha Omega Alpha upon completion of his medical education, he has presented over twenty named lectureships. Among them, the:

- Ruvelson Lectureship, University of Minnesota Medical School (1978)
- Erskine Lecture of the Radiological Society of North America (1979)
- Janeway Lecture of the American Radium Society (1980)
- Maurice Lenz Memorial Lecture of Columbia Presbyterian Medical Center (1983)
- Elis Berven Lectureship of the Swedish Academy of Medicine (1986)
- Patricia Trost Friedler Oncology Lectureship of the Touro Infirmary, New Orleans, LA (1990)
- Probstein Oncology Lecture of the Mallinckrodt Institute of Radiology, St. Louis, MO (1990)
- Jerome M. Vaeth Distinguished Lectureship, W. Coast Cancer Foundation, San Francisco, CA (1991)
- Murray Houser Award and Lectureship, Pennsylvania Hospital, Philadelphia, PA (1992)
- Joseph A. Keelty Lectureship, Union Memorial Hospital, Baltimore, MD (1992)
- Hermann-Holthusen-Institut Lectureship, Hamburg, Germany (1992)
- E. Richard King Lectureship, Medical College of Virginia, Richmond, VA (1993)
- Ruvelson Lectureship in Gynecologic Cancer, University of Minnesota Medical School (1994)
- St. George's Hospital Distinguished Lectureship, University of Eppendorf, Germany (1997)

Dr. Brady has received twenty-eight medals in recognition of his achievement and contributions in his field, many of them gold medals. Thirteen are from societies in the United States:

- Chicago Radiological Society (1977)
- American Radium Society (1981)
- American College of Radiology (1983)
- Gilbert H. Fletcher Society (1984)
- Albert Soiland Society (1985)
- Juan A. del Regato Foundation (1986)
- American Society for Therapeutic Radiology and Oncology (1987)
- Academies of Practice (1988)
- Radiological Society of North America (1989)
- Gold Medal, American College of Radiation Oncology (1996)
- Gold Medal, American Medical Association (AMA) Distinguished Service Award (1999)
- Gold Medal, 1999 Strittmatter Award
- Pennsylvania Medical Society Distinguished Service Award (2011)

Fifteen medals have been granted by societies overseas:

- National Medical Society of Ecuador (1980)
- Catholic University, Rome (1984)
- University of Navarra, Pamplona, Spain (1986)
- Swedish Academy of Medicine (1986)
- Kyushu University, Fukuoka, Japan (1988)
- Georg-August-Universitat Medal of the University of Gottingen (1988)
- International Congress of Radiation Oncology (1989)
- Padre Pio Medal, Casa Sollievo della Sofferenzo, Foggia, Italy (1993)
- Pisa University on occasion of the 650th Anniversary of the School of Medicine, (1993)
- University Medal, Toyama Medical and Pharmaceutical University, Toyama, Japan (1996)
- University Medal, Kanzawa University School of Medicine, Kanazawa, Japan (1996)
- Gold Medal, Fondazaion Giorgio Caleri, Instituto of Poligrafico e Zecca Della State (1996)
- Silver Medal, The Fondazione Internationale, Pisa, Italy (1996)
- Silver Medal for Scientific Excellence, Pisa, Italy (1998)
- Silver Medal, Outstanding Contributions in Medical Education, Pisa, Italy (2000)

As well, Dr. Brady holds honorary fellowships from the Italian Society of Radiologic Medicine (1983), the Royal College of Radiologists (1985), the Deutsche Rontgengesellshaft (1985), and the Academy of Medicine of Belgium (1991). He was awarded Honorary Fellowship in de L'Academie Royale de Medecine de Belgique in Brussels during the occasion of its 150th Anniversary, and represents one of six living Americans who have been elected to the prestigious position as Academician of the Royal Academy. He is the first radiation oncologist to have been elected in its history. Elected a Fellow Member in the Royal Society of Medicine in London (1992), the following year he was elected Member in the Society of Radiology of the Royal Society of Medicine (1993). In 1997 he was elected to receive the

Deutsche Gesellshaft für Radioonkologie Honorary Fellowship, the first such award given by the German Society of Radiation Oncology.

He is also a member of the International Advisory Board of the Austrian/International Club for Radio-Oncologists of the Austrian Society for Radiooncology, Radiobiology & Medical Physics. He served on the Honorary Committee for the 4th International Congress of the International Union Against Cancer, and he has served, nationally and internationally, as chair or co-chair of numerous scientific sessions at conferences on cancer.

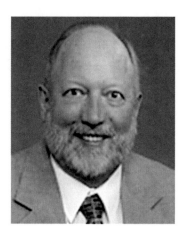

Theodore E. Yaeger
Associate Professor
Department Radiation Oncology
Wake Forest University School of Medicine
Winston-Salem, NC
27157-0001
USA

Dr. Yaeger graduated with a BS degree in biology and chemistry from University of New Mexico, Albuquerque, 1973, and pursued a MS degree in anatomy at Hahnemann University where he was admitted to the class of 1981 Medical School. After graduation with double honors and the Jane Stuart Prize, he completed a radiation oncology residency at Hahnemann in 1985. Dr. Yaeger then began working as a staff radiation oncologist in private practice at the Regional Oncology Center (ROC) in Daytona Beach, FL. He became board certified in Radiotherapy by The American Board of Radiology in 1986 and The American Board of Hyperbaric Medicine in 1988. Over the 20 years at the ROC he worked to successfully develop an outreach cancer center at Bert Fish Hospital in New Smyrna Beach, FL. Eventually he become the Director of Radiation Medicine and then the first Chairman of the Unified Department of Oncology for both centers. In 2006 he accepted a position as Associate Professor for Wake Forest University School of Medicine to become the medical director of radiation oncology at Caldwell Memorial Hospital (CMH). In 2010, Dr. Yaeger was recognized as a 'distinguished alumnus' by Drexel University for his continuing contributions to medicine. He is presently working with CMH to build the first unified cancer center as an outreach facility for Wake Forest/Baptist Medical Center. His ongoing research includes the copyrighted clinical application of a new technique for the least side-effect conservation treatment of primary breast cancer and a team member for the long-term follow-up of patients treated with radiolabeled antibody for primary brain cancer. He is a member of more than a dozen specialty medical organizations, serving on many committees, and is the Radiation Oncology representative member to The North Carolina Radiologic Society. His other contributions include chapters in several books, including the forthcoming 6th edition of 'Principles and Practice of Radiation Oncology', many peer reviewed journals and presentations of primary research at national meetings.

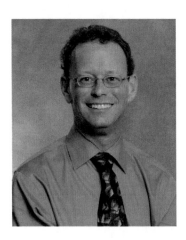

Jay Reiff
Professor and Chief of Physics
Department of Radiation Oncology
Drexel University College of Medicine
Hahnemann University Hospital
Philadelphia, PA
USA
jay.reiff@drexelmed.edu

Jay E. Reiff is a Professor of Radiation Oncology and the Chief of Physics in the Department of Radiation Oncology at Drexel University College of Medicine in Philadelphia, Pennsylvania. He has held this position since 2002.

Dr. Reiff received his B.S. from the University of Rochester in 1982 and his Ph.D. from the University of California, Berkeley in 1989. He completed a postdoctoral fellowship in the Department of Medical Physics at Memorial Sloan-Kettering Cancer Center in New York before joining the staff in the Department of Radiation Oncology at Thomas Jefferson University in Philadelphia in 1991. By 1997 he was in charge of all the medical physics services at the six remote satellite facilities under the TJU umbrella. He remained on staff at Thomas Jefferson University until 2002 having attained the rank of Associate Professor. He received his certification in Therapeutic Radiological Physics by the American Board of Radiology in 1994.

Over the years Dr. Reiff has held leadership positions in various professional societies and committees. He served a three year term on the Board of Directors of the American Association of Physicists in Medicine (AAPM) as the representative from the local Delaware Valley Chapter (DVC-AAPM). In addition, he has served as treasurer, secretary, and president of the Delaware Valley Chapter. He is also a member of the American Society for Radiation Oncology (ASTRO).

Dr. Reiff served on the Radiation Safety Committee of Frankford Hospital – Torresdale Division and was a member of the X-Ray Subcommittee of the Radiation Safety Committee at Thomas Jefferson University. He was a member of the Professional Studies Committee at Drexel University College of Medicine and currently serves on the Radiation Safety Committee of Hahnemann University Hospital.

Dr. Reiff has served as a peer reviewer (referee) for the Medical Physics journal, the International Journal of Radiation Oncology Biology Physics (Red Journal) and the Journal of Applied Clinical Medical Physics. He has authored or co-authored over 20 published peer-reviewed articles, 25 peer-reviewed oral presentations and over 35 peer-reviewed posters presented at national meetings. For four years he wrote questions for the American Board of Radiology for the Therapeutic Radiological Physics written examination. Additionally, he currently serves as a physics consultant to Cianna Medical, Inc. and is on the Editorial Advisory Board of their newsletter "BrachyBytes".

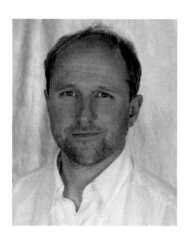

Dr. Reiner Class
Associate Professor
Department of Radiation Oncology
Drexel University
College of Medicine
Philadelphia, PA
USA
and
Head of Target Finding & Biological Profiling
Pharmacelsus GmbH, Science Park 2
66123 Saarbrücken
Germany

Dr. Class is scientific head of Target Finding & Biological Profiling at Pharmacelsus, a pre-clinical CRO located in Germany. Dr. Class received his diploma (1988) and Ph.D. degree (1991) in biology from the University of Saarland, Germany. From 1991-1992, he was visiting scientist in the Experimental Therapeutics group at the Wistar Institute of Anatomy in Philadelphia, PA. In 1992, he became faculty member in the Department of Radiation Oncology at Drexel University School of Medicine in Philadelphia, PA and where he was appointed associate professor. During his tenure at Drexel, he established and headed the Flow Cytometry Core Facility and provided support to the clinical flow cytometry unit of Hahnemann University Hospital. In 2001, Dr. Class accepted a position as Chief Scientific Officer of SymbioTec GmbH, a German biotechnology company developing anti-leukemia drugs. In 2007, he founded C-Square Consulting GbR providing support in all aspects of preclinical and clinical drug development. Dr. Class is (co-)author on more than 50 articles, book chapters and abstracts and holds several patents in the field of oncology, anti-bacterial and anti-viral therapeutics.

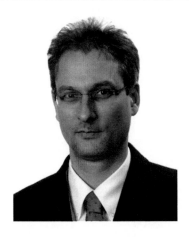

Dr. Stephan Mose
Department of Radiation Oncology
Schwarzwald-Baar-Klinikum
Villingen-Schwenningen
Germany
stephan.mose@sbk-vs.de
www.sbk-vs.de

Stephan Mose is a Professor of Radiation Oncology and since 2003 the Director of the Department of Radiation Oncology at the Schwarzwald-Baar-Klinikum, Villingen-Schwenningen, Germany.

In 1991, he received his M.D. from the Westfälische Wilhelms-University Hospital, Münster. From 1992–2003 he was working at the Johann Wolfgang Goethe–University Hospital, Frankfurt am Main. In 1998 and 2000, he has done experimental research at MCP Hahneman University, Philadelphia, USA. The postdoctorale lecture qualification was awarded to him in 2001. He became Professor in 2008.

Dr. Mose is a member of the Deutsche Gesellschaft für Radioonkologie (DEGRO), the Deutsche Krebsgesellschaft (DKG), the European Society of Radiotherapy and Oncology (ESTRO), and the American Society of Radiation Oncology (ASTRO). He has served as a peer-reviewer for the "International Journal of Radiation Oncology", and "Strahlentherapie und Onkologie". He is author and co-author of more than 100 peer-reviewed oral presentations and posters, and more than 50 peer-reviewed published articles and book-chapters. Furthermore, he is Advisory Editor of the "Journal of Radiation Oncology".

List of Contributors

CHRISTOPHER G. AINSLEY
Department of Radiation Oncology
University of Pennsylvania Hospital
Philadelphia, PA
USA

OGUZ AKIN
Body MRI
Memorial Sloan-Kettering Cancer Center
New York, NY
USA

FIORI ALITE
College of Medicine
Drexel University
Philadelphia, PA
USA

DOUGLAS W. ARTHUR
Department of Radiation Oncology
College of Medicine
Drexel University
Philadelphia, PA
USA

LUTHER W. BRADY
Department of Radiation Oncology
College of Medicine
Drexel University
Philadelphia, PA
USA

JAMES H. BRASHEARS, III
Radiation Oncologist
Venice, FL
USA

D. BOTTKE
Klinik für Radioonkologie und Strahlentherapie
Universitätsklinikum Ulm
Ulm
Germany

ARI D. BROOKS
College of Medicine
Drexel University
Philadelphia, PA
USA

VOLKER BUDACH
Department of Radiotherapy and Radiation
Oncology
Charité - University Hospital Berlin
Berlin
Germany

FELIPE A. CALVO
Department of Oncology
Hospital General Universitario Gregorio
Maranon
Madrid
Spain

JO ANN CHALAL
Department of Radiation Oncology
Fox Chase Cancer Center
Philadelphia, PA
USA

BOK AI CHOO
Department of Radiation Oncology
National University Cancer Institute
Singapore (NCIS)
Singapore

JOHN P. CHRISTODOULEAS
The Perelman Cancer Center
Department of Radiation Oncology
University of Pennsylvania Hospital
Philadelphia, PA
USA

JOHANNES CLASSEN
Department of Radiation Oncology
St. Vincentius-Kliniken Karlsruhe
Karlsruhe
Germany

JAY S. COOPER
Maimonides Cancer Center
New York, NY
USA

LARRY C. DAUGHERTY
Department of Radiation Oncology
College of Medicine
Drexel University
Glenside, PA
USA

ALBERT S. DeNITTIS
Lankenau Institute for Medical Research
Lankenau Hospital
Wynnewood, PA
USA

BERNADINE R. DONAHUE
Department of Radiation Oncology
Maimonides Cancer Center
Brooklyn, NY
USA

LAURA DOYLE
Department of Radiation Oncology
Thomas Jefferson University Hospital
Philadelphia, PA
USA

ANTHONY E. DRAGUN
Department of Radiation Oncology
James Graham Brown Cancer Center
University of Louisville School of Medicine
Louisville, KY
USA

JACQUELINE EMRICH
College of Medicine
Drexel University
Philadelphia, PA
USA

BRANDON J. FISHER
Department of Radiation Oncology
College of Medicine
Drexel University
Philadelphia, PA
USA

ROBERT D. FORREST
Radiation Safety
University of Pennsylvania
USA

JORGE E. FREIRE
Department of Radiation Oncology
Capital Health System – Mercer Campus
Trenton, NJ
USA

A. AL GHAZAL
Urologische Universitätsklinik
Ulm
Germany

ELI GLATSTEIN
Department of Radiation Oncology
University of Pennsylvania Hospital
Philadelphia, PA
USA

MANUEL GONZÁLEZ-DOMINGO
Department of Radiation Oncology
Oncology Institute
Viña del Mar
Chile

GERHARD G. GRABENBAUER
Chairman of the Department of Radiation
Oncology
DiaCura Coburg & Klinikum Coburg
Coburg
Germany

EDWARD J. GRACELY
Department of Epidemiology and Biostatistics
College of Medicine
Drexel University
Philadelphia, PA
USA

PATRIZIA GUERRIERI
Department of Radiation Oncology
Regional Cancer Center "M. Ascoli"
University of Palermo Medical School
Palermo
Italy

BRUCE G. HAFFTY
Department of Radiation Oncology
UMDNJ-Robert Wood Johnson Medical School
Cancer Institute of New Jersey
New Brunswick, NJ
USA

STEPHEN M. HAHN
Department of Radiation Oncology
University of Pennsylvania Hospital
Philadelphia, PA
USA

BRIAN F. HASSON
Department of Radiation Oncology
Abington Memorial Hospital
Abington, PA
USA
and
Department of Radiation Oncology
College of Medicine
Drexel University
Philadelphia, PA
USA

CURT HEESE
Department of Radiation Oncology
Eastern Regional Cancer Treatment Centers of
America
Philadelphia, PA
USA

HANS-PETER HEILMANN
Director of the Hermann-Holthusen-Institute
for Radiotherapy
St. George's Hospital, Hamburg, from 1976 to
2000
Hamburg
Germany

TIMOTHY HOLMES
Department of Radiation Oncology
Sinai Hospital
Baltimore, MD
USA

HEDVIG HRICAK
Department of Radiology
Memorial Sloan-Kettering Cancer Center
New York, NY
USA

M. Saiful Huq
Department of Radiation Oncology
University of Pittsburgh Medical Center Cancer
Pavilion
Pittsburgh, PA
USA

Bradley J. Huth
Department of Radiation Oncology
Philadelphia, PA
USA

Daniel J. Indelicato
Department of Radiation Oncology
University of Florida Proton Therapy Institute
University of Florida College of Medicine
Jacksonville, FL
USA

Lindsay G. Jensen
Center for Advanced Radiotherapy
Technologies
Department of Radiation Oncology
San Diego Rebecca and John Moores Cancer
Center
University of California
La Jolla, CA
USA

Grace J. Kim
Department of Radiation Oncology
University of Maryland
Baltimore, MD
USA

Christin A. Knowlton
Department of Radiation Oncology
Drexel University
Philadelphia, PA
USA

Lydia T. Komarnicky-Kocher
Department of Radiation Oncology
College of Medicine
Drexel University
Philadelphia, PA
USA

Feng-Ming Kong
Department of Radiation Oncology
Veteran Administration Health Center and
University Hospital
University of Michigan
Ann Arbor, MI
USA

Kent Lambert
Radiation Oncology
College of Medicine
Drexel University
Philadelphia, PA
USA

John P. Lamond
Department of Radiation Oncology
Temple University
Crozer-Chester Medical Center
Upland, PA
USA

Rachelle Lanciano
Department of Radiation Oncology
Philadelphia Cyberknife Center
Delaware County Memorial Hospital
Drexel Hill, PA
USA

Johannes A. Langendijk
Department of Radiation Oncology
University of Groningen
University Medical Center Groningen
Groningen
The Netherlands

GEORGE E. LARAMORE
Department of Radiation Oncology
University of Washington Medical Center
Seattle, WA
USA

LINNA LI
Radiation Oncology
Fox Chase Cancer Center
Philadelphia, PA
USA

JAY J. LIAO
Department of Radiation Oncology
University of Washington Medical Center
Seattle, WA
USA

DAVID LIGHTFOOT
Radiation Oncology Department
Grand View Hospital
Sellersville, PA
USA

ERIK VAN LIMBERGEN
Department of Radiation Oncology
University Hospital Gasthuisberg
Leuven
Belgium

JIADE J. LU
Department of Radiation Oncology
National University Cancer Institute, Singapore
(NCIS)
Singapore

CHARLIE MA
Department of Radiation Oncology
Fox Chase Cancer Center
Philadelphia, PA
USA

MICHELLE KOLTON MACKAY
Department of Radiation Oncology
Marshfield Clinic
Marshfield, WI
USA

MARY ELLEN MASTERSON-McGARY
CyberKnife Center of Tampa Bay
Tampa, FL
USA

LOREN K. MELL
Center for Advanced Radiotherapy
Technologies
Department of Radiation Oncology
San Diego Rebecca and John Moores Cancer
Center
University of California
La Jolla, CA
USA

DAREK MICHALSKI
Division of Medical Physics
Department of Radiation Oncology
University of Pittsburgh Cancer Centers
Pittsburgh, PA
USA

PAOLO MONTEMAGGI
Department of Radiation Oncology
Regional Cancer Center "M. Ascoli"
University of Palermo Medical School
Palermo
Italy

WILLIAM F. MORGAN
Biological Sciences Division
Fundamental & Computational Sciences
Directorate Pacific Northwest National
Laboratory
Richland, WA
USA

STEPHAN MOSE
Department of Radiation Oncology
Schwarzwald-Baar-Klinikum
Villingen-Schwenningen
Germany

ARNO J. MUNDT
Center for Advanced Radiotherapy
Technologies
Department of Radiation Oncology
San Diego Rebecca and John Moores Cancer
Center
University of California
La Jolla, CA
USA

CARSTEN NIEDER
Radiation Oncology Unit
Nordlandssykehuset HF
Bodoe
Norway

CASPIAN OLIAI
Department of Radiation Oncology
College of Medicine
Drexel University
Philadelphia, PA
USA

JATINDER PALTA
Department of Radiation Oncology
University of Florida Health Science Center
Gainesville, FL
USA

NISHA R. PATEL
Department of Radiation Oncology
College of Medicine
Drexel University
Philadelphia, PA
USA

CARLOS A. PEREZ
Department of Radiation Oncology
Siteman Cancer Center
Washington University Medical Center
St. Louis, MO
USA

JAGANMOHAN POLI
Department of Radiation Oncology
College of Medicine
Drexel University
Philadelphia, PA
USA

ROBERT A. PRICE, JR.
Department of Radiation Oncology
Fox Chase Cancer Center
Philadelphia, PA
USA

TONY S. QUANG
Department of Radiation Oncology
VA Puget Sound Health Care System
University of Washington Medical Center
Seattle, WA
USA

JAY E. REIFF
Department of Radiation Oncology
College of Medicine
Drexel University
Philadelphia, PA
USA

RAMESH RENGAN
Department of Radiation Oncology
Hospital of the University of Pennsylvania
Philadelphia, PA
USA

JASON K. ROCKHILL
Department of Radiation Oncology
University of Washington Medical Center
Seattle, WA
USA

CLAUS RÖDEL
Department of Radiotherapy and Oncology
Johann Wolfgang Goethe-University Frankfurt
Frankfurt
Germany

CLAUS ROEDEL
Department of Radiotherapy and Radiation
Oncology
University Hospital Frankfurt/Main
Frankfurt
Germany

BRENT S. ROSE
Center for Advanced Radiotherapy
Technologies
Department of Radiation Oncology
San Diego Rebecca and John Moores Cancer
Center
University of California
La Jolla, CA
USA

CLAUDIA E. RÜBE
Department of Radiation Oncology
Saarland University
Homburg/Saar
Germany

RENE RUBIN
Rittenhouse Hematology/Oncology
Philadelphia, PA
USA

IRIS RUSU
Department of Radiation Oncology
Loyola University Medical Center
Maywood, IL
USA

ROBERT H. SAGERMAN
Department of Radiation Oncology
SUNY Upstate Medical University
Syracuse, NY
USA

PAULA R. SALANITRO
Department of Radiation Oncology
Mercy Fitzgerald Hospital
Kimberton, PA
USA

CHENG B. SAW
Division of Radiation Oncology
Penn State Hershey Cancer Institute
Hershey, PA
USA

DANIEL J. SCANDERBEG
Department of Radiation Oncology
John and Rebecca Moores Comprehensive
Cancer Center
University of California
San Diego
La Jolla, CA
USA

PAUL J. SCHILLING
Community Cancer Center of North Florida
Gainesville, FL
USA

M. SCHRADER
Urologische Universitätsklinik
Ulm
Germany

TALHA SHAIKH
College of Medicine
Drexel University
Philadelphia, PA
USA

CAROL L. SHIELDS
Department of Ophthalmology
Thomas Jefferson University
Philadelphia, PA
USA
and
Department of Ocular Oncology
Wills Eye Institute
Philadelphia, PA
USA

JERRY A. SHIELDS
Department of Ophthalmology
Thomas Jefferson University
Philadelphia, PA
USA
and
Department of Ocular Oncology
Wills Eye Institute
Philadelphia, PA
USA

MARIANNE B. SOWA
Biological Sciences Division
Fundamental & Computational Sciences
Directorate Pacific Northwest National
Laboratory
Richland, WA
USA

TOD W. SPEER
Department of Human Oncology
University of Wisconsin School of Medicine and
Public Health
UW Hospital and Clinics
Madison, WI
USA

JEAN ST. GERMAIN
Department of Medical Physics
Memorial Sloan-Kettering Cancer Center
New York, NY
USA

CARMEN STROMBERGER
Department of Radiotherapy and Radiation
Oncology
Charité - University Hospital Berlin
Berlin
Germany

CHARLES R. THOMAS, JR.
Department of Radiation Medicine
Oregon Health Sciences University
Portland, OR
USA

WADE L. THORSTAD
Department of Radiation Oncology
Siteman Cancer Center
Washington University Medical Center
St. Louis, MO
USA

ZELIG TOCHNER
Department of Radiation Oncology
University of Pennsylvania Hospital
Philadelphia, PA
USA

FILIP T. TROICKI
College of Medicine, Drexel University
Philadelphia, PA
USA

SERGEY USYCHKIN
Department of Radiation Oncology
Instituto Madrileño de Oncologia
Madrid
Spain

HEBERT ALBERTO VARGAS
Body MRI
Memorial Sloan-Kettering Cancer Center
New York, NY
USA

SUSAN M. VARNUM
Biological Sciences Division
Fundamental & Computational Sciences
Directorate Pacific Northwest National
Laboratory
Richland, WA
USA

ROBYN B. VERA
Department of Radiation Oncology
University of Michigan
Ann Arbor, MI
USA

LU WANG
Department of Radiation Oncology
Fox Chase Cancer Center
Philadelphia, PA
USA

KEN K.-H. WANG
Department of Radiation Oncology
University of Pennsylvania Medical Center
Philadelphia, PA
USA

JINGBO WANG
Department of Radiation Oncology
Veteran Administration Health Center and
University Hospital
University of Michigan
Ann Arbor, MI
USA

DAVID E. WAZER
Radiation Oncology Department
Tufts Medical Center
Tufts University School of Medicine
Boston, MA
USA
and
Radiation Oncology Department
Rhode Island Hospital
Brown University School of Medicine
Providence, RI
USA

CHRISTIAN WEISS
Department of Radiotherapy and Radiation
Oncology
University Hospital Frankfurt/Main
Frankfurt
Germany

T. WIEGEL
Klinik für Radioonkologie und Strahlentherapie
Universitätsklinikum Ulm
Ulm
Germany

MICHAEL L. WONG
Department of Radiation Oncology
College of Medicine
Drexel University
Philadelphia, PA
USA

JOHN W. WONG
Department of Radiation Oncology and
Molecular Radiation Sciences
Johns Hopkins University
Baltimore, MD
USA

YING XIAO
Radiation Oncology Department
Jefferson Medical College
Philadelphia, PA
USA

CHERIE YAEGER
Department Radiation Oncology
Wake Forest University School of Medicine
Winston-Salem, NC
USA

THEODORE E. YAEGER
Department Radiation Oncology
Wake Forest University School of Medicine
Winston-Salem, NC
USA

DANIEL YEUNG
Department of Radiation Oncology
University of Florida Proton Therapy Institute
Jacksonville, FL
USA

YAN YU
Department of Radiation Oncology
Thomas Jefferson University Hospital
Philadelphia, PA
USA

NING J. YUE
The Department of Radiation Oncology
The Cancer Institute of New Jersey
UMDNJ-Robert Wood Johnson Medical School
New Brunswick, NJ
USA

TIMOTHY C. ZHU
Department of Radiation Oncology
University of Pennsylvania Medical Center
Philadelphia, PA
USA

A

AAPM Task Group

BRIAN F. HASSON
Department of Radiation Oncology, Abington
Memorial Hospital, Abington, PA, USA
Department of Radiation Oncology, College of
Medicine, Drexel University, Philadelphia,
PA, USA

Definition

The AAPM is a scientific, educational, and professional nonprofit organization devoted to the discipline of physics in medicine. A task group of the AAPM is a group of professionals charged with evaluating and divulging specific information in a given specialty of medical physics. See http://www.aapm.org

Cross-References

▶ Stereotactic Radiosurgery – Cranial

Absorbed Dose

CHARLIE MA, LU WANG
Department of Radiation Oncology, Fox Chase
Cancer Center, Philadelphia, PA, USA

Definition

The energy imparted by ionizing radiation per unit mass of medium.

Cross-References

▶ Dose Calculation Algorithms

ACC

▶ Tumor of the Adrenal Cortex

Accelerated Partial Breast Irradiation

DAVID E. WAZER
Radiation Oncology Department, Tufts Medical
Center, Tufts University School of Medicine,
Boston, MA, USA
Radiation Oncology Department, Rhode Island
Hospital, Brown University School of Medicine,
Providence, RI, USA

Definition

An alternative form of adjuvant radiotherapy used when the treatment target is defined as 1–2 cm beyond the lumpectomy cavity allowing treatment to be delivered in an accelerated fashion. Typically, highly conformal treatment techniques deliver the intended dose in ≤5 days.

Cross-References

▶ Cancer of the Breast Tis

L.W. Brady, T.E. Yaeger (eds.), *Encyclopedia of Radiation Oncology*, DOI 10.1007/978-3-540-85516-3,
© Springer-Verlag Berlin Heidelberg 2013

Acceptance Testing

JAY E. REIFF
Department of Radiation Oncology, College of
Medicine, Drexel University, Philadelphia,
PA, USA

Definition
The procedure by which the medical physicist
ensures the medical device is working properly
and is characterized appropriately before it is
used for patient treatment.

Cross-References
▶ Radiation Oncology Physics

Accredited Dosimetry Calibration Laboratory (ADCL)

JAY E. REIFF
Department of Radiation Oncology, College of
Medicine, Drexel University, Philadelphia,
PA, USA

Definition
A laboratory which provides calibration services
for most radiation measurement instrumentation
available in the medical or health physics community. Every piece of equipment used in this
laboratory has its calibration directly traceable
to the National Institute of Standards and
Technology (NIST).

Cross-References
▶ Radiation Oncology Physics

Actinic Keratosis

BRANDON J. FISHER
Department of Radiation Oncology, College of
Medicine, Drexel University, Philadelphia,
PA, USA

Synonyms
Senile keratosis; Solar keratosis

Definition
Actinic keratosis, also known as solar keratosis
and senile keratosis, usually presents as hyperker-
atotic projections from the skin in sun-exposed
areas. They may begin as thick, scaly, or crusty dry
bumps on the skin and are a result of solar damage. These lesions have the potential for malignant transformation to SCCs in about 1% of
cases. They should be treated with excision, cryotherapy, dermabrasion, topical chemotherapy,
and/or laser resurfacing.

Cross-References
▶ Skin Cancer

Activity

TOD W. SPEER
Department of Human Oncology, University
of Wisconsin School of Medicine and Public
Health, UW Hospital and Clinics, Madison,
WI, USA

Definition
Quantity that describes the rate of decay of
a radionuclide. The SI unit of radioactivity is
the becquerel (Bq) and corresponds to one

disintegration per second (dps). The older term, curie (Ci), is still often used and corresponds to 3.7×10^{10} dps.

Cross-References
▶ Targeted Radioimmunotherapy

Acupuncture

JAMES H. BRASHEARS, III
Radiation Oncologist, Venice, FL, USA

Definition
From the Latin *acus* meaning needle and the verb *pungere*, to prick. It is the evaluation of the patient with subsequent insertion and manipulation of needles into the body for therapeutic purposes such as relief of pain or gastrointestinal complaints. This nontraditional or alternative practice is based on Chinese methods that predate modern Western techniques. Broadly, acupuncture may include electric acupuncture, laser acupuncture (photo-acupuncture), microsystem acupuncture (to the ear, face, hand, and scalp), acupressure, and traditional body needling.

Cross-References
▶ Complementary Medicine
▶ Pain Management

Acute Lymphocytic Leukemia (ALL)

▶ Leukemia in General

Acute Myelogenous Leukemia (AML)

▶ Leukemia in General

Acute Radiation Sickness

JOHN P. CHRISTODOULEAS
The Perelman Cancer Center, Department of Radiation Oncology, University of Pennsylvania Hospital, Philadelphia, PA, USA

Synonyms
Acute radiation syndrome

Definition
Acute radiation sickness refers to the constellation of symptoms that may occur after total or near total body radiation exposures. Acute radiation sickness is broken down into three phases: prodrome, latency, and illness. The duration and severity of each of these phases is determined by the total dose of the exposure.

Cross-References
▶ Short-Term and Long-Term Health Risk of Nuclear Power Plant Accident

Acute Radiation Syndrome

▶ Acute Radiation Sickness

Acute Radiation Toxicity

Anthony E. Dragun
Department of Radiation Oncology, James Graham Brown Cancer Center, University of Louisville School of Medicine, Louisville, KY, USA

Synonyms
Radiation dermatitis

Definition
Acute radiation toxicities are side effects that occur on treatment or in the immediate posttreatment period. Onset may be 2–3 weeks after the commencement of a regimen of radiation therapy. Typically, severity and timing are tied to the total biologic dose and the turnover rate of the tissue in question, respectively. It is less dependent on the dose per fraction of treatment. In the case of whole breast radiation therapy, radiation dermatitis usually involves mild puritis and erythema of the skin. Some cases involve patchy moist desquamation in the folds of the axilla and inframammary regions. In the modern era, these side effects are nearly always mild (∼95% of cases are grade 1–2). The degree of dermatitis may be slightly more severe in large-breasted patients and in patients with underlying DNA repair deficits such as ATM heterozygosity. Radiation dermatitis usually resolves rapidly (2–3 weeks post treatment) and results in temporary hyperpigmentation. Mild fatigue is also a common acute radiation–induced toxicity, but has been shown to be mitigated by regular on-treatment exercise.

Cross-References
▶ Collagen Vascular Disease
▶ Early-Stage Breast Cancer

Acute Reactions

Volker Budach
Department of Radiotherapy and Radiation Oncology, Charité – University Hospital Berlin, Berlin, Germany

Definition
Reaction of the healthy tissue due to a radiotherapy treatment occurring during the treatment and up to 90 days post radiotherapy. The type and severity of side effects relate to the area of the body being treated and whether treatment is being given to cure the cancer or to relieve symptoms.

Cross-References
▶ Larynx
▶ Oro-Hypopharynx

Adaptive Radiotherapy

Timothy Holmes
Department of Radiation Oncology, Sinai Hospital, Baltimore, MD, USA

Definition
A method of radiotherapy that uses daily CT localization images to compute estimates of daily dose in order to track the impact of delivered dose on observed anatomical changes (i.e., tumor shrinkage or weight loss), and to adapt the treatment delivery to correct for these deviations. This may result in generating a new treatment plan based on current anatomy.

Cross-References

▶ Image-Guided Radiation Therapy (IGRT): TomoTherapy

▶ Lung Cancer
▶ Nasal Cavity and Paranasal Sinuses
▶ Stomach Cancer

Adenoacanthoma

Filip T. Troicki[1], Jaganmohan Poli[2]
[1]College of Medicine, Drexel University, Philadelphia, PA, USA
[2]Department of Radiation Oncology, College of Medicine, Drexel University, Philadelphia, PA, USA

Definition

Adenocarcinoma where the cells also exhibit squamous differentiation.

Cross-References

▶ Stomach Cancer

Adenocarcinoma

Filip T. Troicki[1], Jaganmohan Poli[2]
[1]College of Medicine, Drexel University, Philadelphia, PA, USA
[2]Department of Radiation Oncology, College of Medicine, Drexel University, Philadelphia, PA, USA

Definition

A cancer derived from glandular tissue within the body.

Cross-References

▶ Bladder
▶ Breast Cancer

Adenocarcinoma of the Colon

▶ Colon Cancer

Adenocarcinoma of the Prostate

▶ Prostate

Adenoid Cystic Carcinoma

Lindsay G. Jensen, Loren K. Mell
Center for Advanced Radiotherapy Technologies, Department of Radiation Oncology, San Diego Rebecca and John Moores Cancer Center, University of California, La Jolla, CA, USA

Definition

Most common malignant tumor of the submandibular, sublingual, and minor salivary glands. Characterized as cribriform, tubular, or solid. Solid subtype has the worst prognosis (Terhaard 2008).

Cross-References

▶ Salivary Gland Cancer

Adipose Tissue Tumors

▶ Soft Tissue Sarcoma

Adrenal Cancer

▶ Carcinoma of the Adrenal Gland

Adrenal Carcinoma

▶ Carcinoma of the Adrenal Gland

Adrenal Cortical Carcinoma

▶ Tumor of the Adrenal Cortex

Adrenal Medulla Tumor

STEPHAN MOSE
Department of Radiation Oncology,
Schwarzwald-Baar-Klinikum,
Villingen-Schwenningen, Germany

Definition

Tumors of the adrenal medulla are very seldom. In contrast to neuroblastoma and ganglioneuroblastoma, the catecholamine-secreting pheochromocytoma is the most common cancer of the adrenal medulla.

Cross-References

▶ Carcinoma of the Adrenal Gland

Adrenocortical Carcinoma

▶ Tumor of the Adrenal Cortex

Afterloading Technique

ERIK VAN LIMBERGEN[1], CHENG B. SAW[2]
[1]Department of Radiation Oncology,
University Hospital Gasthuisberg, Leuven,
Belgium
[2]Division of Radiation Oncology, Penn State
Hershey Cancer Institute, Hershey, PA, USA

Definition

A technique in which catheters and/or applicators are placed in the patient at the time of surgery and radioactive sources are loaded into the patient for treatment at a later time. Loading with the radioactive sources is performed after the dosimetric study. Afterloading can be done manually or with assistance of a remote control afterloading machine. The advantages are full radioprotection of the medical and nursing staff and visitors. It also improves the geometry and hence the quality of the dose distribution of the application/implantation because adjustments of the catheter or needle positioning can be carried out very carefully since there is no radiation exposure involved.

Cross-References

▶ Brachytherapy: High Dose Rate (HDR) Implants
▶ Clinical Aspects of Brachytherapy (BT)
▶ Low-Dose Rate (LDR) Brachytherapy

AGES

Nisha R. Patel, Michael L. Wong
Department of Radiation Oncology, College of
Medicine, Drexel University, Philadelphia,
PA, USA

Definition

Scoring system to predict prognosis that incorporates variables such as age, tumor grade, primary tumor extent, and primary tumor size for papillary thyroid neoplasm.

Cross-References

▶ Thyroid Cancer

AIDS-Related Malignancies

▶ Malignant Neoplasms Associated with Acquired Immunodeficiency Syndrome

Air Kerma Strength

Ning J. Yue
The Department of Radiation Oncology,
The Cancer Institute of New Jersey,
UMDNJ-Robert Wood Johnson Medical School,
New Brunswick, NJ, USA

Definition

The product of air kerma rate in "free space" and the square of the distance of the calibration point from the source center along the perpendicular bisector. The calibration measurement must be performed with a distance between the detector and the source large enough so that the source and the detector can be treated as a point source and a point detector, respectively.

Cross-References

▶ Brachytherapy: Low Dose Rate (LDR) Temporary Implants

Albumin

James H. Brashears, III
Radiation Oncologist, Venice, FL, USA

Definition

Makes up 60% of the total plasma protein in adults. It may be increased with dehydration. Albumin (and prealbumin) will usually be low in those with protein-calorie malnutrition (a catabolic state), liver disease, or severe illness. The normal adult albumin level is 3.5–5.0 g/dL. Prealbumin has a shorter half-life than albumin and so can be used in a more timely fashion to follow the effects of nutritional supports.

Cross-References

▶ Supportive Care and Quality of Life

Alemtuzumab

Curt Heese
Department of Radiation Oncology, Eastern
Regional Cancer Treatment Centers of America,
Philadelphia, PA, USA

Definition

A recombinant DNA-derived humanized monoclonal antibody that is directed against the 21–28 kDa cell surface glycoprotein, CD52.

Cross-References

▶ Cutaneous T-Cell Lymphoma

Algiatry

▶ Pain Management

Alibert-Bazin Syndrome or Granuloma Fungoides

▶ Mycosis Fungoides

Alimta

RAMESH RENGAN[1], CHARLES R. THOMAS, JR.[2]
[1]Department of Radiation Oncology, Hospital of the University of Pennsylvania, Philadelphia, PA, USA
[2]Department of Radiation Medicine, Oregon Health Sciences University, Portland, OR, USA

Definition
Pemetrexed is a novel antifolate that targets critical enzymes in the purine and pyrimidine synthesis pathways.

Cross-References
▶ Pleural Mesothelioma

ALK Inhibitors

RENE RUBIN
Rittenhouse Hematology/Oncology, Philadelphia, PA, USA

Definition
Translocations of the anaplastic large cell lymphoma gene can cause expression of oncogene fusion proteins. This results in increased cell proliferation and survival in tumors expressing these proteins. ALK inhibitors are tyrosine kinase inhibitors that bind to the ALK receptor. ALK overexpression currently is demonstrated in approximately 10% of adenocarcinoma of the lung, especially in the nonsmoking population.

Crizotinib is the first in this class of drugs. It is given orally and should only be used in tumors that demonstrate ALK positivity.

Side Effects
- Pneumonitis
- Hepatic enzyme abnormalities
- QT interval prolongation
- Nausea, vomiting, diarrhea
- Bone marrow suppression

Cross-References
▶ Principles of Chemotherapy

Alkylating Agents

RENE RUBIN
Rittenhouse Hematology/Oncology, Philadelphia, PA, USA

Definition
Alkylation agents are a large group of drugs (altretamine, busulfan, carmusine, chlorambucil, cytoxan, dacarbazine, ifosfamide, lomustine, merchlorethamine, melphalan, procarbazine, temozolamide, thiotepa, streptozocin) which are used in various carcinomas. This group of chemotherapy causes cell damage by alkylating the guanine base of the DNA double helix. Therefore, the affected cells are growth inhibited, and apoptosis (spontaneous cell death) will be stimulated.

Altretamine is an oral agent which is used for ovarian carcinoma.

Busulfan is used for CML and polycythemia vera, but mostly for bone marrow transplantation.

Carmustine is used in brain tumors, Hodgkin's lymphoma, and melanoma.

Chlorambucil is orally dosed and used for CLL and lymphoma.

Cyclophosphamide is used for breast carcinoma, non-Hodgkin lymphoma, and carcinoma of the ovary, leukemia, autoimmune disorders, and bone marrow transplant.

Dacarbazine is helpful in the treatment of malignant melanoma, sarcoma, and lymphomas.

Isophosphamide is given for lung, cervical, and ovarian cancer and soft tissue and osteogenic sarcomas, and it can be used for lymphomas and testicular cancer.

Melphalan is effective in multiple myeloma and ovarian cancer.

Procarbazine is used in Hodgkin's lymphoma and brain tumors (glioblastoma).

Temozoamide (oral BCNU) is especially used in glioblastoma multiforme (alone or together with radiotherapy) and in melanoma.

Thiotepa is mainly used as a conditioning therapy prior to hematopoietic cell transplantation in blood diseases.

Side Effects

- Hemorrhagic cystitis
- Schwarz-Bartter syndrome (SIADH): inappropriate antidiuretic hormone hypersecretion, characterized by excessive release of antidiuretic hormone
- Pulmonary fibrosis
- Severe nausea and vomiting
- Hyperpigmentation
- Liver dysfunction and veno-occlusive disease

Cross-References
- ▶ Hodgkin's Lymphoma
- ▶ Leukemia in General
- ▶ Non-Hodgkin's Lymphoma

- ▶ Ovary Cancer
- ▶ Principles of Chemotherapy

Alternative Medicine

- ▶ Nontraditional Medicine

American Association of Physicists in Medicine (AAPM)

Jay E. Reiff
Department of Radiation Oncology, College of Medicine, Drexel University, Philadelphia, PA, USA

Definition
A scientific, educational, and professional organization made up of over 7,000 medical physicists (http://aapm.org).

Cross-References
- ▶ Radiation Oncology Physics

American Society for Radiation Oncology (ASRO)

Jay E. Reiff
Department of Radiation Oncology, College of Medicine, Drexel University, Philadelphia, PA, USA

Definition
A scientific, educational, and professional organization comprised of more than 10,000 radiation

oncologists, radiation oncology nurses, medical physicists, radiation therapists, dosimetrists, and biologists dedicated to improving radiation therapy as a treatment for cancer (http://astro.org/).

Cross-References
▶ Radiation Oncology Physics

AMES

Nisha R. Patel, Michael L. Wong
Department of Radiation Oncology, College of Medicine, Drexel University, Philadelphia, PA, USA

Definition
Scoring system to predict prognosis for papillary and follicular thyroid malignancy that incorporates age, distant metastases, primary tumor extent, and primary tumor size.

Cross-References
▶ Thyroid Cancer

Ampullary Carcinoma

▶ Liver and Hepatobiliary Tract

Amyloid

Jo Ann Chalal
Department of Radiation Oncology, Fox Chase Cancer Center, Philadelphia, PA, USA

Definition
Extracellular proteinaceous deposit which is birefringent when stained with Congo Red and gives rise to amyloidosis or amyloid-related disorders where there is an accumulation of this material in organs, resulting in diminished functionality. It is also noted in some disease states.

Cross-References
▶ Multiple Myeloma

Anal Cancer

▶ Anal Carcinoma

Anal Carcinoma

Gerhard G. Grabenbauer
Chairman of the Department of Radiation Oncology, DiaCura Coburg & Klinikum Coburg, Coburg, Germany

Synonyms
Anal cancer

Definition/Description
Tumors of the anal region are rare tumors and comprise only 1–2% of all cases with gastrointestinal malignancies. Clinical behavior is mostly characterized by local spread with and without involvement of the regional lymphatics. Primary symptoms include uncharacteristic local irritation of the anal canal or perianal skin, mucous or bloody discharge. Since the vast majority of cases appears to be strongly associated with persistent HPV-infection, particularly immunologically compromised patients like HIV-infected male persons, individuals with a post-transplant status and sexually active female persons with more than ten sexual partners are regarded as being at high risk. Treatment of choice is

a primary chemoradiation approach that will lead to a long-term cure in 80% of the patients. Only in case of persistent and recurrent tumor, salvage surgery is indicated.

Anatomy and Pathology

The anal region is defined as anal canal and anal margin (Fig. 1). The anal canal extends between the upper margin of the internal sphincter muscle down to the skin border with a length between 3 and 4 cm. The anal margin is defined as the region with a diameter of 2–3 cm of the perianal skin; it ends where the anocutaneous line starts. Tumors of the anal region need to be classified according to their initial appearence (or where the maximum of the tumor mass is located) as anal canal or anal margin cancer. This seems specifically important since the primary lymphatic drainage of the anal canal is into the perirectal and presacral nodes (nodi lymphatici pararectales (anorectales) and nodi lymphatici iliaci interni), whereas the perianal skin drainage leads to the superficial inguinal nodes (nodi lymphatici inguinales superomediales).

Epidemiology

Anal cancer is a rare disease with an annual incidence of 1.4–2/100,000 persons. However, the incidence is reported as being in the range of 70-fold increased in patients with HIV-infection and those following organ transplantation. Infection with ▶ HPV accounts for the vast majority of sexually transmitted diseases worldwide with a prevalence between 10% and 50% in sexually active persons. Persistent HPV-infection rates (Types 16, 18, 33) rise with increasing numbers of sexual partners, anal receptive intercourse, and cigarette smoking. HPV-E6 and E7 genome acts as oncogene via inactivation of tumor suppressors like p53 and pRB with the results of the development of anal intraepithelial neoplasia (AIN). The prevalence of AIN in HIV-infected males practicing anal intercourse has been reported to be in the range of 80%.

Clinical Presentation

Clinical inspection, palpation of anal canal, perianal region, and inguinal nodes by digital examination will reveal the most essential information on the primary extension of the disease. Any suspicious induration, ulceration, or exophytic lesion needs further evaluation by excision (perianal skin) or multiple true-cut biopsies (anal canal).

Tumors of the anal region will typically develop as local disease, occasionally spread to regional lymphatics, and rarely develop distant disease. It seems important to distinguish between anal canal and anal margin tumors as depicted by Table 1.

Histopathological classification of tumors arising from the anal canal follows the guidelines as suggested by the WHO (see Table 2). Mostly squamous cell cancer of different subtypes typically arises from the epithelium of the anal canal. Rarely adenocarcinoma will be diagnosed. Anal margin tumor classification follows the classification of skin tumors, including squamous cell cancer, basal cell cancer, and apocrine adenocarcinoma (Le Boit et al. 2006).

Differential Diagnosis

Important differential diagnosis of anal canal carcinoma includes anal intraepithelial neoplasie (AIN), specifically in high-risk patients, since early diagnosis and treatment seems crucial to avoid invasive cancer. Premalignant conditions of the perianal skin are the bowenoid papulosis and Bowen's disease. Other, extremely rare histopathological entities arising in the anal region include lymphoma, melanoma, and leiomyosarcoma. Melanoma contributes to 1–2% of all anal region tumors.

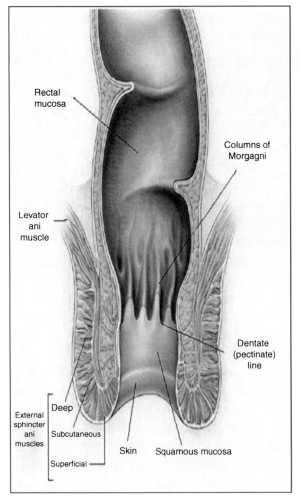

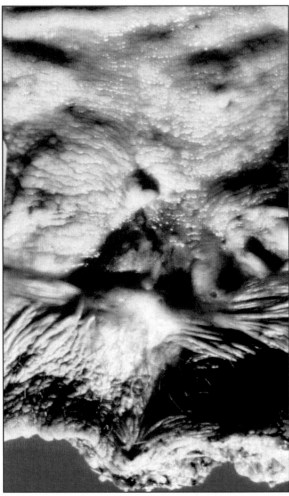

Anal Carcinoma. Fig. 1 Anatomy of anal region

Imaging Studies

Following histopathological diagnosis of malignant disease, clinical examination, endorectal ultrasound (whenever feasible), computed tomography of the abdomen, pelvis and lungs will suffice to have a complete staging according to the UICC classification (2010). The current staging system for anal canal and anal margin cancer is depicted in Tables 3 and 4.

Fluorodeoxyglucose positron emission computed tomography (PET-CT) is helpful to detect the extent of metabolically active disease sites. Moreover, PET-CT appears particularly of value for exact determination of the planning target volume (see Fig. 2) and for assessment of response following chemoradiation (Grabenbauer 2010).

Laboratory Studies

No specific laboratory studies seem helpful for diagnosis or during follow-up.

Treatment

Originally described by Nigro et al. (1974), the combined treatment by external radiation and chemotherapy using mitomycin-C and FU was

Anal Carcinoma. Table 1 Clinical presentation

	Anal canal cancer	Anal margin cancer
Distribution	80%	20%
Gender (m:f)	1:1.2	1:1
Histology	75% squamous cell carcinoma	>90% squamous cell carcinoma
	15–20% adenocarcinoma	
Lymphatics	Perirectal	Inguinal
Treatment for T1	Chemoradiation	Local excision

Anal Carcinoma. Table 2 Classification of anal carcinoma according to WHO (Fenger et al. 2000)

Squamous cell carcinoma	Squamous cell differentiation
	Basaloid differentiation
	Ductal differentiation
Adenocarcinoma	
"Subtypes" with inferior prognosis	Squamous cell carcinoma with mucinous microcysts
	Small cell, non keratinizing squamous cell carcinoma

Anal Carcinoma. Table 3 TNM-staging for anal canal carcinoma (UICC 2010)

T/pT-classification	(p)T0 no evidence of tumor	
	(p)Tis Carcinoma in situ	
	(p)T1 2 cm or less	
	(p)T2 more than 2 cm, less than 5 cm	
	(p)T3 more than 5 cm	
	(p)T4 any dimension, infiltration of adjacent organs (vagina, bladder, etc.)	
N/pN-classification	(p)N0 No regional lymph node metastases	
	(p)N1 Metastase(i)s in perirectal nodes	
	(p)N2 Metastase(i)s in inguinal nodes unilaterally and/or in nodes along internal iliac artery (unilateral)	
	(p)N3 Metastases in perirectal and inguinal nodes and/or in node along bilateral internal iliac and/or in bilateral inguinal nodes	
M/pM-classification	(p)M0 No distant metastases	
	(p)M1 Distant metastases	
Stage groups	M0N0	
	Tis	St.0
	T1	St.I
	T2,3	St.II
	T4	St.IIIA
	M0N1	
	T1-3	St.IIIA
	T4	St.IIIB
	M0N2,3 any T	St.IIIB
	M1 any N any T	St.IV

obviously intended for downstaging and downsizing of advanced disease prior to (sphincter-saving) surgery. However, high rates of complete histopathological response, even after 30 Gy, plus one course of chemotherapy prompted several groups to establish programs of primary chemoradiation that defined the current standard of treatment. Interestingly, Papillon (1974) paralleled with a sphincter-saving treatment using external Co-60 radiation and interstitial implants. During the following years, multiple phase-II studies were published that demonstrated colostomy-free survival rates in the order

Anal Carcinoma. Table 4 TNM-staging for anal margin carcinoma (UICC 2010)

T/pT-classification	(p)T0 no evidence of tumor	
	(p)Tis Carcinoma in situ	
	(p)T1 2 cm or less	
	(p)T2 more than 2 cm, less than 5 cm	
	(p)T3 more than 5 cm	
	(p)T4 any dimension, infiltration of adjacent bone, cartilage, or skeletal muscle	
N/pN-classification	(p)N0 No regional lymph node metastases	
	(p)N1 Metastase(i)s in inguinal nodes	
M/pM-classification	(p)M0 No distant metastases	
	(p)M1 Distant metastases	
Stage groups	M0N0	
	Tis	St.0
	T1	St.I
	T2,3	St.II
	T4	St.III
	M0N1 any T	St.III
	M1 any N any T	St.IV

of 60–80% at 5 years, mostly using chemoradiation with mitomycin-C and FU.

Two randomized phase-III trials addressed the question of whether the addition of chemotherapy would be of benefit since radiation alone obviously induced substantial remission rates. The EORTC-trial was designed to only include patients with advanced disease of the anal canal and anal margin (>4 cm or N+). After randomization of only 110 patients, a significant benefit in the locoregional tumor control rate (52% vs 70%, $p = 0.02$) and in the colostomy-free survival rate (72% vs 40%, p = 0.002) following combined modality treatment as compared to radiation alone was detected (Bartelink et al. 1997).

In addition, the United Kingdom Coordinating Committee on Cancer Research (UKCCCR) trial came to the conclusion that local tumor control rates improved from 39% with radiotherapy alone to 61% following chemoradiation ($p < 0.0001$). This applied specifically for T1N0M0 tumors (Northover et al. 1997). Table 5 gives an overview on the trials.

The RTOG/ECOG-Intergroup study evaluated the question whether mitomycin-C contributed significantly to the improvement in local tumor control and colostomy-free survival. Both colostomy-free survival (59% vs 71%, $p = 0.014$) and NED-survival rates (51% vs 73%, $p = 0.0003$) were markedly enhanced by the addition of mitomycin-C (Flam et al. 1996). Table 6 gives the results.

RTOG/Intergroup study 98-11 evaluated an intensified approach that consisted of induction chemotherapy and concurrent chemoradiation both with FU/cisplatinum in an experimental arm compared to the standard treatment with a chemoradiation using FU/MMC. Primary endpoint was the disease-free survival rate at 5 years. A total of 644 patients with anal canal carcinoma T2-4 N0-3 M0 was randomized (Ajani et al. 2008)

The disease-free survival rate at 5 years following chemoradiation with 5-FU/MMC was 60% (53–67% [95%CI]) and 54% (46–60% [95%CI], p = 0.17) after chemoradiation with 5-FU/Cisplatin. Table 7 gives the detailed results.

Toxicity

Due to the relatively high proportion of elderly patients (>65 years: approximately 40–55%) among the patients that need treatment for anal cancer, early detection, treatment, and possibly prevention of severe acute toxicity seems of paramount interest (Cummings 2006). Life-threatening hematologic toxicity like febrile neutropenia or septicemia was obviously restricted to

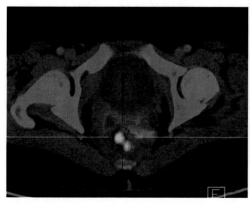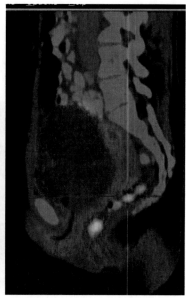

Anal Carcinoma. Fig. 2 FDG-PET-CT in anal canal carcinoma

Anal Carcinoma. Table 5 Results of trials comparing radiotherapy alone (RT) versus chemoradiation (RCT)

Study	Patients	Local control (%)		Overall survival (%)	
		RT	RCT	RT	RCT
EORTC	110	39	58 (p = 0.02)	65	72 (p = 0.2)
UKCCCR	585	39	61 (p < 0.001)	58	65 (p = 0.3)

Anal Carcinoma. Table 6 Impact of mitomycin C (MMC) in addition to flurouracil (FU) with radiation

Treatment	Patients	Colostomy-free survival (%)		NED-survival (%)	
			p-value		p-value
RT + FU	145	59	0.014	51	0.0003
RT + FU/ MMC	146	71		73	

Anal Carcinoma. Table 7 Impact of induction and concurrent chemotherapy with FU/cisplatinum versus standard chemoradiation with 5 FU/MMC

	RCT 5-FU/MMC	RCT 5FU/ cisplatin	p-value
5-year results			
Overall survival	75%	70%	0.10
Locoregional recurrence	25%	33%	na
Distant metastases	15%	19%	na
Colostomy rate	10%	19%	0.02
Toxicity grade 3 + 4	61%	42%	0.001

singular cases in all protocols (Bartelink et al. 1997; Flam et al. 1996; UKCCCR 1996). The impact of mitomycin-C may be well studied with the data of the RTOG study: Grade 4 hematologic toxicity was reported for patients

Tomotherapy

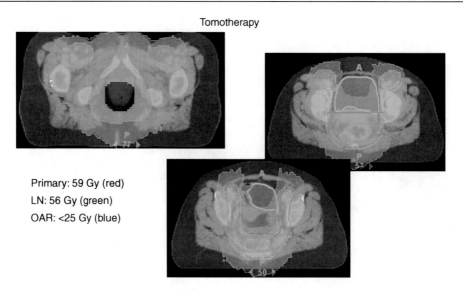

Primary: 59 Gy (red)
LN: 56 Gy (green)
OAR: <25 Gy (blue)

Anal Carcinoma. Fig. 3 IMRT dose distribution

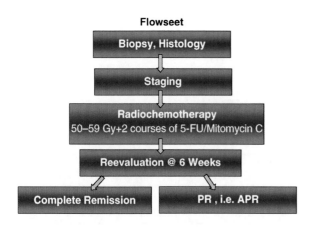

Anal Carcinoma. Fig. 4 Flow-diagram for staging and treatment

participating in the 5-FU arm in 3/145 (2%) cases. However, in the 5-FU/MMC arm, this rate was 18/146 (12%) patients ($p < 0.001$). Accordingly, the treatment-related mortality was significantly higher in the MMC-treated patients than after FU-based chemoradiation alone (3% vs 0.7%). In addition, gastrointestinal toxicity including severe diarrhea with dehydration may be another issue. This is reflected by a marked increase of the grade-4/5-toxicity rate (23% vs 7%, $p < 0.001$) following FU/MMC in the afore-mentioned trial.

Following severe acute toxicity (grade 3–4) after the first course of chemotherapy, a dose reduction of 50% (MMC) was suggested in the RTOG trial. In patients over age 80 years, the UKCCCR trial prescribed only 75% intensity of both drugs.

Treatment Volume and Fractionation

Original techniques as described by Papillon using Co-60 as well as higher single fractions are no longer regarded as state of the art. However, the treated target volumes that included the primary tumor region together with the perirectal and presacral/iliac internal lymphatics has been the standard treatment volume for anal canal carcinoma since the early 1980s. Larger treatment volumes using anterior-posterior field arrangement to the whole pelvis for the first 45 Gy, followed by a local boost of 15–20 Gy were associated with very high acute and chronic toxic effects (UKCCCR-trial: 38–42%, EORTC-trial:29–43%). The application of shrinking-field

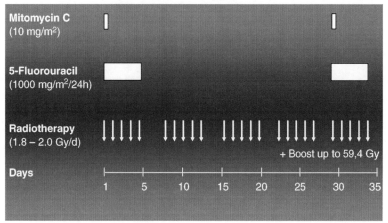

Anal Carcinoma. Fig. 5 Standard chemoradiation protocol

techniques as demonstrated by the RTOG trial (30 Gy by anterior-posterior fields, 45 Gy via 10 × 10 fields, small boost of 50–59 Gy) was then associated with much less toxic late effects of grade 4/5 in the range of 2% only. The treatment of inguinal lymph nodes has been an issue of ongoing debate. Incidence of lymph node metastases may vary from 6% to 23% in different series being only 10% for lesions <4 cm and for larger primaries approaching 15–30%. Tumor involvement of the upper anal canal has merely no inguinal lymphatic drainage, whereas infiltration or ulceration of the perianal skin may almost invariably lead to inguinal disease. Elective treatment of the inguinal lymph nodes was reported to lower the inguinal recurrence rate to 5%. Recent developments including FDG-PET-CT for exact delineation of target volumes and intensity-modulated radiation therapy (IMRT) may overcome this problem (see Fig. 3).

Treatment recommendations for staging and standard chemoradiation protocol are depicted in Figs. 4 and 5.

Cross-References
▶ Clinical Aspects of Brachytherapy (BT)
▶ Rectal Cancer

References

Ajani JA et al (2008) Fluorouracil, mitomycin, and radiotherapy vs fluorouracil, cisplatin, and radiotherapy for carcinoma of the anal canal. A randomized controlled trial. JAMA 299:1914–21

Bartelink H, Roelofsen F, Eschwege F et al (1997) Concomitant radiotherapy and chemotherapy is superior to radiotherapy alone in the treatment of locally advanced anal cancer: results of a phase III randomized trial of the European Organisation for research and treatment of cancer radiotherapy and Gastrointestinal Cooperative Groups. J Clin Oncol 15:2040–2049

Cummings BJ (2006) Anal cancer. In: Gospodarowicz MK, O' Sullivan B, Sobin LH (eds) UICC: prognostic factors in cancer, 3rd edn. Wiley, New York, pp 139–142

Fenger C, Frisch M, Marti NC, Parc R (2000) Tumours of the anal canal. In: Hamilton SR, Aaltonen LA (eds) Pathology and genetics of tumours of the digestive system. WHO classification of tumours. IARC Press, Lyon, pp 145–155

Flam MS, John M, Pajak T, Petrelli N et al (1996) Role of mitomycin C in combination with fluorouracil and radiotherapy, and of salvage chemoradiation in the definitive nonsurgical treatment of epidermoid carcinoma of the anal canal: results of a phase III randomized intergroup study. J Clin Oncol 14:2527–2539

Grabenbauer GG (2010) Analkarzinom. In: Hiddemann W, Bartram C (eds) Die Onkologie. Teil 2: Solide Tumoren, Lymphome, Leukämien. Springer Medizin, Heidelberg, pp 898–906

Le Boit PE, Burg G, Weedon D, Sarasin A (eds) (2006) Pathology and genetics of skin tumours. WHO classification of tumours. IARC Press, Lyon, pp 9–29, 49–65

Nigro ND, Vaitkevicius VK, Considine B (1974) Combined therapy for cancer of the anal canal. Dis Colon Rectum 27:763–766

Northover J, Meadows H, Ryan C (1997) On behalf of UKCCCR anal cancer trial working. The Lancet 349:205–206

Papillon J (1974) Radiation therapy in the management of epidermoid carcinoma of the anal region. Dis Colon Rectum 17:184–187

UICC (2010) TNM Klassifikation maligner Tumoren. 7. Aufl. 2010 (Herausgegeben und übersetzt von Wittekind Ch, Meyer H-J, Bootz F). Springer, Berlin/Heidelberg/New York

Anaplastic Astrocytoma

▶ Primary Intracranial Neoplasms
▶ Spinal Canal Tumor

Anaplastic Ependymoma

▶ Spinal Canal Tumor

Anemia

LINDSAY G. JENSEN, BRENT S. ROSE,
ARNO J. MUNDT
Center for Advanced Radiotherapy Technologies,
Department of Radiation Oncology, San Diego
Rebecca and John Moores Cancer Center,
University of California, La Jolla, CA, USA

Definition
Decreased peripheral red blood cell count, typically Hg <13.5 g/dL in men, <12 g/dL in women.

Cross-References
▶ Bone Marrow Toxicity in Cancer Treatment

Anthroposcopic

▶ Complementary Medicine

Anisotropy Function

NING J. YUE
The Department of Radiation Oncology,
The Cancer Institute of New Jersey,
UMDNJ-Robert Wood Johnson Medical School,
New Brunswick, NJ, USA

Definition
A quantity describing the anisotropy of relative dose distribution around the source.

Cross-References
▶ Brachytherapy: Low Dose Rate (LDR) Temporary Implants

Antiangiogenesis Inhibitors

RENE RUBIN
Rittenhouse Hematology/Oncology,
Philadelphia, PA, USA

Definition
This group describes monoclonal antibodies against vascular endothelial growth factor (VEGF).

It inhibits blood vessel formation in tumors. Avastin is used in carcinoma of the breast, the ovary, the colon, the lung, and brain tumors. Cilengitide, a new antiangiogenic drug, is being tested for glioblastoma multiforme.

Side Effects
- Hypertension
- Worsening of coronary/peripheral artery disease
- Bowel perforation
- Microangiopathy

Cross-References
▶ Principles of Chemotherapy

Antibody

Tod W. Speer
Department of Human Oncology, University of Wisconsin School of Medicine and Public Health, UW Hospital and Clinics, Madison, WI, USA

Definition
A large glycoprotein molecule (immunoglobulin) secreted by B lymphocytes of the immune system that targets antigens on "foreign" objects such as bacteria, viruses, or cancer cells. The targeting takes place with a high degree of specificity and affinity.

Cross-References
▶ Targeted Radioimmunotherapy

Antibody-Dependent Cell-Mediated Cytotoxicity (ADCC)

Tod W. Speer
Department of Human Oncology, University of Wisconsin School of Medicine and Public Health, UW Hospital and Clinics, Madison, WI, USA

Definition
The immune process by which NK cells are targeted to antibody-coated pathogenic cells, causing lysis and death of the antibody-coated cells.

Cross-References
▶ Targeted Radioimmunotherapy

Anti-EGFR (Epidermal Growth Factor Receptor)

Rene Rubin
Rittenhouse Hematology/Oncology, Philadelphia, PA, USA

Definition
This large group of small molecules (gefitinib, erlotinib, cetuximab, panitumumab, sorafenib, sunitinib, pazopanib, vandetanib, cediranib) acts as inhibitor of the EGFR tyrosine kinase. They inhibit the EGFR-signaling and enhance the response to chemotherapy as well as to radiotherapy. K-ras mutations cause resistance. The use is still evolving (colon cancer, renal cell carcinoma,

brain tumors, cancer of the head and neck, lung cancer, and carcinoma of the pancreas).

Side Effects
- Diarrhea
- Skin rash
- Lung toxicity
- Interstitial lung disease
- Transaminitis

Cross-References
▶ Principles of Chemotherapy

Antiemetic Agents

RENE RUBIN
Rittenhouse Hematology/Oncology,
Philadelphia, PA, USA

Definition
Aprepitant: substance P/NK neurokinin 1 receptor antagonist to be used with decadron and ondansetron for highly emetogenic chemotherapy as a prophylaxis.

Dexamethasone: a steroid which works in adjunction to all other antiemetics.

Diphenhydramine: it blocks the chemoreceptor trigger zone.

Dolasetron: 5HT3 receptor antagonist

Granisetron: 5HT3 receptor antagonist

Metoclopramide: stimulates gastrointestinal motility

Ondansetron: 5HT3 receptor antagonist

Palonosetron: 5HT3 receptor antagonist

Cross-References
▶ Principles of Chemotherapy

Antimetabolites/Antifolates

RENE RUBIN
Rittenhouse Hematology/Oncology,
Philadelphia, PA, USA

Definition
This class of drugs works by interfering with normal cell metabolism. They have close structural resemblance to those metabolites required for normal physiologic cell function. They work by competing for the metabolite receptors thus causing cell dysfunction and inhibition (or replication) of the enzymes of a particular metabolic pathway. These drugs include 5-fluorouracil (5-FU), methotrexate, mercaptopurine, thioguanine, cytarabine, cladrabine, gemcitabine, fludarabine, floxuridine, 5-azocytadine, hydroxyurea, clofarabine, and capecitabine.

5-Azocytadine is both a cytotoxic agent and a differentiating agent. It is incorporated into both RNA and DNA. In the DNA it activates silenced genes and allows differentiation of cells. It is used in myelodysplasia.

Capecitabine is an oral prodrug of 5-fluorouracil. It is used in breast and gastrointestinal malignancies.

Cladrabine is a purine deoxyadenosine analog. It is highly specific for lymphoid cells. It is used in hairy cell leukemia, chronic lymphocytic leukemia, and low-grade non-Hodgkin's lymphoma.

Clofarabine is a deoxyadenosine nucleoside analog. It is used in relapsed acute myelogenous leukemia in pediatric patients.

Cytarabine (cytosine arabinoside) inhibits DNA polymerases and DNA repair (s phase specific). It is used in acute myelogenous leukemia, acute lymphocytic leukemia, non-Hodgkin's lymphoma, and for intrathecal in carcinomatous meningitis.

Gemcitabine is a fluorine-substituted deoxycytadine analog. It is incorporated into RNA and causes alterations in RNA processing. It is used in pancreatic, bladder, breast, ovary, and lung carcinoma. It is also a radiosensitizer in that it can increase the effect of radiation delivered simultaneously (and also side effects of both).

Floxuridine is metabolized to 5-FU and is cell cycle specific. It is used specifically for patients with gastrointestinal malignancies and liver metastases. It is given as an intrahepatic infusion.

5-Fluorouracil (5-FU) was first synthesized in 1956. It primarily inhibits DNA synthesis by blocking the conversion of dUMP to dTMP. It is still widely used and frequently concurrently with radiotherapy in gastrointestinal, primary head and neck, and advanced breast tumors, and topically for basal cell carcinomas. It is most commonly given as an infusion over days or with leucovorin, which enhances its antitumor activity.

Fludarabine is resistant to adenosine deaminase. It works both on dividing and resting cells and is used in chronic lymphocytic leukemia, NHL, and cutaneous T cell lymphoma.

Hydroxyurea inhibits RNA and works to lower the white blood count in patients with myeloproliferative syndromes. It is also used in sickle cell disease to induce the production of fetal hemoglobin. It is also a radiosensitizing agent when properly administered to take advantage of the cell cycle (now seldom used).

Mercaptopurine is a purine analog and is phase specific. It is used in acute lymphoblastic leukemia.

Methotrexate is a cell cycle–specific antifolate analog. It is active in s-phase and inhibits the dihydrofolate reductase resulting in depletion of reduced folates. It is in used cancers of the breast, head and neck, sarcoma, acute lymphoblastic leukemia, non-Hodgkin's lymphoma, bladder carcinoma, gestational trophoblastic carcinoma, and for intrathecal use in carcinomatous meningitis. High doses can be given with leucovorin rescue of the bone marrow.

Pemetrexate has a similar action to methotrexate. It inhibits DNA synthesis and is used in mesothelioma and non-small-cell lung carcinoma.

Pentostatin is a purine analog and works by inhibiting the adenosine deaminase. This causes an increase in intracellular dATP and decreased DNA synthesis. Currently, it is used in the treatment of hairy cell leukemia.

Thioguanine is a purine analog which is used in acute myelogenous leukemia.

Side Effects

- Mucositis
- Diarrhea
- Bone marrow suppression
- Liver function abnormalities
- Skin rash/hand foot syndrome
- Hemolytic uremic syndrome (HUS) (gemcitabine)
- Coronary-like syndrome (5-FU)
- CNS cerebellar dysfunction (high-dose cytarabine)
- Non-cardiogenic pulmonary edema (cytarabine)
- Nausea and vomiting
- Hair loss
- Renal dysfunction

Cross-References

▶ Principles of Chemotherapy

Anti-Oncogene

▶ Tumor Suppressor Gene

Apoptosis

TOD W. SPEER
Department of Human Oncology, University of Wisconsin School of Medicine and Public Health, UW Hospital and Clinics, Madison, WI, USA

Definition

A process of rapid cell death that may be initiated by DNA damage caused by irradiation. It has also been called "programmed cell death" due to a progression and cascade of events that result in a rather classic morphology in which the cell nucleus displays densely staining globules, nuclear fragmentation, cell membrane blebbing and asymetry.

Cross-References

▶ Targeted Radioimmunotherapy

ART

▶ cART

Askin's Tumor

DANIEL J. INDELICATO[1], ROBERT H. SAGERMAN[2]
[1]Department of Radiation Oncology, University of Florida Proton Therapy Institute, University of Florida College of Medicine, Jacksonville, FL, USA
[2]Department of Radiation Oncology, SUNY Upstate Medical University, Syracuse, NY, USA

Definition

Originally defined by Askin and Rosai in 1979, this is a peripheral primitive neuroectodermal tumor originating from the soft tissue of the chest wall. The prognosis is typically inferior to Ewing sarcoma arising in the extremities.

Cross-References

▶ Ewing Sarcoma

Astrocytoma with Anaplastic Foci (AAF)

▶ Primary Intracranial Neoplasms

Astrocytomas

▶ Spinal Canal Tumor

Atrial Myxoma

▶ Primary Cardiac Tumors

Atypical (Dysplastic) Nevi

LYDIA T. KOMARNICKY-KOCHER
Department of Radiation Oncology, College of Medicine, Drexel University, Philadelphia, PA, USA

Synonyms

Atypical mole; Atypical nevus; B-K mole; Clark's nevus; Dysplastic melanocytic nevus; Nevus with architectural disorder

Definition

A mole whose features and appearance is different from the common benign mole. These are usually larger and with irregular and indistinct borders, with nonuniform color ranging from pink to dark brown, with an irregular skin surface consisting of flat and raised areas. These lesions are more likely than ordinary moles to develop into melanoma.

Cross-References

▶ Melanoma

Atypical Endometrial Hyperplasia

CHRISTIN A. KNOWLTON[1], MICHELLE KOLTON MACKAY[2]

[1]Department of Radiation Oncology, Drexel University, Philadelphia, PA, USA
[2]Department of Radiation Oncology, Marshfield Clinic, Marshfield, WI, USA

Synonyms

Endometrial hyperplasia with atypia

Definition

Endometrial hyperplasia is abnormal proliferation of the endometrium. Risk factors, symptoms, and workup for endometrial cancer are the same as for cervical cancer. In atypical endometrial hyperplasia, pleomorphic and hyperchromatic nuclei and prominent nucleoli are present in the glandular cells. More than 20% of women with atypical endometrial hyperplasia develop endometrial carcinoma.

Cross-References

▶ Endometrium

Atypical Mole

▶ Atypical (Dysplastic) Nevi

Atypical Nevus

▶ Atypical (Dysplastic) Nevi

Auto Immune Disorders

Definition

Typically a T-cell mediated aberration of the immune system that initiates a destructive process against the host.

Cross-References

▶ Collagen Vascular Disease

Autologous Stem Cell Transplant

JO ANN CHALAL
Department of Radiation Oncology, Fox Chase Cancer Center, Philadelphia, PA, USA

Definition

Immature cells from the patient's bone marrow or peripheral blood are harvested before and returned to the patient after bone marrow ablation in order to restore bone marrow function.

Cross-References

▶ Multiple Myeloma

Autologous Tissue Reconstruction

▶ Post Mastectomy Reconstruction

Average CT Volume

DAREK MICHALSKI[1], M. SAIFUL HUQ[2]
[1]Division of Medical Physics, Department of
Radiation Oncology, University of Pittsburgh
Cancer Centers, Pittsburgh, PA, USA
[2]Department of Radiation Oncology, University
of Pittsburgh Medical Center Cancer Pavilion,
Pittsburgh, PA, USA

Definition
A composite CT volume with voxel values equal
to the mean voxel value of the equivalent voxels
from a given series of other 3D CT volumes.

Cross-References
▶ Four-Dimensional (4D) Treatment Planning/
Respiratory Gating

B

Balanitis Xerotica Obliterans

STEPHAN MOSE
Department of Radiation Oncology,
Schwarzwald-Baar-Klinikum,
Villingen-Schwenningen, Germany

Definition
In male, this disease is thought to be the penile variant of lichen sclerosus et atrophicus involving the prepuce, glans, and/or urethra.

Cross-References
▶ Penile Cancer

Balkan Endemic Nephropathy

STEPHAN MOSE
Department of Radiation Oncology,
Schwarzwald-Baar-Klinikum,
Villingen-Schwenningen, Germany

Definition
This is a familial chronic tubulo-interstitial disease characterized by a slow progression to terminal renal failure with a strong association with upper urothelial carcinoma. In areas where this disease is endemic the incidence of urothelial cancer is significantly higher than in nonendemic regions.

Cross-References
▶ Renal Pelvis and Ureter

Basal Cell Nevus Syndrome

BRANDON J. FISHER
Department of Radiation Oncology, College of Medicine, Drexel University, Philadelphia, PA, USA

Synonyms
Gorlin-Gotz syndrome; Multiple basal cell carcinoma syndrome; Nevoid basal cell carcinoma syndrome

Definition
This condition is an inherited autosomal dominant syndrome that involves defects of many body systems, most notably the nervous system, eyes, endocrine system, skin, and bones. It is also known as nevoid basal cell carcinoma syndrome, multiple basal cell carcinoma syndrome, or Gorlin-Gotz syndrome. Individuals with this syndrome are more sensitive to the carcinogenic effects of radiation, with UV radiation being the main trigger of these cancers. Individuals may

L.W. Brady, T.E. Yaeger (eds.), *Encyclopedia of Radiation Oncology*, DOI 10.1007/978-3-540-85516-3,
© Springer-Verlag Berlin Heidelberg 2013

also have BCCs that occur in areas of the body that are not exposed to sunlight, like the palms or soles. Major criteria for its diagnosis are more than 2 BCCs, or 1 BCC, prior to age 20; odontogenic keratocysts of the jaw; three or more palmar or plantar pits; ectopic calcifications or early calcifications of the falx cerebri; bifid, fused, or splayed ribs; and first-degree relatives with the syndrome.

Cross-References

▶ Skin Cancer

Beam Spoiler

IRIS RUSU
Department of Radiation Oncology,
Loyola University Medical Center, Maywood,
IL, USA

Definition

Used to raise the surface dose to at least 90% of the prescribed dose.

Cross-References

▶ Total Body Irradiation (TBI)

Beamlet

CHARLIE MA, LU WANG
Department of Radiation Oncology,
Fox Chase Cancer Center, Philadelphia,
PA, USA

Definition

Beamlet: The basic small component of a radiation beam.

Cross-References

▶ Dose Calculation Algorithms

Beckwith-Wiedemann Syndrome

LARRY C. DAUGHERTY[1], BRANDON J. FISHER[2],
STEPHAN MOSE[3]
[1]Department of Radiation Oncology, College of
Medicine, Drexel University, Glenside,
PA, USA
[2]Department of Radiation Oncology, College of
Medicine, Drexel University, Philadelphia,
PA, USA
[3]Department of Radiation Oncology,
Schwarzwald-Baar-Klinikum,
Villingen-Schwenningen, Germany

Definition

Clinical constellation of Wilms' tumor (present in 5–10% of cases), gigantism, macroglossia, genitourinary abnormalities, hemihypertrophy, omphalocele, and pancreatic hyperplasia.

This is a syndrome including the diagnosis of Wilms' tumor, neuroblastoma, hepatoblastoma, and ACC.

Cross-References

▶ Carcinoma of the Adrenal Gland
▶ Wilm's Tumor

Benign Skin Tumors

▶ Keloid

Benign Tumors

▶ Radiotherapy of Nonmalignant Diseases

Bifunctional Chelating Agent (BCA)

Tod W. Speer
Department of Human Oncology, University of
Wisconsin School of Medicine and Public Health,
UW Hospital and Clinics, Madison,
WI, USA

Definition
A molecule that incorporates the capacity to
combine a radionuclide to a targeting construct,
creating a single structure.

Cross-References
▶ Targeted Radioimmunotherapy

Bile Duct Cancer

▶ Liver and Hepatobiliary Tract

Binding Site Barrier

Tod W. Speer
Department of Human Oncology, University of
Wisconsin School of Medicine and Public Health,
UW Hospital and Clinics, Madison,
WI, USA

Definition
Phenomenon used to describe the differential
binding of antibody to antigen immediately outside of a vascular wall (vascularized tumor) or in
the periphery of a tumor (preangiogenic tumor).
The differential binding is thought to be due to
very high affinities of the antibody-antigen complex and due to nonspecific binding of normal
tissue. Antibodies, therefore, do not move quickly
"off" of the antigen and therefore do not penetrate into the tumor to any meaningful extent.

Cross-References
▶ Targeted Radioimmunotherapy

Biologic Subtypes

Anthony E. Dragun
Department of Radiation Oncology, James
Graham Brown Cancer Center, University of
Louisville School of Medicine, Louisville,
KY, USA

Synonyms
Luminal subtypes

Definition
Distinct biologic subtypes of breast cancer are
identified by incorporating information obtained
by microarray analysis and traditional immunohistochemistry to stratify breast cancer into risk
categories. The use of biologic subtyping to guide
treatment management is gaining interest in the
radiation oncology and medical oncology communities. Luminal A: This is the most common
subtype making up approximately 40–50% of
breast cancers. It is characteristically estrogen
receptor positive, progesterone receptor positive,
and Her2 negative. It carries the best overall prognosis. Luminal B: This is makes up roughly 20% of
all breast cancers and is characterized as being
estrogen receptor, progesterone receptor, and
Her2 positive. Her2-positive subtype: These constitute 20% of cases, the majority of which are
high-grade tumors. Approximately 40% have
underlying p53 mutations. They are characteristically estrogen and progesterone receptor negative,
Her2 positive. Basal-type ("triple negative"): This
subtype exhibits a distinctive basal gene cluster on

reverse transcriptase polymerase chain reaction. These make up about 15 % of breast cancers, are estrogen receptor, progesterone receptor, and Her 2 negative, and exhibit the worst prognosis. They are linked to carriers of BRCA mutations.

Cross-References
▶ Early-Stage Breast Cancer
▶ Microarray Analysis

Biological Response Modifiers

RENE RUBIN
Rittenhouse Hematology/Oncology,
Philadelphia, PA, USA

Definition
This small group includes interferon and various interleukins. Interferon induces cytotoxicity to T-cells, helper T-cells, and NK cells and also inhibits proliferation. Interleukin induces LAK and NK cell activity and enhances lymphocyte cytotoxicity. Therefore an intact immune system is required. Denileukin difitox is a combination of interleukin and diphtheria toxin. It binds to the CD25 component of the IL-2 receptor. The drugs are used in melanoma, chronic myelocytic leukemia, hairy cell leukemia, myeloma, and in renal cell carcinoma.

Side Effects
- Flu-like symptoms
- Fatigue
- Myelosuppression
- Vascular leak syndrome
- Hepatotoxicity and abnormalities of liver function tests

Cross-References
▶ Principles of Chemotherapy

Biomarkers

CLAUDIA RÜBE
Department of Radiation Oncology,
Saarland University, Homburg/Saar, Germany

Definition
In general are substances used as indicators of a biological state. Biomarkers measured in blood and other samples have been analyzed to potentially predict how certain tissues might respond to radiotherapy.

Cross-References
▶ Predictive In vitro Assays in Radiation Oncology

Biomedicine (also Traditional, Theoretical, Conventional, or Western Medicine)

JAMES H. BRASHEARS, III
Radiation Oncologist, Venice, FL, USA

Synonyms
Conventional medicine; Theoretical medicine; Traditional medicine; Western medicine

Definition
From the Greek *bio* meaning life and the Latin *ars medicina* meaning the art of healing. It comprises the knowledge, research, and practice of medicine as described by the natural sciences. Biomedicine is the predominant mode of understanding taught in modern medical schools.

Cross-References

▶ Allopathic Medicine
▶ Complementary Medicine
▶ Pain Management

Birt–Hogg–Dubé Syndrome

Stephan Mose
Department of Radiation Oncology,
Schwarzwald-Baar-Klinikum,
Villingen-Schwenningen, Germany

Definition

This syndrome (FLCN gene, chromosome 17p11) shows microscopically a chromophobe renal cell carcinoma which is associated with (benign) oncocytomas, transitional tumors, cutaneous fibrofolliculomas, and lung cysts. Worldwide this syndrome has been reported in more than 100 families.

Cross-References

▶ Kidney

Bisphosphonates

James H. Brashears, III
Radiation Oncologist, Venice, FL, USA

Synonyms

Disphosphonates

Definition

Systemic medications that prevent loss of bone mass by interfering with osteoclast activity.

Cross-References

▶ Palliation of Bone Metastases

B-K Mole

▶ Atypical (Dysplastic) Nevi

Bladder

Christian Weiss, Claus Roedel
Department of Radiotherapy and Radiation Oncology, University Hospital Frankfurt/Main, Frankfurt, Germany

Synonyms

Adenocarcinoma; Chemoradiation; Combined modality therapy; Multimodality treatment; Papillary carcinoma; Papilloma; Squamous cell carcinoma; Transitional cell carcinoma; Urinary tract; Urothelial carcinoma

Definition/Description

The term "bladder cancer" comprises a heterogeneous group of bladder neoplasms with different malignant potentials and prognoses. Due to the morphological appearance, bladder cancer can be divided into noninvasive papillary, papillary infiltrating, solid infiltrating, and non-papillary, noninfiltrating, or carcinoma in situ. Depending on the depth of tumor invasion, papillary tumors and flat, high-grade tumors confined to the mucosa are classified as stage Ta or carcinoma in situ (Tis), respectively. Tumors invading the lamina propria are classified as stage T1 according to the 2002 TNM system. These tumors are grouped under the heading of non-muscle-invasive (superficial) bladder cancer (NMIBC). Otherwise, tumors with infiltration into the

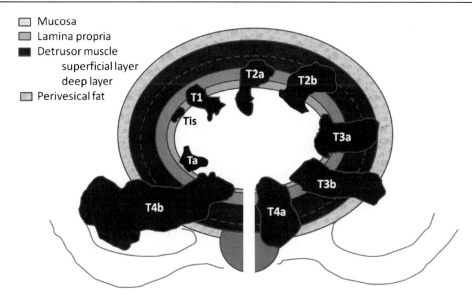

Bladder. Fig. 1 T-stage classification 2002

muscle layer are grouped under the heading of muscle-invasive bladder cancer and staged ≥ T2 according to the 2002 TNM system (Fig. 1, Table 1). After transurethral resection (TUR) for NMIBC, an organ-preserving approach with or without instillation therapy is recommended. Especially in patients with high-risk superficial bladder cancer or in those patients where instillation therapy has failed, radiotherapy or chemoradiation may represent an alternative for a bladder-sparing approach. In case of muscle-invasive disease, radical cystectomy represents the treatment of choice in the last three decades, although organ-preserving regimens, using multimodal approaches, with TUR followed by radiotherapy and concurrent chemotherapy showed to be an alternative to radical surgery in selected patients.

Anatomy

The urinary bladder is a musculomembranous, expendable hollow organ, which lies extra peritoneal in the true pelvis. Only the surface is covered with peritoneum. The form, size, and position of the bladder are strongly dependent on its filling. Bladder capacity has a wide range of about 300–500 mL and more. The bladder can be divided into the corpus vesicae urinariae, representing the body with its walls merging to the vertex vesicae. Its superior surface is covered with peritoneum. The vertex is directed to the pubic symphysis and is joined to the umbilicus by the urachal remnant. The fundus vesicae urinariae contains the bladder trigone defined by the orifices of the ureters and urethra. The collum vesicae ore neck of the bladder refers to the area encompassing the urethral opening. In females, the body of the uterus overhangs the superior surface of the bladder and close to the posterior surface and at base of the bladder lays the anterior wall of the vagina. The bladder neck is directly related to the pelvic fascia surrounding the upper urethra. In males, the upper part of the bladder fundus is separated from the rectum by the rectovesical pouch, the lower part by the seminal vesicles and the deferent duct, while the bladder neck rests on the prostate. The bladder walls are composed of four coats: a serous, a muscular, a submucous, and a mucous coat. The lymphatic drainage is by the external and internal iliac and presacral lymphnodes.

Bladder. Table 1 2002 TNM classification of urinary bladder cancer

T-primary tumor	
Ta	Noninvasive papillary carcinoma
Tis	Carcinoma in situ: "flat tumor"
T1	Tumor invades subepithelial connective tissue
T2	Tumor invades muscle
T2a	Tumor invades superficial muscle (inner half)
T2b	Tumor invades deep muscle (outer half)
T3	Tumor invades perivesical tissue
T3a	Microscopically
T3b	Macroscopically (extravesical mass)
T4	Tumor invades any of the following
T4a	T4a Tumor invades prostate, uterus, or vagina
T4b	T4b Tumor invades pelvic wall or abdominal wall
N-lymph nodes	
N0	No regional lymph node metastases
N1	Metastases in a single lymph node 2 cm or less in greatest dimension
N2	Metastases in a single lymph node more than 2 cm but not more than 5 cm in greatest dimension, or multiple lymph nodes, none more than 5 cm in greatest dimension
N3	Metastases in a lymph node more than 5 cm in greatest dimension
M-distant metastases	
M0	No distant metastases
M1	Distant metastases

Epidemiology

Bladder carcinoma is the second most common genitourinary malignancy. In 2002, bladder cancer was estimated to be the ninth most common cause of cancer worldwide (357,000 cases). In males (274,000 cases), the rates are 3–4 times higher than in females (83,000 cases). In developed countries, bladder cancer is relatively common with high rates in North America and Europe, where 59% of all incident cases occur. The number of deaths was about 145,000 worldwide and makes bladder cancer the 13th most frequent cause of death from cancer. Population-based 5 -year-survival rates range from 40% to 80% depending on whether non-muscle-invasive lesions are included in the computation. In Western countries, more than 90% of bladder cancers are transitional cell carcinomas, about 6–7% are squamous cell carcinomas, and 1–2% are adenocarcinomas. In some African countries, 38% and more of bladder cancers are of squamous histology, which is related to the prevalence of infection with Shistosoma haematobium.

The major risk factor for developing bladder cancer is smoking with a linear relationship between smoking and risk, while quitting smoking reduces the risk. Other factors with elevated risk are associated to occupational exposure with well-known carcinogens such as benzidine, 2-Naphthylamine, hydrocarbons, and petroleum-based chemicals. Moreover, some drugs (phenacetin), ionizing radiation, and chemotherapeutics (cyclophosfamide) have been found to increase the risk of bladder cancer.

Clinical Presentation

The most frequent symptom of bladder cancer is painless, sometimes intermittent, gross hematuria in 75–80% of all cases. About 25% of patients with bladder cancer complain about vesical irritability and dysuria, additionally. In patients without specific symptoms, their cancers are detected because of microscopic hematuria, urine cytology results, pyuria, or so forth. In advanced stages, bladder cancer can cause severe pain because of locoregional invasion or urinary retention due to ureteral obstruction. Signs and symptoms of bone, liver, pulmonary, and central nervous system metastases may be present in disseminated disease.

Differential Diagnosis

In any case of microscopic or macroscopic hematuria, especially when diagnosed in patients with age above 40, it is obligatory to exclude a malignant tumor. The most frequent differential diagnoses of hematuria are inflammation or infection of the prostate or urinary bladder, urinary calculi, and glomerular disorders.

Diagnosis and Imaging Studies

As routine a thorough clinical history, a general physical examination with rectal and pelvic exploration is mandatory. Prior to transurethral resection (TUR), a renal and bladder ultrasonography is recommended.

Cystoscopy with description of the tumor (site, size, number, and appearance) and mucosal abnormalities is the mainstay of diagnosis. If not done in the same session, a cystoscopy with TUR of the tumor under anesthesia is performed. Bimanual examination should be carried out before and after TUR to assess whether there is a palpable mass or the tumor is fixed to the pelvic wall. A fluorescence-guided biopsy, especially when Tis is suspected may be useful (e.g., positive cytology, recurrent tumor with previous history of a high-grade lesion).

A second TUR should be performed at 2–6 weeks after the initial resection when it was incomplete, when a high grade or T1 tumor was detected, or a bladder-sparing approach is planned.

An intravenous pyelogram (IVP) or computer tomography urogram (CTU) should be performed in all patients with at least high-risk NMIBC and muscle-invasive bladder cancer to exclude upper genitourinary tract disease.

In patients suspected to have muscle-invasive disease, a computer tomography scan or magnetic resonance imaging of the pelvis to assess local invasion or regional lymph node metastases may be helpful for subsequent treatment planning. It should be performed prior to TUR. The overall staging accuracy is about 75% for MRI and about 55% for CT concerning the assessment of the primary tumor.

To exclude distant metastases, a CT scan or X-ray of the chest is part of the staging procedure. A bone scan is indicated if levels of alkaline phosphatase are elevated or symptoms are present.

Laboratory Studies

Complete blood count and chemistry profile, including alkaline phosphatase, has to be done routinely.

Urine analysis is commonly used to diagnose a urinary tract or kidney infection, to evaluate causes of kidney failure, and to screen for progression of some chronic conditions such as diabetes mellitus and high blood pressure (hypertension).

Urine cytology is an examination of voided urine or a bladder-washing specimen for exfoliated cancer cells. It has a high sensitivity in high-grade tumors.

Urinary marker tests are based on detection of soluble markers or cell-associated markers. Several tests are available though their benefit for routine use remains to be elucidated.

Treatment

About 70% of newly diagnosed cases of bladder cancer have non-muscle-invasive disease, but as many as 50–70% will recur and, roughly, 10–20% will progress to muscle-invasive disease (T2–4). Standard treatment recommendations differ significantly for non-muscle and muscle-invasive bladder cancer. For most of the NMIBC cases, an organ sparing treatment regimen, including TUR with or without installation therapy, is performed. In localized muscle-invasive cancer, standard therapy remains radical cystectomy with pelvic lymph node dissection. Nevertheless, evidence emerges that multimodality treatment strategies consisting of limited surgery (TUR, partial bladder resection) followed by chemoradiation may represent an alternative to radical cystectomy.

Non-muscle-Invasive Bladder Cancer (NMIBC)

In NMIBC, several risk factors predicting the probability of local recurrence and progression have been identified. Against this background, the European Organization for Research and Treatment of Cancer (EORTC) developed risk tables for predicting recurrence and progression in individual patients with Stage Ta T1 bladder cancer (http://www.eortc.be/tools/bladdercalculator). Similar risk classifications have been published by the National Comprehensive Cancer Network (NCCN). A transurethral resection followed by a single chemoinstillation within 24 h is recommended for all patients regardless of their risk for recurrence or progression. Patients with intermediate-risk NMIBC should receive intravesical chemotherapy (6–12 months) or Bacillus Calmette–Guerin (BCG) as further adjuvant treatment. For high-risk NMIBC, intravesical BCG with maintenance for at least 12 months is indicated. Immediate radical cystectomy may be offered to patients with a very high risk of tumor progression, and salvage radical cystectomy is recommended for patients who fail to respond to BCG.

The rationale for using radiotherapy or chemoradiation for patients with primary or recurrent high-risk non-muscle-invasive bladder cancer stems from the proven efficacy of this approach in more advanced disease. To date, no prospective or randomized trials concerning this issue are available. Long-term results from a single institution series of 141 patients with high-risk NMIBC treated with TUR plus chemoradiation therapy suggest that this selective bladder preservation approach may help to strike a balance between intravesical treatment and

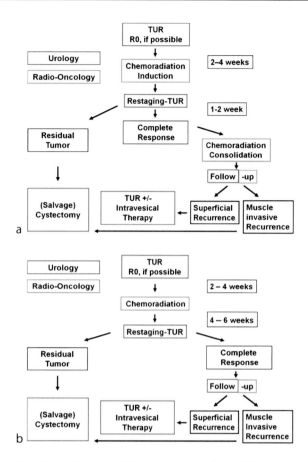

Bladder. Fig. 2 (**a**) Massachusetts General Hospital Boston: Schedule of combined modality therapy. (**b**) University Erlangen: Schedule of combined modality therapy

immediate cystectomy. For these 141 patients, the disease-specific survival was 82% at 5 years, and 70% at 10 years; bladders were preserved in more than 80% of the surviving patients, and more than 70% were very satisfied with their urinary function (see Fig. 2 for treatment schedule).

Muscle-Invasive Bladder Cancer

Surgical Treatment

Standard treatment for muscle-invasive bladder cancer is radical cystectomy with pelvic lymph node dissection. In men, a cystoprostatectomy and in women, an anterior exenteration — including the bladder, urethra, uterus, and ventral vaginal wall has to be performed. After radical cystectomy, urinary diversion is done in either a non-continent or continent way, with a segment of bowel. The simplest form is the non-continent ileal conduit. A continent urinary diversion can be either an orthotopic neobladder or an abdominal pouch. In both diversions, a segment of bowel is made into a detubularized spherical form, with continence in the abdominal pouch relying on a catheterizable continent stoma and on the patient's striated urethral sphincter in the orthotopic neobladder. The reported 5-year overall survival rates from series of radical cystectomy are in the range of 45–54%. In these series, tumor stage and nodal involvement showed to be the only independent predictors of survival.

Limited surgery such as TUR or partial cystectomy as sole treatment should only be used in patients unfit or not willing to undergo radical cystectomy or multimodality treatment.

Multimodality Treatment

The centers that pioneered modern bladder preservation therapy included Harvard University in the United States, the University of Paris in France, and the University of Erlangen in Germany. In the 1980s, studies under the auspices of the US National Bladder Cancer Group showed that irradiation of the bladder tumor could be safely combined with cisplatin in patients who were considered not to be candidates for cystectomy. In 1988, Housset et al. from Paris began a prospective trial of preoperative chemoradiation (CRT), using fluorouracil (FU) and cisplatin with concomitant radiation therapy, followed by cystectomy or additional CRT. Histopathologic examination of the cystectomy specimen revealed complete pathologic response in the first 18 patients after induction therapy. Complete responders were considered candidates

for bladder preservation, and salvage cystectomy was restricted to patients with an incomplete response after induction therapy. This treatment strategy resulted in a 5-year survival of 63%. In 1990, Sauer et al. from Erlangen reported the results of a phase II study of cisplatin with concomitant radiotherapy after TURBT in 67 patients with muscle-invasive bladder cancer. Complete response was obtained in 75% of patients, and overall 3-year survival was 66%. Over the past 15 years, the concept of organ preservation by conservative surgery and combined radiotherapy and chemotherapy has been investigated in several prospective series from single centers and cooperative groups, with more than 1,000 patients included. Five-year overall survival rates in the range of 50–60% have been reported and about three-quarters of the surviving patients maintained their own bladder (Tables 2 and 3).

Clinical criteria helpful in determining patients for bladder preservation include such variables as small tumor size (<5 cm), early tumor stage, a visibly and microscopically complete TURBT, absence of ureteral obstruction, and no evidence of pelvic lymph node metastases. On multivariate analysis, the completeness of TURBT was found to be one of the strongest prognostic factors for overall survival. Thus, a TURBT as thorough as safely possible should always be attempted. Patients at greater risk of new tumor development after initial complete response are those with multifocal disease and extensive associated carcinoma in situ at presentation. Anemia has also been shown to predict reduced local control as well as a higher rate of distant metastases and death from bladder cancer.

The current combined modality treatment regimen for organ preservation in bladder cancer from Massachusetts General Hospital Boston and the University of Erlangen are shown in Fig. 2a and b. The recommended doses and timing of chemoradiation for clinical practice (off study

Bladder. Table 2 MGH and RTOG: Series of combined modality treatment and selective bladder preservation

Series	N	Clinical stage	Treatment	Complete Response pCR (%)	5-Year OS (%)	5-Year OS with bladder (%)
MGH 1986–1993	106	T2-4a	TUR 2 cycles MCV + RT	66	52	43
RTOG 85–12 1986–1988	42	T2-4a	TUR + RT	66	52	42
RTOG 88–02 1988–1990	91	T2-4a	TUR 2 cycles MCV + RT	75	62 (4 years)	44 (4 years)
RTOG 89–03 1990–1993	123	T2-4a	TUR plus 2 cycles MCV vs no chemotherapy + RT	61 vs 55	49 vs 48	36 vs 40
MGH 1993–1994	18	T2-4a	TUR + RCT	78	83 (3 years)	78 (3 years)
RTOG 95–06 1995–1997	34	T2-4a	TUR + RCT	67	83 (3 years)	66 (3 years)
RTOG 97–06 1997–1999	47	T2-4a	TUR + RCT	74	61 (3 years)	48 (3 years)

MGH Massachusetts General Hospital, *RTOG* Radiation Therapy Oncology Group, *TUR* Transurethral Resection of Bladder Tumor, *MCV* Methotrexate, Cisplatin, Vinblastine, *FU* Fluorouracil, *pCR* Pathologic Complete Response, *OS* Overall Survival

protocol) from these institutions are summarized in Fig. 3. In general, radiotherapy planning should be done using a 3D conformal CT-based technique. As a standard, the use of multiple individually shaped fields with high-energy photons > 6MV are recommended. The total radiation dose prescribed to the whole bladder and the pelvic lymph nodes is typically 45–50 Gy followed by a dose escalation between 55 and 70 Gy to the bladder or the tumor area. Single fractionation size is 1.8–2 Gy. It is recommended to plan and treat patients with bladder empty.

Recent developments in irradiation technique, especially intensity-modulated radiotherapy (IMRT) and image-guided radiotherapy (IGRT), promise to improve the treatment ratio by the possibility to deliver a higher dose to the tumor and simultaneously reducing irradiation exposure of healthy tissue. Moreover, the addition, e.g., of deep regional hyperthermia and the integration of novel therapeutic agents potentially will improve the results of multimodality treatment regimen.

In summary, combined modality therapy for bladder preservation has become a safe, tested, and effective alternative to radical cystectomy in selected patients with muscle-invasive bladder cancer who desire to keep their own bladders. There is evidence that radiotherapy alone is less effective than radical surgery or multimodality treatment (Fig. 4).

Neoadjuvant Treatment

In the last decades, various investigators conducted trials or published their experience with protocols using radiotherapy or chemotherapy prior to definitive treatment of muscle-invasive bladder cancer.

Bladder. Table 3 Further series of combined modality treatment for bladder cancer

Series	N	Clinical stage	Treatment	pCR (%)	5-year OS (%)	5-year OS with bladder (%)
Russell et al. (1990)	34	T1-4	TUR + 44 Gy at 2 Gy plus 5-FU and consolidation for patients with pCR with 16 Gy at 2 Gy plus 5-FU	81	64 (4 years)	n.g. (overall rate of cystectomy: 10/34)
Rotman et al. (1990)	20	T1-4	TURBT + 60–65 Gy at 1.8 Gy plus 5-FU	74	39	n.g. (19/20 maintained bladder)
Given et al. (1995)	93	T2-4	TURBT + 2 or 3 cycles MVAC or MCV + 64.80 Gy at 1.8 Gy plus cisplatin (49 patients)	63	39%	n.g.
Housset et al. (1997)	120	T2-4	TURBT + 24 Gy at 3 Gy plus cisplatin/5-FU and consolidation for patients with pCR with 20 Gy at 2.5 Gy plus cisplatin/5-FU	77	63	n.g.
Varveris et al. (1997)	42	T1-4	TURBT + 68–74 Gy at 1.8–2 Gy plus cisplatin and docetaxel	62	78 (median f/u of 25 mo)	n.g.
Fellin et al. (1997)	56	T2-4	TURBT + plus 2 cycles of MCV +40 Gy at 1.8 Gy plus cispaltin and consolidation for patients with pCR with 24 Gy at 2 Gy plus cisplatin	50	55	41
Cervek et al. (1998)	105	T2-4	TURBT + 2–4 cycles MCV + 50 Gy at 2.0 Gy	52	58 (4 years)	45 (4 years)
Zapatero et al. (2000)	40	T2-4	TURBT + plus 3 cycles MCV + 60 Gy at 2.0 Gy	70	84 (4 years)	82.6 (4 years)
Arias et al. (2000)	50	T2-4	TURBT plus 2 cycles MVAC + 45 Gy at 1.80 Gy plus cisplatin and consolidation for patients with pCR with 20 Gy at 2.0 Gy	68	48	-
Rödel et al. (2002)	415	T1-4	TURBT + 50.4–59.4 Gy at 1.8 Gy plus carboplatin/cisplatin (+ 5-FU)	72	50	42
Chen et al. (2003)	23	T3-4	TURBT + 60–61.2 Gy at 1.8/2 Gy plus cisplatin/5-FU/leucovorin	89	69 (3 years)	n.g.
Peyromaure et al. (2004)	43	T2	TURBT + 24 Gy at 3 Gy plus cisplatin/5-FU + Two additional cycles of chemoradiation (doses not given)	74	60 (cancer specific)	n.g. (overall rate of cystectomy: 25.6%)
Danesi et al. (2004)	77	T2-4	TURBT + 2 cycles of MCV (42 pts) + 69 Gy at 1 Gy (three fractions per day) plus cisplatin/5-FU	90	58	47
Hussain et al. (2004)	41	T2-4	TURBT + 55 Gy at 2.75 Gy plus 5-FU and mitomycin-C	69	36%	n.g. (overall rate of cystectomy: 12%)

Bladder. Table 3 (continued)

Series	N	Clinical stage	Treatment	pCR (%)	5-year OS (%)	5-year OS with bladder (%)
Kragelj et al. (2005)	84	T1-4	TURBT + 64 Gy at 1.8–2.2 Gy plus vinblastine	78	25% (9 years)	n.g.
Dunst et al. (2005)	68	T2-4	TURBT + 50.4–59.4 Gy at +1.8 Gy plus cisplatin or paclitaxel	87	45	n.g.

TURBT Transurethral Resection of the Bladder Tumor, *MCV* Methotrexate, Cisplatin, Vinblastine, *MVAC* Methotrexate, Vincristine, Adriamycin, Cisplatin, *FU* Fluorouracil, *pCR* Pathologic Complete Response, *n.g.* Not Given, *OS* Overall Survival, f/u, Follow-up

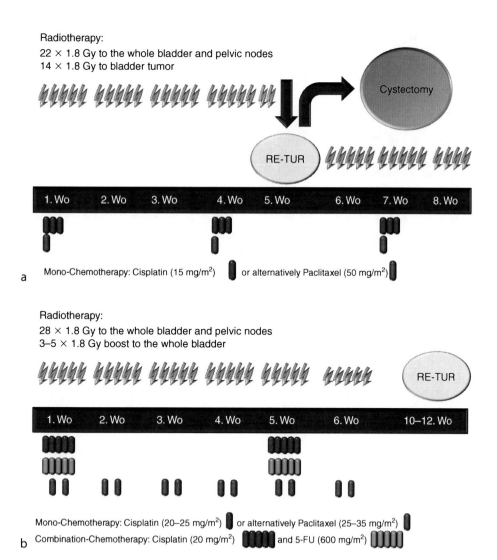

Bladder. Fig. 3 (**a**) Massachusetts General Hospital Boston: Chemoradiation regimen. (**b**) University Erlangen: Chemoradiation regimen

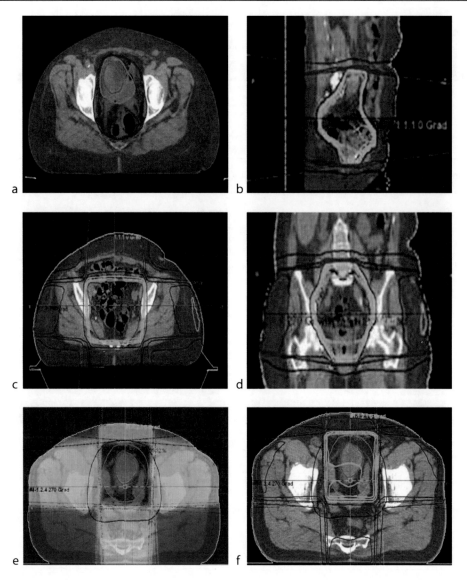

Bladder. Fig. 4 (**a–f**) Radiation technique: Treatment plans to the pelvic lymph nodes and bladder with a total dose of 45–50 Gy (**a–d**), then a cone-down is applied to boost the whole bladder (**e–f**)

Radiotherapy

Both retrospective and randomized trials yielded conflicting data concerning the possible benefit of neoadjuvant radiotherapy in muscle-invasive bladder cancer prior to radical cystectomy. On the other hand, there is evidence that using radiotherapy with a total dose of 45–50 Gy in fractions of 1.8–2 Gy results in down-staging after 4–6 weeks without a significant increase in toxicity following surgery. No long-term experiences or prospective randomized trials addressing the issue of neoadjuvant chemoradiation are available.

Chemotherapy

A recent meta-analysis with independent patient data of 11 randomized trials (3,005 patients) showed a statistically significant 5% absolute improvement in survival at 5 years in favor of neoadjuvant chemotherapy in muscle-invasive bladder cancer. Of note is that the detected survival benefit was only seen with cisplatin-based multi-agent chemotherapy regimens (with at least one additional chemotherapeutic agent) and that it is independent of the kind of definitive treatment applied (radiotherapy or radical cystectomy). Thus, it is recommended to consider neoadjuvant chemotherapy for patients with muscle-invasive bladder cancer.

Adjuvant Treatment

Chemotherapy

Adjuvant chemotherapy is a controversial issue. Neither randomized trials nor a meta-analysis have provided sufficient data to support the routine use of adjuvant chemotherapy.

Radiotherapy

Data are rare on adjuvant radiotherapy. Published in 1992, a randomized trial from Egypt demonstrated a reduction of pelvic recurrences from 50% to 10% in T3 and T4 bladder cancer. But 68% of the patients had histology of squamous cell carcinoma, and it remains unclear if these results are translatable for ▶ transitional cell carcinoma of the urinary bladder.

Metastatic Disease

Chemotherapy

Compared with other solid malignant tumors, transitional cell carcinoma of bladder has shown chemosensitivity. First reports on multi-agent chemotherapy showed response rates of 50–70%. In patients with good performance status, cisplatin-based multi-agent chemotherapy is recommended. Gemcitabine and cisplatin showed similar efficacy to a combination of methotrexate, vinblastine, adriamycine, and cisplatin with a lower toxicity profile and is therefore considered standard of care. In patients unfit to receive cisplatin, use of carboplatin as combination chemotherapy or single agents is a reasonable option. For second-line treatment, single-agent chemotherapy is preferred.

Radiotherapy

Radiotherapy should be offered to patients with local symptoms from recurrent or metastatic disease (e.g., bone metastases, brain metastases). For limited, inoperable, locoregional recurrence after cystectomy, chemoradiation may be an option for patients in good clinical condition.

Cross-References

▶ Concept of Hyperthermia
▶ Conformal Therapy: Treatment Planning, Treatment Delivery, and Clinical Results
▶ Image-Guided Radiotherapy (IGRT)
▶ Intensity-Modulated Proton Therapy (IMPT)
▶ Male Urethra
▶ Molecular Markers in Clinical Radiation Oncology
▶ Principles of Chemotherapy
▶ Renal Pelvis and Ureter

References

Arias F, Dominguez MA, Martinez E et al (2000) Chemoradiotherapy for muscle invading bladder carcinoma. Final report of a single institutional organ-sparing program. Int J Radiat Oncol Biol Phys 47:373–378

Cervek J, Cufer T, Zakotnik B et al (1998) Invasive bladder cancer: our experience with bladder sparing approach. Int J Radiat Oncol Biol Phys 41:273–278

Chao CKS, Perez CA, Brady LW (eds) (2002) Radiation oncology, management decisions, 2nd edn. Wolters Kluwer Lippincott Williams & Wilkins, Philadelphia

Chen WC, Liaw CC, Chuang CK et al (2003) Concurrent cisplatin, 5-fluorouracil, leucovorin, and radiotherapy for invasive bladder cancer. Int J Radiat Oncol Biol Phys 56:726–733

Danesi DT, Arcangeli G, Cruciani E et al (2004) Conservative treatment of invasive bladder carcinoma by transurethral resection, protracted intravenous infusion chemotherapy, and hyperfractionated radiotherapy: long term results. Cancer 101:2540–2548

Dunst J, Diestelhorst A, Kuhn R et al (2005) Organ-sparing treatment in muscle-invasive bladder cancer. Strahlenther Onkol 181:632–637

Fellin G, Graffer U, Bolner A et al (1997) Combined chemotherapy and radiation with selective organ preservation for muscle-invasive bladder carcinoma. A single-institution phase II study. Br J Urol 80:44–49

Given RW, Parsons JT, McCarley D et al (1995) Bladder-sparing multimodality treatment of muscle-invasive bladder cancer: a five-year follow-up. Urology 46:499–504

Gray H (1918) Anatomy of the human body. Lea & Febiger, Philadelphia; Bartleby.com, 2000 www.bartleby.com/107/

Halperin EC, Perez CA, Brady LW (eds) (2007) Principles and practice of radiation oncology, 5th edn. Wolters Kluwer, Lippincott Wiliams & Wilkens, Philadelphia

Housset M, Dufour B, Maulard-Durdux C, Chretien Y, Mejean A (1997) Concomitant fluorouracil (5-FU)-cisplatin (CDDP) and bifractionated split course radiation therapy (BSCRT) for invasive bladder cancer. Proc Am Soc Clin Oncol 16:319a (abstract)

Hussain SA, Stocken DD, Peake DR et al (2004) Long-term results of a phase II study of synchronous chemoradiotherapy in advanced muscle invasive bladder cancer. Br J Cancer 90:2106–2111

Kaufman DS, Shipley WU, Feldman AS (2009) Bladder cancer. Lancet 374:239–249

Kragelj B, Zaletel-Kragelj L, Sedmak B et al (2005) Phase II study of radiochemotherapy with vinblastine in invasive bladder cancer. Radiother Oncol 75:44–47

Parkin DM (2008) The global burden of urinary bladder cancer. Scand J Urol Nephrol Suppl 218:12–20

Peyromaure M, Slama J, Beuzeboc P et al (2004) Concurrent chemoradiotherapy for clinical stage T2 bladder cancer: report of a single institution. Urology 63:73–77

Rödel C, Grabenbauer GG, Kuhn R et al (2002) Combined-modality treatment and selective organ preservation in invasive bladder cancer: long-term results. J Clin Oncol 20:3061–3071

Rodel C et al (2006) Trimodality treatment and selective organ preservation for bladder cancer. J Clin Oncol 24:5536–5544

Rotman M, Aziz H, Porrazzo M et al (1990) Treatment of advanced transitional cell carcinoma of the bladder with irradiation and concomitant 5-fluorouracil infusion. Int J Radiat Oncol Biol Phys 18:1131–1137

Russell KJ, Boileau MA, Higano C et al (1990) Combined 5-fluorouracil and irradiation for transitional cell carcinoma of the urinary bladder. Int J Radiat Oncol Biol Phys 19:693–699

Varveris H, Delakas D, Anezinis P et al (1997) Concurrent platinum and docetaxel chemotherapy and external radical radiotherapy in patients with invasive transitional cell bladder carcinoma. A preliminary report of tolerance and local control. Anticancer Res 17:4771–4780

Weiss C et al (2006) Radiochemotherapy after transurethral resection for high-risk T1 bladder cancer: an alternative to intravesical therapy or early cystectomy? J Clin Oncol 24:2318–2324

Zapatero A, Martin de Vidales C, Marin A et al (2000) Invasive bladder cancer: a single-institution experience with bladder-sparing approach. Int J Cancer 90:287–294

Zietman AL, Shipley WU (2007) Bladder Cancer. 60. In: Gunderson LL, Tepper JE (eds) Clinical radiation oncology, 2nd edn. Elsevier Churchill Livingstone, Philadelphia

Bladder Cancer

CHRISTIAN WEISS, CLAUS ROEDEL
Department of Radiotherapy and Radiation Oncology, University Hospital Frankfurt/Main, Frankfurt, Germany

Definition

Any kind of malignant growths of the urinary bladder. In the Western world, transitional cell carcinoma is the predominant histology. In regard to the infiltration depth of the tumor non-muscle-invasive and muscle-invasive bladder cancer can be differentiated.

Cross-References

▶ Renal Pelvis and Ureter

Blinding

EDWARD J. GRACELY
Department of Epidemiology and Biostatistics, College of Medicine, Drexel University, Philadelphia, PA, USA

Definition

Ensuring that individuals (subjects or researchers) do not have information about the status or assignment of individual subjects that might bias them in their evaluations.

Cross-References

▶ Statistics and Clinical Trials

Bone Marrow Rescue Agents

RENE RUBIN
Rittenhouse Hematology/Oncology,
Philadelphia, PA, USA

Definition

G-CSF and GM-CSF stimulate granulocytes and macrophages to proliferate and prevent chemotherapy-induced neutropenia. These agents should be used in chemotherapy regimens that are known to cause neutropenia or after patients demonstrate low bone marrow tolerance. Side effects include fevers, chills, and bone pain.

Erythropoeitin is a hormone secreted in the kidney which induces red blood cell production. Chemotherapy can induce induced anemia and often the erythropoietin level is low. Keeping the hemoglobin in the normal ranges appears to improve quality of life and to reduce chemotherapy-induced fatigue. Side effects include thrombosis and bone pain.

Thrombopoietin stimulates megakaryocyte production. It may cause thrombosis and possibly bone marrow fibrosis.

Cross-References

▶ Principles of Chemotherapy

Bone Marrow Toxicity in Cancer Treatment

LINDSAY G. JENSEN, BRENT S. ROSE, LOREN K. MELL,
ARNO J. MUNDT
Center for Advanced Radiotherapy Technologies,
Department of Radiation Oncology, San Diego
Rebecca and John Moores Cancer Center,
University of California, La Jolla, CA, USA

Definition/Description

Bone marrow is a highly radiosensitive tissue, which is made up of hematopoietically active (red) marrow and relatively hematopoietically inactive (yellow) marrow. The distribution of active bone marrow changes with age. In childhood, active bone marrow is found in the sternum, ribs, pelvis, spine, skull, femur, humerus, and other long bones. This distribution contracts to the axial skeleton, proximal femur, and humerus later in life (Mauch et al. 1995).

Approximately half of active bone marrow in adults is located in the pelvic bones and lumbar spine, making bone marrow radiation dose an important consideration when treating pelvic or abdominal tumors (Roeske et al. 2005). Bone marrow toxicity from radiation results from damage to ▶ Hematopoietic Stem Cells as well as bone ▶ Microenvironment. The degree of bone marrow toxicity during and after radiotherapy depends on a number of factors, including volume of bone marrow within the field, dose, fractionation, and concurrent chemotherapy regimen (Mauch et al. 1995). This entry focuses on bone marrow toxicity from radiation therapy. For further discussion of radiation for stem cell transplant, please see ▶ Total Body Irradiation (TBI).

Acute Bone Marrow Toxicity

Hematologic toxicity (HT) is a relatively common high-grade toxicity in patients treated with pelvic irradiation and chemotherapy, with grade 3 or greater hematologic toxicity occurring in approximately 27% of women being treated for ▶ Cervical Cancer (Rose et al. 2011). Hematologic toxicity puts patients at an increased risk of infection, fatigue, hemorrhage, and hospitalization. Patient instability and hospitalization can lead to radiation treatment breaks and missed doses of chemotherapy, which may adversely affect disease control and survival.

Hematologic toxicity is monitored using peripheral blood counts, though these do not immediately reflect damage to the bone marrow due to variation with the lifetime of circulating cells, time to maturation, and radiosensitivity of precursor cells (Mauch et al. 1995). Lymphocytes are particularly radiosensitive and peripheral counts fall almost immediately following even low doses of radiation. Neutropenic nadir occurs next, within 1 week, followed by ▶ Thrombocytopenia at 2–3 weeks and ▶ Anemia at 2–3 months (Hall and Giaccia 2006; Mauch et al. 1995). Patients with severe hematologic toxicities may require transfusions, ▶ Erythropoietin, or growth factors to increase proliferation of hematopoietic stem cells.

Chronic Bone Marrow Toxicity

The long-term effects of high doses (30 Gy cumulative or 20 Gy in one dose) of irradiation to the bone marrow have been shown to vary according to what percent of bone marrow is within field. When less than 50% of the bone marrow is irradiated, the surrounding nonirradiated bone marrow is able to increase hematopoietic activity to compensate for decreased activity in the irradiated region and in-field regeneration does not occur. When 50–75% of the bone marrow is irradiated, the surrounding nonirradiated bone marrow becomes more active and extends into previously inactive regions such as the femur.

At higher doses of 35–40 Gy, in-field regeneration has been shown to occur, which may be related to increased growth factors being released from the surrounding nonirradiated bone marrow (Constine et al. 2008; Mauch et al. 1995).

Bone Marrow Sparing

A significant percentage of active bone marrow falls within most conventional pelvic and abdominal radiation fields. The application of highly conformal techniques, such as ▶ Intensity Modulated Radiation Therapy (IMRT), is one potential strategy to reduce bone marrow irradiation and, consequently, HT. In a study by Brixey and colleagues, patients initially treated with pelvic IMRT for gynecologic malignancies received lower bone marrow radiation doses and were found to have lower rates of grade 2 or greater hematologic toxicity (31%) compared with patients treated using conventional whole pelvic RT (60%) (Brixey et al. 2002). Several recent studies of patients treated with IMRT for cervical (Rose et al. 2011; Albuquerque et al. 2010) and anal cancer (Mell et al. 2008) reported that patients with lower bone marrow radiation dose-volume parameters were less likely to develop hematologic toxicity.

Bone marrow sparing in radiation therapy is challenging due to the large volume of the pelvic bone marrow and the close proximity of the bone marrow to the pelvic organs and lymph nodes. Radiation planning studies with bone marrow–sparing IMRT and proton therapy have demonstrated the ability to further reduce bone marrow irradiation compared to conventional radiation techniques, but the extent of bone marrow sparing is limited. A possible solution to this challenge is to identify and spare only hematopoietically active bone marrow, which is not well visualized on CT.

Magnetic resonance imaging (MRI), single photon emission CT (SPECT), and positron emission tomography (PET) have been used previously to reveal locations of active bone marrow. MRI relies on the difference between the relative proton density in the highly cellular, active bone marrow, versus the inactive bone marrow which is largely composed of hypocellular adipose tissue. Technetium-99 sulfur colloids used in SPECT imaging are taken up by macrophages in the red marrow. PET imaging employs a positron-emitting radionuclide which is incorporated into a biological molecule. Fluorine-18 (F-18) fluorodeoxyglucose (FDG), is a PET tracer that is taken up by metabolically active cells and is commonly used in pelvic malignancies for cancer staging. F-18 deoxyfluorothymidine (FLT) is a newer PET tracer that is taken up by cells undergoing DNA synthesis which may be a better marker for proliferation than metabolic activity alone. These functional imaging modalities may help to identify a smaller hematopoietically active bone marrow volume. Sparing this active subregion could be more feasible and effective than total bone marrow sparing, though future studies will be required to identify the clinical impact of functional bone marrow sparing.

Future Directions

The reduction of radiation-associated hematologic toxicity could improve tolerance to chemoradiotherapy or allow additional systemic agents, potentially enhancing disease control in patients with pelvic malignancies. Understanding the effects of radiation in active bone marrow subregions, and refining efforts to selectively spare active bone marrow, could help optimize bone marrow–sparing radiation techniques. Prospective evaluation of bone marrow sparing is ongoing and will be helpful to establish the role of bone marrow–sparing radiation therapy for pelvic and other malignancies in the future.

Cross-References

▶ Anal Carcinoma
▶ IMRT
▶ Proton Therapy
▶ Total Body Irradiation (TBI)
▶ Uterine Cervix

References

Albuquerque K, Giangreco D, Morrison C et al (2010) Radiation-related predictors of hematologic toxicity after concurrent chemoradiation for cervical cancer and implications for bone marrow-sparing pelvic IMRT. Int J Radiat Oncol Biol Phys 79:1043–1047

Brixey CJ, Roeske JC, Lujan AE, Yamada SD, Rotmensch J, Mundt AJ (2002) Impact of intensity-modulated radiotherapy on acute hematologic toxicity in women with gynecologic malignancies. Int J Radiat Oncol Biol Phys 54:1388–1396

Constine L, Milano M, Friedman D et al (2008) Late effects of cancer treatment on normal tissues. In: Halperin EC, Perez CA, Brady LW (eds) Principles and practice of radiation oncology, 5th edn. Wolters Kluwer, Lippincott Williams and Wilkens, Philadelphia

Hall EJ, Giaccia AJ (2006) Clinical response of normal tissues. In: Hall EJ, Giaccia AJ (eds) Radiobiology for the radiologist, 6th edn. Lippincott Williams and Wilkins, Philadelphia

Mauch P, Constine I, Greenberger J et al (1995) Hematopoietic stem cell compartment: acute and late effects of radiation therapy and chemotherapy. Int J Radiat Oncol Biol Phys 12:1861–1865

Mell LK, Schomas DA, Salama JK et al (2008) Association between bone marrow dosimetric parameters and acute hematologic toxicity in anal cancer patients treated with concurrent chemotherapy and intensity-modulated radiotherapy. Int J Radiat Oncol Biol Phys 70:1431–1437

Roeske J, Lujan A, Mundt A (2005) Bone marrow-sparing IMRT: emerging technology. In: Mundt A (ed) Intensity modulated radiation therapy: a clinical perspective, 1st edn. BC Decker, Toronto

Rose BS, Aydogan B, Liang Y et al (2011) Normal tissue complication probability modeling of acute hematologic toxicity in cervical cancer patients treated with chemoradiotherapy. Int J Radiat Oncol Biol Phys 79:800–807

Bone Marrow Transplantation

IRIS RUSU
Department of Radiation Oncology, Loyola University Medical Center, Maywood, IL, USA

Definition

Offered to patients with malignant diseases as well as autoimmune and genetic disorders.

Cross-References

► Total Body Irradiation (TBI)

Boost to Breast

Anthony E. Dragun
Department of Radiation Oncology, James
Graham Brown Cancer Center, University of
Louisville School of Medicine, Louisville,
KY, USA

Definition

This refers to the addition of a focused dose of radiation therapy to the 1–2 cm of breast tissue surrounding the lumpectomy cavity. It is usually delivered after a regimen of conventionally fractionated or hypofractionated whole breast radiation therapy. A typical dose is approximately 10–20 Gy delivered over 1–2 weeks. Randomized trials show a benefit to local regional control with the addition of a boost in patients with invasive breast cancer. It is most beneficial for premenopausal patients and in patients with close surgical margins. It has been shown to have no significant impact on cosmetic outcome. Its utility is generally in question for elderly patients and those with ductal carcinoma in situ. External beam radiation therapy is most commonly used to deliver the boost, and techniques usually involve electrons or three-dimensional conformal radiation therapy to target the lumpectomy cavity with ultrasound or CT guidance. Other techniques include intraoperative radiation therapy, brachytherapy, or intensity-modulated radiation therapy with simultaneous integrated boost.

Cross-References

► Brachytherapy
► Early-Stage Breast Cancer

► Intensity Modulated Radiation Therapy (IMRT)
► Intraoperative Radiation Therapy (IORT)

Bowel Cancer

► Colon Cancer

Bowel Resection

► Colectomy

Brachial Plexopathy

► Brachial Plexus Dysfunction

Brachial Plexus Dysfunction

Anthony E. Dragun
Department of Radiation Oncology, James
Graham Brown Cancer Center, University of
Louisville School of Medicine, Louisville,
KY, USA

Synonyms

Brachial plexopathy

Definition

This entity refers to injury of the brachial plexus and is a rare late complication of regional lymph node irradiation for the treatment of locally advanced or recurrent breast cancer. The risk is less than 1% in properly treated patients. Symptoms include painful paresthesias and immobility. These symptoms must be distinguished from lymphedema and recurrent breast cancer. The incidence is significantly higher with mismatched or overlapping radiation therapy portals, which result in an overdose of the supraclavicular fossa. Also, risk is significant if lymph node irradiation dose is higher than 50 Gy or if two-dimensional radiation therapy techniques or concurrent chemotherapy is employed. Treatment of brachial plexopathy includes medical therapy as well as oral analgesics, steroids, anticonvulsives, and tricyclic antidepressants. Electrical nerve stimulation and neurolytic procedures along with physical therapy may also be used. Hyperbaric oxygen has been shown to be ineffective in the treatment of brachial plexopathy in randomized controlled trials.

Cross-References

▶ Stage 0 Breast Cancer

Brachytherapy

ALBERT S. DENITTIS
Lankenau Institute for Medical Research, Lankenau Hospital, Wynnewood, PA, USA

Definition

Radiation delivered from inside or near a tumor. The advantage of brachytherapy centers on the exploitation of the inverse square law and quick dose fall-off, thus sparing surrounding tissues from radiation while providing focal dose escalation. The radioactive source of choice is usually ^{192}Ir. High-dose-rate (HDR) techniques can deliver 100–400 Gy per hour, and treatment to brachytherapy can be given in 5–10 min on a weekly basis.

Cross-References

▶ Brachytherapy: Low Dose Rate (LDR) Permanent Implants (Prostate)
▶ Esophageal Cancer
▶ Vagina

Brachytherapy-GyN

CHRISTIN A. KNOWLTON[1], MICHELLE KOLTON MACKAY[2], YAN YU[3], LAURA DOYLE[3]
[1]Department of Radiation Oncology, Drexel University, Philadelphia, PA, USA
[2]Department of Radiation Oncology, Marshfield Clinic, Marshfield, WI, USA
[3]Department of Radiation Oncology, Thomas Jefferson University Hospital, Philadelphia, PA, USA

Synonyms

Carcinoma of the uterine cervix; Uterine neoplasm; Uterus

Definition

Brachytherapy, derived from the Greek term for "close" therapy, refers to placing a radiation source in or close to the tumor region. In cervical cancer, brachytherapy is used to boost the tumor region of an intact cervix or to treat the vaginal cuff in some postoperative patients to allow a higher dose to the region with limited side effects. Specialized instruments are placed in and around the region to allow for implantation of the radioactive source. Commonly used radiation sources include cesium-137 in low-dose-rate brachytherapy and iridium-192 in high-dose-rate brachytherapy.

Cross-References

▶ Accelerated Partial Breast Irradiation
▶ Esophageal Cancer
▶ Uterine Cervix

Brachytherapy: High Dose Rate (HDR) Implants

CHENG B. SAW
Division of Radiation Oncology, Penn State
Hershey Cancer Institute, Hershey, PA, USA

Definition

High dose rate (HDR) brachytherapy refers to the delivery of a high dose of radiation in a relatively short time compared to ▶ low dose rate (LDR) brachytherapy. This technology uses a single high-activity radioactive source inserted close to or directly into the tumor site. In accordance to ICRU Report No. 38 (1985), radiation treatments performed with dose rates higher than 12 Gy/h equivalent to 0.2 Gy/min are considered HDR brachytherapy. The pathways for the insertion of the radioactive source are created using catheters inserted into the tumor or tumor bed, through luminal regions, or by an applicator inserted into a body cavity or mold. The external access of the pathways allows the radioactive source to be inserted at anytime postsurgery and hence is referred as ▶ afterloading technique. Due to the high activity, the radioactive source is inserted remotely into the patient using a remote afterloader unit. This mode of radiation treatment has the advantage of rapid dose falloff and minimizes the exposure of surrounding normal healthy tissues compared to ▶ external beam radiation therapy (EBRT). After the treatment is complete, the radioactive source is retracted from the patient making the treatment a ▶ temporary implant. Additional information on HDR technology can be obtained from Glassgow (Glassgow 1999), Khan (Khan 2003) and Nag (Nag 1994).

Background

High dose rate brachytherapy evolved from manual preloading brachytherapy techniques. In the early 1950s, the practice of brachytherapy seriously declined due to the concern of harmful effects of radiation to professional personnel. Although the brachytherapy modality using radium and radon sources was well established for over 50 years, the procedures were complicated and time consuming. The procedure involved direct insertion of preloaded applicators and radioactive sources with the patient under general anesthesia, thus creating potential radiation hazards to hospital personnel. The introduction of man-made radionuclides and the development of manual afterloading techniques contributed to the renaissance of the brachytherapy practice. The afterloading techniques allow radioactive sources to be inserted after surgery in the patient's room. Manual afterloading techniques eliminate radiation exposure to personnel in the operating room but not to the nursing staff caring for the patient. The natural extension of the manual afterloading technique is the development of remote afterloading techniques, which were initiated by the radiation oncology group at Memorial Hospital in New York. The remote afterloading technique eliminates the manual insertion of radioactive sources and allows the retraction of radioactive sources at will, thereby reducing exposure to the professional and nursing staff. The high dose rate remote afterloading technique was also investigated at Memorial Hospital starting in 1961. The final version of the remote HDR afterloader unit was installed in 1964 and later commercially marketed as Brachytron (Hilaris 1994). Remote HDR afterloader units must be housed in a shielded and secured room.

Remote HDR afterloader units that represent technological advances in brachytherapy offer a number of advantages over manual afterloading techniques. This includes improved radiation protection to the professional and nursing staff. Because the loading of the radiation source is done remotely and the radiation source can be retracted at will, the radiation exposure to personnel while attending the patient's needs is eliminated. As compared to manually loaded sources, there is less probability of misplacing sources or actually losing sources. Because of the use of the computer system, the high dose rate technique also reduces human error. With modern treatment planning systems, the dwell positions and dwell times can be easily adjusted to optimize the dose distributions to conform to the tumor while reducing the dose to the surrounding normal tissue. With the relatively short treatment times, prolonged bed confinement of the patients is not necessary. This is particularly favorable for elderly patients who are prone to confinement complications and reduces patient discomfort as well. In addition, patients can be treated on an outpatient basis and this procedure is well suited for large patient populations. Generally, the applicators used with remote HDR afterloaders are smaller and hence the placement in the patient can be done without anesthesia. As a result of this offering, the radiation therapy staff, radiation oncologist, and medical physicist do not need to leave the department (for the surgical suite) for a long period of time.

However, remote afterloading technology has its disadvantages as well. It requires large capital expenditure for both the purchase of the equipment as well as housing the remote afterloader unit. As mentioned above, the afterloader unit must be housed in a secured and shielded room. Although the hospitalization of the patient is not required, the treatment itself may be more costly.

Remote HDR Afterloader Unit

The essential components of an HDR brachytherapy system are (a) operating console of the remote afterloader unit, (b) remote afterloader unit, (c) radioactive source, (d) transfer tubes, (e) afterloading catheters and applicators, and (f) treatment planning system. The objective of the HDR brachytherapy system is to move the radioactive source through the prescribed channels and applicators to the planned dwell positions with the source dwelling for a defined time. The longer the source

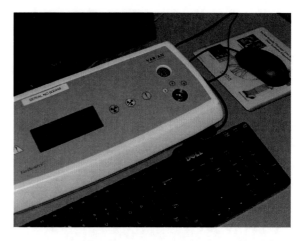

Brachytherapy: High Dose Rate (HDR) Implants.
Fig. 1 The afterloader unit operating console

dwells in a particular ▶ dwell position, the dose delivered from that particular position will increase. The positioning accuracy of the source is specified to within 1 mm. The dwell times are determined to within 0.1 s resolution.

The remote afterloader unit operating console (Fig. 1) is a computer system that is capable of accepting data either through network or transportable media from the treatment planning system. The data will have instructions for the afterloader unit to set the dwell positions and dwell times along the catheters or applicators during dose delivery. During dose delivery, the operating console is used to monitor the status of the afterloader unit as well as the movement of the source, detection of any obstructions, or any other errors that may occurred.

The remote afterloader unit (Fig. 2) consists of (a) a primary safe, (b) a source control/drive mechanism to move the source out to applicators and return to the safe, and (c) a precisely calibrated counter to determine the distance traveled by the source from the afterloader unit. The purpose of the primary safe is to store the radioactive source when it is not in use. The radioactive source that looks like a small metallic pellet (also called seed) is commonly welded to the

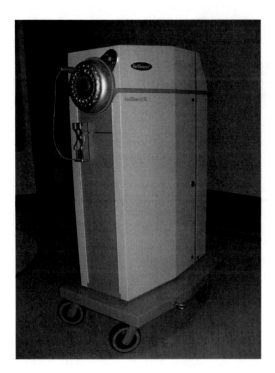

Brachytherapy: High Dose Rate (HDR) Implants.
Fig. 2 The afterloader unit

end of a metallic cable which is wound over a drive. The cable with attached source is called source wire. For afterloader unit with multiple channels, an indexer motor is used to move the source to the prescribed channel as planned.

The three radionuclides that have been used in HDR units are cobalt-60, cesium-137, and iridium-192. Because of its initial availability, cobalt-60 was the first isotope used in HDR afterloader units. The long half-life of cobalt-60 (5.26 years) and high specific activity (200 Ci/g) are the advantages of this radioisotope. However, the high energies of the emitted gamma rays (1.17 and 1.33 MeV) result in a higher half-value layer of 1.1 cm in lead, and this is a distinct disadvantage. On the other hand, cesium-137 has a low specific activity (10 Ci/g) and its low gamma ray energy of 0.66 MeV is less penetrating with 0.65 cm half-value layer in lead. The half-life of cesium-137 is 30 years. The HDR sources of cobalt-60 and cesium-137 generally have large diameters (2.5–4 mm) and are unsuitable for interstitial treatments but acceptable for intraluminal and intracavitary treatments. Iridium-192 is the source most commonly used in the HDR afterloaders today. The disadvantage of the short half-life of 73.83 days is offset by its low average gamma ray energy of 0.38 MeV. This requires source replacement every 3–4 months. In addition to its low half-value layer of 0.3 cm in lead, it has high specific activity (about 450 Ci/g) allowing it to be constructed at high activity (10 Ci) with the smallest diameter source of about 0.6–1.1 mm and length (3.5–10 mm) and is suitable for all interstitial, intraluminal, and intracavitary treatments.

Transfer tubes or transfer guides are critical components of the remote HDR brachytherapy system. The function of the transfer tubes is to connect the catheters and applicator systems to the afterloader unit. It guides the source to the tumor site. Improper input of the transfer tube length or connection to the incorrect channel will lead to mistreatment so it is crucial that the correct length be verified for each transfer tube–catheter combination, and that the transfer tube connects the appropriate afterloader channel to the corresponding catheter.

Prior to performing the treatment, a dummy wire is extended into the catheters or applicators to make sure the path is not obstructed. The movement of the source wire and dummy wire through the individual channel and applicators is controlled by a driving mechanism consisting of stepping motors inside the afterloader. The positioning of the source at the programmed dwell positions in the applicators is achieved in precise increments by the stepper motors.

A number of safety features are incorporated into every HDR brachytherapy system. This includes the door interlocks such that the source will automatically retract if the room door is opened. In addition, for rooms

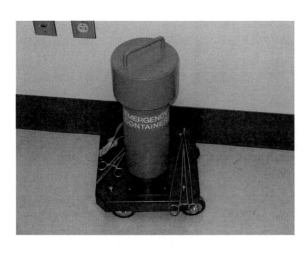

Brachytherapy: High Dose Rate (HDR) Implants.
Fig. 3 The emergency response equipment

containing other radiation-producing machines such as a simulator or CT scanner, a manual key is used to activate only one unit at a time. Other interlocks will ensure that transfer tubes are properly attached to the afterloader unit and also the applicators. Batteries backup are provided to take over the operation should there be a power failure. A manual source retraction mechanism is available to withdraw the source into the safe should it get stuck and cannot be retracted using emergency switch. An emergency response kit is available to handle exposed source (Fig. 3). The treatment is aborted if the system detects blockage or excessive friction during source transits.

HDR Brachytherapy Applicators
The ability to deliver the radiation dose to the tumor is highly dependent on the availability of specially designed catheters and applicators. For example, the Fletcher-Suit or Fletcher-Suit-Delclos applicator is specially designed with a configuration suitable to treat gynecological malignancies of the uterus, cervix, and pelvic side-walls. Likewise, a simple long catheter of approximately 100 cm in length is used for the treatment of endobronchial cancer in the lung. Similarly, there are several applicators on the market used to treat

early stage breast cancer via ▶ accelerated partial breast irradiation (APBI). Many specially designed applicators are available to treat various anatomical sites from the vendors of the afterloader units as well as from third-party vendors.

Regulatory Compliance
In the USA, the medical use of remote HDR brachytherapy is regulated by the Nuclear Regulatory Commission (NRC) guidelines under Part §35, subpart H or Department of Environment Protection (DEP) of the individual states for those agreement states. Agreement states are states that have entered into a contractual agreement with the NRC to administer as well as to comply with the NRC guidelines. A license is therefore required from the regulatory agency prior to the use of the HDR afterloader units for patient treatments. The license application must demonstrate the existence of a safety program that includes an appropriately shielded facility, emergency procedures, patient treatment procedures, quality assurance programs, training, and qualification of personnel, in particular authorized users (AU) and authorized medical physicists (AMP).

NRC Part §35.610 and NRC Part §35.615 address the safety procedures and safety precautions, respectively, in the use of the HDR afterloader units. The safety procedures address the need (a) to secure the afterloader unit, (b) to limit access to the treatment room during patient treatment, (c) to limit the operation to one radiation-producing machine at a time in a room where two or more radiation-producing machines are available, and (d) to have written procedures for responding to abnormal situations. Examples of abnormal situations are the inability to return the source to the storage safe and the inability to control the afterloader unit from the operating console. The safety precaution aspects point to the need to (a) control access to the entrance to the treatment room, (b) have interlocking interruption that prevents radiation exposure if access tools such as the door is inadvertently opened, (c) have written procedures to deal with jammed source, and (d) assure the physical presence of specified personnel, in particular authorized user (AU), authorized medical physicist (AMP), and, if applicable, a trained physician at the initiation of and for the duration of patient treatments.

In addition, the regulatory guidelines mandate the performance of periodic spot checks (NRC Part §35.643) and full calibration measurements (NRC Part §35.633). The periodic spot-checks should be performed (a) prior to first use on a given day and (b) following each source installation. The periodic spot checks aim at assuring the proper operation of the safety features and the consistency of the timing devices including the timer and clock which is used to correct decay to current source activity on the afterloader unit. The full calibration measurements should be performed (a) prior to first clinical use, (b) following source replacement, (c) following afterloader unit reinstallation, and (d) following major repairs involving the source assembly. The full calibration measurements should be performed at intervals not to exceed a calendar quarter for sources with half-life exceeding 75 days. The calibration measurements must comply with published protocols under nationally recognized bodies.

Quality Assurance

The quality assurance (QA) program for the remote HDR brachytherapy must be designed by a qualified medical physicist in accordance with the regulatory guidelines. In order to ensure compliance with the regulation, QA should include specific tasks as outlined in the regulatory guidelines discussed above.

The daily quality assurance (QA) for the remote HDR brachytherapy should include specific tasks as identified in the periodic spot checks (NRC Part §35.643) as listed in Table 1. The daily

Brachytherapy: High Dose Rate (HDR) Implants.
Table 1 Daily quality assurance for HDR afterloader unit

No	Description	Tolerance
1	Electrical interlocks	Functional
2	Source indicator	Functional
3	Audiovisual system	Functional
4	Emergency response equipment	Availability
5	Radiation monitor	Functional
6	Timer accuracy	±1 s
7	Afterloader clock (date and time)	±1 s
8	Afterloader activity	±1%
9	Simulator/HDR switch	Functional
10	Emergency switches	Functional
11	Stepper motor error detection	Functional
12	Distance source travels	±1 mm

QA checks for the proper operation of the safety features and timing devices, consistent with the regulatory guidelines. These include the functionality of the interlocks, light indicator, audiovisual system, and radiation monitors. The timing devices being checked are the timer and the computer clock, which is used to compute the current physical activity of the radioactive source. This, in turn, affects the ▶ dwell time in each dwell position for the current treatment. In addition, the daily QA verifies the availability of emergency response equipment and checks the functioning of the emergency switches. The ability of the mechanism to detect obstruction is also verified. Lastly, the physical distances traveled by the dummy and active sources are checked.

For remote afterloaders using an iridium-192 source, full calibration measurements as listed in Table 2 are performed at the time of source exchange which is typically done quarterly. This source exchange QA incorporates the specific

Brachytherapy: High Dose Rate (HDR) Implants.
Table 2 Source exchange QA for HDR afterloader unit

No	Description	Tolerance
1	Output measurements	±5%
2	Source (dwell) position accuracy	±1 mm
3	Source retraction under backup battery	Functional
4	Timer accuracy and linearity under the useful range	
5	Length, integrity, and functionality of transfer tubes	Baseline
6	Length, integrity, and functionality of applicators	Baseline
7	Physical decay correction	±1%

tasks outlined in the regulatory guidelines (NRC Part §35.633). The primary purpose of the source exchange QA is to calibrate the radioactive source and verifies the proper function of the dose delivery system. This includes the integrity and functionality of (a) the transfer tubes, (b) the applicators, and (c) connecting devices. In addition, the QA also checks for dwell times and dwell positions accuracy. Lastly, this QA checks for the proper operation of the battery backup system.

Clinical Applications

The clinical implementation of HDR brachytherapy involves (a) the insertion of catheters and/or applicators into the patient, (b) radiographic simulation or CT scanning to acquire the applicator geometries with respect to the patient anatomy, (c) treatment planning in order to plan appropriate dose distributions, (d) equipment spot checks, and (e) dose delivery to the patient. The insertion of catheters and/or applicators are most often performed in the surgical suite but in some cases are performed in a CT room or in a simulator room under the guidance of a fluoroscopic system. In the past, orthogonal radiographs were used for dosimetry; however today, three-dimensional (3D)-based images are more commonly used. The image-based treatment planning offers the visualization of the dose distributions in three dimensions including doses to critical anatomical structures. The availability of inverse planning and the option of varying dwell positions and dwell times offer greater flexibility of treatment planning to optimize individualized dose distributions. The dose distribution is typically generated using a dedicated treatment planning system for the remote afterloader unit. The dose calculation formalism follows that recommended by the AAPM Task Group 43. (Nath et al. 1995) The treatment plan is often manually verified using simple dose calculations. The dwell positions and dwell times for each channel are downloaded from the treatment planning system for each patient to the operating console of the remote afterloader unit for dose delivery.

Prior to initiating treatment, the written directives must be signed and dated by the authorized user. In addition, the patient identity must be verified using two independent methods as the individual named in the treatment plan. Before initiating dose delivery, a dummy wire is sent out to all the channels used by the afterloader unit to ensure that there are no obstructions. Under the regulatory guidelines, an authorized medical physicist must be present throughout the patient treatment while the authorized user must be present at the initiation of the treatment and can be supported during the treatment by other trained physicians. After the completion of the treatment, the patient and the afterloader unit must be surveyed before releasing the patient in accordance to regulatory guidelines NRC Part §35.604.

Technically, HDR brachytherapy may be used to treat any anatomical site; however, it has been used primarily for the treatment of the prostate, gynecological diseases, breast, lung, and skin diseases.

Cross-References

References

Glasgow GP (1999) Brachytherapy. In: Van Dyk J (ed) The modern technology of radiation oncology. Medical Physics, Madison

Hilaris BS (1994) Evolution and general principles of high dose rate brachytherapy. In: Nag S (ed) High dose rate brachytherapy – a textbook. Futura Publishing, Armonk

ICRU Report No. 38 (1985) Dose and volume specification for reporting intracavitary therapy in gynecology, International Commission on Radiation Units and Measurements, Bethesda, MD

Khan FM (2003) The physics of radiation therapy. Lippincott Williams & Wilkins, Philadelphia

Nag S (ed) (1994) High dose rate brachytherapy – a textbook. Futura Publishing, Armonk, NY

Nath R, Anderson LL, Luxton G et al (1995) Dosimetry of interstitial brachytherapy sources: recommendations of the AAPM radiation therapy committee task group no. 43. Med Phys 22:209–234

Brachytherapy: Low Dose Rate (LDR) Permanent Implants (Prostate)

YAN YU, LAURA DOYLE
Department of Radiation Oncology, Thomas Jefferson University Hospital, Philadelphia, PA, USA

Synonyms

Prostate seed implants (PSI)

Definition

A low dose rate (LDR) permanent prostate implant is a ▶ brachytherapy procedure in which radioactive seeds are permanently implanted into the prostate to deliver radiation to treat low-grade prostate cancers.

Background

Brachytherapy is a technique for delivering radiation at close distances to the target. LDR permanent implants involve a sealed source of radiation, specifically in a seed form, to be placed within or in close proximity to the tumor. Although LDR brachytherapy implants may be used to treat many sites of disease, permanent prostate implants are among the most common types of brachytherapy procedures. This type of procedure is commonly referred to as a prostate seed implant (PSI). The purpose of this procedure is to eradicate tumor cells within the prostate while sparing surrounding healthy tissues.

LDR ▶ permanent implants for prostate cancer is an outpatient procedure that serves as an alternative treatment option to radical prostatectomy, high dose rate (HDR) brachytherapy implants, or external beam radiotherapy. The short duration of the procedure, minimal invasiveness, and fast recovery make this an appealing treatment option to many patients. The technique has been in practice for many years and has been proven a safe and effective treatment option for prostate cancer when performed by an experienced team with an established quality assurance program. It involves team members from multiple disciplines including radiation oncologists, medical physicists, urologists, anesthesiologists, and nurses, and takes place in an operating room or a dedicated brachytherapy suite.

This type of brachytherapy procedure is considered an ▶ interstitial implant, where radioactive seeds are inserted directly into the tumor and surrounding tissue. This low dose rate (LDR) implant involves radioactive isotopes that deliver radiation at an initial dose rate in the range of 7–21 cGy/h.

Brachytherapy: Low Dose Rate (LDR) Permanent Implants (Prostate). Table 1 Characteristics of common isotopes used for prostate seed implants

Isotope	I-125	Pd-103	Cs-131
Mean energy	28 keV	21 keV	30 keV
Half-life	59.4 days	17 days	9.7 days
Prescription dose	145 Gy	110 Gy	115 Gy
Activity per seed	0.3–0.8 mCi	1.1–1.7 mCi	2.5–3.5 mCi
Radiation form	Photon	Photon	Photon

Isotopes

Common radioactive isotopes for this procedure include iodine (I-125) and palladium (Pd-103). Cesium (Cs-131) was introduced as an option for prostate seed implants in 2004 (Bice et al. 2008). All isotopes are in the low-energy range for therapeutic radiation and have short half-lives. The low energy minimizes the amount of tissue that the radiation is able to penetrate. A ► half-life is the length of time it takes for the amount of activity to be reduced to half of the original amount. The short half-life is an attractive characteristic since the seeds will be permanently left in the prostate. Specifics about each isotope are listed in Table 1.

All isotopes are manufactured in the form of tiny seeds approximately 5 mm in length and 1 mm in diameter. These seeds are produced by a number of different companies. The amount of radiation emitted per seed is measured by the total activity or number of decays per unit time. Activity is expressed in units of millicurie (mCi) or as air kerma strength in units of $\mu Gy\ m^2\ h^{-1}$ (U). The average activity for prostate seed implants range from 0.3–0.7 mCi per seed for I-125 depending upon user preferences. The total number of seeds per implant varies from approximately 40–120 seeds depending on the activity per seed and prostate size (Fig. 1) Nath et al. (1995).

Procedure/Technique

Prostate seed implants require dosimetric planning to determine the number of seeds and needle/seed locations needed to provide adequate dose to the target volume. The implementation of planning varies among institutions. The American Brachytherapy Society (ABS) has defined three different levels of planning from static preplanning to true dynamic planning (Nag et al. 2001). Although the complete range of techniques is listed in Table 2, this chapter will focus on the general characteristics of preoperative planning and real-time intraoperative dosimetry outlining the procedures for each technique.

Prostate seed implants were traditionally performed as a preplan technique. This requires the patient to undergo a preimplant volume study a few weeks before the implant date. During the volume study, the patient must be placed in the lithotomy position with legs secured in stirrups. Anesthesia is not necessary for this procedure. A transrectal ultrasound (► TRUS) probe is inserted into the rectum. A TRUS study is conducted to determine the volume and position of the prostate. The TRUS probe usually has both sagittal and axial crystals for imaging the prostate in biplanes. Once the prostate is clearly visualized, ultrasound images of the prostate are captured, digitally or via printer, for planning purposes.

The TRUS images are usually acquired at 5 mm step increments encompassing the entire prostate, including a slice superior to the base and inferior to the apex of the prostate. If digital transfer of the images is not possible, the images may be printed to hard copy for the physician to outline the contour of the prostate on each slice. More commonly, images are digitally captured and transferred to a planning system. Using digital images, all contouring of the prostate and critical structures can be performed using a computerized treatment planning system. The medical physicist will determine the location, number, and activity of seeds necessary to achieve

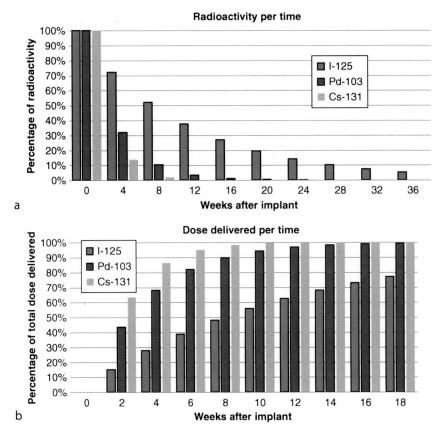

Brachytherapy: Low Dose Rate (LDR) Permanent Implants (Prostate). Fig. 1 (**a**) Percentage of source activity and (**b**) percentage of total dose delivered as a function of time for I-125, Pd-103, and Cs-131 with half-lives of 59.4, 17, and 9.7 days, respectively

adequate radiation dose coverage of the prostate. The appropriate seed activity/quantity is ordered for the date of the implant. The treatment plan displays isodose lines superimposed over the contours of the prostate on each slice. The plan also provides dosimetric information such as dose volume histograms (DVH) for the prostate, urethra, rectum, and any other contoured structures. The main objectives of the treatment plan are to provide optimal coverage of the entire target volume, including the prostate and desired margin, by the prescribed dose while limiting the dose to the rectum and urethra. The dosimetric planning goals include adequate coverage of the entire prostate plus a 2–3 mm margin by the prescription dose. The most common dose constraint for

the urethra is the D10 (dose received by 10% of the volume) aimed to be less than 200 Gy. Likewise, the rectal dose should be limited, specifically the D5 less than prescription dose Yu et al. (1999).

During the seed implant procedure, the patient is positioned in the same position as the volume study and placed under general anesthesia. The entire procedure usually lasts between 1 and 3 h. The first part of the procedure involves reproducing the position of the prostate and matching images to those used for the preoperative plan. The ultrasound apparatus is positioned on a stand at the foot of the bed to provide stability and consistency during the implant. A ▶ template, or grid-like device, is placed at the end of the ultrasound stand. This device has

Brachytherapy: Low Dose Rate (LDR) Permanent Implants (Prostate). **Table 2** The ABS terminology for elements of intraoperative planning

Level	Terminology	Definition
0	Preplanning	None
1	Intraoperative preplanning	Creation of a plan in the OR just before the implant procedure with immediate execution of the plan
2	Interactive planning	Stepwise refinement of the treatment plan using dose calculations derived from image-based needle position feedback
3	Dynamic dose calculation	Constant updating of dose calculations of implanted sources using continuous seed position feedback

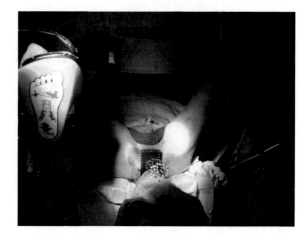

Brachytherapy: Low Dose Rate (LDR) Permanent Implants (Prostate). **Fig. 2** Depiction of prostate seed implant procedure, including patient positioning and necessary equipment

numerous holes equally spaced for needles to be guided through. Each position is labeled by a letter and/or number system. See Fig. 2 for an example of a template. A virtual template or grid pattern is displayed on the ultrasound and treatment planning system which correlates to the physical template. The virtual template must be calibrated by the medical physicist to ensure precise correspondence to the physical template as measured in prostate tissue-like imaging conditions. The preplan lists the needle locations with respect to the template and the depth of needle insertion. Most preplan techniques use preloaded needles with seeds placed in specific locations. This expedites the seed delivery portion of the implant procedure.

There are some limitations to the preplan technique, including patient positioning challenges and inability to adapt to changes in the prostate or adjustments in the previously calculated treatment plan. Today, many centers are moving away from the preplan technique and employing real-time or intraoperative planning

in which all of the planning takes place in the OR at the time of the seed implant procedure. ▶ Real-time planning still involves some preparatory work prior to the date of implant. This includes obtaining the volume of the prostate most commonly by use of CT or ultrasound. This volume is necessary to estimate the total activity needed to deliver the prescribed dose to the prostate. The relationship between total activity and volume of the prostate is given in various nomograms. Wu et al. (2000) constructed a ▶ nomogram for (Model 6711) I-125 seeds based on a peripheral loading technique. Peripheral loading implies most of the radiation distributed toward the edges of the prostate, minimizing high dose regions closer to the center of gland surrounding the urethra.

Seeds may be obtained in a number of forms. The most common forms are loose or stranded seeds. Loose seeds are appealing to physicians who prefer to use a ▶ Mick applicator to insert the seeds one at a time from a cartridge. Stranded seeds are convenient when placing multiple seeds with regular interspacing in a needle at one time.

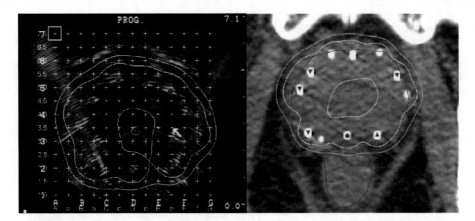

Brachytherapy: Low Dose Rate (LDR) Permanent Implants (Prostate). Fig. 3 (*Left*) TRUS image with needles inserted displays contour of prostate (*red*), rectum (*blue*), and urethra (*green*) and isodose lines (*green* = prescription dose, *yellow* = 150% of prescription dose); (*right*) CT image for post-implant analysis with contours (prostate, rectum, and urethra) and isodose lines (*green* = prescription dose, *yellow* = 150% of prescription dose). The *red marks* indicate needle or seed locations. The template is with 5 mm grid spacing (labeled with letters horizontal axis and numbers across the vertical axis) is evident on the TRUS image on the left

Cystoscopy

At the conclusion of the implant, the urologist usually performs a cystoscopy. The purpose of this procedure is to check for any seeds that may have punctured the bladder or migrated through the urethra. Radioactive seed in the bladder or urethra causes unnecessary radiation, and whenever possible should be removed during cystoscopy.

Post-Implant Dosimetry

To evaluate the dosimetric quality of a prostate seed implant, it is recommended that the patient receive a post-implant CT scan approximately 30 days after the implant. CT-based evaluation of post-implant dosimetry is recommended by the American Brachytherapy Society (Nag et al. 2000). The timing of 30 days allows for the edema from the trauma associated with the implant to subside and for the prostate to return approximately to its previous volume. Since the radioactive seeds will continue to deliver radiation for many months, exponentially decreasing in activity as time passes, this 30-day mark is a good indication of the effective locations of the seeds within the prostate and their contribution of dose to the target volume. The pelvic region of the patient is imaged at sufficiently thin slices so as not to miss any seeds. The scan area must be large enough to include possible locations for seed migration. Occasionally, seeds migrate distantly within the patient by ways of blood vessels, such as to the lung. There has been no report of serious consequences due to such distant migrations.

The CT image set is transferred to a treatment planning system for dosimetric review. Much like preplanning or intraoperative planning, the target and surrounding critical structures are contoured. The radioactive seeds have a much higher contrast and are easier to locate on CT image than on TRUS. Due to artifacts, the seed may appear on the CT slice in a star-like shape. All seeds should be identified, and the total number of seeds should agree with the number of seeds implanted during the procedure. Implants are judged based on the dosimetric criteria discussed in the treatment planning section. Specifically, a quality I-125 implant is characterized by a V100 greater than 90% of the prostate and D90 value equal to or greater than the prescribed dose. Doses to the surrounding critical structures including the urethra and rectum are also verified during this post-implant analysis (Fig. 3).

Radiation Safety

Due to the low energy of the radioactive seeds and the location within the body, very little radiation is detectable outside the patient. Radiation survey of the patient must be conducted and must comply with standards set by the Nuclear Regulatory Commission (NRC) or state-governing body before the patient may be discharged. This exposure rate measurement is obtained with a calibrated ▶ ion chamber.

Cross-References

▶ Clinical Aspects of Brachytherapy (BT)
▶ Prostate

References

Bice WS, Prestidge BR, Kurtzman SM, Beriwal S, Moran BJ, Patel RR, Rivard MJ (2008) Recommendations for permanent prostate brachytherapy with 131Cs: a consensus report from the Cesium Advisory Group. Brachytherapy 7:290–296

Nag S, Bice W, DeWyngaert K, Prestidge B, Stock R, Yu Y (2000) The American Brachytherapy Society recommendations for permanent prostate brachytherapy post implant dosimetric analysis. Int J Radiat Oncol Biol Phys 46:221–230

Nag S, Ciezki JP, Cormack R, Doggett S, DeWyngaert K, Edmundson GK, Stock RG, Stone NN, Yu Y, Zelefsky M (2001) Intraoperative planning and evaluation of permanent prostate brachytherapy: report of the American Brachytherapy Society. Int J Radiat Oncol Biol Phys 51:1422–1430

Nath R, Anderson LL, Luxton G, Weaver KA, Williamson JF, Meigooni AS (1995) Dosimetry of interstitial brachytherapy sources: recommendations of the AAPM Radiation Committee Task Group No. 43. Med Phys 22:209–234

Wu A, Lee C, Johnson M, Brown D, Benoit R, Miler R, Cohen J, Geis P, Chen ASJ, Kalnicki S (2000) A new power law for determination of total ^{125}I seed activity for ultrasound-guided prostate implants: clinical evaluations. Int J Radiat Oncol Biol Phys 47:1397–1403

Yu Y, Anderson LL, Li Z, Mellenberg DE, Nath R, Schell MC, Waterman FM, Wu A, Blasko JC (1999) Permanent prostate seed implant brachytherapy: report of the American Association of Physicists in Medicine Task Group No. 64. Med Phys 26:2054–2076

Brachytherapy: Low Dose Rate (LDR) Temporary Implants

Ning J. Yue
The Department of Radiation Oncology, The Cancer Institute of New Jersey, UMDNJ-Robert Wood Johnson Medical School, New Brunswick, NJ, USA

Definition/Description

▶ Brachytherapy is the use of sealed radioactive sources to treat cancers and other benign diseases by placing the sources inside the target volume or within close proximity to the target volume. ▶ Low dose rate (LDR) ▶ temporary implant is the type of brachytherapy in which radioactive source placement is temporary and the dose rate delivered to a prescription point ranges from 4 to 200 cGy per hour. In the LDR temporary brachytherapy implants, radioactive source placement is normally performed through manually or automatically controlled after-loading applicators. The radioactive sources, along with the after-loading applicators, are removed from the treatment site after achieving desired dose coverage.

Background and Basic Characteristics

Radiotherapy is an effective treatment modality in the management of various malignant and benign diseases. The success of radiation treatment is highly dependent on the ability to deliver a radiation dose high enough to sterilize tumor cells without severely damaging adjacent normal structures. In this respect, due to its relatively high dose gradient, brachytherapy offers the potential of a high degree of localized dose distribution in the tumor with the radioactive sources implanted directly inside the tumor or placed near the tumor. With LDR brachytherapy, the relatively lower dose rate may reduce potential damages to adjacent critical organs and may contribute to the effectiveness of treatment for certain tumor sites (Hall 1972). The LDR temporary brachytherapy distinguishes itself from the LDR permanent brachytherapy in that the radioactive sources are removed from patients after desired dose coverage is achieved while for the permanent brachytherapy the sources are placed and permanently left inside or around the tumor volume.

LDR temporary brachytherapy has been used in treating head and neck, breast, cervical, skin, endometrial, esophageal, and bronchial cancers since the early 1900s, shortly after the discovery of radioactivity. Although the treatment of breast, skin, esophageal, and bronchial cancers with LDR temporary brachytherapy is becoming less common and has been gradually replaced with other treatment modalities such as the high dose rate (HDR) brachytherapy and external beam radiotherapy, the LDR temporary brachytherapy is still being routinely used in the treatment of head and neck, cervical, and endometrial cancers in many medical centers.

LDR temporary brachytherapy can be classified into three categories based on the forms and anatomic pathways the therapy is delivered: (1) intracavitary (intraluminal), (2) interstitial, and (3) external surface brachytherapy. The intracavitary (intraluminal) LDR brachytherapy is to deliver radiation doses by placing radioactive sources inside anatomic cavities through specially designed applicators. This type of treatment is applied to tumors that are located inside or near

body cavities such as uterus, vagina, and esophagus (intraluminal). The interstitial LDR brachytherapy is conducted by placing sources inside needles and catheters which are directly inserted into the tissues and positioned near or in the tumor or tumor bed. This form of treatment can be used for diseases such as breast and head and neck cancers. The external surface (mold) LDR brachytherapy is another form of treatment in which external applicators or molds loaded with radioactive sources are positioned near or on patient's body surface to treat superficial diseases.

A variety of photon emitting radionuclides has been applied in LDR temporary brachytherapy in the form of encapsulated sources. These radionuclides include radium (^{226}Ra), radon (^{222}Rn), cesium (^{137}Cs), iridium (^{192}Ir), iodine (^{125}I), and palladium (^{103}Pd). They have different energy spectra and half-lives, and their respective radioactive characteristics are tabulated in Table 1 (Nath et al. 1995; Chu et al. 1999). ^{226}Ra and ^{222}Rn are sources emitting photons of relatively high energies, and have been mostly replaced by ^{137}Cs sources to avoid safety hazard of radon gas and are now readily available in the USA for the purpose of LDR temporary brachytherapy treatments. ^{125}I and ^{103}Pd sources are low energy photon emitters with relatively short half-lives. Their usage in LDR temporary implants is not as common as in LDR permanent implants. The most commonly used radionuclides in LDR temporary implants are ^{137}Cs and ^{192}Ir.

For LDR temporary implants, radioactive sources are normally available in cylindrical shape, which individual size ranges from less than 1 mm to a few millimeters in diameter and a few millimeters to a few centimeters in length. In many cases, for the convenience of implantation, the sources may also be made commercially available in ribbons, in which individual sources of the same strength are evenly spaced. The ribbons can be easily cut into different lengths based

Brachytherapy: Low Dose Rate (LDR) Temporary Implants. Table 1 Radioactive characteristics of a variety of radioactive sources that are used in LDR temporary brachytherapy. The exposure rate constants in the table are for unfiltered sources except for ^{226}Ra. These values are subject to change with source encapsulation, structural design, and radioactivity distribution

Radionuclide	Half-life	Average energy (keV)	Exposure rate constant for an ideal point source
^{226}Ra	1,600 years	830	8.25 R cm^{2}mg^{-1}h^{-1}
^{222}Rn	3.82 days	830	10.15 R cm^{2}mCi^{-1}h^{-1}
^{137}Cs	30.07 years	662	3.26 R cm^{2}mCi^{-1}h^{-1}
^{192}Ir	73.83 days	380	4.69 R cm^{2}mCi^{-1}h^{-1}
^{125}I	59.4 days	28	1.45 R cm^{2}mCi^{-1}h^{-1}
^{103}Pd	16.99 days	21	1.48 R cm^{2}mCi^{-1}h^{-1}

on clinical needs. Typically, ^{125}I or ^{103}Pd brachytherapy seeds are 4.5 mm long and 0.8 mm in diameter, and are most likely used in interstitial and external applicator (mold) brachytherapy treatments. They are more commonly used in permanent brachytherapy than in temporary brachytherapy. ^{192}Ir seeds are available in diameters ranging from 0.3 mm to 0.8 mm (including nylon ribbon encapsulation) and in length of about 3 mm. ^{192}Ir seeds, in the form of ribbons or strands, are often used in LDR breast and head and neck temporary implants, and they can be applied to treatments of many other disease sites, too. The physical size of ^{137}Cs sources is around 2 cm in length and about 3 mm in diameter although the size may slightly vary among different models. The ^{137}Cs sources are normally placed inside applicators (e.g., Fletcher Suit applicator and Henschke applicator) to treat GYN cancers in LDR temporary implants.

The strength of a brachytherapy source can be specified in different ways: air kerma strength, activity, apparent activity, exposure rate at a specified distance, and equivalent mass of radium. The current trend is to use air kerma strength as the standard specification of brachytherapy sources. The air kerma strength is defined as the product of air kerma rate in "free space"

and the square of the distance of the calibration point from the source center along the perpendicular bisector. The air kerma rate should be contributed from photons greater than a cutoff energy, below which the photons increase the air kerma strength but do not contribute significantly to the dose at distances greater than 0.1 cm in tissue (Rivard et al. 2004). The calibration measurement must be performed with a distance between the detector and the source large enough so that the source can be treated as a point source and the detector can be treated as a point detector. Recommended unit for air kerma strength is μGy m^{2}h^{-1} (U) (Nath et al. 1987).

In general, the dose calculations from a single brachytherapy source in temporary LDR brachytherapy follow the formalisms recommended by Task Group No. 43 of the American Association of Physicists in Medicine (▶ The AAPM TG-43) (Nath et al. 1995; Rivard et al. 2004). There are five basic quantities or functions in the formalisms: source strength, dose rate constant, geometric function, radial dose function, and anisotropy function. As mentioned previously, the source strength is recommended to be expressed in air kerma strength. The dose rate constant is the ratio of dose rate at a reference position and source strength. The dose rate constant has a unit of cGy per hour per U (cGyh^{-1} U^{-1}), and the reference position is 1 cm from the center of source along the source central transverse axis. The geometry function accounts for the impacts of spatial radionuclide distribution within the source on the source relative dose distribution, ignoring photon absorption and scattering in the source structure (Nath et al. 1995; Rivard et al. 2004). For a point source, the geometry function is inversely proportional to the square of distance from point of interest to the source. The radial dose function describes the relative dose change due to photon attenuation and scatter in the medium along the source central transverse axis. The anisotropy function describes the anisotropy of relative dose distribution around the source. For brachytherapy sources made of low energy photon emitters, such as ^{125}I and ^{103}Pd, the dose rate constant, the radial dose function, and the anisotropy function are sensitive and susceptible to construction structure, encapsulation, and internal radionuclide distribution, and are normally different among different models. Given the five physical quantities, the dose rate at a point (r, θ) can be calculated as:

$$\dot{D}(r,\theta) = S_k \bullet \Lambda \bullet \frac{G_L(r,\theta)}{G_L(r_o, \theta_o)} \bullet g_L(r) \bullet F(r,\theta)$$

Where S is the source strength, Λ is the dose rate constant, G_L is the geometry function, g_L is the radial dose function, F is the anisotropy function, (r_o, θ_o) is the reference point, and L represents active source distribution (normally active length).

Although exposure rate constant is less and less used for dosimetry calculations, familiarity with its numerical values of various radionuclides is helpful in estimating exposures for the purpose of ▶ radiation safety. The numerical values of exposure rate constant for radionuclides used in LDR temporary brachytherapy are tabulated in Table 1.

Clinical Process

LDR temporary brachytherapy can be an invasive procedure that may require hospitalization of the patient. The process also involves radioactive materials, and requires comprehensive program that pays detailed attention to radiation safety, personnel trainings, equipment quality assurance, patient education, etc. It also highly requires team efforts since the process involves personnel from different disciplines including radiation oncologists, medical physicists, medical dosimetrists, radiation therapists, nurses, and radiation safety officer (s). Detailed guidelines and policies should be established to define the roles and responsibilities of each of the team members in the clinical process and be strictly enforced. According to the practice guideline of American College of Radiology (ACR) for the performance of LDR brachytherapy (ACR 2005), a well-defined LDR brachytherapy process should consist of the following components (quoted from the ACR guideline):

1. Clinical evaluation
   The initial evaluation of the patient includes history, physical examination, review of pertinent diagnostic studies and reports, and communication with the physicians involved in the patient's care. The extent of the tumor must be determined and recorded for staging.
2. Establishing treatment goals
   The goal of treatment should be documented as clearly as possible. Treatment options and their relative merits and risks should be discussed with the patient. Integration of brachytherapy with external beam therapy should be defined. A summary of the consultation should be communicated to the referring physician.
3. Informed consent
   Informed consent must be obtained and documented.
4. Applicator/source insertion
   The brachytherapy team should operate according to an established system of

procedural steps that have been developed by the radiation oncologist and brachytherapy team members. This systematic approach to applicator or source insertion should include a description of preimplantation steps, sedation or anesthesia procedures, the specific applicators used, and the insertion techniques.

5. Treatment planning

LDR brachytherapy is administered according to the written, signed, and dated prescription of the radiation oncologist. Before loading, the prescription must designate the treatment site, the isotope, the number of sources, the planned dose, and the dose rate to designated points. The treatment planning is preferably performed based on images of CT, MRI, and other types of imaging modalities on which applicator geometry, anatomic structures, and isotope positions can be defined. The plan should be conducted by a qualified medical physicist or his/her designee, and approved by the radiation oncologist. Independent verification of brachytherapy parameters should also be done pretreatment.

6. Treatment delivery

LDR sources are manually or remotely loaded into applicators to deliver the prescribed treatment. If treatment modification is required, such modification must be documented.

7. Radiation safety considerations

Patients should be provided with written descriptions of the radiation protection guidelines, including, but not limited to, discussion of potential limitations of patient contact with minors and pregnant women.

8. Patient evaluation during temporary implants

The radiation oncologist evaluates patients on a regular basis during their brachytherapy treatment. The patient's progress through therapy should be documented. At the end of treatment, the patient and room must be surveyed to ensure that all radiation sources have been retrieved.

9. Treatment summary

A written summary of the treatment delivery parameters should be generated, including the total dose of brachytherapy and the total dose of external beam therapy if given, treatment technique, treatment volume, acute side effects, clinical course, and patient disposition.

10. Follow-up evaluation

Patients should be evaluated after treatment at regular intervals for response and early and late effects on normal tissues.

Training, Education, Quality Assurance, and Radiation Safety

Team effort and good training are critical to the success of an LDR temporary brachytherapy implant program. Before starting such a program, a team should be formed and should include the radiation oncologist, medical physicist, dosimetrist, therapist, nurse, and radiation safety officer. The team members should meet the qualification criteria set forth by recognized national organizations. Extensive trainings should be provided to the radiation oncologist, the medical physicist, the medical dosimetrist, the nurse, and the therapist. The training should cover all aspects of brachytherapy, including applicator insertion and placement, equipment and treatment planning system operation, radioactive source handling, and radiation safety requirements and regulations. Responsibilities of each member should be clearly defined and understood.

A comprehensive quality assurance program should be established and maintained to ensure the integrity and accuracy of delivery equipment (e.g., applicators and catheters), treatment planning computer systems (software and hardware), radiation survey meters, source strength measurement and assay systems (electrometers, chambers, cables, etc.), and other treatment-related equipment. Periodical inspections and evaluations should be conducted on the equipment. For the equipment related to source strength measurement and assay, such as chamber, electrometer, thermometer, and barometer, periodical calibrations are required and the calibrations should adhere to national or international standards.

The "hot lab" should be secured and labeled following radiation safety guidelines. An active source inventory procedure, permanent documentation mechanism, and in-use logging system should be implemented for a LDR temporary brachytherapy program. Source inventory should be periodically updated for information such as radionuclide and source type, number and strength of sources, clinical usage, etc. Permanent documentation should be maintained and contain details of source descriptions. An in-use logging system should exist to document current clinical usage of sources. The logging system should contain information about patients, clinicians, sources, date and time of source-in and source-out, brief description, and location of the clinical procedures. Wipe tests should also be periodically conducted on radioactive sources to ensure source integrity.

A comprehensive radiation safety program should be maintained for the purpose of radiation protection of patients, staff, and the general public. Radiation safety regulations should be strictly followed and their appropriate implementation should be periodically evaluated. The radiation safety program should include radiation monitoring system, necessary radiation storage and shielding devices, appropriate radiation signs and labels, radiation safety education of patient and staff, procedures for radioactive source transportation and disposal, and continued education of staff on clinical procedures (techniques and new technologies) and equipment. Appropriate procedure rooms should be identified with radiation safety and convenience of shielding taken into consideration.

As additional new technologies become available in radiotherapy, some of LDR temporary brachytherapy implant procedures are being replaced by some alternative treatment modalities. However, it is still very important for radiation oncologists, medical physicists and other radiotherapy personnel to understand the principles and characteristics of the procedures. In some clinical cases, LDR temporary implant offers its unique advantages and can provide various benefits to patients. The LDR temporary brachytherapy is still a viable treatment modality and plays an important role in radiotherapy.

Cross-References

▶ Brachytherapy: High Dose Rate (HDR) Implants
▶ Brachytherapy: Low Dose Rate (LDR) Permanent Implants (Prostate)
▶ Clinical Aspects of Brachytherapy (BT)
▶ Eye Plaque Physics
▶ Intensity Modulated Radiation Therapy (IMRT)
▶ Radiation Oncology Physics

References

American College of Radiology (ACR) (2005) ACR practice guideline for the performance of low-dose-rate brachytherapy. American College of Radiology (ACR), Reston, p 5

Chu SYF, Ekström LP, Firestone RB (1999) The Lund/LBNL Nuclear Data Search. http://nucleardata.nuclear.lu.se/nucleardata/toi/index.asp

Hall EJ (1972) Radiation dose rate: a factor of importance in radiobiology and radiotherapy. Brit J Radiol 45:81

Nath R, Anderson LL, Jones D, Ling C, Loevinger R, Williamson JF, Hanson W, Khan FM (1987) Specification of brachytherapy source strength: recommendations of the AAPM radiation therapy committee task group No. 32. AAPM Report 21, AAPM, College Park

Nath R, Anderson LL, Luxton G, Weaver KA, Williamson JF, Meigooni AS (1995) Dosimetry of interstitial brachytherapy sources: recommendations of the AAPM Radiation Therapy Committee Task Group No. 43. Med Phys 22:209–234

Rivard MJ, Coursey BM, DeWerd LA, Hanson WF, Huq MS, Ibbott GS, Mitch MG, Nath R, Williamson JF (2004) Update of AAPM task group No. 43 report: a revised AAPM protocol for brachytherapy dose calculations. Med Phys 31(3):633–674

BRAF Inhibitors

RENE RUBIN
Rittenhouse Hematology/Oncology, Philadelphia, PA, USA

Definition

BRAF is a human protein (serine/threonine-protein kinase B-Raf) encoded by the BRAF gene that sends signals in cells and is responsible for cell growth. Mutations in this gene may cause cancer; 60% of melanomas and 10% of colon cancer cells have BRAF mutations. Furthermore, these mutations are found in papillary thyroid carcinoma. BRAF enzyme inhibition (vemurafenib, oral agent, used in melanoma) is only useful in tumors that have the mutation. It may actually promote tumor growth in BRAF non-mutated tumors.

Side Effects
- Anapyhlaxis
- Rashes
- Myalgia/athralgia
- Diarrhea
- Liver function abnormalities
- Skin lesions, including squamous cell carcinoma of the skin

Cross-References
▶ Principles of Chemotherapy

BRAF-V600E

NISHA R. PATEL, MICHAEL L. WONG
Department of Radiation Oncology, College of Medicine, Drexel University, Philadelphia, PA, USA

Definition
Point mutation involving the RAF kinase protein within the RAS–RAF–MEK–ERK pathway associated with aggressive papillary thyroid cancer.

Cross-References
▶ Thyroid Cancer

Bragg Peak

BRIAN F. HASSON[1,2], DANIEL YEUNG[3], JATINDER PALTA[4]
[1]Department of Radiation Oncology, Abington Memorial Hospital, Abington, PA, USA
[2]Department of Radiation Oncology, Drexel University, College of Medicine, Philadelphia, PA, USA
[3]Department of Radiation Oncology, University of Florida Proton Therapy Institute, Jacksonville, FL, USA
[4]Department of Radiation Oncology, University of Florida Health Science Center, Gainesville, FL, USA

Definition
A region of large energy transfer from a proton or heavy ion. It is seen as a region of high-dose deposition at the end of the particle's range in tissue. The peak in dose occurs when the energy of the particles in the beam have declined to approximately 0.15 MeV. The characteristic peak in a depth-dose curve near the end of the range for a (near) monoenergetic proton beam traveling through a medium.

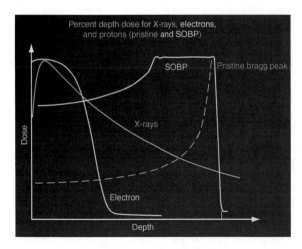

Bragg Peak. Fig. 1 Percent depth dose for X-Rays, electrons and protons (Pristine peak and spread out Bragg peak – SOBP)

Cross-References

▶ Proton Therapy
▶ Stereotactic Radiosurgery – Cranial

BRCA1 and BRCA2

Christin A. Knowlton[1], Michelle Kolton Mackay[2]
[1]Department of Radiation Oncology, Drexel University, Philadelphia, PA, USA
[2]Department of Radiation Oncology, Marshfield Clinic, Marshfield, WI, USA

Definition

BRCA1 and *BRCA2* are tumor suppressor genes that when mutated place a patient at higher risk of breast and ovarian cancer. Genetic testing can be performed to evaluate for the presence of a *BRCA1* or *BRCA2* mutation. Patients with a strong family history of breast and ovarian cancer may benefit from genetic counseling and testing, as there are options to address their cancer risk.

Cross-References

▶ Ovary

Breakthrough Pain

James H. Brashears, III
Radiation Oncologist, Venice, FL, USA

Definition

Acute pain exacerbation that occurs despite the suppression measures or maintenance dose of long-acting, usually opioid, medication. This may occur during repositioning, with exertion, or at the end of a long-acting opioid dosing interval.

Cross-References

▶ Pain Management

Breast Cancer Risk Models

Anthony E. Dragun
Department of Radiation Oncology, James Graham Brown Cancer Center, University of Louisville School of Medicine, Louisville, KY, USA

Synonyms

Gail; International Breast Cancer Intervention Survey (IBIS) models; Luminal subtypes; Tyrer-Cuzick

Definition

These are statistical tools to estimate breast cancer risk by incorporating known risk factors of an individual patient. The Gail model was the first widely used and validated system. It incorporates age, obstetric history, family history, and breast health history. A Gail model score of greater than or equal to 1.6 is considered high enough risk to justify the consideration of chemoprevention in some patients. Newer models incorporate body mass indices and the patient's history of exogenous hormone use.

Cross-References

▶ Early-Stage Breast Cancer
▶ Hormonal Agents

Breast Cancer: Locally Advanced and Recurrent Disease, Postmastectomy Radiation and Systemic Therapies

ANTHONY E. DRAGUN
Department of Radiation Oncology, James Graham Brown Cancer Center, University of Louisville School of Medicine, Louisville, KY, USA

Definition

Locally advanced breast cancer is a term applied to variable entities with a wide range of prognoses. Generally speaking, primary breast tumors that are T3 or T4 and/or disease that has extensively spread to the regional nodal basins (the axilla, supraclavicular fossa, and/or internal mammary chain) are included (Fig. 1). A particularly aggressive subtype of locally advanced breast cancer is "inflammatory breast cancer," which presents with rapid onset of erythema, warmth, and significant swelling of the breast (Fig. 2). Inflammatory breast cancer may or may not have an associated underlying mass. The histologic hallmark is dermolymphatic invasion and biologically, these cancers are typically high grade and estrogen and progesterone receptor negative.

Recurrent breast cancer is also a term that encompasses a wide variety of clinical scenarios. It is usually divided into the following: ipsilateral breast tumor recurrence (for patients who have under gone a previous breast conserving therapy), chest wall recurrence (for patients who have under gone a previous mastectomy), and regional lymph node recurrence (in either of the aforementioned two groups). Ipsilateral breast tumor recurrence is usually divided into two subgroups. So-called "true recurrences" make up the overwhelming majority of ipsilateral breast tumor recurrences. These cancers recur within 1–2 cm of the original lumpectomy cavity or within the same quadrant of the original index lesion. They have a relatively early occurrence (5–7 years) following primary therapy. "Elsewhere breast failures" are rarer and occur later in the time course of follow-up in treatment for breast cancer. They generally occur with the same frequency as contralateral breast cancers (approximately 0.5–1% per year) after the treatment of a primary breast cancer.

Chest wall recurrences indicate disease that has relapsed in the skin, subcutaneous tissue, or muscle of the chest wall in the postmastectomy setting. The most common site of the chest wall recurrence is in the original mastectomy scar. Lymph node recurrences may manifest in the axilla, supraclavicular fossa, infraclavicular or internal mammary chain (in that order of frequency).

Etiology

The etiology of locally advanced breast cancer is similar to that described for ▶ early-stage breast cancer; however, advanced disease is usually more

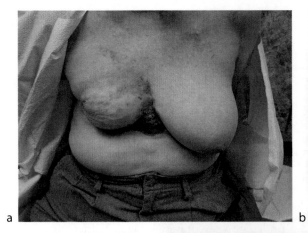
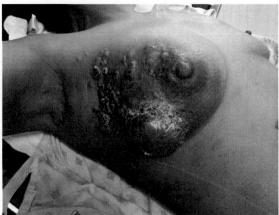

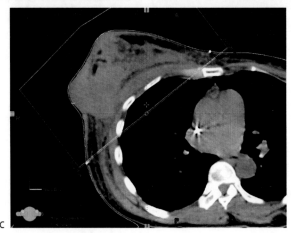

Breast Cancer: Locally Advanced and Recurrent Disease, Postmastectomy Radiation and Systemic Therapies. Fig. 1 (**a**) A 62-year-old female who presented with locally advanced infiltrating ductal carcinoma of the right breast. The patient sought medical attention approximately 4 years after she first detected a small mass in her right breast. This depicts an "endophytic" growth pattern, with the right breast completely replaced by a firm, fixed cancerous mass with contiguous spread to the dermis in the lower inner quadrant. The carcinoma has caused near complete involution of the breast with consumption of the nipple-areolar complex, a phenomenon referred to as "autoamputation." (**b**) A 54-year-old female presented with a fungating infiltrating ductal carcinoma of the right breast. This is an example of "exophytic" growth pattern, with multiple masses erupting through the skin as well as dermal nodules and fixed axillary lymph nodes. (**c**) An axial CT image of the patient shown in (**b**), showing multiple necrotic masses in the breast

biologically aggressive, with early spread to regional lymphatics. These cancers are also the result of a delay in treatment due to misdiagnosis, neglect, or fear. The etiology of recurrent breast cancer has mainly to do with risk factors for recurrence after previous treatment. The main risk factor for an ipsilateral breast tumor recurrence is lack of the use of adjuvant radiation therapy and systemic therapy after breast conservation surgery. Otherwise, the incidence depends heavily on age, margin status, tumor size, and nodal status at the time of the original diagnosis. There is also an association of true recurrence with lymphovascular space invasion, perineural

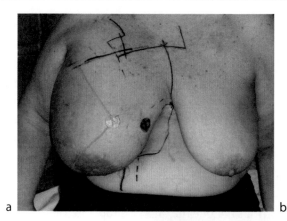

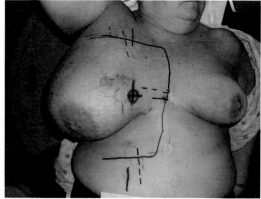

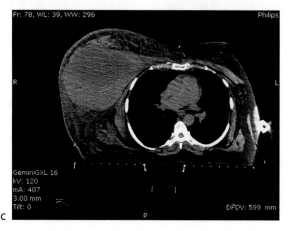

Breast Cancer: Locally Advanced and Recurrent Disease, Postmastectomy Radiation and Systemic Therapies. Fig. 2 A 49-year-old presented with inflammatory breast carcinoma, with rapid enlargement, engorgement, and erythema (in the upper outer quadrant) of the right breast. (**a**) A biopsy of her large breast mass returned infiltrating ductal carcinoma, estrogen receptor, and progesterone receptor negative. A punch biopsy of the skin showed dermolymphatic invasion. The patient was started on neoadjuvant therapy, but her disease rapidly progressed during administration of combination cytotoxic chemotherapy. The patient underwent radiation therapy for disease control and was ultimately able to undergo modified radical mastectomy with negative margins; (**b**) shows the patient's clinical radiotherapy setup; and (**c**) shows an axial CT image of the underlying necrotic mass at the time of therapy initiation

invasion, extensive intraductal component as well as biologic subtype. With regard to recurrences in the chest wall and regional lymph nodes (following mastectomy), patients are at higher than average risk if they originally presented with inflammatory breast cancer, or involvement of the skin or nipple-areolar complex. In addition, close or positive margins at the time of surgery, multicentric disease, involvement of the pectoralis fascia, and tumor size greater than approximately 4–5 cm are risk factors. Lymph node involvement – including the overall number of lymph nodes involved with tumor and the percentage of involved lymph nodes – is an important factor. Additionally, lymphovascular space invasion and extracapsular lymph node extension place patients at a high risk for locoregional recurrence.

Clinical Presentation

Presenting symptoms for patients with locally advanced breast cancer include a mass detected by either a breast self-exam or clinical breast exam, edema of the breast, skin retraction, or ulceration, nipple inversion, or bleeding. Axillary masses, swelling of the breast and/or upper extremity, pain or parathesias of the upper extremity are also possible. Inflammatory breast cancer involves the rapid development of skin rash, edema, and the sensation of "fullness" of the breast. A detailed clinical history should focus on the onset, duration, characteristics, and course of these aforementioned symptoms.

Clinical signs of locally advanced breast cancer include the long-established "Haagensen's Grave Signs" (first described in the 1940s), a group of clinical presentations of advanced breast carcinoma that indicate inoperability and generalized poor prognosis. These include skin ulceration, fixation of the tumor to the chest wall, axillary lymph nodes greater than 2.5 cm in diameter, edema of the breast, and presence of fixed axillary lymph nodes. On physical exam, the breast exam should focus on the size and mobility of the dominant breast mass as well as any overlying skin changes. Edema of the breast, resulting in a prominence of skin appendages is usually termed peau d'orange. Edema of the upper extremity must be quantified as well as any clinically apparent lymph nodes including those in the axilla, supraclavicular fossa, and internal mammary chain.

Presentation of recurrent breast cancer varies, but the majority of recurrences occur within the first two years from completion of treatment. Ipsilateral breast tumor recurrence usually presents as a new abnormality on surveillance mammogram, which includes microcalcifications or spiculated appearance similar to those described on breast screening. Additionally, these may present as a new mass on breast self-exam or clinical breast exam. Chest wall recurrences most commonly present as a new abnormality in the mastectomy scar. This is usually described as a "pimple," ulceration, or skin rash. The majority of chest wall recurrences occur within the first two years from completion of treatment. Lymph node recurrences usually present as a painless mass in the axilla, or supraclavicular fossa. Parasternal tenderness may be indicative of a recurrence in the internal mammary chain. Other, less common presentations include the onset of upper extremity edema, pain, or brachial plexopathy.

Diagnostics

In terms of radiologic workup of locally advanced disease, diagnostic mammogram and ultrasound are useful for characterizing any new lesion. Furthermore, MRI may be helpful in defining possible chest wall invasion as well as assisting with operative planning. Ultrasound of the axilla may help to define lymph node disease and assist in obtaining tissue diagnosis. Additionally, all new skin rashes should be biopsied if suspicious. Metastatic workup consists of routine blood counts and serum chemistries. CT scans of the chest, abdomen, and pelvis along with a bone scan are routinely employed for radiologic staging. Although not currently standard of care, whole body PET-CT scan is being used more commonly in place of these aforementioned tests. For breast cancer recurrence, a complete restaging workup is recommended to determine if the local and/or regional recurrence is isolated or associated with synchronous distant metastatic disease.

Differential Diagnosis

Locally Advanced Breast Cancer. The differential diagnosis of a large breast mass includes a breast abscess, hematoma, fat necrosis, hamartoma, phylloides tumor, breast lymphoma, and sarcoma. Differential diagnosis of a new breast rash includes infectious mastitis, trauma, inflammatory conditions, and connective tissue disorders such as systemic lupus erythematosus. *Recurrent Breast Cancer.* Differential diagnosis of suspicious findings after a treatment for breast cancer should be considered cancer until proven otherwise. Ipsilateral breast tumor recurrence is usually detected mammographically on surveillance images and as such, differential diagnosis is similar to that of a new screening-detected primary. Considerations include fibroadenoma, fat necrosis, and breast seroma. Chest wall recurrences may be confused with a late radiation toxicity including skin ulceration and/or necrosis. Fibrosis may be mimicked by carcinoma "en cuirasse" (diffuse involvement of the skin and subcutaneous tissue with recurrent carcinoma). Lymph node recurrences: palpable masses in the supraclavicular fossa or axillary region may indicate underlying seroma or fibrosis, especially if painful. Parasternal or pain may indicate a costochondritis or osseous metastatic disease involving the ribs or sternum.

Prophylaxis

For locally advanced breast cancer, prophylactic treatment is similar to that for early-stage breast cancer. The most common strategy to avoid locally advanced breast cancer is early detection with routine screening mammography, self breast exam, and clinical breast exam. Breast cancer awareness by the patient and her primary caretakers is also crucial, as complete workup of any new dominant breast mass or rash is a must.

Prevention of recurrent breast cancer involves appropriate up front primary and adjuvant therapies. Ipsilateral breast tumor recurrence is most often prevented with clear surgical margins on primary surgery, postoperative radiation therapy integrated with proper systemic treatment with cytotoxic chemotherapy and/or hormonal therapy. Preventative strategies in the postmastectomy setting include the judicious use of postmastectomy radiotherapy and tailored systemic treatment.

Therapy

Combined modality therapy with surgery, radiotherapy, and systemic treatment is the standard for both locally advanced breast cancers and recurrent breast cancers. These entities, like early-stage breast cancer, are best treated in a multidisciplinary setting. Treatment may vary by institution and may be individualized based on the patient's presentation and general overall medical comorbidites. General principles are as follows:

Locally Advanced and Recurrent Breast Cancer

Primary surgery for locally advanced breast cancer may involve a modified radical mastectomy or breast conserving surgery. Breast conserving surgery is most often performed after neoadjuvant ("up front") chemotherapy. If neoadjuvant chemotherapy is a consideration, then it is important to place a radioopaque marker at the time of the initial workup and biopsy of the primary breast mass. This assists with localization of the lesion in the postchemotherapy period. Selection criteria for breast conserving surgery and overall volume of tissue removed varies by surgeon. Principles of breast conserving surgery are the same as those outlined for early-stage breast cancer.

Modified radical mastectomy involves removal of the entire mammary gland from the clavicle superiorly to rectus sheath inferiorly, as well as to the sternal border medially and the latisimus dorsi laterally. The nipple areola complex is typically removed and the deep resection is performed to include the removal of pectoralis fascia. Skin flaps may be dissected and created to assist with reconstructive efforts ("▶ skin-sparing mastectomy"). Newer techniques of skin-sparing mastectomy also include sparing the nipple areola complex.

Radiation Therapy: Whole breast radiation therapy is carried out in a fashion similar to that described in early-stage breast cancer, if breast conserving surgery is performed. In the

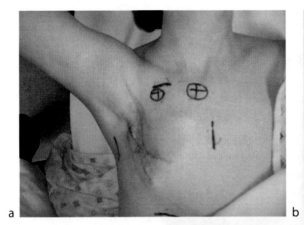

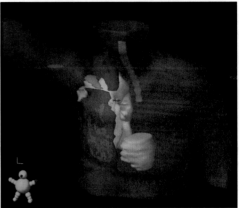

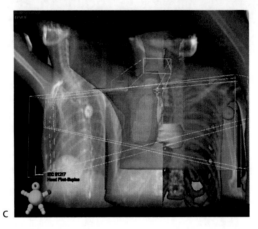

Breast Cancer: Locally Advanced and Recurrent Disease, Postmastectomy Radiation and Systemic Therapies. Fig. 3 Typical supine setup for a 58-year-old patient with locally advanced breast cancer (status-post modified radical mastectomy conserving surgery) who is to be treated with chest wall and regional lymphatic irradiation using a monoisocentric setup (**a**). Three-dimensional treatment planning techniques (**b**) are used to define the chest wall (*red*), levels 1 (*green*), 2 (*yellow*), and 3 (*orange*) of the axilla, supraclavicular fossa (*violet*), and internal mammary chain (*light blue*). The adjacent organs at risk, the ipsilateral lung, heart, and cervical spinal cord are shown in light yellow. Distribution of radiation dose in three dimensions (**c**) shows the chest wall and regional nodal volumes covered by the 95% dose cloud (*pink*)

postmastectomy setting, radiation therapy is directed to the chest wall, and in most cases, the selective regional lymphatics. A total dose of 45–50 Gy delivered to these targets using conventional fractionation is recommended. There are multiple described techniques to "match" fields in order to encompass the chest wall and regional lymphatic targets in order to avoid overlap and the resultant increased toxicity. These techniques include alignment of the gantry, couch, and collimator to best match beam penumbra, or the use of independent jaws and multileaf collimation for the more modern, monoisosentric technique (Fig. 3). Chest wall radiation therapy includes treating the entire chest wall from the clavicle superiorly to the sternal border medially, the midaxillary line laterally, and inferiorly to match the contralateral inframmary fold. Customarily, a boost to the mastectomy scar using electrons delivers an additional 10–16 Gy.

In terms of radiotherapy to the regional lymph nodes, the decision on which lymph node basins to include under which circumstance depends on the overall number of lymph nodes involved, the percentage of positive lymph nodes, the presence of extracapsular extension, and the adequacy of the lymph node resection. These factors must be balanced with the risk of additional morbidity in the context of modern systemic therapies. Treatment of the axilla (levels I and II) are generally included within the chest wall tangent fields. Modification of the supraclavicular fossa field may be used to supplement the axilla. Irradiation of the lymph nodes of the supraclavicular fossa is generally not complicated and can be done with little risk of morbidity. The use of three-dimensional treatment planning helps guide therapy and usually eliminates the need for the so-called "posterior axillary boost" which has been associated with increased risk of ipsilateral upper extremity ▶ lymphedema.

Routine inclusion of the internal mammary lymph nodes is highly controversial in terms of the estimations of therapeutic benefit in the age of modern systemic therapy. Postmastectomy trials that showed an overall survival benefit to postmastectomy radiation therapy included the radiation of comprehensive nodal sites including the internal mammary chain. These trials were initiated in the late 1970s and early 1980s and thus did not include anthracycline, taxane-based chemotherapy, nor targeted systemic therapies such as trastuzimab, all of which are cardiotoxic. Irradiation of the internal mammary chain typically results in higher radiotherapeutic doses to the heart and coronary vessels, and the substantial risk of cardiotoxicity from trials which included internal mammary nodal irradiation is well documented. All these factors must be balanced with the fact that isolated internal mammary chain recurrence is very rare. Treatment to the internal mammary chain is mandated if lymph nodes are involved clinically or radiographically; otherwise, the risks of electively irradiating the internal mammary chain must be weighed carefully especially for patients with left-sided breast cancers where doses to the heart may be significant. When treated, the internal mammary chain may be targeted with a separate "patched" field with electrons or included with the chest wall tangent fields (partial deep tangent technique).

With regard to timing of radiotherapy, multiple studies have shown that sequencing radiation therapy after systemic therapy is ideal and does not compromise local regional control, even after a long sequence of multiagent combination chemotherapy (Sartor et al. 2005). Radiation therapy usually commences 2–4 weeks after the final cycle of cytotoxic chemotherapy.

Systemic Treatment: Cytotoxic chemotherapy is routine in the adjuvant treatment of nonmetastatic locally advanced breast cancer. The first widely established combination regimen to show a disease-free survival and overall survival benefit in this setting was CMF (cyclophosphomide, methotrexate, and 5-fluorouacil). Over time, anthracycline-continuing regimens have generally replaced CMF. Of the anthracycline family, adriamycin is favored in the United States; epirubicin is the agent of choice in Canada and Europe. The taxane family of drugs (microtubule stabilizers), when used in addition to anthracycline-containing regimens, have been shown to increase disease-free survival and overall survival, especially in lymph node positive patients (Mamounas EP, et al. 2005). The taxanes (docetaxel and paclitaxel) are also gaining popularity in substitution regimens for anthracyclines.

In terms of novel targeted agents, herceptin (trastuzumab) is a humanized monoclonal antibody tyrosine kinase inhibitor. It has also been shown to increase disease-free survival and overall survival in patients with ► Her2 overexpression when added to these aforementioned modern cytotoxic chemotherapy regimens. (Romond et al. 2005). Hormonal therapy is also a mainstay for the estrogen and progesterone receptor positive patient. Treatment strategy for administration of hormonal therapy is similar to that of early-stage breast cancer.

Neoadjuvant chemotherapy, the utilization of cytotoxic therapy for cytoreduction of large breast cancers prior to definitive surgery, is a treatment strategy that is gaining in popularity. The major advantage of neoadjuvant chemotherapy is that it increases the availability of patients to choose breast conservation. In addition, assessing the chemosensitivity of the primary tumor may help predict overall prognosis. A disadvantage of this approach is that it delays the local therapy and interferes with proper traditional pathologic staging. Modern studies that include the use of anthracyclines and taxanes in the neoadjuvant setting show an approximately 60% conversion rate of patients from mastectomy to breast conserving techniques (Rastogi et al. 2008). Modern regimens also show a clinical complete response rate at approximately 60–75% and a pathologic complete response rate at approximately 20–25%. In the case of patients who have undergone neoadjuvant chemotherapy and subsequently require a mastectomy, radiation therapy is indicated if the patient was clinically lymph node positive or clinically stage T3 at diagnosis. Current controversy exists as to whether postmastectomy radiation therapy is necessary in all patients who have a pathologic complete response after neoadjuvant chemotherapy.

In terms of inflammatory carcinoma of the breast, the standard of care for patients is to undergo neoadjuvant chemotherapy followed by mastectomy and axillary clearance. Postmastectomy radiation therapy is always indicated in cases of patients treated for inflammatory

carcinoma. Some accelerated fractionation schedules of postmastectomy radiation therapy (twice daily radiotherapy) have been shown to be associated with increased local regional control.

Recurrent Breast Cancer. The current standard of care for the treatment of ipsilateral breast tumor recurrence is salvage mastectomy followed by systemic chemotherapy and/or hormonal therapy. Newer strategies include the use of repeat breast conservation surgery with ► accelerated partial breast irradiation for continued breast preservation. The strategy for controlling chest wall recurrence is individualized based on patients' overall performance status and prior treatment. Wide local excision of the recurrent lesion is indicated if possible, because it has been shown to add a local control benefit especially for small, singular lesions. Following this, radiation therapy to the chest wall and regional lymphatics is recommended with the addition of systemic chemotherapy either concurrently or adjuvantly. Radiotherapy involves treatment of the entire chest wall with inclusion of the regional lymph nodes to reduce the risk of metachronous lymph node recurrence. In patients who have been previously irradiated, ► re-irradiation should be considered if the patient is otherwise healthy and the disease-free interval has been significant.

Lymph Node Recurrence. The utility of surgery for isolated lymph node recurrence is limited, beyond establishing the diagnosis. Radiation therapy is generally recommended to treat the comprehensive locoregional area including the chest wall, especially if no prior radiation therapy has been given. Lymph node recurrence also mandates an assessment of the patient for systemic therapy.

Prognosis

Locally Advanced Breast Cancer: Modern combination therapy improves outcomes compared to historical studies, which show very few patients surviving 10 years or greater. Today, greater than 60% overall survival at 10 years is commonly achieved. Multidisciplinary therapy continues to increase cure rates with the adoption of anthracycline-based chemotherapy, taxanes, hormonal therapy, and targeted systemic therapy. The addition of postmastectomy radiotherapy for high-risk, locally advanced patients improves overall survival by as much as 10%. This benefit is mainly due to the fact that overall locoregional recurrence rates for patients with T3 or T4 primaries and N2 or N3 disease is as high as 35–50%, and radiotherapy reduces this risk to less than 10–15%. As with early-stage breast cancer, it is estimated that for every four local recurrences prevented, one life is saved. In the case of inflammatory breast cancer, historically, very few patients were expected to live after this diagnosis. Modern series, however, show 3 year overall survival rates approaching 70% and 3 year disease-free survival rates at approximately 45%.

Recurrent Breast Cancer. The prognosis after recurrence of breast cancer varies widely. Generally, depending on the volume of recurrent disease, the absence of distant disease, and the ability of the patient to undergo aggressive salvage treatment, overall survival rates of approximately 60% may be achieved. Factors that influence prognosis include the disease-free internal, presence of multiple sites of involvement, volume of disease recurrence, tumor biology (tumor grade, estrogen receptor, and Her2 status), and the prognostic factors of the patient's original index tumor. Ten-year overall survival rates for patients with ipsilateral breast tumor recurrence, chest wall recurrence, and lymph node recurrence are approximately 75%, 45%, and 30%, respectively.

Epidemiology

The incidence of locally advanced breast cancer is significantly decreasing due to early detection and overall higher levels of breast cancer awareness regarding the importance of breast cancer screening. Approximately 10,000 new cases of locally advanced breast cancer occur per year in the United States. The incidence is higher in underserved minority populations. Inflammatory breast cancer comprises approximately 2% of all new breast cancers in the United States.

The epidemiology of recurrent breast cancer is somewhat more difficult to estimate. Overall, the estimate of ipsilateral breast tumor recurrence in the appropriately treated patient is 5–10% at 10 years. This translates to a 0.5–1% annual risk of local recurrence. Chest wall relapse after mastectomy makes up approximately two-thirds of local regional recurrences after initial therapy with mastectomy. The overall risk is approximately 10–25% and is decreased with the use of adjuvant radiation therapy and chemotherapy. Isolated lymph node recurrences are less frequent, with the most common site being the axilla followed by the supraclavicular fossa, and rarely the internal mammary chain. Relapse in multiple concurrent sites (in the chest wall or breast as well as the lymph nodes) occurs in approximately 20% of cases of locoregional recurrence.

Cross-References

▶ Early-Stage Breast Cancer

References

Mamounas EP, Bryant J, Lembersky B et al (2005) Paclitaxel after doxorubicin plus cyclophosphamide as adjuvant chemotherapy for node-positive breast cancer: results from NSABP B-28. J Clin Oncol 23(16):3686–3696

Rastogi P, Anderson SJ, Bear HD et al (2008) Preoperative chemotherapy: updates of national surgical adjuvant breast and bowel project protocols B-18 and B-27. J Clin Oncol 26(5):778–785

Romond EH, Perez EA, Bryant J et al (2005) Trastuzumab plus adjuvant chemotherapy for operable HER2-positive breast cancer. N Engl J Med 353(16):1673–1684

Sartor CI, Peterson BL, Woolf S et al (2005) Effect of addition of adjuvant paclitaxel on radiotherapy delivery and locoregional control of node-positive breast cancer: cancer and leukemia group B 9344. J Clin Oncol 23:30–40

Breast Conservation Therapy

DAVID E. WAZER
Radiation Oncology Department, Tufts Medical
Center, Tufts University School of Medicine,
Boston, MA, USA
Radiation Oncology Department, Rhode Island
Hospital, Brown University School of Medicine,
Providence, RI, USA

Definition

There are three variants of noninvasive breast disease: lobular carcinoma in situ (LCIS); Paget's disease; and ductal carcinoma in situ (DCIS).

A multidisciplinary approach of breast conserving surgery and adjuvant radiotherapy with the goal of achieving in-breast disease control while preserving breast cosmesis.

Cross-References

▶ Cancer of the Breast Tis
▶ Early-Stage Breast Cancer

Breast Lymphoma

ANTHONY E. DRAGUN
Department of Radiation Oncology, James
Graham Brown Cancer Center, University of
Louisville School of Medicine, Louisville,
KY, USA

Synonyms

Diffuse large B cell lymphoma of the breast

Definition

Primary lymphomas of the breast account for approximately 2% of extranodal lymphoma and 1% of all breast neoplasms. They are usually diffuse large B cell ▶ non-Hodgkin's lymphomas. The role of surgery is limited to establishing the diagnosis of breast lymphoma. Mastectomy offers no benefit to disease control. Standard systemic therapy for non-Hodgkin's lymphoma with rituximab, cyclophosphomide, doxorubicin, vincristine, and prednisone (R-CHOP), together with involved field radiation therapy, is the standard of care.

Cross-References

▶ Early-Stage Breast Cancer

Breast Tumor Markers

ANTHONY E. DRAGUN
Department of Radiation Oncology, James
Graham Brown Cancer Center, University of
Louisville School of Medicine, Louisville,
KY, USA

Synonyms
CA 15-3; CA 27-29

Definition

These are serum tumor markers identified in breast cancer patients. The use of these tumor markers and the routine management of early stage breast cancer is controversial due to concerns regarding false positives and false negatives. CA 15-3 has been shown to be sensitive in early detection of osseous metastatic disease. CA 27-29 may eventually become useful in detecting early posttreatment recurrence.

Cross-References

▶ Early-Stage Breast Cancer

Bronchopulmonary Carcinoma

▶ Lung

Budd-Chiari Syndrome

STEPHAN MOSE
Department of Radiation Oncology,
Schwarzwald-Baar-Klinikum, Villingen-
Schwenningen, Germany

Definition

This syndrome is defined as an occlusion of the hepatic veins which could be caused by a variety of different diseases. The classical symptoms are abdominal pain, ascites, hepatomegaly, elevated liver enzymes, and jaundice.

Cross-References

▶ Carcinoma of the Adrenal Gland

Bystander Effects

SUSAN M. VARNUM, MARIANNE B. SOWA,
WILLIAM F. MORGAN
Biological Sciences Division, Fundamental &
Computational Sciences, Directorate Pacific
Northwest National Laboratory, Richland,
WA, USA

Definition

Bystander effects describe the ability of an irradiated cell to send a signal capable of eliciting a response in a nonirradiated cell. This signal may be communicated via cell-to-cell gap junction communication and/or from secreted or shed factors from irradiated cells.

Cross-References

▶ Radiation-Induced Genomic Instability and Radiation Sensitivity

C

CA-125

Christin A. Knowlton[1], Michelle Kolton Mackay[2]
[1]Department of Radiation Oncology, Drexel University, Philadelphia, PA, USA
[2]Department of Radiation Oncology, Marshfield Clinic, Marshfield, WI, USA

Synonyms
Cancer antigen 125

Definition
CA-125 is a protein that is considered a tumor marker, or biomarker, found in greater concentration in tumor cells than in normal tissues. Ovarian cancer demonstrates a higher concentration of CA-125 in most cases. The role of CA-125 is not well understood. This blood test is performed at diagnosis and can be helpful for following disease status.

Cross-References
▶ Endometrium
▶ Ovary

CA 15-3

▶ Breast Tumor Markers

CA 27-29

▶ Breast Tumor Markers

CAMPEP

▶ Commission on Accreditation of Medical Physics Education Programs, Inc.

Cancer Antigen 125

▶ CA-125

Cancer Colon

▶ Colon Cancer

Cancer Immunome

Tod W. Speer
Department of Human Oncology, University of Wisconsin School of Medicine and Public Health, UW Hospital and Clinics, Madison, WI, USA

Definition
Complete set of all known immunogenic tumor antigens. Theoretically it is a infinite challenge.

L.W. Brady, T.E. Yaeger (eds.), *Encyclopedia of Radiation Oncology*, DOI 10.1007/978-3-540-85516-3,
© Springer-Verlag Berlin Heidelberg 2013

C

It is currently under ongoing research and development.

Cross-References

▶ Targeted Radioimmunotherapy

Cancer Intestine

▶ Colon Cancer

Cancer of the Breast Tis

ROBYN B. VERA[1], DOUGLAS W. ARTHUR[2],
DAVID E. WAZER[3,4]
[1]Department of Radiation Oncology, University of Michigan, Ann Arbor, MI, USA
[2]Department of Radiation Oncology, College of Medicine, Drexel University, Philadelphia, PA, USA
[3]Radiation Oncology Department, Tufts Medical Center, Tufts University School of Medicine, Boston, MA, USA
[4]Radiation Oncology Department, Rhode Island Hospital, Brown University School of Medicine, Providence, RI, USA

Synonyms

Carcinoma in situ; Noninvasive breast cancer; Stage 0 breast cancer; TisN0M0

Definitions

Breast Conservation Therapy. A multidisciplinary approach of breast-conserving surgery and adjuvant radiotherapy with the goal of achieving in-breast disease control while preserving breast cosmesis.

Paget's Disease. A clinical presentation of nipple eczema and superficial epidermal scaling, which can progress to crusting, erosion, and exudates. Histologically characterized by the presence of Paget's cells, described as large, round to oval cells that contain hyperchromatic nuclei and prominent nucleoli, scattered throughout the epidermis, this process is often associated with underlying DCIS or invasive carcinoma.

Lobular Carcinoma In Situ (LCIS). Non-infiltrating lobular proliferation of loosely cohesive carcinoma cells filling the acinar space.

Ductal Carcinoma In Situ (DCIS). A proliferation of ductal carcinoma cells that arise within and are confined to the ductal lumens of the breast and that do not infiltrate the basement membrane.

In Situ Carcinoma. A proliferation of malignant-appearing cells without evidence of invasion through the epithelial basement membrane, variants arising from the breast include LCIS, Paget's disease, or DCIS.

Lumpectomy/Segmental Mastectomy. The removal of breast disease with the goal of complete excision with negative surgical margins while conserving the breast.

Simple Mastectomy. The removal of the entire breast tissue, from the clavicle to the rectus abdominus muscle, between the sternal edge of the latissimus dorsi muscle, with the removal of the fascia of the pectoralis major muscle.

Modified Radical Mastectomy. An axillary nodal dissection, levels I and II, in addition to the removal of the entire breast tissue, from the clavicle to the rectus abdominus muscle, between the sternal edge of the latissimus dorsi muscle, including the removal of the fascia of the pectoralis major muscle.

Multicentric Disease. At least two areas of discontinuous disease within the breast that are separated by more than 4 cm signifying the inability to remove known disease in one lumpectomy specimen. Multicentric disease is a contraindication to breast conservation therapy.

Multifocal Disease. At least two areas of discontinuous disease that are within 4 cm of one another and removable within in one lumpectomy specimen. Multifocality is not a contraindication to breast conservation therapy.

Accelerated Partial Breast Irradiation. An alternative form of adjuvant radiotherapy used when the treatment target is defined as 1–2 cm beyond the lumpectomy cavity allowing treatment to be delivery in an accelerated fashion. Typically, highly conformal treatment techniques deliver the intended dose in ≤5 days.

Whole Breast Radiation. Treatment of the all ipsilateral breast tissue with external beam irradiation utilizing a conventional or hypofractionated treatment scheme.

Background

Lobular Carcinoma In Situ

Histologically, LCIS is a non-infiltrating lobular proliferation of loosely cohesive epithelial cells that fill the acinar space. A distinguishing feature is that LCIS lacks E-cadherin gene expression in over 95% of cases. E-cadherin is a cell–cell adhesion molecule that contributes to epithelial organization and its absence results in the microscopic discohesive nature of LCIS. The presence or absence of E-cadherin positivity aids in distinguishing LCIS from DCIS. LCIS specimens are typically estrogen receptor positive and rarely Her2Neu positive or p53 mutated.

Paget's Disease

Histologically, scattered throughout the epidermis of patients presenting with a crusting, bleeding and/or ulcerative nipple, are characteristic Paget's cells. Paget's cells are described as large, round to oval cells with hyperchromatic nuclei, prominent nucleoli with frequent mitosis. In about half of the cases, an appreciable mass is present of which most are invasive carcinoma. Without an associated palpable mass, 66–86% of patients will have an underlying component of DCIS.

DCIS

Out of the estimated 192,370 new breast cancers diagnosed in 2009, 62,280 will be noninvasive of which 85% will be DCIS. DCIS represents a continuum of histologic clonal proliferations that arise within and are confined to the ductal lumens. DCIS lacks the ability to metastasize. Associated axillary nodal metastasis or distant metastasis are rarely reported and most likely represent undetected invasive carcinoma. Risk factors associated with the development of DCIS are akin to those established for invasive breast cancers and include female gender, older age, benign breast disease, family history, nullparity, and unopposed exposure to estrogen. Historically an architectural classification system has been used, dividing DCIS into five classic histologic subtypes: comedo, solid, cribiform, papillary, and micropapillary. Often, there are mixed architectural subtypes within one specimen. Limited prognostic significance has been associated with these descriptors suggesting limited value in this architectural division. However, alternative features have been shown to be important and should be reported: nuclear grade, necrosis, polarization. Additional features that are of prognostic and therapeutic significance include margin status, size of the lesion, and a description of the relationship of the lesion to any microcalcifications, specimen x-rays, and mammography findings.

Initial Evaluation

The incorporation of mammograms as a standard screening for invasive breast cancers has resulted in the increased diagnosis of *in situ* breast. Once detected, biopsy confirmation of *in situ* disease should be pursued. Biopsy can be obtained under ultrasound or needle-localized guidance using a fine-needle aspiration, core-cutting needle biopsy, or excisional biopsy. In addition, a thorough history and physical exam should be completed with a medical history documenting family history of associated cancers as well as obstetric and gynecological histories including the age at first menarche, age at first pregnancy, number of pregnancies, duration of breast feeding, any hormone replacement therapies, and the use of oral contraceptives. The physical exam should include examination of bilateral breasts, supraclavicular, infraclavicular, and axillary nodal basins with staging documentation.

Once all biopsies have been evaluated and the specific disease entity is identified, therapeutic options that should be considered include observation, breast-conserving therapy, and mastectomy. Suitable management recommendations will depend on details of diagnosis, patient characteristics, and patient preferences.

Differential Diagnosis

The skin and nipple changes characteristic of the clinical presentation of Paget's disease can mimic that of contact dermatitis, eczema, superficial-spreading melanoma, pagetoid squamous cell carcinoma *in situ*, and the histologic clear cells of Toker.

Mammographic abnormalities that signal the presence of DCIS and/or LCIS are not specific to these pathologic entities, and a biopsy is required to distinguish from papilloma, atypical ductal hyperplasia, atypical lobular hyperplasia, invasive lobular carcinoma, and invasive ductal carcinoma.

Imaging Studies

Mammography plays an essential role in the early detection of noninvasive lesions. Patients with suspected or known Paget's disease require bilateral mammograms to evaluate for evidence of underlying disease and to rule out additional multicentric and contralateral disease processes. The distinctive mammographic features of DCIS and LCIS are the presence of microcalcifications and the specific character of these calcifications are suggestive of the pathologic disease process.

Linear branching microcalcifications are associated with high-grade DCIS and comedo necrosis. Heterogeneous granular calcifications are associated with moderately differentiated DCIS. Fine granular microcalcifications are found with low-grade, non-comedo DCIS. The mammographic extent of the abnormality guides the planned extent of surgical excision; however, the imaging size typically underestimates the pathologic disease spread by 1–2 cm.

Increasingly, bilateral breast magnetic resonance imaging (MRI) studies are ordered prior to surgery, yet their role as screening study remains controversial.

In patients presenting with nipple discharge and negative mammography, a galactography can be employed to distinguish the presence of a papilloma from an underlying DCIS.

Laboratory Studies

There are no specific laboratory studies needed in the workup and evaluation of noninvasive disease but it is anticipated that patients will have the appropriate blood work and metabolic panel analyzed in anticipation of surgery.

Treatment

Paget's Disease

Treatment for Paget's disease is started with the resection of the affected nipple-areolar complex, skin, and underlying breast tissue. This can be accomplished with a total mastectomy or a breast-conserving surgical resection achieving negative pathologic margins. Breast-conserving surgery should be followed by whole breast radiotherapy. Further treatment details are dictated by the presence and characteristics of any underlying invasive or noninvasive disease.

LCIS

Typically, LCIS is an incidental biopsy finding. Patients with a diagnosis of LCIS only managed with biopsy only have an increased risk for developing invasive ipsilateral and contralateral carcinomas. The risk for subsequent development of invasive disease is less than 15% at 12 years; therefore, observation alone is the standard management for pure LCIS. Biopsy evidence of pure LCIS should be followed by lumpectomy to rule out adjacent DCIS or invasive disease. There is no benefit to achieving pathologically negative margins and thus no role for re-excision to obtain margins clear of LCIS. Patients should be followed regularly with routine bilateral mammograms and physical exams. If there is an additional histology identified in the tissue, that is, DCIS or invasive carcinoma, the accepted approach is to disregard the presence of LCIS and accordingly manage the *in situ* or invasive breast component. Patients who are young, with a strong family history, and with diffuse disease are a subset of the population with LCIS who are considered high risk for subsequent development of invasive disease. Prophylactic intervention with the use of tamoxifen or bilateral mastectomies is an appropriate consideration in this group of patients.

DCIS

Once other invasive components of disease have been excluded, the primary focus becomes local management of DCIS in the breast. There are several approaches ranging from whole breast therapy to the treatment of a partial breast target. All presentations of DCIS can be successfully managed with total mastectomy. Mastectomy series report disease control rates approaching 100% and a cancer-specific mortality rate of less than 4%. In cases of multicentric disease presentations, diffuse DCIS processes, in patients with contraindications to radiotherapy, or when anticipated cosmetic results are unacceptable, mastectomy is the standard of care. There is no phase III trial comparing total mastectomy to lumpectomy plus radiation for patients with pure DCIS;

however, parallel phase III trials for invasive carcinomas demonstrate comparable local control rates and equivalent overall survival between breast conservation treatment with post-lumpectomy radiation and mastectomy. Providing the additional psychological benefit of organ preservation, breast-conserving therapy has been accepted as standard of care. There are four randomized trials with similar outcomes that aggregately demonstrate the locoregional benefit of adjuvant radiation by comparing surgical excision to surgical excision with the addition of whole breast radiation. The role of tamoxifen has also been established in breast conservation therapy with several phase III trials (see Table 1).

The National Surgical Adjuvant Breast and Bowel Project (NSABP) protocol B-17 was the first prospective randomized trial to evaluate the role of adjunctive radiotherapy for patients with DCIS who had undergone a local excision with tumor-free margins (Fisher et al. 2001). After lumpectomy, 814 patients were randomized to either postoperative whole breast radiotherapy to 50 Gy, or no further therapy. With a median follow-up of 12 years, the in-breast tumor recurrence rate with lumpectomy alone was 31.7% and reduced to 15.7% with the addition of radiation. The benefit was realized within patient groups that presented clinically and mammographically and in those ≤49 years old and >49 years old. Evaluation of pathologic features that included comedonecrosis, histologic type, margin status, lymphoid infiltrate, nuclear grade, focality, stroma, and tumor size revealed only comedonecrosis as a significant predictor for in-breast recurrence. It should be noted that despite higher failure rates in those with comedonecrosis whole breast radiotherapy reduced the risk of in-breast failure and supporting breast conservation therapy as an appropriate approach in this group of patients.

A randomized phase III trial, contemporary to the NSABP B-17, was launched by the European Organization for Research and Treatment of

Cancer of the Breast Tis. Table 1 Results from five randomized trials comparing breast conservation therapies for DCIS

	No of patients	XRT dose	Median follow-up (months)	IBTR after excision alone	IBTR after excision + XRT
NSABP B-17 (12 year follow-up)	818	50 Gy	128	32%	16%
EORTC 10853 (10 year follow-up)	1,010	50 Gy (5% boosted)	126	26%	15%
NSABP B-24 (7 years follow-up)	1,804	50 Gy	87	–	11.1% (7.7% + TAM)
UKCCCR (4.4 year follow-up)	1,030	50 Gy	53	14% (11% + TAM)	6% (2% + TAM)
SweDCIS (8 year follow-up)	1,067	50–54 Gy	96 (mean)	27%	12%

XRT radiation, *IBRT* in-breast tumor recurrence, *TAM* tamoxifen, *NSABP* National Surgical Breast and Bowel Project, *EORTC* European Organization for Research and Treatment of Cancer, *UKCCCR* United Kingdom Coordinating Committee on Cancer Research

Cancer (EORTC) evaluating the role of radiotherapy after complete local excision of DCIS with histologically confirmed tumor-free margins (Bijker et al. 2008). The 1,002 patients were randomized to local excision with or without whole breast radiotherapy to 50 Gy. Out of these patients, 5% received a boost to the surgical bed. After a median follow-up of 10.5 years, the in-breast recurrence rate of 26% is reported in the excision alone arm, whole breast radiotherapy reduced this rate to 15%. Subgroup analysis revealed the benefit of radiation was equivalent for all entrants. However, two groups with an exceptionally low risk of recurrence, less than 10%, were those with well-differentiated DCIS with either a clinging or micropapillary growth pattern. The absolute benefit of radiotherapy remained consistent for these patients but the relative benefit of radiotherapy was less. This was further confirmed in an intergroup trial run by the Eastern Cooperative Oncology Group and North Central Cancer Treatment Group in

a population of conservatively selected patients with DCIS and treated with wide excision only. This experience was reported with a median follow-up of 6.2 years. Five hundred and sixty-five patients were evaluable and the 5 year rate of ipsilateral in-breast failure was 6.1% in the low-intermediate grade group and 15.3% in the high-grade group.

From the conclusions drawn from B-17, the NSABP initiated a follow-up trial to determine the benefit of tamoxifen after postoperative radiotherapy (Fisher et al. 1999). The criteria were expanded from B-17 to include women with DCIS and LCIS, with one or more masses or calcification clusters, provided that all disease was excised. Of note, 15% of the patients had microscopically positive margins on histologic evaluation. After local excision, 1,804 women were randomized to whole breast irradiation and placebo or whole breast irradiation followed by tamoxifen for 5 years. Postoperative radiotherapy was delivered with tangential fields to 50 Gy in 25 fractions. Patients were administered either placebo or tamoxifen at 10 mg, twice daily for 5 years. At 7 years of follow-up, the in-breast failure rate following lumpectomy, radiotherapy and placebo was 11.1% and reduced to 7.7% when tamoxifen was added to lumpectomy and radiotherapy. The addition of tamoxifen reduced the contralateral breast occurrence rate from 4.9% to 2.3%.

To further examine the role of tamoxifen, The United Kingdom Coordinating Committee on Cancer Research (UKCCCR) DCIS Working Group designed a protocol comparing excision alone, excision plus tamoxifen, excision plus radiotherapy, and excision plus radiotherapy and tamoxifen (Houghton et al. 2003). Tamoxifen was prescribed as 20 mg/day, and radiotherapy was delivered through whole breast tangential fields to a total dose of 50 Gy. Boost was not recommended. To qualify for enrollment, the 1,030 patients underwent an excision with free histologic margins. Randomization in this 2 × 2 factorial design was optional, and the patient and surgeon were able to select portions of their adjuvant treatment. When reported with 52.6 month follow-up, local recurrence was documented in 14% of the patients treated with excision only and reduced to 6% when the excision was followed by radiotherapy. The addition of tamoxifen offered minimal benefit toward overall ipsilateral local control rates when added to radiotherapy; however, it did appear to reduce the ipsilateral recurrence rate of DCIS in the absence of radiotherapy.

The SweDCIS study from the Swedish Breast Cancer Group randomized 1,067 patients between lumpectomy followed by radiotherapy and lumpectomy alone for the treatment of DCIS (Holmberg et al. 2008). Patients underwent a sector resection with the goal of achieving a 1 cm gross surgical margin, yet microscopic clear resection was not required. The majority of patients received 50 Gy in 25 fractions to the whole breast. In a separate series, a split course of 54 Gy in 27 fractions, separated by a 2 week break was allowed. No boost dose was delivered. At a mean 8 year follow-up, the in-breast failure risk reduction was 16.0%. Subgroup analysis by age, lesion size, focality, completeness of excision, and having a screening detected lesion confirmed radiation provided a benefit to all groups.

The results from these phase III randomized trials report relatively similar outcomes. In summary, they demonstrate lumpectomy plus adjuvant radiation durably reduces the ipsilateral breast cancer recurrence rates by approximately 50–60% compared to lumpectomy alone. After excision only, one half of the local recurrences are DCIS and the other half are invasive tumors; radiation reduces each of these recurrence rates by 50%. None of the randomized trials demonstrate an overall survival benefit. The addition of adjuvant radiation reduces the rate of invasive breast cancer recurrence to 0.5–1%/year.

Excision Alone for DCIS

Considerable effort has been made to identify a subset population within DCIS patients for whom adjuvant radiation does not offer a benefit. The Van Nuys Prognostic Index is a scoring index that was developed through retrospective analysis, to select patients for whom lumpectomy alone was sufficient to control local disease. It is based on tumor grade, size, and surgical margin. Rigorous obtainment of surgical margins greater than 1 cm was an important predictor of this index that required meticulous evaluation of the entire surgical specimen. This exhaustive pathologic evaluation is not a routine practice at most facilities. The Van Nuys Prognostic Index opens up the possibility of lumpectomy alone to control DCIS once the requisite 1 cm circumferential pathologic margin are achieved, yet this index has yet to be independently validated.

Accelerated Partial Breast Irradiation

In much the same way as excision only, the goal of APBI is to treat a limited aspect of the breast; surgical cavity, plus a 1–2 cm margin. Several techniques are in use and being evaluated all with their own pros and cons. The treatment time is most frequently 5 days, but shorter courses and intraoperative treatment is also being evaluated. Several small studies have reported good results using APBI in the treatment of DCIS; however, definitive data is awaited.

In summary, accepted treatment approaches for DCIS are directed to the whole breast with either mastectomy or breast conservation therapy with whole breast radiotherapy. Partial breast treatments with wide excision only or lumpectomy followed by APBI appear to have a role but additional data is awaited. Size, margin status, and grade appear to be important factors in determining the needed extent of treatment. The use of tamoxifen is a decision balanced between the benefit of reducing recurrence and the toxicity from taking the medication realizing that no overall survival benefit is associated with reduced recurrence rates.

Cross-References
▶ Brachytherapy: High Dose Rate (HDR) Implants
▶ Conformal Therapy: Treatment Planning, Treatment Delivery, and Clinical Results
▶ Stage 0 Breast Cancer

References

Bijker N, Meijnen P, Peterse JL et al (2008) Breast-conserving treatment with or without radiotherapy in ductal carcinoma-in-situ: ten-year results of European Organisation for Research and Treatment of Cancer randomized phase III trial 10853 – a study by the EORTC breast cancer cooperative group and EORTC radiotherapy group. J Clin Oncol 24:3381–3387

Fisher B, Dignam J, Wolmark N et al (1999) Tamoxifen in treatment of intraductal breast cancer: National Surgical Adjuvant Breast and Bowel Project B-24 randomised controlled trial. Lancet 353:1993–2000

Fisher B, Land S, Mamounas E et al (2001) Prevention of invasive breast cancer in women with ductal carcinoma in situ: an update of the National Surgical Adjuvant Breast and Bowel Project Experience. Semin Oncol 28:400–418

Holmberg L, Garmo H, Granstrand B et al (2008) Absolute risk reductions for local recurrence after postoperative radiotherapy after sector resection for ductal carcinoma in situ of the breast. J Clin Oncol 26:1247–1252

Houghton J, George WD, Cuzick J et al (2003) Radiotherapy and tamoxifen in women with completely excised ductal carcinoma in situ of the breast in the UK, Australia, and New Zealand: randomized controlled trial. Lancet 362:95–102

Cancer of the Colon

▶ Colon Cancer

Cancer of the Large Intestine

▶ Colon Cancer

Cancer of the Pancreas

RACHELLE LANCIANO
Department of Radiation Oncology, Philadelphia Cyberknife Center, Delaware County Memorial Hospital, Drexel Hill, PA, USA

Synonyms

Ductal adenocarcinoma; Exocrine pancreatic neoplasms; Pancreatic cancer

Definition

Carcinoma arising within the exocrine or endocrine cells of a centrally located gland in the epigastrum of the abdomen called the Pancreas.

Description

In the USA, pancreas cancer is the second most common malignant tumor of the gastrointestinal tract and the fourth leading cause of cancer deaths in adults surpassed only by lung, colon, and breast cancers. Pancreas cancer is difficult to diagnose in early stages with only 15–20% resectable for cure at presentation. Even for those patients able to have surgery with pancreaticoduodenectomy, long-term survival rate remains poor with median survival of 13 months and 5-year survivals of 15–30% for node negative and 10% for node positive disease. Forty percent of patients present with metastatic disease with median survival of less than 8 months and 30–40% of patients present with locally advanced unresectable tumors with median survival of 8–12 months. Most tumors arise in the head of the pancreas, often causing bile duct obstruction with jaundice.

The majority of pancreas cancers (85%) are adenocarcinoma arising from the ductal epithelium and more than 95% arise from the exocrine elements including the ductal and acinar cells.

Only 5% of pancreatic neoplasms arise from the endocrine pancreas or islet cells.

Surgery, if possible, is the first treatment approach for pancreatic cancer.

Adjuvant treatment with chemotherapy and radiation following surgery has improved survival over surgery alone. If the cancer is unresectable or the patient is medically inoperable, local and systemic treatments can provide palliation.

Anatomy

The pancreas is a lobulated transverse retroperitoneal gland located in the upper abdomen extending from the duodenum to the spleen divided into the head, neck, body, and tail. The transverse colon passes in front of the pancreas while the posterior surface is in contact with the inferior vena cava, common bile duct, right diaphragm, and aorta (Fig. 1).

The head of the pancreas is lodged within the curve of the duodenum and includes the medial and inferior uncinate process. Tumors of the head

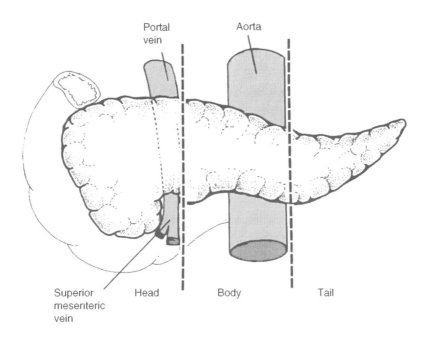

Cancer of the Pancreas. Fig. 1 Anatomy of the Pancreas

of the pancreas are those arising to the right of the superior mesenteric-portal vein confluence. Tumors of the body and neck of the pancreas are defined as those arising between the left edge of the superior mesenteric-portal vein confluence and the left edge of the aorta. The body of the pancreas is in contact with the pylorus and stomach anteriorly and the aorta, left adrenal gland, and kidney posteriorly. The tail is narrow and extends to the gastric surface of the spleen and left colic flexure. Tumors of the tail are those arising to the left edge of the aorta.

The pancreas is intimately related to the origin of the superior mesenteric and celiac arteries and portal vein posterior. Invasion of these vessels determines resectability. The pancreatic duct passes from the tail to head emptying the pancreatic juices through the Ampulla of Vater into the duodenum. Regional drainage is to the superior and inferior pancreaticoduodenal, portahepatic, celiac, and superior mesenteric and paraaortic lymph nodes. Venous drainage of the pancreas is through the portal system to the liver. In addition to the liver, lung and peritoneum are common sites of metastatic disease.

The ductal and acinar cells secrete digestive enzymes and bicarbonate through the pancreatic duct which helps break down carbohydrates, fats, and acids in the duodenum. In the interstitium of the ductal and acinar cells lie the "Islets of Langerhans" which secrete hormones such as insulin, glucagon, and somatostatin into the systemic circulation for glucose control.

Epidemiology

Pancreas cancer is rare before age 45, and the incidence increases with age.

Studies suggest that a small proportion of pancreas cancers have a genetic etiology ranging from 5% to 10%. Hereditary pancreatitis is associated with a markedly increased risk of pancreas cancer and the risk increases with age with a cumulative risk of 40–50% at age 70 years. Pancreas cancer is associated with Ashkenazi Jews and BRCA mutations, Peutz-Jeghers syndrome (hereditary intestinal polyposis), atypical multiple-mole melanoma syndrome, ataxia-telangiectasia, and possibly adenomatous polyposis and Lynch syndrome (hereditary non-polyposis colon cancer). Other associations with pancreas cancer include non-O blood group, nonhereditary chronic pancreatitis and atypical diabetes mellitus (onset in a thin older patient). Cigarette smoking, high body mass, and lack of physical activity are considered additional risk factors for development of pancreas cancer. Spiral CT and endoscopic ultrasound are suggested for patients at significant risk of developing pancreas cancer such as those with a strong family history of pancreas cancer and hereditary pancreatitis.

Clinical Presentation, Initial Evaluation, and Imaging/ Laboratory Studies

Mortality rates for pancreas cancer parallel incidence because of locally advanced unresectable and metastatic disease at presentation. Patients present with pain, weight loss, and jaundice. On exam, ascites or abdominal mass may be appreciated. Workup includes CT of the abdomen and pelvis which may detect dilated ducts, pancreatic mass, or evidence of metastatic disease to the liver, peritoneum, or retroperitoneal lymph nodes. Contrast-enhanced CT scan with thin sections can also determine resectability. Many patients require endoscopic retrograde cholangiopancreatography (ERCP) with stent placement to bypass biliary obstruction and for cytology. Endoscopic ultrasound is used to stage the primary tumor, evaluate for peripancreatic adenopathy, assess vascular invasion, and obtain biopsy of tumor if ERCP cytology is nondiagnostic. In most patients with pancreas cancer, CA 19-9 serum tumor marker can be prognostic with values $\geq$130 units/ml associated with a higher rate of unresectable disease. CA 19-9 can also be used to follow patients after surgery if positive preoperatively to detect recurrent disease and for chemotherapy response in patients who are unresectable. Patients are generally considered unresectable for cure if there is extensive peripancreatic and distant lymph nodes or metastases, encasement of the superior mesenteric vein (SMV), or SMV-portal vein confluence, or involvement of the superior mesenteric artery (SMA), inferior vena cava, aorta, celiac axis, or hepatic artery. Small peritoneal and liver metastases can be detected by laparoscopy in high-risk patients including those with CA 19-9 >1,000 units/ml selecting out those who benefit most from pancreas resection.

Clinical staging utilizes all clinical testing including CT scans and endoscopic ultrasound, and patients are classified into localized resectable (Stage I and II), locally advanced (Stage III), and metastatic (Stage IV) pancreas cancers. Pathologic staging requires resection of the pancreatic cancer with at least 12 regional lymph nodes assessed. To record T stage, tumor size (≤2 cm vs. >2 cm), extra-pancreatic extension, and involvement of the celiac axis or superior mesenteric artery must be assessed from the surgical specimens.

Treatment

Surgery is the standard treatment for pancreas cancer if resectable. Approximately one third of patients will have positive margins following surgery (usually retroperitoneal) and two thirds lymph node metastases. Following surgery alone, more than one half of patients develop locoregional recurrence without distant metastases.

Adjuvant chemotherapy and chemoradiotherapy have been shown to increase survival in randomized and uncontrolled trials following surgery for pancreas cancer. Two-year survival rate from the Gastrointestinal Tumor Study Group trial utilizing 40 Gy to the tumor bed with concurrent and adjuvant 5FU chemotherapy increased from 10% with surgery alone to 20% with combined modality adjuvant treatment. In a series of 1,092 patients with pancreas cancer

treated with chemotherapy and radiation (50.4 Gy) following surgery at Johns Hopkins Hospital and Mayo Clinic between 1985 and 2005, 2-year survival rate increased from 31% with surgery alone to 45% with adjuvant combined modality treatment.

An alternative adjuvant approach preferred in Europe is chemotherapy alone with 5FU or Gemcitabine regimens since European randomized trials did not show a benefit to postoperative radiation. The most recent European trial found no difference in survival between 5FU and Gemcitabine in the adjuvant setting; however, Gemcitabine had less toxicity and is the favored regimen. The current Radiation Therapy Oncology Group (RTOG#0848) randomized trial for adenocarcinoma of the pancreas following pancreaticoduodenectomy randomizes patients with pancreatic head lesions to Gemcitabine+/-erlotinib for five cycles with a second randomization to 5FU/radiation 50.4 Gy versus an additional cycle of chemotherapy. This international study should elucidate the benefit of adjuvant radiation and erlotinib in resected pancreatic head adenocarcinoma.

For patients that have marginally or borderline resectable cancer, preoperative chemoradiotherapy has been used to improve resectability, identify those patients who are unlikely to benefit from surgery due to development of metastatic disease, and hopefully improve survival by the early and intensive use of chemotherapy. For patients with locally advanced unresectable disease, radiation and concurrent 5FU chemotherapy improved survival and performance status and decreased hospital days compared to supportive care alone.

Radiation can be delivered with conventional fractionation (50.4 Gy over 5.5 weeks) with conformal or intensity-modulated radiation therapy (IMRT) techniques. Treatment planning includes a CT in the treatment position with immobilization to include the entire liver and kidneys for dose volume analysis. Bowel contrast may be used to help identify the stomach and duodenum as well as large and small bowel within the treatment fields. IV contrast can be helpful to outline the celiac axis, portal vein, aorta, and superior mesenteric artery. The tumor volume is contoured if the tumor is not resected and considered gross tumor volume (GTV). In the postoperative setting there is no GTV. The location of the pancreatic tumor prior to resection must be contoured based on preoperative CT with axial images, the operative note, and pathology report. The most proximal 1–1.5 cm of celiac axis, 2.5–3.0 cm of superior mesenteric artery and portal vein segment that runs anterior to the IVC should be contoured. In addition the aorta from the level of the highest contoured vessel/tumor bed to the bottom of L2 and the pancreaticojejunostomy should be contoured separately. The clinical tumor volume (CTV) includes the above structures with variable expansion depending on the structure contoured. The planning tumor volume (PTV) includes the CTV with 0.5 cm expansion. In addition, normal tissues that should be contoured include liver, right and left kidneys, small and large bowel, stomach, and spinal cord. The goal of radiation treatment planning is to treat the PTV with the prescribed dose, minimize dose to normal structures, and maximize dose homogeneity.

Stereotactic body radiotherapy (SBRT) and intraoperative radiation therapy (IORT) have been explored as alternative techniques for radiation delivery. Unfortunately the available data has not shown a survival advantage for these techniques over standard fractionated radiation.

Chemotherapy for metastatic disease includes gemcitabine, 5-fluorouracil, and oxaliplatin. Radiation therapy can also be useful in palliation of pain or alternative symptoms related to metastatic disease.

Cross-References

▶ Colorectal Cancer
▶ Hepatic Metastasis
▶ Intraoperative Radiation Therapy (IORT)
▶ Primary Cancer of The Duodenum

References

American Joint Committee on Cancer (AJCC) (2010) Exocrine and endocrine pancreas, Chapter 24. In: Edge SB (ed) Cancer staging manual, 7th edn. Springer, New York

Fernandez-del Castillo C (2012) Clinical manifestations, diagnosis and surgical staging of exocrine pancreatic cancer. www.uptodate.com

Fernandez-del Castillo C, Jimenez R (2012) Epidemiology and risk factors for exocrine pancreatic cancer. www.uptodate.com

Jemal A, Siegel R, Xu J et al (2010) Cancer statistics, 2010. CA Cancer J Clin 60:277

Lim JE, Chien MW, Earle CC et al (2003) Prognostic factors following curative resection for pancreatic adenocarcinoma: a population-based, linked database analysis of 396 patients. Ann Surg 237:74

Longnecker D (2012) Pathology of exocrine pancreatic neoplasms. www.uptodate.com

National Comprehensive Cancer Network, Practice guidelines in oncology. Version 2.2012. Pancreatic adenocarcinoma. www.nccn.org

Pancreatic cancer radiation atlas for treatment planning. www.rtog.org/atlas/pancreasAtlas/main.html. RTOG 0848 A phase III trial evaluating both erlotinib and chemoradiation as adjuvant treatment for patients with resected head of pancreas adenocarcinoma. www.rtog.org/members/protocols/0848/0848.pdf

Ryan D, Mamon H (2011) Adjuvant and neoadjuvant therapy for exocrine pancreatic cancer. www.uptodate.com

Ryan D, Mamon H (2012) Management of locally advanced and borderline resectable exocrine pancreatic cancer. www.uptodate.com

Willett CG, Czito BG, Bendell JC (2008) Cancer of the pancreas, Chapter 56. In: Perez CA, Brady LW (eds) Principles and practice of radiation oncology, 5th edn. Lippincott Williams and Wilkins, Philadelphia

Cancer Quality of Life

▶ Pain Management
▶ Palliation
▶ Supportive Care and Quality of Life

Cancer-Related Fatigue

JAMES H. BRASHEARS, III
Radiation Oncologist, Venice, FL, USA

Definition

A persistent sense of physical, emotional, cognitive, and/or spiritual tiredness or exhaustion that interferes with normal functioning of the individual. It is worse than might be expected from recent activity, frequently does not improve with rest, and is linked with malignancy or its management.

Cross-References

▶ Supportive Care and Quality of Life

Carboplatin (Carboplatinum)

CHRISTIN A. KNOWLTON[1], MICHELLE KOLTON MACKAY[2]
[1]Department of Radiation Oncology, Drexel University, Philadelphia, PA, USA
[2]Department of Radiation Oncology, Marshfield Clinic, Marshfield, WI, USA

Definition

Carboplatin is a chemotherapy agent in the class of platinum medications that works by creating intra- and interstrand DNA cross-links and DNA to protein cross-links, therefore interfering with cell division. Carboplatin is commonly administered in the treatment of ovarian cancer, often in combination with paclitaxel. Side effects of carboplatin include nausea and vomiting, myelosuppression, brittle hair, and fatigue.

Cross-References

▶ Ovary
▶ Principles of Chemotherapy

Carcinoid Tumor

FILIP T. TROICKI[1], JAGANMOHAN POLI[2]
[1]College of Medicine, Drexel University, Philadelphia, PA, USA
[2]Department of Radiation Oncology, College of Medicine, Drexel University, Philadelphia, PA, USA

Definition

Slow-growing, hormone-producing tumor that exists within various sites of the body, most commonly within the gastrointestinal tract.

Cross-References

▶ Colon Cancer
▶ Lung Cancer
▶ Stomach Cancer

Carcinoma In Situ

THEODORE E. YAEGER
Department Radiation Oncology, Wake Forest University School of Medicine, Winston-Salem, NC, USA

Definition

Non-invasive cancers that are typically small and confined to the primary tissues of commencement within the organ of initiation.

Cross-References

► Cancer of the Breast Tis
► Melanoma
► Stage 0 Breast Cancer
► Uterine Cervix

Carcinoma of Lungs

THEODORE E. YAEGER
Department Radiation Oncology,
Wake Forest University School of Medicine,
Winston-Salem, NC, USA

Definition

Malignancies arising from pulmonary tissues or resultant from metastasis to lung tissue.

Cross-References

► Lung

Carcinoma of the Adrenal Gland

STEPHAN MOSE
Department of Radiation Oncology,
Schwarzwald-Baar-Klinikum,
Villingen-Schwenningen, Germany

Synonyms

Adrenal carcinoma; Adrenal cancer

Description

Tumors of the adrenal gland are rare tumors with mostly aggressive local and metastatic spread and – in case of advanced and metastatic disease – disappointing overall survival rates. They are characterized by adrenal gland-specific hormonal dysfunction, which often lead to the diagnosis, and/or non-specific abdominal symptoms. Adrenal cancer which pathogenesis is largely unknown is found in every age. Treatment of choice is the radical surgical approach which also should be discussed in an actual inoperable situation to reduce tumor burden and hormone induced symptoms. Although literature data provide little information, chemotherapy and radiotherapy may be recommended for adjuvant and palliative treatment.

Anatomy

Both of the adrenal glands are located between the superior part of the kidney and the diaphragmatic crura. The triangular right gland is related to the inferior vena cava and the liver, whereas the semilunar left one is placed in the near of the spleen, pancreas, and stomach. Embedded by perinephric tissue and still separated from the kidney itself, they are enclosed by the renal fascia. The blood supply is derived from the inferior phrenic artery, the abdominal aorta, and the renal artery (superior, middle, and inferior suprarenal arteries). A large central hilar vein drains to the inferior vena cava (right) and to the renal vein (left). The lymphatic drainage follows the arterial vessels and drains predominately to the lumbar nodes (celiac plexus, lateroaortic nodes above the renal pedicle).

The adrenal gland is a hormone producing organ which consists of two functionally separate units with different embryologic origins. The central part of the gland (medulla, 10–20% of the organ) produces catecholamines. The cortex (80–90% of the organ) secrets steroids: mineralocorticoids (e.g., aldosterone), glucocorticoids (e.g., cortisol), sex hormones (e.g., androgen).

Epidemiology

Most of the adrenal carcinomas are cortex tumors. However, the adrenocortical carcinoma (ACC) is a very seldom neoplasia (1–2 per 1 million inhabitants), which could occur in every age with a peak before the age <5 years and in the fourth and fifth decades. Bilateral tumors are discovered in 2.4%. Whereas hormonal inactive tumors are more common in men (3:2 ratio) and in older patients (>30 years of age) hormonal active carcinomas are more often diagnosed in female (7:3 ratio) and younger patients. Carcinomas of the adrenal medulla are divided into neuroblastoma which is the most common tumor of the adrenal gland in children (90%) originating from the sympathetic nervous system, and malignant pheochromocytoma with an incidence of 5–46% of all diagnosed pheochromocytomas. Most of the extra-adrenal discovered pheochromocytomas are malignant as well.

There is only little information about the pathogenesis of adrenal tumors. In case reports, the transformation from adenomas into carcinomas is discussed ("second hit theory") but the long-term follow-up of so-called incidentalomas demonstrated no further advices. Most cases present as sporadic tumors. However, adrenal carcinoma has been described as a part of hereditary cancer syndromes (e.g., ▶ Li–Fraumeni syndrome, ▶ Beckwith–Wiedemann syndrome, ▶ multiple endocrine neoplasia type I, and ▶ SBLA syndrome) (Allolio & Fassnacht 2006; Coen 2008).

Clinical Presentation

Tumors of the adrenal gland (Table 1) are very malignant tumors with aggressive local and multilocal metastatic spread (liver, lung, bone, lymph nodes). Because of its retroperitoneal location and – in case of hormonal inactivity – their nonspecific symptoms (back pain, abdominal fullness, seldom weakness, and fever), they are often diagnosed at a late date. However, 95% of tumors are hormonal active and in more than 60% the patient is diagnosed with a hormonal excess while these tumors are mostly diagnosed at an earlier stage.

In adrenocortical tumors, most frequently a ▶ Cushing's syndrome alone or together with

Carcinoma of the Adrenal Gland. Table 1 Classification of adrenal tumors

Adrenal cortex	Adenoma (hormonal active/inactive) Carcinoma (hormonal active/inactive)
Adrenal medulla	Ganglioneuroma Pheochromocytoma (benign/malignant) Neuroblastoma Mixed type (ganglioneuroblastoma)
Connective tissue tumors	Myelolipoma, lipoma Myoma, angioma Fibroma, fibrosarcoma

virilization is presented. Virilization is more common in children (adrenogenital syndrome). In women, the overproduction of androgens leads to hirsutism. The overproduction of aldosterone is very seldom. Likewise, estrogen producing tumors that are commonly malignant are seldom; in men the tumor leads to testicular atrophy and gynecomastia.

In adrenal medulla tumors (pheochromocytoma), which in 90% occurs in inherited syndromes (▶ multiple endocrine neoplasia type II (MEN II A), association with Hippel–Lindau's disease, neurofibromatosis, von Recklinghausen's disease), patients present with a wide range of hypertensive disease and associated symptoms (e.g., headache, tachycardia, palpitations, weakness) as well as cardiac failure and infarction which are caused by excessive catecholamine production of the tumor.

Macroscopically, carcinomas often show hemorrhage and necrosis. However, to finally differentiate between benign and malignant tumors, histopathological and immunohistological discrimination is necessary (larger nuclear size, numerous and atypical mitotic figures, invasion of vessels, and invasion of the capsule) (Weiss et al. 1989; Saeger 2000; Johanssen et al. 2008).

Differential Diagnosis

Benign tumors of the adrenal gland (e.g., adenomas, ganglioneuromas) are more common (1–8% of the general population). Most of them are incidentally diagnosed. Laboratory and imaging studies are very important with regard to the therapeutic procedure to differentiate these benign tumors from carcinoma.

A rare tumor of the adrenal medulla is the benign pheochromocytoma, which produces catecholamines causing hypertension (prevalence of 0.1% of hypertensive patients) and may be associated with various endocrine- and nonendocrine-inherited disorders. The minimally invasive adrenalectomy by the transperitoneal or retroperitoneal lateral approach has become the treatment of choice.

Imaging Studies

Tumors larger than 6 cm are suspected to be malignant (NIH-consensus). Carcinomas are often irregularly shaped with potential invasion into local structures and demonstrate inhomogeneous contrast enhancement in imaging studies. However, although there may be no symptoms, with modern imaging studies more tumors of the adrenal gland tend to be incidentally discovered in an earlier stage (<3–6 cm). Computed tomography (CT) and the magnetic resonance imaging (MRI) are quite equivalent with an advantage for the MRI (T2-weighted images) toward the diagnosis of venous invasion. This may be completed by an angiography. The evaluation of the fat content as well as the wash out of contrast media after 10 min could help to discriminate tumors. It has to be evaluated if the fluorodeoxyglucose positron emission tomography is helpful to better differentiate between benign and malignant lesions. Furthermore, CT (chest, abdomen) and bone scan are useful regarding the diagnosis of metastases (see Tables 2 and 3) (Coen 2008; Johanssen et al. 2008).

Carcinoma of the Adrenal Gland. Table 2 TNM-staging (WHO 2004)

Stage	T	N	M
I (T1 N0 M0)	≤5 cm without invasion	–	–
II (T2 N0 M0)	>5 cm without invasion	–	–
III (T3 N0 M0, T1–2 N1 M0)	Outside adrenal fat	+	–
IV (T3–4 N1 M0, T1–4 N0–1 M1)	Invading adjacent organs	+	+

Laboratory Studies

The evaluation of hormonal changes is mandatory in all patients with an adrenal mass. The results could give strong advices and could lead to the diagnosis of cancer (e.g., estrogen production in men, secretion of steroid precursor). Furthermore, the evaluation before therapy may have influence on the extent of surgery (open versus minimal invasive surgery) as well as on postoperative strategies (e.g., postoperative insufficiency of the adrenal gland in case of Cushing's syndrome). However, the evaluation before therapy is important to enable the early diagnosis of recurrence during the follow-up of patients.

Besides taking the history and doing the physical examination, preoperative hormonal diagnostic studies are recommended (Table 3).

Treatment

Nowadays, approximately two-thirds of patients are diagnosed in tumor stages in which surgery is the treatment of choice (stage I 5%, stage II 39%, stage III 27%). In the other patients, a metastatic disease has to be treated. The overall 5-year-survival of all stages ranges from 16% to 47% (stage I 80%, stage II 57%, stage III 40%, stage IV 15%). The median survival in metastatic disease is less than 12 months. However, despite

Carcinoma of the Adrenal Gland. Table 3 Preoperative hormonal diagnostic studies in suspicion of cancer of the adrenal gland (Recommendations of the "European Network for the Study of Adrenal Tumors," ENSAT)

Laboratory studies	
Glucocorticoids	Dexamethason suppression test (24 h) Twenty-four hour urinary cortisol Basal level of serum cortisol Basal level of plasma ACTH (adrenocorticotrophic hormone)
Mineralocorticoids	Serum potassium Quotient of aldosterone/ renin (in case of hypertension and/or hypokaliemia)
Sex hormones, steroid precursors	Dehydroepiandrosterone (DHEA) (serum) 17-hydroxyprosterone (serum) Androstendione (serum) Testosterone (serum) Estradiole (in men and postmenopausal women)
Evaluation of pheochromocytoma	Twenty-four hour urinary control of catecholamine Metanephrine (plasma)

radical surgery 70–85% of patients develop both local recurrent and/or metastatic disease, which gives rise to the evaluation of adjuvant therapies.

Surgery

Surgery is the treatment of choice in adrenal tumors giving the best chance to cure the patient. Hereby, a margin-free resection is a strong prognostic factor; if there is macroscopic tumor left, a second surgical approach has to be discussed. Even if the tumor seems to be inoperable predominately in hormone active tumors as well as in metastatic tumors, surgery could be performed to reduce the tumor mass and its associated symptoms, and to control the excessive production of hormones. Likewise, in case of local recurrence, surgery should be discussed for the same reason. Especially in pheochromocytoma, the surgical approach is a high-risk procedure because of possible catecholamine excess during surgery. Therefore, the patients have to be monitored very carefully.

Beyond studies, the open radical adrenalectomy is the standard procedure that is often combined with a lymphadenectomy. In case of invasion of adjacent organs, these organs have to be (partially) removed. To reduce peri- and postoperative complications, tumor spillage has to be avoided. The lateral retroperitoneal approach represents the standard procedure in localized adrenal tumors whereas the transabdominal anterior approach is usually performed in tumors with invasion of adjacent organs and/or lymph nodes (Allolio et al. 2006; Johanssen et al. 2008).

Chemotherapy

In advanced and/or metastastic disease, the adrenolytic agent mitotane is clearly effective with objective response rates of 14–36%. Unfortunately, most studies failed to demonstrate a survival benefit and despite a response to mitotane approximately 50% of patients had a recurrence within 5 years. Nevertheless, because of the results in metastatic disease and despite limiting data mitotane is recommended in the adjuvant setting.

To reduce the hormonal excess serum, levels of 10–14($-$20) mg/L have to be obtained based on the knowledge that higher levels are associated with better tumor response. Because of the increased metabolic clearance of glucocorticoids during the mitotane therapy, the patient has to be substituted with cortisol. Unfortunately, therapy is often limited by the side effects of mitotane (e.g., gastrointestinal symptoms, diarrhea, and nausea, less often: lethargy, somnolence, ataxia, dizziness). Therefore, besides an evaluation of

ACTH, aldosterone, and rennin, a strong monitoring (blood count, cholesterol, triglyceride, transaminases) is mandatory.

A lot of other chemotherapeutic agents were studied in ACC but only a few patients responded to those treatments. A regimen with a promising potential might be the combination of mitotane, etoposide, cisplatin, and doxorubicin; in the first worldwide phase III trial (FIRM-ACT-study), this regimen will be actually compared to a combination of mitotane and streptomycin in metastatic disease. Furthermore, efforts are made to evaluate the efficiency of monoclonal antibodies and tyrosine kinase inhibitors (Terzolo & Berruti 2008; Veytsman et al. 2009).

Radiotherapy

The role of radiotherapy in the treatment of the carcinoma of the adrenocortical gland is controversial because the tumor was formerly considered to be radioresistant. However, some small trials reported some objective local tumor responses especially in a palliative setting (40–57%). Likewise, there is only little information about the role of radiotherapy in an adjuvant situation where in 25–86% a local control was obtained. Unfortunately, the number of patients locally treated in the primary tumor area is small and details about the delivered dose and the target volume definition are mostly missing. On the other hand, there are some reports demonstrating that radiotherapy is effective regarding symptom reduction in case of bone and brain metastases as well as in vena cava obstruction (50–77%). In malignant pheochromocytoma, it may be assumed that radiotherapy is limited to palliative treatment (Coen 2008).

After reviewing literature data and taking into account the limited number of retrospectively published trials, the European Network for the Study of Adrenal Tumors (ENSAT) actually stated that the role of radiotherapy should not be neglected regarding the prevention of a local recurrence (Cerquetti et al. 2008; Polat et al. 2009). The following recommendations are given:

1. In patients with localized tumors and microscopically complete resection (R0 resection) postoperative radiotherapy does not seem to be beneficial and may be only discussed in tumors larger than 8 cm with histopathologic evidence of invasion in blood vessels and a Ki-67 index >10%.
2. Postoperative radiotherapy is recommended in all patients in whom a microscopically incomplete resection (R1 resection) was performed. If there is doubt about the resection status, radiotherapy should be considered as well. Furthermore, patients with a stage III tumor may have a benefit from postoperative local treatment as long as there is no tumor thrombus in the vena cava.
3. If the tumor capsule is intraoperatively harmed or if tumor spillage into the abdominal cavity could not be avoided, the effectiveness of radiotherapy is questionable and should not be indicated.
4. Palliative radiotherapy of symptomatic metastatic lesions is well known. As literature data demonstrate, ACC is not radioresistant; therefore, radiotherapy is an option in both local symptomatic tumor and metastatic lesions (e.g., bone lesions, cerebral metastases, vena cava obstruction).
5. Because of the new promising results of mitotane in cell culture models as well as in the adjuvant setting, a combined treatment is recommended whereas there are no data about the combination with other cytotoxic drugs. When mitotane is simultaneously given, the daily dose should not be higher than 3 g/day because of limiting liver toxicities.
6. Radiotherapy should be started within 6–12 weeks after surgery. Of course, an individualized three-dimensional planning using modern technique has to be used to shield organs at risk

(especially kidney, liver, small bowel). The recommended target volume includes (a) the diaphragm and – in case of invasion – the part of the thoracic wall, (b) the para-aortic/paracaval lymph nodes (if involved or at high risk to be involved), (c) the anterior border of the tumor, (d) the border of the diaphragm crus, and (e) caudally at least the kidney hilum. A dose of 40 Gy (1.8–2.0 Gy, 5×/week) should be administered and followed by a boost to the tumor region with 10–20 Gy (1.8–2.0 Gy, 5×/week). In palliative treatment, the well-known dose schedules should be used based on an individualized decision (e.g., 1×8, 5×4, 10×3 Gy).

Based on literature data as well as on these recommendations, acute and late side effects induced by radiotherapy should be only mild with a low incidence of grade III and IV toxicities. Kidney and liver functions have to be monitored during therapy as well as during follow-up. Very seldom, a ▶ Budd–Chiari syndrome is diagnosed. It has to be taken into account that in ACC per se a high incidence of secondary malignancies (12–24%) is reported. Restaging is recommended every 3 months for the first 2 years; afterwards the intervals could be prolonged.

The results of treatment depend on the early diagnosis followed by excellent surgery. The limited data including our knowledge about adjuvant therapies lead to the actual recommendation that – if indicated – the combination of radiotherapy and mitotane could gain a better local control as well as a lower incidence of metastases. This might possibly cause a survival benefit. In palliative treatment, radiotherapy is a helpful option in most patients with a metastatic adrenal gland carcinoma. Further efforts are needed to transfer these recommendations into evidence-based therapy.

Cross-References

▶ Neuroblastoma
▶ Thyroid Cancer

References

Allolio B, Fassnacht M (2006) Clinical review: adrenocortical carcinoma: clinical update. J Clin Endocrinol Metab 91:2027–2037

Cerquetti L, Bucci B, Marchese R, Misiti S, De Paula U, Miceli R, Muleti A, Amendola D, Piergrossi P, Brunetti E, Toscano V, Stigliano A (2008) Mitotane increases the radiotherapy inhibitory effect and induces G2-arrest in combined treatment on both H295R and SW13 adrenocortcal cell lines. Endocr Relat Cancer 15:623–634

Coen JJ (2008) Adrenal Gland. In: Halperin EC, Perez CA, Brady LW (eds) Principles and practice of radiation oncology, 5th edn. Wolters Kluwer/Lippincott Wiliams & Wilkens, Philadelphia

Johanssen S, Fassnacht M, Brix D, Koschker AC, Hahner S, Riedmiller H, Allolio B (2008) Das Nebennieren-karzinom – Diagnostik und Therapie. Urologe 47:172–181

Polat B, Fassnacht M, Pfreudner L, Guckenberger M, Bratengeier K, Johanssen S, Kenn W, Hahner S, Allolio B, Flentje M (2009) Radiotherapy in adrenocortical carcinoma. Cancer 115:2816–2823

Saeger W (2000) Histopathological classification of adrenal tumours. Eur J Clin Invest 30(Suppl 3):58–62

Terzolo M, Berruti A (2008) Adjunctive treatment of adrenocortical carcinoma. Curr Opin Endocrinol Diabetes Obes 15:221–226

Veytsman I, Nieman L, Fojo T (2009) Management of endocrine manifestation and the use of Mitotane as a chemotherapeutic agent for adrenocortical carcinoma. J Clin Oncol 27:4619–4629

Weiss LM, Medeiros LJ, Vickery AL Jr (1989) Pathologic features of prognostic significance in adrenocortical carcinoma. Am J Surg Pathol 13:202–206

Carcinoma of the Colon

▶ Colon Cancer

Carcinoma of the Male Urethra

▶ Male Urethra

Carcinoma of the Penis

▶ Penile Cancer

Carcinoma of the Upper Urinary Tract

▶ Renal Pelvis and Ureter

Carcinoma of the Uterine Cervix

▶ Brachytherapy-GyN
▶ Uterine Cervix

Carcinomas: Basal Cell Carcinoma

▶ Skin Cancer

Cardia of Stomach

Filip T. Troicki[1], Jaganmohan Poli[2]
[1]College of Medicine, Drexel University, Philadelphia, PA, USA
[2]Department of Radiation Oncology, College of Medicine, Drexel University, Philadelphia, PA, USA

Definition
Most proximal section of the stomach which is attached to the esophagus.

Cross-References
▶ Stomach Cancer

Cardiac Toxicity

Anthony E. Dragun
Department of Radiation Oncology, James Graham Brown Cancer Center, University of Louisville School of Medicine, Louisville, KY, USA

Definition
The risk of cardiotoxicity due to radiation therapy is mainly a historical phenomenon, correlated to the use of crude radiotherapy planning and delivery techniques. Modern radiation planning techniques allow exclusion of the majority of cardiac tissue and, thus, this is exceedingly rare in the modern era. In multidisciplinary management, increased risks of premature cardiac disease including decreased left ventricular ejection fraction, congestive heart failure, cardiomyopathy, and acute myocardial infarction are mainly incurred by the increased use of cardiotoxic systemic therapies, such as anthracycline, taxane, and trastuzimab-containing chemotherapeutic regimens. Radiation techniques that exclude treatment of the internal mammary chain and utilize novel methods such as forward planning, respiratory gaiting, and deep inspiration breath hold techniques are all useful in reducing the irradiated heart volume and reducing overall risk.

Cross-References
▶ Stage 0 Breast Cancer

Carney Complex

RAMESH RENGAN[1], CHARLES R. THOMAS, JR.[2]
[1]Department of Radiation Oncology, Hospital of the University of Pennsylvania, Philadelphia, PA, USA
[2]Department of Radiation Medicine, Oregon Health Sciences University, Portland, OR, USA

Definition
An autosomal dominant syndrome with varying penetrance characterized by cardiac myxomas, cutaneous myxomas, spotty pigmentation of the skin, endocrinopathy, and both endocrine and nonendocrine tumors.

Cross-References
▶ Primary Cardiac Tumors

cART

BERNADINE R. DONAHUE[1], JAY S. COOPER[2]
[1]Department of Radiation Oncology, Maimonides Cancer Center, Brooklyn, NY, USA
[2]Maimonides Cancer Center, New York, NY, USA

Synonyms
ART

Definition
Combined antiretroviral therapy (also called ART or HAART)

Cross-References
▶ HAART
▶ Malignant Neoplasms Associated with Acquired Immunodeficiency Syndrome

CD20 Surface Antigen

TOD W. SPEER
Department of Human Oncology, University of Wisconsin School of Medicine and Public Health, UW Hospital and Clinics, Madison, WI, USA

Definition
It is an activated-glycosylated phosphoprotein that is expressed as a cell surface antigen on mature B lymphocytes. It has no known natural ligand and its function is not fully elucidated. It is the antigenic target for anti-lymphoma TRIT.

Cross-References
▶ Targeted Radioimmunotherapy

Celiac Axis

FILIP T. TROICKI[1], JAGANMOHAN POLI[2]
[1]College of Medicine, Drexel University, Philadelphia, PA, USA
[2]Department of Radiation Oncology, College of Medicine, Drexel University, Philadelphia, PA, USA

Definition
Branch of vessels originating from the aorta just below the diaphragm that supply the liver, stomach, part of the esophagus, spleen, part of the duodenum, and the pancreas.

Cross-References
▶ Cancer of the Pancreas
▶ Esophageal Cancer
▶ Hodgkin's Lymphoma
▶ Stomach Cancer
▶ Testes

Centigray (cGy)

Tod W. Speer
Department of Human Oncology, University of
Wisconsin School of Medicine and Public Health,
UW Hospital and Clinics, Madison, WI, USA

Definition
Gray is the SI unit of absorbed dose for ionizing
radiation. It represents the energy (joule; J)
absorbed by one kilogram (kg) of matter. One
hundred cGy is equal to one Gy.

$$1Gy = 1J/kg$$

Cross-References
▶ Radiation Oncology Physics

Cervical Cancer

▶ Brachytherapy-Gyn
▶ Uterine Cervix

Cervical Intraepithelial Neoplasia (CIN)

Patrizia Guerrieri, Paolo Montemaggi
Department of Radiation Oncology, Regional
Cancer Center "M. Ascoli", University of Palermo
Medical School, Palermo, Italy

Definition
The term "cervical intraepithelial neoplasia"
(CIN) was introduced by Richart (1973) to
present the concept of cervical neoplasia as
a disease continuum. Dysplasia and CIS, rather
than representing separate diseases, were part of
the spectrum of disease progression to invasive
squamous cell carcinoma. In Richart's system,
CIN 1 corresponds to mild dysplasia, and CIN
2 to moderate dysplasia. CIN 3 encompasses
both severe dysplasia and carcinoma in situ
(CIS). The National Cancer Institute in 1988
worked on developing a uniform terminology
system that could be reproducible, would
correlate with the histology of the lesion,
and would facilitate communication between
the laboratory and the clinician. The result
was the Bethesda Nomenclature system for
cervicovaginal cytology (National Cancer Institute Workshop 1989). By this time, the role of
human papilloma virus (HPV) as an etiologic
agent in the development of cervical intraepithelial
neoplasia and cervical carcinoma was well
established. The data, coupled with the lack of
reproducibility in assigning lesions to the categories
of CIN 1, CIN 2, CIN 3, and CIS led the
introduction of only two categories: low-grade
squamous intraepithelial lesion (LSIL) and high-
grade squamous intraepithelial lesion (HSIL).
The classification LSIL encompassed HPV,
mild dysplasia, and CIN 1; HSIL encompassed
moderate dysplasia, severe dysplasia, CIS, CIN 2,
and CIN 3.

Cross-References
▶ Vagina

References
National Cancer Institute Workshop (1989) The 1988
    Bethesda System for reporting cervical/vaginal
    cytological diagnoses. J Am Med Assoc 262:
    931–934
Richart RM (1973) Cervical intraepithelial neoplasia. Pathol
    Annu 8:301–328

Cervical Malignancy

▶ Uterine Cervix

Cetuximab

Carsten Nieder[1], Tod W. Speer[2]
[1]Radiation Oncology Unit, Nordlandssykehuset HF, Bodoe, Norway
[2]Department of Human Oncology, University of Wisconsin School of Medicine and Public Health, UW Hospital and Clinics, Madison, WI, USA

Synonyms
Erbitux

Definition
Monoclonal antibody interfering with the epidermal growth factor receptor (EGFR) pathway. Many tumors overexpress EGFR, and in head and neck cancer, administration of cetuximab plus radiotherapy has been shown to be superior to radiotherapy alone.

Cross-References
▶ Monoclonal Antibodies
▶ Targeted Radioimmunotherapy
▶ Total Body Irradiation (TBI)

Chemoradiation

▶ Bladder
▶ Esophageal Cancer

▶ Lung
▶ Sarcomas of the Head and Neck

Chernobyl Nuclear Reactor Accident

John P. Christodouleas
The Perelman Cancer Center,
Department of Radiation Oncology, University of Pennsylvania Hospital, Philadelphia, PA, USA

Definition
The Chernobyl nuclear reactor accident which occurred on April 26, 1986, in what is now the Ukraine, is widely considered the worst powerplant accident in history. The power plant at Chernobyl lacked many safety features including an adequate containment structure.

Cross-References
▶ Short-Term and Long-Term Health Risk of Nuclear Power Plant Accident

Chest, Abdominal, and Pelvic Tumor Metastases

▶ Palliation of Visceral Recurrences and Metastases

Chiropractic

▶ Complementary Medicine

Chloroma

Caspian Oliai[1], Theodore E. Yaeger[2]
[1]Department of Radiation Oncology, College of Medicine, Drexel University, Philadelphia, PA, USA
[2]Department Radiation Oncology, Wake Forest University School of Medicine, Winston-Salem NC, USA

Definition

A chloroma is also known as a granulocytic sarcoma or myeloblastoma, as it is usually a solid but extramedullary tumor that is mainly comprised of myeloid precursors.

Solid collection of leukemic cells composed mostly of myeloblasts occurring outside of the bone marrow. Simply stated, it is an extramedually manifestation of AML, but can also be found in MDS and MPD. Also known as myeloid sarcoma or granulocytic sarcoma.

Chloromas are usually associated with acute myelocytic leukemia mostly presenting in the orbit and extracranial bone structures (Chapman 1980). The term "Chloroma" is derived from the Greek root of "Chloros" (similarly *chloro*phyll) because the cells produce a myeloperoxidase that can cause a greenish hue to the tumor. The alternate term "granulocytic sarcoma" (GS) is often applied when the tint is not produced. As such, a GS only represents about 3% of patients actually seen with a diagnosis of acute or chronic granulocytic, polycythemia vera, hypereosinophilia, and myeloid metaplasia. Without these associated hemopoietic events, the presentation of GS alone is typically a precursor to acute myelocytic leukemia and blast crisis (Neiman 1986). Interestingly, increased survival of the acute leukemias are allowing increasing numbers of patients that develop GS (Neiman 1981).

GS is usually found in the first decade of life and is associated with M4 and M5 acute myeloid subtypes and 8:21 translocations.

Cross-References
► Hodgkin's Lymphoma
► Leukemia in General
► Sarcoma
► Sarcomas of the Head and Neck

References
Chapman P (1980) Johnson S Mastoid chloroma relapse in acute myeloid leukemia. J Laryngol Otol 94:1423–1427
Neiman RS (1986) The peripheral cell lymphomas come of age. Mayo Clin Proc 61:504–506
Neiman RS et al (1981) Granulocytic sarcoma: a clinico-pathologic study of 61 biopsied cases. Cancer 48: 1426–1437

Cholangiocarcinoma

► Liver and Hepatobiliary Tract

CHOP

Curt Heese
Department of Radiation Oncology, Eastern Regional Cancer Treatment Centers of America, Philadelphia, PA, USA

Definition

Multidrug chemotherapy regimen consisting of Cyclophosphamide (brand names *c*ytoxan, neosar), Adriamycin (doxorubicin/*h*ydroxydoxorubicin), Vincristine (*O*ncovin), *P*rednisone (sometimes called Deltasone or Orasone).

Cross-References
► Cutaneous T-Cell Lymphoma

Chordomas

CARLOS A. PEREZ, WADE L. THORSTAD
Department of Radiation Oncology, Siteman Cancer Center, Washington University Medical Center, St. Louis, MO, USA

Definition

A tumor arising from the primitive notochord (chorda dorsalis) that typically involves the clivus and notochord along the cervical vertebrae in the head and neck region.

Epidemiology

Chordomas are more common in patients in the fifth to sixth decade.

Although slowly growing, they are locally invasive. Basisphenoidal chordomas tend to cause symptoms earlier and may be difficult to differentiate histologically from chondromas and chondrosarcomas and radiographically from craniopharyngiomas, pineal tumors, and hypophyseal and pontine gliomas. The incidence of metastasis has been reported to be as high as 25%. Lymphatic spread is uncommon.

Clinical Presentation

Chordomas tend to originate from the clivus and chondrosarcomas from the temporal bone. In the head, extension may be intracranial or extracranial, into the sphenoid sinus, nasopharynx, clivus, and sellar and parasellar areas, with a resultant mass effect. In chordomas of the sphenooccipital region, the most common presenting symptom is headache. Other presentations include symptoms of pituitary insufficiency, nasal stuffiness, bitemporal hemianopsia, diplopia, and other cranial nerve deficits.

Diagnostic Workup

Most patients have significant bony destruction, and some may have calcifications in the tumor; hence, plain films and, specifically, CT scans or MRI are very useful. In most cases, the soft tissue component is much more extensive than initially appreciated, and a CT scan with contrast enhancement is required. MRI is inferior to CT to demonstrate bony destruction and intratumoral calcification, but MRI is superior to CT regarding the delineation of the exact extent of the tumor, which allows for better treatment planning. Because of availability and lower cost, CT appears to be the technique of choice for routine follow-up of previously treated patients (Perez and Thorstad 2008).

General Management

The management of the patient, which is challenging, is dictated by the anatomic location of the tumor, the direction, and extent of spread. A surgical approach is recommended (when feasible) but complete surgical extirpation alone is unusual. Intracranial spread usually requires steroid coverage and therapy directed to correction of neurologic deficits, which may be present. Because of the high incidence of local recurrence, combined surgical excision and irradiation is frequently used. No effective chemotherapeutic agent or combination of drugs has been identified.

Radiation Therapy

Irradiation techniques vary, depending on the location of the tumor. Basisphenoidal tumors were treated by a combination of parallel-opposed lateral fields, anterior wedges, and photon and electron beam combinations, depending on the extent of the neoplasm. Precision radiation therapy planning, using CT and MRI, is required because high doses of external-beam radiation therapy are needed. 3D CRT or IMRT provide optimal dose distributions, with sparing of normal tissues (Fig. 1).

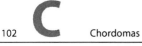

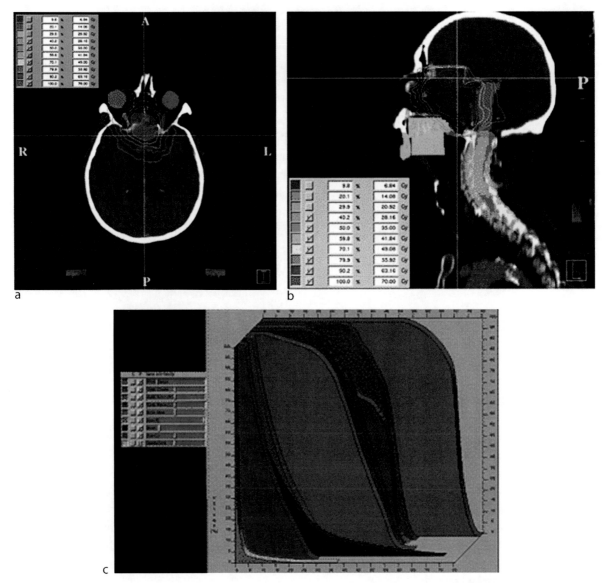

Chordomas. Fig. 1 Chordoma of clivus in 81-year-old man treated with 70 Gy in 2 Gy fractions. Example of IMRT plan: (**a**) cross section in upper portion of PTV demonstrating coverage of target volume (PTV) with sparing of ocular structures. (**b**) Sagittal plane dose distribution with excellent coverage of PTV. (**c**) Dose-volume histogram:

Structure	Dose range (Gy)	Mean dose (Gy)
PTV (including left neck)	60–75	70
Optic nerves/chiasm	25–50	41
Ocular globe	3–30	12

Source: Reproduced with permission from LeVay J, O'Sullivan B, Catton C, et al (1994)

The tumor usually surrounds the spinal cord and infiltrates vertebral bones. A combined technique using protons or electrons to boost the initial photon fields has been generally applied. In the treatment of chordomas surrounding the spinal cord, IMRT can provide high-dose homogeneity and PTV coverage. Frequent digital portal image-based setup control reduces random positioning errors for head and neck cancer patients immobilized with conventional thermoplastic masks (Gabriele et al. 2003). Image-guided radiation therapy with daily setup correction and verification using megavoltage or kilovoltage CT imaging may be useful as well.

Because of the slow proliferative nature of chordomas, high linear energy transfer (LET) may prove useful in their management. Rutz et al. (2007) reported a 77% 3-year progression-free survival in 26 patients treated with spot-scanning proton irradiation (median dose 72 ▶ Co Gray Equivalent. Four grade 2–5 late effects were observed. Brachytherapy can be used for recurrent tumors of the base of skull or adjacent to the spine when a more aggressive surgical exposure is offered.

Results of Therapy

Photons

Forsyth and colleagues (1993) reported on 51 patients with intracranial chordomas (19 classified as chondroid) treated surgically (biopsy in 11 patients and subtotal removal or greater in 40); 39 patients received postoperative irradiation. The 5- and 10-year survival rates were 51% and 35%, respectively; 5-year survival was 36% for biopsy patients and 55% for those who had resection. Tai and associates (1995) reviewed the results of irradiation combined with surgery, irradiation alone, and surgery alone in 159 patients reported in the literature. Analysis of the optimal biologically equivalent dose was performed using the linear-quadratic formula on 47 patients treated with photons; no dose–response relationship was shown. Keisch and coworkers (1991) reported on 21 patients with chordoma treated at our medical center. The 5- and 10-year actuarial survival was significantly better in patients treated with surgery alone or surgery and irradiation than in those treated with radiation therapy alone (52%, 32%, and 0%, respectively) ($P = 0.02$).

Protons

The best results in the treatment of chordomas have been obtained with radical surgical procedures followed by high-dose proton irradiation. Berson et al. (1988) described 45 patients with chordomas or chondrosarcomas at the base of the skull or cervical spine treated by subtotal resection and postoperative irradiation. Twenty-three patients were treated definitively by charged particles, 13 patients with photons and particles, and nine were treated for recurrent disease. Doses ranged from 36 to 80 Gy equivalent. Patients with smaller tumor volumes had better survival rate at 5 years (80% vs. 33% for larger tumors). Patients treated for primary disease had a 78% actuarial local control rate at 2 years, versus 33% for patients with recurrent disease.

Fagundes and colleagues (1995) updated the Massachusetts General Hospital experience with 204 patients treated for chordoma of the base of the skull or cervical spine. Sixty-three patients (31%) had treatment failures, which were local in 60 patients (29%) and the only site of failure in 49 patients. Two patients had regional lymph node relapse, and three developed surgical pathway recurrence. Thirteen patients relapsed in distant sites (especially lungs and bones). The 5-year actuarial survival rate after any relapse was 7%. Two patients (1.4%) with local tumor control developed distant metastases in contrast with 10 of 60 (16%) who failed locally and distantly.

Terahara et al. (1999) reported on 132 patients with skull base chordoma treated with combined photon and proton irradiation; in 115 patients dose-volume data and follow-up were available. Doses ranged from 66.6 to 79.2 ► CGE (median 68.9 ► CGE). The dose to the optic structures (optic nerves and chiasm), the brain stem surface, and the brain stem center was limited to 60, 64, and 53 ► CGE, respectively. Local failure developed in 42 of 115 patients 36%), with actuarial local tumor control rates at 5 and 10 years being 59% and 44%, respectively.

A report on proton therapy for base of skull chordoma was published by the Royal College of Radiologists (2000). They concluded that outcome after proton therapy is superior to conventional photon irradiation.

Cross-References

► Conformal Therapy: Treatment Planning, Treatment Delivery, and Clinical Results
► Image-Guided Radiation Therapy (IGRT): kV Imaging
► Image-Guided Radiation Therapy (IGRT): MV Imaging
► IMRT
► Pediatric Ovarian Cancer
► Proton Therapy
► Renal Pelvis and Ureter
► Sarcomas of the Head and Neck

References

Berson AM, Castro JR, Petti P et al (1988) Charged particle irradiation of chordoma and chondrosarcoma of the base of skull and cervical spine: the Lawrence Berkeley Laboratory experience. Int J Radiat Oncol Biol Phys 15:559–565

Fagundes MA, Hug EB, Liebsch NJ et al (1995) Radiation therapy for chordomas of the base of skull and cervical spine: patterns of failure and outcome after relapse. Int J Radiat Oncol Biol Phys 33:579–584

Forsyth PA, Cascino TL, Shaw EG et al (1993) Intracranial chordomas: a clinicopathological and prognostic study of 51 cases. J Neurosurg 78:741–747

Gabriele P, Macias V, Stasi M et al (2003) Feasibility of intensity-modulated radiation therapy in the treatment of advanced cervical chordoma. Tumori 89:298–304

Keisch ME, Garcia DM, Shibuya RB (1991) Retrospective long-term follow-up analysis in 21 patients with chordomas of various sites treated at a single institution. J Neurosurg 75:374–377

LeVay J, O'Sullivan B, Catton C et al (1994) An assessment of prognostic factors in soft tissue sarcoma of the head and neck. Arch Otolaryngol Head Neck Surg 120:981–986

Perez CA, Thorstad WL (2008) Unusual non-epithelial tumors of the head and neck. In: Halperin EC, Perez CA, Brady LW (eds) Perez and Brady's principles and practice of radiation oncology, 5th edn. Wolters Kluwer Lippincott Williams & Wilkins, Philadelphia, p 996

Royal College of Radiologists Proton Therapy Working Party (2000) Proton therapy for base of skull chordoma: a report for the Royal College of Radiologists. The proton therapy working party. Clin Oncol (R Coll Radiol) 12:75–79

Rutz HP, Weber DC, Sugahara S et al (2007) Extracranial chordoma: outcome in patients treated with function-preserving surgery followed by spot-scanning proton beam irradiation. Int J Radiat Oncol Bio Phys 67:512–520

Tai PT, Craighead P, Bagdon F (1995) Optimization of radiotherapy for patients with cranial chordoma: a review of dose–response ratios for photon techniques. Cancer 75:749–756

Terahara A, Niemierko A, Goitein M et al (1999) Analysis of the relationship between tumor dose inhomogeneity and local control in patients with skull base chordoma. Int J Radiat Oncol Biol Phys 45:351–358

Chronic Lymphocytic Leukemia

► Leukemia in General

Chronic Myelogenous Leukemia (CML)

Definition

Also known as chronic granulocytic leukemia is a white blood cell line malignancy of predominately a myeloid stem cell line. It characteristically exhibits a chromosome translocation commonly called 'The Philadelphia Syndrome' which has a 9 and 22 translocation. CML can evolve into an acute phase or blast phase which represents a bone marrow crisis with shortened survival.

Cross-References

▶ Leukemia in General

Cine CT

DAREK MICHALSKI[1], M. SAIFUL HUQ[2]
[1]Division of Medical Physics, Department of Radiation Oncology, University of Pittsburgh Cancer Centers, Pittsburgh, PA, USA
[2]Department of Radiation Oncology, University of Pittsburgh Medical Center Cancer Pavilion, Pittsburgh, PA, USA

Definition

A stationary volume scanning mode in planar geometry with patient being consecutively scanned in space and continuously in time.

Cross-References

▶ Four-Dimensional (4D) Treatment Planning/ Respiratory Gating

Cisplatin

CHRISTIN A. KNOWLTON[1], MICHELLE KOLTON MACKAY[2]
[1]Department of Radiation Oncology, Drexel University, Philadelphia, PA, USA
[2]Department of Radiation Oncology, Marshfield Clinic, Marshfield, WI, USA

Synonyms

Cisplatinum

Definition

Cisplatin is a platinum-based chemotherapy agent frequently used in cervical cancer. Its mechanism of action is to cross-link strands of DNA and thereby interfere with mitotic cell division. It is frequently administered on a weekly basis with radiation therapy as a definitive treatment for advanced cervical cancer or as postoperative treatment with concurrent radiation. Possible side effects of cisplatin include nausea, nephrotoxicity, neurotoxicity, ototoxicity, alopecia, and electrolyte disturbances.

Cross-References

▶ Principles of Chemotherapy
▶ Uterine Cervix

Cisplatinum

▶ Cisplatin

Clark Level

BRANDON J. FISHER
Department of Radiation Oncology, College of Medicine, Drexel University, Philadelphia, PA, USA

Definition

The Clark level is a measure of depth of invasion into the skin used as a prognostic indicator for skin cancers: level I: confined to the outermost layer of the skin, epidermis; level II: penetration into the dermis; level III to IV: invasion through the dermis into deeper dermal layers, yet still confined to the skin; level V: penetration through the dermis and into the fat and hypodermis.

Cross-References

▶ Skin Cancer

Clark's Nevus

▶ Atypical (Dysplastic) Nevi

Class I Hysterectomy

▶ Total Abdominal Hysterectomy

Class II Hysterectomy

▶ Modified Radical Hysterectomy

Class III Hysterectomy

▶ Radical Hysterectomy

Class IV Hysterectomy

▶ Extended Radical Hysterectomy

Clinical Aspects of Brachytherapy (BT)

Erik Van Limbergen
Department of Radiation Oncology, University
Hospital Gasthuisberg, Leuven, Belgium

Synonyms

Curietherapy

Definition/Description

Brachytherapy (BT) is a technique of radiation therapy delivery where the radioactive sources are placed very close or even inside the target volume. The name is derived from the Greek word βραχυσ which means short as this is opposed to other techniques of radiotherapy: teletherapy or external beam radiation therapy.

Background

Brachytherapy is the earliest method of radiotherapy which was developed soon after the discovery of radioactivity by Becquerel in 1896 and development of radium sources by Marie Curie. During the first decade of the twentieth century, the first treatments with radium were performed by Danlos and Bloc (1901) in Paris and Abbe (1905) in the USA.

Modern brachytherapy uses artificial isotopes (Iridium-192, Cobalt-60, Iodine-125, Palladium-103), remote control afterloading machines with stepping source facilities, 3D dose planning based on 3D imaging (ultrasound, CT, MRI) to optimize dose distribution and deliver high doses more and more conformal to the planning target volume (PTV) and low doses to the surrounding organs at risk.

Basic Characteristics

Brachytherapy is able to deliver a very localized radiation, since sources have a very steep fall off of the doses and are applied very close to the target volume (intracavitary, endoluminal, endovascular, or surface contact brachytherapy) or implanted in the target (▶ interstitial brachytherapy). In most cases when adequate techniques are applied, uncertainties in dose delivery are small and no or no large PTV to CTV margins have to be taken. This reduces significantly the treated volume and thus also the side effects of high radiation doses.

Since the doses are delivered in small volumes, radiation can be delivered in a short overall treatment duration which reduces the risk of tumor repopulation (Joiner and van der Kogel 2009).

The dose can be delivered by temporary or permanent implants.

▶ Temporary implants can deliver the dose at classical low dose rate, but with stepping source technology ▶ High Dose Rate (HDR) brachytherapy and more recently ▶ Pulsed Dose Rate (PDR) brachytherapy has been developed. PDR brachytherapy like HDR brachytherapy utilizes a single miniaturized source which moves step by step through implanted afterloading devices to achieve the desired dose distribution. In PDR such a sequence of steps, also called a pulse, is repeated a number of times to obtain the prescribed total dose. By choosing an appropriate number of pulses one can simulate, from a radiobiological point of view, a continuous low dose rate treatment (Fowler and Van Limbergen 1997). This and other newly developed techniques allow brachytherapy to be used in a very wide variety of tumor types and sites (Gerbaulet Poetter et al. 2002 and Devlin 2007).

▶ Permanent implants: The most common radionuclides used for permanent implants are iodine-125, palladium-103, and gold-198 encapsulated in seeds. These sources have a relatively short half-life and are left implanted in the tissue for gradually delivering the dose while the activity decays. The photon energy used in permanent seed implants is low so that radiation protection can be achieved with relatively simple measures (Fig. 1).

Different Dose Rates in Brachytherapy

Depending on the source strength, brachytherapy can deliver the target dose at classical low dose rate, high dose rate, medium dose rate, or pulsed dose rate (Joiner and van der Kogel 2009). At low dose rate (LDR) the dose is delivered at 0.4–1 Gy/h (+/−10 Gy/day). The sources

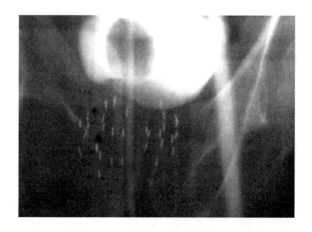

Clinical Aspects of Brachytherapy (BT). Fig. 1 Permanent seed implant with I-125 sources for the curative treatment of early prostate cancer

commonly used for LDR are cesium-137 (LDR afterloaders), or iridium-192 as LDR wires. Irradiation is continuous and can take 1–6 days depending on the dose.

At ▶ medium dose rate (MDR) the dose is delivered at 1–12 Gy/h usually by cesium-137 sources in 1–3 days depending on the dose.

At high dose rate (HDR) the dose is delivered by a stepping source afterloader (iridium-192 or cobalt-60) at >12 Gy/h (>10 Gy/min) in one or several fractions. As in external beam irradiation, enough time is kept in between fractions (>6 h) to allow for full repair.

At pulsed dose rate (PDR) the dose is delivered by a stepping source afterloader iridium-192 at >12 Gy/h (>10 Gy/min) in hyperfractionated hourly or two hourly pulses with incomplete repair in between fractions (Fowler and Van Limbergen 1997).

At very low dose rate (VLDR) the dose is delivered by low-activity, low-energy seed sources (iodine-125, palladium-103, gold-198) which are implanted permanently in the clinical target volume.

▶ Afterloading technique implies implantation of nonradioactive source carriers: dedicated applicators such as gynecological (Fig. 2) or endobronchial or endoesophageal (Fig. 3) brachytherapy, guide needles (Figs. 4 and 5), catheters or tubes (Fig. 6) which later after dosimetric study are loaded with radioactive sources. Because the application itself is with nonradioactive material a meticulous and very precise positioning of the source carriers allows a high geometric quality of application, and an effective radioprotection.

Manual afterloading is possible with plastic tubes, guide gutters, hypodermic and guide needles, plastic needles, silk threads (for interstitial brachytherapy); applicators (for intracavitary or surface brachytherapy); and catheters (for intraluminal applications).

Remote afterloading machines: these projectors can be used with interstitial, intracavitary, intraluminal as well as with contact brachytherapy (Fig. 7). Afterloading equipment is connected to various types of applicators and catheters. Remote afterloading is mandatory for MDR, HDR, as well as PDR brachytherapy for reasons of radiation protection.

Stepping source afterloaders contain a high activity source mounted on a cable. Dwell positions and dwell times are calculated in 3D planning systems and allow for optimization of the dose distribution (Fig. 8). They can be used for HDR (with a 10 Ci source) as well as PDR (with a 0.5–1 Ci source) brachytherapy (Fig. 9).

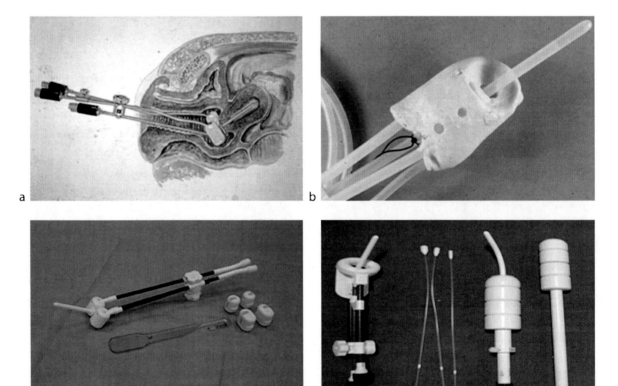

Clinical Aspects of Brachytherapy (BT). Fig. 2 (**a**) Fletcher-type applicator for intrauterine–intravaginal brachytherapy for cervix cancer. (**b**) Chassagne–Pierquin individually designed mold applicator. (**c**) MRI-compatible IU-IV applicator for MR image-guided BT. (**d**) Different MRI compatible applicators for intracavitary brachtherapy: Stockholm-type ring IU-IV applicator, Norman Simon capsules for endometrial cancer combined intrauterine and vaginal applicator

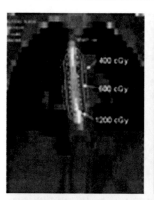
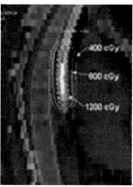
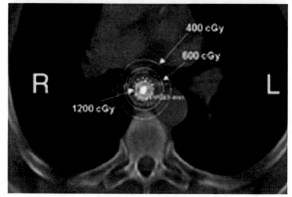

Clinical Aspects of Brachytherapy (BT). Fig. 3 Endoesophageal brachytherapy with a dedicated endoesophageal applicator of appropriate diameter

Indications for Brachytherapy

Over the past two decades, technical developments, new radioactive sources, modern afterloading machines using different dose rates and 3D dose distribution optimization, and great progress in imaging have opened new fields for brachytherapy.

The target volumes to be implanted should be relatively small and accessible, and the target limits should be well defined.

Brachytherapy Alone

It is used for small tumors of the skin in small areas of the skin such as eyelids, nose, ear, lip, oral cavity, as an alternative to mutilating surgery. It is also an established treatment technique used for early low-risk prostate cancer.

Brachytherapy as Boost After External Beam Irradiation

For larger tumors which measure 40 mm or more, frequently because of poorly defined tumor limits, radiation treatment should start with external beam radiation, delivering 45–50 Gy in

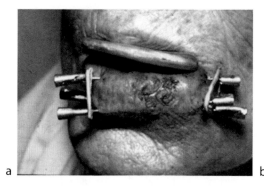
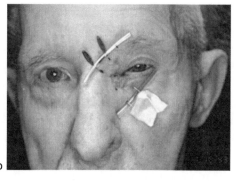

Clinical Aspects of Brachytherapy (BT). Fig. 4 Hypodermic needles: small (length 20–80 mm, external diameter 0.8 mm) hypodermic needles are used in small-size implants in sensitive structures like lip (Fig. 4a), inner canthus and eyelids (Fig. 4b), nose vestibulum and penis. These small needles have to be afterloaded manually with Iridium 192 wires

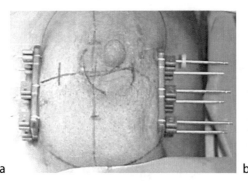
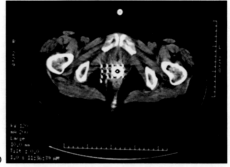

a   b

Clinical Aspects of Brachytherapy (BT). **Fig. 5** Larger (100–200 mm, external diameter 1.6–2 mm) guide needles are used in breast (**a**), prostate, anus, interstitial pelvis (**b**). When made of titanium they are compatible with CT and MRI imaging and can be connected to a remote control afterloader

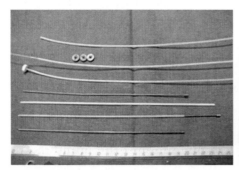
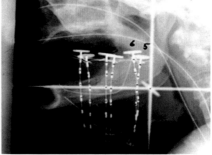

Clinical Aspects of Brachytherapy (BT). **Fig. 6** Semiflexible to rigid plastic needles and tubes with an external diameter of 1.6–2 mm, which are compatible with CT and MRI imaging, are used in prostate, anus, rectum, gynecology, brain, head and neck, and soft tissue sarcomas. They can be connected via transfer tubes to a HDR or PDR remote control afterloading machine

5 weeks. Brachytherapy is used as a boost for dose escalation following as soon as possible after the end of the external beam therapy.

Brachytherapy in Combination with Surgery

Perioperative or postoperative implants can be indicated after surgery with positive or doubtful margins. This strategy is used as barrier brachytherapy in oral cavity cancers, bladder cancers, soft tissue sarcomas (especially in children for gynecological, urological, or intraorbital localizations) or as ▶ accelerated partial breast irradiation (APBI) as alternative to whole breast irradiation after breast conservative surgery in selected small and low-risk breast cancer (Polgár et al. 2010).

Brachytherapy for Reirradiation in Previously Irradiated Area

Because the treatment volumes are small and conformal to the clinical target volume, brachytherapy is also used as retreatment technique for recurrences or new secondary tumors in irradiated areas in head and neck, breast or prostate cancer.

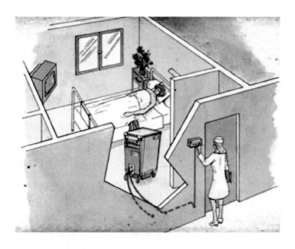

Clinical Aspects of Brachytherapy (BT). Fig. 7
Treatment with a remote control afterloader secures radioprotection

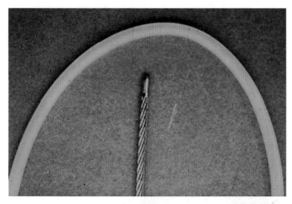

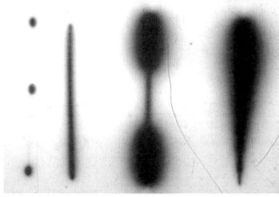

Clinical Aspects of Brachytherapy (BT). Fig. 8 The Ir-192 stepping source mounted on a cable allows dwell position and dwell time optimization by the programmed stepping motor

Many technical innovations have made this change possible, based on a more frequent use of new dose rates: high dose rate, medium dose rate, and pulsed dose rate brachytherapy. The technological aspects of brachytherapy are more and more sophisticated, allowing the integration of 3D imaging data and 3D dose distributions. Examples are: 3D navigation for interstitial stereotactic brachytherapy, scanner simulation and 3D virtual planning, MRI- and ultrasound-assisted brachytherapy treatment planning, and CT-based software for clinical evaluation.

Other technologies are developed for adapted and effective brachytherapy when combined with other treatment modalities, such as radiosensitizers, hyperthermia, external beam irradiation, chemotherapy, and surgery.

Contraindications to Brachytherapy

Brachytherapy is not indicated in target volumes that are not accessible enough to perform a geometrically correct source positioning in order to obtain a good dose distribution.

Since the lower energy radiation of the brachytherapy sources is absorbed by photoelectric absorption, which is proportional to Z^3, positioning of sources close to bone, for instance, the mandibula in head and neck cancer, should be avoided, and use of leaded mandibular protectors is advocated. If this is not feasible without compromising target covering, BT is contraindicated.

LDR or PDR BT is contraindicated in patients who are mentally unfit or too confused to stay alone in a treatment room for a longer time to avoid displacement or removal of the source carriers by the patient.

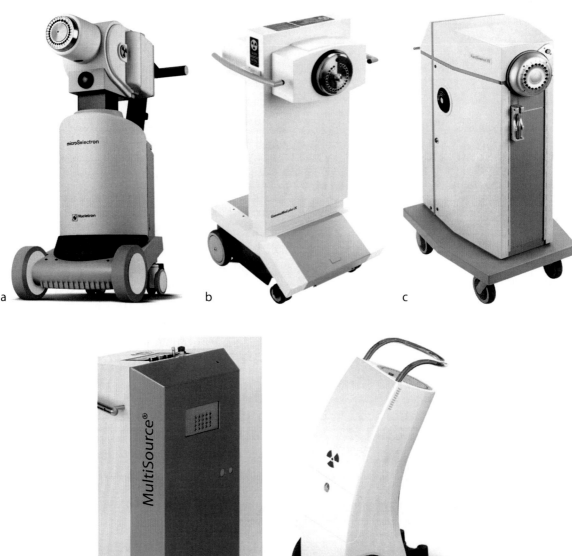

Clinical Aspects of Brachytherapy (BT). Fig. 9 Modern stepping source afterloaders: (**a**) Nucletron Microselectron (PDR or HDR), (**b**) Varian GammaMed (HDR or PDR), (**c**) Varian Varisource (HDR), (**d**) Bebig Multisource (HDR), and (**e**) Nucletron Flexitron (HDR or PDR)

Cross-References

▶ Anal Cancer
▶ Brachytherapy
▶ Carcinoma of the Uterine Cervix
▶ Endometrium
▶ Esophageal Cancer
▶ Female Urethra
▶ Male Urethra

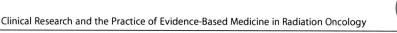

▶ Penile Cancer

▶ Prostate

▶ Sarcomas of the Head and Neck

▶ Soft Tissue Sarcoma

▶ Stage 0 Breast Cancer

▶ Vagina

References

Devlin P (2007) Brachytherapy: applications and techniques. Lippincott Williams and Wilkins, Philadelphia

Gerbaulet Poetter R, Mazeron JJ et al (2002) The GEC-ESTRO handbook of brachytherapy. ESTRO, Brussels

Fowler JF, Van Limbergen E (1997) Biological effect of pulsed dose rate brachytherapy with stepping sources if short half-times of repair are present in tissues. Int J Radiat Oncol Biol Phys 37:377–383

Joiner M, van der Kogel A (2009) Basic clinical radiobiology. Hodder Arnold, London

Polgár C et al (2010) Patient selection for accelerated partial breast irradiation (APBI) after breast-conserving surgery: recommendations of the Groupe Européen de Curiethérapie-European Society for Therapeutic Radiology and Oncology (GEC-ESTRO) Breast Cancer Working Group based on clinical evidence. Radiother Oncol 94: 264–273

Clinical Evidence

▶ Clinical Research and the Practice of Evidence-Based Medicine in Radiation Oncology

Clinical Research

▶ Clinical Research and the Practice of Evidence-Based Medicine in Radiation Oncology

Clinical Research and the Practice of Evidence-Based Medicine in Radiation Oncology

Bok Ai Choo[1], Jiade J. Lu[1], Luther W. Brady[2]
[1]Department of Radiation Oncology, National University Cancer Institute, Singapore (NCIS), Singapore
[2]Department of Radiation Oncology, College of Medicine, Drexel University, Philadelphia, PA, USA

Synonyms

Clinical evidence; Clinical research; Evidence-based medicine; Laboratory biology; Translational research

Introduction

Shortly after the discovery of X-rays by Roentgen in 1895, the first use of radiotherapy in the treatment of cancer was reported in 1902 and 1903 for the treatment of lymphoma and leukemia (Pusey 1902; Senn 1903). Clinical research at that time involved treating the patient and assessing the response with loose ethical considerations. This formed the basis of the earliest clinical research using radiation in the field of oncology. The exploratory use of radium by Marie Curie improved the understanding of using radioisotopes to treat cancer. However, due to its long half-life and difficulty in targeting the dose, radium was not deemed an ideal source. In 1950, cobalt and cesium sources were used and radiotherapy was established as a definitive treatment for cancer. Similarly, in late 1940s, nitrogen mustard became the first form of chemotherapy used in the treatment of cancer (Rhouds 1946). Since then, over 70 chemotherapy agents have been developed and more than 10 targeted therapy drugs are in routine use today; many are used in combination with radiation therapy. As the older orthovoltage energy X-ray machines and the cobalt and cesium units are phased out, they are being replaced by megavoltage linear accelerators which do not contain a radioactive source.

Parallel to the use of radiotherapy, the field of diagnostic radiology has expanded with the invention of computerized tomography (CT) scanners in 1971 (Hounsfield 1973), magnetic resonance (MRI) scanners in 1977 (Mansfield and Maudsley 1977), and positron emission tomography-computerized tomography (PET-CT) scanners in 2000 (Beyer et al. 2000). With advancements in technology in both the hardware and software realms, it is now possible to accurately localize the treatment targets and use advanced treatment modalities such as ▶ intensity-modulated radiotherapy (IMRT) to deliver high doses of radiation to the tumor while minimizing doses to adjacent organs at risk.

The effectiveness of radiotherapy will continue to improve as techniques which use higher precision for both targeting and delivery result in an improved therapeutic index. Such techniques include ▶ image-guided radiation therapy (IGRT), stereotactic ablative radiotherapy, and ▶ proton therapy. Improved treatment strategies, especially ▶ multimodality therapy, have also been shown to improve the therapeutic index. However, it is imperative to demonstrate reproducible clinical evidence before any new technology or strategy is routinely used in the clinical setting.

This entry focuses on the commonly used research modalities in the field of radiation oncology, as well as their application in the practice of evidence-based radiation oncology.

Definition of "Clinical Research"

Clinical research is defined by the National Institutes of Health as "research conducted with human subjects that is patient oriented. The research could include the pathophysiology of human disease, epidemiology, and therapeutic interventions with clinical outcomes." (http://grants.nih.gov/grants/policy/hs/glossary.htm).

Definition of "Evidence-Based Medicine"

As proposed by Dr. David Sackett and colleagues at McMaster University in Hamilton, Ontario, Canada, evidence-based medicine may be defined as "the judicious use of the best current evidence in making decisions about the care of the individual patient. Evidence-based medicine (EBM) is meant to integrate clinical expertise with the best available research evidence and patient values" (Sackett et al. 1996).

Purpose of Clinical Research

The purpose of clinical research is to investigate, test, and establish new treatments, or to validate existing clinical practices. It seeks to improve the understanding of molecular biology, genetics, and proteomics in the laboratory setting using cancer cell lines in animal subjects. Once the therapy shows promising results, this is further tested in human subjects through different phases according to established protocols.

Types of Clinical Research in Radiation Oncology

Research in radiation oncology can be categorized in a number of ways. It can be broadly categorized as either experimental or observational research based on whether researchers assign radiation doses to the subjects (Fig. 1), or the research may be classified based on what the researchers are studying, for example, therapeutic treatment regimes, diagnostic and screening studies, disease prevention, epidemiology, quality of life, genetics, or behavioral studies to name a few (Table 1). As in any other medical field, scientific research provides the foundation for the practice of evidence-based radiation oncology.

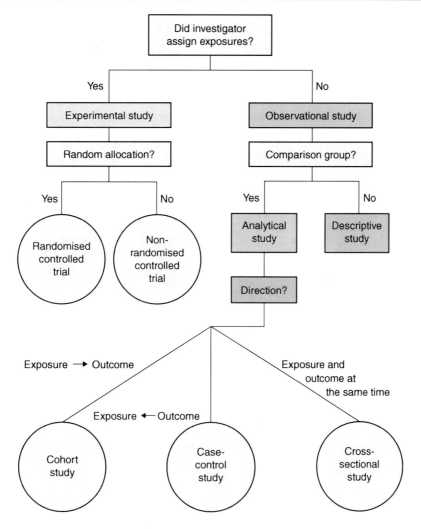

Clinical Research and the Practice of Evidence-Based Medicine in Radiation Oncology. Fig. 1
Classification of types of clinical research (Schulz KF, Grimes DA. The Lancet Handbook of Essential Concepts in Clinical Research)

In experimental studies, the investigators assign the radiation dose to be delivered either in a randomized or nonrandomized fashion. The commonly read "phase III randomized trial" and "single arm phase II trial" are examples of experimental studies.

In observational studies, delivered doses are not usually assigned by the study investigators. An analytical study has a comparison or control group, but a descriptive study does not. Observational studies dominate the literature in the field

of radiation oncology. Most retrospective studies in radiation oncology such as case series, case–control, and surveillance studies are observational in nature. Cohort, cross-sectional studies, and case reports are less commonly used in radiation oncology.

Therapeutic, diagnostic, and quality-of-life studies, all of which can be either experimental or observational, are more commonly observed in the field of radiation oncology than epidemiological, behavioral, and screening studies. Recently,

Clinical Research and the Practice of Evidence-Based Medicine in Radiation Oncology. Table 1 Classification of clinical research in radiation oncology

Type	Description
Therapeutic	Assigning differential doses and fractionation and radiobiology concepts to achieve a higher therapeutic ratio
	Use of radiosensitizer such as chemotherapy or targeted agent in concurrent treatment
	Outcome measured in response, local control, and survival
Diagnostic	Exploring better quality and accuracy of imaging to help define the radiation target
	Example: PET-CT or MRI fusion with CT simulation scan to define PTV (planning target volume)
Screening and disease prevention	Early detection of organ damage related to background or therapeutic radiation exposure
	Example : measurement of DNA microarray in sudden radiation exposure due to a nuclear plant leakage
Epidemiology	Exposure of low background dose or sudden overexposure or therapeutic radiation in causal of diseases ranging from end-organ failure, gestation abnormality and causal of cancer
	Example: Prolonged radon gas contact/inhalation from granite stones used in the building industry
Quality of life	Study on the early and late side effects of radiotherapy by charting the time of onset, frequency, severity, and long-term outcome on daily activities/living
	Often in parallel with therapeutic research using validated questionnaire scoring system
Genetics	Radiobiology and clinical studies in genetic effect on DNA repair, mutation, and apoptosis after radiation exposure
	Exploring genetic interaction with radiation can be both therapeutic as cancer treatment or preventative in limiting radiation exposure damage
	Example: Radiosensitivity in ataxic-telangiectasia or radioresistance in certain cancer cell lines
Behavioral study	Physical, cognitive, or psychological response to changes in adaptive or adverse response to radiotherapy

translational studies with emphasis on genetics and proteomics are increasingly utilized in clinical research studies in radiation oncology, particularly with aims which will predict treatment outcomes. In addition, dosimetry studies can be considered a form of clinical research, and their results are commonly incorporated in decision making in radiation therapy.

Studies in radiation physics and radiation biology are important health service research areas in radiation oncology. Most studies of radiation biology are laboratory or animal studies. Likewise, most radiation physics studies do not involve human subjects. Technically speaking, radiation biology and radiation physics studies are not considered to be clinical research;

however, these studies often provide the important fundamentals on which clinical research in radiation oncology is based.

Clinical Trials

Clinical trials are usually experimental therapeutic research which involves an intervention such as radiation therapy or chemotherapy. They are designed to evaluate and test new treatment modalities (e.g., combined chemoradiation therapy for advanced NSCLC), novel techniques (e.g., brachytherapy for prostate cancer), or innovative treatment devices (e.g., a stereotactic body radiotherapy device for a metastatic focus in the spinal cord). Clinical trials are often conducted in "phases," each one with a different purpose.

Phase 1

Phase 1 trials are usually the initial studies involving human subjects that study the tolerability (side effects) of a particular type of treatment (e.g., intracavitary brachytherapy for unresectable bile duct cancer). A continual escalation of radiation (or medication) dose to the maximum tolerance or a preset high value is usually performed. The treatment schedule and safety dose can usually be determined in phase 1 trials, and such doses/schedules can be used in a subsequent phase 2 clinical trial to test its efficacy. The early potential effectiveness of the new therapy may be available as well, and phase 1 trials can be continuous with a subsequent phase 2 trial (hence a phase 1/2 study).

Phase 1 clinical trials are often offered to cancer patients who have exhausted standard treatment and are willing to explore new treatments in oncology. Although not commonly observed in radiation oncology, the study subjects of a phase 1 trial could also be healthy volunteers as long as the subjects understand the potential risks involved. The study numbers are usually small involving no more than 20 subjects.

Phase 2

Phase 2 clinical trials explore the efficacy of a particular type of treatment as well as the short- and long-term side effects. In a preset protocol, the primary and secondary objectives of the trial are clearly defined. In radiation oncology, the objectives of phase 2 trials are usually clinical outcomes such as response to treatment, local control, progression-free survival, overall survival, etc. The results of a phase 2 clinical trial provide knowledge on the effectiveness of a treatment and whether the therapy is effective enough such that it may be compared with the current standard of care treatment in a randomized phase 3 trial.

To demonstrate a clear clinical benefit in a phase 2 trial (e.g., 10% or more in control), a sufficient sample size is usually needed. Sample sizes can be calculated using a number of methods, including the Simon's two-stage design (Simon 1989).

Phase 3

Phase 3 clinical trials are usually performed in a randomized, controlled manner with large sample sizes. These studies test the null hypothesis that a new treatment is superior to a treatment that is considered the current standard (including best supportive care).

Although single- or double-blinded phase 3 randomized clinical trials (RCT) are commonly used in studies involving drug treatment, sham radiation therapy is not commonly utilized in phase 3 trials in radiation oncology. RCT is now the preferred method and gold standard of testing and validating the benefits of new therapies.

Sufficient sample size is required to demonstrate a clear clinical benefit in a phase 3 randomized clinical trial. In a well-designed randomized controlled trial, bias is reduced to a minimum. It is not uncommon to randomize hundreds of cases to detect a small difference in clinical outcome in an RCT in radiation oncology. Therefore, time and effort for patient accrual to a randomized trial can be substantial and costly.

Phase 4

Continuous post-research collection of information after a regimen has been granted an approval for use in human subjects is important so that researchers may generate a large database of the expected as well as unexpected long-term side effects. This is commonly also known as a phase 4 trial. Phase 4 clinical trials are less commonly performed in radiation oncology.

Meta-analysis

Meta-analysis is a statistical analysis of multiple studies which have related hypotheses that is used to determine the benefits of a therapy. Meta-analysis itself is not clinical research per se, but a statistical tool by which to overcome reduced statistical power in studies with small sample sizes. However, there remains a risk of selection bias as the studies may not be 100% comparable; there may be different end points as well as different inclusion and exclusion criteria in the various studies under consideration. Although a meta-analysis may raise multiple questions as to whether there is a definite benefit of a given therapy, the overall trend of the potential effects of a therapy can be charted out.

Case Reports

Case reports contain information and knowledge about a specific diagnosis, investigation, treatment, and outcome of a disease. The purpose is to report rare or unusual cases by generating hypotheses about the disease and discussing specific learning points. Case reports have been used in radiation oncology to report rare and/or adverse effects of treatment.

Quality-of-life studies

Also known as "supportive care," this avenue of research explores ways to improve patient comfort and the quality of life for individuals with a chronic illness.

Genetic studies

Genetic studies aim to improve the prediction of disorders by identifying and understanding how genes and illnesses may be related. Research in this area may explore ways in which a person's genes make him or her more or less likely to develop a disorder. This may lead to development of tailor-made treatments based on a patient's genetic makeup.

Epidemiological studies

Epidemiological studies seek to identify the patterns, causes, and control of disorders on a population-based scale.

Commonly Measured Outcomes in Clinical Research of Radiation Oncology

Overall Survival

Overall survival is an indication of the proportion (in percentage) of patients within a specific group who are expected to be alive after a specified time. Overall survival (OS) takes into account death due to any cause, both related and unrelated to the disease in question. Overall survival is the primary end point in clinical trials, particularly phase 3 randomized studies, which is used to evaluate the benefits of a treatment.

Median Survival

Median survival is the measure of how long (in length of time) patients will live with a certain disease or therapy. The probability of surviving beyond the median survival time is 50%.

Disease-Free Survival

Disease-free survival (DFS) measures the proportion (in percentage) of patients among those treated for a specific cancer who remain disease free for a specified length of time after the completion of treatment. DFS provides a short-term surrogate end point to overall survival, and allows treatment comparisons that could significantly speed the translation of results into clinical practice. Although not universal, DFS and OS are usually correlated.

Progression-Free Survival

Progression-free survival (PFS) measures the proportion (in percentage) of patients treated for a malignancy whose disease remains stable, that is, without progression after a specified time after completing the prescribed course of treatment. Progression-free survival is likely to be more useful for providing information about the control of a disease that is deemed incurable (palliative care) than any of the other survival measures discussed.

Metastasis-Free Survival

Metastasis-free survival measures the proportion (in percentage) of patients among those treated for a specific cancer who remain free of distant metastases. Unlike disease-free survival, MFS excludes local recurrence. Metastasis-free survival is a less commonly used measurement in radiation oncology research.

Event-Free Survival

Another less commonly used measurement in radiation oncology research, event-free survival measures the proportion (in percentage) of patients who remain free of an "event" after treatment. An "event" may be any adverse effect, local recurrence, or distant metastasis.

Cancer-Specific Survival

Another less commonly used measurement in radiation oncology research, cancer-specific survival (CSS) measures the proportion (in percentage) of patients who are expected to decease due to the cancer under study at a specified time. CSS excludes death due to causes unrelated to the cancer.

Local Control

Local control in radiotherapy is the most common measure of the effectiveness of radiotherapy. It is useful in measuring cure in terms of local-regional control in early stage cancer, for example, the efficacy of the use of local radiotherapy in T1N0M0 lung cancer. However, optimum local control cannot be associated with improvement in survival in patients whose cancer has a high rate of early metastasis.

The use of the measure of local control in radiotherapy is also seen in the adjuvant setting such as after wide local excision in breast cancer. Locally, the effect of radiation is not limited to direct DNA damage in cancer cells, but may also increase tumor-mediated cell kill by immunogenicity. In the Oxford overview meta-analysis of the use of adjuvant radiotherapy in breast cancer, improved local-regional control translated into an improved overall survival and breast cancer–specific survival independent of systemic therapies.

Local palliation for the relief of adverse symptoms such as pain and bleeding is a common indication for the use of radiotherapy. For example, in the case of a fungating breast cancer, local control can be measured in terms of reduction in pain, bleeding, infection, or fungation. Effective local control is commonly translated into improvement in quality of life with the absence of significant side effects.

Clinical research in optimization of local control depends on understanding of the 5 R's of radiobiology. Dose and fractionation studies with radiosensitizers exploit the potential benefits of altering repopulation, redistribution, reoxygenation, repair, and radiosensitivity of cancer cells. These represent the most common basic science and clinical research activities in radiotherapy.

Adequate local control may or may not closely correlate to overall, disease-free, or other survival measures, and should not be used as a surrogate for overall survival after a treatment.

However, it may be an important indicator in palliative settings for symptomatic control.

Quality of Life

Quality of life has become an important end point in recent clinical trials. It is no longer acceptable to give a therapy purely for its effectiveness if it causes unacceptable reduction in functional activity of daily living. Knowledge of quality of life is usually collected using Quality of Life questionnaires, which provide information and data to the investigators. The European Organization for Research and Treatment of Cancer (EORTC) group has devised multiple validated questionnaires for different cancer sites to standardize the quality of life measurement in clinical trials. The details can be found at http://groups.eortc. be/qol/index.htm. Quality of life is particularly crucial in palliative therapy when the treatment is intended to alleviate cancer-caused symptoms and not to cure the patient of the disease itself.

Therapeutic Index

The therapeutic index is defined as the ratio of improvement to the side effects of the treatment. A narrow therapeutic index means the benefit (improvement after treatment) is small when compared to the cost (side effects) from the treatment. For example, ambitious dose escalations in radiotherapy with hypofractionated treatment schedules may cause a negative impact in therapeutic index, particularly if surrounding normal tissues/organs cannot be adequately differentiated from the tumor/target(s).

The Practice of Evidence-Based Medicine in Radiation Oncology

Evidence-based medicine aims to utilize scientifically obtained evidence for use in everyday medical practice. According to its definition, it involves integrating the best available scientific evidence from systematic research on patients' disease (mostly malignancies in the field of radiation oncology), expectations, and value, as well as the oncologists' expertise in clinical decision making as depicted in Fig. 2.

Often, the science is structured into guidelines, or a systematically developed statements to assist practitioner and patient decisions about appropriate health care for specific clinical circumstances.

Clinical evidence is one of the most important elements of evidence-based medicine. However, clinical evidence alone, even obtained correctly through systematic and exhaustive research, is not sufficient for effective clinical decision making. It must be integrated with the clinical expertise of the attending oncologists as well as the patients' expectations and value. Thus, the evidence-based practice of radiation oncology involves the active participation of patients in making decisions about their cancer care. Although it is a daunting concept, the premise for using evidence to make medical decisions is simple. However, making treatment decisions based on available and accepted scientific evidence requires that consumers of medical care comprehend their

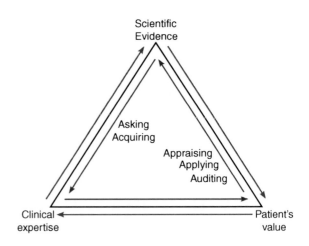

Clinical Research and the Practice of Evidence-Based Medicine in Radiation Oncology. Fig. 2 The triad of evidence-based medicine (Adapted from Radiation Oncology: An Evidence-Based Approach)

diagnosis. They must participate in a reasoned assessment of the available treatment options with an understanding of the benefits and risks associated with each.

The "5A" Practice of Evidence-Based Medicine

Radiation oncology is an ever-changing field. With the development of new technology and treatment techniques, the management of cancer using ionizing or particle radiation is evolving on a monthly, if not daily, basis. Like any other forms of therapy, applying newly developed radiation techniques (such as image-guided radiation therapy and particle therapy) or treatment strategies (such as combined chemoradiotherapy) to a particular type of malignancy, or applying existing treatment techniques proven for one type of disease to a different type of cancer, requires vigorous testing and verification before it can be considered standard of care. As a result, the field of radiation oncology is flooded with publications and literature.

While it is encouraging to observe the exponential growth in scientific research papers and literature published in this field, it is important to recognize that evaluating and understanding the scientific evidence such that one can utilize it in decision making requires proficient skills and knowledge of evidence-based medicine, as well as sufficient time and effort. Scientific evidence is one of the three integral parts of evidence-based medical practice; thus, understanding and being able to apply pertinent and best available evidence for a particular clinical question is crucial in the practice of evidence-based medicine in radiation oncology. To achieve this purpose, the following five key steps (the "5As" cycle) should be considered sequentially as shown in Fig. 3. These five steps are:

1. Formulating a clinical question (Asking)
2. Acquiring relevant and complete information (Acquiring)

3. Critically appraising the quality (including validity and importance) of available evidence, or identifying the lack of evidence (Appraising)
4. Applying the knowledge in the clinical management of patients (Applying)
5. Evaluating the results of practice (Auditing)

Critical Appraisal of Studies and Rating Clinical Evidence

Scientific evidence plays a major role in decision making of cancer management. However, the nature and quality of scientific evidence vary substantially. Results from basic science, animal, translational, as well as clinical research mentioned above can all be used as medical evidence. Further observations made in a clinician's daily practice are also considered clinical evidence. Clearly, not all evidence is created equal and sound medical judgment should be used in decision making in cancer treatment.

Evidence-based medicine, including the practice radiation oncology, seeks to assess the quality of scientific evidence relevant to the risks and benefits of treatment or lack of treatment, with the purpose of improving the health of patients by means of decisions that will maximize the quality of life and life span. Merely applying study results without critical appraisal may not only be less useful, but can be harmful or even dangerous to patients.

Evidence used in any clinical decision-making process can be categorized according to its quality based on the probability of freedom from error, and is usually classified by critical appraisal (see Fig. 4 and Table 2). The most basic aspects of critical appraisal include relevance, validity, consistency, and significance of the results. The quality of a piece of clinical evidence can be categorized based on these elements of quality.

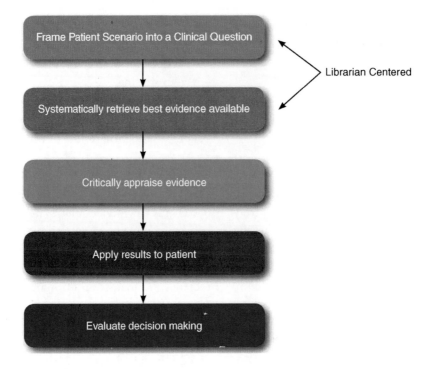

Clinical Research and the Practice of Evidence-Based Medicine in Radiation Oncology. Fig. 3 Five key steps of effective evidence-based medical practice (Adapted from UBC Health Library (2008))

Issues in the Practice of Evidence-Based Radiation Oncology

The basic principles of evidence-based medicine can largely be applied to any of the specialties in healthcare, including public health and policy making. However, specific issues encountered by clinicians in their own specialties, including radiation oncologists, affect how they practice evidence-based medicine.

Formulating a Clinical Question in Oncology

Clinical questions encountered in the practice of radiation oncology are usually individualized based on the diagnoses, patients' medical conditions, and preferences, as well as the availability of medical resources. However, as a disease category, cancer has been effectively categorized based on pathological diagnosis, differentiation, and staging. The value of the AJCC/UICC staging system on predicting outcome, thus facilitating the choice of treatment strategy for most types of cancers, has been repeatedly proven. In addition, with the development of molecular biology and genetics, other disease characteristics have been continuously discovered.

At the present time, a clinical question in cancer management can be formulated on the basis of pathologic diagnosis and cancer staging, combined with patients' characteristics and other disease-associated prognostic factors. For the purpose of knowledge development and learning, the clinical question of focus in the practice of evidence-based radiation oncology is usually "What is the most effective treatment of this malignancy at the current stage?"

Acquiring Relevant and Complete Information

Once the target question is formulated, the next step in the practice of evidence-based radiation oncology is to search for the relevant evidence.

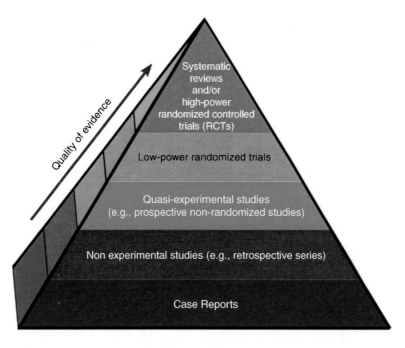

Clinical Research and the Practice of Evidence-Based Medicine in Radiation Oncology. **Fig. 4** Hierarchy of evidences. (Adapted from Radiation Oncology: An Evidence-Based Approach)

With the development of information technology and the internet, obtaining an exhaustive amount of information through literature searches using databases such as PubMed and ScienceDirect is no longer an issue. However, the problem that perturbs most practicing radiation oncologists is usually not the lack of data, but rather excessive amounts of information, often of varying quality. While all professionals aim to keep abreast of developing research, differentiating the "relevant" and "complete" information in a flood of publications usually requires an enormous amount of time and effort, and is hardly achievable.

It is usually not feasible for a clinician to find, read, and appraise all available evidence on his/her own. The time and effort needed to acquire and then critically appraise information is currently an insurmountable obstacle standing between individual clinicians and the practice of evidence-based medicine, including radiation oncologists.

Evaluating the Quality of the Evidence

As mentioned previously, not all evidence is created equal. Much of the available evidence is not clinically relevant for decision making. The quality (i.e., validity and importance) of relevant and pertinent clinical evidence varies significantly. As the practice of evidence-based medicine involves the integration of the best available scientific evidence with expertise and patients' value in patient care, the critical appraisal of evidence obtained from systematic research is crucial for identifying the best available and most relevant evidence.

To evaluate the quality of a piece of evidence, basic knowledge and skills in critical appraisal of medical publications are usually required. Often, formal training in literature research and review is necessary to attain proficiency in appraising scientific evidence. However, critical appraisal of scientific evidence is extremely time consuming

Clinical Research and the Practice of Evidence-Based Medicine in Radiation Oncology. Table 2 Levels of evidence and grade of recommendations

Level	Type of evidence
I	Evidence obtained form meta-analysis of multiple, well-designed, controlled studies. Randomized trials with low false-positive and low false-negative errors (high power)
II	Evidence obtained from at least one well-designed experimental study. Randomized trials with high false-positive and/or negative errors (low power)
III	Evidence obtained from well-designed, quasi-experimental studies such as nonrandomized, controlled, single group, pre-post, cohort, and time or matched case-control series
IV	Evidence from well designed, nonexperimental studies such as comparative and correlational descriptive and case studies
V	Evidence from case reports
Grade	Grade of recommendation
A	There is evidence of type I or consistent findings from multiple studies of type II, III, or IV
B	There is evidence of type II, III, or IV and findings are generally consistent
C	There is evidence of type II, III, or IV but findings are inconsistent
D	There is little or no systemic empirical evidence

and, as with the process of acquiring relevant and complete information, the time and effort required to critically appraise the literature comprises yet another obstruction to the practice of evidence-based radiation oncology.

It is important for clinicians to understand that, in many instances, the only evidence available is of low quality. For example, the majority of available evidence used in guiding radiation therapy for rare tumors (such as cancer of the ▶ fallopian tube, cancer of urachus) is retrospective in nature. A lack of high-quality evidence does not preclude the feasibility of practicing evidence-based medicine in the treatment of these malignancies. One can always use the current best evidence after critical appraisal, bearing in mind that even the best may be flawed.

Cross-References

▶ Evidence-Based Medicine
▶ History of Radiation Oncology
▶ Short-Term and Long-Term Health Risk of Nuclear Power Plant Accident
▶ Statistics and Clinical Trials

References

Beyer T, Townsend DW, Brun T et al (2000) A combined PET/CT scanner for clinical oncology. J Nucl Med 41:1369–1379

Hounsfield GN (1973) Computerized transverse axial scanning (tomography): part 1. Description of system. Br J Radiol 46:1016–1022

Mansfield P, Maudsley AA (1977) Medical imaging by NMR. Br J Radiol 50:188–194

Pusey WA (1902) Report of cases treated with Roentgen rays. J Am Med Assoc 38:911

Rhouds CP (1946) Nitrogen mustards in the treatment of neoplastic disease. Official statement. J Am Med Assoc 131:656–658

Sackett DL, Rosenberg WM, Gray JA et al (1996) Evidence based medicine: what it is and what it isn't. BMJ 312(7023):71–72

Senn N (1903) Case of splenomedullary leukaemia successfully treated by the use of Roentgen rays. Med Record 64:281

Simon R (1989) Optimal two-stage designs for phase II clinical trials. Control Clin Trials 10:1–10

Clinical Target Volume (CTV)

BRANDON J. FISHER[1], LARRY C. DAUGHERTY[2]
[1]Department of Radiation Oncology, College of Medicine, Drexel University, Philadelphia, PA, USA
[2]Department of Radiation Oncology, College of Medicine, Drexel University, Glenside, PA, USA

Definition
CTV includes the GTV as well as the regions of direct, local subclinical spread of disease that must be treated. The CTV often has a high tumor cell density nearest the GTV with decreasing density toward the periphery. The CTV volumes may not contain demonstrable tumor but are considered at risk, such as regional lymph nodes and their volumes, for subclinical spread.

Cross-References
▶ Nasopharynx

Clonogenic Survival Assay

CLAUDIA RÜBE
Department of Radiation Oncology,
Saarland University, Homburg/Saar, Germany

Definition
The clonogenic cell survival assay determines the ability of a cell to proliferate indefinitely, thereby retaining its reproductive ability to form a large colony or a clone. In this test, cells are grown in vitro in soft agar, which reduces cell movement and allows individual cells to develop into cell clones that are identified as single colonies.

Cross-References
▶ Predictive In vitro Assays in Radiation Oncology

Cobalt Gray Equivalent (CGE)

DANIEL YEUNG[1], JATINDER PALTA[2]
[1]Department of Radiation Oncology, University of Florida Proton Therapy Institute, Jacksonville, FL, USA
[2]Department of Radiation Oncology, University of Florida Health Science Center, Gainesville, FL, USA

Definition
An "unofficial" unit which states the equivalent biological dose and includes the RBE factor of 1.1 for protons. ICRU 78 does not recommend using CGE; instead it recommends using D_{RBE} because RBE is a dimensionless quantity and therefore the unit of dose remains unchanged (Gy).

Cross-References
▶ Chordomas
▶ Proton Therapy

Colectomy

BRADLEY J. HUTH
Department of Radiation Oncology,
Philadelphia, PA, USA

Synonyms
Bowel resection

Definition
This describes surgical resection of one more portions of the colon. Traditionally, this was performed through an open laparotomy. More recently, minimally invasive techniques including laparoscopic, single-port access and robotic-assisted procedures have become readily available. Minimally invasive techniques have resulted in

less blood loss, less time under anesthesia, quicker recovery, and shorter hospitalization. A steep learning curve remains in this highly technical trade.

Cross-References

► Colon Cancer
► Rectal Cancer

Collagen Vascular Disease

ANTHONY E. DRAGUN
Department of Radiation Oncology, James Graham Brown Cancer Center, University of Louisville School of Medicine, Louisville, KY, USA

Synonyms

Connective tissue disorders

Definition

This is a group of diseases, such as rheumatoid arthritis, systemic lupus erythematosus, scleroderma, dermatomyositis, and others, thought to impart an increased risk of acute and late radiation-induced sequelae. Single institution studies conflict with regard to the risk or degree of increased toxicity. Caution is advised in patients under active treatment for collagen vascular disease at the time of breast cancer therapy, but these disorders are not, in and of themselves, an absolute contraindication for breast-conserving therapy.

Cross-References

► Acute Radiation Syndrome
► Breast Conservation Therapy
► Early-Stage Breast Cancer
► Late Radiation Toxicity

Collimator-Based Tissue Compensation

Definition

Devices attached to linear accelerators to develop beam dose manipulations to increase dose homogeneity over varied tissue densities or surfaces.

Cross-References

► Conformal Therapy: Treatment Planning, Treatment Delivery, and Clinical Results
► Electron Dosimetry and Treatment
► Forward-Planning
► Intensity Modulated Radiation Therapy
► Proton Therapy
► Radiation Oncology Physics

Colon Cancer

BRADLEY J. HUTH
Department of Radiation Oncology, Philadelphia, PA, USA

Synonyms

Adenocarcinoma of the colon; Bowel cancer; Cancer colon; Cancer intestine; Cancer of the Colon; Cancer of the large intestine; Carcinoma of the colon; Colonic cancer; Colorectal cancer; Intestinal cancer

Definition

The colon and rectum form the terminal portions of the gastrointestinal tract. The colorectum begins at ileocecal valve and ends at the anus. This entry will focus on the colon extending from the ileocecal valve to the distal sigmoid colon junction with the rectum. The colon can be subdivided, from proximal to distal, into the cecum and appendix, ascending colon, hepatic flexure, transverse colon, splenic flexure, descending colon, and sigmoid colon. The appendix is a blind pouch arising from the cecum. The appendix normally measures 10 cm but can range from 2 to 20 cm. The colon commonly measures 1.5 m in length. One variation on the normal anatomy of the colon occurs when extra loops form, resulting in a longer than normal organ. This condition, referred to as redundant colon, typically has no direct major health consequences. The colon is mainly responsible for storing waste, reclaiming water, maintaining the water balance, absorbing some vitamins, and providing a location for flora-aided fermentation. As stool moves through the bowel, water is absorbed and stool becomes firm and formed. Over its course through the abdomen, the colon has both intraperitoneal and retroperitoneal portions. Blood to the colon is primarily supplied through the superior and inferior mesenteric arteries, which drain into the portal vein. The vast majority of colorectal cancers arise from the mucosa. More than 90% of these mucosal lesions are adenocarcinomas, but carcinoid, small cell, and lymphoid tumors are not unheard of. Metastases most commonly spread to regional mesenteric lymph nodes, the liver, peritoneal cavity, and lung.

Background

Colorectal cancer is the third most common cancer diagnosed in the USA in both men and women, excluding skin cancers. In 2009, there were an estimated 106,100 new cases of colon cancer and 40,870 new cases of rectal cancer deaths in the USA, with a lifetime risk of 1 in 19 (American Cancer Society, 2011). There were an estimated 49,920 deaths from colorectal cancer. Worldwide, nearly one million new cases of colorectal cancer are diagnosed with approximately 529,000 deaths. Colon cancer is a disease of adults. Ninety percent of new patients are over 50 years. The median age at diagnosis is 72 years.

The molecular progression from normal to benign polyposis to malignant tumor has been well described. The multifactorial process ultimately leads to inactivation of ▶ tumor suppressor gene adenomatous polyposis coli (APC) and tissue-protein 53 (P53), and activation of ▶ proto-oncogene, such as ras. The specific environmental causes of colon cancers are unclear in the vast majority of cases. Increased risk may be associated with increasing age, male sex, increasing body mass index, processed meats, high alcohol intake, inflammatory bowel disease, tobacco usage, family and personal history of gastrointestinal polyposis or cancer, and a low consumption of fruits and vegetables. Prevention may be possible through dietary means, increased activity, and abstinence from tobacco and alcohol consumption. Chemoprevention through carentenoids, aspirin, and nonsteroidal anti-inflammatory drugs is currently under investigation.

Nearly 10% of colon cancers arise as part of a hereditary syndrome. The two most common syndromes are ▶ Familial Adenomatous Polyposis (FAP) and ▶ Hereditary Nonpolyposis Colorectal Cancer (HNPCC). FAP is an autosomal dominant disorder of the APC gene with variable penetrance. Nearly 50% of carriers will develop adenomas by age 15 years and greater than 90% by age 35 years. Classic cases present with hundreds of polyps throughout the colorectum. Treatment is total ▶ colectomy and is done during the teenage years. If untreated, all patients will develop carcinoma. HNPCC is also autosomal dominant and is more common than APC. The disorder is associated with a germ-line mutation in at least one mismatch repair gene (MSH2, MSH6, MLH1, PMS1, or PMS2). HNPCC results in ▶ microsatellite instability (MSI), which may be associated with a more favorable prognosis. In addition to the risk of colon malignancy, HNPCC-carriers have an increased risk of developing endometrial, ovarian, gastric, urothelial, and small bowel malignancies. Screening colonoscopy is performed every 2–3 years beginning at age 20 years then annually at age 40 years.

Detection and removal of benign polyps leads to prevention of progression to malignancy. Early detection can be performed though a variety of measures. Colonoscopy is the gold standard of screening and is recommend beginning at age 50 years in the general population. Following a thorough bowel cleansing, the colon is inflated with air and the colonoscope is advanced through the anus to the ileocecal valve. Working channels on the instrument permit biopsy, resection, and tattooing of concerning lesions. Following a normal exam, patients may go for 10 years without another assessment. If benign lesions are identified, repeat colonoscopy is performed after 2–3 years. ► Fecal occult blood test is quite sensitive for blood but less specific than direct visualization methods. Fecal occult testing should be combined with either flexible ► sigmoidoscopy or double contrast barium enema. If abnormalities are found, colonoscopy should be performed. Virtual colonoscopy may be performed using either high-resolution computed tomography (CT) imaging with three-dimensional reconstruction or by swallowing an encapsulated digital camera and strobe light fitted with a radiofrequency transmitter. Both methods are performed in selected patients in whom colonoscopy is contraindicated or technically unfeasible. Such can occur in patients with redundant colon where additional pediatric instruments and tools may be helpful.

Initial Evaluation

The initial work-up of patients with suspected colon cancer should include a complete history and physical exam, detailed family history, digital rectal exam, fecal occult blood testing, and complete colonoscopy with biopsy. A complete colonoscopy is important to assess for synchronous primaries found in 3% of patients. For female patients with suspected advanced disease, a complete gynecologic examination should be performed.

The signs and symptoms of colon cancer vary by stage and location within the organ. Early disease is often asymptomatic, while some patients describe ill-defined abdominal discomfort, flatulence, minor changes in bowel movements, or blood in the stool. Frequently, occult blood is found on routine stool testing. Left-sided cancers frequently result in alternating diarrhea and constipation and obstructive symptoms, such as nausea and vomiting. Right-sided lesions are more subtle causing anemia due to chronic blood loss, weight loss, or a palpable abdominal mass. Radiating back or pelvic pain is indicative of local extension into extra peritoneal nerves. Abdominal ascites or palpable abdominal wall adenopathy, such as ► Sister Mary Joseph's node, raise the suspicion of peritoneal carcinomatosis. Hepatomegaly and disturbance of liver functions are common in patients with metastatic disease.

Differential Diagnosis

The differential diagnosis varies by the presenting symptoms. Positive fecal occult tests could indicate parasitic infection, benign hemorrhoids, anal fissure, arteriovascular malformations, or contamination from menstrual bleeding or urinary tract disorders. Obstructive symptoms could be caused by benign strictures, volvulus, stool impaction, bezoars, or hernias. Colonic lesions found at routine colonoscopy could be hyperplastic polyps, inflammatory polyps, benign hamartomas, or neoplastic polyps such as tubular, tubulovillous, and villous adenomas. Abdominal distention with ascites raises the question of hepatobiliary disease, ovarian cancer in women or primary peritoneal cancer in both men and women, or infection.

Imaging Studies

Prior to definitive therapy, a chest X-ray and CT imaging of the abdomen and pelvis with both intravenous and oral contrast agents is recommended. Areas concerning for metastatic disease may further be evaluated by positron emission tomography (PET), magnetic resonance imaging (MRI) with and without gadolinium, or ultrasound to determine feasibility of curative resection.

Laboratory Studies

Prior to definitive treatment, laboratory blood analysis should include a complete blood count, liver enzymes, renal functions, and carcinoembryonic antigen level (CEA). The CEA is prognostic as values under 5 ng/mL carry a more favorable outcome and lower disease burden. A serum beta-human chorionic gonadotropin (β-hcg) should be drawn in women of child-bearing age.

Treatment

The sequence of definitive therapy and role of neoadjuvant or adjuvant therapy is established by the stage. Current staging is based on the American Joint Committee on Cancer (AJCC) seventh edition enacted in January 2010 (American Joint Commission on Cancer 2010). This staging system follows the tumor, node, and metastasis (TNM) algorithm. Discussion of the nuances of the TNM staging is beyond the scope of this book and readers are referred to the AJCC staging manual for full details. The basic principles of staging for all lumenal organs of the gastrointestinal (GI) track are listed in Table 1. Stage I includes T1/T2 tumors without nodal spread. Stage II includes T3/T4 tumors without nodal spread. Stage III includes T1 through T4 tumors and is subdivided by the number of lymph nodes evaluated, involved, and the presence of extranodal mesenteric tumor deposits. Stage IV includes any tumor and any amount of nodal involvement with metastatic disease. Stage IV is also subdivided by the number of metastatic foci.

Surgery remains the definitive therapy for colon carcinomas and is done with curative intent in more than 75% of patients. Open laparotomy with partial bowel resection is the current standard of care. Both laparoscopic and robotic procedures are becoming more common in experienced hands. Both procedures boast less blood loss and faster recovery time as compared to open procedures. Curative resection requires wide proximal and distal margins as mucosal carcinomas may track along the submucosa. Resection of the bowel along named blood vessels including the regional lymphatics removes potential disease spread. The number of resected lymph nodes correlates with survival. A minimum of 12 lymph nodes should be evaluated from which the ratio of positive to negative nodes is

Colon Cancer. Table 1 Colon cancer tumor stage

Tumor stage	
Tis	Carcinoma in situ
T1	Invades submucosa
T2	Invades muscularis propria
T3	Invades through muscularis propria into pericolorectal tissue
T4a	Penetration to visceral peritoneum
T4b	Invades adjacent structures
Nodal stage	
N0	No nodal metastasis
N1	One to three nodal metastasis or peritoneal tumor deposits without involved nodes
N2	Four or more nodal metastasis
Distant metastasis	
M0	No distant metastasis
M1	Metastasis to one or more sites

prognostic. In the setting of limited metastatic disease, most commonly to the liver, a sequential, or staged, resection of the primary tumor and metastatic disease can be done.

Disease-specific survival at 5 years following surgery alone for T1 tumors is greater than 95% and greater than 85% for T2 tumors. Survival drops quickly to approximately 70% with deeper extension of tumor or limited nodal spread with surgery alone raising the need for adjuvant therapy. For more extensive disease, adjuvant therapy has shown benefit in overall and disease-free survival. The backbone of adjuvant therapy in colon carcinomas is systemic chemotherapy. 5-fluorouracil (5FU) based chemotherapy has long been the gold standard. 5FU is intravenously infused, generally over a long, continuous infusion. Continuous infusion 5FU requires patients to wear a pump for up to 96 h while therapy is delivered. More recently, an oral 5FU equivalent, capecitabine, has become widely available with equivalent outcomes to infusional 5FU. 5FU is commonly combined with either platinum agents, such as oxaliplatin, topoisomerase inhibitors, such as irinotecan, or biologic agents that target aberrant growth factors, receptors, or their downstream molecular cascades. Overall survival at 5 years ranges from 73% for patients with T1/T2, N1 disease to 28% for T4, N2, and 5% for Stage IV. Five-year survival rates and the associated stage are listed in Table 2.

The predominant site of relapse in colon cancer is distant from the primary site so the role of radiotherapy is limited. The risk of local failure correlates with the ability for the surgeon to achieve wide surgical margins. The risk of local recurrence increases with deeper invasion, retroperitoneal location in the bowel, extension into adjacent tissues, and amount of mesentery present for resection. Multiple single-institution, retrospective series have shown that following surgery alone there is a greater than 30% risk of local failure in deeply invasive lesions and those

Colon Cancer. Table 2 Overall survival at 5 years by AJCC seventh edition stage

Stage	Overall survival (%)
I	74
IIa	67
IIb	59
IIc	37
IIIa	73
IIIb	46
IIIc	28
IV	6

adherent to adjacent tissues (Czito & Willett 2007). For patients treated with surgery followed by adjuvant radiation had a 20% absolute benefit in local control. This translated to a statistically significant improvement in relapse-free survival in patients with T4 tumors. The Intergroup began a prospective, cooperative study in the late 1990s to evaluate the role of the addition of radiotherapy to adjuvant systemic therapy. The trial closed early due to poor accrual. The results of the trial were published, despite being severely underpowered, and failed to show a benefit of the addition of radiotherapy.

Radiotherapy planning is accomplished using CT-based simulation and immobilization to limit motion to 5 mm or less. Oral contrast delineates the bowel. Intravenous contrast is encouraged for identification of the vascular structures. The field design will vary depending on the location within the bowel. The tumor bed is outlined on the axial imaging. An additional 3–4 cm margin is applied to the tumor bed. For right-sided tumors, surgical resection of the mesentery is limited by a shared blood supply between the colon and small intestine. Here, an additional margin covering the mesentery may be employed, if an adequate number of lymph nodes could not be removed. A dose of 45 Gray (Gy) is prescribed. An additional boost of 5–9 Gy may be delivered to the remaining gross disease if one can meet dose constraints to the surrounding small bowel and kidney (Mohiuddin et al. 2008). Small portions of the small bowel can tolerate 50 Gy, but the risks of ulceration, bleeding, and bowel obstruction rises quickly with increasing volumes of bowel. Two-thirds of one kidney should receive less than 20 Gy. The liver may receive 30 Gy to less than two-thirds of the organ. The number of fields and design will vary depending on the location in the abdomen and proximity to surrounding normal structures.

Patients suffering from limited metastatic disease to the liver may undergo ablation of the malignant spread through multiple means. Surgical resection, chemo-embolization, radio-frequency ablation, cryotherapy, infusion of Yttrium-90 microspheres, and external beam radiotherapy have all been shown to be effective. More recently, stereotactic body radiotherapy (SBRT) delivering doses up to 60 Gy in three treatments has been shown to be effective in multi-institutional prospective trials. General use of SBRT in nonacademic centers has not been accepted for the treatment of liver lesions.

Following completion of the initial treatment course, patients are followed closely for signs of recurrence and to manage late complications of therapy. Routine office evaluation and serum CEA level are performed every 3–6 months for the first 2 years then every 6 months for 5 years. CT imaging of the abdomen and pelvis is performed annually for the first 3 years. A colonoscopy is done 1 year following the completion of therapy (National Comprehensive Cancer Network 2010).

Cross-References

▶ Cervical Cancer
▶ Conformal Therapy: Treatment Planning, Treatment Delivery, and Clinical Results
▶ Liver and Hepatobiliary Tract
▶ Ovarian Cancer
▶ Principles of Surgical Oncology
▶ Stereotactic Radiosurgery: Extracranial

References

American Cancer Society (2011) Colorectal cancer. American Cancer Society, Atlanta
American Joint Commission on Cancer (2010) Colon and rectum. In: Edge SB, Byrd DR, Compton CC, Fritz AG, Greene FL, Trotti A (eds) AJCC cancer staging manual, 7th edn. Springer, New York
Czito BG, Willett CG (2007) Colon Cancer. In: Gunderson LL, Tepper JE (eds) Clinical radiation oncology, 2nd edn. Elsevier/Churchill/Livingstone, Philadelphia
Mohiuddin M, Czito BG, Willett CG (2008) Colon and rectum. In: Halperin EC, Perez CA, Brady LW (eds) Principles and practice of radiation oncology, 5th edn. Wolters Kluwer/Lippincott Williams & Wilkins, Philadelphia
National Comprehensive Cancer Network (2010) NCCN clinical practice guidelines in oncology: uterine neoplasms, V.1.2010. http://www.nccn.org/professionals/physician_gls/PDF/colon.pdf. Accessed 20 February 2010

Colonic Cancer

▶ Colon Cancer

Colonoscopy

BRADLEY J. HUTH
Department of Radiation Oncology, Philadelphia, PA, USA

Synonyms
Endoscopy

Definition
Colonoscopy is a minimally invasive procedure during which a long endoscope is used to examine the rectum and colon from the distal rectum to the ileocecal valve. Direct visualization of the bowel is done following thorough bowel cleansing and inflation with air. The scope has multiple

channels which permit biopsy, resection, and tattooing of concerning lesions for easy identification during follow-up or surgery.

Cross-References

▶ Colon Cancer
▶ Rectal Cancer

Colorectal Cancer

▶ Colon Cancer

Colorectal Metastases to Liver

▶ Palliation of Metastatic Disease to the Liver

Combined Modality Therapy

Definition

Utilization of multiple interventions to treat a disorder or disease state.

Cross-References

▶ Concurrent Chemoradiotherapy
▶ Induction Chemotherapy
▶ Radioimmunotherapy (RIT)

Comet Assay

CLAUDIA E. RÜBE
Department of Radiation Oncology, Saarland University, Homburg/Saar, Germany

Definition

Electrophoresis technique for the detection of single-strand and double-strand breaks at the single cell level. It involves the encapsulation of cells in low-melting-point agarose suspension, lysis of the cells in neutral or alkaline conditions, and electrophoresis of the suspended lysed cells.

Cross-References

▶ Predictive In vitro Assays in Radiation Oncology

Commission on Accreditation of Medical Physics Education Programs, Inc.

JAY E. REIFF
Department of Radiation Oncology, College of Medicine, Drexel University, Philadelphia, PA, USA

Synonyms
CAMPEP

Definition

A body jointly sponsored by the American College of Radiology (ACR), the American Association of Physicists in Medicine (AAPM), and the American College of Medical Physics (ACMP) which accredits graduate education programs, residency education programs, professional degree programs, private practice education programs, and continuing education programs in medical physics (http://campep. org/).

Cross-References

▶ Radiation Oncology Physics

Complementary and Alternative Medicine (CAM)

THEODORE E. YAEGER
Department Radiation Oncology,
Wake Forest University School of Medicine,
Winston-Salem, NC, USA

Definition

Nontraditional medicine (also alternative, complementary, nonconventional, or complementary and alternative medicine [CAM]).

Cross-References

▶ Complementary Medicine

Complementary Medicine

THEODORE E. YAEGER
Department Radiation Oncology,
Wake Forest University School of Medicine,
Winston-Salem, NC, USA

Synonyms

Acupuncture; Anthroposcopic; Chiropractic; Complementary and Alternative Medicine (CAM); Herbalism; Homeopathy; Naturopathy

Definition

Also known as alternative medicine commonly practiced based on historical or cultural traditions rather than on rigorous scientific evidence as in allopathic or modern medicine. More recently becoming 'integrative medicine' when used in conjunction with allopathic treatments.

Cross-References

▶ Conventional Medicine
▶ Supportive Care

Complement-Dependent Cytotoxicity (CDC)

TOD W. SPEER
Department of Human Oncology, University of Wisconsin School of Medicine and Public Health, UW Hospital and Clinics, Madison, WI, USA

Definition

The immune process by which the antibody–antigen complex activates a cascade of proteolytic enzymes that ultimately results in the formation of a terminal lytic complex that is inserted into a cell membrane, resulting in lysis and cell death.

Cross-References

▶ Targeted Radioimmunotherapy

Concept of Hyperthermia

ANTHONY E. DRAGUN[1], CARSTEN NIEDER[2]
[1]Department of Radiation Oncology, James Graham Brown Cancer Center, University of Louisville School of Medicine, Louisville, KY, USA
[2]Radiation Oncology Unit, Nordlandssykehuset HF, Bodoe, Norway

Definition

Hyperthermia therapy is temperature created artificially for the treatment of various cancers often in conjunction with chemotherapy and radiotherapy.

Microwave hyperthermia (to a temperature of approximately 43-C for approximately 10 min) concurrent with the administration of external beam radiotherapy results in clinical complete response rates approaching 70% for patients with chest wall recurrence treated nonsurgically. Hyperthermia may also be combined with concurrent systemic chemotherapy. The response rates to microwave hyperthermia, as a radiosensitizing technique, are generally highest for patients with low volume, noninflammatory breast cancer recurrences.

Cross-References
► Hyperthermia
► Sarcoma
► Sarcomas of the Head and Neck
► Stage 0 Breast Cancer

Concomitant Treatment

FILIP T. TROICKI[1], JAGANMOHAN POLI[2]
[1]College of Medicine, Drexel University, Philadelphia, PA, USA
[2]Department of Radiation Oncology, College of Medicine, Drexel University, Philadelphia, PA, USA

Definition
Different therapies that occur simultaneously, as in simultaneous use of chemotherapy and radiation.

Concurrent Chemoradiation

VOLKER BUDACH
Department of Radiotherapy and Radiation Oncology, Charité - University Hospital Berlin, Berlin, Germany

Definition
The use of chemotherapy delivered concurrently with radiation. Either chemotherapy can act as a radiosensitizer, improving the probability of local control and potentially the survival, by aiding the destruction of radio-resistant clones, or it can be used with organ-preserving intent, resulting in improved function and/or cosmetic results compared with surgical resection with/without adjuvant treatment. In addition, chemotherapy given as part of concurrent chemoradiation may act systemically and potentially prevent distant metastases.

Cross-References
► Hodgkin's Lymphoma
► Larynx
► Lung
► Oro-Hypopharynx
► Uterine Cervix

Confidence Interval

EDWARD J. GRACELY
Department of Epidemiology and Biostatistics, College of Medicine, Drexel University, Philadelphia, PA, USA

Definition
An interval around a sample statistic intended to have a certain (often 95%) probability of containing the population value of that statistic.

Cross-References
► Statistics and Clinical Trials

Conformal

TIMOTHY HOLMES
Department of Radiation Oncology, Sinai Hospital, Baltimore, MD, USA

Definition
This refers to conformal radiotherapy (CRT), a form of external beam radiotherapy that uses

multiple (typically 3–6) non-coplanar radiation beams shaped to the tumor volume to deliver a high dose to the tumor while reducing dose to the surrounding non-tumor tissues.

Cross-References

▶ Image-Guided Radiation Therapy (IGRT): TomoTherapy

Conformal Therapy: Treatment Planning, Treatment Delivery, and Clinical Results

DANIEL J. SCANDERBEG
Department of Radiation Oncology, John and Rebecca Moores Comprehensive Cancer Center, University of California, San Diego, La Jolla, CA, USA

Definition

Three dimensional conformal radiotherapy (3DCRT) is targeted radiotherapy based on three dimensional (3D) imaging of the patient and is the basis for advanced treatment modalities available today.

Background

Despite the advent of these advanced treatment techniques, such as intensity modulated radiation therapy (IMRT) and stereotactic radiosurgery (SRS), three-dimensional conformal radiotherapy remains a common and effective treatment modality used in most clinics today. Using 3D imaging, a physician can assess the disease (target) extent while identifying normal organs in close proximity to the target that are at risk of damage from radiotherapy. The dosimetry and physics team can then create a treatment plan that conforms to the target, while minimizing exposure to the surrounding normal tissues, or organs at risk (OARs). Radiation therapists use immobilization devices to accurately reproduce patient setup from the initial imaging study and deliver the prescribed treatment plan. Working together, the radiation oncology team can prepare a highly conformal treatment to maximize target coverage while minimizing dose to normal tissue.

The major advantage of 3DCRT is the conformal dose that allows high doses to be given to the target while not overdosing surrounding normal tissue. Most experts would agree that a major disadvantage to a conformal treatment is the uncertainty in the true spatial extent of the disease. However, since this is true for all conformal treatments, this drawback is not specific to 3DCRT, but is also present in IMRT and SRS treatments. Even with advanced imaging techniques, it can be difficult to discern the clinical target volume (CTV), which includes both the visible and microscopic disease. Often, imaging will only show the gross tumor volume (GTV), or visible disease, and so if care is not taken and proper margins are not added to the GTV, disease could be missed.

There are several key components for 3DCRT that include 3D imaging, patient immobilization devices, 3D planning software, and a teletherapy machine capable of delivering the planned treatment; each of these ingredients are described below.

Basic Characteristics

Imaging

Imaging is a key component of 3DCRT, with the current standard being computed tomography (CT) for each patient. Additional imaging modalities that can aid in target localization and delineation include, but are not limited to, magnetic resonance imaging (MRI), ultrasound (US), and positron emission tomography (PET). These additional imaging studies can be registered, or fused, with the planning CT scan. With this information, 3D anatomy, including the target and surrounding normal tissue, can be mapped and used to create an optimal treatment plan.

Each of the modalities listed above are succinctly described in the following sections; however, the reader is referred to Bushberg (Bushberg et al. 2003) for more detailed descriptions of the techniques.

Computed Tomography (CT)

Computed tomography allows individual cross-sectional planes of a patient to be constructed. Typically, a patient is setup on the CT table with some immobilization devices used to reproducibly position the patient for future therapy and also to help keep any patient motion to a minimum. The table then moves through the gantry, which contains an x-ray source, along with a circular array of detectors. The x-ray source will make one revolution around the patient at each indexed position of the table, before the table moves to the next position, followed by another revolution of the x-ray source around the patient. Helical, or spiral, CT scans are also available on modern machines, which speed up the scan time by moving the table continuously through the gantry while the x-ray source revolves around the patient. Helical scanners can be used to take scans as a function of time, which allows tumor tracking as a function of the respiratory cycle (4D CT or respiratory gating).

The three dimensional data can be used to reconstruct images in any plane, thus it is necessary to take images with sufficiently small slice thickness to allow high quality interpolation and reconstruction. In addition to localization of the disease, the CT scan can also be used for tissue inhomogeneity corrections in the treatment planning process. A CT calibration curve can be established in order to associate CT numbers (or Hounsfield units) with linear attenuation coefficients. Hounsfield units are defined as:

$$HU = (\mu_{tissue} - \mu_{water})/\mu_{water} \times 1,000$$

The Hounsfield unit scale ranges from –1,000 for air to +1,000 for bone, with water in between those two values at 0.

Some of the advantages of CT scans are the fast scan times, the relationship to linear attenuation coefficients, and imaging of bony anatomy. One of the biggest drawbacks is poor soft tissue imaging, which can lead to the necessity of the complimentary imaging modalities listed below for certain disease sites. These additional modalities can be fused with a CT scan and most modern treatment planning systems allow contouring on any of the images (Fig. 1).

Magnetic Resonance Imaging (MRI)

Magnetic resonance imaging uses high magnetic fields coupled with radiofrequency signals to image a patient. It is usually used in combination with computed tomography scanning (Fig. 2). The biggest advantage of MRI is the soft tissue imaging capability that is especially useful for imaging disease sites such as those in the brain, neck, or prostate. Additionally, it does not expose the patient to ionizing radiation. However, some of the drawbacks to MRI are long scan times and no information related to tissue heterogeneity.

Ultrasound (US)

Ultrasound imaging utilizes sound waves to probe the areas of interest in the patient and produce images; hence, one of the big advantages to US, like MRI, is the lack of exposure to ionizing radiation. Ultrasound imaging is also less

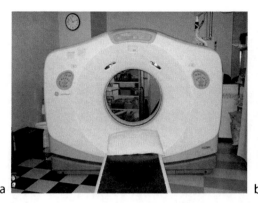
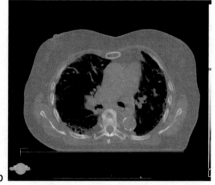

a   b

Conformal Therapy: Treatment Planning, Treatment Delivery, and Clinical Results. Fig. 1 Computed tomography. (**a**) GE Lightspeed RT CT scanner. (**b**) Axial image from a CT scan

expensive than computed tomography or magnetic resonance imaging. Drawbacks include poor imaging near bony structures or air interfaces (Fig. 3).

Positron Emission Tomography (PET)

Positron emission tomography is a nuclear medicine procedure that is growing in popularity and is regularly coupled with a CT scanner system to produce PET/CT data sets that are automatically fused at a common user origin. PET images can be difficult to register with CT images if taken separately, since PET images show areas of high metabolic activity and not anatomic information. However, when coupled with the anatomical information from a CT scan, a PET/CT is a powerful tool in radiation oncology (Fig. 4).

Immobilization Devices

Accurate patient positioning is a major component to successful patient treatment. In order to achieve accurate patient positioning and reproducibly over the course of imaging and treatment, there is a need for immobilization devices. These devices keep a patient secure and in a well defined geometry and minimize any patient movement (excluding internal organ motion). There are advantages and disadvantages to all devices and it is important to research all of the types on the market with clinical implementation in mind. Before investing in a certain technology, there should be discussions between all parties (therapists, dosimetrists, physicists, and physicians) to hear all aspects of the treatment process and how a particular device will fit the clinic. A large number of treatment devices exist because of the many factors involved in choosing an appropriate device for a certain tumor in a certain patient. Several factors include type of tumor and location, positional accuracy desired, and patient comfort and support. Additional factors include connectivity and integration with existing departmental equipment, budget for equipment (initial outlay and recurring costs), and setup time, to name a few. Device complexity can also vary widely from something as simple as tape and/or Velcro straps to as elaborate as invasive standoffs or screws into a patient's skull to affix a head frame. Khan (Khan 2007) provides a good overview and description of many types of devices and their suppliers as the list is quite vast and too numerous to list or describe here.

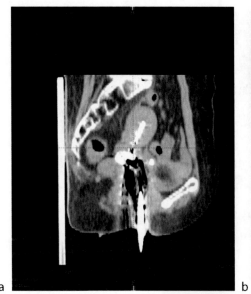

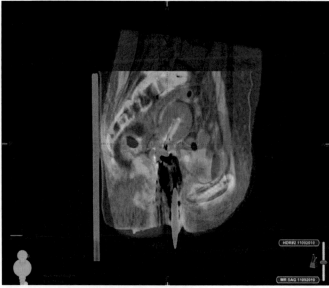

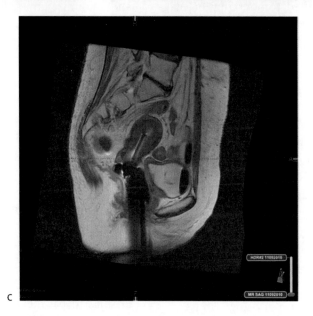

Conformal Therapy: Treatment Planning, Treatment Delivery, and Clinical Results. Fig. 2 CT and MRI images. (**a**) Sagittal CT images. (**b**) CT/MRI images fused and blended. (**c**) Sagittal MRI images

The following is a list of a variety of popular devices used:

Polyurethane foam casts

Vacuum bags

Thermoplastics

Foam wedges

Neck rolls

Tilt/slant/breast boards

Prone breast board

Belly board

Bite-block

Stereotactic head frames

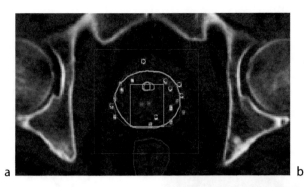 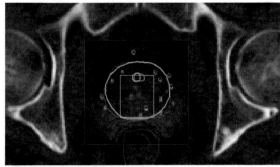

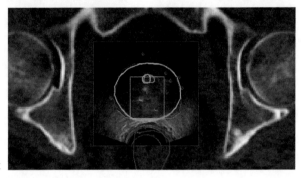

Conformal Therapy: Treatment Planning, Treatment Delivery, and Clinical Results. Fig. 3 Computed tomography and ultrasound images. (**a**) Axial CT image. (**b**) CT/US images fused and blended. (**c**) Axial US image

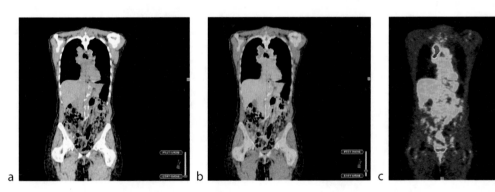

Conformal Therapy: Treatment Planning, Treatment Delivery, and Clinical Results. Fig. 4 Computed tomography and positron emission tomography images. (**a**) Coronal CT scan. (**b**) CT/PET images registered and blended. (**c**) PET image

These immobilization devices are introduced to the patient at the time of imaging. Patients are placed in the treatment position and the devices are made or molded to the patient's anatomy before imaging. The devices are stored in the clinic and retrieved for each treatment visit. The patient is then setup on the treatment unit based on the immobilization device and patient marks.

Structures

There are broadly two classes of structures in 3DCRT: the target(s) and organs at risk. Organs at risk include all of the surrounding normal tissue near the target. The primary goal of 3DCRT is to maximally dose the target, or targets, while giving the minimal possible dose to the OARs.

Target

The target can be broken down into a number of components, which are listed and defined below (ICRU 1993; ICRU 1999):

GTV – Gross Tumor Volume – Any palpable mass or visible tumor on imaging

CTV – Clinical Target Volume – Tumor volume that includes GTV, plus a margin to include any microscopic disease not visible on imaging

PTV – Planning Target Volume – Tumor volume that includes CTV, plus a margin to include any patient setup errors

GTV + margin = CTV and CTV + margin = PTV

After imaging, it is necessary to contour the gross tumor volume on the CT images. Once the tumor volume is segmented, the CTV can be constructed by adding a margin to include any areas with a high probability of disease that is not readily apparent on the images. Finally, the CTV can be transformed to the PTV by adding additional margin to account for interfraction variability in patient setup as well as intrafraction motion, such as that caused by patient breathing (Fig. 5).

Organs at Risk (Oars)

Organs at risk are any organs surrounding the target that are at risk of receiving a high dose of radiation. With modern linear accelerators, it is possible to shape the beam to accurately conform to the tumor volume and thus spare, or limit dose to, the OARs (Fig. 6). OARs vary with disease site and need to be contoured to produce a dose volume histogram (DVH) that aids in evaluation of a treatment plan.

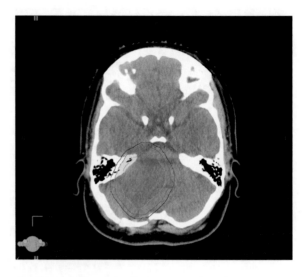

Conformal Therapy: Treatment Planning, Treatment Delivery, and Clinical Results. Fig. 5 Axial CT image showing the gross tumor volume (GTV) (*orange*), clinical target volume (CTV) expansion (*blue*), and planning target volume (PTV) expansion (*red*) for a patient with a glioblastoma multiforme

Treatment Planning

Treatment planning is a complex topic with multiple variations depending on type of disease, location of disease, available treatment modalities, and therapy equipment. The reader is referred to Khan for a more thorough introduction to treatment planning (Khan 2007) and also the physics behind dose calculations and treatment (Khan 2010). In general, there are several necessary components to treatment planning: simulation, beam configuration, dosimetric calculation, and plan evaluation.

Simulation

Before CT-based simulations, there were conventional simulators. A conventional simulator is a radiographic/fluoroscopic machine that looks similar to the therapy unit. It has a gantry and collimator that mimic the motion of the therapy machine. However, they are equipped with a diagnostic (kV) x-ray tube. In this way, once

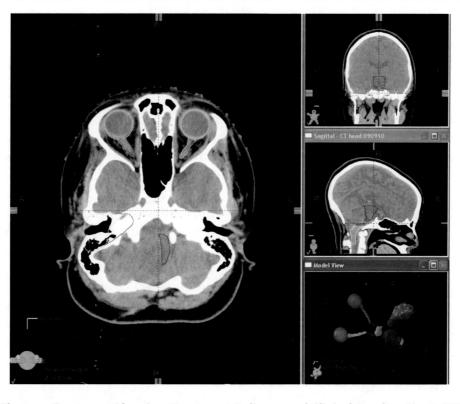

Conformal Therapy: Treatment Planning, Treatment Delivery, and Clinical Results. Fig. 6 CT images and model view displaying the target structure and OARs in the brain of a patient treated for glioblastoma multiforme

gantry angles were determined, a patient could be setup on the simulator and the gantry/collimator angles could be simulated and imaged. This allowed direct visualization of the treatment field with internal and external patient anatomy. A therapy machine can also be used to image the treatment fields with port films (see also section Treatment Planning); however, this takes time that could otherwise be used to treat patients and the MV therapy beam produces a poorer quality image than the diagnostic beam. Despite some advantages of having a conventional simulator, many radiation oncology departments have replaced their conventional simulators, as they take a considerable amount of room, and replaced them with CT scanners.

Beam Configuration

Beam configuration refers to the process by which the treatment planner determines the optimal beam angles by which to treat the disease site. Modern treatment planning systems have virtual simulations that can aid in this process. Beams eye view (BEV) allows the planner to look at the patient from the perspective of the beam entering the patient. This makes it possible to optimize the gantry angle(s) in order to avoid sensitive normal tissue surrounding the target. Some treatment planning systems also display a virtual treatment room so it is possible to visualize the patient on the table and avoid gantry angles that could cause problems; for example, angles that could lead to a collision between the gantry and couch or patient.

Field shaping is achieved through the use of collimator jaws, blocks, and multileaf collimators (MLCs) (Boyer 1996). The collimator jaws can be set for rectangular field shapes. Blocks are not commonly used as multileaf collimators are standard on modern linear accelerators and allow for precise field shaping to almost any size or shape.

Dose Calculations

Once the beams have been designed and prescription entered, it is possible to calculate the dose distribution. There are three broad types of dose calculation algorithms: correction based, model based, and direct calculation. Correction based algorithms are based on measured data but are infrequently used with the advancement of model-based and direct calculation methods. Model based (example: Convolution-superposition) is the most common method used by commercial planning systems. However, vendors are moving toward integrating more direct calculations in commercial software. One example is Acuros, which is commercially available from Varian Medical Systems, Inc., and directly solves radiation transport equations. This numerical method combines the accuracy of Monte Carlo with the speed of a model based calculation. The reader is referred to Mackie et al. for discussion of dose calculations (Mackie et al. 1996; Mackie et al. 2007).

Plan Evaluation: Dose Volume Histogram (DVH)

Plan evaluation is typically carried out by evaluating the dose volume histogram, which is a graph summarizing the dose delivered to any defined structure. There are two types of DVHs used, differential and cumulative, with the cumulative type being the most commonly used. It plots structure volume versus dose and an example is shown in Fig. 7. With a DVH, it is easy to identify structures that are getting doses that are too high or too low. However, the DVH does not give any spatial information about the location of those hot or cold spots. Therefore to make an accurate assessment of the treatment plan as a whole, the DVH and dose distributions on multiple slices in multiple orientations must be evaluated simultaneously.

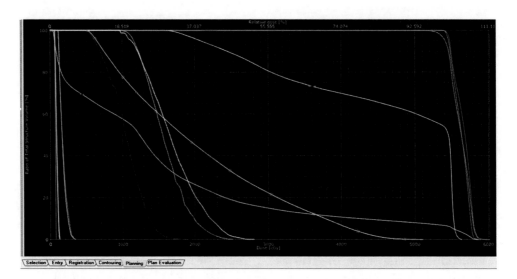

Conformal Therapy: Treatment Planning, Treatment Delivery, and Clinical Results. Fig. 7 Typical dose volume histogram (DVH) displaying dose coverage for target (GTV and CTV) and various OARs

Treatment Delivery

Accurate patient positioning prior to treatment delivery is essential for a quality conformal treatment as well as overall patient care. This can be accomplished with patient marks put on the patient at the time of their imaging study along with any immobilization devices made at that time. The patient can then be aligned to the marks while on the treatment couch. The treatment beam on the linear accelerator can be used to image the patient and verify patient position and alignment prior to treatment. It can also be used to take portal films, or port films, that can show the field shape in relation to patient anatomy, which is a particularly important quality assurance (QA) step in static field delivery.

While using the treatment beam for imaging is relatively simple, necessary for treatment field verification (port films), and doesn't require any additional equipment, it does have a drawback. The main drawback is that this technique is limited to the mega-voltage (MV) energies used by the clinic. Mega-voltage energies have an increased dose delivery to the patient compared to kilovoltage (kV) energies as well as reduced subject contrast. Some linear accelerators have on-board imaging (OBI), shown in Fig. 8, which does not use the MV beam as it consists of a separate kV x-ray source and detector that can be used for orthogonal films or cone-beam computed tomography (CBCT). This technology also has its pros and cons. Kilo-voltage imaging has increased subject contrast and reduced dose to the patient compared with MV imaging. A consequence of this is that, similar to CT images, artifacts may be produced by dental fillings, artificial joints, etc., which may obscure the region that needs to be evaluated.

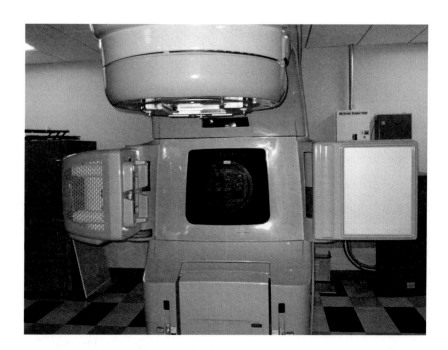

Conformal Therapy: Treatment Planning, Treatment Delivery, and Clinical Results. Fig. 8 Varian on-board imaging (OBI) system

A kV imaging system is a separate system that has its own characteristics separate from that of the linear accelerator and therefore needs its own separate quality assurance regimen. Additionally, the kV imaging system cannot take port films.

Treatment Verification

Three-dimensional conformal radiation therapy is an excellent tool to maximize tumor coverage while minimizing dose to surrounding normal tissue. However, since the field margins are much smaller than traditional fields, it is important to have a quality assurance (QA) program in place to ensure patient safety. A comprehensive QA program should verify the entire 3DCRT program from imaging, through treatment planning, and finally to treatment delivery. There are many different approaches to quality assurance along with many tools and tests for a comprehensive program. However, these are too numerous to list for this entry, and hence, the reader is referred to the task group report from the American Association of Physicists in Medicine (AAPM): TG-40 – Comprehensive QA for Radiation Oncology for suggestions on a comprehensive QA program (Kutcher et al. 1994). For updates on recommendations on quality assurance procedures for linear accelerators, the reader is referred to the AAPM TG-142 report entitled Quality Assurance of Medical Linear Accelerators (Klein et al. 2009).

Cross-References

▶ AAPM Task Group
▶ American Association of Physicists in Medicine (AAPM)
▶ Clinical Target Volume (CTV)
▶ Dose Calculation Algorithms
▶ External Beam Radiation Therapy
▶ Four-Dimensional (4D) Treatment Planning/ Respiratory Gating
▶ Gross Tumor Volume (GTV)
▶ Image-Guided Radiotherapy (IGRT)
▶ Imaging in Oncology
▶ Linear Accelerators (LINAC)
▶ Planning Target Volume (PTV)

References

Boyer AL (1996) Basic applications of a multileaf collimator. In: Palta J, Mackie TR (eds) Teletherapy: present and future. AAPM, Wisconsin

Bushberg JT et al (2003) The essential physics of medical imaging. Lippincott Williams & Wilkins, Philadelphia

International Commission on Radiation Units and Measurements (ICRU) Report 50 (1993) Prescribing, recording, and reporting photon beam therapy. ICRU, Maryland

International Commission on Radiation Units and Measurements (ICRU) Report 62 (1999) Prescribing, recording, and reporting photon beam therapy (Supplement to ICRU Report 50). ICRU, Maryland

Khan FM (ed) (2007) Treatment planning in radiation oncology, 2nd edn. Lippincott Williams & Wilkins, Philadelphia

Khan FM (2010) The physics of radiation therapy, 4th edn. Lippincott Williams & Wilkins, Philadelphia

Klein EE et al (2009) American association of physicists in medicine (AAPM) task group 142. Quality assurance medical linear accelerators. Med Phys 36:4197–4212

Kutcher GJ et al (1994) American association of physicists in medicine (AAPM) task group 40. Comprehensive QA for radiation oncology. Med Phys 21:581 618

Mackie TR et al (1996) Photon beam dose computation. In: Palta J, Mackie TR (eds) Teletherapy: present and future. AAPM, Wisconsin

Mackie TR et al (2007) Treatment planning algorithms. In: Khan FM (ed) Treatment planning in radiation oncology, 2nd edn. Lippincott Williams & Wilkins, Philadelphia

Connective Tissue Disorders

▶ Collagen Vascular Disease

Containment Structure

JOHN P. CHRISTODOULEAS
The Perelman Cancer Center, Department of
Radiation Oncology, University of Pennsylvania
Hospital, Philadelphia, PA, USA

Definition
Containment structure is a thick (typically 1 m)
steel-reinforced concrete enclosure surrounding
a nuclear reactor. The shell is gas-tight and built
to minimize the risk of environmental releases of
radiation should the reactor malfunction.

Cross-References
▶ Short-Term and Long-Term Health Risk of
Nuclear Power Plant Accident

Conventional Medicine

▶ Biomedicine (also Traditional, Theoretical,
Conventional, or Western Medicine)

Convolution-Superposition Dose Model

TIMOTHY HOLMES
Department of Radiation Oncology, Sinai
Hospital, Baltimore, MD, USA

Definition
A highly accurate three-dimensional dose computation method used for CT-based external
beam treatment planning applications including
conformal and intensity modulated radiotherapy
techniques.

Cross-References
▶ Image-Guided Radiation Therapy (IGRT):
TomoTherapy

Corpus Uteri

▶ Endometrium

Cranial Nerve Palsy (CNP)

BRANDON J. FISHER[1], LARRY C. DAUGHERTY[2]
[1]Department of Radiation Oncology, College of
Medicine, Drexel University, Philadelphia,
PA, USA
[2]Department of Radiation Oncology, College of
Medicine, Drexel University, Glenside, PA, USA

Definition
CNP is a dysfunction of one or more of the following cranial nerves (CN): CN I, the olfactory nerve
responsible for smell; CN II, the optic nerve
responsible for visual transmission to the brain;
CN III, the oculomotor nerve, which innervates
the levator palpebrae superioris, superior rectus,
medial rectus, inferior rectus, and inferior oblique
muscles of the eye; CN IV, the trochlear nerve,
which innervates the superior oblique muscles of
the eye; CN V, the trigeminal nerve, receives sensation from the face and innervates the muscles of
mastication; CN VI, the abducens nerve, innervates
the lateral rectus muscle of the eye; CN VII, the
facial nerve, responsible for movements of the
face; CN VIII, the vestibulocochlear nerve, senses
sound, rotation, and gravity; CN IX, the
glossopharyngeal nerve, responsible for taste from
the posterior one-third of the tongue; CN X, the
vagus nerve, innervates most laryngeal and

pharyngeal muscles; CN XI, the accessory nerve, innervates the sternocleidomastoid and the trapezius muscles; CN XII, the hypoglossal nerve, innervates the tongue.

Cross-References

▶ Nasopharynx

Crossfire Effect

TOD W. SPEER
Department of Human Oncology, University of Wisconsin School of Medicine and Public Health, UW Hospital and Clinics, Madison, WI, USA

Definition

The deposition of ionizing radiation in cells or tissue that are not specifically targeted by the radioconjugate. Due to an emitted radiation particle path length that is longer than at least several cell diameters, cells and tissue not expressing the target antigen will still be impacted upon by the incidental radiation.

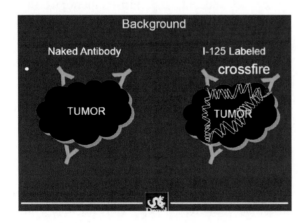

Cross-References

▶ Targeted Radioimmunotherapy

Cryptorchidism

JOHANNES CLASSEN
Department of Radiation Oncology, St. Vincentius-Kliniken Karlsruhe, Karlsruhe, Germany

Definition

Maldescensus testis.

Cross-References

▶ Testes

Curettage

▶ Dilation and Curettage

Curietherapy

▶ Clinical Aspects of Brachytherapy (BT)

Cushing's Syndrome

STEPHAN MOSE
Department of Radiation Oncology, Schwarzwald-Baar-Klinikum, Villingen-Schwenningen, Germany

Definition

This syndrome is defined as an overproduction of glucocorticoids leading to, for example, moonshaped face, steroid induced diabetes, and adrenocortical obesity.

Cross-References

▶ Adrenal Cancer
▶ Carcinoma of the Adrenal Gland
▶ Primary Intracranial Neoplasms

Cutaneous Melanoma

▶ Melanoma

Cutaneous T-Cell Lymphoma

CURT HEESE
Department of Radiation Oncology, Eastern
Regional Cancer Treatment Centers of America,
Philadelphia, PA, USA

Definition/Description

Cutaneous T-cell lymphoma (CTCL) refers to a spectrum of closely related malignant T-cell lymphoproliferative disorders in which the predominant clinical manifestations involve the skin. There are two major subgroups within the CTCL spectrum: ▶ mycosis fungoides (MF) and Sezary's syndrome, in which the distinction is based solely on the absence (MF) or presence (Sezary's) of peripheral blood malignant T-cells. The malignant cells have an immunophenotype characteristic of mature T-cells, usually with CD4 positivity, and show a propensity to infiltrate the epidermis (epidermotropism). The malignant nature of CTCL has been established by autopsy findings showing widespread infiltration of almost every organ system by malignant T-cells in advanced disease and by DNA cytophotometric and cytogenetic studies of the abnormal cells. Treatment can involve radiation, ▶ PUVA (*p*soralen sensitization of the skin to *u*ltra*v*iolet *A* light), or chemotherapy.

Epidemiology

According to data from the Surveillance, Epidemiology and End Results Program of the National Cancer Institute (NCI), the incidence of CTCL in the USA has increased 3.2-fold during the period 1973–1984 and currently exceeds 0.4 new cases per 100,000 population. This reported increase was probably the result of improved and earlier diagnosis. CTCL occurs more frequently in men than in women by a ratio of approximately 2:1, and blacks are twice as likely to be affected as whites. As with other lymphomas, the incidence of CTCL increases sharply with age.

Clinical Presentation

Most cases of MF evolve slowly and progressively through three clinical phases: patch or premycotic phase, infiltrated plaques or mycotic phase, and tumor or fungoid phase. This typical evolution is referred to as the *classic* or *Alibert–Bazin form*. The plaque and tumor phases of classic MF are characterized by clinically perceptible accumulations of atypical lymphoid cells in the skin to produce palpable lesions. Individual lesions tend to regress spontaneously in areas and merge with adjacent lesions to form lesions with irregular shapes. The magnitude of infiltration varies from lesion to lesion, which, with the characteristic configurations, produces a virtually diagnostic clinical appearance (Fig. 1). Tumorous lesions may develop gradually from preexisting plaques or may appear suddenly in an eruptive manner, indicating a biologically more aggressive clone of malignant cells. Cutaneous ulceration and secondary infections are frequently encountered in this phase. Approximately 17% of patients with CTCL present with generalized ▶ erythroderma, and approximately 50% of these have clear-cut Sezary's syndrome. Extracutaneous involvement is present in >80% of cases of CTCL at autopsy. Skin-associated peripheral lymph nodes are involved preferentially, if not initially,

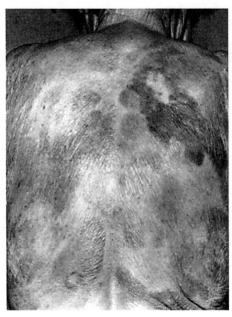

Cutaneous T-Cell Lymphoma. Fig. 1 Classic mycosis fungoides, plaque phase

Diagnostic Work-Up and Pathology

Punch biopsy specimens should be taken from the most infiltrated lesions for routine and immunopathologic processing to establish the diagnosis and define the characteristics of the malignant infiltrate. Blood smear for presence and quantitation of atypical mononuclear (Sezary) cells should be performed. Bone marrow biopsy should also be performed. Bone scans are done when clinically indicated.

The status of lymph nodes in the cervical, axillary, and inguinal regions in the staging and evaluation of patients is of primary importance. If lymph nodes are palpable, a biopsy should be obtained. If the nodes are nonpalpable, it is less certain that a lymph node biopsy should be performed at random. CT scans of the visceral organs to confirm or exclude extracutaneous involvement should be performed, and the presence of any questionable abnormalities by scan should be confirmed by histopathologic diagnosis if reasonable.

The cellular infiltrate of CTCL consists of malignant T-cells admixed with varying numbers of normal lymphocytes, histiocytes, eosinophils, plasma cells, and other cells (a polymorphous cellular infiltrate.) The cytomorphology of the atypical lymphoid cells varies from small cells with hyperchromatic, convoluted nuclei (referred to as *cerebriform cells*), to large cells with pale-staining vesicular nuclei and prominent nucleoli. Many intermediary cellular forms with pleomorphic nuclei may occur, including the so-called mycosis cell, a mononuclear cell with a large, hyperchromatic nucleus. In patch, plaque, and erythrodermic lesions of CTCL, the cellular infiltrate is located predominantly in the superficial part of the dermis, often arranged in a bandlike distribution immediately beneath the epidermis. However, it may extend into deeper regions around hair follicles and eccrine glands. With tumor formation, the infiltrate penetrates between the collagen bundles of the reticular

during the process of dissemination and are considered a poor barrier against further spread. Any organ system can be infiltrated by MF. The most common extracutaneous sites at autopsy are the lymph nodes (68%), spleen (56%), liver (49%), lungs (50%), and bone marrow (42%). The median survival of patients with histopathologically confirmed lymph node involvement is <2 years. Patients with visceral disease have a more ominous prognosis, with median survival of <1 year.

The median duration from the onset of skin lesions to histologic diagnosis of CTCL is approximately 8–10 years, with considerable variation from patient to patient. After the histologic diagnosis is established, the median survival for all patients has been reported to be <5 years. However, more recent series record a median survival after histopathologic confirmation of approximately 10 years, which may reflect earlier diagnosis or improvement in treatment approaches.

dermis and into the subcutaneous fat; the depth may range from a few millimeters to several centimeters, an important factor in treatment planning. Characteristically, atypical lymphoid cells in classic MF and Sezary's syndrome invade the epidermis and follicular epithelium to form small groups surrounded by a halolike clear space (Pautrier's microabscess).

The histopathologic appearance of CTCL in organ systems other than the skin may be confused with that of other lymphomas. The presence of clusters and sheets of mononuclear cells with convoluted nuclei is highly suggestive of CTCL. Lymph node involvement is underestimated by routine methods because early nodal involvement cannot be easily differentiated from dermatopathic lymphadenitis or other nonspecific changes.

Staging

The staging system proposed originally by Fuks and Bagshaw at Stanford has particular significance to the radiation oncologist because it concerns data generated from patients treated with total skin electron beam (► TSEB) irradiation (Table 1). A unifying staging system based on the tumor–node–metastasis (TNM) format was proposed initially at a Mycosis Fungoides Cooperative Group workshop on CTCL at the NCI (Table 2). Both the Stanford and Mycosis Fungoides Cooperative Group staging systems recognize the prognostic importance of cutaneous tumors, lymphadenopathy, and extracutaneous involvement.

Treatment

Because CTCL may originate in the skin, intensive therapy directed at the skin alone seems to offer the possibility of cure mostly for patients with early, limited involvement (stage Ia). The goal of therapy in early disease is to induce complete remission, reduce tumor burden, reduce symptoms, and prevent disease progression. Frequent remissions and sustained long-term disease-free intervals have occurred in such patients treated with TSEB

Cutaneous T-Cell Lymphoma. Table 1 Stanford staging system

Stage	Description
I	Mycosis fungoides limited to the skin; no tumors, ulcers, significant adenopathy, or visceral involvement (clinical or pathologic)
Ia	Eczematous or limited plaque disease with involvement of <25% of the total skin surface
Ib	Involvement of >25% of the total skin surface; includes the generalized plaque, lichenoid and generalized erythroderma variants
II	The presence of skin tumors or biopsy-proven dermatopathic lymphadenopathy; no extracutaneous involvement
III	Mycosis fungoides involving the skin with biopsy-proven involvement of the lymph nodes or spleen; no other visceral involvement
IV	Cutaneous and extracutaneous mycosis fungoides with documented visceral involvement

(Total Skin Electron Beam) irradiation, topically applied solutions of mechlorethamine, photochemotherapy using oral methoxsalen followed by intensive exposure to long-wave ultraviolet light, and ultraviolet B (UVB) phototherapy using either broadband or narrowband UVB without oral methoxsalen. The determination of "cure" requires considerable follow-up intervals because of the characteristically indolent time course of early MF. Patients with stage IIB disease have T3 tumor involvement and tend to have aggressive disease with poor prognosis, despite being free of visceral or nodal disease. Most patients with this stage require more aggressive therapy to clear tumors. TSEB therapy, oral bexarotene, and the recombinant fusion protein denileukin diftitox are relatively well tolerated and effective options, although systemic treatment may be required in

Cutaneous T-Cell Lymphoma. Table 2 TNM classification of cutaneous T-cell lymphoma

Magnitude of skin involvement (T)	
T0	Clinically or pathologically suspect lesions
T1	Premycotic lesions; papules, or plaques involving <10% of the skin
T2	Premycotic lesions; papules, or plaques involving >10% of the skin
T3	One or more tumors on the skin
T4	Extensive, often generalized erythroderma
Status of peripheral lymph nodes (N)	
N0	Clinically normal; pathologically not involved
N1	Clinically abnormal; pathologically not involved
N2	Clinically normal; pathologically involved
N3	Clinically abnormal; pathologically involved
Status of peripheral blood (B)	
B0	Atypical circulating cells not present (<1,000 ▶ Sezary cells/mL)
B1	Atypical circulating cells present (>1,000 Sezary cells/mL)
Status of visceral organs	
M0	Pathologically not involved
M1	Pathologically involved

patients with disease refractory to treatment. Oral bexarotene, which is a retinoid, and denileukin diftitox, which is a fusion toxin protein, have been approved by U.S. Food and Drug Administration for treatment of CTCL in patients who have disease that is refractory or resistant to treatment or who are unable to tolerate other therapies.

Patients with stage III disease or Sezary's syndrome who have leukemic involvement are often best treated with extracorporeal photopheresis with addition of biologic response modifiers as needed. Another option in these patients is oral low-dose methotrexate, which is also active in erythrodermic CTCL. Alemtuzumab is a humanized recombinant monoclonal antibody specific for the CD52 cell surface glycoprotein, found on normal and malignant B-cells and T-cells. A phase 2 trial has shown some potential efficacy of this antibody, although severe neutropenia was seen and severe cardiac toxicity may be a significant complication of treatment.

Chemotherapy

Pathologically confirmed extracutaneous involvement usually means that systemic chemotherapy must be provided to control CTCL. Several single agents produce beneficial, albeit temporary, responses in most patients. These include several alkylating agents (mechlorethamine, cyclophosphamide, chlorambucil, and temozolomide), antimetabolites (methotrexate, gemcitabine, and pentostatin), and antitumor antibiotics (bleomycin and doxorubicin). Attention also has been directed to combinations of drugs, and preliminary results have been encouraging. ▶ CHOP (cyclophosphamide, doxorubicin, vincristine, prednisone) has been the most frequently used multiagent regimen in advanced CTCL, and can produce a complete response in up to 38% of patients. However, most cytotoxic chemotherapies with either single or multiple drugs result in complete responses in only 20–25% of patients with advanced CTCL, and there are no long-term disease-free survivors who underwent chemotherapy alone.

Failure of systemic drugs to control advanced CTCL usually is the result of incomplete responses of cutaneous lesions, whereas extracutaneous foci of disease often respond completely. For this reason, additional treatment for cutaneous lesions (e.g., topical mechlorethamine chemotherapy or TSEB irradiation) would be expected to have additive beneficial effects for patients treated primarily with systemic drugs and should be considered for every patient. Depsipeptide, a histone deacetylase inhibitor, has been used in a small number of CTCL patients with some success. Systemic drugs, denileukin diftitox, and serotherapy with ^{90}Y-tagged murine monoclonal anti–T-cell antibodies against CD5 antigen are potential additional therapeutic measures that can be used in advanced CTCL.

Radiation Therapy

Superficial irradiation (80–140 kVp) with a half-value layer of 0.7–1 mm aluminum and a target–skin distance of 15–30 cm can be used for most infiltrated plaques. For markedly infiltrated plaques and tumors, higher-energy orthovoltage irradiation (200–280 kVp) or local-field electron beam irradiation (10–15 MeV) is recommended. Discrete lesions may be treated satisfactorily with a variety of protraction–fractionation schedules, ranging from 10 to 12 Gy in three or four treatment fractions during a 3- to 4-day period, up to 20–30 Gy in 10–15 fractions during 2–3 weeks. Generous portals should be used to cover defined anatomic areas. Because of the possible need for subsequent treatment in adjacent areas, it is important to document the treated areas with photographs, accurate portal drawings, and, if feasible, tattooing of the corners of the fields with India ink. In most patients, the lesions do not clear during or at the completion of irradiation, and it may take up to 6–8 weeks for complete response.

In general, the uniformity of dose distribution improves as the number of fields increases, but at the expense of complexity and increased machine time for the treatment of each patient. The optimal technique with reasonable uniformity of dose appears to be a six dual-field technique. The electron beam with an effective central

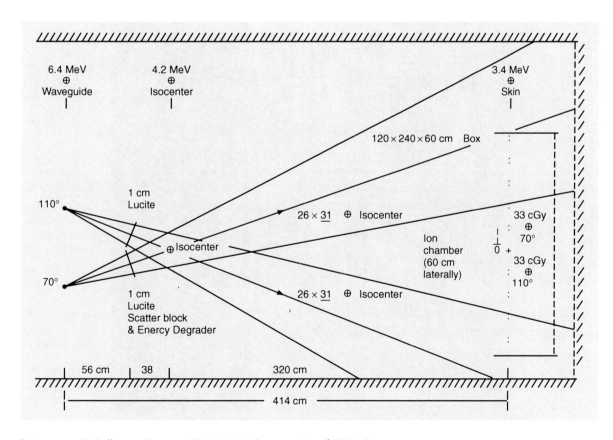

Cutaneous T-Cell Lymphoma. Fig. 2 Portal geometry of TSEB therapy

axis energy of 3–6 MeV and, rarely, 9 MeV is used to treat three anterior and three posterior stationary treatment fields, each having a superior and inferior portal with beam angulation 20° above and 20° below the horizontal axis (Fig. 2). The patient is placed in front of the beam in six positions during treatment (Fig. 3). The straight anterior, right posterior oblique, and left posterior oblique fields are treated on the first day of each treatment cycle, and the straight posterior, right anterior oblique, and left anterior oblique fields are treated on the second day of each cycle.

The entire wide-field skin surface receives 1.5–2 Gy each 2-day cycle. The majority of patients can tolerate 2 Gy/cycle. However, patients with previous course of TSEB irradiation or atrophic skin tolerate 1.5 Gy/cycle better. Irradiation usually is administered on a 4-day/week dose schedule; the total dose depends on the intent (curative versus palliative). Doses of 30–40 Gy are delivered during an 8- to 10-week interval with a 1- to 2-week break at 18–20 Gy for patients treated with curative intent; 10–20 Gy is administered for palliation. The average skin dose is calculated as the

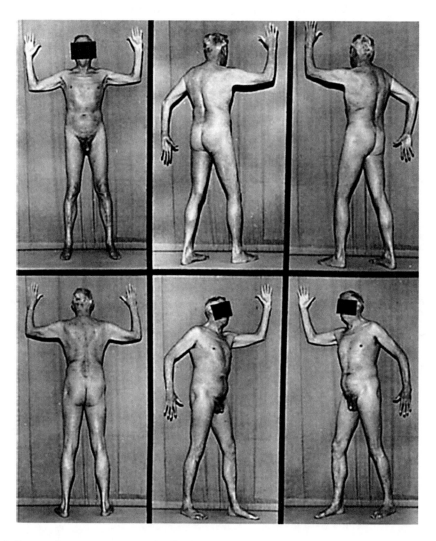

Cutaneous T-Cell Lymphoma. Fig. 3 Positions assumed by the patient for TSEB, six-field technique

product of the dose delivered to the center of the treatment plane for one of the dual fields multiplied by a correction factor (F). Factor F represents the fact that any given point on the surface receives some radiation from at least two of the six dual-exposure fields and is calculated from phantom measurements. The percentage of photon contamination for a single dual-field cycle should not exceed 0.3%. Machine calibration is performed daily, as are point-of-dose prescription and side-to-side flatness. Verification of delivered doses should be performed routinely using thermoluminescent dosimeters placed on skin surfaces.

During wide-field skin irradiation, internal or external eye shields are used routinely to protect the cornea and lens. The globe of the eye must not receive more than 15% of the prescribed skin surface dose. If internal eye shields are used, the energy build-up at the surface of the eye shields (if metallic uncoated shields are used) could result in significant overdosage of the eyelids. Shielding of the digits and lateral surfaces of the hands or feet may be necessary because of local skin reaction from overlapping treatment fields in these areas. In palliative setups, shielding of uninvolved skin is recommended. Areas not directly exposed to the path of the electron beam (soles of feet, perineum, medial upper thighs, axillae, posterior auricular areas, inframammary regions, vertex of scalp, and areas under the skin folds) are treated with separate electron beam fields (with appropriate energy) or individual 100-kV orthovoltage x-rays (0.4-mm aluminum filtration), usually at a rate of 1 Gy daily to a total dose of 20 Gy. Markedly infiltrated tumors may be treated with supplemental orthovoltage irradiation or higher-energy electrons to bring the total dose to 36–40 Gy.

Radiation Sequelae

Mild erythema in some normal regions of skin with greater skin reaction in areas of prior ultraviolet exposure; the lesions of mycosis fungoides become erythematous, then pigmented:

- Complete, temporary scalp alopecia (100%)
- Temporary nail stasis (100%)
- Some edema of hands and feet (<50%)
- Minor nosebleeds (<10%)
- Blisters on fingers and feet (<5%)
- Self-limiting anhidrosis, minor parotiditis, and gynecomastia in men (<3% each)
- Corneal tears from internal eye shields (<1%)
- Chronic nail dystrophy, chronic xerosis, partial but permanent alopecia of the scalp, and fingertip dysesthesias that persist for more than a year (<1% each)
- Acute or late mortality attributable to total skin electron-beam irradiation (0%)

Cross-References

▶ Electron Dosimetry and Treatment
▶ Total Skin Electron Therapy (TSET)

References

Bunn PA Jr, Lamberg SI (1979) Report of the committee on staging and classification of cutaneous T-cell lymphomas. Cancer Treat Rep 63:725

Fuks ZY, Bagshaw MA, Farber EM (1973) Prognostic signs and the management of the mycosis fungoides. Cancer 32:1385

Heese C et al Chapter 77. In: Halperin EC, Perez CA, Brady LW (ed) Principles and practice of radiation oncology, 5th edn. Wolters Kluwer, Lippincott Williams & Wilkins, Philadelphia

Jones GW, Kacinski BM, Wilson LD et al (2002) Total skin electron radiation in the management of mycosis fungoides: consensus of the European Organization for Research and Treatment of Cancer (EORTC) Cutaneous Lymphoma Project Group. J Am Acad Dermatol 47:364–370

Maingon P, Truc G, Dalac S et al (2000) Radiotherapy of advanced mycosis fungoides: indications and results of total skin electron beam and photon beam irradiation. Radiother Oncol 54:73–78

Meyler TS, Blumberg AL, Purser P (1978) Total skin electron beam therapy in mycosis fungoides. Cancer 42:1171

Micaily B, Campbell O, Moser C et al (1991) Total-skin electron beam and total nodal irradiation of cutaneous T-cell lymphoma. Int J Radiat Oncol Biol Phys 20:809

Micaily B, Moser C, Vonderheid EC et al (1990) The radiation therapy of early stage mycosis fungoides. Int J Radiat Oncol Biol Phys 18:1333

Micaily B, Vonderheid EC, Brady LW (1983) Combined moderate dose electron beam radiation and topical chemotherapy for cutaneous T-cell lymphoma. Int J Radiat Oncol Biol Phys 9:475

Patterson JAK, Edelson RL (1982) Interactions of T cells with the epidermis. Br J Dermatol 107:117

Samman PD (1976) Mycosis fungoides and other cutaneous reticuloses. Clin Exp Dermatol 1:197

Weinstock MA, Horm JW (1988) Mycosis fungoides in the United States. JAMA 260:42

Cyclotron

GEORGE E. LARAMORE, JAY J. LIAO, JASON K. ROCKHILL
Department of Radiation Oncology, University of Washington Medical Center, Seattle, WA, USA

Definition

A device which accelerates charged particles by applying multiple accelerations as the particles move in confined circular orbits due to the presence of a high-strength magnetic field. Neutrons are produced by accelerating protons or deuterons to approximately 20–50 MeV and then impacting them onto an appropriate target such as beryllium.

Cross-References

▶ Neutron Radiotherapy

Cystectomy

Definition

Surgical removal of bladder tissues, whole or in part.

Cross-References

▶ Bladder

Cytokines

CLAUDIA RÜBE
Department of Radiation Oncology, Saarland University, Homburg/Saar, Germany

Definition

Proteins, peptides, or glycoproteins secreted by specific cells of the immune system that carry signals locally between cells, and thus have an effect on other cells (Cellular Communication). Cytokines bind to specific receptors and cause a change in the function or development of the target cells. Cytokines are involved in the response to radiation-induced injury.

Cross-References

▶ Predictive In vitro Assays in Radiation Oncology
▶ Targeted Radioimmunotherapy

Cytoreductive Surgery

▶ Debulking Surgery

D

3DCRT

▶ Three-Dimensional Conformal Radiation Therapy

D&C

▶ Dilation and Curettage

Dalton (Da)

TOD W. SPEER
Department of Human Oncology, University of Wisconsin School of Medicine and Public Health, UW Hospital and Clinics, Madison, WI, USA

Definition
This is the unit used to represent mass on a molecular scale. It is one-twelfth the rest mass of carbon-12 atom (in its ground state) and is $1.660538782 \times 10^{-27}$ kg.

Debulking Surgery

CHRISTIN A. KNOWLTON[1], MICHELLE KOLTON MACKAY[2]
[1]Department of Radiation Oncology, Drexel University, Philadelphia, PA, USA
[2]Department of Radiation Oncology, Marshfield Clinic, Marshfield, WI, USA

Synonyms
Cytoreductive surgery

Definition
Debulking surgery is used in patients with more advanced ovarian cancer often in addition to a total abdominal hysterectomy and bilateral salpingoopherectomy. The goal is to achieve maximum cytoreduction with less than 1 cm of residual disease. To achieve maximum debulking, surgery may need to include procedures such as radical pelvic dissection, bowel resection, stripping of diaphragm or peritoneal surfaces, or splenectomy.

Cross-References
▶ Ovary

L.W. Brady, T.E. Yaeger (eds.), *Encyclopedia of Radiation Oncology*, DOI 10.1007/978-3-540-85516-3,
© Springer-Verlag Berlin Heidelberg 2013

Denotology

▶ Kantianism

Density Correction/ Inhomogeneity Correction/ Heterogeneity Correction

CHARLIE MA, LU WANG
Department of Radiation Oncology, Fox Chase
Cancer Center, Philadelphia, PA, USA

Definition
The correction that accounts for the effect of the
difference in tissue density and composition
between human body and water when simple
dose calculation methods are used.

Cross-References
▶ Dose Calculation Algorithms

Denys Drash Syndrome

LARRY C. DAUGHERTY[1], BRANDON J. FISHER[2]
[1]Department of Radiation Oncology, College of
Medicine, Drexel University, Glenside, PA, USA
[2]Department of Radiation Oncology, College of
Medicine, Drexel University, Philadelphia,
PA, USA

Definition
A rare disorder of infants with abnormal development of sex organs and increased risk of
cancers, notably Wilms tumor.

Cross-References
▶ Pediatric Ovarian Cancer
▶ Rectal Cancer
▶ Wilm's Tumor

Detective Quantum Efficiency (DQE)

JOHN W. WONG
Department of Radiation Oncology and
Molecular Radiation Sciences, Johns Hopkins
University, Baltimore, MD, USA

Definition
The square of the ratio of the output ▶ Signal-to-
Noise Ratio (SNR) to the input SNR of
a detection system.

Cross-References
▶ Electronic Portal Imaging Devices (EPID)

Diffuse Large B Cell Lymphoma of the Breast

▶ Breast Lymphoma

Digitally Reconstructed Radiograph (DRR)

BRIAN F. HASSON
Department of Radiation Oncology, Abington
Memorial Hospital, Abington, PA, USA
Department of Radiation Oncology, College of
Medicine, Drexel University, Philadelphia,
PA, USA

Definition
A reconstructed image or set of images
in planes other than the original plane of

image acquisition that are generated by a computer system.

Cross-References

▶ Stereotactic Radiosurgery – Cranial

Dilation and Curettage

CHRISTIN A. KNOWLTON[1], MICHELLE KOLTON MACKAY[2]
[1]Department of Radiation Oncology, Drexel University, Philadelphia, PA, USA
[2]Department of Radiation Oncology, Marshfield Clinic, Marshfield, WI, USA

Synonyms

Curettage; D&C

Definition

In this procedure, the cervix is widened (dilated) and part of the endometrium is removed. The endometrium may be scraped with a curette or extracted via suction. This procedure is often performed in the setting of postmenopausal or abnormal uterine bleeding. It may also be used to clear the uterine contents following an incomplete miscarriage.

Cross-References

▶ Endometrium

Disphosphonates

▶ Bisphosphonates

Display Window Setting

DAREK MICHALSKI[1], M. SAIFUL HUQ[2]
[1]Division of Medical Physics, Department of Radiation Oncology, University of Pittsburgh Cancer Centers, Pittsburgh, PA, USA
[2]Department of Radiation Oncology, University of Pittsburgh Medical Center Cancer Pavilion, Pittsburgh, PA, USA

Definition

Setting for the CT scan radiodensity range for visual rendition to specify the image brightness and contrast in given display units.

Cross-References

▶ Four-Dimensional (4D) Treatment Planning/ Respiratory Gating

Dissemination or Involvement

▶ Palliation of Bone Metastases

Dissociation Constant (Kd)

TOD W. SPEER
Department of Human Oncology, University of Wisconsin School of Medicine and Public Health, UW Hospital and Clinics, Madison, WI, USA

Definition

Mathematical representation of the strength of binding between the antigen-binding site and the antigen (affinity)

$$K_d = [Ab][An]/[C]$$

where [Ab] is the concentration of unbound anti-body, [An] is the concentration of unbound antigen, and [C] is the concentration of the Ab-An complex. The smaller the K_d, the more tightly bound is the Ab-An complex and higher the affinity. The association constant (K_a) may also be used and is the inverse of K_d.

Cross-References

▶ Targeted Radioimmunotherapy

dmax

JAY E. REIFF
Department of Radiation Oncology, College of Medicine, Drexel University, Philadelphia, PA, USA

Definition

The depth of maximum dose for a given radiation beam.

Cross-References

▶ Stereotactic Radiosurgery: Extracranial

DNA Damage

CLAUDIA E. RÜBE
Department of Radiation Oncology, Saarland University, Homburg/Saar, Germany

Definition

DNA is under constant siege from a variety of damaging agents. Damage to DNA and the ability of cells to repair that damage have broad health implications, from aging and heritable diseases to cancer.

Cross-References

▶ Predictive In vitro Assays in Radiation Oncology

Dose Calculation Algorithms

LU WANG, CHARLIE MA
Department of Radiation Oncology, Fox Chase Cancer Center, Philadelphia, PA, USA

Absorbed dose is a physical quantity routinely used in the clinical radiation therapy prescription. It is defined as the energy imparted by ionizing radiation per unit mass of medium (SI unit: gray or Gy; 1 Gy = 1 J/kg). The calculation of absorbed dose (or simply dose) is a critical component in radiation therapy treatment planning, and dose calculation algorithms are the fundamental tools to facilitate this process.

Commonly used dose calculation algorithms can be generally divided into three categories. The first category is referred to as correction-based algorithms, which employ semiempirical approaches to account for tissue heterogeneity and surface curvature based on measured dose distributions in water. The second category is referred to as model-based algorithms, which predict patient dose distributions from primary particle fluence and a dose kernel. The third category is Monte Carlo simulations, which calculate dose distributions based on computer simulations of particle transport and energy deposition in patient geometry.

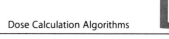

Correction-Based Algorithms

Correction-based algorithms were widely used in conventional radiation therapy, which involved minimal computation. There are generally two steps in dose calculation using a correction-based algorithm: (1) establishing dose calculation data; and (2) reconstructing patient dose distribution by applying corrections.

Establishing Dose Calculation Data

The basic dose calculation parameters (or data library) and dose distribution functions are measured in a water phantom under standard conditions that include a flat phantom surface, a fixed source-to-surface distance (SSD), and normal beam incidence. The phantom has to be large enough in volume to provide full electron equilibrium. The dose measurements under those conditions include:

- Central-axis depth doses, normalized to the maximum dose value, for various square fields.
- Lateral dose profiles at a reference depth or several depths, which extend outside of the square field, normalized to the central-axis value, to give the off-axial ratios (OAR).
- Beam output factors for various square fields relative to a reference field (typically $10 \times 10 \text{ cm}^2$), which can be decomposed into phantom scatter factors, S_p, and collimator scatter factors, S_c.
- Beam modifier factors (f) as a function of depth and field size to account for the attenuation and scattering effect of a beam modifier such as a wedge or a compensator.

Another commonly used dose quantity similar to depth dose is the tissue-air ratio (TAR), which is defined as the ratio of the dose at a given point in a phantom to that at the same point in free air in the absence of the phantom. For photon energies above 4 MV, it becomes impractical to measure dose in air for TAR. A tissue-phantom ratio (TPR) is used, which is defined as the ratio of the dose at any depth in the phantom to that at a fixed reference depth measured at the same spatial point (e.g., isocenter). If this reference depth is chosen to be at the depth of the maximum dose, the ratio is called tissue-maximum ratio (TMR).

Theoretically, using the above beam data, the dose at any point in a radiation field that satisfies those standard conditions can be calculated by the following formula:

$$D = C \times MU \times TMR \times OAR \times S_p \times S_c \times f \quad (1)$$

where, MU is the monitor chamber reading of a clinical accelerator (or the beam-on-time of a ^{60}Co unit) and C is the machine calibration factor, which specifies the dose delivered to a reference point for a monitor unit (MU) (or a unit of beam-on-time). This formula is still widely used by medical physicists to perform a "hand calculation" to check the MUs of individual beams of a treatment plan for a given prescription dose.

However, the situations encountered in clinical radiotherapy often impose limitations on the use of "standard" distribution functions and dose calculation parameters. Therefore, various correction methods have been proposed and applied to dose calculation under nonstandard conditions (Fig. 1).

Reconstructing Dose Distribution

Correction for Irregular Fields

The Clarkson method can be used for calculating dose in an irregularly shaped radiation field by summing up or integrating the individual contributions of each decomposed fan beamlet (a small sector of the beam), which constitutes the irregular field (Clarkson 1941).

This method is based on the principle that the scattering component of the dose depends on the field size and shape, while the primary component of the dose is independent of the field size

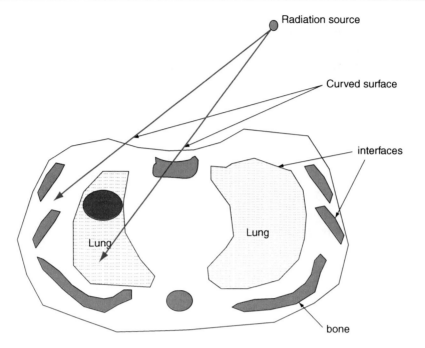

Dose Calculation Algorithms. Fig. 1 Schematic diagram showing nonstandard calculation conditions due to oblique incidence, curved surface, and heterogeneities

and shape. Thus, the primary and scattered dose at any point in an irregular field can be calculated separately using an effective TMR, that is:

$$TMR(r, d) = TMR(0, d) + \sum_{i} SMR(d, r_i) \quad (2)$$

where, $TMR(0, d)$ is the primary component and $SMR(d, r_i)$ is the scatter-maximum ratio at the depth of d for a narrow fan beamlet with a radius r_i, which is defined as the ratio of the scattered dose at a given point in phantom to the effective primary dose at the same point at the depth of maximum dose.

Correction for Contour Irregularities

A convenient, yet effective method to make contour corrections to account for oblique beam incidence or surface curvature is the TMR method. This method is based on the principle that TMR does not depend on SSD but only on

the depth of interest and the field size at that depth. Therefore, if the tissue is missing underneath the surface denoted by the dotted dash line SS at the standard SSD (Fig. 2), the correction factor (*CF*) will be

$$CF = \frac{TMR(d - t, r_P)}{TMR(d, r_P)} \quad (3)$$

where r_P is the field size projected at point P (i.e., at a distance of $SSD + d$ from the surface).

The corrected dose D_c at the point P is thus given by:

$$D_c = D \times CF \quad (4)$$

where D is the uncorrected dose.

Correction for Tissue Heterogeneities

Traditionally, the effects of tissue heterogeneities are corrected using semiempirical methods, such

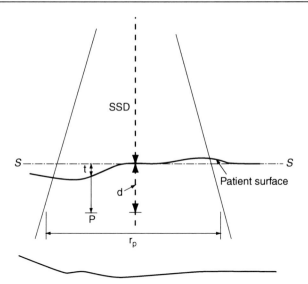

Dose Calculation Algorithms. Fig. 2 An example of patient surface irregularities

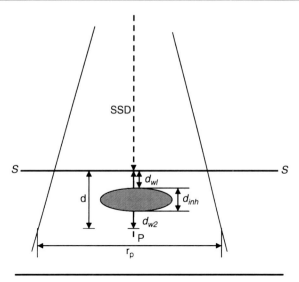

Dose Calculation Algorithms. Fig. 3 An illustration of tissue heterogeneity correction

as the TAR method. The key to this correction is to employ an effective depth by scaling the physical depth using the relative electron density, ρ_e (with respect to that of water). The principle of physics (rationale) for this approach is that, for megavoltage photon beams, Compton Effect is the dominant mode of interaction, so that the attenuation of the beam in any medium is dictated primarily by the electron density of the medium. Thus, the correction factor for tissue heterogeneities is

$$CF = \frac{TAR(d_e, r_d)}{TAR(d, r_d)} \quad (5)$$

where d is the actual depth of P from the surface, d_e is the equivalent water depth, that is, $d_e = d_{w1} + \rho_e d_{inh} + d_{w2}$, and r_d is the field size projected at the point P (Fig. 3).

One of the limitations of this correction method is that it does not take into account the location of the inhomogeneity relative to the point of interest P. This limitation was removed by the power law method (Batho 1964), in which the correction factor is given by

$$CF = \left[\frac{TAR(d_{inh} + d_{w2}, r_d)}{TAR(d_{w2}, r_d)} \right]^{\rho_e - 1} \quad (6)$$

where the variables are defined as in Fig. 3, except that the power law method assumes the heterogeneity is a slab larger than the radiation field.

Another improvement was proposed to predicate scattered dose by scaling the field size using relative electron density (Sontag and Cunningham 1977). The correction factor based on the "equivalent" tissue-air ratio (ETAR) is

$$CF = \frac{TAR(d_e, r_e)}{TAR(d, r_d)} \quad (7)$$

where $r_e = r_d \cdot \bar{\rho}$ is the scaled field size dimension, and $\bar{\rho}$ is the weighted average density of the inhomogeneities.

Overall, the existence of irregular fields, surface irregularities, and tissue heterogeneities not only changes the attenuation and scattering of the primary radiation but also alters the secondary electron transport. However, intrinsically, correction-based algorithms assume the existence of electronic equilibrium and neglect the effects of electron transport, which could result in appreciable errors near beam edges or within the heterogeneities.

Model-Based Algorithms

A class of deterministic model-based algorithms is called the convolution-superposition method. First proposed by Dean (1980), this method has been developed and implemented clinically in various forms (Boyer and Mok 1985; Mackie et al. 1985; Mohan et al. 1986). The common feature of this class of algorithm is the use of dose kernels to model dose distributions resulting from interactions of primary radiation particles at a point or along a ray line in the dose calculation geometry. Generally, dose kernels at different locations in a human body should not be the same due to the existence of various tissue compositions and densities. For efficiency, however, simplified dose kernels have been used in commercial treatment planning systems. Thus, the accuracy of a convolution-superposition algorithm depends critically on how the kernel variation is implemented for heterogeneous geometry.

Convolution-Superposition with Point Dose Kernels

Mathematically, for a monoenergetic photon field, the dose $D(\vec{r})$ at a point $\vec{r}$ (a vector that consists of x, y, z component, that is, $\vec{r} = x\vec{i} + y\vec{j} + z\vec{k}$) is given by:

$$D(\vec{r}) = \int_F \frac{\mu}{\rho} \Psi_p(\vec{r}')k(\vec{r} - \vec{r}')d\vec{r} \qquad (8)$$

where μ/ρ is the mass attenuation coefficient, $\Psi_p(\vec{r}')$ is the primary photon energy fluence, and $k(\vec{r}')$ is the point dose kernel. The product of mass attenuation coefficient and the primary energy fluence is the total energy released per unit mass (TERMA), $T_p(\vec{r}')$. The point dose kernel represents the dose distribution in water resulting from both scattered photons and secondary

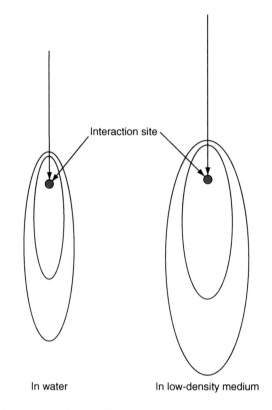

In water   In low-density medium

Dose Calculation Algorithms. Fig. 4 Schematic diagrams showing point dose kernels in water and in a low-density medium for the same photon beam

electrons set in motion by the primary photon interactions (Figs. 4 and 5).

Since both the primary photon energy fluence and point dose kernels are functions of energy, for a clinical photon beam, the total dose is given by the integration of the product of TERMA and the point dose kernel over the photon field for the energy spectrum.

The Fast Fourier Transform (FFT) Algorithm

Calculation of the dose distribution in homogeneous geometry by (8) can be performed very efficiently using the FFT method, in which the convolution of two functions with three variables each in the physical space can be transformed into the product of the two functions in the frequency

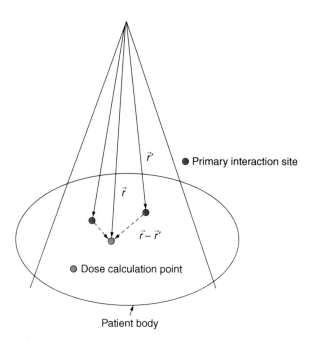

Dose Calculation Algorithms. Fig. 5 The relationship between primary interaction sites and the calculation point

space. The FFT method is similar to correction-based algorithms in accuracy for heterogeneous geometry because it ignores the spatial variation of the point dose kernel variation completely.

The Superposition Algorithm

When dose calculation is performed in heterogeneous geometry, the point dose kernels vary spatially and the dose at a point has to be summed up by superposition of the variable point dose kernels, which are typically approximated by stretching or compressing the point dose kernel based on the electron density of the local medium. Mathematically, the dose at a point (i,j,k) is given by

$$D(i,j,k) \propto \sum_{i'} \sum_{j'} \sum_{k'} T_p(i',j',k') k_e(i,j,k,i',j',k')$$

$$(9)$$

where $k_e(i,j,k,i',j',k')$ represents the scaled point dose kernel based on local electron density. The

point dose kernels can be represented in a Cartesian grid or discretized using collapsed cones (Ahnesjo 1987); the latter are more computationally efficient (e.g., for kernel tilting and density scaling). It is also more efficient to separate the point dose kernel into a primary kernel for secondary electrons and a scatter kernel for scattered photons with a different spatial resolution. Due to kernel scaling, the superposition method is more accurate and time consuming than the FFT convolution method for calculating dose in a heterogeneous geometry.

Convolution-Superposition with Pencil-Beam Dose Kernels

The pencil-beam dose kernel represents the dose distribution resulting from scattered photons and secondary electrons set in motion by a single ray of primary photons. Thus, the dose distribution can be calculated by

$$D(x,y,z) = \int\int_F T_p(x',y') k_{PB}(x-x',y-y',z) dx' dy'$$

$$(10)$$

where $T_p(x',y')$ is energy-integrated TERMA at the surface of the patient, and $k_{PB}(x',y',z)$ is the pencil-beam dose kernel.

For heterogeneous geometry, the depth coordinate z is scaled with electron density, which is equivalent to stretching or compressing the pencil-beam dose kernel longitudinally. The effect of lateral density variation from the considered ray is often ignored or approximated using the ETAR correction. From this point of view, a pencil-beam algorithm is very similar to a correction-based dose algorithm.

The Finite-Size Pencil-Beam (FSPB) Algorithm

In this algorithm, the pencil-beam dose kernel is replaced with a three-dimensional dose distribution resulting from a photon beam of a finite field size that typically corresponds to a beamlet used in intensity-modulated radiation therapy (IMRT). The advantage of FSPB is its high computation efficiency, as the convolution-superposition is performed in two dimensions, which is essential to pre-optimization dose calculations when hundreds or even thousands of beamlets are needed to achieve an optimal dose distribution. However, due to its approximation in heterogeneity corrections, pencil-beam algorithms may show significant uncertainties in the vicinity of heterogeneities (Wang et al. 1998; Krieger and Sauer 2005). Therefore, more accurate dose algorithms (e.g., convolution-superposition methods using point dose kernels) are often used in the post-optimization dose calculation for IMRT and other advanced treatment techniques.

The Anisotropic Analytical Algorithm (AAA)

The AAA algorithm is an improved pencil-beam algorithm, which uses multiple pencil-beam dose kernels to describe the dose contributions from various radiation sources of a clinical beam (Van Esch et al. 2006). In particular, the pencil-beam dose kernels for the photon sources are further separated into a depth component and a lateral component. The heterogeneity correction is incorporated in the dose summation stage by scaling the depth dose component using the equivalent path length and the lateral component anisotropically according to the local electron density. This has significantly improved the accuracy of dose calculations for heterogeneous geometry compared to other pencil-beam algorithms (Bragg et al. 2008).

Monte Carlo Simulations

The Monte Carlo method is theoretically the most complete and rigorous dose calculation method, since it simulates the radiation transport and energy deposition of individual particles following the fundamental laws of physics. In fact, it is the only method that takes into account electronic disequilibrium at medium interfaces and in tissue heterogeneities, as well as particle backscattering from dense materials such as teeth, bones, and metal prostheses in a patient.

Monte Carlo dose calculation consists of using a computer program to simulate the transport and interaction of individual particles in a patient by random sampling from probability distribution functions that govern the underlying physical processes (Rogers and Bielajew 1990). The patient's geometry is reconstructed from CT data with different biological media and mass densities. The dose distribution is calculated by tallying the ionization events that give rise to energy deposition in individual calculation voxels. In order to obtain statistically meaningful dose distributions, a large number ($>10^8$) of radiation particles have to be simulated for a radiation treatment, resulting in long CPU times. This situation has been improved with the availability of fast computers and various variance-reduction and efficiency-improvement techniques such as photon interaction forcing, particle splitting, Russian roulette, and electron track repeating (Ma et al. 2002).

Accurate Monte Carlo dose calculation requires the precise knowledge of the phase-space information (i.e., the angle, position, and energy) of the radiation particles impinging on the patient. This can be achieved by directly simulating the radiation beams from the clinical accelerator or using source models with parameters derived from measurements or Monte Carlo simulated phase space data (Ma and Jiang 1999; Verhaegen and Seuntjens 2003). Patient-specific beam modifiers such as wedges, blocks, and multileaf collimators can be directly simulated in the patient dose calculation to account for their attenuation and scattering effects.

Currently, Monte Carlo dose calculation has been used extensively for assessing existing dose calculation algorithms, investigating novel treatment modalities, and treatment techniques prior to their widespread clinical applications, and validating treatment dose delivery in combination with advanced image guidance and in vivo dosimetry measurements (Chetty et al. 2007; Reynaert et al. 2007). Several commercial treatment planning systems have implemented Monte Carlo algorithms for electron therapy, photon IMRT, and stereotactic radiosurgery/therapy (Cygler et al. 2004; Heath et al. 2004; Pemler et al. 2006; Ma et al. 2008). Monte Carlo algorithms are expected to be the dose engine for the next generation of treatment planning systems.

Cross-References

▶ Conformal Therapy: Treatment Planning, Treatment Delivery, and Clinical Results
▶ Electron Dosimetry and Treatment
▶ History of Radiation Oncology
▶ Imaging in Oncology
▶ Intensity-Modulated Proton Therapy (IMPT)
▶ Intraoperative Irradiation
▶ Linear Accelerators (LINAC)
▶ Proton Therapy
▶ Radiation Detectors
▶ Radiation Oncology Physics
▶ Radiation Therapy Shielding
▶ Re-Irradiation
▶ Stereotactic Radiosurgery? Cranial
▶ Stereotactic Radiosurgery: Extracranial
▶ Total Body Irradiation (TBI)
▶ Total Skin Electron Therapy (TSET)

References

Ahnesjo A, Andreo P, Brahme A (1987) Calculation and application of point spread functions for treatment planning with high energy photon beams. Acta Oncol 26:49–56

Batho HF (1964) Lung corrections in cobalt 60 beam therapy. J Can Assoc Radiol 15:79–83

Boyer AL, Mok EC (1985) A photon dose distribution model employing convolution calculations. Med Phys 12:169–177

Bragg CM, Wingate K et al (2008) Clinical implications of the anisotropic analytical algorithm for IMRT treatment planning and verification. Radiother Oncol 86:276–284

Chetty IJ, Curran B, Cygler J et al (2007) Report of the AAPM Task Group No. 105: issues associated with clinical implementation of Monte Carlo-based photon and electron external beam treatment planning. Med Phys 34:4818–4853

Clarkson J (1941) A note on depth doses in fields of irregular shape. Br J Radiol 14:265

Cygler JE, Daskalov GM, Chan GH et al (2004) Evaluation of the first commercial Monte Carlo dose calculation engine for electron beam treatment planning. Med Phys 31:142–153

Dean RD (1980) A scattering kernel for use in true three-dimensional dose calculations. Med Phys 7:429

Heath E, Seuntjens J, Sheikh-Bagheri D (2004) Dosimetric evaluation of the clinical implementation of the first commercial IMRT Monte Carlo treatment planning system at 6 MV. Med Phys 31:2771–2779

Krieger T, Sauer OA (2005) Monte Carlo- versus pencil-beam-/collapsed-cone-dose calculation in a heterogeneous multi-layer phantom. Phys Med Biol 50:859–868

Ma C-M, Jiang SB (1999) Monte Carlo modelling of electron beams from medical accelerators. Phys Med Biol 44: R157–R189

Ma C-M, Faddegon BF, Rogers DWO et al (1997) Accurate characterization of Monte Carlo calculated electron beams for radiotherapy. Med Phys 24:401–416

Ma C-M, Li JS, Pawlicki T et al (2002) A Monte Carlo dose calculation tool for radiotherapy treatment planning. Phys Med Biol 47:1671–1689

Ma C-M, Li JS, Deng J et al (2008) Implementation of Monte Carlo dose calculation for CyberKnife treatment planning. J Phys Conf Ser 102:012016

Mackie TR, Scrimger JW, Battista JJ (1985) A convolution method of calculating dose for 15-MV X rays. Med Phys 12:188–196

Mohan R, Chui C, Lidofsky L (1986) Differential pencil beam dose computation model for photons. Med Phys 13:64–73

Pemler P, Besserer J, Schneider U et al (2006) Evaluation of a commercial electron treatment planning system based on Monte Carlo techniques (eMC). Med Phys 16:313–329

Reynaert N, van der Marcka SC, Schaarta DR et al (2007) Monte Carlo treatment planning for photon and electron beams. Radiat Phys Chem 76:643–686

Rogers DWO, Bielajew AF (1990) Monte Carlo techniques of electrons and photons for radiation dosimetry. In: Kase K, Bjarngard BE, Attix FH (eds) Dosimetry of ionizing radiation (V3). Academic, New York, pp 427–539

Sontag MR, Cunningham JR (1977) Corrections to absorbed dose calculations for tissue inhomogeneities. Med Phys 4:431–436

Van Esch A, Tillikainen L, Pyykkonen J et al (2006) Testing of the analytical anisotropic algorithm for photon dose calculation. Med Phys 33(1):4130–4148

Verhaegen F, Seuntjens J (2003) Monte Carlo modelling of external radiotherapy photon beams. Phys Med Biol 48:R107–R164

Wang L, Chui CS, Lovelock M (1998) A patient-specific Monte Carlo dose-calculation method for photon beams. Med Phys 25:867–878

Dose Rate

DAREK MICHALSKI[1], M. SAIFUL HUQ[2]
[1]Division of Medical Physics, Department of Radiation Oncology, University of Pittsburgh Cancer Centers, Pittsburgh, PA, USA
[2]Department of Radiation Oncology, University of Pittsburgh Medical Center Cancer Pavilion, Pittsburgh, PA, USA

Definition

Dose delivered per unit time.

Cross-References

▶ Four-Dimensional (4D) Treatment Planning/ Respiratory Gating

Dose Rate Constant

NING J. YUE
The Department of Radiation Oncology,
The Cancer Institute of New Jersey,
UMDNJ-Robert Wood Johnson Medical School,
New Brunswick, NJ, USA

Definition

The ratio of dose rate at a reference position and source strength.

Cross-References

▶ Brachytherapy: Low Dose Rate (LDR) Temporary Implants

Dose Volume Histogram (DVH)

BRIAN F. HASSON
Department of Radiation Oncology, Abington Memorial Hospital, Abington, PA, USA
Department of Radiation Oncology, College of Medicine, Drexel University, Philadelphia, PA, USA

Definition

A graphical representation of the dose that is received by normal tissues and target volumes within a 3-D radiation therapy plan. They provide information on the volume of a structure receiving a given dose over a range of doses. There are two general types of DVHs, namely, differential and cumulative.

Cross-References

▶ Conformal Therapy: Treatment Planning, Treatment Delivery, and Clinical Results
▶ Stereotactic Radiosurgery – Cranial

Ductal Adenocarcinoma

THEODORE E. YAEGER
Department Radiation Oncology,
Wake Forest University School of Medicine,
Winston-Salem, NC, USA

Definition

Cancers arising from the tissues lining glandular ducts of various organs but not invasive.

Cross-References

▶ Cancer of the Pancreas

▶ Stage 0 Breast Cancer

Ductal Carcinoma In Situ (DCIS)

DAVID E. WAZER
Radiation Oncology Department, Tufts Medical Center, Tufts University School of Medicine, Boston, MA, USA
Radiation Oncology Department, Rhode Island Hospital, Brown University School of Medicine, Providence, RI, USA

Definition

A proliferation of ductal carcinoma cells that arise within and are confined to the ductal lumens of the breast and that do not infiltrate the basement membrane.

Cross-References

▶ Cancer of the Breast Tis

▶ Stage 0 Breast Cancer

Duodenum

FILIP T. TROICKI[1], JAGANMOHAN POLI[2]
[1]College of Medicine, Drexel University, Philadelphia, PA, USA
[2]Department of Radiation Oncology, College of Medicine, Drexel University, Philadelphia, PA, USA

Definition

First section of the small intestine that is connected to the stomach via the pylorus.

Cross-References

▶ Cancer of the Pancreas

▶ Colon Cancer

▶ Liver and Hepatobiliary Tract

Dwell Position

CHENG B. SAW
Division of Radiation Oncology, Penn State Hershey Cancer Institute, Hershey, PA, USA

Definition

The position at which the afterloader source is placed to deliver the radiation dose.

Cross-References

▶ Brachytherapy: High Dose Rate (HDR) Implants

Dwell Time

CHENG B. SAW
Division of Radiation Oncology, Penn State Hershey Cancer Institute, Hershey, PA, USA

Definition

The time set for the afterloader source to deliver the radiation dose.

Cross-References

▶ Brachytherapy: High Dose Rate (HDR) Implants

Dyscrasias

Jo Ann Chalal
Department of Radiation Oncology, Fox Chase
Cancer Center, Philadelphia, PA, USA

Definition
Disorders of the blood where the components are
abnormal or are present in abnormal quantities.

Cross-References
▶ Leukemia in General
▶ Lymphoma
▶ Multiple Myeloma

Dysplastic Melanocytic Nevus

▶ Atypical (Dysplastic) Nevi
▶ Melanoma

E

Early-Stage Breast Cancer

ANTHONY E. DRAGUN
Department of Radiation Oncology, James
Graham Brown Cancer Center, University of
Louisville School of Medicine, Louisville,
KY, USA

Synonyms

Breast cancer risk models; Gail

Definition

Early-stage breast cancer refers to stage I or II
disease (T1-2, N0-1), with the most common
histologies generally referred to as "the carcinomas." Adenocarcinoma of the breast is by far the
most common and represents a heterogeneous
group of diseases with a wide variety of prognosis
and natural history. The overwhelming majority
(90–95%) of breast cancers are epithelial in origin, with infiltrating ductal carcinoma (IDC)
making up about 80% of this group of diseases.
Many times, it is associated with preinvasive disease (ductal carcinoma in situ). A second histology which is rarer, but not unusual in clinical
practice is invasive lobular carcinoma (ILC). The
hallmark of ILC is that it is generally mammographically occult. Other histologies which generally
portend a better prognosis with a less risk of
systemic spread include tubular carcinoma, medullary carcinoma, mucinous carcinoma, and
adenoidcystic carcinoma.

Etiology

Breast cancer is thought to originate from
a combination of germ-line and somatic gene
mutations that lead to dysregulated cell growth
and oncogenesis. Specific germ-line mutations
are identified in approximately 10% of all breast
cancers. The most common of these is BRCA1 or
2. These are tumor suppressor genes which are
more common in women with Ashkenazi Jewish
heritage and generally either gene results in
a lifetime risk of breast cancer that is 65–85%.
The BRCA1 mutation is also associated with
a high risk of ovarian cancer (approximately 40–
50% lifetime risk) and with colorectal and prostate cancers. BRCA2 is also associated with a risk
of ovarian cancer albeit slightly lower (approximately 15–20% lifetime risk) and with male
breast cancer and pancreatic cancer. Another
common germ-line mutation is the p53 mutation
(▶ Li-Fraumeni syndrome). Mutations in this
tumor suppressor gene are associated with
an 80–90% of lifetime risk of breast cancer.
Other less-common germ-line mutations include
PTEN (Cowden syndrome) and ATM (ataxia-
telangectasia). Genetic testing should be considered when family history suggests an underlying
genetic susceptibility and the results of the genetic
tests will influence the overall management of
the patient. Genetic counseling should be offered
to all patients with strong family history prior
to genetic testing, and to all patients with an
identified germ-line mutation.

Despite the growing body of medical knowledge regarding the aforementioned germ-line

L.W. Brady, T.E. Yaeger (eds.), *Encyclopedia of Radiation Oncology*, DOI 10.1007/978-3-540-85516-3,
© Springer-Verlag Berlin Heidelberg 2013

mutations, approximately 85% of breast cancer patients have no significant family history or identifiable genetic abnormality. These breast cancers are thought to arrive mainly from somatic mutations which are the result of an accumulation of environmental and personal risk factors. Age is the most important risk factor for the development of breast cancer. The incidence of breast cancer increases significantly with age and the increase in incidence is highest in premenopausal women. A personal history of previous breast disease is also an identifiable risk factor, with a risk of metachronous contralateral breast cancer of approximately 0.5–1% per year after the treatment of a previously diagnosed breast cancer. Atypical hyperplasia of the breast portends an approximately fourfold increase in risk of breast cancer. Family history: the risk depends on the number of relatives affected, the age of these relatives at diagnosis, and the degree of relationship to the patient. Obstetric history: risk of breast cancer is increased both with early onset of menses and late menopause. Young age at first parity is significantly protective as is multiple pregnancies. Breast feeding has been shown to have a small but significant protective effect.

Hormone Replacement Therapy

Long-term postmenopausal use of hormone replacement therapy has been shown to increase risk. Oral contraceptive pill use: the data regarding the risk of breast cancer is currently conflicting on this subject. Prior radiation exposure: patients who have had multiple exposures of either diagnostic or therapeutic radiation including tuberculosis screening and/or radiation therapy for diseases such as Hodgkin's lymphoma fall into this category. Life style factors: the risk of breast cancer has been shown to increase with obesity, high body mass index, heavy alcohol use as well as smoking. Data regarding dietary specifics such as the influence of red meat, dairy and soy products have been conflicting.

Clinical Presentation

The emergence of early-stage breast cancer as a common clinical entity is a direct result of the significant impact of routine screening mammography, clinical and self breast exam, along with public awareness campaigns. Mammography and physical exam detect early-stage breast cancer prior to the onset of any symptoms, and the majority of lesions detected by screening mammography have no corresponding clinical sign. Screening mammography has been shown to reduce the relative risk of mortality from breast cancer for women aged 40–75. The benefits of screening mammography in the elderly are less known. There have been no randomized trials to evaluate the comparative effectiveness of different screening intervals, but an interval of approximately 1–2 years between screenings is generally recommended.

Regarding location, nearly half of newly diagnosed breast cancers occur in the upper outer quadrant of the breast, with the remainder presenting in equal rates in upper inner, lower inner, lower outer, and central locations. Mammographically, new lesions present as a new density or cluster of microcalcifications on an interval screening mammogram. When early breast cancers are clinically detectible, they are generally present on physical exam as a firm, nontender, mobile mass. Overlying skin changes and/or nipple discharge are relatively rare. Once a new abnormality is detected, the strategy is to avoid any delays in further evaluation or treatment. Generally, patients have a better prognosis when treated within 3 months of their diagnosis or onset of symptoms.

Diagnostics

A thorough clinical history of breast symptoms is a crucial component of the diagnostic workup of any new breast abnormality. The initial focus should be on the onset, duration, characteristics, and course of all breast symptoms. History of prior diagnostic tests including any abnormal screening mammograms or previous biopsies is helpful. Identification of any of the aforementioned risk factors including family history and obstetric history is also required. On physical examination, it is important to distinguish thickening and nodularity, which can occur normally in heterogeneous breast tissue versus any suspicious dominant masses. It is important to note that breast self-exam and clinical breast exam have been shown to be an effective complement to screening mammography, detecting approximately 10–15% of cancers that are not well visualized on mammograms.

Mammography is the foundation of screening for the early detection of breast cancer and is also used as the first diagnostic tool of choice in any newly detected palpable mass (Fig. 1a). Mammography has a sensitivity of approximately 90% and a specificity of approximately 95%. New early-stage disease usually presents an ill-defined or speculated mass. New lesions may be described as lobulated or smooth and may have associated architectural distortion of the breast. Compression views are helpful for distinguishing subtle changes of the breast from suspicious lesions (Fig. 1b). Microcalcifications (approximately 200 μm in size) in heterogeneous clusters are characteristic of associated intraductal disease.

Ultrasound is used to supplement mammography, but it is not an established first-line screening tool. It is best at distinguishing cystic from solid lesions and can also assist with biopsy guidance (Fig. 1c). Ultrasound has a sensitivity of approximately 70% and a specificity of approximately 95%. The hallmark of suspicious breast abnormalities on ultrasound is "posterior acoustic shadowing" which occurs deep to a hypoechoic, ill-defined lesion.

Breast MRI is not established as a screening tool or in the initial diagnosis of the palpable mass, due to concern regarding false positives and expense. Despite this, routine use of breast MRI is increasing, especially in the United States. More studies have shown that women with a known ipsilateral breast cancer have an approximately 5% rate of detection of contralateral "occult" disease. These studies have also shown that the use of MRI correlates with increased rates of mastectomy with no associated disease-free or overall survival benefit. MRI may be useful for targeted population such as younger women with dense breasts on mammography or women at high risk (BRCA or other germ-line mutations), where sensitivity and specificity approach 80% and 90%, respectively (Fig. 2). MRI is also useful in the detection of an occult breast primary in patients who present with a positive axillary lymph node and no clinically or mammographically detectable breast lesion. Novel imaging techniques that are not currently in routine use include breast CT, thermography, microwave imaging, and optical imaging.

Breast Biopsy

Biopsy is obligatory for any suspicious breast mass. Fine-needle aspiration is routine in the workup of cystic masses. Cytology for malignant cells should be performed for any lesion that is identified as complex on ultrasound. Core biopsy is the most common initial invasive procedure for the diagnosis of breast cancer and may be performed with the guidance of stereotactic mammography or ultrasound. Excisional biopsy is acceptable for palpable lesions when core biopsy or fine-needle aspiration is not feasible. Needle-localization is used to assist with excisional biopsy for lesions that present as a nonpalpable group of microcalcifications on screening mammography. Specimen radiograph of tissue removed under needle localization assures complete removal of any mammographic abnormalities.

Differential Diagnosis

New calcifications on a screening mammogram are usually classified as suspicious or benign.

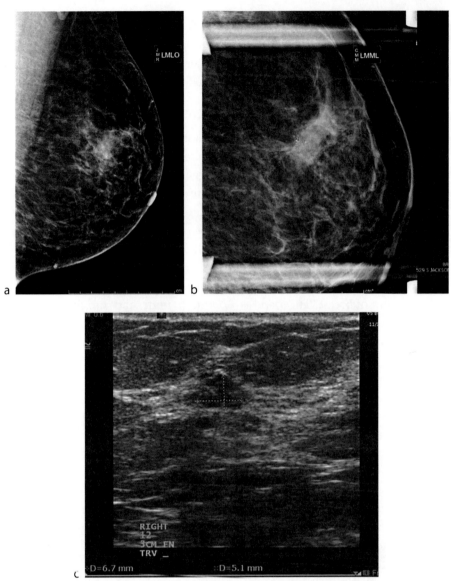

Early-Stage Breast Cancer. Fig. 1 Digital radiographic images from a 47-year-old female who presented with a new abnormality of the left breast on screening mammogram (**a**) which led to further diagnostic mammography with spot compression and magnification views (**b**), detailing a cluster of microcalcifications and architectural distortion. Subsequent ultrasound (**c**) showed a 6–7 mm lesion in the upper outer quadrant of the left breast. A core biopsy was obtained under ultrasound guidance which revealed infiltrating ductal carcinoma, estrogen and progesterone receptor positive, Her2 negative

Suspicious microcalcifications are characterized as pleomorphic, heterogenous, microcalcifications. These suggest an underlying preinvasive (ductal carcinoma in situ) or invasive process. Other types of calcifications which are larger and more regular in size and appearance suggest nonmalignant processes such as fibroadenoma, benign ductal ectasia, fat necrosis, or calcified cysts.

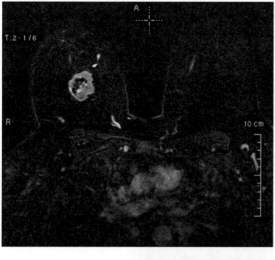

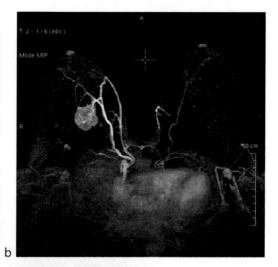

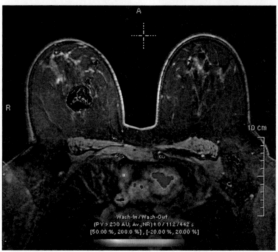

Early-Stage Breast Cancer. Fig. 2 Magnetic resonance imaging (*MRI*) of a 32-year-old female with heterogeneous breast tissue and a new abnormality in the right breast which was found on self-breast exam. The lesion was obscured by dense breast tissue on diagnostic mammogram. On breast magnetic resonance (*MR*), the lesion is seen as a ring enhancing 3.4 cm mass in the right breast near the 12:00 location (**a**). Additional vascular phase views show increased vascular flow very characteristic of malignancy (**b, c**). No additional ipsilateral or contralateral lesions were found. Biopsy was consistent with infiltrating ductal carcinoma, estrogen, progesterone receptor and Her2 negative (triple negative). The patient was subsequently found to be a carrier of BRCA1

The new appearance of a painless breast mass either by physical exam or screening mammography should never be dismissed by the evaluating physician. New breast masses may be a sign of a new invasive carcinoma or unusual breast malignancies such as lymphoma or sarcoma.

Preinvasive cancer may also, on rare occasion, present as a mass. Benign causes of painless breast masses include, but are not limited to, fibroadenoma, cysts, hematoma, fat necrosis, lipoma, breast abscess, galactocle, seroma, and gynecomastia (in male patients).

Prophylaxis

Preventive therapy with either medical (hormonal therapy) or surgical (prophylactic mastectomy) therapy is highly debated in terms of appropriate candidates as well as the risk–benefit profile. Medical prophylaxis of breast cancer is usually termed "chemoprevention." The largest national trial of chemoprevention in the United States was NSABP P-01, which was a randomized placebo-controlled trial of nearly 14,000 women conducted to evaluate the effect of tamoxifen for the prevention of breast cancer in women at the "elevated risk." Women who were over the age of 60, had lobular carcinoma in situ (LCIS) or a relative risk of 1.6 by the Gail model were judged to be eligible. Although tamoxifen reduced the relative risk of invasive and noninvasive breast cancers by approximately 50%, the absolute reduction in risk was approximately 2% at 5 years (Fisher et al. 1998). In addition, tamoxifen increased the relative risk of endometrial cancer and had an associated risk of deep venous thrombosis. Other similar studies from the United Kingdom and Europe suggest that tamoxifen does not reduce the relative risk of breast cancer in similarly studied patients.

The mainstay of surgical prevention of breast cancer is the prophylactic mastectomy. It is usually offered to women at extremely high risk for breast cancer such as women with the aforementioned germ line mutations (BRCA1 or 2), strong family history, diffuse LCIS, or contralateral prophylactic mastectomy in patients who have had a mastectomy for a previously diagnosed breast cancer. Patients who are BRCA1 or 2 positive have a cumulative risk for contralateral breast cancer at 25 years of approximately 45% after the diagnosis of ipsilateral breast cancer. Multiple studies have shown that the incidence of prophylactic mastectomy, especially contralateral prophylactic mastectomy, is on the rise in the United States. The reasons for this are uncertain although the growing use of breast MRI is thought to be a major factor. Prophylactic mastectomy reduces breast cancer risks by approximately 90% in women at high risk and should be a consideration in women with genetic mutation, strong family history, and/or dense breast tissue that makes routine mammographic surveillance difficult. The use of prophylactic mastectomy is highly influenced by surgeon and patient biases. Patients should be counseled in a multidisciplinary breast cancer center with all of their therapeutic options prior to proceeding with surgical prophylaxis.

Therapy

Breast Conservation Therapy

This is the preferred method of management for the overwhelming majority of women who present with early-stage breast cancer. The underlying rationale is that multiple randomized trials from the United States, United Kingdom, and Europe have shown no advantage of more radical surgery (mastectomy). Breast conservation therapy involves a multidisciplinary approach involving the breast surgeon, radiation oncologist, and medical oncologist. Ideally, patients should be evaluated by these aforementioned specialists after a biopsy-proven diagnosis of breast cancer prior to therapeutic decision making. Discussion in the multidisciplinary setting should include the pros and cons of breast conservation therapy and mastectomy including the toxicities and logistics of surgery, radiation therapy, and possible breast reconstruction. Psychological implications of posttreatment mammographic surveillance of patients who undergo breast conservation as well as the body image implications of mastectomy should be fully discussed. Patients should be counseled that mastectomy does not always eliminate the need for the addition of radiation therapy, as indications for postmastectomy radiation therapy continue to evolve. Discussion should also focus on the cosmetic outcome of breast conservation therapy, which is good to excellent in approximately 85% of patients, as well as any potential contraindications to radiation therapy.

Breast Conservation Surgery

Breast conserving therapy is, at its foundation, a minimally invasive surgery. Surgery for the breast primary in this regard is essentially an oncologic procedure that involves a wide local excision of the primary tumor. This is most often termed a partial or segmental mastectomy (synonyms: lumpectomy, tylectomy, tumorectomy, quantrantectomy). For patients who present with nonpalpable disease, needle-localization by mammographic guidance prior to the definitive procedure is necessary. Complete excision with negative margins is the overall goal. It is generally agreed that wide surgical margins are preferred and that positive surgical margins should be reexcised to clear residual tumor. Significant controversy exists on what constitutes "close" surgical margins. It has been suggested that surgical margins greater than or equal to 2 mm can be managed without reoperation. It should be noted that cosmetic outcome depends heavily on the volume of normal breast tissue removed and this may have an implication on the choice and technique of surgery.

Sentinel lymph node biopsy is performed for patients with biopsy-proven invasive disease or those with preinvasive disease with high suspicion for occult invasive component. It has been estimated that approximately 10–40% of clinically lymph node negative patients contain pathologically positive disease. Sentinel lymph node biopsy has largely replaced axillary lymph node dissection for most patients in order to minimize the risk of lymphedema and other long-term morbidity. The sentinel lymph node biopsy is generally performed at the same time as the surgery for the primary tumor and consists of an injection of vital blue dye and/or technetium-99m sulfur colloid. The objective is to identify 1–4 sentinel lymph nodes for removal. If any of these are positive, then complete axillary lymph node dissection is subsequently performed with approximately 50% of patients having additional lymph nodes positive.

Adjuvant Radiation Therapy

Treatment with breast conservation therapy requires the use adjuvant radiation therapy to reduce the risk of in-breast recurrence and improve overall survival. Addition of radiation therapy to breast conserving surgery results in an absolute risk reduction of 25–30% for local recurrence and an absolute improvement in overall survival of 5–7% at 15 years (Clarke et al. 2005). As a result, for every four local recurrences that are prevented, one life is saved. The magnitude of benefit is higher in younger patients. Patients should begin adjuvant radiation therapy in a timely manner once final surgical pathology has been obtained. Whole breast radiation therapy has been the mainstay of adjuvant radiation therapy techniques for the better part of 30 years. Patients are usually placed in the supine position with their arm abducted and extended (Fig. 3a). Other techniques involve using prone positioning especially for larger breasted women. The target of therapy is the breast tissue as it extends from the clavicle to the inframammary fold and from midsternum to the midaxillary line. Custom planning using computed tomography is essential and segmental tissue compensation to homogenize radiation dose is essential to minimize toxicity (Fig. 3b). Ideally, the entire breast is treated with doses between 95% and 105% of prescription dose (Figs. 3c and 3d). Conventional dose fractionation schedules involve delivering approximately 45–50 Gy to the whole breast in daily fractions of 1.8–2 Gy over 5–6 weeks using megavoltage x-rays, usually in the range of 6–18 MV.

A " ► boost to the breast" dose is conventionally performed for most patients to deliver additional radiation to the breast tissue at highest risk – the 1–2 cm of tissue immediately adjacent

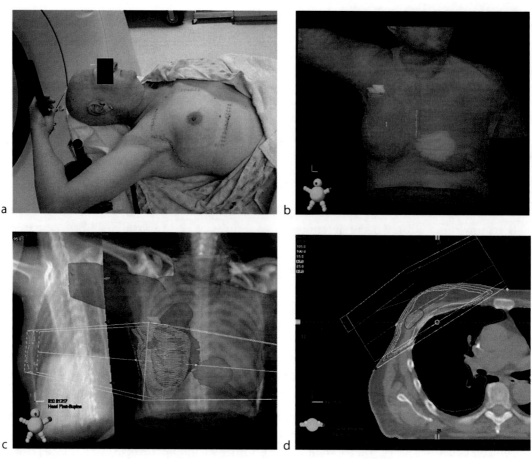

Early-Stage Breast Cancer. Fig. 3 Typical supine setup for a 52-year-old patient with early-stage breast cancer (status-post breast conserving surgery) who is to be treated with whole breast irradiation (**a**). Three-dimensional treatment planning techniques (**b**) are used to define the breast (*red*), lumpectomy cavity (*blue*), levels 1 (*green*) and 2 (*yellow*) of the axilla, the ipsilateral lung (*pink*), and heart (*orange*). Distribution of radiation dose in three dimensions (**c**) shows the breast volume and lower axilla covered by the 95% dose cloud (*green*). Axial view of breast dosimetry (**d**) shows locations of isodose lines in relation to the lumpectomy cavity (*bold blue*)

to the lumpectomy cavity. The evidence for reduction in local recurrence by employing a boost is strongest for younger patients. For the boost, an additional 10–20 Gy in conventional fractions is given using a combination of appositional electrons and/or megavoltage photons (Fig. 4a). Image-guided radiation planning using CT or ultrasound to target the postsurgical lumpectomy cavity for this boost dose is customary (Fig. 4b). Other techniques of lumpectomy

cavity boost involve interstitial brachytherapy or ▶ intraoperative radiation therapy (IORT) at the time of lumpectomy.

Hypofractionated whole breast radiation therapy is designed to accelerate therapy and compress overall treatment time in half. Doses between 2.5 and 3 Gy per fraction are given in daily fractions over approximately 3 weeks. Recent data has shown that this schedule is equivalent in terms of disease control and toxicity and

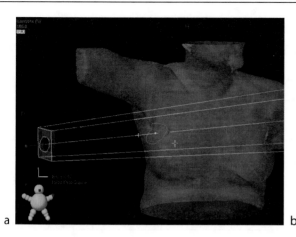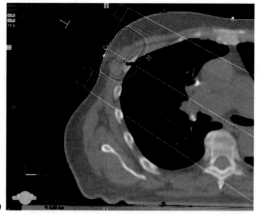

a   b

Early-Stage Breast Cancer. Fig. 4 Computed tomography (*CT*)-guided electron boost plan for the same patient shown in Fig. 3. A three-dimensional reconstructed skin rendering (**a**) shows the field shape within the linear accelerator, as well as the shape of the field on the skin of the breast (*yellow line*) in order to encompass the lumpectomy cavity tissue target (*blue*). Axial view of dosimetry (**b**) shows the lumpectomy cavity tissue target (*blue*) within the therapeutic isodose curves

cosmetic outcome when compared to conventionally fractionated techniques (Whelan et al. 2008).

Accelerated partial breast irradiation (APBI) is a strategy to target radiation therapy only to the area at highest risk for in-breast recurrence. The strategy involves an accelerated treatment regimen (5 days) to deliver focused radiotherapy to the 1–2 cm of breast tissue surrounding the lumpectomy cavity. The selection of patients for the proper use of APBI is currently a matter of controversy; however, recent consensus guidelines have been proposed (Table 1) to triage and select appropriate patients (Smith et al. 2009). APBI may be delivered using brachytherapy or external-beam techniques. Brachytherapy techniques for APBI have been developed over the course of approximately the last 20 years. Clinical experience from multiple institutions was initially reported for multicatheter brachytherapy techniques, where approximately 20–30 parallel brachytherapy catheters are inserted under CT or mammographic guidance. The objective is to deliver approximately 34 Gy in ten fractions of 3.4 Gy twice daily to a 1–2 cm volume of pericavity breast tissue. Balloon-based brachytherapy techniques were developed approximately 9 years ago and greatly simplify the multicatheter technique and provide a therapy that is much less user dependent and easier for patients to endure (Fig. 5). With either technique, avoiding excessive skin dose (>125%) is crucial to achieving good cosmetic outcome.

Three-dimensional conformal radiation therapy (3D-CRT) may also be used and can be delivered using a 4–5 field noncoplanar technique or "mini-tangent" technique with or without electron supplementation. The total dose is approximately 38.5 Gy in ten fractions delivered twice daily. The popularity of three-dimensional conformal radiation therapy stems from its ability to be noninvasive. Concerns include the relatively scant amount of clinical experience compared to brachytherapy and the potential increase in integral radiation dose to the lung and normal breast tissue. In summary, APBI is an emerging technology that is currently the subject of randomized controlled trials in the United States and Europe. Careful patient selection using the aforementioned guidelines is crucial to proper treatment.

Early-Stage Breast Cancer. Table 1 General guidelines and selection criteria for evaluation of patients for accelerated partial breast irradiation (*APBI*), adopted from the 2009 ASTRO Consensus Statement (Smith et al. 2009)

Criterion			
ASTRO consensus definition	*"Suitable"*	*"Cautionary"*	*"Unsuitable"*
Age	≥ 60 years	50–59 years	<50 years
T-stage	T1	T0 or T2 (<3 cm)	T2 (>3 cm), T3/4
N-stage	N0 (i–, i+)	N0	≥N1
Margins	Wide (>2 mm)	Close (≤2 mm)	Positive
Histology	Invasive ductal, mucinous, tubular, colloid carcinoma	DCIS, invasive lobular carcinoma	Any
ER status	Positive	Negative	Any
LVSI	None	Limited	Extensive
EIC	None	≤3 cm	>3 cm
Focality	Unifocal	Microscopic multifocality	Clinical multifocality
Centricity	Unicentric	Unicentric	Multicentric

ASTRO American Society for Radiation Oncology, *LVSI* lymphovascular space invasion, *EIC* extensive intraductal component

Regional Nodal Irradiation

Irradiation of the regional lymph nodes is usually omitted in early-stage breast cancer due to the low risk of regional lymph node relapse (approximately 2–8%). Lymph node irradiation may be considered with patients at high risk, where estimated local failure is 15% or greater. Regional lymph node irradiation is also considered in patients who have extracapsular extension or inadequate lymph node dissection.

Contraindications to Radiation Therapy

This is currently an area of therapeutic investigation. The majority of the contraindications encountered in clinical practice are "relative," and one can easily find published institutional experience involving irradiation of such patients. Most absolute contraindications are due to unexpected extent of underlying disease. Absolute contraindications include: diffuse microcalcifications on mammography, persistent positive margins despite multiple attempts at breast conservation surgery, and multicentric disease (disease in multiple breast quadrants). All of these situations indicate a volume of gross and occult breast disease that likely precludes acceptable cosmetic outcome with attempted breast conservation. Additionally, pregnancy is almost always an absolute contraindication to radiation therapy. Relative contraindications include: ▶ collagen vascular disease, recurrent disease, prior breast radiation, or BRCA 1 and 2.

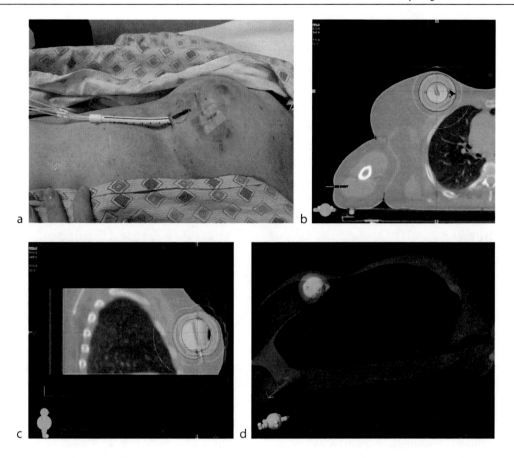

Early-Stage Breast Cancer. Fig. 5 Typical positioning for balloon brachytherapy (**a**) shown for a 54-year-old patient with early-stage breast cancer (status-post breast conserving surgery). The original lumpectomy scar is superior to the multicatheter balloon device, which was placed under ultrasound guidance after confirmation of the final pathologic stage. Dose distribution is shown in the axial (**b**), sagittal (**c**), and three-dimensional (**d**) views. The breast tissue target is represented in all three views (*shaded green*), and is covered by the therapeutic isodose line (*yellow*) as seen in (**b**) and (**c**)

Mastectomy

The most common indication for mastectomy in early-stage disease is patient choice. Other indications include diffuse microcalcifications on mammography, and the inability to obtain partial mastectomy with negative margins with an acceptable cosmetic result. Recommendations for postmastectomy radiation therapy generally include lymph node positive disease, larger than expected tumor size (more than 4–5 cm), close or positive margins at the time of mastectomy, where the addition of radiotherapy has been shown to both reduce locoregional recurrence and improve overall survival (Clarke et al. 2005).

Systemic Therapy

Hormonal Therapy

Antiestrogenic therapy is a mainstay in the treatment of early-stage breast cancer to both improve disease-free survival and to add to local regional control in the estrogen receptor or progesterone receptor positive patient. This therapy is usually delivered after the completion of radiation therapy, and there is no proven benefit of offering it concurrent with radiotherapy. The standard treatment for premenopausal patients is usually 5 years of tamoxifen. In postmenopausal patients, there exists data for more options including the use of aromatase inhibitors (letrozole or anastrozole) alone for 5 years, or 5 years of tamoxifen followed by 5 additional years of letrozole.

Chemotherapy

Cytotoxic chemotherapy is used selectively in the treatment of early-stage breast cancer (EBCTCG 2005). Treatment selection largely depends on age, biologic subtype of tumor, menopausal status, and/or results of ► microarray analysis. Combinations of chemotherapeutic agents and sequencing are similar to that described for locally advanced breast cancer.

Prognosis

Available evidence from single institutions series and large randomized trials in the United Kingdom and Europe suggest improvement in disease-free survival and overall survival in patients with early-stage breast cancer as therapies have evolved over time. All endpoints have improved over time due to earlier detection and patient selection with mammographic screening, breast cancer awareness, and the use of systemic therapy including hormonal therapy and cytotoxic chemotherapy.

Local Control

The most recent data suggests that the 10 year overall local regional control of early-stage breast cancer is in the range of roughly 90% (stage I disease: 95%, stage II disease: 85%). It is important to delineate a true recurrence from an elsewhere breast failure in the cases of patients treated with breast conservation therapy. True recurrences are located within 1–2 cm of the original lumpectomy cavity (within the same quadrant of the initial index lesion). The incidence depends heavily on age, margin status, the use of systemic treatment, tumor size, and nodal status. There is also an association of true recurrence with lymphovascular space invasion, perineural invasion, extensive intraductal component, biologic subtype, radiation therapy dose, and radiation therapy delay. True recurrences typically reoccur within the first 2–5 years following treatment for breast cancer.

Elsewhere Breast Failures

These are clinically different entities from true breast recurrences and appear later in the time course of follow-up in the patient with breast cancer. They appear to occur with the same frequency as contralateral breast cancer (0.5–1% per year) and the incidence is decreased by use of antiestrogenic therapy. Overall, the disease-free survival at 10 years for early-stage breast cancer patients is approximately 80% (85% for stage I, 75% for stage II). Overall survival numbers at about 20–25 years is approximately 60% with a wide range accounting for patient age and comorbid conditions at diagnosis.

Epidemiology

Incidence

Overall, there are approximately 180–190 thousand new cases of breast cancer per year in the United States, making breast cancer the number one nonskin malignancy to occur in women. The average lifetime risk of breast cancer is approximately 12%, or 1 out of 8 women. The incidence has decreased slightly over time due to the decreased use of sustained hormone replacement therapy in postmenopausal patients. There are 40,000 deaths due to breast cancer in the United States every year. Mortality has decreased significantly over the last decade due to earlier detection (screening) and improvements in treatments (especially with regard to systemic therapy).

With regard to demographics, age is the most significant predictor for incidence of breast cancer. There is a steep increase in incidence after age 40 and incidence continues to rise in perimenopausal years. With regard to race, incidence in the United States is highest for white women; however, African American women are likely to have an earlier age of onset and present with more advanced disease. Other demographic influences on the epidemiology of breast cancer include family history (especially first-degree relatives), early menarche, late menopause, older age at first pregnancy, nulliparity, use of hormone replacement therapy, and obesity. Geographically, breast cancer is more common in the United States and in Europe compared to Asia and Africa.

Cross-References
▶ Breast Cancer: Locally Advanced and Recurrent Disease, Postmastectomy Radiation and Systemic Therapies
▶ Breast Conservation Therapy

References
Clarke M, Collins R, Darby S et al (2005) Effects of radiotherapy and of differences in the extent of surgery for early breast cancer on local recurrence and 15-year survival: an overview of the randomised trials. Lancet 366(9503):2087–2106

Early Breast Cancer Trialists' Collaborative Group (EBCTCG) (2005) Effects of chemotherapy and hormonal therapy for early breast cancer on recurrence and 15 year survival: an overview of the randomized trials. Lancet 365(9472):1687–1717

Fisher B, Constantino JP, Wickerman DL et al (1998) Tamoxifen for the prevention of breast cancer: report of the National Surgical Adjuvant Breast and Bowel Project P-1 study. J Natl Cancer Inst 90:1371–1388

Smith BD, Arthur DW, Buchholz TA et al (2009) Accelerated partial breast irradiation statement from the American Society for Radiation Oncology (ASTRO). Int J Radiat Oncol Biol Phys 74(4):987–1001

Whelan TJ, Kim DH, Sussman J (2008) Clinical experience using hypofractionated radiation schedules in breast cancer. Semin Radiat Oncol 18(4):257–264

EBRT
▶ External Beam Radiation Therapy

Economics

PAUL J. SCHILLING
Community Cancer Center of North Florida, Gainesville, FL, USA

Economics of Loco-Regional Failure
In 2010, 562,340 deaths from cancer were recorded (American Cancer Society 2010). Of these, half had a component of local or regional failure. As systemic therapy improves, consequences of local failure become more pronounced (Regaz et al. 1997; GITSG 1985). Improving systemic therapy may lead to a longer lifetime free of systemic metastasis during which local failure can occur. This is one reason that postoperative radiation treatment improves survival in breast cancer, small cell lung cancer, prostate cancer, and rectal cancer (Regaz et al. 1997; GITSG 1985; Schilling 2007). The cost of regional failure in terms of human life and tragedy is staggering.

Economic Profiling: Insurance Companies Determine Who Provides the Least Expensive Care
Economic profiling tracks physician care expenditures including specialty referrals, laboratory testing, and utilization of other costly resources. Physicians are allowed to continue on the panel of certain insurance plans based on their level of utilization and cost to the insurance plan. Yet, expenditures to provide care to individual patients are variable (Schilling 2003a). Patients who have complex cancers have a higher average

cost of care, which may institute multiple inquiries from the insurance company about specialist referral, prescribing habits, and overall resource utilization. Higher average costs of care may lead to deselection from insurance plans for "outlier" utilization. When comprehensive care is provided in a single geographic setting, insurance companies know that patient compliance in the stated plan of disease management is enhanced, leading to fewer episodes of missed testing or treatment. This "dropout rate" is calculated as care prescribed by a physician but not undertaken by a patient (Schilling 2003a). Physicians with high dropout rates reduce costs to the insurance company, but only temporarily.

Economic Credentialing: Hospitals Seek to Prevent Patient Choice

Economic credentialing is defined by the American Medical Association as the "use of economic criteria unrelated to the quality of care or professional competency to determine an individual physician's qualifications for granting or renewal of medical staff privileges" (Schilling 2003a). The goal of economic credentialing in radiation oncology is to capture a revenue stream by denying hospital privileges to a group or terminating hospital privileges and thereby limiting competition. Hospital bylaws are considered by many states to be a contract between a hospital and medical staff, serving as a guideline for actions against physicians, as well as outlining due process provisions for physicians (Schilling 2003a). Read your hospital bylaws carefully and watch for hospital proposed changes. The Medical Staff should have its own legal representation, separate from the hospital, when hospital bylaws changes are proposed.

Hospitals may seek to institute differential credentialing to keep qualified physicians from becoming members of the medical staff, and thus limiting competition. One example is requiring radiation oncologists to complete 4 years of residency, whereas before 1994 radiation oncology residencies were only 3 years (Schilling 2003a).

Contracts between physician groups and hospitals establish a business relationship to provide radiation oncology services. Traditionally, exclusive contracts assured patient access to care that would otherwise not be available. Because of increased access to cancer treatment in the United States, this is almost never the case today. Most hospitals enter into an exclusive contract strictly for financial reasons, which put the physicians in the position of being controlled by the hospital master financial plan. Exclusive contracts may deprive patients of choices and limit the establishment of new physician practices. Some exclusive contracts contain "clean sweep" provisions that stipulate when a group loses an exclusive contract with a hospital, that each physician simultaneously forfeits clinical privileges without the benefit of due process afforded by the hospital bylaws (Schilling 2003a).

The peer review process may be misused to further a hospital's economic goals. Because in most states peer review proceedings are protected from legal discovery, peer review affords an opportunity for physicians to evaluate their care and remediate their knowledge if necessary. Protection from legal discovery also invites hospitals to target and eliminate physicians who are economic threats to their service lines. This is particularly true for hospital-based specialists including radiation oncologists. Some radiation oncologists find themselves excluded from equipment or facilities when a health-care institution changes radiation oncology from a hospital inpatient service to an outpatient service. This may occur with no change in location of building, equipment, or staffing. There is an entire consulting industry that teaches hospitals how to displace existing radiation oncologists and put their replacement physicians on salary. We are not the only target; physical medicine, diagnostic radiology, and cardiothoracic surgery are also vulnerable to these tactics (Schilling 2003a).

The American Medical Association has a long, continuous interest in fighting economic credentialing, and has a litigation department with years of accumulated information and experience and will assist physicians who challenge health-care institutions about these issues (Schilling 2003a).

Radiation Oncology's Socioeconomic Ties with Diagnostic Radiology

In previous years, delivery of radiation treatment was both crude and considerably simpler. "Therapeutic radiology" was a discipline of diagnostic radiology. As radiation treatment became more sophisticated and as megavoltage linear accelerators became available, it was clear that separate training was necessary for radiation oncologists to treat cancer patients. Eventually, new CPT codes were created for radiation oncology and governmental payers began to recognize us as being separate from diagnostic radiology. Diagnostic radiologists seemed to be embroiled in a campaign to close the "in-office ancillary exemption" which allows non-radiologist physicians to perform imaging within their offices. Currently, obstetricians perform pregnancy-related ultrasounds, cardiologists perform cardiac catheterizations and nuclear cardiac procedures, and family physicians perform bone densitometry within their offices. With the advent of image-guided radiation treatment, PET/CT simulators and MRI simulators for treatment planning, radiation oncologists continue to fight for the ability to image our patients for diagnosis, staging, and treatment planning related to cancer. Our objective is to show CMS that imaging is necessary for treating cancer patients appropriately (Schilling 2009a).

In 2009, Medicare proposed a 95% "usage rate" for diagnostic imaging equipment and then extended this to all equipment costing more than $1 million. This proposal was advanced by the Medicare Payment Advisory Commission and was based on a sample size of only six urban diagnostic radiology centers but because of the cost of linear accelerators, was extended to radiation oncology (Schilling 2009). If enacted for radiation oncology it would force the closure of many rural practices, making patients travel longer distances for cancer treatment. Fortunately, this proposal was defeated because radiation oncologists like you told congress that we are different from diagnostic imaging. Radiation oncologists need to continue to fight for the ability to image and treat their patients appropriately for cancer therapy now and into the future. We also need to show CMS that we treat cancer patients and are separate from diagnostic radiology (Schilling 2009a).

Medical Physicists: Should They Bill Medicare Directly for Their Services?

Many medical physicists maintain that they are Board Certified professionals so should be able to bill Medicare directly. In 1960, lists of providers that could bill Medicare directly were formulated, and physicists were not among these professionals. Because of this, a congressional act is required to give billing status to medical physicists (Schilling 2008). Currently, there are only two codes recognized for the contribution of medical physicists: Code 77336 continuing medical physicist services and code 77370 special medical physics consultation. There is no other methodology in Medicare Part A or Part B that identifies a medical physicist component of work in any other codes (Schilling 2008). At Florida Medicare rates, code 77336 reimburses at $50.43 and code 77370 reimburses at $105.55. In a busy department with 30 patients under continuous radiation treatment, there would be 30 continuing medical physicist services provided at a Medicare reimbursement level of $50.93 for 50 weeks per year, for a total reimbursement of

$75,645. If 50% (this is high) of patients under treatment required a special medical consultation, this would mean a yearly reimbursement of $15,833. The total for these services, $91,478, is dramatically below what the average medical physicist makes in the United States (Schilling 2008). Professional self-determination appears to be important to the medical physicist. If we examine published literature available to the public on the process of radiation treatment, very few of them mention medical physicists as a member of the patient care team. This is unfortunate. This is true of the National Cancer Institute Manual on radiation therapy as the American Cancer Society's publication on the process of care for radiation oncology. There is certainly room for improvement to include medical physicists in the process of care because they are an integral component. The patient should understand their role and perhaps additional efforts can be directed toward recognizing the contributions of medical physicists in the care of cancer patients (Schilling 2008).

Health-care Reform

In 2010, 54 million Americans were without health insurance. Approximately one-third of those people held jobs which offered health insurance coverage but they chose not to take this coverage due to cost considerations. As we grapple with the need for health-care reform, the Congressional Budget Office estimated that tort reform with a $250,000 cap on noneconomic damages would save the US $54 billion over 10 years and reduce national health-care spending by 1/2 of 1% annually and save $41 billion in tests ordered due to physicians' needs to practice defensive medicine (AMA 2009). Medicaid expansion during a time when fewer doctors accept Medicare patients may not be an answer that is palatable to many physicians. The government continues to study bundled "bulk" payments for hospital and physician care. One proposal would be to negotiate a bundled fee

paid to hospitals for an episode of care (i.e., lung cancer). The physicians would then negotiate with the hospital for their component. As always, greater bargaining power is in the hands of the entity that receives the check.

There has been a tremendous push for independent practice of nurse practitioners (without physician supervision) and for nurse anesthetists (Schilling 2009b). These physician extenders may close the gap in primary care due to the lack of physicians choosing primary care as a profession due to low reimbursement.

The AMA has requested insurance market reform with elimination of denials for preexisting conditions, health insurance for all Americans, and with health-care decisions remaining in the hands of patients and their physicians, as well as repealing the Medicare sustainable growth formula that triggers deep cuts in Medicare and threatens seniors' access to care. The AMA also desires proven medical liability reforms to reduce the cost of defensive medicine (AMA 2009).

Radiation Oncologists' Lobbying and Political Activity

Americans place a high value on the quality and availability of medical care. In this country, we have massive government programs that provide the funds to pay for the health care of the poor, disabled, and elderly. Unfortunately, payment rules are created by the legislature for a large portion of all physicians' practices in the United States (Schilling 2007; Pcady 2006). The importance of interfacing with governmental payers as well as in influencing the process that benefits our patients and brings them new technologies cannot be underestimated. This can be accomplished through membership and in financial support of organized medicine at all levels. Select the organizations that you support carefully and specifically with an eye toward those that provide lobbying power for you and for your patients (Rubenstein 2004, 2002; Woods 2003a; Woods 2003b). There are multiple organizations which interact with the Centers for Medicare and Medicaid Services. These include the American College of Radiation Oncology, the American Brachytherapy Society, the Association of Freestanding Radiation Oncology Centers, and the American Society for Radiation Oncology (Rubenstein 2004, 2002; Woods 2003b).

Starting a Freestanding Cancer Center

Starting a freestanding cancer center requires substantial time, effort, and diligence. The population area served by the freestanding center must be clearly defined by the radiation oncologist. In an area where there is no cancer program, the population data for the area can be gathered, complete with the age range of the population, and the number of potential patients within defined age ranges. The SEER data can then be applied using population-based cancer incidence. In 2005, the age-adjusted incidence of new cancers diagnosed was 4.7 cases per thousand of population (Schilling 2007; Gillette 2005). The raw cancer incidence provided by the SEER data does not tell us how many patients may undergo radiation treatment during the course of their illness. Take the number of estimated patients and then apply a yield ratio of approximately 50%, which should estimate the total number of patients that the new cancer center would serve. An additional 25% of patients will need to be retreated for other metastases or other new primary cancers (Gillette 2005). Model radiation oncology courses of treatment must be developed to estimate reimbursement per course of treatment (see Table 1) (Schilling 2007). A certain percentage of patients will receive a palliative treatment course, a 3-D conformal treatment, and an intensity-modulated radiation treatment. If an average length of treatment (including palliative treatment and definitive treatment) is approximately 5 weeks, to have 20 patients under continuous treatment per day will require 200 new patients per year (Schilling 2007).

Economics. **Table 1** Model radiation oncology treatment courses to estimate professional/technical split

IMRT prostate		
CPT Code	**Professional RVUs**	**Technical RVUs**
99245	5.89	
77263	4.40	
76370	1.18	3.09
77280	1.94	7.24
77290	4.24	13.60
77417		8.82
77300	15.48	25.20
77336		24.96
77427	36.16	
77334	23.66	47.46
77470	2.85	11.64
77301	21.46	58.34
77418		754.32
	117.26	954.67
	10.93%	89.10%
3-D conformal treatment		
99245	5.89	
77263	4.40	
76370	1.18	3.00
77280	0.97	3.60
77290	4.24	13.60
77295	6.22	29.17
77417		6.30
77300	5.16	8.40
77336		21.84
77427	31.64	6.80
77334	8.45	16.95
77414		80.52
77470	2.85	11.64
77315	2.12	2.78

Economics. Table 1 (continued)

	73.12	197.80
	27%	73%
Palliative treatment		
99245	5.89	
77263	4.40	
76370	1.18	3.09
77290	2.12	6.80
77417		1.89
77300	7.72	2.80
77336		6.24
77427	9.04	
77334	3.38	6.78
77414		24.40
77315	2.12	2.78
	35.85	54.78
	35.30%	64.70%

A second way to estimate the population served is to count the number of occupied beds of hospitals serving the area. Each permanently filled hospital bed yields approximately one cancer patient per year, of which half will require radiation treatment (Schilling 2007).

For a cancer center in a competitive market, one must establish exactly how many patients would be treated in the new cancer center and specifically how the physicians plan to obtain these referrals. If a hospital-based group of physicians builds its own freestanding cancer center, some of the patients may follow because referring physicians will continue to refer. There are always surprises and changes in referral patterns when hospital-based radiation oncologists open a competing freestanding center (Schilling 2007).

Once the numbers of patients to be treated are established, along with their treatment length, the reimbursement for an "average course of treatment" can then be calculated. This average course of treatment should take into account intensity-modulated radiation treatment, palliative treatments, and 3-D conformal therapy. When one uses a conservative estimate and sets the total reimbursement at Medicare rates, this seems to be a reasonable approach to many lending institutions. Once total collections for the population to be served are established, the total expenses need to be established as well. This includes the costs of debt service, interest, principle, sales tax on equipment when installed, electric bills, costs of physics and dosimetry, costs of personnel including nursing and therapists, costs of water, building maintenance, professional liability, building insurance, employee benefits, physics equipment, accelerator maintenance, etc.

All of this can be packaged together as a pro forma to take to your financial institution. Generally, banks require a down payment between 5% and 20% of the total amount borrowed. In addition, working capital will be needed for approximately 6 months of operation (Schilling 2007). The pro forma should be conservative. The goal should be to exceed the numbers that are projected, not to just meet them. This will give the bank a substantial amount of comfort as well. The carrying cost of maintaining a center, maintaining a competitive edge with equipment, and attracting and maintaining high-quality personnel are substantial. There is often an underestimation of the cost of running a cancer center (Schilling 2007). If medical oncology is to be added, the costs of the monthly drug bill need to be calculated.

Marketing a Radiation Oncology Practice

Marketing for radiation oncology is directed toward the referring physician. Determine the physicians most likely to refer to you and make a list. Any physician can be a referring physician (Schilling 2007; Gillette 2005). I have received two referrals from psychiatrists who had cancer patients that were unhappy with their care, underscoring this premise.

Presenting patient cases at cancer conference at your local hospitals is a time honored and useful form of individual marketing for your practice (Gillette 2005). Nursing staff usually attend, and they can be a referral source. Radiation oncology images can be rewarding to present at tumor boards. Outlines of isodose plans and other imaging studies, MammoSite depictions, high-dose-rate brachytherapy plans, etc., form an image in referring physicians' minds that medical oncologists cannot accomplish (Gillette 2005).

Giving talks to civic organizations and cancer support groups is also beneficial, but requires patience for the long term (Schilling 2007; Gillette 2005). Although I give multiple talks to groups, there has never been an instance where someone in the audience decided that they would change to me as a physician as the result of my presentation. Nonetheless, there have been multiple times when family members of new patients have said that they have heard me give a presentation. This underscored another physician's referral choice.

Advertising to the public generally does not yield new patients alone. Advertising advanced technology may be helpful, but usually only bolsters the understanding and familiarity with the physicians and facility when another primary physician makes a referral. In some larger urban markets, advertising advanced technology may make a difference, or get some patients to call, ask questions, and possibly self-refer.

If your hospital has a teaching program, it is often rewarding to give a lecture or two within this program (Gillette 2005). Physicians who attend will soon become your referring physicians, especially if they stay in the area.

Develop a telephone answering on-hold message that showcases your technology as well as the talents of your physicians. Thus, when the patients and physicians call, they are given an explanation of exactly what your practice does while they are waiting for the receptionist.

Developing an immediate fax or e-mail form to let referring physicians know what is being done for a new patient facilitates communication and gives them immediate information about the workup and progress about a patient that you have seen for an opinion (Schilling 2007).

Internet website development can also be helpful. Again, this usually does not yield new patients, but rather reinforces the choice that other physicians have made to refer patients. Patients can find out about your practice on the internet, as well as fill out their intake forms, etc. Some of these techniques may be helpful. None of these techniques will be useful unless outstanding patient care is delivered, both socially and medically.

Selling a Freestanding Cancer Center

In recent years, there has been much interest in private or publically traded groups for purchasing radiation oncology centers. Publically held or private corporations may seek to purchase radiation oncology centers to induce an economy of scale, dominate a certain region or state (and thereby exact additional reimbursement from the area insurers), or ultimately to go public (issue stock certificates that can be purchased by the public). Generally, a sale is based on earnings before depreciation interest, taxes, and amortization (EBDITA). A multiple of this number is paid to the owner, generally in the 4–7.5 range. This range may decrease as cuts in reimbursement occur. Generally, purchasers ask for the owner to retain minority percentage of the original cancer center that they built. Sometimes this can be as small as a few percent, sometimes up to 49%. Many purchasers require a reduction in the ultimate purchase price based on the prospect of reduced reimbursement for some procedures. For example, an IMRT or stereotactic radiosurgery "earn out" may be a reduction in payment price based on the future of reimbursement for these two modalities, with a portion of purchase price paid at a later date. Predicting in the future of reimbursement is beyond the scope of most of our readers.

Nonprofit Hospitals and Radiation Oncologists

Earnings from many nonprofit hospitals have soared with a combined income of the 50 largest nonprofit hospitals in the United States increasing eightfold to $4.27 billion between 2001 and 2006, according to a *Wall Street Journal* analysis updated from the American Hospital Directory. Nonprofit hospitals' "excess cash flow" (we call this profit in the for-profit sector) is spent on new facilities, generous executive pay, and often new and lavish cancer centers (Schilling 2009a). The largest nonprofit hospitals Chief Executive Officer pay ranged from $3.3 to $16.4 million per year (Schilling 2009a). Historically, most nonprofit hospitals in America have been recognized as Charitable Organizations and are exempt from taxes under Section 501 (C) (3) of the US tax code. In return for a generous tax exemption, the US Internal Revenue Service has previously required a nonprofit hospital to provide substantial amount of charity care for the poor. However, in 1965 when Medicare and Medicaid were created, the hospital industry felt there would not be enough demand for charity care to satisfy the IRS exemption standards. With substantial lobbying, the nonprofit hospital industry pushed for more flexible exemptions that became known as the Community Benefits Standard adopted by the Internal Revenue Service in 1969. This allowed hospitals to provide local "community benefit" consistent with any other nonprofit hospital in their area (Schilling 2009a). Unlike for-profit hospitals, nonprofit hospitals do not pay dividends to

shareholders. Instead, they use "excess cash flow," (profits) earned from operations, to pay for new facilities. Among these include proton treatment centers, under construction in the Midwest and located within minutes of each other, and various cancer centers being built by nonprofit hospitals without paying any taxes. These compete with those facilities that do pay taxes. While nonprofit hospitals have a charity obligation to the communities that they serve, do they compete with physician practices by using an unfair tax advantage? (Schilling 2009a).

Federal STARK Regulations Affecting Radiation Oncology

Current STARK laws prohibit self-referral to designated health services, which includes radiation oncology. Radiation oncologists who own their own facilities and equipment do not fall under violations of the STARK rule because it is not considered self-referral when the referring physician personally performs a designated health service (Woods 2004).

There is also an in-office ancillary exemption, which applies to ownership and investment interest for ancillary services. The in-offices ancillary service must be provided in a building in which the referring physician also furnishes substantial physician services (Woods 2004). This loophole exploited by some urologists to create a "group practice" with radiation oncologists and add a linear accelerator to their building. Curiously enough, the very radiation oncologists who join these ventures are often the displaced victims of hospital tactics of economic credentialing.

Congress based some of their conclusions and wrote portions of the Stark law based on studies that examined the effects of ownership of freestanding radiation oncology facilities by referring physicians who were not radiation oncologists and did not directly provide services. These "joint ventures" yielded a utilization rate 40% higher in these facilities in Florida than the rest of the United States, and cost of radiation treatment that was 60% higher than the rest of the United States (Mitchell 1992). In addition, these studies showed that there was less access to poorly served populations without any reduction in mortality among cancer patients that indicated improved quality of care (Woods 2004; Mitchell 1992). State laws may strengthen current existing federal laws, and it is important to understand the laws in your state concerning self-referral (Schilling 2007; Woods 2004; Mitchell 1992).

"Group Practices" Including Radiation Oncology

Radiation oncologists have become increasingly concerned about the growing trend of self-referral for radiation treatment services by other specialty physicians seeking to create a group practice for apparent economic gain. Physician-driven financial arrangements may be consummated specifically to facilitate the delivery of intensity-modulated radiation treatment and have caused concern for the quality and cost of radiation treatment delivery. These arrangements have caused proliferation of "multispecialty groups" with the objective of delivering IMRT to prostate cancer patients that the groups' urologist diagnosed. Prior to the initiation of the STARK Laws, studies of radiation oncology facilities owned by referring physicians reported higher costs for cancer treatment without improved outcomes (Schilling 2010). Radiation oncology is a designated health service under Section 1877 of the Social Security Act which prohibits financial arrangements between the physicians and entities providing these services. Congress created an "in-office ancillary exemption" to protect medical services for which a test result is immediately needed for in-office patient care. As part of a program to address and study this growing trend, the American College of Radiation Oncology issued a physician statement on self-referrals specifically addressing the formation of urology and radiation

oncology radiation groups for apparent financial reasons. We then surveyed radiation oncologists who identified themselves as having a financial relationship with urologists. After telephone verification, there were 75 radiation oncologists who identified themselves as having a practice model that included urologists. The radiation oncologists were both employed and were also a financial partner in the group. No radiation oncologists responded that their practice model included "block leasing" linear accelerator time to urologists. For all respondents, the radiation oncologists received the professional component of treatment. All 75 respondents were economically displaced in a geographic region by either existing radiation oncology groups and/or were economically displaced by a hospital in their region (Schilling 2010). All respondents were unable to achieve professional partnership status within a radiation oncology group and 98.6% were unable to achieve a share of the technical component for radiation treatment within a radiation oncology group. Sixty-six of 75 physicians provided a daily total of prostate cancer patients treated in their facility (Schilling 2010). The range was one prostate cancer patient treated per day (newly started practice) to 48 patients per day (for a mature practice) (Schilling 2010). The mean was 17.1 prostate cancer patients per day treated. Eighty-six percent of radiation oncologists within this model were treating both prostate and non-prostate cancer patients. The average combined urology radiation oncology practice treated 33 patients per day with non-prostate malignancies. Thus, the radiation oncologists responding to our survey who treated both prostate and non-prostate cancer patients treated 1.9 times more non-prostate cancer patients than prostate cancer patients (Schilling 2010). This may possibly indicate that urologists seek radiation oncologists in an area where radiation oncologists already have an established referral base and bring non-prostate cancer referrals with them (Schilling 2010). On August 19,

2008, the Office of the Inspector General (OIG) issued an opinion on the relationships between urologists and radiation oncologists that addressed leasing radiation equipment to provide IMRT to prostate cancer patients that urologists diagnose. The OIG expressed concern that urology groups are in a position to choose IMRT instead of other forms of radiation and assure economic success of a joint venture while assuming minimal business risk. The radiation oncologist would then be able to reward the referring urologist with a profit. The opinion as written states, "We conclude the proposed arrangement could potentially generate prohibited remuneration under the anti-kickback statute" (Schilling 2010).

Some medical oncologists, general surgeons, and neurosurgeons have also chosen a variation of this business model when they combine with radiation oncologists to provide radiation treatment including robotic radiosurgery (Schilling 2010).

Economic Issues Specific to New Graduates of Residency Programs

Most new graduates are largely concerned about mastering the amount of medical knowledge necessary to become a specialist as well as passing their radiation oncology boards. Few articles have been written on contracting specific to radiation oncology (Schilling and Woods 1997). A contract is simply a promise between two parties which the law recognizes as a duty. Five elements are required to create a valid contract: two competent parties, mutual consent, consideration, a legal purpose and duty, and a mutual obligation. When evaluating a first contract, obtaining legal advice from a health-care attorney is essential.

The terms and conditions of the contract should set forth working conditions, provision of nursing service, transcription, ancillary help, on-call arrangements, vacation time, and coverage. Arrangements should be spelled out for professional liability insurance coverage including

term limits and a tail policy in the event that termination of employment occurs. Duties should be specific to the practice of radiation oncology and not be vaguely worded so the new physician is expected to "perform all duties as the board of directors may assign" (Schilling and Woods 1997). The employer should also spell out the terms of potential termination. Reasonable terms of automatic contract termination include loss of your medical license, loss of hospital privileges for patient care issues, loss of a drug enforcement agency license, loss of ability to prescribe controlled substances, conviction of a felony, etc. If there is a provision for termination of the contract prior to the end of the term, it should be clear and available to both parties. For example, "either party may terminate this agreement with 90 days written notice with or without cause" (Schilling and Woods 1997). Written performance reviews should be given at least quarterly. This assists the employer and the employee to identify potential areas of conflict and allow resolution.

Restrictive covenants protect employers by placing limitations on the rights of the employee to compete with the employer. They should include the period of time the restriction shall remain in effect as well as the geographic restriction. Because some of these restrictive covenants are not enforceable in certain states, liquidated damages for terminating employment and remaining in an area to compete has also been used by some practices (Schilling and Woods 1997). A liquidated damage clause provides a payment to the practice owner, negotiated in advance, that allows the employed physician to work in the area and compete after the contract is terminated (Schilling and Woods 1997).

Associates are invited to become partners after some period of time which varies from region to region. Traditionally, this has meant financial parody with the senior partners. Many physicians are being offered positions without a partnership track. Partnership has also traditionally meant voting and decision making parody. Some groups offer graduated financial parody: the first two years may be salaried, and during the next three years they may gradually reach financial parody with senior partners in percentage increments. Formulas for buying into the practice are similarly variegated. In a hospital-based practice with an exclusive contract to provide professional services, the buy-in should be minimal, simply because the costs of maintaining the contract and capital equipment costs are minimal. One should only purchase assets that have real value or cover the cost of maintaining the contract over time. The accounts receivable are usually generated by the physician during the years of non-partnership. One questions a "buy-in" for these accounts receivable that the new physician helped to generate. Goodwill is augmented by the employed physician as well. It is my opinion that these particular items are not worth a great deal financially (Schilling 2007; Schilling and Woods 1997).

Less than one-third of radiation oncologists are still in their first job post residency 5 years later (Schilling and Woods 1997). If negotiated into the contract, arbitration or mediation can be an effective and cost efficient means to negotiate a dispute and avoid litigation between parties, should you decide to separate (Schilling and Woods 1997).

Economics of Medical Oncology

As a way to achieve the prescription drug coverage for our seniors, chemotherapy drug payments were the source of some revenue (Schilling 2003b). The target is huge: Medicare spends 70 billion dollars each year for chemotherapy drugs and administration. Compare that to the amount spent on radiation oncology professional and technical fees which totals 7 billion dollars per year, and our services appear very cost effective (Schilling 2003b; Schilling 2004). Outpatient

drug reimbursement has changed from paying a percentage of the average wholesale price (AWP) to paying a percentage of the average sales price (ASP). ASP is the sales price that is actually paid by outpatient practices with a tiny margin added, only 5–6%. Medical oncologists argue appropriately that the administration of chemotherapy does not cover the cost of nursing time, waste disposal, and supplies. Medicare responded to this reality by increasing the fee for administration of the first hour of chemotherapy infusion by over 270% between 2003 and 2004 (Schilling 2004). Because reimbursement for the first hour of chemotherapy has had the most dramatic increase in reimbursement for medical oncology, this makes any regimen that requires multiple days of therapy profitable for our medical oncology colleagues. These include daily or weekly chemoradiation protocols (Schilling 2004). There is a new drug reimbursement update by Medicare every 12 weeks as the average sales price for chemotherapeutic drugs is recalculated by the Centers for Medicare and Medicaid.

Consulting groups are letting medical oncologists know that they can profit from incorporating positron emission tomography scanners, CT scanners, and radiation oncology equipment into their practices. Perhaps more realistically, medical oncologists will be looking for reduction in their overhead through combining with radiation oncologists and being able to enhance patient care by giving daily chemotherapy sensitization protocols within a combined cancer center. Do not build a new cancer center without at least considering adding space for them.

Medical Oncology Supply and Demand, How Will This Affect Radiation Oncology in the Future?

The demand for medical oncologists will rise by 48% by the year 2020 but the supply will only rise 14%, creating a 34% shortfall in the number of medical oncologists needed in the workforce. These conclusions were drawn from a study performed by the American Association of Medical Colleges and reported in the *Journal of Oncology Practice* (Erickson 2007; Schilling 2009b). The number of patient visits for medical oncology was determined by the National Cancer Institute Analysis of Survey Epidemiology and End Results (SEER) database. There was no adjustment for the ever-lengthening regimens of palliative or adjuvant chemotherapy nor is there any adjustment for patients with metastatic cancer who may live longer as a result of palliative treatment and thus require increased patient visits in the future. In his article, Dr. Erickson proposes increased use of nurse practitioners, physician assistants, and delays in retirement for current medical oncologists. He also proposed increased use of primary care physicians to monitor patients during and after chemotherapy (Erickson et al. 2007; Schilling 2009b). With the shortage of primary care doctors in the United States, this does not seem likely. One of our most respected mentors and longtime leader in radiation oncology, Dr. Luther Brady teaches residents that we are first and foremost cancer physicians who use radiation as a tool to treat cancer patients. Radiation oncologists are trained in all aspects of solid tumor oncology and can easily direct medical care for cancer patients during their disease process. Given the need, there is every reason for radiation oncologists to see cancer patients for consultation, design a program for workup, and management of their malignancy, even if it did not include delivery of radiation treatment. We encourage radiation oncologists to step up to the plate and provide more consultative services, more direct patient care, more inpatient care, and more general oversight than ever before. This new and important role may be one of the most important challenges for our specialty. However, if realized, it will benefit countless cancer patients by the year 2020 (Schilling 2009b).

Pay for Performance

The Centers for Medicare and Medicaid (CMS) are moving toward a system of Pay for Performance. Under this system, a physician practice meeting a certain benchmark of quality in patient care does not receive a reduction in Medicare payments. This movement, in its various combinations and permutations, started in 1999 when the Institute of Medicine released a report called "To Err is Human" (Kohn et al. 1999). This report documented quality of care concerns in our health-care system and pointed out that 98,000 people die each year due to preventable medical errors from health-care professionals. Subsequently, a Rand study found that many hospital deaths were preventable (Hayward and Hofer 2000). In our legislators' minds, the findings of these studies sharpened their resolve to improve the quality of care delivered in our health-care system. "Pay for Performance" has the objective of improving the quality of care by linking physician reimbursement to quality measures and outcomes. Pay for Performance was first instituted in hospitals. Under the Deficit Reduction Act of 2005, hospitals receive a 2% reduction if they do not report to CMS on ten quality measures and have acceptable performance targets. This pilot project with hospitals has been viewed by Congress to be successful. The results in quality of care measures for these areas are available on the CMS web site for any hospital that participates.

Certain specialties lend themselves better to Pay for Performance measures than others. For example, diabetic patients should have retina exams as a component part of their care, and not doing so would not be optimal care for them. The care of cancer patients is, however, quite variegated. As we all know, some patients with brain metastasis live only a few months and others live for a year or more. Thus, outcome measures for patients who have cancer would probably not be appropriate. It is the physicians themselves within each specialty that should shape the compliance program linked to Pay for Performance. In this regard, likely the better measure of quality of care would be practice accreditation. Practice accreditation is currently required in several states in the United States (ASTRO 2006; Dobelbower et al. 2003).

Radiation Oncology Department: Appropriate Staffing and Personnel

Radiation treatment consists of a series of steps and involves a number of different professionals. Each radiation oncology department should establish a staffing program consistent with the level of patient care complexity and other factors within that department. Radiation oncologists can manage 30–40 patients per day under continuous radiation treatment. When considering new patient visits, treatment simulation, and follow-up visits, this translates to 65–90 patient encounters per week and allows us sufficient time for treatment planning and clinical functions (Cotter and Dobelbower 2007). Medical physicists should be available when necessary for consultation with the radiation oncologists and to provide advice and direction of the technical staff when treatments are being planned or patient treatment initiated. Chart checks by the physicists should be performed at least once per week. Generally, one medical physicist is needed for every 30–40 patients under continuous radiation treatment (Cotter and Dobelbower 2007). Medical dosimetrists act under the supervision of the radiation oncologist and medical physicist. There should be one full-time equivalent dosimetrist per 40 patients under continuous treatment. More dosimetrists may be needed if a larger proportion of patients receive higher complexity care. Radiation therapy technologists practice under the direction of the radiation oncologists. They should have achieved American Registered Radiologic Technologist (ARRT) certification in radiation oncology (Cotter and Dobelbower 2007). One radiation therapist is needed for 20 patients under continuous treatment (Cotter and Dobelbower 2007). It is ideal to have two therapists per treatment machine and to allow for vacations, meetings, absences, etc. Radiation oncology support staff may include radiation therapist treatment aides. These work under the direct supervision of the radiation therapist and radiation oncologist and are generally trained on site to assist and facilitate patient transport and patient flow.

Radiation Oncology Staff Recruiting and Retention

In the United States, currently there is a critical manpower shortage in radiation therapy personnel. Regional shortage of therapists, dosimetrists, and physicists create a musical chair job market: the bell rings and everyone changes position (Schilling 2007, 2005). This situation is neither beneficial to patient care nor fiscally sound for our shrinking health-care dollar. For those of us who have depended on temporary workers, we know that this is both an expensive proposition and seriously disruptive to employee morale (Schilling 2005).

The U.S. Bureau of Labor Statistics predicted that by the year 2010, there would be a shortage of 7,000 radiation therapists (Schilling 2007, 2005; Cotter and Dobelbower 2007). One way to stabilize your workforce, create goodwill, and create excellence in our field is to start a scholarship program for radiation therapy professionals. Currently, most scholarship programs support radiographers to take an additional year of training to become radiation therapists. During the time of training, the student can receive a stipend as well as have their tuition and books paid for. In exchange, the candidate agrees to work for the cancer center for a period of time after graduation. One source of candidates can be a local radiography training program. Contact the director of the program and let them know that you are offering a scholarship program to qualified candidates. For students who receive monthly stipend support, the best way to ensure that they are serious about accepting the obligation is to have them sign a promissory note. If they fail to honor their contract or pass the registry within a specified period of time, the amount that the practice advanced them becomes due with interest (Schilling 2007, 2005).

Although many dosimetrists today are trained "on the job," there are 1-year programs that enroll therapists in full-time dosimetry training. If you have a candidate willing to relocate to one of the cities that has these programs, it is worth the investment to train them outside of your facility and hopefully bring back some fresh ideas.

Opening your practice to scholarship programs and scholarship support creates a unique marketing opportunity for your facilities (Schilling 2007, 2005). This also augments cancer center morale where the seasoned employees can teach the new graduates the tricks of the trade (Schilling 2007, 2005).

Practice Accreditation

Practice accreditation is a way to demonstrate the quality of your radiation oncology practice to the public as well as third-party payers. Practice accreditation may be one avenue whereby a practice that demonstrates quality does not receive payment reduction under "Pay for Performance." Currently, the American College of Radiation Oncology (ACRO) and the American College of Radiology (ACR) are the two practice accreditation bodies for radiation oncology practices. Some states (Alabama, New Jersey, and New York) require practice accreditation for state certification (Schilling 2007; ASTRO 2006; Cotter and Dobelbower 2005).

Most importantly, practice accreditation constitutes a mechanism to accomplish quality assurance and assess compliance with recognized standards for hospital or freestanding radiation oncology practices (Schilling 2007; ASTRO 2006; Cotter and Dobelbower 2005). Practice accreditation can also be a value-added qualification for third-party payers.

Standards for accreditation should include external review of randomly selected radiation oncology treatment courses, peer review, and quality assurance activities performed regularly, physics and dosimetry standards consistent with drafted standards for external beam radiation treatment, brachytherapy, and medical physics quality assurance (ASTRO 2006; Dobelbower 2003; Cotter and Dobelbower 2005). An on-site verification visit by both physicists and physicians is essential to practice accreditation (Cotter and Dobelbower 2005).

Economics of Radiation Oncology: Selected International Perspectives

The rate of installation of megavoltage radiation therapy equipment was compared in Canada, Germany, and the United States (Schilling 2007; Rublee 1994). Rublee et al. concluded that the higher proliferation of radiation equipment in the United States promoted rapid access to advanced medical services but was not necessarily associated with improved outcomes, more patient utilization, or efficient use of health-care funds. He noted an average rate of growth of 10.3 radiation therapy units per million persons in the United States, 4.6 units per million persons in Germany, and 4.8 units per million persons in Canada (Schilling 2007; Rublee 1994).

Canada's socialized health-care system creates some access problems for cancer patients. Currently, Canada has a scoring system that lists the severity of each curative cancer patient and urgency in starting radiation treatment. Curable head and neck cancers received the highest score, whereas curable prostate cancers the lowest. This system sorts access to radiation treatment (Schilling 2007).

Radiation oncologists in China note that they have a single governmental payer system with socialized medicine and staggering cost increases. Patients in China who require chemotherapy are required to pay cash up front for their medication prior to its delivery. With respect to radiation oncology, radiation oncologists note a dearth of intensity-modulated radiation treatment, image-guided radiation treatment, and access to 3-D conformal radiation treatment as well.

Calvo and Santos describe monetary limits on the investment in innovative radiation treatment techniques in Western Europe (Calvo and Santos 1999). These authors note that the need for cost containment in the public health-care system in Western European countries has slowed investment in stereotactic radiosurgery, conformal radiation treatment, high-dose-rate brachytherapy, and intraoperative radiation treatment. They reported on cost-benefit analysis of each of these technologies. Their conclusion was that Western Europe was not adopting new technology rapidly enough (Calvo and Santos 1999).

Radiation oncologists responding to our survey in England felt that access to curative radiation oncology was good. However, access to palliative radiation oncology was suboptimal (Schilling 2007).

Radiation oncologists in the Netherlands felt that their cancer programs limited neither access nor the development of new technology. Dutch radiation oncologists reported limited waiting times for patients to start radiation treatment (Schilling 2007).

Radiation oncologists in South America and Latin America cite too few radiation oncology installations particularly in Mexico, Bolivia, and Venezuela. They also note a rapidly growing number of radiation oncology installations especially in Argentina. The latter have tended to be for profit centers. Latin American radiation oncologists also point with pride to the Organization of Radiation Oncologists which currently serves their members needs, and also seeks to engage more Latin American patients in cooperative prospective randomized trials (Schilling 2007).

Radiation oncologists in Scandinavian countries of Denmark and Sweden point with pride to their innovative and large cancer centers. They do point out that they are geographically distant from each other but there appears to be minimal to no limit in their access to new technology nor long waiting times for patient treatment (Schilling 2007).

Practice accreditation is uncommon internationally. However, the American College of Radiation Oncology currently has accredited a number of international facilities and practice accreditation in other countries continues to be in greater demand and is growing (Schilling 2007; Cotter and Dobelbower 2005).

In general, countries with socialized medicine have certain defined limits on capital investment each year. As our technology grows ever more costly, these issues will need to be dealt with both at home as well as in the international community (Schilling 2007).

References

AMA (2009) AMA meeting policy, November 2009

American Cancer Society (2010) Cancer prevention and early detection facts and figures 2009. American Cancer Society, Atlanta, pp 14–26

ASTRO (2006) American Society of Therapeutic Radiology and Oncology Government Relations update: pay for performance and quality of care, white paper

Calvo FA, Santos M (1999) Innovative techniques in modern radiation oncology: the economic and organizational impact. Rays 24(3):379–389

Cotter GW, Dobelbower RR (2005) The American College of Radiation Oncology practice accreditation program. Crit Rev Oncol Hematol 55:93–102

Cotter GW, Dobelbower RR (2007) American College of Radiation Oncology red book: ACRO practice accreditation program

Dobelbower RR, Cotter GW, Schilling PJ (2003) Radiation oncology practice accreditation. Rays 26(3): 191–198

Erickson S et al (2007) Future supply and demand for oncologists: challenges to assuring access to oncology service. J Clin Oncol 3:79–86

Gastrointestinal Study Group (1985) Prolongation of the disease free interval in surgically treated rectal carcinoma. New Engl J Med 312:1465–1472

Gillette R (2005) Marketing a practice. American College of Radiation Oncology Practice Management Guide, pp 39–46

Hayward RA, Hofer TP (2000) Estimating hospital deaths due to medical errors. JAMA 285:415–420

Kohn LT, Corrigan JM, Donalson MS et al (1999) To err is human: building a safer healthcare system. National Academy, Washington, DC

Mitchell JM (1992) Consequences of physician ownership of healthcare facilities – joint ventures in radiation therapy. New Engl J Med 327:1497–1501

Pcady DN (2006) American Medical Association Board of Trustees report 19-A-06 health plan and insurer transparency

Regaz J, Jackson SM, Le N (1997) Adjuvant radiotherapy and chemotherapy in node-positive premenopausal woman with breast cancer. New Engl J Med 337:956–962

Rubenstein J (2002) ACRO responds to proposed CMS payment cuts. American College of Radiation Oncology ACRO Alert, 6 Oct 2002

Rubenstein J (2004) Political activity. American college of radiation oncology practice management guide, pp 87–88

Rublee DA (1994) Medical Technology in Canada, Germany and the United States: an update. Health Affair 13(4):113–117

Schilling PJ (2003a) Economic profiling and economic credentialing: the increasing challenge for organized medicine. J Fla Med Assoc 5:33–35

Schilling PJ (2003b) Radiation oncology and the prescription drug program: what does it mean to us? American College of Radiation Oncology ACROGRAM, 18 Sep 2003

Schilling PJ (2004) AWP and ASP: what does the alphabet soup of medical oncology mean to the practicing radiation oncologist? ACROGRAM, June 2004

Schilling PJ (2005) Your cancer center can benefit from starting a scholarship program for radiation therapy professionals. American College of Radiation Oncology Practice Management Guide

Schilling PJ (2007) Economics of radiation oncology, chapter 98. In: Halperin EC, Perez CA, Brady LW (eds) Perez and Brady's principles and practice of radiation oncology, 5th edn. Philadelphia, Lippincott Williams & Wilkins, pp 2043–2049

Schilling PJ (2008) ACRO ALERT: should medical physicists bill governmental payers directly? ACRO Alert American college of radiation oncology

Schilling PJ (2009a) ACRO ALERT more imaging limits: administration proposes a 95% usage rate for diagnostic imaging equipment; how will this affect radiation oncology?

Schilling PJ (2009b) ACRO ALERT: nurse doctors

Schilling PJ (2009a) ACRO ALERT: nonprofit hospitals exploit tax breaks to outperform for-profit facilities, 2009

Schilling PJ (2009b) ACRO ALERT: shortfall in the number of medical oncologists to reach 34% in the year 2020

Schilling PJ (2010) Formation of combined urology and radiology practices: objective data from radiation oncologists for rationale. Am J Clin Oncol, manuscript (in press)

Schilling PJ, Woods A (1997) Anatomy of a professional services' contract for radiation oncology. American College of Radiation Oncology website

Woods A (2003a) ACRO supports Quality Care Preservation Act. ACRO Alert, 23 April 2003

Woods A (2003b) The American College of Radiation Oncology lobbies Washington: our specialty succeeds in reversing payment cuts. ACROGRAM, 1 Dec 2003

Woods A (2004) The impact of federal stark laws on radiation therapy. American College of Radiation Oncology practice management guide

Effective Half-Life

Tod W. Speer
Department of Human Oncology, University of Wisconsin School of Medicine and Public Health, UW Hospital and Clinics, Madison, WI, USA

Definition

The time it takes for a biological system to eliminate one-half of the injected radioactivity. It takes into account the interaction between the physical half-life of the radionuclide and the biological half-life of elimination (metabolism, diffusion, excretion) of the radiolabeled targeting construct.

Cross-References

▶ Targeted Radioimmunotherapy

Elective Nodal Irradiation

FENG-MING KONG, JINGBO WANG
Department of Radiation Oncology, Veteran
Administration Health Center and University
Hospital, University of Michigan, Ann Arbor,
MI, USA

Synonyms
ENI; Total nodal irradiation

Definition
Elective nodal irradiation field encompasses hilar
and whole mediastinal nodes, occasionally to
supraclavicular areas besides the primary tumor,
regardless of whether these regions are involved.

Cross-References
▶ Hodgkin's Lymphoma
▶ Lung
▶ Sarcomas of the Head and Neck

Electromagnetic Radiation

HEDVIG HRICAK[1], OGUZ AKIN[2], ALBERTO VARGAS[2]
[1]Department of Radiology, Memorial Sloan-
Kettering Cancer Center, New York, NY, USA
[2]Body MRI, Memorial Sloan-Kettering Cancer
Center, New York, NY, USA

Definition
Self-propagating waves in a vacuum or in matter. It
comprises electric and magnetic field components,
which oscillate in phase perpendicular to each
other and perpendicular to the direction of energy
propagation. Electromagnetic radiation is classified
into several types according to the frequency of its
wave, including (in order of increasing frequency
and decreasing wavelength): radio waves, microwaves, infrared radiation, visible light, ultraviolet
radiation, X-rays, and gamma rays.

Cross-References
▶ Imaging in Oncology

Electron Beam Dosimetry

PAULA R. SALANITRO
Department of Radiation Oncology, Mercy
Fitzgerald Hospital, Kimberton, PA, USA

Definition
The scientific determination of amount, rate, and
distribution of radiation dose emitted from a
source of ionizing radiation in this case, electrons.

Cross-References
▶ Electron Dosimetry and Treatment

Electron Beam Therapy

PAULA R. SALANITRO
Department of Radiation Oncology, Mercy
Fitzgerald Hospital, Kimberton, PA, USA

Definition
The use of electrons for the treatment of lesions,
whose depth of interest is not more than the
depth of the 90% isodose line. The rationale for
using electron beams, rather than conventional
photon beams, is based on the fact that electron
beams allow one to achieve a fairly uniform dose
distribution to a well-defined depth.

Cross-References
▶ Electron Dosimetry and Treatment

Electron Dosimetry and Treatment

PAULA R. SALANITRO
Department of Radiation Oncology, Mercy
Fitzgerald Hospital, Kimberton, PA, USA

Synonyms

Electron beam dosimetry; Electron beam therapy

Description

The treatment of cancer with ionizing radiation is an effective way of disrupting the reproductive process of diseased tissue without undermining the resilience of adjacent healthy tissue. The biological effect of ionizing radiation arises from the ionization of the chemical substances within cells. When a substance such as DNA is damaged directly or indirectly by radiation, the cells die because the damaged DNA prevents successful cell division.

Several modalities are available, electrons being effective in the superficial regions extending from skin to an approximate depth of 8 cm, depending on the beam energy. The properties of clinical electron beams allow delivery of a high dose of radiation to superficial and moderately deep tumors without damaging deeper-situated healthy tissue. The dosimetric accuracy obtainable with high-energy electron beams is highly dependent upon the knowledge of physical properties of the particular electron beam. This in turn determines the accuracy of the absorbed dose distribution in a patient. The International Commission of Radiation Units and Measurements (ICRU) have published two reports (ICRU 1984, 2004) on the subject of electron dosimetry.

Background

The first publication by the ICRU on electrons in radiation therapy was in 1984 (ICRU Report 35). The earliest reference cited in that document was from 1927. High-energy electrons were first produced from a betatron in 1947. They were being used successfully in a few institutions for routine patient treatment by the 1950s. A 10-year study was published in 1962 on the use of low-megavolt electron therapy (Smedal et al. 1962). Although medical accelerators were capable of producing an electron beam, the quality of the beam generated was not generally acceptable. By the 1970s a thorough study of the problem was undertaken in Germany, the USA, and elsewhere. An incongruity existed, however, in that the technological advances preceded dosimetric techniques for assessment of the dose distribution and dose delivery. In the mid-1970s text books on radiological physics addressed the calibration and dosimetry of electron beams but as of 1977 no method was available to calculate dose distributions for non-rectangular fields. Prominent institutions in the USA and elsewhere diligently pursued researching ▶ Electron Beam Dosimetry in the late 1970s and 1980s. Extensive literature on various aspects of electrons in radiation therapy appeared. In 1984, the ICRU published an exhaustive report on all aspects of electron beam dosimetry. Though not practical for clinical use, it is an essential document of study. The state of the art of ▶ Electron Beam Therapy is such that the standard of practice in today's radiation oncology facilities demands it as a treatment option where appropriate.

Basic Characteristics

In medicine, commonly used sources of radiation are of two types: electromagnetic and particulate. The distinguishing characteristic of particulate radiation, such as electrons, is that it carries a rest mass. The electron has a rest mass (m_e) of 9.109×10^{-31} kg and one unit of negative charge.

One unit of electrical charge is equal to 1.602×10^{-19} coulomb (C). When electrons impinge on a medium they interact with atoms by one of four processes: (1) inelastic collisions with atomic electrons (ionization and excitation); (2) inelastic collisions with nuclei (bremsstrahlung); (3) elastic collisions with atomic electrons, and (4) elastic collisions with nuclei. These Coulomb force interactions result in a loss or a redistribution of kinetic energy as the electron traverses the medium depositing energy along its path. The most important quantitative data on electron energy loss and scattering characteristics can be described by parameters known as the total mass stopping power, the mass collision stopping power, the restricted mass stopping power, the mass radiative stopping power, and the continuous-slowing-down range (practical range). It is beyond the scope of this discussion to adequately define these parameters. The reader is referred to the reference section for further reading.

This work will address the main topics of interest which are the physical issues of **beam generation**, of **radiation dosimetry**, and of **dose planning**.

Generation of Clinical Electron Beams

Beam Flattening and Collimation

Of particular importance in the clinical setting are the scattering characteristics of electrons. In order to obtain high-quality electron beams for radiation therapy, the initial electron beam must be broadened and **flattened** (see Fig. 1). Accelerators with magnetically scanned beams do not require scattering foils.

It is known that electrons suffer multiple scattering between the incident electrons and, predominantly, the nuclei of the atoms in a medium. As the nearly monoenergetic beam traverses the exit window of the accelerator tube and the monitoring ionization chamber, it

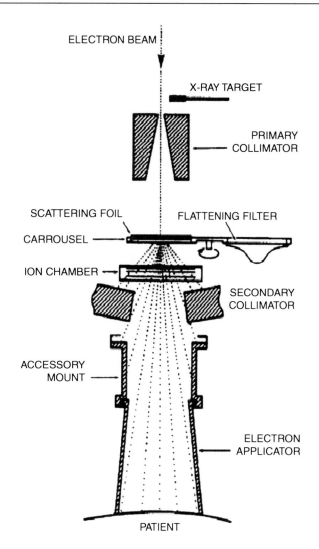

Electron Dosimetry and Treatment. Fig. 1
Schematic diagram indicating path electrons take from wave guide to patient. Scattering foil, collimators, accessory mount and applicator contribute to achieving a uniform electron field suitable for therapeutic use

experiences random energy degradation, and angular and spatial spread. By inserting a thin foil of known high atomic number (e.g., lead) and scattering power (scattering power varies as the square of the atomic number and inversely as the square of the kinetic energy of the electron), the beam characteristics can be manipulated. A second, shaped foil adds further control of angular spread of the beam as it is designed to make the beam uniform in cross section. Other methods include magnetic defocusing, scanning magnets, electromagnetic beam scanning quadrupoles, and defocusing diffusers. The latest methods have been developed to overcome the considerable energy loss, energy spread, and photon contamination.

Acceptable field flatness and symmetry still is not achieved without proper **collimation**. After passing through the scattering foil, the electron field size is only limited by the photon collimators. The width of the beam beyond the secondary collimators increases very rapidly due to the accumulated scattering interactions in the air. The primary function of beam defining collimators (electron applicator) is to limit the size of the flattened field at the surface of the patient. Additionally, the design of the electron applicator aids in maintaining or improving flatness of the beam. Such designs may include an open structure where there is a primary frame closer to the source to define maximum field size and then a secondary frame closer to the patient to limit the broad angular distribution of wall-scattered electrons reaching the patient. In some designs, the applicator is solid. In these cases the wall-scattered electrons are used to improve flatness at the surface. In either case, air is an integral part of the collimator system having a significant influence on planar fluence due largely to the fact that there is a lack of side scatter equilibrium in air.

The quality of resultant therapeutic beam including output factor, depth dose, and field flatness, as it enters the patient is heavily dependent on the design of the collimation system.

For additional beam shaping lead may be used either on the skin or inside the electron applicator; however careful attention must be paid to the energy used for treatment versus lead thickness. To provide adequate shielding, that is, <5% transmission, 3 mm of lead is sufficient for energies less than 10 MeV, and 8 mm for energies 10 MeV or greater. If Lipowitz metal (trade name: Cerrobend) is used, generally a uniform thickness of approximately 16 mm is used for all energies. See Table 1.

Dose Measurements

TG-51, the AAPM protocol for clinical reference dosimetry of high-energy photon and electron beams (Almond et al. 1999), describes the steps required to calibrate megavoltage clinical electron beams of nominal energy ranging from 4 MeV through 50 MeV. It defines a procedure for determining the absorbed dose to water at the specified reference depth d_{ref} in a water phantom. As with all protocols, exact adherence to the recommended procedure is essential in obtaining the correct dose per monitor unit at the calibration point. The full calibration must be done in water but output constancy measurements can be done in plastic phantom materials provided that a transfer factor has been established.

Electron Dosimetry and Treatment. Table 1 Calculation of Pb (lead) shielding per electron energy for patient field shaping

Nominal energy, E^0	6 MeV	9 MeV	12 MeV	15 MeV	18 MeV
Average incident energy, $E^0 = 2.33\,R_{50}$	6.01	8.8	11.7	14.0	16.0
Calculated Pb thickness (mm), t, $t = E^0/2$ mm	3	4.4	6.0	7.0	8.0
In use					
Cerrobend thickness (mm), t	16	16	16	16	16

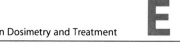

Beam Quality Specification

Beam quality is specified by R_{50} (see Table 2), the depth in water in cm at which the absorbed dose falls to 50% of the maximum dose for a beam which has a field size on the phantom surface $\geq 10 \times 10$ cm^2 ($>20 \times 20$ if $R_{50} >8.5$ cm) at a nominal source-to-surface distance (SSD) of 100 cm. Acceptable methods of determining R_{50} using ionization chambers, plane-parallel chambers, diode detectors, or radiographic film are described in the TG-51 report.

Dosimetry Equipment

Ionization chambers are the gold standard when it comes to measuring relative dosimetry for clinical electron beams. Cylindrical chambers rather than plane-parallel chambers are more widely used for measurement of central axis depth–dose distributions although the advantages offered by plane-parallel chambers should not be overlooked.

Diode detectors and radiographic film can also be used for the collection of beam data. Their use has been described in the TG-25 report (Khan et al. 1991; Gerbi et al. 2009) and its supplement.

Phantoms

Water is the required medium for absolute dose calibration. The water phantom should extend at least 5 cm beyond all four sides of the largest field size employed at the depth of measurement. Beam scanning systems used to obtain clinical electron beam percentage depth–dose measurements consist of a large water phantom, a scanning ion chamber or a diode, a 2D or 3D scanning arm, and the required electronics. AAPM Task Group Report 105 (Report of the AAPM Task Group No.105: Issues associated with clinical implementation of Monte Carlo-based photon and electron external beam treatment planning, Medical Physics, Vol 34, Issue 12) (Chettya et al. 2007) has a comprehensive description of scanning and data collecting methods for both electrons and photons.

Measurement of Central Axis Depth Dose

The variation of output (absorbed dose at a reference point in phantom) with field size differs considerably not only from one accelerator to another, but from one energy to another on a given accelerator. The output of each electron applicator should be measured with one in particular (e.g., 10×10) being selected as the standard to which other output measurements are referred. The reference water equivalent depth, d_{ref}, for measurement should be 0.6 R_{50} -1 (cm) on the central axis.

Electron Dosimetry and Treatment. Table 2 Typical beam characteristics for five commonly used electron beams including d_{max}, the depth of maximum dose and R_{50}, the depth where the dose is 50% of the maximum dose

Beam (MeV)	Surface dose (%)	Pre-d_{max} 90%	d_{max} (cm)	Post-d_{max} 90% (cm)	R_{50} (cm)	R_{10} (cm)
6	75	0.8 cm	1.5	2.0	2.5	3
9	83	1.0 cm	2.0	3.0	3.5	4.5
12	88	0.5 cm	3.0	4.0	5	6
16	94	N/A	3.5	5.0	6.5	8
20	95	N/A	2.3	6.0	8.5	10.5

The electrons contributing to the dose at d_{max} along the central axis originate from several sources:

(a) Most come directly from the scattering foils which then undergo scattering in the air and the phantom before reaching d_{max}

(b) Some are scattered off the x-ray collimator jaw faces

(c) Some are scattered off the electron applicators and shielding blocks

Some useful "rules of thumb" of clinical electron beams (see Fig. 2):

1. Depth of maximum dose and the 80% isodose line shift toward the surface as the field size decreases.

2. Surface dose increases as energy increases.

3. The rate of energy loss of megavoltage electrons in water is about 2 MeV/cm.

4. The mean energy of a beam in MeV at the phantom surface is $\overline{E}_0 = 2.33 * R_{50}$.

5. The energy at depth is approximately $E_z = \overline{E}_0 * [1-(z/R_p)]$, where R_p is the practical range in centimeters and z is the depth of interest in centimeters.

6. The range of electrons may be estimated as: $R = 0.6 \text{g/cm}^2 * (E \text{ in MeV})/(\text{density of medium})$ or $0.5 \text{ cm} * (E \text{ in MeV})$.

7. The useful depth in centimeters where electrons deliver a dose to the 80–90% isodose line is equal to about one third to one fourth of the electron energy in MeV.

A step-by-step method for determining percentage depth doses along the central axis in water using integrated charge readings is covered in the report written by the TG-70. The calculative methods are discussed in detail for data collected using cylindrical ion chambers in water, plane-parallel ion chambers in water, and diodes in water. The raw charge measurements are collected at a reference point in water and corrected for various parameters, namely, P_{ion}, P_{pol}, P_{wall}, P_{tp}, P_{repl} as appropriate to energy and detector.

Output Factors

The output factor for a particular electron field size and treatment distance, SSD, is defined as the ratio of dose per monitor unit on the central axis at the depth of maximum dose for the field to the dose per monitor unit for the reference applicator and SSD. Electron beam output factors are a function of field size, and are needed for each standard applicator and energy over the range of SSDs in clinical use. The change in output is primarily due the scattering variations of the electrons off the x-ray collimator jaw faces and off the electron applicator. This effect is most significant at low electron energies since the angular scattering power for electrons is approximately inversely proportional to the square of the electron energy.

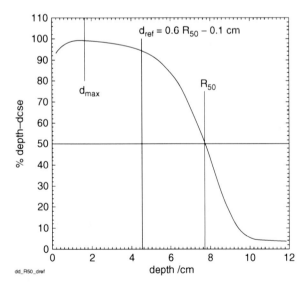

Electron Dosimetry and Treatment. Fig. 2 Depth dose curve illustrating the definitions of d_{max}, d_{ref}, and R_{50}

Electron Source Position

For purposes of clinical dosimetry and treatment planning, it is desirable to represent the geometry of the actual beam as emanating from a point source in a vacuum, so that correction factors based on the inverse square law can be applied. This "point" source is called the virtual point source, which is located at the virtual source position. It simulates an electron beam that is not influenced by interactions with air, monitor chambers, foils, etc., as is the actual beam. The method of collecting the required data for the exact calculation of this location is impractical. A simpler method uses measurements made at a number of small distances from the end of the cone, gap = 0, to a gap distance of approximately 20 cm. A plot of the square root of the ratio of reading at zero gap to the measured gap distance versus the air gap in cm will yield a line whose slope may be interpreted as the virtual source distance. This is shown in Fig. 3. Virtual source positions must be measured for each energy and field size.

Electron Beam Dose Planning

In the clinical application of electron beams, it is the task of the treatment planner to meld together all that is known about electron interactions with matter for the express purpose of controlling disease. The optimal treatment planning system would (1) calculate absolute dose per monitor unit throughout the calculation volume under all treatment conditions and (2) calculate absolute dose per monitor unit at the central-axis (or field center) d_{max} point in a water phantom with the same SSD as for the patient. This would also take into account the use of beam modifiers and absorbers, air gaps, beam obliquity, inhomogeneities, and adjacent fields.

Selection of Energy and Field Size

The choice of energy will be determined by the depth of the target volume, the minimum target dose needed, and the acceptable dose to critical organs (see Table 2). Optimally, the target volume would be enveloped by the 90% isodose line but not less than the 80% line.

Field size selection is based on the isodose coverage of the target volume. It cannot be assumed that the size at the surface is representative of the coverage at the depth of interest. Electron beam isodose lines both constrict and broaden depending on the energy, collimation, and depth in tissue.

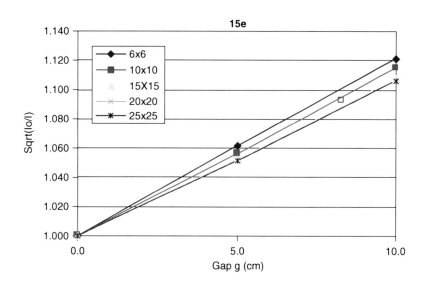

Electron Dosimetry and Treatment. Fig. 3 Virtual source distance measurements

Special attention must be paid to small fields as well as irregularly shaped fields. Unpredicted and unwanted changes in dose rate and dose distribution may occur in treatment fields which are not large enough to provide lateral equilibrium scatter. The rule of thumb here is that the minimum field opening measured in cm needs to be at least one half the beam energy measured in MeV. The magnitude of the deviations from the standard tables of electron dosimetry is dependent upon the extent of the blocking, the location of the blocking (on skin or in applicator), the thickness of the block, and the electron energy. For example, if the blocked field is smaller than the minimum size required for lateral dose buildup, the dose will differ significantly from that of the open (unblocked) applicator opening. In heavily blocked and severely irregular fields, the entire isodose distribution as well as the output factor needs to be measured (see Fig. 4).

The characteristics of *very small electron fields*, 1 × 1 and 2 × 2 are of particular interest because there is a high risk of underdosing the target volume due to a decrease in depth dose and lateral coverage. The "rules of thumb" mentioned in V.C. cannot be applied. Beam flatness decreases with field size. The depth of maximum dose as well as the depth of 80% dose shifts toward the surface. For example, the distal depth of the 80% depth dose for a 7 MeV beam and a 10 × 10 field size may be 2.3 cm. This value decreases to 1.2 cm for 1 × 1 field size. In other words, a target that is 1.5 cm in maximum dimension in the direction parallel to the central axis would be underdosed at its greatest depth.

To assure adequate coverage of the lesion, the isodose curves in a plane perpendicular to the beam axis should be obtained at the therapeutic depth of interest. The "uniformity index" is a value defined as the ratio of the cross sectional area where the dose exceeds 90% of the central axis dose at a reference depth to the beam's cross-sectional area at the phantom surface. For a 10 × 10 field size at d_{max} the uniformity index ranges from

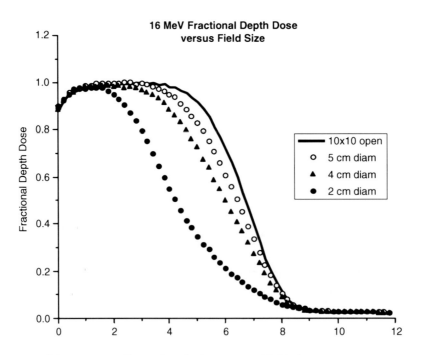

Electron Dosimetry and Treatment. Fig. 4 Depth dose versus Field size

0.77 to 0.90 for energies ranging from 5 to 18 MeV, respectively. When a field is blocked down to a 1 × 1 on the surface, the uniformity index for the same energies averages 0.60 ± .03. In other words, a target that is 8 mm in maximum dimension in the direction perpendicular to the central axis would be underdosed at the edges of the lesion. Using the target dimensions of 1.5 cm deep by 0.8 cm wide, the minimum field size for a 7 MeV beam would have to be 3 × 3 cm². Although this data can be found in the literature, it is recommended that each facility gather data on individual treatment units.

Corrections

Beam modifiers and absorbers are used to intentionally affect the beam shape in order to achieve a desired distribution. Bolus, a tissue equivalent material with equivalent stopping power and scattering power, is a modifier used to flatten out irregular patient surfaces, increase surface dose, or reduce electron penetration in selected parts of the treatment field. Placed on the skin surface, conformity to surface contours is important since air gaps between the bolus and skin surface would produce an unwanted dose reduction on the skin surface.

Adjacent Fields

Treating electron fields that are adjacent to each other also requires special attention. The fields may be abutting, gapped, or overlapping depending on the energy chosen, the specific site and extent of disease, nearby critical structures, etc. There is danger in delivering excessively high doses or seriously underdosing parts of the tumor if the geometry of the fields is not chosen appropriately. The decision as to where to locate multiple beams should be based on the uniformity of the combined dose distribution across the target volume. When using electron-photon adjacent beam orientations, similar considerations must be taken into account.

Inhomogeneities

Small Inhomogeneity

The effect of a small tissue inhomogeneity is predominately due to changes in the scattering of electrons (See Fig. 5).

Dense Inhomogeneity

If a small dense inhomogeneity is present (e.g., bone), it scatters electrons laterally due to its greater mass scattering power. This leads to a cold spot directly beyond the inhomogeneity and hot spots lateral to the inhomogeneity.

Air Cavity

If a small, non-dense inhomogeneity is present (e.g., lung), then electrons passing through will have minimal scattering interactions. There will be a loss of electronic equilibrium in the tissue on each side of the cavity. Beyond the inhomogeneity, there will be a hot spot due to scatter from the tissue lateral to the inhomogeneity combined with the unscattered electrons that have passed through the cavity.

Edges

The edge of an inhomogeneity can cause difficulties with dose distribution. This includes the air–tissue

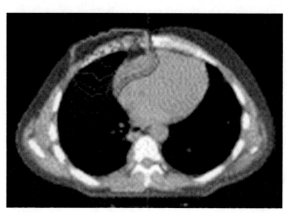

Electron Dosimetry and Treatment. Fig. 5 Isodose distribution includes effect on electrons passing through air (lung) and dense material (bone)

interface on the surface, as discussed in the contour section above. Increased scatter from the denser material into the less dense material leads to a cold spot beneath the dense material and a hot spot in the adjoining less dense material. The effect is most pronounced at the edge itself, but blurs at increasing depth.

The increased attenuation in bone leads to loss of dose in structures beyond bone and an increase in absorbed dose within the bone itself. Thus, bone limits the utility of electrons in treating deeper structures (i.e., brain, oral cavity).

Another important feature of bone inhomogeneities is that it causes **backscattering** of electrons. Backscattering occurs due to the higher atomic number and density of bone, causing a larger than expected number of electrons to deposit dose on the soft tissue side of the inhomogeneity.

Special Cases

Total skin electron treatment (TSET) is used for treating large areas of very superficial disease such as mycosis fungoides. Specialized equipment is necessary to position the patient. The goal is to irradiate the total skin to as homogeneous a dose as possible. Beam modifiers such as a spoiler and an energy degrader may be used to improve dose uniformity. AAPM Report 23 describes the irradiation requirements, irradiation techniques, linac operating conditions, dosimetry and instrumentation, and patient setup.

Current Knowledge

The treatment of cancer with ionizing radiation is an effective way of disrupting the reproductive process of diseased tissue without undermining the resilience of adjacent healthy tissue. Several modalities are available, electrons being effective in the superficial regions.

Cross-References

▶ Linear Accelerators (LINAC)
▶ Melanoma
▶ Mycosis Fungoides
▶ Skin Cancer
▶ Total Skin Electron Therapy (TSET)

References

Almond PR, Biggs PJ, Coursey BM, Hanson WF, Saiful Huq M, Nath R, Rogersa DWO (1999) Report of the AAPM Task Group 51: protocol for clinical dosimetry of high-energy photon and electron beams. Med Phys 26(9):1847

Bruinvis I (1987) Electron beams in radiation therapy: collimation, dosimetry and treatment planning. Thesis (doctoral), Universiteit van Amsterdam

Chettya IJ, Curran B, Cygler JE, DeMarco JJ, Ezzell G, Faddegon BA, Kawrakow I, Keall PJ, Liu H, Charlie Ma C-M, Rogers DWO, Seuntjens J, Sheikh-Bagheri D, Siebers JV (2007) Report of the AAPM Task Group No.105: issues associated with clinical implementation of Monte Carlo-based photon and electron external beam treatment planning. Med Phys 34(12):4818

Gerbi BJ, Antolak JA, Deibel FC, Followill DS, Herman MG, Higgins PD, Huq MS, Mihailidis DN, Yorke ED, Hogstrom KR, Khan FM (2009) Recommendations for clinical electron beam dosimetry: supplement to the recommendations of Task Group 25. Med Phys 36(7):3239

International Commission of Radiation Units and Measurements (ICRU) (1984) ICRU Report 35 radiation dosimetry: electron beams with energies between 1 and 50 MeV. ICRU, Bethesda

International Commission on Radiation Units and Measurements (2004) Prescribing, recording, and reporting electron beam therapy (ICRU Report 71). J ICRU 4(1):21–24. doi:10.1093/jicru/ndh007. © International Commission on Radiation Units and Measurements

Khan FM, Dopphe KP, Hogstrom KR, Kubcher GJ, Nadh R, Prasad SC, Pordy JA, Rozenfeld M, Wesner BL (1991) Med Phys 18(1):73

Khan FM (2010) The physics of radiation therapy, 4th edn. Williams and Wilkins, Baltimore

Klein EE, Hanley J, Bayouth J, Yin F-F, Simon W, Dresser S, Serago C, Aguirre F, Ma L, Arjomandy B, Liu C, Sandin C, Holmes T (2009) Task Group 142 report: quality assurance of medical accelerators. Med Phys 36(9):4197

Niroomand-Rad A et al (1986) Film dosimetry of small electron beams for routine radiotherapy planning. Med Phys 13(3):416–421

Rustgi SN et al (1992) Dosimetry of small field electron beams. Med Dosim 17:107–110

Smedal MI et al (1962) Ten year experience with low megavoltage electron therapy. Am J Roentgenol Radium Ther Nucl Med 88:215–228

Electronic Portal Imaging Devices (EPID)

John W. Wong
Department of Radiation Oncology and
Molecular Radiation Sciences, Johns Hopkins
University, Baltimore, MD, USA

Definition

Electronic portal imaging devices (EPIDs) are used to measure the x-ray intensity transmitted through a patient from a radiation port during a treatment session. The radiation signal is converted electronically into a two-dimensional (2D) digital radiographic image to verify the correct beam placement in relation to the patient's anatomy.

Background

Accurate placement of the radiation beam at the prescribed location on the patient is the hallmark of external beam radiation therapy. Portal imaging, i.e., the imaging of the radiation exiting the patient, is the critical, final step in the treatment process to ensure accurate beam placement. The rapid advance of technologies used for portal imaging is testimony to its important role.

The first practical means to acquiring portal images was the introduction in the mid-1970s of "ready pack" films that could be developed automatically. Many film studies soon followed emphasizing the need for frequent portal imaging to reduce errors in patient setup. Unfortunately, there was a practical limit to the frequency with which port films could be acquired, given the manual nature of film exposure and review. That led to the wide adoption of the weekly port film practice and the related prescription of a safety margin for setup on the order of 10 mm. Clearly, such margins impeded the desire to escalate dose with advanced treatment methodologies, such as three-dimensional (3D)

conformal radiation therapy (CRT) in the late 1980s and intensity modulated radiation therapy (IMRT) in the late 1990s. The need for more accurate setup with reduced margin has been, and continues to be, the underlying motivation in the advancement of electronic portal imaging devices (EPIDs).

In place of film, an EPID is used to generate high-quality portal images expeditiously for *online* evaluation at the time of patient treatment and efficiently for frequent, or even daily, review. Importantly, they are acquired in a digital format that is amenable for computerized and distributed analysis. Since their commercial introduction in the early 1990s, the technology has continued to evolve. This entry provides an overview of the evolution of EPIDs and their clinical utility. The reader is referred to several excellent and comprehensive reviews on the broad spectrum of technical and clinical topics pertaining to EPIDs (Munro 1999; Herman et al. 2001; Antonuk 2002; Kirby and Glendinning 2006).

Basic Principles of Portal Imaging

Performance of an imaging device is often made in reference to the image quality it produces. Image quality is a ubiquitous term used to describe the detectability of objects, and is comprised of several physical quantities. It is useful to briefly review the underlying physics of portal imaging so as to understand the image quality achievable with portal imaging.

The detection of an object in portal imaging, as with all radiographic imaging, is related to its contrast with its surrounding. The concept of ▶ subject contrast, C, is given by the following equation and illustrated in the schematic of Fig. 1,

$$C(\%)=\frac{I_1-I_2}{(I_1+I_2)/2} \times 100\%$$

where I_1 and I_2 are the radiation intensities transmitted through a medium with and without an object in place respectively. In the ideal noise-free

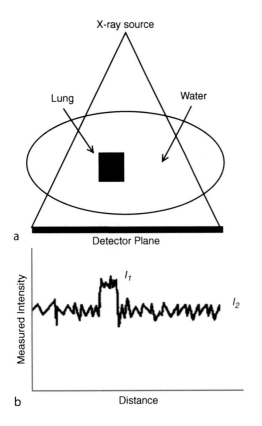

a   Detector Plane

b   Distance

Electronic Portal Imaging Devices (EPID). Fig. 1
Example figure for EPID. (**a**) Schematic representing
of the definition of contrast in the imaging process.
(**b**) Graph depicting the presence of noise in the
imaging signal

detection of an object. A fundamental quantity
that contributes to image quality is the ▶ signal-
to-noise ratio (SNR) in the image. Simplistically,
signal is related to subject contrast whereas noise
pertains to all detected events that do not contribute to the signal. There are many sources of
imaging noise. Intrinsic to the x-ray detection
process is quantum, or photon, noise. Because
photon interaction with matter is a stochastic
process, its behavior is described by the Poisson
statistics, where the variance of the detected photons is equal to the mean number of detected
photons. An ideal detector will exhibit only photon noise in its signal.

Both the primary signal and the photon
noise propagate through the process of detection,
and will be affected by the performance of the
detection system. A detector with high quantum
efficiency is most desirable for producing a large
signal. However, many downstream events, such
as the generation of electric charges or light photons, will also add noise. These combined effects
are described by the ▶ detective quantum efficiency (DQE) of the detection system, which is
the square of the ratio of output SNR to the input
SNR. DQE is a function of spatial frequency of the
detected object, generally decreasing with
decreasing object dimension.

There are many sources of noise that affect
image quality. Inherent to the radiographic imaging process, scattered x rays arising mostly from
the patient obscure the primary signal at the
detector and contribute as noise. The scatter fraction, i.e., the ratio of scattered to primary photons, at the detector is less with MV portal
imaging than with diagnostic kV imaging. Other
noises include electronic noises that are intrinsic
to the detection system, such as amplifier noise,
and also extrinsic ones, such as interference arising from the medical accelerator. There can also
be undesirable processing noise or artifacts when
the detection system is not optimally calibrated.
Many of the undesirable elements, however, can

scenario, the contrast of a 1 cm thick bone in
a 20 cm thick soft tissue medium decreases from
50% for a diagnostic kilovoltage (kV) x-ray beam
to 4% for a therapeutic megavoltage (MV) x-ray
beam; whereas, the contrast of a 1 cm lung in the
same geometry decreases from 17% to 4%. The
subject contrast of an object is a function of photon
energy and decreases as photon energy increases. It
is noteworthy that the subject contrast of bone is
similar to that of lung at the MV energies; but is
much higher at the kV energies where photoelectric
interactions play a more significant role.

As can be seen on the profile in Fig. 1, noise
in the measured x-ray intensities can affect the

be greatly alleviated with proper system design, commissioning, and maintenance.

Spatial resolution is also used to compare the performance of various portal imaging systems. While it seems intuitive that a system with smaller pixels is better equipped for detecting small objects, a more appropriate descriptor is its ▶ modulation transfer function (MTF). The MTF shows how well the system passes spatial (frequency) information such as the point spread function it produces for an ideal point signal. MTF of the imaging system is, in turn, embedded in its DQE which is characterized as a function of spatial frequency. Finally, it should be noted that the ability of an imaging system to resolve an object depends not only on its MTF or DQE but also on the size of the x-ray source and image magnification. As the image receptor is moved further from the source, the projected anatomic features are magnified, but as well as the blurring due to the x-ray source. For MV imaging, a reasonable magnification factor ranges from 1.3 to 2.

Electronic Portal Imaging Devices

In the 20 years since the commercial introduction of EPID, much has evolved in the technologies of portal imaging. As the display and evaluation of digital images become more prevalent in radiation oncology, there is significant decline in the use of the film media for portal imaging. For those clinics that prefer the compact, lightweight, and mobile format of film, computed radiography (CR) systems based on photo-stimulable phosphor technology have become the imaging system of choice, an example of which is shown in Fig. 2. The phosphor plate, encased in a cassette like holder, is handled very much like film. Upon exposure to x-rays, the phosphor stores a latent image which can be converted directly into a high-quality, high-resolution digital image with a laser readout system. The digital format is readily amenable to all the advantages of computer analysis and distribution. That CR phosphor

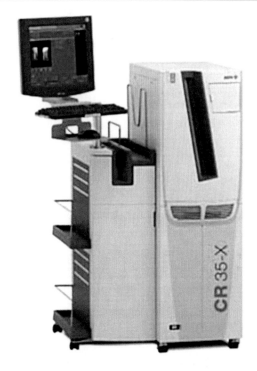

Electronic Portal Imaging Devices (EPID). Fig. 2 A picture of Agfa CR 35 system

plates are reusable is also a highly attractive feature. CR systems thus constitute a class of EPID tailored for *off-line* use, and are available from Agfa, Fuji, and Kodak. However, they do not represent mainstream EPIDs which are increasingly associated with advanced treatment methodologies that require online image guidance.

Two approaches made up the first-generation EPIDs: the matrix ionization chamber system and the camera-based systems. They have been mostly supplanted by the flat panel technology during the past decade, although a camera-based system, Theraview, is still available commercially from Cablon Medical. The matrix liquid ionization EPID was pioneered by the group at Netherland Cancer Institute and commercialized by Varian in 1990. The device is no longer available commercially although a brief review is useful for historical perspective. The matrix detector consists of two planes of linear electrodes separated by 0.8 mm and orientated perpendicular to each other to make up a matrix of 256×256 ionization detector cells. X-rays interact with a 1 mm thick plasto-ferrite plate also in the liquid medium of the matrix to produce ionizations. The DQE of the device is at best 0.5%. Through row-by-row switching of high voltage to one plane of electrodes, the ionization signal in each cell is read one at a time. The image acquisition is thus inherently inefficient as ionizations occurring in the rest of the matrix are not collected. Nevertheless, the compact design of the device was attractive to many users.

In the camera-based system, a 2 mm thick copper plate bonded to an underlying gadolinium oxy-sulfide (Gd_2O_2S) phosphor screen is used to detect the x-rays and produce an optical signal. Within a light-tight housing, a 45-degree mirror redirects the optical image for acquisition with a digital camera. The Theraview system employs a cooled CCD camera, capable of acquiring four image frames per second and integrating multiple frames as a single image acquisition. The display matrix of the standard camera is selectable from a $512 \times 512 \times 12$-bit (binned mode), $1,024 \times 1,024 \times 12$-bit (non-binned). In practice, acquired images are optimized to display in a 512×512 pixels 8-bit format. The field of view of the system spans 28 cm $\times$ 28 cm at isocenter. Indicative of photon interaction cross sections at MV energies, the maximum DQE achievable with the camera-based system is less than 1%. The DQE also decreases significantly with increasing spatial frequency. Much of degradation is due to the loss of signal in the transfer from the large phosphor plate to the camera sensor. Figure 3 shows a picture of the retractable Theraview system with the housing deployed. While the camera-based EPID technology is not new, it performance and reliability is well understood. It remains a viable and low cost alternative to the flat panel EPID for some clinics. At the time of writing, there are about 70 Theraview systems in clinical use in the USA and 600 worldwide.

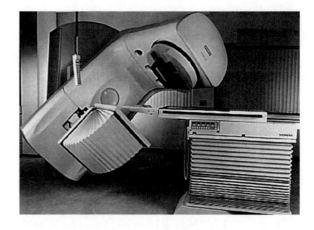

Electronic Portal Imaging Devices (EPID). Fig. 3
The commercial Theraview system with its retractable phosphor-mirror assembly deployed

The present generation of EPIDs is based on the active matrix flat panel imager pioneered by the University of Michigan and Xerox PARC beginning in the late 1980s. The first commercial system was available in 2000, and has since supplanted the matrix ionization system. Using noncrystalline, amorphous silicon (a:Si-H), a large 2D grid of thin film pixel switches is deposited on a 1 mm thick glass substrate. Each pixel switch on the array can be addressed by a 2D grid of voltage control and data lines. For MV portal imaging, all commercially a:Si-H flat panel imager presently operates in the indirect detection mode. X-rays interact with an overlying copper/Gd_2O_2S phosphor plate to produce optical photons that are detected by a photosensor at each pixel element. With voltage lines inactive and the switches off during irradiation, the photosensors hold the charge signals as capacitive elements. The switches are then turned on in between radiation pulses to facilitate row-by-row readout of all data lines. The DQE of the a:Si-H flat panel imager is about 1%, but is superior than that of the camera-based system at higher spatial frequencies.

The a:Si-H flat panel imager represents a major technological advance for portal imaging.

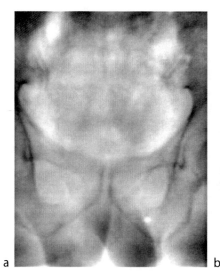 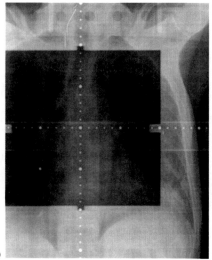

Electronic Portal Imaging Devices (EPID). Fig. 4 (**a**) A 6 MV open-field image of the pelvic region acquired with the Theraview camera-based system. (**b**) A double exposed 6MV setup image of the thorax acquired with an a:Si-H flat panel EPID. Both images have been processed to enhance visualization

Similar to the matrix ionization chamber EPID, the device is compact. The image receptor is large, from 30 cm × 40 cm to 41 cm × 41 cm, consisting of up to 1,024 × 1,024 pixels, operating with a dynamic range from 14-bit to 16-bit. Images can be acquired as fast as 15 frames per second. Compared with the earlier EPIDs, equivalent or better image quality can be produced at lower imaging doses. Figure 4a shows a 6 MV open-field image of the pelvic region acquired with the Theraview camera-based system. Figure 4b shows a double exposed 6MV image of the thorax acquired with an a:Si-H flat panel EPID for patient setup. Typically, 2–4 cGy is employed for clinical imaging. With the use of an advanced CCD camera, the images of the Theraview system are comparable to that of the flat panel imager. However, the compact form factor of the flat panel imager, as well as its availability from all major manufacturers of medical accelerators, has resulted in its prevalent adoption in the community, albeit at about twice the cost of the camera-based system. Figure 5 shows pictures of the EPID products from Elekta, Varian, and Siemens, respectively.

Clinical Applications

The use of EPID particularly the online varieties, is commonplace in the USA, if not, in the world. No doubt, the rapid advances in computer technology and network environment have helped its adaptation. There are more than 500 scientific publications listed in Pubmed (http://www.ncbi.nlm.nih.gov/pubmed/) since 1986 pertaining to the use of EPID; and close to 400 appeared since the year 2000. There were initial expectations that EPIDs would revolutionize treatment verification and improve patient setup accuracy. Early studies indicated that analysis of a few electronic portal images early on in the treatment course would be very useful to minimize the more detrimental systematic setup error. Unfortunately, to this date, many clinics still apply EPIDs according to the age-old practice of weekly MV portal reviews. This is because, to a large degree, the clinical workflow has not been modified to support more frequent acquisition and analysis of portal images. Commercial workflow management software products have utilities for analyzing images from a single fraction for field placement error,

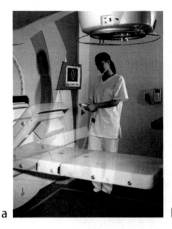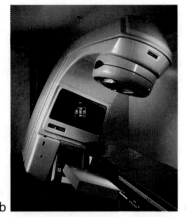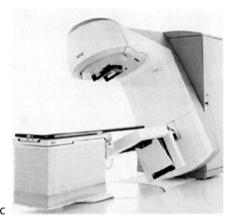

a b c

Electronic Portal Imaging Devices (EPID). Fig. 5 The a:Si-H flat panel imaging systems from (**a**) Elekta, (**b**) Varian, and (**c**) Siemens

but lack the necessary "trending" tools to characterize the setup errors of patients as individuals, or as a population. Almost all efforts made to improve patient setup accuracy using EPIDs, such as determining the appropriate margin for setup errors, have been in-house projects at a few centers.

On the other hand, the deployment of advanced treatment technologies such as multileaf collimators (MLCs) and IMRT has led to changes in how the EPIDs are used. Insofar that the MLCs are under computer control and can be checked independently, or in the case of IMRT where reviews of portal images of MLC segments become convoluted, more and more clinics are using EPID to acquire orthogonal open-field MV images to check isocenter location in the patient, bypassing the traditional practice of double exposure imaging. However, for sites where patient positioning is inherently difficult, such as a breast treatment that involves fields for tangents, supraclavicular and axilla regions, MV portal imaging remains invaluable to ensure proper patient positioning with respect to the fields.

It is noteworthy that EPIDs had made possible the many portal imaging studies of treatment accuracy and led to the advent of image guided

radiation therapy. It is recognized that the customary two to four portal images acquired of bony structures do not provide sufficient information to resolve setup variations that have nonrigid components. They also do not contain information about soft tissues that may vary during the course of treatment. But with the availability of a:Si-H flat panel imagers, it soon became obvious and practical to apply them for in-room kV imaging to overcome the inherent poorer quality of MV images. It follows that the lower kV imaging dose would allow the acquisition of more images for tracking motion of tumor or its surrogates; and when mounted on board the medical accelerator, kV cone-beam CT imaging can be performed to show setup error in 3D and volumetric soft tissue information. It is worth noting that EPID has also been used for acquiring MV cone-beam CT on the Siemens accelerator, although such utility is much less commonly used than the kV version.

The increasing adoption of in-room kV imaging, as well as other guidance methods, for patient setup is altering the portal imaging practice. Many clinics that employ daily or weekly kV imaging for patient localization simply forgo MV portal imaging, while some still retain the weekly practice either out of habit or as additional measure for clinical quality assurance (QA). It should not be forgotten that a portal image provides the most direct means to verify the correctness of a treatment port with respect to the patient's anatomy; albeit little information may be available without double exposure. EPIDs, nevertheless, are playing an increasingly larger role in QA procedures. The more common applications include periodic evaluation of MLC positioning and verification of MLC segments for IMRT treatment. The most advanced, and less common, application is the measurement of exit dosimetry to verify in vivo dosimetry with analysis tools that are mostly developed in-house (van Elmpt et al. 2008).

The Evolving Practice of Imaging in Radiation Therapy

There are several ongoing developments that hold potential to further advance electronic portal imaging. The technological focus is to improve image quality by improving the DQE of the EPID. There are investigations into promising direct detection methods using amorphous selenium and gaseous amplification. Another area of investigation is to improve the efficiency of indirect detection. For kV imaging, CsI scintillator is the detector of choice for the a:Si-H flat panel at present. For MV imaging, the use of thicker scintillating BGO and CsI crystals improve zero-frequency DQE by 10- to 20-fold. Such improvements can have profound effect as it makes possible high-quality low-dose MV cone-beam CT. However, commercial adoption of these in-house efforts is necessary to supplant the current a:Si-H flat panel imager.

More important, however, is the evolving role of imaging in radiation therapy. The development of EPID had originally focused on periodic treatment verification and the characterization of setup variation. With the advent of complex treatment methodologies, such as stereotactic body radiation therapy, the new emphasis is on image guided

radiation treatment (IGRT). Along with emerging imaging modalities, such as detection of implanted markers, ultrasound imaging for soft tissue localization, and MRI on-board the medical accelerator, EPIDs will be part of the technological arsenal to support IGRT. EPID, nevertheless, will remain uniquely matched to the radiographic and dosimetric QA of radiation therapy.

Cross-References
▶ Imaging in Oncology
▶ Image-Guided Radiation Therapy (IGRT): kV Imaging
▶ Image-Guided Radiation Therapy (IGRT): MV Imaging

References
Antonuk L (2002) Electronic portal imaging devices: a review and historical perspective of contemporary technologies and research. Phys Med Biol 47:R31–R65
Herman M, Balter J, Jaffray D et al (2001) Clinical use of electronic portal imaging: report of AAPM radiation therapy committee task group 58. Med Phys 28:712–737
Kirby M, Glendinning A (2006) Developments in electronic portal imaging systems. Br J Radiol 79:S50–S65
Munro P (1999) Megavoltage radiography for treatment verification. In: van Dyk J (ed) The modern technology of radiation oncology – A compendium for medical physicists and radiation oncologists. Medical Physics Publishing, Madison
Van Elmpt W, McDermott L, Nijsten S et al (2008) A literature review of electronic portal imaging for radiotherapy dosimetry. Radiat Oncol 88:289–309

Endoluminal Brachytherapy

Erik van Limbergen
Department of Radiation Oncology, University Hospital Gasthuisberg, Leuven, Belgium

Definition
Sources are contained by dedicated applicators for esophageal, bronchial, or bile duct cancers'

indications: bronchus, esophagus biliary duct, endovascular brachytherapy.

Cross-References
▶ Clinical Aspects of Brachytherapy (BT)
▶ High-Dose Rate (HDR) Brachytherapy
▶ Low-Dose Rate (LDR) Brachytherapy

Endometrial Carcinoma

▶ Endometrium

Endometrial Hyperplasia with Atypia

▶ Atypical Endometrial Hyperplasia

Endometrium

CHRISTIN A. KNOWLTON[1], MICHELLE KOLTON MACKAY[2]
[1]Department of Radiation Oncology, Drexel University, Philadelphia, PA, USA
[2]Department of Radiation Oncology, Marshfield Clinic, Marshfield, WI, USA

Synonyms
Corpus uteri; Endometrial carcinoma; Uterine cancer; Uterine lining; Uterine neoplasm; Uterus

Definition
The endometrium is the inner epithelial lining of the uterus. In premenopausal women, the endometrium proliferates during the menstrual cycle and is shed every 28 days in the absence of a fertilized egg. The endometrium becomes atrophic in postmenopausal women. Endometrial cancer arises in this inner lining of the uterus. The most common histologic type is endometrioid adenocarcinoma. Uterine sarcomas that arise from the myometrium or uterine stroma are not endometrial cancers; however, they are tumors of the corpus uteri. They account for approximately 2% of uterine corpus tumors.

Background
In 2009, there were 42,160 new cases of cancer of the uterine corpus and 7,780 deaths in the USA, accounting for 6% of all cancer diagnoses in women and 3% of cancer-related deaths (American Cancer Society 2011). Endometrial cancer is the most common gynecologic malignancy in the USA. Worldwide, endometrial cancer accounts for 4% of new cancer diagnoses and less than 2% of cancer-related deaths (Boyle and Levin 2008). It is more common in developed countries. Most cases are diagnosed in postmenopausal women aged 50–69 years. Endometrial cancer most commonly presents with postmenopausal bleeding. Other presenting symptoms may include irregular vaginal bleeding in premenopausal women, vaginal discharge, pelvic pressure or pain, pelvic mass, and weight loss.

Endometrial cancer is associated with elevated estrogen levels relative to progesterone. Risk factors related to increased estrogen exposure include obesity, nulliparity, menarche before age 12, menopause after age 50, anovulation, infertility, history of polycystic ovarian syndrome, tamoxifen use (an estrogen agonist), unopposed estrogen therapy, atypical endometrial hyperplasia, and a history of breast or ovarian tumors. Other risk factors include diabetes mellitus, hypertension, and a family history of endometrial cancer or hereditary nonpolyposis colorectal cancer (HNPCC). The use of oral contraceptives containing progesterone has a protective effect against the development of endometrial cancer (American Cancer Society 2011).

There is no screening test for endometrial cancer. The Papanicolaou test, used for screening of cervical cancer, has a low yield for endometrial cancer. Women with HNPCC have 40–60% risk of developing endometrial cancer in their lifetime. Screening for these women should begin at age 35 with yearly hysteroscopy and endometrial biopsy. Prophylactic hysterectomy and bilateral salpingo-oophorectomy can be considered in these women after childbearing is complete.

The most common histologic type of endometrial cancer is endometrioid adenocarcinoma, which accounts for 80% of cases. It includes villoglandular/papillary, secretory, and ciliated subtypes as well as adenocarcinoma with squamous differentiation. Less common but more aggressive histologic types include uterine papillary serous carcinoma (~10%), clear cell carcinoma (4%), undifferentiated carcinoma, pure squamous cell carcinoma, uterine carcinosarcoma (also referred to as malignant mixed mesodermal/müllerian tumors), and adenosarcoma. Other rare histologic types of endometrial cancer include mucinous carcinoma and transitional cell carcinoma. Subtypes of uterine sarcoma include endometrial stromal sarcoma, which arises from uterine stroma (connective tissue), and leiomyosarcoma, which arises from the myometrium. These latter uterine sarcomas comprise less than 3% of all cancers of the uterine corpus.

Histologic grade of endometrial carcinoma is an important factor in both prognosis and treatment decision making. The grade is based upon the ratio of the amount of nonsquamous solid component relative to the amount of glandular tissue. Grade 1 tumors, referred to as well differentiated, demonstrate ≤5% of nonsquamous solid growth pattern; grade 2 (moderately differentiated) have 6–50% nonsquamous solid growth pattern; grade 3 (poorly differentiated) tumors have >50% nonsquamous solid growth pattern. Higher-grade

tumors are more aggressive with increased incidence of recurrence and metastatic spread. All uterine papillary serous carcinomas, clear cell carcinomas, and uterine carcinosarcomas are considered grade 3 (Cardenes et al. 2008; American Joint Committe on Cancer 2010).

Endometrial cancer is divided into types I and II based on etiology and prognosis. Type I tumors are estrogen-dependent tumors that are considered low-grade and relatively slow-growing and have a more favorable prognosis. Type I tumors include grade 1 and 2 endometrioid carcinomas. They constitute 80–85% of all endometrial cancers. They are associated with mutations in the K-*ras* oncogene and the *PTEN* tumor suppressor gene (phosphatase and tensin homolog) as well as microsatellite instability in DNA mismatch repair genes. Type II tumors are more aggressive tumors and are not associated with estrogen exposure. They include grade 3 endometrioid adenocarcinomas, papillary serous, clear cell carcinoma, and squamous cell carcinoma. They are associated with *p53* tumor suppressor mutation and have a higher risk of relapse and metastatic disease (Boyle and Levin 2008).

Approximately, 80% of women with endometrial cancer present with disease that is confined in the uterus. Five-year overall survival for these patients is 75–95%. With cervical stromal involvement, 5-year overall survival is 69%. Lymph node involvement or spread to the uterine serosa, adnexae, or vagina decreases 5-year overall survival to 47–58%. Invasion of the bladder or rectum or distant metastasis correlates with 5-year overall survival of <20% (American Joint Committee on Cancer 2010).

Initial Evaluation

The first step in evaluation of endometrial cancer is a thorough patient history and examination, including evaluation for vaginal bleeding or discharge, pelvic pain or pressure, the sensation of a pelvic mass, or weight loss. The medical history should also include evaluation for risk factors for endometrial cancer. Physical examination, including speculum examination, bimanual examination, and rectovaginal examination, is performed to assess clinically evident involvement of the cervix, vagina, adnexa, rectum, and regional lymph nodes. Initial workup also includes a complete blood count including platelets. β-Human chorionic gonadotropin (β-hCG) levels should be measured in pre- or perimenopausal patients. Chest radiography is performed to assess for metastatic disease and is part of the standard preoperative evaluation. Endometrial biopsy is the gold standard for diagnosis. Biopsy is often performed in the gynecologist's office although for patients with a stenotic cervical os, dilatation and curettage (D&C) may be required. D&C and/or hysteroscopy should be performed in patients with negative biopsy findings who remain symptomatic. If cervical involvement is seen or suspected on examination, a dedicated cervical biopsy and/or pelvic magnetic resonance imaging (MRI) should be performed (National Comprehensive Cancer Network 2010).

Differential Diagnosis

The differential diagnosis for endometrial cancer includes dysfunctional uterine bleeding, uterine fibroid, uterine polyps, endometritis, endometrial hyperplasia, cervical polyps, other gynecologic malignancy, and metastasis from other malignancy (rare).

Imaging Studies

Transvaginal ultrasound (sonography) may be performed as part of the initial workup. A thickened endometrial stripe of ≧5 mm is consistent with a diagnosis of endometrial cancer. In women with continued postmenopausal bleeding, an endometrial biopsy should be performed irrespective of endometrial thickness; therefore, transvaginal sonography is not necessary for these patients. Chest radiography should be performed

to evaluate for pulmonary metastasis and as part of preoperative assessment.

Hysteroscopy may be performed if endometrial biopsy is inconclusive. It allows for visualization of the endocervix and endometrial cavity. It may be used to help guide the practitioner in performing a biopsy of abnormal areas. Curettage may be performed without utilization of hysteroscopy.

If the patient presents with symptoms that suggest local extension to the bladder, cystoscopy may be performed. Proctoscopy, sigmoidoscopy, colonoscopy, or barium enema may be performed if symptoms suggest rectal or bowel involvement. These studies are becoming less common in the setting of endometrial cancer with the availability of computed tomography (CT) scanning and MRI.

Abdominal and pelvic imaging via CT scan or MRI is indicated when extrauterine disease is suspected. Pelvic MRI is the preferred study to assess for cervical involvement. These imaging modalities are indicated for patients who present with symptoms, physical examination findings, and/or laboratory values that are indicative of extrauterine or metastatic disease. Practitioners should have a lower threshold for ordering imaging studies of the abdomen, pelvis, and chest in the setting of high-grade tumors. The role of positron emission tomography (PET) in endometrial cancer has not been clearly defined (Cardenes et al. 2008; American Cancer Society 2011).

Laboratory Studies

A complete blood count, including platelet count, is performed on all patients to evaluate for anemia as well as coagulopathy in the setting of vaginal bleeding. β-hCG measurements should be considered for all pre- and perimenopausal patients. A metabolic panel, kidney function (blood, urea, nitrogen, and creatinine) tests, and liver function tests are commonly performed because patients in this age group often have comorbid illnesses. These tests also serve to provide a thorough preoperative evaluation.

Cancer antigen 125 (CA-125) is not considered clinically relevant in patients with early-stage disease. A value >40 U/mL may be indicative of locally advanced or metastatic disease. CA-125 can also be used to monitor clinical response in patients with suspected or proven extrauterine disease, although it is falsely elevated in the setting of infection, inflammation, and local tissue damage due to radiation (Cardenes et al. 2008).

Treatment

Surgery is the main treatment modality for endometrial cancer. Staging for endometrial cancer is surgically based as clinical staging has been shown to understage the extent of disease in up to 20% of patients. Surgical staging allows for thorough examination of multiple prognostic factors, including regional lymph node involvement, depth of myometrial invasion, tumor grade, and lymphovascular space involvement. The International Federation of Gynecology and Obstetrics (FIGO) staging system is the primary staging system for gynecologic cancers. Changes in staging made by FIGO are presented to the American Joint Commission on Cancer (AJCC) and the International Union Against Cancer (UICC) for approval. The most recent FIGO staging of endometrial cancer, which includes uterine carcinosarcoma, is provided in Table 1. Note that leiomyosarcoma, endometrial stromal sarcoma, and adenosarcoma have separate FIGO staging classifications (Pecorelli 2009).

Comprehensive surgical staging includes total abdominal hysterectomy with bilateral salpingo-oophorectomy (TAH-BSO), peritoneal washings, inspection and palpation of abdominal organs with tumor debulking (if present), and pelvic and para-aortic lymph node evaluation and resection for pathologic examination. There is controversy regarding the necessity of pelvic and para-aortic lymph node resection in low-grade endometrioid carcinoma that is confined to the uterus. In addition, there is no standardized method for staging

Endometrium. Table 1 FIGO staging of endometrial cancer, 2009

FIGO stage	
I	Tumor confined to the corpus uteri (including endocervical glandular involvement)
IA	Tumor limited to endometrium or invades less than one-half of the myometrium
IB	Tumor invades one-half or more of the myometrium
II	Tumor invades stromal connective tissue of the cervix but does not extend beyond uterus
III	Local and/or regional spread
IIIA	Tumor involves serosa of the corpus uteri and/or adnexa(e) (direct extension or metastasis)
IIIB	Vaginal involvement (direct extension or metastasis) and/or parametrial involvement
IIIC1	Metastasis to pelvic lymph node(s)
IIIC2	Metastasis to para-aortic lymph node(s)
IVA	Tumor invades bladder mucosa and/or bowel mucosa
IVB	Distant metastasis

lymphadenectomy. At minimum, visual inspection and palpation of the bilateral pelvic and para-aortic lymph nodes should be performed on all patients and suspicious nodes should be removed. However, practitioners commonly forego lymph node sampling in patients with low-grade endometrioid adenocarcinoma with less than 50% myometrial invasion on frozen section and no visibly enlarged lymph nodes, particularly in pre- or perimenopausal women. Laparoscopic-assisted vaginal hysterectomy with bilateral salpingo-oophorectomy (LAVH-BSO) has been shown to be a feasible alternative to TAH-BSO for select patients, although survival data from a Gynecologic Oncology Group phase III trial are forthcoming. The role of sentinel lymph node sampling in endometrial cancer for staging purposes requires further investigation.

Patterns of failure indicate that patients with uterine-confined disease are most likely to have disease recurrence at the vaginal apex. Following surgical staging, patients with early-stage grade 1 or 2 tumors limited to the endometrium and grade 1 tumors with ≦50% myometrial invasion are considered to be at a low risk for recurrence and no adjuvant therapy is given. Patients with grade 3 tumors limited to the endometrium, grade 2 or 3 tumors with ≦50% myometrial invasion, and grade 1 or 2 tumors with >50% myometrial invasion are considered to be at intermediate risk for recurrence. For these patients, postoperative intracavitary brachytherapy alone delivered via vaginal cylinder (Fig. 1) can be offered, using either a low dose rate (LDR) or a high dose rate (HDR) source. Common dosing schemes for HDR brachytherapy when used alone in the postoperative setting include 7 Gy × 3 fractions prescribed to a depth of 0.5 cm from the vaginal mucosa and 6 Gy × 5 fractions prescribed to the vaginal surface. LDR dosing is 50–60 Gy to the vaginal surface. Typically, the prescription covers the proximal one half to two thirds of the vagina.

If complete surgical staging including lymphadenectomy was not performed or if adverse risk factors for recurrent disease are present, including age ≥60 years, positive lymphovascular

invasion, grade 3 histology, or deep myometrial invasion, pelvic radiotherapy may be given in lieu of or in addition to vaginal brachytherapy. When delivered following pelvic radiotherapy, vaginal brachytherapy is usually delivered in two to three treatments of 5–6 Gy each (HDR) or to a dose of 30 Gy (LDR). For stage IB (>50% myometrial invasion) and grade 3 tumors, pelvic radiotherapy is often followed by vaginal brachytherapy or an external beam boost to the vaginal cuff. Pelvic radiotherapy fields are designed to cover the common iliac, external iliac, and internal iliac lymph nodes, the pre-sacral nodes (in patients with cervical involvement), plus the parametria and proximal one-half of the vagina (Figs. 2 and 3). Typically, 45–50.4 Gy is prescribed in 1.8 or 2.0 Gy fractions (National Comprehensive Cancer Network 2010).

Pelvic radiotherapy has greater toxicity than vaginal brachytherapy. Common acute side effects of pelvic radiotherapy include fatigue, diarrhea, and increased urinary frequency or urgency, which may persist after treatment is completed. Additional late side effects may include small bowel obstruction, femoral head necrosis, and vaginal shortening or narrowing. The latter can be

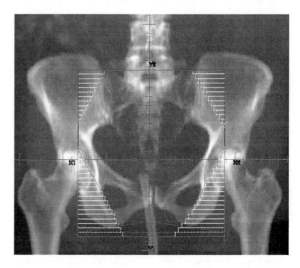

Endometrium. Fig. 2 Anteroposterior (AP) pelvic 3D external beam radiotherapy field for endometrial cancer

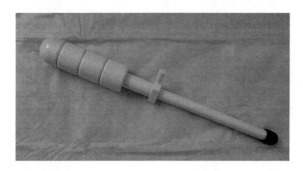

Endometrium. Fig. 1 Vaginal cylinder used for brachytherapy

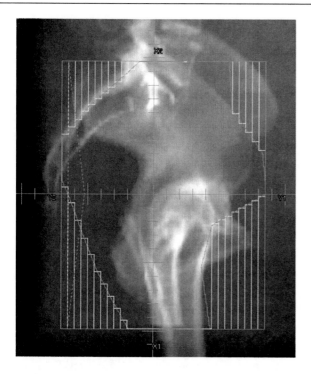

Endometrium. Fig. 3 Lateral pelvic 3D external beam radiotherapy field for endometrial cancer

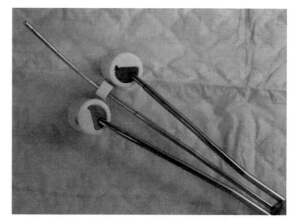

Endometrium. Fig. 4 Tandem and ovoids brachytherapy applicator

prevented with the use of a vaginal dilator or regular sexual intercourse following the completion of therapy. Serious long-term side effects are experienced in less than 10% of patients. The use of intensity-modulated radiation therapy (IMRT) is increasing due to reports of reduced radiation-induced toxicity. For IMRT planning, the above target volumes are contoured and a 7-mm margin is added for the planning target volume (PTV). The plan is designed to limit dose to the small bowel, bladder, and rectum.

Involvement of the cervical stroma designates stage II disease. Disease extension to the endocervical glandular tissue without inclusion of the stroma is classified as stage I disease and is treated as described above. For patients with gross cervical involvement or cervical involvement seen on imaging, a radical hysterectomy–bilateral salpingo-oophorectomy should be performed as part of the initial staging procedure. Postoperative pelvic radiation therapy plus vaginal brachytherapy

are recommended. For patients with gross cervical involvement that hinders a radical hysterectomy with negative margins, preoperative radiotherapy is given. Preoperative treatment technique includes a combination of whole pelvic external beam radiotherapy to 45–50 Gy followed by an intracavitary brachytherapy boost to the endometrial cavity and cervix (National Comprehensive Cancer Network 2010). For the brachytherapy boost, tandem and ovoids (see Fig. 4) are commonly used. Chemotherapy may also be considered for patients with grade 3 tumors.

For patients with stage IIIA–C and stage IVA disease, external beam radiation therapy and vaginal brachytherapy are given. Extended-field radiation therapy (EFRT), which includes the pelvis and para-aortic lymph nodes, is given to patients with positive para-aortic lymph node(s). Dose to the kidneys should be limited. With vaginal involvement, vaginal brachytherapy should encompass the entire vaginal extension, although dose should be limited at the introitus due to increased toxicity to the distal mucosa. Chemotherapy, given concurrently and/or following radiotherapy, may be considered for these patients. Commonly used chemotherapeutic agents include cisplatin, doxorubicin, and paclitaxel. Bevacizumab is currently under investigation as an adjuvant agent. In cases of distant metastatic disease (stage IVB), aggressive therapy consists of maximal debulking with chemotherapy and/or radiation therapy. Palliative treatment may include TAH-BSO, hormonal therapy, and/or radiotherapy reserved for control of symptoms. Hormone therapy with a progestin has been shown to slow the growth of endometrioid adenocarcinoma and offer palliation; however, progestins have not been shown to increase survival and are associated with the low risk of a thromboembolic event. Progestational agents also have a role in the treatment of patients with grade 1 endometrial cancer who wish to preserve fertility, with the goal of forestalling hysterectomy until childbearing is complete. The role of tamoxifen and aromatase inhibitors is less clear.

With clear cell carcinoma, serous papillary carcinoma, and carcinosarcoma, rates of abdominal recurrence outside of the radiation field range from 30% to >50%. Whole abdominal radiotherapy (WART) may be offered to these patients, including patients with stage I disease at some institutions. WART is delivered using an anteroposterior (AP) and a posteroanterior (PA) field including 1 cm above the diaphragm superiorly, 1 cm lateral to the peritoneal reflection (at the interior abdominal wall), and below the obturator foramen inferiorly to a dose of 30.0 Gy in 1.5 Gy fractions. The para-aortic region is boosted to 42–45 Gy and the pelvis is treated to a dose of 50.4–54 Gy. The liver is blocked after 25 Gy and the kidneys are blocked after 15 Gy. IMRT can also be used to limit dose to critical structures. Due to toxicity, chemotherapy plus pelvic radiotherapy with or without para-aortic radiotherapy is often used in lieu of WART. These patients should be offered a clinical trial.

For medically inoperable patients, MRI is recommended to delineate depth of myometrial invasion and cervical involvement. For patients with stage IA, grade 1 or 2 disease, intrauterine brachytherapy alone using an intrauterine device (tandem with ovoids, ring, or cylinder; double or triple tandem; Heyman's capsules) can be offered. The American Brachytherapy Society has published detailed guidelines regarding HDR brachytherapy for medically inoperable patients. LDR dosing is 70–75 Gy to point A, which is located 2 cm superior to cervical os along the tandem and 2 cm lateral to the plane of the tandem. For more advanced disease (stages II–III), external beam radiation therapy to the pelvis or EFRT is given in conjunction with brachytherapy or with an external beam conedown (Cardenes et al. 2008). Chemotherapy may be offered. Due to patient comorbidities, palliative measures alone may be appropriate.

Follow-up consists of physical examination every 3–6 months for 2 years, then every 6–12 months for 5 years, then annually. Papanicolaou test is performed every 6 months for the first 2 years, then annually. CA-125 levels may be followed if initially elevated at diagnosis (National Comprehensive Cancer Network 2010). For an isolated vaginal cuff recurrence, treatment includes surgical resection and/or radiation therapy. Treatment may be curative. For more locally advanced recurrent disease, surgical resection plus radiotherapy, if not previously administered, should be performed. Intraoperative radiotherapy may be considered for patients who have previously undergone radiation treatment, although availability may be limited. Hormonal therapy or chemotherapy may be offered. For recurrent disease with distant spread, systemic treatment is the mainstay of treatment with radiotherapy reserved for palliation as needed. Typically, a shorter course of radiotherapy is offered for palliative treatment.

Cross-References

▶ Brachytherapy: High Dose Rate (HDR) Implants

▶ Brachytherapy: Low Dose Rate (LDR) Temporary Implants

▶ Cervical Cancer

▶ Intensity-Modulated Proton Therapy (IMPT)
▶ Ovarian Cancer
▶ Vagina

References

American Cancer Society (2011) Endometrial (uterine) cancer. American Cancer Society, Atlanta
American Joint Committee on Cancer (2010) Corpus uteri. In: Edge SB, Byrd DR, Compton CC, Fritz AG, Greene FL, Trotti A (eds) AJCC cancer staging manual, 7th edn. Springer, New York
Boyle P, Levin B (eds) (2008) Endometrial cancer. In: World cancer report 2008. International Agency for Research on Cancer, Lyon
Cardenes HR, Look K, Michael H, Cerezo L (2008) Endometrium. In: Halperin EC, Perez CA, Brady LW (eds) Principles and practice of radiation oncology, 5th edn. Wolters Kluwer/Lippincott Williams & Wilkins, Philadelphia
National Comprehensive Cancer Network (2010) NCCN clinical practice guidelines in oncology: uterine neoplasms, V.1.2010. http://www.nccn.org/professionals/physician_gls/PDF/uterine.pdf. Accessed 30 January 2010
Pecorelli S (2009) Revised FIGO staging for carcinoma of the vulva, cervix, and endometrium. Int J Gynaecol Obstet 105(2):103–104

Endoscopic Ultrasonography (EUS)

FILIP T. TROICKI[1], JAGANMOHAN POLI[2]
[1]College of Medicine, Drexel University, Philadelphia, PA, USA
[2]Department of Radiation Oncology, College of Medicine, Drexel University, Philadelphia, PA, USA

Definition

An ultrasound visualization of the esophagus, rectum and stomach for diagnostic/ staging purposes looking at depth of tumor invasion.

Cross-References

▶ Esophageal Cancer
▶ Rectal Cancer
▶ Stomach Cancer

Endoscopy

FILIP T. TROICKI[1], JAGANMOHAN POLI[2]
[1]College of Medicine, Drexel University, Philadelphia, PA, USA
[2]Department of Radiation Oncology, College of Medicine, Drexel University, Philadelphia, PA, USA

Definition

A fiber-optic visualization of a hollow organ (usually pharynx, vocal cords, esophagus, and stomach) for diagnostic or therapeutic purposes.

Cross-References

▶ Cancer of the Pancreas
▶ Colonoscopy
▶ Esophageal Cancer
▶ Sarcomas of the Head and Neck
▶ Stomach Cancer

ENI

▶ Elective Nodal Irradiation

Enteral Nutrition

FILIP T. TROICKI[1], JAGANMOHAN POLI[2]
[1]College of Medicine, Drexel University,
Philadelphia, PA, USA
[2]Department of Radiation Oncology, College of
Medicine, Drexel University, Philadelphia,
PA, USA

Definition
Tube feeding directly into the stomach or small intestine, bypassing the oral cavity.

Cross-References
▶ Esophageal Cancer
▶ Sarcomas of the Head and Neck
▶ Stomach Cancer

Ependymomas

▶ Spinal Canal Tumor

Epidermal Growth Factor Receptor (EGFR)

CLAUDIA E. RÜBE
Department of Radiation Oncology, Saarland
University, Homburg/Saar, Germany

Definition
Activating of the EGFR signalling pathway has been linked with important mechanisms of tumor progression such as proliferation, angiogenesis, metastasis and decreased apoptosis. EGFR is frequently expressed at elevated levels in multiple cancers, affecting adversely the treatment outcome and prognosis of patients.

Cross-References
▶ Predictive In vitro Assays in Radiation Oncology

Epidermoid Intradermal Carcinoma

▶ Skin Cancer

Epidural Spinal Cord Compression (Also Epidural Spinal Cord Metastases)

JAMES H. BRASHEARS, III
Radiation Oncologist, Venice, FL, USA

Synonyms
Epidural spinal cord metastases

Definition
It is the most frequently diagnosed form of spinal cord compression and requires compression of the contents of the dural sac by an extrinsic mass for diagnosis. Often, the offending tumor's epicenter is a nearby vertebra and the patient complains of worsening back pain with or without other symptoms.

Cross-References
▶ Palliation of Brain and Spinal Cord Metastases

Epidural Spinal Cord Metastases

Definition

A tumor developing along or adjacent to the spinal tract causing invasion, pressure or volume compromise of the spinal canal which produces localized pain, radiating neuropathy and/or neurologic dysfunctions leading to paralysis.

Cross-References

▶ Palliation of Brain and Spinal Cord Metastases

Epigenetics

Susan M. Varnum, Marianne B. Sowa, William F. Morgan
Biological Sciences Division, Fundamental & Computational Sciences Directorate Pacific Northwest National Laboratory, Richland, WA, USA

Definition

Epigenetics – the study of inherited changes in gene function caused by mechanisms other than changes in the underlying DNA sequence.

Cross-References

▶ Radiation-Induced Genomic Instability and Radiation Sensitivity

Episcleral Plaque Therapy

▶ Eye Plaque Physics

Epitope

Tod W. Speer
Department of Human Oncology, University of Wisconsin School of Medicine and Public Health, UW Hospital and Clinics, Madison, WI, USA

Definition

The specific molecular region on an antigen that binds to the antigen-binding site of an antibody and is capable of eliciting an immune response. A single antigen typically can have different epitopes.

Cross-References

▶ Targeted Radioimmunotherapy

Epothilones

Rene Rubin
Rittenhouse Hematology/Oncology, Philadelphia, PA, USA

Definition

Epothilones are a new class of chemotherapeutic agents (ixabebilone, erubulin). They work similar to the taxanes, but are also active in taxane-resistant cells. Currently, they are only approved for metastatic breast carcinoma and being evaluated in lung cancer also. They work by interfering with microtubule function. This inhibits cell division by stabilizing the microtubules. They are better tolerated than taxanes and have fewer side effects.

Side Effects

- Prolonged QT interval
- Nausea/vomiting
- Hair loss

- Neuropathy (especially in patients who have had taxanes)
- Neutropenia
- Anemia

Cross-References

▶ Principles of Chemotherapy

Eppendorf Microelectrode

CLAUDIA E. RÜBE
Department of Radiation Oncology,
Saarland University, Homburg/Saar, Germany

Definition

Allows direct measurement of the oxygen tension in tumor tissue.

Cross-References

▶ Predictive In vitro Assays in Radiation Oncology

Epstein-Barr Virus (EBV)

BRANDON J. FISHER[1], LARRY C. DAUGHERTY[2]
[1]Department of Radiation Oncology, College of Medicine, Drexel University, Philadelphia, PA, USA
[2]Department of Radiation Oncology, College of Medicine, Drexel University, Glenside, PA, USA

Definition

EBV, also known as human herpesvirus 4 (HHV-4), is a cancer-causing virus of the herpes family. It is found worldwide and has been linked to Burkitt's lymphoma and nasopharyngeal carcinomas. When the EBV infects B lymphocytes in in-vitro models, the cells become capable of indefinite growth, a consequence of viral protein expression. Infection with EBV usually causes no symptoms and is indistinguishable from other mild, brief illnesses. The virus has been linked to mononucleosis and is associated with chronic fatigue syndrome.

Cross-References

▶ Nasopharynx

Equivalent Path Length

CHARLIE MA, LU WANG
Department of Radiation Oncology, Fox Chase Cancer Center, Philadelphia, PA, USA

Definition

The distance that is equivalent to that measured in water. It is usually calculated as the product of the distance in the considered materials and the ratio of electron density of the materials to that of water.

Cross-References

▶ Dose Calculation Algorithms

ERBB2

▶ Her-2

Erbitux

▶ Cetuximab

ERG Gene

DANIEL J. INDELICATO[1], ROBERT H. SAGERMAN[2]
[1]Department of Radiation Oncology, University of Florida Proton Therapy Institute, University of Florida College of Medicine, Jacksonville, FL, USA
[2]Department of Radiation Oncology, SUNY Upstate Medical University, Syracuse, NY, USA

Definition

The *ERG* gene (*Ets Related Gene*) encodes the transcriptional regulator ERG protein. It may participate in transcriptional regulation through the recruitment of SETDB1 histone methyltransferase and subsequent modification of local chromatin structure. In Ewing sarcoma, a chromosomal translocation generates a fusion of the 5′ transactivation domain of EWS with the 3′ Ets domain of ERG.

Cross-References

▶ Ewing Sarcoma

Erythroderma

CURT HEESE
Department of Radiation Oncology, Eastern Regional Cancer Treatment Centers of America, Philadelphia, PA, USA

Definition

Also known as "exfoliative dermatitis," "dermatitis exfoliativa," and "red man syndrome" is an inflammatory skin disease with erythema and scaling that affects nearly the entire cutaneous surface.

Cross-References

▶ Cutaneous T-Cell Lymphoma

Erythroplasia de Queyrat

STEPHAN MOSE
Department of Radiation Oncology, Schwarzwald-Baar-Klinikum, Villingen-Schwenningen, Germany

Definition

Erythroplasia de Queyrat is an in situ variable of squamous cell carcinoma resembling Bowen′s disease; however, it is limited to the epithelial cells of the glans penis and the inner prepuce. Symptoms are redness, itching, pain, ulceration, dysuria, penile discharge, and difficulties retracting the foreskin.

Cross-References

▶ Penile Cancer

Erythropoiesis-Stimulating Agent (also ESA or Exogenous Erythropoietin)

JAMES H. BRASHEARS, III
Radiation Oncologist, Venice, FL, USA

Synonyms

ESA; Exogenous erythropoietin

Definition

Pharmaceutically similar in structure to erythropoietin that is normally produced by the kidney and promotes red blood cell production in the bone marrow. These medications include epoetin alfa, epoetin beta, and darbepoetin alfa.

Cross-References

▶ Supportive Care and Quality of Life

Erythropoietin

LINDSAY G. JENSEN, BRENT S. ROSE,
ARNO J. MUNDT
Center for Advanced Radiotherapy Technologies,
Department of Radiation Oncology, San Diego
Rebecca and John Moores Cancer Center,
University of California, La Jolla, CA, USA

Definition
A hormone that stimulates red blood cell production.

Cross-References
▶ Bone Marrow Toxicity in Cancer Treatment

ESA

▶ Erythropoiesis-Stimulating Agent (also ESA or Exogenous Erythropoietin)

Esophageal Cancer

ALBERT S. DENITTIS
Lankenau Institute for Medical Research,
Lankenau Hospital, Wynnewood, PA, USA

Definition
Esophageal carcinoma is an extremely deadly disease, and in spite of major advances in cancer treatment, prognosis is poor. The use of radiation therapy in the treatment of esophageal carcinoma was first described in France in the early 1900s; radium was used as a local treatment and provided palliation. ▶ External-Beam Radiation Therapy (EBRT) was then introduced with the development of orthovoltage; however, the depth of penetration was not sufficient to produce tumoricidal doses without causing major morbidity. With the advent of cobalt and the linear accelerator, dose delivery has been increased to the megadose range. This new technology allows radiation oncologists to have an impact on treatment outcomes with a decrease in treatment-related side effects. This chapter describes the behavior of esophageal cancer, its risk factors and proper staging, and the advances in radiation and chemotherapy.

Anatomy
The esophagus is a thin-walled, hollow tube with an average length of 40 cm. The normal esophagus is lined with stratified keratinized squamous epithelium, which extends from the cricoid cartilage inferiorly to the gastroesophageal junction. In the lower third (5–10 cm) of the esophagus, there are glandular elements, and the columnar epithelium frequently replaces the stratified squamous epithelium, especially at the gastroesophageal junction. There are four layers to the esophagus. The innermost layer consists of epithelium, followed by the inner circular muscle layer, the outer longitudinal muscle layer, and an adventitia. No serosa is present.

There are many methods of subdividing the esophagus, all of which are arbitrary. The esophagus is usually divided into cervical and thoracic components. The cervical esophagus begins at the cricopharyngeal muscle (C7 level or 18 cm from the incisors) and extends to the thoracic inlet (T3 level or 24 cm from the incisors). The thoracic esophagus represents the remainder of the organ, extending from the level of T3 to T10 or T11 (38–40 cm from the incisors). The American Joint Committee on Cancer (AJCC) divides the esophagus into four regions: cervical, upper thoracic, midthoracic, and lower thoracic. The esophagus has an extensive longitudinal interconnecting system of lymphatics. The lymphatic channels in the mucosa and submucosa communicate with the lymphatic channels in the muscle layers extending through the esophagus. As a result of this system, lymph can travel the entire length of the esophagus before draining into the lymph nodes, and thus the entire esophagus is at risk for lymphatic metastasis. Lymphatics of the esophagus drain into nodes that usually follow arteries, including the inferior thyroid artery, the bronchial and esophageal arteries, and the left gastric artery (celiac axis).

Epidemiology

Esophageal carcinoma is relatively rare representing approximately 1% of all malignancies and rarely occurs before the age of 65 years. Before 65 years of age, the incidence is 1.9/100,000 persons, and over 65 years, the incidence is 22.3/100,000 persons. In the United States, there are an estimated 14,520 new patients diagnosed with esophageal cancer yearly. The majority of these occurred in men, with a rate of 3.5:1 over women. There were an estimated 13,570 deaths per year with an overall mortality rate of 4.0/100,000 persons. The incidence and mortality rates vary between races. The incidence in white men is 4.39/100,000, whereas the incidence in African-American men is 8.63/100,000. Age-adjusted mortality for African-American although showing a declining trend, was nearly twice that of whites (7.79 vs. 3.96, p = 0.05).

In the United States, there has been a rise in the incidence of adenocarcinoma of the esophagus and a decline in squamous cell carcinoma. In 1987, adenocarcinoma represented 34% and 12% of esophageal cancers in white men and women, respectively. The numbers were 3% and 1% for African-American men and women, respectively. However, over the last 20 years, there has been an increase in adenocarcinoma of almost 5–10% per year. This is a faster increase than for any other cancer. As of 1998, esophageal adenocarcinoma accounted for almost 55% of all diagnosed cases in white men.

The incidence of esophageal carcinoma varies greatly worldwide, ranging from rare to almost epidemic proportions. The international incidence in men and women ranges from 2.5 to 5.0 per 100,000 and from 1.5 to 2.5 per 100,000, respectively. Some of the highest rates in the world are found in northern China, Iran, and the Soviet Union, near the Caspian Sea, and can be as high as 100 + per 100,000 persons. High-risk clusters can also be seen in South Africa, northern France, Hong Kong, and Brazil. The international mortality rates have been relatively stable.

In North America and Western Europe, alcohol and tobacco use are the major risk factors and are associated with 80–90% of all cases of squamous cell carcinoma. Blot has demonstrated a relative risk of 155 to 1 when consuming greater than 30 g/day of tobacco along with 121 g/day of alcohol. As for adenocarcinoma, the risk actually has been shown to decline with the drinking of wine.

In high-risk populations, diets limited to corn, wheat, millet, small amounts of fruits, vegetables, and animal products correlate to increases in squamous cell carcinoma. Other risk factors associated with esophageal carcinoma include achalasia, caustic burns (especially lye corrosion), and tylosis.

The risk factors for adenocarcinoma are not as well known. Most esophageal adenocarcinomas tend to rise from the metaplastic columnar-lined epithelium known as *Barrett's esophagus*. In a report by Cameron et al., it was demonstrated that most adenocarcinomas of the esophagus occur in the short-segment Barrett's esophagus. Severe and long-standing gastro- esophageal reflux disease has also been shown to be a cause for Barrett's esophagus, which therefore could indirectly lead to adenocarcinoma. Last, obesity has been linked to a threefold to fourfold risk of adenocarcinoma.

Clinical Presentation

Symptoms of esophageal cancer usually start 3–4 months before diagnosis, and the location of the primary tumor can influence the presenting symptoms. Dysphagia is seen in more than 90% of patients regardless of location. Odynophagia (pain on swallowing) is present in up to 50% of patients. Weight loss is also a presenting finding in patients 40–70% of the time. There is a better prognosis if weight loss is limited to less than 5% of total body weight. Other, less frequent symptoms may include hoarseness, cough, and glossopharyngeal neuralgia.

Advanced lesions can produce signs and symptoms from tumor invasion into local structures. Hematemesis, hemoptysis, melena, and persistent cough secondary to esophagotracheal or esophagobronchial fistula may occur. Compression or invasion of the left recurrent laryngeal nerve or the phrenic nerves can cause dysphonia or paralysis of a hemidiaphragm. Superior vena cava syndrome and Horner's syndrome can also appear. Pleural effusion and exsanguination resulting from aortic communication can occur. Tumors in the lower third of the esophagus can invade the aorta or pericardium, causing a mediastinitis, massive hemorrhage, and empyema. Distant metastasis may be detected at diagnosis at almost any site.

Differential Diagnosis

Squamous cell carcinoma and adenocarcinoma account for 95% of all esophageal tumors, although there are other rare histologic subtypes that are occasionally seen.

Pseudosarcoma is a variant of a poorly differentiated squamous cell carcinoma with spindle-shaped cells in the stroma resembling fibroblasts. Verrucous carcinoma is another variant of squamous cell carcinoma. It is well differentiated and papillary in appearance. Adenocarcinoma is the other major cell type and is becoming increasingly common. Adenocarcinoma may arise from foci of ectopic gastric mucosa, intrinsic esophageal glands, or Barrett's esophagus. Submucosal spread is not as common as in squamous cell carcinoma, and metastasis usually occurs by transverse penetration through the full thickness of the wall. If a small focus of squamous cell metaplasia is found in an adenocarcinoma, the tumor is called an *adenoacanthoma.*

Adenoid cystic carcinomas have an incidence of 0.75% and occur in the sixth decade of life. Mucoepidermoid tumors (adenosquamous carcinomas), although similar to their salivary gland counterpart, are more aggressive and have a poor prognosis. Small cell carcinoma has a prevalence of 1.7–2.4%, presents in the sixth to eighth decades of life, and is found predominantly in the middle and lower esophagus in men. Small cell carcinomas are thought to originate in the argyrophilic cells in the esophagus. They are highly malignant and may produce paraneoplastic syndromes, such as antidiuretic hormone secretion and hypercalcemia.

Nonepithelial tumors of the esophagus are rare. Among these, leiomyosarcomas are the most common. In patients with Kaposi's sarcoma, gastrointestinal involvement of the esophagus can be seen. Malignant melanoma is very rare as well as lymphoma, occuring in 1% of esophageal diagnoses. Metastases to the esophagus do occur. The most common source is the breast, but other reported sites include the pharynx, tonsil, larynx, lung, stomach, liver, kidney, prostate, testis, bone, and skin.

Imaging Studies

After a thorough history and physical examination, all patients should have a workup.

Although the esophagogram may be used to define lesion extent, endoscopy is the key diagnostic procedure and of vital importance to accurately diagnose and define the lesion. During flexible endoscopy, biopsies and brushings should be taken on the primary site and any areas suspected of containing satellite or submucosal spread. Examination with panendoscopy of the oral cavity, pharynx, larynx, and tracheobronchial tree should also be performed at the time of esophagoscopy because of the high incidence of second tumors in the head and neck and upper airway. Computed tomography (CT) of the thorax can demonstrate extramucosal extension of disease, and should be extended below the diaphragm to include the liver, upper abdominal nodes, and adrenals. The CT scan may not adequately assess periesophageal lymph node involvement or accurately show the true length of the primary tumor. To assess periesophageal and celiac lymph node involvement and the transmural extent of disease, endoscopic ultrasonography (EUS) should be performed. EUS provides an accuracy of 85% for tumor invasion (T stage) compared with surgical pathology, and 75% for the assessment of lymph node metastases.

Surgical staging procedures, including thoracoscopy, mediastinoscopy, and laparoscopy, can add valuable information regarding primary tumor penetration, lymph node involvement, and distant spread and should be considered in appropriately selected patients.

Another useful test that should be used to evaluate the extent of esophageal cancer is positron emission tomography (PET). Recent studies have shown that the addition of PET to standard staging studies such as CT can improve the accuracy of detecting stage III and stage IV disease by 23% and 18%, respectively When comparing PET, CT, and EUS, PET has only a 22% sensitivity in determining N1 disease compared to 83% for EUS and CT scans. PET has also been shown to upstage patients by 15% and downstage patients by 7%. When using PET as a staging tool, overall survival can be predicted more accurately. Separating patients into nonmetastatic and metastatic disease shows a 1- and 2-year survival of 77% and 65% versus 35% and 17%, respectively.

Staging can be either pathologic or clinical. A pathologic stage can be established if invasive procedures are performed such as surgery consisting of mediastinotomy and thoracotomy. Clinical staging is usually performed and is less precise. Table 1 presents the recommended AJCC clinical and pathologic staging system.

Treatment

Curative Surgery

Curative surgery of the esophagus is the treatment of choice in Stage I and II disease, and involves a subtotal or total esophagectomy, and is usually performed for lesions of the mid and lower thoracic, as well as the gastroesophageal junction. The issue of how to treat early stage adenocarcinoma of the esophagus is not yet resolved. The traditional approach has been curative surgery, but data suggest that double or triple-modality therapy may improve local control and survival. Postoperative radiation therapy is recommended in all patients in whom a microscopically incomplete resection (R1 resection) was performed. Squamous cell carcinoma of the cervical esophagus presents a very difficult situation. If surgery is performed, it usually requires removal of portions of the pharynx, the entire larynx and thyroid gland, and the proximal esophagus. Radical neck dissections are also carried out. For this reason, radiation therapy to this portion of the esophagus is preferable.

Curative Combination Therapy

For patients with Stage III or IVa disease, an approach with radiation and chemotherapy with or without surgery should be used. Currently, multiagent chemotherapy is used, with cisplatin, 5-fluorouracil (5-FU), being the most frequently used drugs. There are newer chemotherapeutic regimens using the taxanes either alone or in combination with the current standard therapies, but they are still being used on trials. The best results are seen with patients who have esophageal tumors that are truly localized. Survival rates range from 25% to 35% at 5 years, and these results have been attained using various types of preoperative treatment. In the 2005 patterns of care study, the

Esophageal Cancer. Table 1 TNM staging for cancer of the esophagus (Adapted from American Joint Committee on Cancer 2010)

Primary tumor (T)	
TX	Primary tumor cannot be assessed
T0	No evidence of primary tumor
Tis	Carcinoma in situ
T1	Tumor invades lamina propria or submucosa
T2	Tumor invades muscularis propria
T3	Tumor invades adventitia
T4	Tumor invades adjacent structures
Regional lymph nodes (N)	
NX	Regional lymph nodes cannot be assessed
N0	No regional lymph node metastasis
N1	Regional lymph node metastasis
Distant metastasis (M)	
MX	Presence of distant metastasis cannot be assessed
M0	No distant metastasis
M1	Distant metastasis
Tumors of the lower thoracic esophagus	
M1a	Metastases in the celiac lymph nodes
M1b	Other distant metastases
Tumors of the midthoracic esophagus	
M1a	Not applicable
M1b	Nonregional lymph nodes and/or distant metastases
Tumors of the upper thoracic esophagus	
M1a	Metastases in the cervical nodes
M1b	Other distant metastases

Stage grouping			
Stage 0	Tis	N0	M0
Stage I	T1	N0	M0
Stage IIA	T2	N0	M0
	T3	N0	M0
Stage IIB	T1	N1	M0
	T2	N1	M0

Esophageal Cancer. Table 1 (continued)

Stage III	T3	N1	M0
	T4	Any N	M0
Stage IV	Any T	Any N	M1
Stage IVA	Any T	Any N	M1a
Stage IVB	Any T	Any N	M1b

national practice standards for patients receiving radiation therapy for esophageal cancer were evaluated. The authors found that patients treated between 1996 and 1999 had a decreased risk of death with a hazards ratio of 0.32 if treated with concurrent chemoradiatherapy followed by surgery compared with chemoradiotherapy-alone.

Palliative Treatment

Palliative treatment is chosen only for the relief of symptoms of esophageal carcinoma, especially dysphagia. Dilatation is a reasonable alternative. When the lumen of the esophagus is dilated to 15 mm, dysphagia is no longer experienced. Esophageal stenting with either conventional plastic stents or metallic self-expanding stents can also be used to maintain patency. Palliative irradiation can be used to control the primary disease as well as distant metastasis. Resolution of symptoms, especially pain and dysphagia, can be accomplished in as much as 80%.

Radiation Therapy

Radiotherapy should be started concurrently with chemotherapy. Before starting, either three-dimentional treatment planning or ▶ Intensity-Modulated Radiation Therapy should be utilized. Target volumes include all areas of subclinical disease which includes at least a 5 cm margin both cephalad and caudad and a 2 cm radial margin. The fusion of CT-PET has been shown to cause a treatment modification in the gross tumor volume (GTV). The target treatment

volume changed in 56% of patients. Escalating doses seem to increase tumor response; however, no dose regimen has been shown to be superior when comparing overall survival. Based on data from squamous cell carcinoma of the upper aerodigestive tract, 50 Gy at 1.8 to 2 Gy per fraction over 5 weeks should control more than 90% of subclinical disease. At least 60–70 Gy are needed to treat gross disease in fractions of 1.8–2 Gy per day, 5 days per week. Intracavitary High-Dose-Rate (HDR) ▶ Brachytherapy can be used as part of a curative or palliative treatment plan. High-dose-rate (HDR) technique can deliver 100–400 Gy per hour, and treatment can be given in 5–10 min after placement of an intraluminal catheter. Doses of 5–20 Gy are usually delivered to a depth of 1 cm from the center of the catheter. Local control rates with any technique range from 40% to 95%, with a 4–20% risk of stricture and a 2–10% risk of fistula formation.

Cross-References

▶ Stomach Cancer

References

American Cancer Society (1997) Cancer facts and figures – 2005. American Cancer Society, Atlanta

American Joint Committee on Cancer (2010) Esophagus. In: Edge SB, Byrd DR, Compton CC et al (eds) AJCC cancer staging manual, 7th edn. Springer, New York, p 103

Blackstock AW, Farmer MR, Lovato J et al (2005) A prospective evaluation of the impact of 18-F-fluor-deoxy-d-glucose positron emission tomography staging on survival for patients with locally advanced esophageal cancer. Int J Radiat Oncol Biol Phys 64(2):455–460

Czito B, De Nittis AS, Willet C (2008) Esophageal cancer. In: Halperin EC, Perez C, Brady LW (eds) Principles and practice of radiation oncology, 5th edn. LWW, Philadelphia, p 1131

Konski A, Doss M, Milestone B et al (2005) The integration of 18-fluoro-deoxy-glucose positron emission tomography and endoscopic ultrasound in the treatment planning process for esophageal carcinoma. Int J Radiat Oncol Biol Phys 61(4):1123–1128

Lerut T, Flamen P, Ectors N et al (2000) Histopathologic validation of lymph node staging with PET scan in cancer of the esophagus and gastroesophageal junction: a prospective study based on primary surgery with extensive lymphadectomy. Ann Surg 232:743–752

Parkin M, Muir L, Whelan S et al (1992) Cancer incidence in five continents, vol 6. International Agency for Research on Cancer, Lyon, France

Posner M, Minsy B, Ilson D (2008) Cancer of the esophagus. In: De Vita VT, Hellman S, Rosenberg SA (eds) Cancer: principles and practice of oncology, 8th edn. JB Lippincott, Philadelphia, p 993

SEER cancer statistics review, 1973–1998. Bethesda, MD: National Cancer Institute, 1998.

Seydel HG, Wichman L, Byhhardt R et al (1988) Preoperative radiation and chemotherapy for localized squamous cell carcinoma of the esophagus: an RTOG study. Int J Radiat Oncol Biol Phys 14:33

Suntharalingham M, Moughan J, Coia LR et al (2005) Outcome results of the 1996–1999 patterns of care survey of the national practice for patients receiving radiation therapy for carcinoma of the esophagus. J Clin Oncol 23(10):2325

Zabotto L, Touboul E, Lerouge D et al (2005) Impact of CT and 18F-deoxyglucose positron emission tomography image fusion for conformal radiotherapy in esophageal carcinoma. Int J Radiat Oncol Biol Phys 63(2):340

Esophagogastroduodenoscopy

Filip T. Troicki[1], Jaganmohan Poli[2]
[1]College of Medicine, Drexel University, Philadelphia, PA, USA
[2]Department of Radiation Oncology, College of Medicine, Drexel University, Philadelphia, PA, USA

Definition

Endoscopic evaluations of the upper digestive tracts including the esophagus, stomach, duodenum and Ampulla of Vater.

Cross-References

▶ Cancer of the Pancreas
▶ Endoscopy
▶ Esophageal Cancer
▶ Stomach Cancer

Esthesioneuroblastomas

Carlos A. Perez, Wade L. Thorstad
Department of Radiation Oncology, Siteman Cancer Center, Washington University Medical Center, St. Louis, MO, USA

Definition

Rare tumor arising from the olfactory receptors within the cribriform plate in the ethmoid bone anterior to the fossa of Rosenmuller.

Esthesioneuroblastomas (ENBs) are rare tumors thought to arise in the olfactory receptors in the mucosa or the cribriform plate of the ethmoid bone (Cole and Beiler 1994).

Epidemiology

ENB constitutes 3% of all endonasal neoplasms About 945 cases have been reported in the world literature. There appears to be a slight male predominance. The age incidence has a bimodal distribution, with peaks at 11–20 years and 40–60 years, the highest incidence at 51–60 years.

Most of these tumors occur high in the nasal cavity or in the lateral wall adjacent to the ethmoids. The tumor may spread to the opposite ethmoid, superiorly to the frontal sinus and anterior cranial fossa, posteriorly to the sphenoid sinus, nasopharynx, and base of skull, laterally to the orbits, forward to the frontonasal angle, or inferiorly to the nasal cavity and antrum. Lymphatic spread may be to the subdigastric, posterior cervical, submaxillary, or preauricular nodes, as well as to the nodes of Rouviere. The exact incidence of distant metastases is uncertain; it has been quoted to be as high as 50%, but this rate is influenced by the use of chemotherapy in high-risk patients.

Clinical Presentation

The most common clinical symptoms are epistaxis and nasal blockage. Patients also may have local pain or headache, visual disturbances, rhinorrhea, tearing, proptosis, or swelling in the cheek. The symptoms may be associated with a mass in the neck.

Diagnostic Workup and Staging

Physical examination may show the inferior aspect of a polypoid friable mass in the nasal cavity. Ocular findings or a mass in the nasopharynx may be present. With early lesions, radiographs or CT or MRI may show only nonspecific opacification, soft tissue swelling, and occasionally bone destruction. Octreotide scintigraphy (OS) may be useful in confirming the preoperative diagnosis of certain head and neck NET, such as paragangliomas, Merkel cell carcinomas, medullary thyroid carcinomas, and esthesioneuroblastomas.

MRI, especially with gadolinium contrast, may be used as a supplement or alternative to CT scanning as CT provides the best information about the tumor and its local invasion into surrounding bone structures. MRI allows an estimate of tumor spread into surrounding soft tissue areas, such as the anterior cranial fossa and the retromaxillary space. Bone scintigraphy scan detects distant metastases.

A staging system has been proposed by Kadish and associates (Table 1). Esthesioneuroblastomas may be confused with lymphoma or anaplastic carcinoma and have diffuse, regular distribution. Esthesioneuroblastomas contain many fibrils, which fill the central space of the rosette (called a pseudorosette).

Argiris et al. (2003) reported on 16 patients with ENB. Craniofacial resection was performed in 13 patients (81%); 14 received either

Esthesioneuroblastomas. Table 1 Kadish system for staging of esthesioneuroblastoma

Stage	Characteristic
A	Disease confined to the nasal cavity
B	Disease confined to the nasal cavity and one or more paranasal sinuses
C	Disease extending beyond the nasal cavity or paranasal sinuses; includes involvement of the orbit, base of skull or intracranial cavity, cervical lymph nodes, or distant metastatic sites

Source: Kadish et al. (1976)

preoperative or postoperative therapy; (radiation therapy in 11 and chemotherapy in 4). The actuarial 5-year survival was 60%, disease-free survival 33%, with a median follow-up of 4.3 years. The first site of failure was locoregional alone in 10 of 12 patients who progressed, and in 6 patients involved the brain or the meninges. Two patients were successfully salvaged.

General Management

Surgery alone appears to be adequate treatment for small, low-grade tumors confined to the ethmoids in which negative surgical margins are obtained. An ethmoidomaxillary resection with or without orbital sparing is usually necessary but in some patients a craniofacial approach is adequate. These procedures are combined with preoperative or postoperative irradiation (Foote et al. 1993).

Dias et al. (2003) reported on 35 patients with ENB treated with gross tumor resection through a transfacial approach with postoperative radiotherapy (RT) in 11 patients, craniofacial resection (CFR) and postoperative RT in 7, exclusive RT in 14, CFR alone in 1, and a combination of chemotherapy and RT in 2. Radiation therapy median dose is 48 Gy. Craniofacial resection plus postoperative RT provided a better 5-year disease-free survival (86%) compared with the other therapeutic options used ($p = .05$). The 5-year disease-specific survival rate was 64% and 43% for the low- and high-grade tumors, respectively ($p = .20$). Disease-free survival was 46% and 24% at 5 and 10 years, respectively. Overall survival was 55% and 46% at 5 and 10 years of follow-up, respectively.

Early lesions involving the ethmoids with little or no bony destruction or nerve invasion can be treated adequately by high-energy (photon or electron) radiation therapy with good cosmetic and functional results (Foote et al. 1993). Those with more extensive local disease benefit from surgery, adjuvant irradiation, and chemotherapy, although some have spoken against combined surgery and radiation therapy because of complications.

Treatment, which could be classified in 898 reported cases, consisted of surgery alone in 24% (226 cases), radiation therapy alone in 18.4% (165 cases), combined surgery and radiation therapy in 43.2% (388 cases), chemotherapy in 13.2% (119 cases), and in 11 cases (1.2%) bone marrow transplant. In the reported cases, follow-up could be evaluated in 477 cases, while in only 234 cases a 5-year follow-up was done; on these 20.5% had surgery only, 11.1% radiation therapy, and 68.4% combined surgery and radiation therapy. The best survival rates were obtained by combined therapy (72.5%) versus 62.5% with surgery alone and 53.8% with radiation therapy (Broisch et al. 1997).

Radiation Therapy

Contrast-enhanced CT or MRI scans before initiation of treatment are crucial to demarcate extension of the tumor and to aid in treatment planning (Fig. 1).

A combination of photons and electrons with anterior fields provides good coverage for limited ethmoidal disease when the tumor is confined anteriorly. Beam arrangement can be modified for disease extending into the orbit or maxillary sinus. Obturator or bolus may be needed postoperatively to compensate for tissue deficit. When intracranial or posterior extension is present or tumor has spread into the maxillary sinus, a pair of perpendicular (anteroposterior and lateral) portals with wedges or two lateral wedge fields in conjunction with an open anterior photon field will give good coverage of the

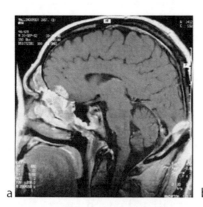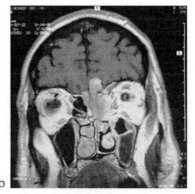

Esthesioneuroblastomas. Fig. 1 (**a** and **b**) The sagittal and coronal views of a preoperative MRI of a 56-year-old patient who was initially seen with a Kadish stage C esthesioneuroblastoma involving left nasal cavity and extending intracranially (Reproduced with permission, Chao KSC, Kaplan C, Simpson JR, et al (2001) Esthesioneuroblastoma: The impact of treatment modality. Head Neck 23:749–757)

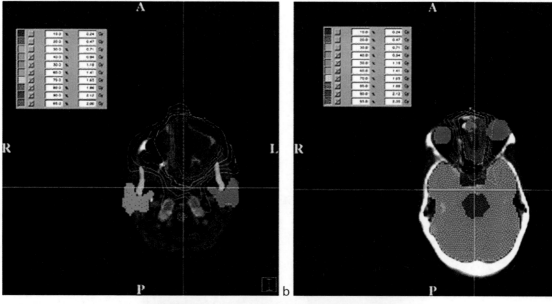

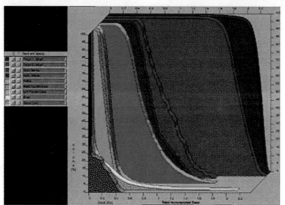

Esthesioneuroblastomas. Fig. 2 Esthesioneuroblastoma in a 35-year-old female, initially treated with a craniofacial surgical resection. Patient received postoperative IMRT (2 Gy fractions). (**a**) Cross section illustrating coverage of ethmoid-nasal and left maxillary antrum volume. (**b**) Cross section showing dose distribution in target volume with excellent sparing of ocular structures. (**c**) Dose volume histogram:

Structure	Dose range (Gy)	Mean dose (Gy)
PTV 1	30–70	65
PTV 2 (+RT nasal cavity)	40–70	58
Optic chiasm and nerves	13–42	24

Source: Reproduced with permission, from LeVay J, O'Sullivan B, Catton C, et al (1994)

treatment volume with the dose inhomogeneity around 10–20%. Incorporation of a vertex field eliminates the high inhomogeneous dose along the junction line of the conventional three-field technique. Treatment techniques are similar to those described for treatment of paranasal sinuses. The orbits can be spared or treated as the degree of extension dictates. Occasionally, an anterior electron beam field may be needed to supplement low-dose areas. When the electron beam is used over air cavities, some dosimetry problems result. Eye blocks must be positioned precisely to avoid undesirable side effects.

Three-dimensional CRT or intensity-modulated radiation therapy (IMRT) provides an alternative to the conventional three-field technique frequently used to treat these tumors (Fig. 2). Special attention should be directed to reduce unnecessary irradiation to ocular and nerve structures. Because of the proximity of esthesioneuroblastoma to the optic nerves, optic chasm, and the brain stem, the precision of treatment setup, target volume definition, and dose homogeneity dictate tumor control and the sequelae of treatment. Treatment techniques similar to those for paranasal sinuses may create "hot spots" along the optic tracks. High doses per fraction (exceeding 2 Gy) increase the possibility of late sequelae such as blindness and bone and brain necrosis.

When combined therapy is used, preoperative doses of 45 Gy and postoperative doses of 50–60 Gy are indicated, depending on the status of the surgical margins. Doses of 65–70 Gy are delivered with irradiation alone in patients with inoperable tumors.

Cross-References

► Palliation of Brain and Spinal Cord Metastases

References

Argiris A, Dutra J, Tseke P et al (2003) Esthesioneuro-blastoma: the Northwestern University experience. Laryngoscope 113:155–160

Broisch G, Pagliari A, Ottaviani F (1997) Esthesioneuro-blastoma: a general review of the cases published since the discovery of the tumour in 1924. Anticancer Res 17:2683–2706

Chao KSC, Kaplan C, Simpson JR et al (2001) Esthesioneur-oblastoma: the impact of treatment modality. Head Neck 23:749–757

Cole JM, Beiler D (1994) Long-term results of treatment for glomus jugulare and glomus vagale tumors with radiotherapy. Laryngoscope 104:1461–1465

Dias FL, Sa GM, Lima RA et al (2003) Patterns of failure and outcome in esthesioneuroblastoma. Arch Otolaryngol Head Neck Surg 129:1186–1192

Foote RL, Morita A, Ebersold MJ et al (1993) Esthesioneur-oblastoma: the role of adjuvant radiation therapy. Int J Radiat Oncol Biol Phys 27:835–842

Kadish S, Goodman M, Wang CC (1976) Olfactory neuro-blastoma: a clinical analysis of 17 cases. Cancer 37:1571–1576

LeVay J, O'Sullivan B, Catton C et al (1994) An assessment of prognostic factors in soft tissue sarcoma of the head and neck. Arch Otolaryngol Head Neck Surg 120:981–986

Ethmoid Sinus

FILIP T. TROICKI
College of Medicine, Drexel University, Philadelphia, PA, USA

Definition

Ethmoid Sinus is a mucous membrane–lined cavity located behind the bridge of the nose.

Cross-References

► Nasal Cavity and Paranasal Sinuses

Evidence-Based Medicine

► Clinical Research and the Practice of Evidence-Based Medicine in Radiation Oncology

Ewing Family of Tumors (Including Ewing's Sarcoma of Bone, Extraosseous Ewing's [EOE] Sarcoma, Primitive Neuroectodermal Tumor [PNET], and Askin's Tumor)

▶ Ewing Sarcoma

Ewing Sarcoma

DANIEL J. INDELICATO
Department of Radiation Oncology, University of Florida Proton Therapy Institute, University of Florida College of Medicine, Jacksonville, FL, USA

Synonyms

Ewing family of tumors (including Ewing's sarcoma of bone, extraosseous Ewing's [EOE] sarcoma, primitive neuroectodermal tumor [PNET], and Askin's Tumor); Ewing tumor

Definition

Diverse group of small, round, blue-cell tumors arising from mesenchymal stem cells usually characterized by a translocation between the ▶ EWS gene on chromosome 22 and the ▶ FLI1 gene on chromosome 11 (t[11;22][q24;q12]) or the ▶ ERG gene on chromosome 21 (t[21;22] [q22;q12]).

Etiology

The etiology of Ewing sarcoma is unclear. No definite patient or environmental factors have been identified.

Clinical Presentation

Ewing sarcoma can occur anywhere in the body but arise most frequently in the lower extremity. The most common symptoms are pain and swelling in the primary site, whether it is bone or soft tissue. The symptoms often wax and wane, sometimes leading to a long delay in diagnosis. Ewing sarcomas have been shown to have the longest lag time in diagnosis of any pediatric solid tumor (mean, 146 days). Occasionally a patient may present with systemic symptoms such as low-grade fevers, malaise, or weakness due to widespread metastases. Pathologic fracture is rarely a presenting symptom.

Ewing sarcoma spreads by direct extension from the primary lesion into the adjacent bone or soft tissue. Therefore, tumors may be characterized by both an intraosseous component and extraosseous component (Fig. 1a). Tumors in the thorax or abdomen may grow quite large and exhibit a "pushing margin" into body cavities. Following a good tumor response to chemotherapy, normal tissues within the cavity may return to their natural position (Fig. 1b). Metastases generally spread through the blood stream, with the most common sites being the lung and nonadjacent bones, and approximately 25% are metastatic at diagnosis (Nesbit et al. 1990; Donaldson et al. 1998; Paulussen et al. 2001; Grier et al. 2003; Yock et al. 2006). Lymph node metastases are uncommon, except in ▶ peripheral primitive neuroectodermal tumors (PNETs). Organ involvement, such as brain or liver, is rare and usually occurs only in end-stage disease.

Diagnostics

Diagnostic radiograph may show characteristic "onion skin" or "sunburst" periosteal reaction. In a suspected case of Ewing sarcoma, a computed tomography (CT) and magnetic resonance imaging (MRI) of the primary site should be performed. An incisional biopsy or complete resection should be performed, depending on

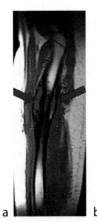
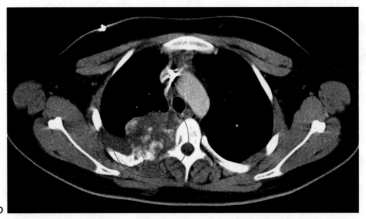

a b

Ewing Sarcoma. Fig. 1 Ewing sarcoma of the (a) femur with extraosseous soft tissue extension as indicated by arrows and (b) the posterior chest wall prior to chemotherapy demonstrating an intrathoracic "pushing margin"

site and degree of infiltration, followed by cytogenetic analysis of the specimen. Upon confirming the pathologic diagnosis, a complete blood count and serum chemistry, including lactate dehydrogenase (LDH), should be obtained. A CT of the chest and a bone scan are indicated to evaluate for metastatic disease. Positron emission tomography (PET)-CT may also be considered.

Differential Diagnosis

- Osteosarcoma
- Mesenchymal chondrosarcoma
- Soft tissue sarcoma
- Giant cell tumor
- Lymphoma
- Neuroblastoma
- Bone metastases from primary tumor elsewhere

Therapy

The standard therapeutic pathway has been outlined in guidelines from the National Comprehensive Cancer Network (NCCN) (Fig. 2).

In contrast to earlier eras where most tumors were treated with definitive radiation, today local management is primarily guided by tumor resectability (Table 1).

Radiation Therapy Techniques

Imaging for Planning/Simulation

The patient may be treated in the supine, prone, or lateral position. Volumetric CT-based planning is necessary to optimize the dose to the target volume while protecting normal tissues. MRI fusion is recommended. If MRI is utilized, axial T1-gadolinium and T2-weighted sequences should cover the entire area of tumor (intra- and extraosseous) and the entire involved bone.

Timing of Radiation

Radiation is typically undertaken at week 13 from the start of chemotherapy. The sequencing of radiation relative to surgery is variable (Table 2). The target definition (GTV, CTV) depends on tumor presentation (Table 3).

Special Sites

Vertebral Body Lesions

- The gross tumor volume (GTV)1 and GTV2 are defined in Table 3. At a minimum, clinical target volume (CTV)1 is defined as the entire vertebral body. For the field-reduction boost, CTV2 is defined as GTV2 plus an additional

Ewing Tumor Treatment Schema (modified from NCCN guidelines)

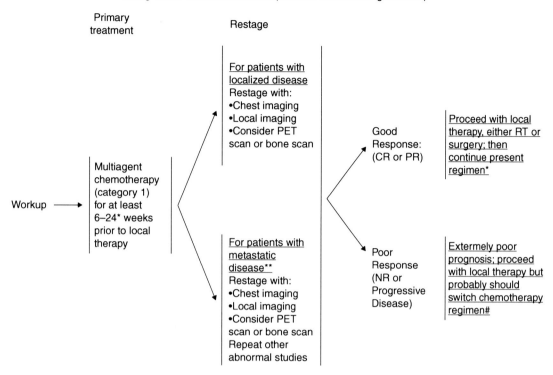

*Most protocols give 12 or more weeks of induction chemotherapy now; however, data from Schuck et al indicates that the shorter the length of time before radiation therapy begins the better the local control and survival.

#Patients who have less than a PR to induction chemotherapy (50% shrinkage in volume of soft tissue mass or poor histologic response at surgery) almost universally die.

**For patients with many metastatic lesions, it may be preferable to wait until the end of chemotherapy to proceed with radiation therapy to the metastatic lesions, including lung irradiation if indicated.

Ewing Sarcoma. Fig. 2 Ewing tumor treatment schema (modified from NCCN guidelines)

Ewing Sarcoma. Table 1 Treatment by tumor resectability

Surgical Status	Example	Treatment
Unresectable lesions	Maxilla, base of skull, vertebral bodies	RT alone
Lesions in expendable bones	Scapula, rib, clavicle, fibula, ilium	Surgery with wide margins
Borderline lesions	Long bones, mandible	Can be treated with surgery alone and reconstruction; can also be treated with RT alone. Lesions with positive margins, close margins, or expected positive margins should receive pre- or post-op RT

RT radiotherapy

Ewing Sarcoma. Table 2 Advantages and disadvantages to radiotherapy sequencing

Sequence	Advantages	Disadvantages
Preoperative RT	• Lowest dose • Smaller field size • May decrease tumor seeding at surgery	• Risk of overtreatment • Increased postoperative infection rate • Impaired bony union
Postoperative RT	• Allows pathologic response and margin status to inform RT recommendations	• Intermediate dose • Larger field size • May be associated with inferior late functional outcome
Definitive RT	• Historical standard • Option for large, unresectable tumors • Less delays in chemotherapy	• Highest dose • May be associated with inferior local control compared to combined modality treatment

RT radiotherapy

Ewing Sarcoma. Table 3 Target definition according to presentation

Target volume		Definition	Margin
GTV1	Definitive and preoperative radiation	Visible gross tumor consisting of prechemotherapy bone and soft tissue	N/A
	Postoperative radiation	Surgical tumor bed consisting of the margin of bone initially involved with tumor, the soft tissue tumor bed, and soft tissue contiguous with the tumor prior to surgical resection	N/A
GTV2	Definitive and preoperative radiation	Visible gross tumor consisting of (1) bone initially involved with tumor (prechemotherapy) and (2) residual soft tissue tumor prior to radiotherapy (post-chemotherapy) including the surfaces of normal tissues in contact with tumor, now returned to normal anatomic position	N/A
CTV1		Standard-risk CTV	GTV1 plus a 1.5-cm anatomic margin of tissue, respecting anatomic barriers that limit tumor spread. Scar, drain site, and contaminated surgical sites should also be included

Ewing Sarcoma. Table 3 (continued)

Target volume	Definition	Margin
CTV2	High-risk CTV	GTV2 plus a 1-cm anatomic margin of tissue, respecting anatomic barriers that limit tumor spread
PTV1/PTV2	PTVs	CTV1/CTV2 plus an institutional specified margin to account for day-to-day setup variation related to the ability to immobilize the patient and physiologic motion of the CTV1

CTV clinical target volume, *GTV* gross target volume, *PTV* planning target volume, *N/A* Not applicable

1.5-cm margin to account for subclinical areas of residual disease but confined by anatomic boundaries (e.g., CTV2 does not enter the spinal canal if initial disease did not enter the canal).

Tumors Within a Body Cavity (e.g., Abdominal, Pelvic, or Chest Wall Tumors)
- Regardless of GTV, CTV1 and CTV2 will be limited by the "pushing margin" of the tumor within the peritoneal or thoracic cavity where infiltration by microscopic disease is not suspected (Fig. 3).

Radiation Dose
The recommended radiation dose to PTV1 and PTV2 depends on tumor site and presentation (Table 4).

Radiation Modality
There are different approaches to the technical delivery of radiation for Ewing sarcoma. Each has its advantages and disadvantages.

Two- and Three-Dimensional Conformal Photon Radiotherapy
- Historical standard in Ewing sarcoma
- Technique utilized in the vast majority of randomized trials to date

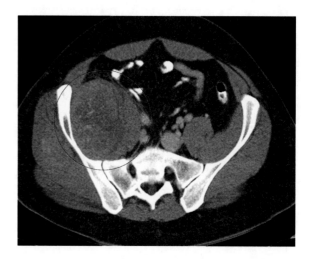

Ewing Sarcoma. Fig. 3 Ewing sarcoma of the pelvis extending into the pelvic cavity. Note that CTV1 and CTV2 would both be defined by the postinduction disease extent along the peritoneal surface of the tumor

- Relatively homogeneous dose distribution
- Dose conformality often suboptimal for tumors near critical tissue

Brachytherapy
- Excellent dose conformality
- Efficient and convenient
- Risk of heterogeneous dose distribution
- Limited to certain subsites and resectable tumors

Ewing Sarcoma. Table 4 Recommended radiation dose according to tumor site and presentation

Tumor site and presentation	PTV1	PTV2
Definitive RT or residual gross disease following incomplete resection	45 Gy	≤8 cm: 10.8 Gy
		>8 cm: 16.2 Gy
Definitive RT for vertebral body where spinal cord will receive the prescription dose (i.e., spinal cord cannot be avoided)	45 Gy	5.4 Gy
Definitive RT – unresected, involved lymph nodes	45 Gy	10.8 Gy
Preoperative RT	45 Gy	5.4 Gy
Postoperative RT – inadequate margins; microscopic residual	50.4 Gy to 55.8 Gy	N/A

Doses above at 1.8 Gy per fraction daily using external beam radiotherapy
RT radiotherapy, *PTV* planning target volume

Intensity-Modulated Radiation Therapy (Photon)
- Improved high isodose conformality relative to 2- and 3-D conformal therapy
- Heterogeneous dose distribution
- High integral body dose
- Poor low isodose conformality

Proton Therapy
- Excellent dose conformality
- Low integral body dose
- Limited availability

Normal Tissue Tolerance Guidelines
Radiation dose-effect for the various elements of the musculoskeletal system is poorly characterized. Table 5 represents the best available guidelines on normal tissue toxicity. It is well-recognized, however, that the growth of long

Ewing Sarcoma. Table 5 Normal tissue toxicity for musculoskeletal elements

Toxicity	Recommendations
Long bone fracture	Bone V40 <64% Bone mean dose <37 Gy 1 cm³ max dose <59 Gy
Flat bone hypoplasia	Minimize V35
Slippage of an upper femoral or humeral epiphysis	Minimize epiphyseal V25
Muscular hypoplasia	Minimize compartmental V20
Scoliosis	"All or none" irradiation of vertebral body
Lymphedema	Keep dose to longitudinal 2–3-cm strip of extremity <15 Gy
Radiation-induced sarcoma	Minimize normal-tissue V60
Long bone growth	Minimize growth plate V2[a]

[a]The severity of this effect is dependent on the radiation dose, the patient's age at irradiation, and the epiphysis irradiated. The skeleton is particularly sensitive to radiation effects during the periods of most active bone growth in early childhood and during puberty

Ewing Sarcoma. Table 6 Proportional contribution of long bone epiphyses to overall bone growth

	Proportional contribution to overall bone growth	
Long bone	Proximal epiphysis	Distal epiphysis
Femur	30%	70%
Tibia	60%	40%
Humerus	80%	20%

bones depends on the proportional contribution of their respective epiphyses to overall length (Table 6).

Follow-Up
Refer Table 7.

Ewing Sarcoma. Table 7 Recommended baseline imaging

Site	Anatomic imaging	Functional imaging	Timing
Recommended baseline imaging after local management			
Primary	AP and lateral radiographs	–	Within 2 weeks of surgery
Primary	MRI with gadolinium or CT scan with IV contrast (in patients without significant metallic artifact at primary tumor site)	–	3 to 4 months after local control
Surveillance on chemotherapy and end-of-therapy evaluations			
Primary	AP and lateral radiographs	–	After 10 cycles of chemotherapy (about half way through treatment)
Chest	CT	–	After 10 cycles of chemotherapy (about half way through treatment)
Whole body	–	MDP bone scintigraphy	At end of cytotoxic chemotherapy (unless bone scintigraphy negative and FDG-PET positive at presentation)
Whole body	–	FDG-PET	At end of cytotoxic chemotherapy (unless bone scintigraphy positive and FDG-PET negative at presentation)
Primary	MRI with gadolinium or CT scan with IV contrast	–	If symptoms or abnormal imaging (and surgical intervention or radiation therapy contemplated)
Primary	AP and lateral radiographs	–	After 10 cycles of chemotherapy (about half way through)
Chest	CT	–	After 10 cycles of chemotherapy (about half way through)
Recommended surveillance post chemotherapy			
Primary and chest	AP and lateral radiographs	–	q 3 months × 8, then q 6 months × 6, then q 12 months × 5
Primary	MRI with gadolinium or CT scan with IV contrast	–	If symptoms or abnormal imaging (and surgical intervention or radiation therapy contemplated)
Chest	CT	–	If abnormal chest radiographs
Whole body	–	MDP bone Scintigraphy	If symptoms or abnormal imaging (and primary tumor positive on prior bone scintigraphy AND surgical or other intervention contemplated)

Ewing Sarcoma. Table 7 (continued)

Site	Anatomic imaging	Functional imaging	Timing
Whole body	–	FDG-PET	If symptoms or abnormal imaging (and primary tumor positive on prior FDG-PET AND surgical or other intervention contemplated)
Primary and chest	AP and lateral radiographs	–	q 3 months × 8, then q 6 months × 6, then q 12 months × 5

MRI magnetic resonance imaging, *AP* anteroposterior, *CT* computed tomography, *IV* intravenous, *FDG-PET* fludeoxyglucose-positron emission tomography, *q* every

Prognosis

There is no standard accepted staging system for Ewing sarcoma. The prognosis of Ewing sarcoma depends on the location of the primary tumor, the size of the primary tumor, and whether or not there are metastases present at diagnosis (Nesbit et al. 1990; Donaldson et al. 1998; Paulussen et al. 2001; Grier et al. 2003; Yock et al. 2006):

- Primary site: Extremity primaries (particularly distal extremity) versus axial lesions (unfavorable).
- Volume of tumor: Small primary versus larger lesion (unfavorable). Both a maximum tumor size of larger or smaller than 8 cm has been used, as well as a volume cutoff of 200 cm^3.
- Extent of disease: Localized disease versus metastatic disease (unfavorable).
- Site of metastasis: Lung metastases versus bone/bone marrow (unfavorable) versus both bone and lung metastases (worst).

These prognostic factors are probably related, since axial lesions are usually larger than extremity lesions, particularly those in the distal extremity bones. It is important to realize that most of the data for Ewing sarcoma is based

Ewing Sarcoma. Table 8 Survival estimates according to presentation (Nesbit et al. 1990; Donaldson et al. 1998; Paulussen et al. 2001; Grier et al. 2003; Yock et al. 2006)

Extent of disease	Approximate 5-year survival
Localized disease	55%
Extremities	60%
Axial	45%
Metastases at diagnosis	20%
Lung metastases only	30% (40% for patients receiving whole-lung RT)
Bone metastases only	20%
Bone and lung metastases	10%

RT radiotherapy

primarily on the prognosis of bone primary lesions (Table 8).

Epidemiology

The overall incidence of ESFT is approximately one per one million in the US population. The median age at diagnosis is 13 years old, and

80% of tumors occur within the first 2 decades of life (Nesbit et al. 1990; Donaldson et al. 1998; Paulussen et al. 2001; Grier et al. 2003; Yock et al. 2006).

Cross-References

► Brachytherapy
► Clinical Target Volume (CTV)
► Conformal Therapy: Treatment Planning, Treatment Delivery, and Clinical Results
► External Beam Radiation Therapy
► Gross Tumor Volume (GTV)
► Intensity-Modulated Proton Therapy (IMPT)
► Planning Target Volume (PTV)
► Proton Therapy
► Radiation-Induced Sarcoma

References

Donaldson SS, Torrey M, Link MP et al (1998) A multidisciplinary study investigating radiotherapy in Ewing's sarcoma: end results of POG #8346. Int J Radiat Oncol Biol Phys 42:125–135

Grier HE, Krailo MD, Tarbell NJ et al (2003) Addition of ifosfamide and etoposide to standard chemotherapy for Ewing's sarcoma and PNET of bone. N Engl J Med 348:694–701

Nesbit ME Jr, Gehan EA, Burgert EO Jr et al (1990) Multimodal therapy for the management of primary nonmetastatic Ewing's sarcoma of bone: a long-term followup of the first intergroup study. J Clin Oncol 8:1664–1674

Paulussen M, Ahrens S, Dunst W et al (2001) Localized Ewing tumor of bone: final results of the cooperative Ewing's sarcoma study CESS 86. J Clin Oncol 19:1818–1829

Yock TI, Krailo M, Fryer CJ et al (2006) Local control in pelvic Ewing sarcoma: analysis from INT-0091 – a report from the children's oncology group. J Clin Oncol 24:3838–3843

Ewing Tumor

► Ewing Sarcoma

EWS Gene

DANIEL J. INDELICATO[1], ROBERT H. SAGERMAN[2]
[1]Department of Radiation Oncology, University of Florida Proton Therapy Institute, University of Florida College of Medicine, Jacksonville, FL, USA
[2]Department of Radiation Oncology, SUNY Upstate Medical University, Syracuse, NY, USA

Definition

The *EWS* gene (EWSR1, Ewing sarcoma breakpoint region 1), which maps to band q12 of human chromosome 22, is involved in a wide variety of human solid tumors including Ewing sarcoma, related primitive neuroectodermal tumors, clear cell sarcoma, malignant melanoma of soft parts, and desmoplastic small round cell tumors. Ewing sarcoma is characterized by recurrent translocations that fuse EWS to one of the following genes FLI1 (>90% of cases), ERG, ETV1, E1AF, and FEV.

Cross-References

► Ewing Sarcoma

Exocrine Pancreatic Neoplasms

► Cancer of the Pancreas

Exogenous Erythropoietin

► Erythropoiesis-Stimulating Agent (also ESA or Exogenous Erythropoietin)

Extended Radical Hysterectomy

CHRISTIN A. KNOWLTON[1], MICHELLE KOLTON MACKAY[2]
[1]Department of Radiation Oncology, Drexel University, Philadelphia, PA, USA
[2]Department of Radiation Oncology, Marshfield Clinic, Marshfield, WI, USA

Synonyms
Class IV hysterectomy

Definition
An extended radical hysterectomy is the surgical removal of the uterus, cervix, upper portion of the vagina, portions of the ureters and bladder, and superior vesicular artery. This procedure is performed for the removal of extensive disease.

Cross-References
▶ Uterine Cervix

External Beam Radiation Therapy

CHRISTIN A. KNOWLTON[1], MICHELLE KOLTON MACKAY[2], ALBERT S. DeNITTIS[3], CHENG B. SAW[4]
[1]Department of Radiation Oncology, Drexel University, Philadelphia, PA, USA
[2]Department of Radiation Oncology, Marshfield Clinic, Marshfield, WI, USA
[3]Lankenau Institute for Medical Research, Lankenau Hospital, Wynnewood, PA, USA
[4]Division of Radiation Oncology, Penn State Hershey Cancer Institute, Hershey, PA, USA

Synonyms
EBRT

Definition
External beam radiation therapy uses high-energy x-rays to target rapidly dividing cancer cells and destroy their ability to divide. External beam radiation is used in combination with chemotherapy for cervical cancer stage IA2 or higher. It is generally administered to a pelvic field encompassing the cervix, uterus, and regional lymph nodes. An extended field of external beam radiation may be designed to also treat the para-aortic lymph nodes. The course of external beam radiation therapy is administered in daily treatments for approximately 5–6 weeks.

The treatment of patients using teletherapy or radiation generated from OUTside a patient. Most common is photon radiation generated by a linear accelerator but can also be electron beam or proton beam.

Cross-References
▶ Brachytherapy: High Dose Rate (HDR) Implants
▶ Conformal Therapy: Treatment Planning, Treatment Delivery, and Clinical Results
▶ Esophageal Cancer
▶ Intensity Modulated Radiation Therapy

Extracranial Meningioma

THEODORE E. YAEGER
Department Radiation Oncology, Wake Forest University School of Medicine, Winston-Salem, NC, USA

Definition
A very rare meningioma tumor usually presenting in the sinonasal tract areas.

About 30 recorded cases are reviewed in the Armed Forces Institute of Pathology. There is an equal distribution of male and females with an average presentation age of about 50 years (range 13–88). Patients present with nasal symptoms such as epistaxis, mass displacement and nasal obstruction, painful sinusitis, and/or visual changes. The nasal cavity and all anterior sinuses can be affected with possible direct erosion of the facial bones and extension into the central nervous system. Immunohistochemistry is needed to confirm epithelial cell origins with positive reaction to epithelial membranes and vimentin. The differential diagnosis is paraganglioma, melanoma, psammomatoid ossifying fibroma, angiofibroma and, of course, carcinoma either primary or metastatic.

The overall prognosis is consistent with benign to atypical meningioma and surgical excision with appropriate reconstruction is the primary intervention. Early recurrence is considered a poor prognostic sign and there can be latent recurrences so long-term follow-up of these patients is appropriate.

Cross-References

► Benign Tumors
► Nasopharynx
► Primary Intracranial Neoplasms
► Sarcomas of the Head and Neck

Reference

Tidwell TJ, Montague ED (1975) Chemodectoma involving the temporal bone. Radiology 116:147–149

Extrafascial Hysterectomy

► Total Abdominal Hysterectomy

Extragonadal Germ Cell Tumor

► Mediastinal Germ Cell Tumor

Extramedullary Mass

Jo Ann Chalal
Department of Radiation Oncology, Fox Chase Cancer Center, Philadelphia, PA, USA

Definition

Arising outside the bone marrow, this is a localized mass of monoclonal B-cells. Plasmacytomas can occur outside the bone and are considered extramedullary when this occurs.

Cross-References

► Multiple Myeloma

Extramedullary Plasmacytomas

Carlos A. Perez, Wade L. Thorstad
Department of Radiation Oncology, Siteman Cancer Center, Washington University Medical Center, St. Louis, MO, USA

Definition

Solitary plasmacytomas are rare tumors of plasma cell origin making up 4% of all plasma cell tumors. Multiple myeloma occurs about 40 times more frequently than solitary plasmacytomas. Monoclonal extramedullary plasmacytomas (EMPs) are rare, low-grade lymphomas found predominantly in the head and neck region.

Epidemiology

Extramedullary plasmacytomas (EMPs) constitute only 0.5% of all upper respiratory tract malignancies. Male patients exceed female patients by a ratio of 4:1, and 75% of patients are 40 and 60 years of age. The most common sites in the head and neck are the nasopharynx, nasal cavity, paranasal sinuses, and tonsils.

Clinical Presentation and Diagnostic Workup

EMP of the head and neck area should be considered a separate entity because of its clinical behavior. The most common symptoms are nasal obstruction, local pain and swelling, and epistaxis.

Grossly, plasmacytomas tend to be sessile in the nasal cavity and paranasal sinuses and pedunculated in the nasopharynx and larynx. The masses are soft, pliable, and pale gray. The lesion may remain localized or may infiltrate and destroy the surrounding soft tissue and bone. The usual criteria for solitary plasmacytomas, either medullary or extramedullary, include a biopsy-proven plasma cell tumor with one or, at the most, two solitary foci, absence of Bence-Jones protein in the urine, bone marrow taken some distance from the primary site not involved by tumor (less than 10% of plasma cells), hemoglobin of 13 g/ml or more, and a normal serum protein level or serum electrophoresis at the time of the diagnosis. Basically, the diagnosis of solitary plasmacytoma is made by exclusion, by eliminating the possibility of multiple myeloma. Diagnosis is based on histology along with special immunoperoxidase staining for immunoglobulin lambda and kappa light chains.

Many patients enjoy prolonged disease-free survival, but the incidence of systemic relapse is high. Bone destruction is not a particularly bad prognostic sign, although some investigators report that it adversely affects prognosis.

Cervical lymph node metastasis from EMP varies with the site of the primary lesion and follows the same pattern of spread as squamous cell carcinoma arising in a similar site. The reported incidence of lymph node metastasis ranges from 12% to 26%.

The exact relationship between EMP and multiple myeloma is unclear; however, approximately 20–30% of EMP cases will convert to multiple myeloma (MM).

The extent of the tumor and bone destruction is accurately detected by CT scanning with contrast or with MRI (Fagundes et al. 1995). F-Fluorodeoxyglucose PET scanning was found to be of value in the radiation treatment planning and posttreatment evaluation of 21 patients with isolated head and neck plasmacytoma (Kim et al. 2009).

General Management

Pedunculated EMP lesions may be treated by surgical excision because the chance of local recurrence is low. The treatment of choice for all other lesions is radiation therapy alone or combined with other modalities. In a review of 714 cases in the literature, the following therapeutic strategies were used to treat patients with EMP of the upper aerodigestive tract: radiation therapy alone in 44.3%, combined therapy (surgery and irradiation) in 26.9%, and surgery alone in 21.9%. The median overall survival or recurrence-free survival was longer than 20 years for patients who underwent combined intervention (surgery and irradiation), for surgical intervention alone (median survival time, 156 months), and for radiation therapy alone (median survival time, 114 months). Overall, after treatment for EMP in the upper aerodigestive tract, 61% of all patients had no recurrence or conversion to systemic involvement; however, 22% had recurrence of EMP, and 16.1% had conversion to multiple myeloma.

Radiation Therapy Techniques

Irradiation techniques vary with the location of the primary tumor. The techniques are similar to those used for primary tumors in comparable locations (i.e., nasopharynx, tonsil, paranasal sinuses). Solitary plasmacytomas respond well to doses of 50–60 Gy in 2-Gy fractions. The local tumor control rate with radiation therapy alone is about 85%. There is a high risk of local recurrence with tumor doses below 30 Gy and a negligible risk for those treated at or above 40 Gy.

Michalski et al. (2003) described ten patients with EMP treated with radiotherapy. Median follow-up period was 29 months. All nine patients who received definitive radiation therapy (40–50 Gy) achieved a complete response. Four patients relapsed, three died of their disease. Two patients with paranasal sinus disease subsequently relapsed with multiple myeloma at 10 months and 24 months, respectively. The relapse rate in neck nodes of 10% does not justify elective irradiation of the uninvolved neck.

Creach et al. (2009) reported on 18 patients with solitary head and neck plasmacytoma treated with irradiation. One patient developed a marginal recurrence and six (33%) multiple myeloma or plasmacytoma at distant sites. Ten-year overall survival was 55%. Two patients developed a radiation-induced malignancy at 6.5 and 6.9 years after treatment.

Ozsakin et al. (2006) published a compilation of solitary plasmacytoma (42 in the head and neck), 258 patients with bone ($n = 206$) or extramedullary ($n = 52$) without evidence of multiple myeloma (MM). Most ($n = 214$) of the patients received radiotherapy (RT) alone; 34 received chemotherapy and RT; and eight surgery alone. The median radiation dose was 40 Gy. Median follow-up was 56 months (range 7–245). The median time for MM development was 21 months (range 2–135), with a 5-year probability of 45%. (Fig. 1a) The 5-year overall survival, disease-free survival, and local control rate was 74%, 50%, and 86%, respectively (Fig. 1b). On multivariate analyses, favorable factors were younger age and tumor size <4 cm for survival; age, extramedullary localization, and RT for disease-free survival; and small tumor and RT for local control. Bone localization was the only predictor of MM development. No dose-response relationship was found for doses >30 Gy, even for larger tumors.

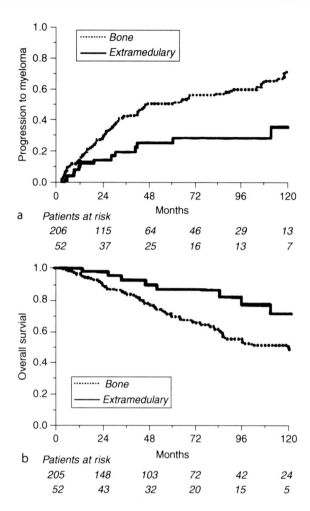

Extramedullary Plasmacytomas. Fig. 1 (a) Probability of progression to multiple myeloma according to bone (*dotted line*) or extramedullary (*solid line*) solitary plasmacytoma ($p = 0.0009$). (**b**) Overall survival correlated with bone (*dotted line*) or extramedullary (*solid line*) solitary plasmacytoma ($p = 0.04$) (Reproduced with permission, Ozsakin M, Tsang RW, Poortmans P et al (2006) Outcomes and patterns of failure in solitary plasmacytoma: a multicenter rare cancer network study of 258 patients. Int J Rad Oncol Biol Phys 64:210–217)

On the other hand, Tournier-Rangeard et al. (2006) in an analysis of 17 patients showed that those who received less than 45 Gy to the clinical target volume (CTV) had a tumor control of 50%

Extramedullary Plasmacytomas. Table 1 Extramedullary plasmacytoma of head and neck treated by radiation therapy

Author	Number of patients	Number of males/ number of females	Number <50 years of age	Local control	Number with multiple myeloma	Recommended tumor dose (Gy)[a]
Wiltshaw[65]	14	10/4	10	11/14	N/A	–
Woodruff et al.[66]	15	8/7	11	14/15	1	40–50
Harwood et al.[27]	22	18/4	16	18/22	4	35 for 3 weeks
MD Anderson Hospital[b]	15	12/3	12	13/15	4	50
Total	119	53/23 (2.5:1)	54 (71%)	64/76 (84.9%)	23 (19.3%)	40–50

[a]10 Gy/week unless otherwise stated
[b]Updated data of Corwin J, Unpublished data

versus 100% for the patients treated to higher doses ($p = 0.034$).

Table 1 summarizes the doses of irradiation and probability of tumor control reported by various investigators. Our limited experience confirms the efficacy of tumor doses of 45–50 Gy for local tumor control. In patients who had extensive disease, a higher dose (50–60 Gy) was used, as recommended by several investigators (Perez and Thorstad 2008).

Cross-References

▶ Hodgkin's Lymphoma
▶ Multiple Myeloma
▶ Plasmocytoma
▶ Sarcomas of the Head and Neck

References

Creach KM, Foote RL, Neben-Wittich MA et al (2009) Radiotherapy for extramedullary plasmacytoma of the head and neck. Int J Radiat Oncol Bio Phys 73:789–94

Fagundes MA, Hug EB, Liebsch NJ et al (1995) Radiation therapy for chordomas of the base of skull and cervical spine: patterns of failure and outcome after relapse. Int J Radiat Oncol Biol Phys 33:579–584

Kim PJ, Hiks RJ, Wirth A et al (2009) Impact of 18F-fluorodeoxyglucose positron emission tomography before and after definitive radiation therapy in patients with apparently solitary plasmacytoma. Int J Radiat Oncol Bio Phys 74:740–46

Michalski VJ, Hall J, Henk JM et al (2003) Definitive radiotherapy for extramedullary plasmacytomas of the head and neck. Br J Radiol 76:738–41

Ozsakin M, Tsang RW, Poortmans P et al (2006) Outcomes and patterns of failure in solitary plasmacytoma: A multicenter rare cancer network study of 258 patients. Int J Rad Oncol Biol Phys 64:210–217

Perez CA, Thorstad WL (2008) Unusual non-epithelial tumors of the head and neck. In: Halperin EC, Perez CA, Brady LW (eds) Perez and Brady's principles and practice of radiation oncology, 5th edn. Wolters Kluwer/Lippincott Williams & Wilkins, Philadelphia, p 996

Tournier-Rangeard L, Lapeyre M, Graff-Caillaud P et al. (2006) Radiotherapy for solitary extramedullary plasmacytoma in the head-and-neck region: A dose greater than 45 Gy to the target volume improves the local control. Int J Radiat Oncol Bio Phys 64:1013–1017

Extraskeletal Small Cell Tumors

► Neuroblastoma
► PNET tumor
► Small Cell Lung Cancer
► Soft Tissue Lymphoma
► Soft Tissue Sarcoma

Eye and Orbit

Jorge E. Freire[1], Carol L. Shields[2,3],
Jerry A. Shields[2,3], Luther W. Brady[4]
[1]Department of Radiation Oncology, Capital
Health System – Mercer Campus, Trenton,
NJ, USA
[2]Department of Ophthalmology, Thomas
Jefferson University, Philadelphia, PA, USA
[3]Department of Ocular Oncology, Wills Eye
Institute, Philadelphia, PA, USA
[4]Department of Radiation Oncology, College of
Medicine, Drexel University, Philadelphia,
PA, USA

Synonyms
Eye brachytherapy; Eye plaque therapy

Introduction
Intraocular and orbital tumors are rare in the field of ophthalmology and oncology consequently those patients are usually referred to specialized centers for the proper management.

The American Cancer Society (American Cancer Society 2007) estimated 2,400 new diagnoses of ocular and orbital tumors in the United States during 2009–2010 with 10% deaths during the same period.

Of these, seventy-five percent are classified as choroidal or uveal melanomas. Lymphomas of the conjunctiva and orbit are the next most common ocular tumors.

Retinoblastoma, predominately a pediatric tumor, accounts for a minority of cases. The remainder include metastatic tumors to the eye, particularly from breast, lung, colon, and other sites. Other tumors include orbital cavernous hemangioma, tumors such as rhabdomyosarcoma, optic nerve glioma, and lacrimal gland tumors, as well as conjunctival and eyelid malignancies.

Anatomy
The ocular adnexae consist of structures including the eyelids, cilia, lacrimal glands, lacrimal drainage apparatus, conjunctiva and orbit.

The eyeball, or globe, is a spherical organ composed of three tunicae. The outer coat consists of the clear cornea anteriorly and the sclera posteriorly.

The uvea is comprised of the choroid, ciliary body, and iris, all of which contain a high concentration of melanocytes as well as vascular tissue.

The retina is the innermost sensory layer composed of photoreceptors cones and rods that perceive light and through a complex mechanism transmit light signals through nine layers of retina into the neural tissue of the optic disc, then to the nerve, the chiasm and into the occipital lobe. The retina extends from the ora serrata retinae anteriorly to the optic nerve posteriorly.

The vascular supply to the retina derives from the central retinal artery, which enters the globe through the optic nerve.

The lens is suspended from the ciliary body by the zonule and is located posterior to the iris.

The orbit is composed of seven bones: frontal, maxilla, lacrimal, palatine, ethmoid, sphenoid, and zygomatic.

The bony orbit contents include the ocular globe, vessels, nerves, orbital fat, lacrimal gland, and extra ocular muscles consisting of: superior, inferior, medial, and lateral recti as well as superior and inferior oblique muscles. The six muscles insert on the sclera, anteriorly, and at the orbital apex, posteriorly.

Ocular Malignant Tumors

Choroidal Metastases

Metastatic carcinoma is probably the most common intraocular malignant tumor.

Metastatic uveal lesions develop in approximately 15% of cases, as synchronous metastases in 4% and metachronous in most of the remaining cases.

Uveal metastases most commonly originate from primary breast and lung cancers in women, and lung and gastrointestinal tract cancers in men.

Uveal metastases may be unifocal or multifocal within the eye or may be bilateral. Shields and associates (Depotter et al. 1994b; Freire et al. 2008) found 88% in the posterior uvea, 9% in the iris, and 2% in the ciliary body.

The aim of therapy is to preserve visual function. Observation for small lesions may be appropriate if the patient is receiving an effective systemic chemotherapy.

The treatment of uveal metastasis depends on the systemic condition of the patient. If the patient has visual symptoms, in order to improve and preserve quality of life, treatment should be offered as soon as possible.

Choroidal metastases, depending on the primary tumor, may be treated with chemotherapy, hormone therapy, external beam radiotherapy (EBRT), brachytherapy or laser therapy such as photodynamic therapy (PDT).

Palliative response is achieved in 90% with EBRT by delivering a dose of 30–36 Gy over 3–3½ weeks to the globe.

Brachytherapy with I-125 plaque and a prescribed dose of 36–40 Gy to the tumor apex is prescribed at Wills Eye Hospital and the Department of Radiation Oncology, Drexel University College of Medicine in Philadelphia (see "▶ Eye Plaque Physics").

Shields and associates, reported globe preservation of 98% of 188 patients, and 43% experienced improvement in visual acuity using this technique.

Currently, hypofractionated CyberKnife radiosurgery is being explored for the treatment of uveal metastasis, although no dose recommendations are available at the time of this manuscript (Fig. 1) (see "▶ Eye Plaque Physics").

Choroidal Melanoma

Choroidal melanoma is the most common primary intraocular tumor in adults. The incidence in the United States is six cases per million per year or 2000 new cases per year.

Uveal melanoma affects all ages, mostly older than 50 years and both sexes, with a slight predominance in males.

Uveal melanoma has one tenth the incidence of cutaneous melanomas (see "▶ Melanoma").

Risk factors for uveal melanoma include suspicious choroidal nevus: choroidal nevi, or the presence of oculodermal melanocytosis, a condition that manifests with pigmented skin, sclera and heterochromia (different colored iris).

The diagnosis of malignant uveal melanoma has become easier and more accurate with a variety of techniques: indirect ophthalmoscopy, fundus photography, autofluorescence photography, fluorescein and indocyanine angiography, ultrasound, both A and B modes, optical coherence tomography (OCT), MRI, and CT scan.

The most important means of diagnosis is the measurement of tumor thickness over three millimeters. Other features that assist in the diagnosis, include detection of subretinal fluid surrounding the lesion and orange pigment on the surface of the tumor. History of a nevus with signs of growth over time may indicate transformation into melanoma. The prognosis of choroidal

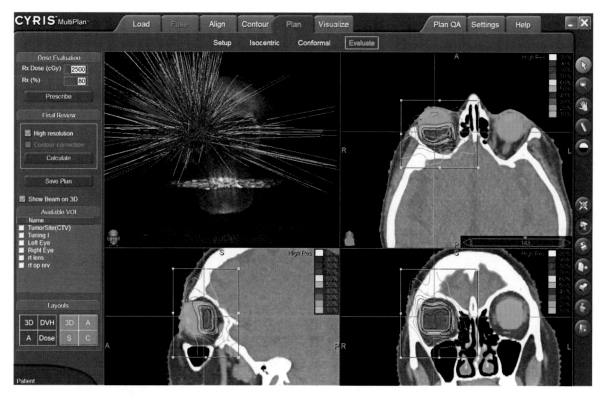

Eye and Orbit. Fig. 1 CyberKnife plan for choroidal metastases

melanoma depends on tumor size. Every millimeter increase promotes 5% up to 20% risk of metastases (Sagoo et al. 2011).

Management of choroidal or uveal melanoma continues to be controversial. Several options for management have been advocated: local surgical resection; laser photocoagulation; thermotherapy; plaque brachytherapy; charged particle radiotherapy; and CyberKnife radiosurgery, observation, and enucleation (see "▶ Brachytherapy – Low Dose Rate (LDR) Temporary Implants," "▶ Proton Therapy," "▶ Stereotactic Radiosurgery – Cranial," "▶ Robotic Radiosurgery").

Several factors influence the management of uveal melanoma and include tumor size, activity, location, growth pattern, patient's general health, age, and status of opposite eye.

If the melanoma is large and the chances for functional visual acuity are minimal or intraocular pressure is elevated causing pain, enucleation is warranted.

Choroidal nevus (less than 10 mm in diameter and less than 2 mm thickness) are usually observed. High-risk small melanomas are commonly managed with thermotherapy, charged particle radiotherapy, or plaque brachytherapy.

Medium-size uveal melanomas (3–8 mm in thickness and 10–15 mm in diameter) can be managed with plaque brachytherapy, charged particle radiotherapy, local resection, or enucleation depending on particular factors.

Large tumors (more than 8 mm in thickness and greater than 15 mm in base) are managed with local resection, plaque brachytherapy, or enucleation.

Uveal melanoma with involvement of the iris, ciliary body, or the posterior choroid and are managed accordingly (Shields et al. 2003; Sagoo et al. 2011).

Tumors that are diffuse, have fast growth pattern, and have extrascleral extension are amenable to be treated with enucleation or plaque brachytherapy.

Iris melanoma could be treated with excision, brachytherapy, or enucleation. Ciliary body and choroidal melanoma are treated by either brachytherapy or excision.

With regards to brachytherapy, the closer the tumor to the optic disk and fovea, the higher the risk of irreversible visual impairment.

The concept of enucleation has been questioned. Some investigators believe that tumor seeding is effected by the manipulation of the globe during the surgical procedure and advocate a "no-touch" approach to enucleation. Others suggest that enucleation alters the immune capacity and micrometastases begin to grow.

In the United States and Canada, this controversy lead to the Collaborative Ocular Melanoma Study (COMS) a prospective randomized study to compare survival in patients treated with either brachytherapy or enucleation (Combs et al. 2005).

COMS report #28, published in December 2006, evaluated 1,317 patients accrued from 1987 to 1998. Patients were randomized to enucleation ($n = 660$) or to ^{125}I plaque brachytherapy ($n = 657$) (Fig. 2) (Combs et al. 2005; Depotter et al. 1994b). The conclusion of this study showed that mortality rates following ^{125}I brachytherapy did not differ from enucleation through 12 years of follow-up. The power of the study indicated that neither treatment was likely to increase or decrease mortality rates by as much as 25% relative to the other.

At present, ^{125}I is predominantly used in the United States, Canada, and the United Kingdom, whereas ^{106}Ru is popular in Germany and other European countries.

The current indications for plaque radiation therapy are as follows: (1) small melanomas that

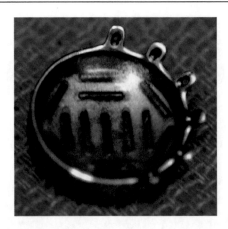

Eye and Orbit. Fig. 2 COMS plaque with I-125 seeds and inset

are documented to be growing or show signs of activity on the first visit, (2) most medium-sized, some large choroidal and ciliary body in an eye with potential salvageable vision, or (3) almost all actively growing melanomas that occur in the patient's only useful eye.

If a melanoma exceeds 15 mm in diameter and 10 mm in thickness, one should anticipate visual morbidity from radiation therapy, and enucleation should be strongly advised.

There does not appear to be a major difference in local tumor control among the various brachytherapy techniques. Local tumor relapse after plaque radiation therapy occurs in up to 16% of cases.

Local tumor recurrence constitutes an important post-treatment clinical indicator of the tumor's great malignant potential and the patient's increased risk of melanoma-specific mortality.

Sagoo and associates in a recently published paper, report the analysis of 650 patients with juxtapapillary melanoma treated with plaque brachytherapy, 80% showed local tumor control (Sagoo et al. 2011).

In an analysis of 270 patients with choroidal melanoma treated with custom-designed plaque radiotherapy combined with transpupillary thermotherapy, long-term tumor control was achieved in 97% of eyes. The excellent control was attributed to the custom design of the plaque by the radiation oncology team and precise plaque placement by the surgical ocular oncology team. Patients with juxtapapillary choroidal melanoma achieved 95% long-term control in this series (Brady et al. 1984; Freire et al. 1997; Freire et al. 2008; Shields et al. 2002).

The visual outcome with brachytherapy depends mainly on tumor size and location as well as on the development of radiation retinopathy and papillopathy.

Patients with tumors located near the fovea or optic disk and those with larger tumors have the worst visual outcome.

Combined plaque irradiation and laser photocoagulation has been used recently to increase local tumor control, particularly juxtapapillary tumors. Shields and associates achieved a recurrence rate of 3% in 8 years in 100 patients treated with plaque and transpupillary thermotherapy.

Brachytherapy for Choroidal Melanoma

Iris, ciliary body, posterior uveal, and juxtapapillary tumors require a surgical episcleral application of a radioactive plaque (Figs. 3–5). There are different types of plaques with standard or customized I-125 seed distributions (Freire et al. 1997; Shields et al. 2002; Sagoo et al. 2011). The most common are: round, standard notched, deep notched, and semicircular also called "boomerang." Sizes: 10, 15, 18, 20, and 22 mm in diameter (Figs. 6–11). The prescribed isodose line should extend about 2 mm around the tumor (Fig. 12).

The dose used by the Wills Eye Hospital and Hahnemann University Hospital Department of Radiation Oncology team in several thousand patients, as outpatients or admitted to the hospital for other medical reasons, has been 80 Gy to the apex in 4–5 days.

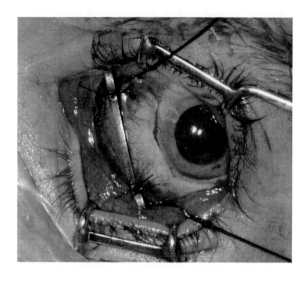

Eye and Orbit. Fig. 3 Surgical plaque insertion

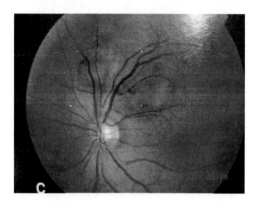

Eye and Orbit. Fig. 4 Choroidal melanoma before plaque

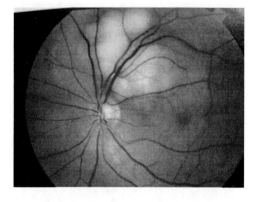

Eye and Orbit. Fig. 5 Choroidal melanoma after plaque

E

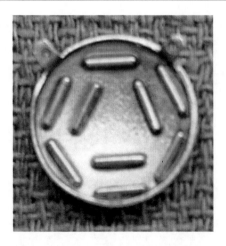

Eye and Orbit. Fig. 6 Round plaque

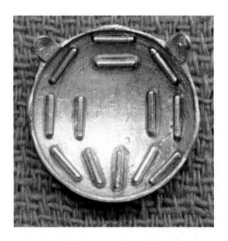

Eye and Orbit. Fig. 7 Customized round plaque

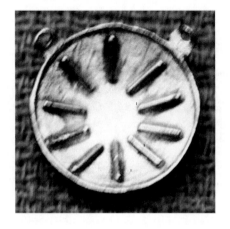

Eye and Orbit. Fig. 8 Iris radial plaque

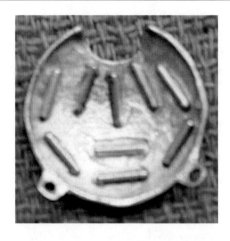

Eye and Orbit. Fig. 9 Customized notched plaque

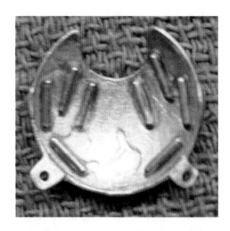

Eye and Orbit. Fig. 10 Deep notched standard plaque

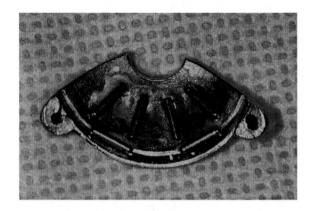

Eye and Orbit. Fig. 11 Iris boomerang plaque

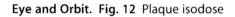

Eye and Orbit. Fig. 12 Plaque isodose

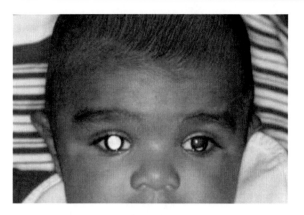

Eye and Orbit. Fig. 13 Bilateral RB

Retinoblastoma

Retinoblastoma is the most common intraocular malignancy of childhood, making approximately 4% of pediatric malignancies. The incidence is approximately one in 15,000–18,000 live births, and 250–300 new cases per year in the United States.

The disease is bilateral in 20–30% of patients. Of newly diagnosed children, 10% have a family history of retinoblastoma and these are always heritable cases. The remaining 90% are sporadic, of which 20–30% are bilateral, these become heritable cases (Figs. 13 and 14).

Of the remaining 70–80% of apparent unilateral, sporadic cases, 10–12% are heritable. Therefore, of all cases diagnosed in the United States annually, approximately 40–50% are heritable.

Retinoblastoma (RB) can arise in hereditary, nonhereditary, and chromosome-deletion forms, the last occurring on the long arm of chromosome 13, locus 14 (13q14): a tumor suppressor RB gene.

The hereditary form is diagnosed earlier than the sporadic form of the disease a risk for other malignancies, and can affect the offspring of the affected individual. The disease may be bilateral or unilateral. The chromosomal abnormality can

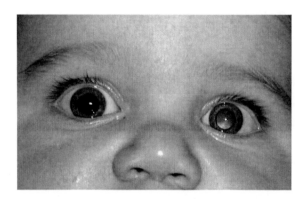

Eye and Orbit. Fig. 14 Unilateral RB

result from a germinal mutation or may be inherited.

The nonhereditary form is unilateral; offspring of the affected individual are normal. This form of the disease has low risk of other malignancies. The chromosomal abnormality is caused by a somatic mutation.

The hereditary form is carried as a germ cell mutation in every cell in the body and the sporadic, as somatic cell mutation, only in the retinal cells.

The disease may be present at birth, but most children with retinoblastoma are diagnosed before age 3 or 4 years, and rarely beyond the age of 6 years (Depotter et al. 1994a).

The most common presenting signs and symptoms are leukocoria (Figs. 13–15) strabismus, or a mass in the fundus noticed during ocular examination.

Accurate diagnosis is paramount because several nonmalignant conditions can present similarly.

Evaluation begins with an accurate history that emphasizes prenatal and parturition information, prematurity, oxygen therapy, family history of RB, whether leukocoria was present at birth or later, whether the child had contact with puppies or other animals.

Most common sign of RB is leukocoria or strabismus at birth, usually noticed at 6–24 months of age.

Frequently, parents or other relatives notice a whitish papillary reflex at a certain angle, a "white eye" instead of the usual "red eye" in photographs raises the suspicion and prompts to seek medical attention.

A careful ophthalmologic examination of the child must be performed to rule out other diagnoses compatible with pseudoretinoblastoma.

Diagnostic tests include slit-lamp biomicroscopy, binocular indirect ophthalmoscopy, B-mode ultrasonography, CT scan to rule out extrascleral extension, MRI of orbits and brain that helps to determine pineal involvement, particularly in bilateral RB cases.

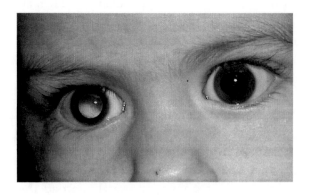

Eye and Orbit. Fig. 15 Leukocoria

The final ophthalmologic procedure is accurate mapping and sizing of tumor deposits in both eyes, which is best accomplished by indirect bilateral ophthalmoscopy with the child under general anesthesia.

Staging studies consist of lumbar puncture with cytospin analysis of the cerebrospinal fluid and bone scan if indicated. The child's siblings and parents should also undergo bilateral indirect ophthalmoscopy to detect current or regressed disease.

Therapy of bilateral disease is complex and traditionally has consisted of enucleation of the eye with more advanced disease and radiation therapy for the less involved eye (Depotter et al. 1994a; Eng et al. 1993; Freire et al. 1997; Freire et al. 2008).

At present, chemoreduction using casboplatin, vincristine, and etoposide has rendered many advanced cases to spare enucleation and this may be considered as salvage. Intra-arterial chemotherapy has become popular for unilateral retinoblastoma with dramatic control, as reported by Shields and associates in a recent paper in press.

Laser photocoagulation, cryotherapy, thermotherapy, or plaque brachytherapy may be indicated after chemoreduction for persistent or recurrent tumor.

External beam radiotherapy is reserved for selected group cases.

According to the International Classification of Retinoblastoma, successful treatment with chemoreduction was achieved in 100% of group A, 93% of group B, 90% of group C, and 47% of group D.

External Beam Radiotherapy

The first successful treatment of retinoblastoma by x-rays was reported by Hilgartner in 1903. Other techniques that spared the lens were developed since. All of them resulted in underdosing the anterior and posterior chamber, increasing the risk for recurrence and cataract formation.

At present, EBRT is less common and indicated only in selected patients with chemorefractory vitreal or retinal tumor seeds or tumors next to the optic disk.

At Drexel University College of Medicine/Hahnemann University Hospital we have discouraged lens-sparing techniques for external beam irradiation of retinoblastoma. We attempted uniform treatment of the entire retina using a hinged wedge technique, accepting the potential for ultimate cataract formation. Other radiation oncologists have confirmed this philosophy (Eng et al. 1993; McCormick et al. 1988).

3-D Conformal Radiotherapy Technique

Freire et al. at Drexel/Hahnemann University Hospital, in cooperation with Wills Eye Hospital, have developed and used 3-D conformal radiotherapy in patients with unilateral or bilateral retinoblastoma (Figs. 16 and 17).

Prior the megavoltage era, orbital bone hypoplasia was quite frequent as a long-term side effect, mostly due to treatment with orthovoltage machines. These equipments generate photons of relatively low energy and the process by which energy is absorbed by tissue is called photoelectric effect and is dependent on atomic number (Z); therefore, the bone in the orbit that is in process of growth becomes stunted causing orbital hypoplasia causing a cosmetic defect that may require, in some cases, reconstructive plastic surgery.

Currently, megavoltage linear accelerators of 4 or 6 MV lack this property, for the predominant absorption mechanism is the Compton effect that is independent of the atomic number, and consequently orbital hypoplasia is extremely rare (Freire et al. 2008).

Treatment of unilateral retinoblastoma cases consists of four noncoplanar fields. All fields are anterior oblique: superior, inferior, medial, and lateral. A 0.5 cm bolus may be used.

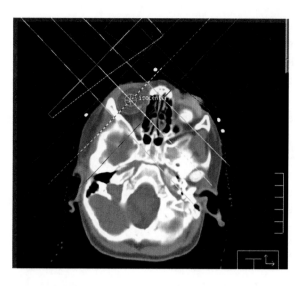

Eye and Orbit. Fig. 16 Fields for unilateral RB

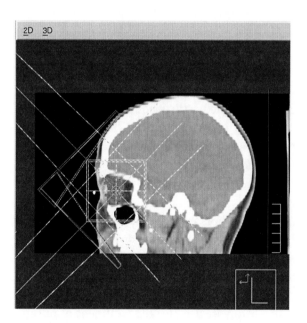

Eye and Orbit. Fig. 17 Fields for bilateral RB

Caution must be taken to minimizing the dose to critical structures such as contralateral eye, chiasm, pituitary gland, brain stem, posterior-most upper teeth, and upper cervical spine.

The entire retina should be treated, including 5–8 mm of proximal optic nerve. With this technique, the tumor volume is treated approximately to the 95% line, whereas the 50% line encompasses the orbit and lower doses to the above-mentioned tissues.

Bilateral disease requires treatment to both eyes with six noncoplanar fields: two lateral opposing and two anterior oblique fields to each eye following the same criteria described above. The authors recommend a dose of 40–44 Gy in daily fractions of 1.8 Gy over a period of 4½–5 weeks, and after chemotherapy, 36–40 Gy (Eng et al. 1993; McCormick et al. 1988).

Conscious sedation administered by an anesthesiologist may be necessary in small children during the treatment planning CT scan, simulation, and daily treatments.

Brachytherapy for Retinoblastoma

Plaque brachytherapy can be used as primary or secondary treatment of retinoblastoma.

Carefully selected retinoblastomas, even juxtapapillary and macular tumors, can be successfully treated with plaque radiation therapy. The procedure is identical to the application of plaque for choroidal melanoma. In children there is need for general anesthesia.

Visual outcome varies with tumor size and location.

The authors from the Hahnemann/Wills Eye Hospital team prescribe a dose of 40 Gy prescribed to the apex or deepest point of a conglomerate of seeds, delivered over 4 days.

Plaques of different size, shape, and seed distribution are used for the treatment of retinoblastoma similar to those described in choroidal melanoma.

Intraocular Lymphomas

Primary intraocular lymphoma is a rare disease which can involve the retina, vitreous, or optic nerve with or without extension to the CNS. Histologically, they are commonly diffuse large B-cell and, rarely, T-cell lymphomas.

The initial manifestation is usually blurred vision or floaters resulting from a cellular infiltration of the vitreous cavity. In many cases, there appears to be no systemic manifestation, and the diagnosis is made either by enucleation or by vitreous biopsy.

At Hahnemann University Hospital, ocular lymphoma patients are being treated with 3-D conformal radiotherapy using four oblique fields, with a dose of 30–36 Gy in 1.8–2.0 Gy fractions.

Choroidal Hemangiomas

Choroidal hemangiomas are rare, congenital, benign vascular tumors of the choroid. There are two types of choroidal hemangiomas: circumscribed and diffuse.

Circumscribed choroidal hemangiomas are small tumors with a mean diameter of 7 mm located within 3 mm of the fovea and occasionally in the subfoveal region.

The subfoveal tumors tend to cause visual loss early in life due to the anterior displacement of the retina. Patients with parafoveal tumors remain asymptomatic until the third or fourth decade of life. External ocular examination in these patients is usually unremarkable.

Circumscribed choroidal hemangiomas of the diffuse variety is large, and extends anterior to the equator associated with facial nevus flammeus or other manifestations of the Sturge-Weber Syndrome (SWS).

Diffuse tumors are usually diagnosed in young patients either due to examination of the fundus prompted by a facial hemangioma, visual impairment secondary to serous retinal detachment, or hyperopic amblyopia.

Choroidal hemangiomas do not transform into malignant tumors.

The indication for treatment is loss of visual acuity, due to extensive retinal detachment and associated glaucoma.

Treatment alternatives include laser photocoagulation, thermotherapy, photodynamic therapy, and radiotherapy. Radiotherapy is typically reserved for eyes with extensive subretinal fluid. Circumscribed hemangiomas may be treated with plaque brachytherapy and a dose of 30–36 Gy over 4 days.

Diffuse hemangiomas are treated by the authors, with 3-D conformal radiotherapy to the whole globe and a dose of 36 Gy in 2 Gy daily fractions at Hahnemann University Hospital.

Patients have generally shown partial flattening of the hemangioma, complete resorption of subretinal fluid, and reattachment of the retina within 6–12 months (Kivela et al. 2003).

Orbital Tumors

Orbital Prelymphoma, Lymphoid Hyperplasia, and Lymphoma

Benign primary lymphoreticular tumors, if localized to the orbit, have a good prognosis with a 5-year survival rate of 70% ("▶ Non-Hodgkins Lymphoma").

Approximately 20–25% of cases of apparent pseudolymphoma can convert to malignant lymphoma. It is often difficult to differentiate between pseudolymphoma and true lymphoma by biopsy. Immunophenotypic and molecular genetic analysis are necessary in some cases.

Steroids can be effective, but radiation therapy appears to be more effective and can control cases that have been refractory to steroids (Fig. 21).

At Drexel University College of Medicine, Hahnemann University Hospital, we elect to treat the orbit with 20–26 Gy given in fractions of 1.8–2.0 Gy a day, which can cause to dramatically resolve along with reabsorption of subretinal fluid.

It could also be treated with CyberKnife radiosurgery.

Graves' Ophthalmopathy

Patients with hyperthyroidism may develop exophthalmus. The primary tissues involved are the intraocular muscles. They become thickened as a result of lymphocytic infiltration and edema, which subsequently causes the eye globe to protrude forward.

Indications for therapy include corneal exposure, which may cause corneal ulceration and can progress to cause scarring and compression of the optic nerve, thus rendering partial or permanent visual loss.

The diagnosis is aided by CT imaging, which may demonstrate thickened muscles.

Steroid therapy is considered the first line of treatment given during a minimum of 2–8 weeks, but radiation therapy can be beneficial if these treatments fail.

The great majority of cases are bilateral.

Patients with a history of more than 6 months of exophthalmus and failure to steroids tend to fail to radiation due to fibrosis formation within the muscles and internal decompression is the best alternative.

At Drexel/Hahnemann University Hospital, for bilateral disease, we recommend two lateral opposing fields encompassing the muscles up to the insertion at the orbital apex, designed through CT planning with an anterior edge just posterior to the lens. We recommend using a dose of 20 Gy in 2 Gy fractions.

Optic Nerve Glioma

Optic (nerve) glioma is most common in children under 15 years of age.

The name is justified by the mixture of astrocytic-dominant and oligodendroglial cell lines.

The incidence is about 1% of all central nervous system tumors. A significant number of patients with neurofibromatosis type I or II contract this tumor.

Optic glioma is a slow-growing tumor. Symptoms often predate diagnosis by about 2 years.

Tumors often affect the optic chiasm (more than 50% of cases), and some exhibit extension into the hypothalamus.

Unilateral proptosis and vision defects indicate chiasmal involvement. Hypothalamic symptoms produce endocrine defects and increased intracranial pressure. Optic atrophy or nystagmus can also be a presenting symptom ("▶ Stereotactic Radiosurgery – Cranial") (Collaborative Ocular Melanoma Study Group 2006).

CT and MRI imaging are needed for an anatomic diagnosis.

Visual acuity and field examinations indicate severity and progress of defects. Tumor extension into the hypothalamus may cause enlargement of the sella.

Radiation therapy is indicated when intracranial or progressive symptoms are evident.

Bilateral temporal or multiportal beam arrangements are preferred for lesions involving both the posterior optic nerve and chiasm. A dose of 50 Gy in 1.8- to 2-Gy fractions is generally recommended for adults and 45 Gy in 1.6- to 1.8-Gy daily fractions for children less than 15 years of age.

CyberKnife radiosurgery could be an alternative to be explored using hypofractionation for the treatment of optic gliomas; however, there is no dose recommendation as yet and more studies are needed.

Numerous reports have documented the value of radiation therapy for patients with optic glioma. Long-term survival rates range from 80% to 100%. Improvement or stabilization of symptoms can be expected in a majority of patients.

Radiation therapy complications (calcification, necrosis, and chiasmal damage) are rare except for endocrine disorders in children.

Primary malignant tumors of the orbit are rare.

Among them, tumors arising from the eyelids, conjunctiva, Meibomian gland carcinomas, malignant lymphoma, rhabdomyosarcoma, and lacrimal gland tumors account for most cases. Of these, rhabdomyosarcoma has generated the most interest.

Eyelid Basal and Squamous Cell Carcinomas

For basal cell and squamous cell carcinomas of the eyelids, radiation therapy can achieve an overall 90–95% cure rate with a dose of 50–60 Gy (depending on histology and size of the tumor) using photon- or electron-beam techniques. An internal eye shield may be used to protect the globe ("▶ Skin Cancer").

Although surgery is the treatment of choice, radiation therapy may be able to provide more acceptable cosmetic outcome in selected cases while providing similar cure rates.

Conjunctival Tumors

The conjunctiva can be the site of squamous cell carcinoma, melanoma, or lymphomas.

Squamous cell carcinomas arise in most cases at the inner canthus and may infiltrate the eyelids, lacrimal duct, and cornea (Figs. 18 and 19).

Treatment of choice is surgical resection followed by cryotherapy to the surrounding healthy conjunctiva.

Brachytherapy after resection has been used by the authors, with episcleral plaque applied weekly in order to deliver 10 Gy at 1–2 mm depth for a total dose of 50 Gy in 5 weeks, longer follow-up results are pending at present. Preliminary response is satisfactory.

Another brachytherapy alternative is to use a specially constructed conformer with customized

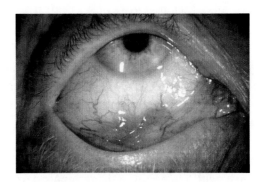

Eye and Orbit. Fig. 18 Conjunctiva lymphoma

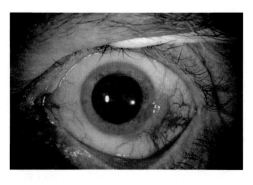

Eye and Orbit. Fig. 19 Conjunctiva squamous cell carcinoma

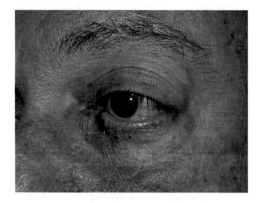

Eye and Orbit. Fig. 20 Metastatic melanoma to orbit

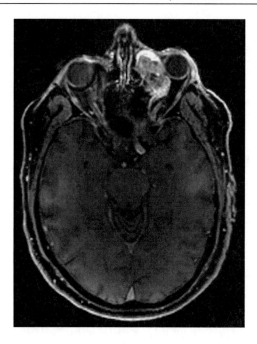

Eye and Orbit. Fig. 21 MRI of patient with met. Melanoma

seed distribution, with or without lead shielding on one side, depending on tumor extent or conjunctiva at risk, and deliver 50 Gy over 7 consecutive days.

Conjunctival melanoma requires similar procedure as squamous cell carcinoma: cryotherapy and weekly plaque therapy for 6 weeks for a total dose of 60 Gy in fractions of 10 Gy, or a conformer with a dose of 60 Gy in 7 consecutive days.

The authors have also used CyberKnife radiosurgery for selected cases. The dose is still debatable. Preliminary results are satisfactory.

Conjunctival lymphoma occasionally presents as an isolated site in 2% of patients with extranodal non-Hodgkin's lymphoma.

Approximately, 25–30% of lymphomas are mucosal associated lymphoma tumors (MALT) and involve the stomach, intestine, tonsils or adenoids, and skin.

Some of these tumors respond to a short course of antibiotics against *Chlamydia trachomatis* or *Helicobacter pilorii*, but most of the time they require systemic chemotherapy and/or local treatment with irradiation in the form of 3-D conformal external beam, electron therapy with a dose of 30–36 Gy, or CyberKnife radiosurgery.

Sebaceous Carcinoma

Meibomian gland (sebaceous) carcinomas make up 1–5.5% of eye malignancies and have a mortality rate of 30%. Surgery is considered the main treatment option followed by radiation for partial resection or positive margins ("▶ Skin Cancer").

These tumors can be multicentric, which may lead to local recurrences. Radiation therapy may be used for the treatment of these tumors in selected cases, particularly if surgery would not provide acceptable cosmesis or for recurrence after surgery. High doses of irradiation (60–65 Gy in 6–7 weeks) are required. They may also be treated with CyberKnife SRS.

Rhabdomyosarcoma

Rhabdomyosarcoma (RMS) is the most common soft tissue sarcoma (STS) in children with an incidence of 50–60% of all STS ("▶ Rhabdomyosarcoma").

There are three main histological types: embryonal, alveolar, and botrioid.

The former is frequently found in the head and neck area, either in the orbit or as parameningeal tumor ("▶ Rhabdomyosarcoma").

Alveolar and botrioid types are most commonly seen in the genitourinary system and extremities.

Rhabdomyosarcoma of the orbit is most often seen in young children and carries a favorable prognosis. Has a rapid onset with marked proptosis and swelling of the adnexal tissue (Forstner et al. 2006).

Previously, the recommended treatment was orbital exenteration because many ophthalmologists thought that the tumor was radioresistant.

Current recommendations are for combined radiation therapy and chemotherapy as the initial management, limiting surgical intervention to biopsy or local excision.

According to the most recent recommendations of the International Rhabdomyosarcoma Group (IRSG), the IRS-IV trial for orbital RMS was reported to be superior to IRS-III.

The former had a 100% successful outcome compared to 83% in the latter.

A dose of 50.4 Gy or higher is given using IMRT or 3-D conformal radiotherapy and chemotherapy: vincristine and actinomycin-D with or without cyclophosphamide.

Lacrimal Gland Tumors

Adenoid cystic carcinoma is the most common in the lacrimal gland and is a challenge to control properly, caused by the difficult surgical approach and the tendency of these tumors to infiltrate the orbital nerves and travel along to the base of the skull.

Although relatively radioresistant, lacrimal gland tumors should routinely be irradiated after surgery to reduce postoperative recurrences.

Tumor doses of 50–60 Gy are necessary, after surgical resection and/or enucleation in cases where there is compromise of the optic nerve by tumor around the nerve extending to the orbital apex and beyond.

The authors have attempted to control microscopic adenoid cystic carcinoma post enucleation in a 16-year-old boy who had post-surgery recurrence with the use of CyberKnife robotic radiosurgery. Twelve months posttreatment MRI showed no evidence of orbital or intracranial tumor activity. A formal investigative protocol, IRB approved is necessary for more extensive analysis of patients treated with this modality to obtain reliable results in terms of efficacy as well as toxicity.

Metastatic Orbital Tumors

Metastatic tumors to the orbit may be treated with 40 Gy fractionated over 4 weeks. We advocate 3-D conformal or IMRT.

Orbital metastasis is also amenable to be treated palliatively with focused radiation using CyberKnife radiosurgery (Fig. 22). Further research with this technique is necessary on an IRB-approved protocol.

Sequelae of Therapy

Skin and Adnexae

Skin changes include erythema, hyperpigmentation, depigmentation, atrophy, telangiectasia, and ectropion or entropion of the eyelid.

Loss of the cilia from the eyebrow or eyelashes may occur after radiation therapy.

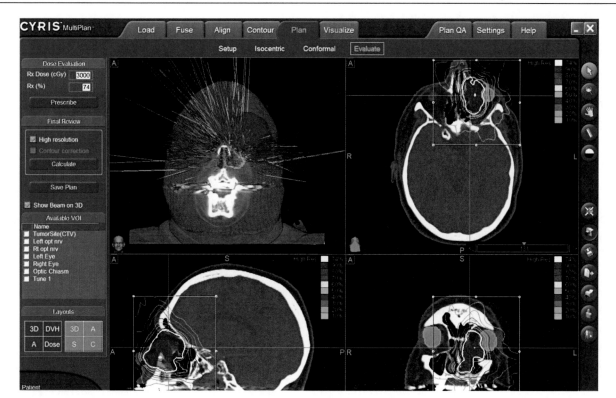

Eye and Orbit. Fig. 22 CyberKnife plan for same patient

Hair loss from the scalp may occur at an exit area of an external beam portal.

Cornea

Direct corneal injury may result from high doses of irradiation with ulceration, opacification, or scar fibrosis.

Lens

Cataract formation occurs with a minimum dose of 2 Gy, and consequently, if the lens is in the field, the risk of cataract is 100%; however, it could be operated in about 2 years.

Retina and Choroid

Changes in the retina and choroid are observed after doses of 45–60 Gy. Vascular damage leads to infarction of tissue with the formation of exudates and hemorrhages. Decreased visual acuity may result from damage to the retinal tissue or from atrophy of the optic nerve.

Sclera

Because of the extreme radioresistance of the sclera, which may tolerate doses to 750 Gy or more, only a few cases of scleral necrosis have been reported.

Lacrimal Gland

Radiation damage to the lacrimal gland may decrease tear production and produce xerostomia with corneal changes.

Optic Nerve

Optic nerves that received doses of 60 Gy or higher, the 15-year actuarial risk of optic neuropathy was 11% with fraction of 1.8 Gy, compared to 47% with larger fractions.

Hypothalamus and Pituitary Dysfunction

Hypothalamus or pituitary function in children with optic glioma may be impaired by the tumor itself and by high radiation doses, greater than 50 Gy.

Growth hormone deficiency is rare at doses of 50 Gy. Precocious puberty is rarely seen with these doses.

Cross-References

▶ Brachytherapy: Low Dose Rate (LDR) Temporary Implants
▶ Eye Plaque Physics
▶ Melanoma
▶ Non-Hodgkins Lymphoma
▶ Proton Therapy
▶ Rhabdomyosarcoma
▶ Robotic Radiosurgery
▶ Skin Cancer
▶ Stereotactic Radiosurgery – Cranial

References

American Cancer Society (2007) Detailed guide: eye cancer. www.cancer.gov

Brady LW, Shields JA, Augsburger JJ et al (1984) Posterior uveal melanomas. In: Phillips TL, Pistenmaa DA (eds) Radiation oncology annual, vol 1. Raven, New York, pp 233–245

Collaborative Ocular Melanoma Study Group (2006) COMS report 28. Arch Ophthalmol 124:1684–1693

Combs SE, Schulz-Ertner D, Moschos D et al (2005) Fractionated stereotactic radiotherapy of optic pathway gliomas: tolerance and long-term outcome. Int J Radiat Oncol Biol Phys 62:814

DePotter P, Shields CL, Shields JA (1994a) Clinical variation of trilateral retinoblastoma: a report of 13 cases. J Pediatr Ophthalmol Strab 31:26–31

DePotter P, Shields CL, Shields JA et al (1994b) Impact of enucleation versus plaque radiotherapy in the management of juxtapapillary choroidal melanoma on patient survival. Br J Ophthalmol 78:109–114

Eng C, Li FP, Abramson DH et al (1993) Mortality from second tumors among long-term survivors of retinoblastoma. J Natl Cancer Inst 85:1121–1128

Forstner D, Borg M, Saxon B (2006) Orbital rhabdomyosarcoma: multidisciplinary treatment experience. Australas Radiol 50:41

Freire JE, Brady LW et al (1997) Brachytherapy in primary ocular tumors. Semin Surg Oncol 13:167–176

Freire JE, Kolton MM, Brady LW, Shields JA, Shields CL (2008) Eye and orbit. Chapter 35. In: Principles and practice of radiation oncology, 5th edn. Lippincott, Williams and Wilkins, Philadelphia, pp 778–799

Kivela T, Tenhunen M, Joensuu T et al (2003) Stereotactic radiotherapy of symptomatic circumscribed choroidal hemangiomas. Ophthalmology 110:1977–1982

McCormick B, Ellsworth R, Abramson D et al (1988) Radiation therapy for retinoblastoma: comparison of results with lens-sparing versus lateral beam techniques. Int J Radiat Oncol Biol Phys 15:567

Sagoo S, Shields CL, Mashayekhi A, Freire JE, Emrich J, Reiff J, Komarnicky L (2011) Plaque radiotherapy for juxtapapillary choroidal melanoma: tumor control in 650 consecutive cases. Ophthalmology 118:402–407 (American Association of Ophthalmology)

Shields CL, Cater J, Shields JA, Chao A, Krema H, Materin M, Brady LW (2002) Combined plaque radiotherapy and transpupillary thermotherapy for choroidal melanoma in 270 consecutive patients. Arch Ophthalmol 120:933–940

Shields CL, Naseripour M, Shields JA, Freire J, Cater J (2003) Custom designed plaque radiotherapy for non-resectable iris melanoma in 38 patients. Tumor control and ocular complications. Am J Ophthalmol 135:648–656

Shields CL et al (2009) Metastasis of uveal melanoma millimeter-by-millimeter in 8033 consecutive eyes. Arch Ophthalmol 127(8):989–998

Eye Brachytherapy

▶ Eye and Orbit

Eye Plaque Physics

LUTHER W. BRADY, JAY E. REIFF
Department of Radiation Oncology, College of Medicine, Drexel University, Philadelphia, PA, USA

Synonyms

Episcleral plaque therapy; Radioactive plaque therapy

Definition

Episcleral plaque therapy is one modality of treating various intraocular malignancies such as choroidal melanoma, retinoblastoma, and various conjunctival tumors. This brachytherapy technique consists of fabricating a small (10–22 mm in diameter), spherically curved metal (typically gold) plaque onto which radioactive sources are adhered. After immobilizing the patient's eye, the plaque is sutured onto the sclera over the tumor where it remains for 3–10 days.

Background

The most common primary intraocular tumor in adults is uveal melanoma with approximately 2,000 new cases per year being diagnosed in the United States (Margo 2004). One of several treatment options for this disease that has been employed is radioactive plaque therapy. Over the years, various radionuclides have been used as the sources of radiation in these plaques. The external surface of the gold plaque shields the bony orbit surrounding the eye, and by manipulating the seed orientation on the plaque in the planning process, one can minimize the dose to the normal structures in the vicinity such as the optic nerve and the macula. Because of the close proximity of the radioactive sources to the tumor, a highly localized and intense dose of radiation is delivered to the tumor while sparing more normal tissues and structures than is possible by conventional external beam radiation therapy techniques. Brachytherapy is competitive with the precision that one can achieve using heavy particle therapy.

Historically, eye plaque brachytherapy was performed using ^{60}Co as the isotope of choice. Developed by Stallard in the early 1960s, his plaques ranged in diameter from 8 to 12 mm (Stallard 1961). Illustrated in Fig. 1 are the axial views of the standard Stallard plaques where the ^{60}Co was encapsulated in a platinum sheath and distributed evenly over the blackened rings. The

semicircular plaques with notches were used to treat posterior tumors abutting the optic nerve. Although these plaques were fairly easy to prepare, the limited size range of the plaques severely hampered the flexibility that one had in treating larger size tumors. Also, they did not allow for the customization of the dose distribution, the shielding of nearby critical structures, or permit patient treatment on an outpatient basis.

Over the years, a variety of radionuclides have been used in the brachytherapy management of ocular diseases including ^{60}Co, ^{106}Ru/^{106}Rh, ^{192}Ir, and ^{125}I (Bedford et al. 1970; Lommatzsch 1974; Lommatzsch 1977; Bergman et al. 2005; Luxton et al. 1988; COMS Report 22 2004). These studies showed that the ^{125}I allows the greatest degree of flexibility in terms of achieving the prescribed dose to the tumor as well as limiting the dose to the nearby critical structures. The long-term outcome comparing all the radionuclides in terms of tumor control was essentially the same, but the complications associated with the utilization of brachytherapy plaques was least in those individuals who were treated with the ^{125}I.

In 1987, a multi-institutional randomized clinical trial was organized through the Collaborative Ocular Melanoma Study (COMS) group. The aim of this study was to compare eye plaque brachytherapy to enucleation using survival and preservation of vision as the endpoints. A group of 1,317 patients from 43 clinical centers in the United States and Canada were randomly assigned to receive either enucleation (660 patients), or ^{125}I brachytherapy (657 patients). To be enrolled in this study the patients had to be diagnosed with a choroidal melanoma which ranged from 2.5 to 10 mm in apical height, and had a basal diameter of no more than 16 mm in any dimension. Patients with peripapillary tumors were eligible only when the tumor was contained within a 90° angle between the apex and the optic disk, and when the enrolling ophthalmologic oncologist was confident that an

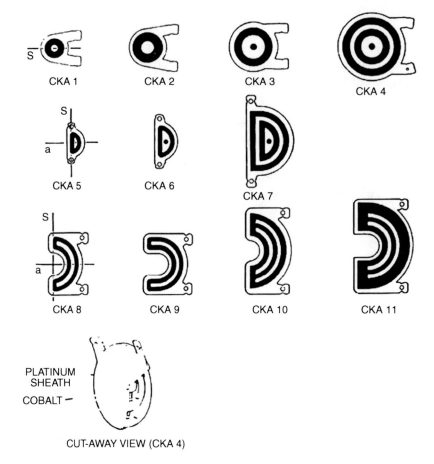

CKA 1   CKA 2   CKA 3   CKA 4

CKA 5   CKA 6   CKA 7

CKA 8   CKA 9   CKA 10   CKA 11

PLATINUM SHEATH
COBALT —

CUT-AWAY VIEW (CKA 4)

Eye Plaque Physics. Fig. 1 Axial views of the standard Stallard plaques where the ^{60}Co was encapsulated in a platinum sheath and distributed evenly over the blackened rings

episcleral plaque could be placed to cover the entire base of the tumor plus an additional 2.0 mm margin beyond the tumor extent, while also providing adequate and appropriate distance from the optic disk.

In the COMS study, the 5-year survival rates were 81% for enucleation group and 82% for patients who underwent brachytherapy (COMS Report 19 (2002)). The risk of treatment failure after brachytherapy was estimated to be 10.3% in this study. Treatment failure was the most common reason for enucleation within 3 years of the treatment. Beyond 3 years, ocular relapses were the most common cause for enucleation. It was identified that risk factors for treatment failure

were older age, greater tumor thickness, and proximity of the tumor to the foveal avascular zone. Local treatment failure was weakly associated with reduced survival. Almost all surviving patients enrolled in the COMS study regained good visual acuity in the treated eyes throughout 10 years of follow-up (COMS Report 22 2004). It was also found that through 10 years of follow-up there was no evidence that the treated eye was at a greater risk for loss of visual acuity or new ophthalmologic diagnoses than eyes of patients treated with enucleation alone (Krintz et al. 2003).

Major criticisms have been made of the COMS study because many patients refused to be randomized once they knew the parameters of the study and were therefore treated off protocol. It was never possible to acquire the 2,000 patients thought necessary to show a statistical difference between these two therapies.

At the meetings prior to the onset of the COMS study, suggestions were made to accumulate all the available data relative to ocular melanomas and then decide which treatment regimens would be pursued. However, that recommendation was not followed. A second protocol that was developed as a consequence of those meetings compared enucleation with preoperative radiation therapy with 20 Gy being given in five fractions of 4 Gy each followed by local resection the following week. No survival differences were noted between those two groups.

Today, patient selection for episcleral plaque therapy has evolved such that most patients with a clinical diagnosis of malignant melanoma of the uvea are candidates for the procedure. Also, patients with retinoblastoma, vasoproliferative tumors, conjunctival lesions, and ocular metastases may be treated with plaque brachytherapy. Contraindications for this procedure include tumors with gross extrascleral extension, ring melanoma, and tumor involvement of more than half of the ciliary body.

Plaque Construction and Dosimetry

Prior to plaque fabrication, the ophthalmologist must provide relevant clinical tumor data to the radiation oncology department. These data include the tumor location and tumor size, specifically, the basal diameters and tumor height. These measurements should be measured clinically and verified by A-mode and/or B-mode ultrasound studies. Fluorescein angiograms are helpful in determining the posterior boundary of the tumor. Once the location and dimensions of the tumor have been determined, a detailed fundus diagram with the orientation of the tumor

borders relative to the surrounding structures must be provided. These structures include the optic nerve, foveola, equator, ora serrata, and the center of the lens. The fundus diagram typically serves as the primary data set from which the plaque design and subsequent dosimetry is based. Such a diagram is shown in Fig. 2.

The next step in the treatment planning process is to transfer all the data from the fundus diagram to a computerized treatment planning program. Not only must the location and dimensions of the tumor be accurately represented, the proximity of the plaque to the macula and optic disk structures must be known because these data will not only provide an accurate estimation of the doses to these structures, they will help determine whether a round or notched plaque is to be used.

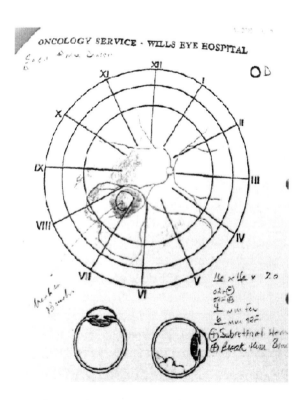

Eye Plaque Physics. Fig. 2 A fundus diagram which typically serves as the primary data set on which the plaque design is based

Before developing a treatment plan, one must next select which isotope is to be used. As previously noted, ^{125}I is the most commonly used isotope for eye plaque brachytherapy in the United States. Major disadvantages of using ^{60}Co and ^{192}Ir include the fact that they emit high-energy gamma rays which deliver large doses to unaffected structures and present radiation exposures hazards to caregivers. [125]I and [103]Pd emit much lower energy radiation and thus present less radiation exposure hazards to surrounding personnel. In fact, [103]Pd emits lower energy radiations than ^{125}I and has been recommended for very shallow tumors as the more rapid dose falloff could better protect nearby critical structures. The gold plaque absorbs the low energy radiation from both ^{125}I and [103]Pd and therefore protects the extraocular structures. The major disadvantage of using [103]Pd is its short half-life of 17 days. This short half-life implies a relatively large difference in dose rate over the course of the implant, assuming the dose will be delivered in the standard 4–5 day time period. [131]Cs has been suggested as an appropriate radionuclide to be used for eye plaques (Rivard et al. 2008). Its emitted gamma rays are quite similar in energy to ^{125}I, but with its short 9.7 day half-life, one runs into the same dose rate issues as for [103]Pd. [106]Ru, which is a beta emitter, has a more rapid dose falloff than [103]Pd. Widely used in Europe for several decades, its large dose gradient has made it the preferred isotope to treat small melanomas (apical height less than 5 mm). However as the tumor height increases, so do the scleral complications and local failure rate.

The most common eye plaque styles used in the United States are rimmed plaques and unrimmed plaques. The COMS study employed rimmed plaques which allow for the placement of a silastic insert. This insert has precut channels for reproducibly positioning the seeds in concentric circles ranging from 12 to 20 mm in diameter. Once the seeds are positioned in the insert, they are glued to the plaque so that the seeds are sandwiched between a 1 mm thick layer of plastic and the gold backing of the plaque. These plaques can be assembled within a very short period of time after computer-derived preplanning has been carried out and it eliminates almost completely the potential for seed loss during the treatment. Even though the seeds are in a rigid geometry they can be placed in such a way that one has a major degree of individualization.

Unrimmed custom-made plaques may be used to better optimize the dosimetric coverage of irregularly shaped tumors or for tumors located close to or abutting a critical structure. The inner surface of unrimmed plaques is raised from the surface of the sclera to reduce the dose to the sclera and increase the depth dose to the tumor apex. Unrimmed plaques may be circular, notched, oval, or kidney shaped. They are often fabricated in diameters ranging from 10 mm to 22 mm. Sources are glued onto the concave surface of the plaque using a cyanoacrylate adhesive in the pattern determined from the plan. A photograph of a 20 mm round, unrimmed plaque with ^{125}I seeds adhered to its surface is shown in Fig. 3.

Once in the operating room, the patient may be placed under either general or local anesthesia, or conscious sedation. Anterior tumors and those with visible anterior margins can be localized by transillumination. More posterior tumors are localized by point source illumination, scleral indentation ophthalmology around the plaque, or ultrasound imaging. A plastic dummy plaque of identical size and shape to the radioactive plaque is used to position sutures on the sclera and to verify the plaque position on the eye before the radioactive plaque is applied. A photograph of a plaque and its associated plastic dummy plaque is shown in Fig. 4. A thin lead foil of 0.2 mm thickness is placed over the patient's eye afterward to substantially reduce the radiation exposure to family, nurses, physicians, etc. This makes it

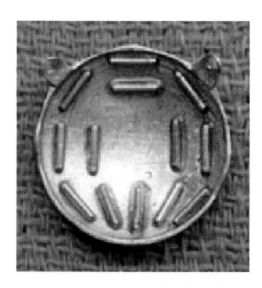

Eye Plaque Physics. Fig. 3 A 20 mm diameter, round, unrimmed plaque showing the ^{125}I sources glued onto the concave surface

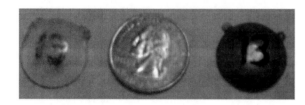

Eye Plaque Physics. Fig. 4 A picture of a round plaque and its associated plastic dummy. The coin is shown for size reference

possible to treat patients with plaques on an outpatient basis.

When using ^{125}I plaques, physicists and clinicians should be aware that recent data show that conventional ^{125}I data overestimate the dose rate in water at 1.0 cm from a model 6711 seed by 13–20% (Williamson 1988; Weaver et al. 1989; Nath et al. 1990). The American Association of Physicists in Medicine (AAPM) has incorporated these differences into an interstitial brachytherapy dosimetry protocol studies for all tumor sites (AAPM 1995). Weaver demonstrated that the gold backing of the plaque would significantly reduce the volume of tissue contributing scatter dose to the tissue anterior to the plaque, and may reduce doses to points on the plaque axis by an additional 5–8% (Weaver 1986). Chiu-Tsao et al. have shown that the 1.0 mm thick silastic insert which has an effective atomic number of 11.2 is higher that of tissue, may reduce doses to the central axis of the plaque by 10% (Chiu-Tsao et al. 1986). Because the dosimetry algorithms originally used in the COMS study did not take these dosimetric effects into account, the minimum tumor dose delivered by these plaques is probably no greater than 75% of the normally prescribed values.

Krintz et al. (Krintz et al. 2003) recalculated the dosimetric data of the brachytherapy arm for patients enrolled in the COMS study. A plaque radiotherapy planning system (plaque simulator) that incorporates all these dosimetric corrections including line source approximations, anisotropy, silastic attenuation, and gold shield attenuation has shown that the dose delivered to structures within the eye that was significantly lower (7–21%) than the prescribed dose. Astrahan used an ophthalmic plaque planning system modified to incorporate additional scatter and attenuation correction factors that take into account the path length of primary radiation in the silastic seed carrier and the distance between the dose calculation point and the eye–air interface. He found that dose to critical ocular structures ranged from 16% to 50% less than would have been calculated using the standard COMS dose calculation protocol (Astrahan 2005).

The development of distant metastases as well as melanoma-related mortality is associated with low dose rates to the tumor apex. Current data suggest that dose rates to the tumor apex of less than 70 cGy/h reduce systemic control. Dose rates higher than 90 cGy/h are associated with worse results regarding residual ocular function. The ideal dose and dose rate for achieving local and systemic control without incurring a high risk of decreased visual acuity remains undefined. However in the United States, the ^{125}I episcleral applicator has become the primary choice for brachytherapy.

Cross-References

▶ Brachytherapy: Low Dose Rate (LDR) Temporary Implants
▶ Clinical Aspects of Brachytherapy (BT)
▶ Eye and Orbit
▶ Melanoma

References

American Association of Physicists in Medicine (1995) Dosimetry of interstitial brachytherapy sources. Recommendations of the AAPM radiation therapy committee task group No. 43. Med Phys 22:209

Astrahan MA (2005) Improved treatment planning for COMS eye plaques. Int J Radiat Oncol Biol Phys 61(14):1227

Bedford MA, Bedotto C, MacFaul PA (1970) Radiation retinopathy after application of a cobalt plaque: report of three cases. Br J Ophthalmol 54:505

Bergman L, Nilsson B, Lundell G (2005) Ruthenium brachytherapy for uveal melanoma 1979–2003. Survival and functional outcomes in the Swedish population. Ophthalmology 112(5):834

Chiu-Tsao S-T, Tsao HS, Vialotti C et al (1986) Monte Carlo dosimetry for ^{125}I and ^{60}Co in eye plaque therapy. Med Phys 13:678

Collaborative Ocular Melanoma Study Group (2002) COMS randomized trial of iodine 125 brachytherapy for choroidal melanoma, IV: local treatment failure and enucleation of the first 5 years after brachytherapy. COMS report 19. Ophthalmology 109(12):2197

Collaborative Ocular Melanoma Study Group (2004) Ten-year follow-up of fellow eyes of patients enrolled in COMS randomized trials. COMS report no. 22. Ophthalmology 111(5):966

Krintz AL, Hanson WF, Ibbot GS et al (2003) A reanalysis of the collaborative ocular melanoma study medium tumor trial eye plaque dosimetry. Int J Radiat Oncol Biol Phys 56(3):889

Lommatzsch P (1974) Treatment of choroidal melanomas with ^{106}Rh beta-ray applicators. Surv Ophthalmol 19:85

Lommatzsch P (1977) Beta-irradiation of retinoblastoma with ^{106}Ru/^{106}Rh applicators. Mod Probl Ophthalomol 18:128

Luxton G, Astrahan MA, Liggett PE et al (1988) Dosimetric calculations and measurements of gold plaque ophthalmic irradiators using ^{192}Ir and ^{125}I seeds. Int J Radiat Oncol Biol Phys 15:167

Margo CE (2004) The collaborative ocular melanoma study: an overview. Cancer Control 11:304

Nath R, Meigooni AS, Meli JA (1990) Dosimetry on the transverse axes of ^{125}I and ^{192}Ir interstitial brachytherapy sources. Med Phys 18:1032

Rivard MJ, Melhus CS, Sioshansi S et al (2008) The impact of prescription depth, dose rate, plaque size, and source loading on the central axis using ^{103}Pd, ^{125}I, and ^{131}Cs. Brachytherapy 7:327

Stallard HB (1961) Malignant melanoma of the choroid treated with radioactive applicators. Ann R Coll Surg Engl 29:180

Weaver K (1986) The dosimetry of ^{125}I seed eye plaques. Med Phys 13:78

Weaver K, Smith V, Huang D et al (1989) Dose parameters of ^{125}I and ^{192}Ir seed sources. Med Phys 16:636

Williamson JF (1988) Monte Carlo evaluation of specific dose constant in water for ^{125}I seeds. Med Phys 15:686

Eye Plaque Therapy

▶ Eye and Orbit

F

Fallopian Tube

Patrizia Guerrieri, Paolo Montemaggi
Department of Radiation Oncology, Regional
Cancer Center "M. Ascoli", University of
Palermo Medical School, Palermo, Italy

Definition/Description

Tumors of the Fallopian tube are a rarely presenting cancer, highly aggressive, like tumors of the ovary, even though, thanks to a frequently earlier diagnosis, less dramatic in the figures of the overall survival. They are characterized by the presence of pain and bleeding even in a relatively early stage of the disease, which helps for an early disease detection. Treatment of choice is a surgical approach, followed, if negative prognostic factors are present, by chemotherapy. Radiotherapy is arguably used as adjuvant postsurgical treatment with indication criteria, treatment techniques, and risk for adverse events similar to those of ovarian cancer. As far as today, even if the available data are controversial, chemotherapy and radiotherapy must be taken into account as a valuable postsurgical approach in specific clinical and pathologic situations.

Anatomy

The Fallopian tubes are hollow, muscular structures lying in the superior part of the broad ligament, extending from the correspondent ovary into the peritoneal cavity. They project outward, backward, and finally downward opening in the uterus corpus, communicating with the endometrial cavity. The tubal wall consists of four layers: mucosa, submucosa, muscularis (external longitudinal and internal circular) and outer serosa, the latter continuous to the visceral uterine peritoneum.

The mucosa is extremely folded, with an epithelium mainly composed of ciliated and secretory cells. Hormonal cycle impacts the tubal epithelium as it does with the uterus, due to the estro-progestinic stimuli. Most of the tubal malignancies arise from the epithelium, possibly somehow relating to the periodic hormones-induced changes.

Vascular supply derives from the ovarian artery, with anastomoses to the uterine artery. Venous drainage is through the pampiniform plexus to the ovarian vein. Lymphatic circulation drains into the ovarian lymphatics and lumbar lymphonodes. Para-aortic and iliac nodes may be infected directly from the lymphatic network of the mucosa.

Epidemiology

Cancer of the Fallopian tube is the rarest female genital tract malignancy; only 1,500 cases have been so far reported in the medical literature. They account for 0.15–1.8% of all gynecological malignancies, averaging 0.3% (Hanton et al. 1990), with a higher prevalence in white than in black women (Rosenblatt et al. 1989).

The age range of this disease has been reported as wide as 18–87 years, with a peak of incidence in the fifth and sixth decades of life. Patients with Fallopian tube cancer tend to be women with a low parity rate, and more frequently in postmenopause (Nordin 1994).

L.W. Brady, T.E. Yaeger (eds.), *Encyclopedia of Radiation Oncology*, DOI 10.1007/978-3-540-85516-3,
© Springer-Verlag Berlin Heidelberg 2013

Clinical Presentation

Several symptoms and signs, sometimes in an early phase of the disease, characterize Fallopian tubes cancers. Classically, triad of pelvic pain, pelvic mass, and leucorrhea or the other one consisting of vaginal bleeding, vaginal discharge, and lower abdominal pain has been associated with these tumors (1). Another frequent sign of a Fallopian tubes cancer is the hydrops tubae profluens, which is a sudden emptying of fluid accumulated in the distended Fallopian tubes causing profuse, watery serosanguinous vaginal discharge, followed by a decrease in pelvic mass size on physical examination (Nordin 1994). Regardless of these reported early symptoms and sign, there is no general agreement on their real value in helping an early diagnosis and the disease might present with nonspecific symptoms (Sedlis 1978; Roberts and Lifshitz 1982).

Imaging Studies

Because of its rarity and because the presenting signs are similar to those of other pelvic inflammatory, infectious, and neoplastic conditions, the correct diagnosis of Fallopian tube cancer is frequently missed until the surgical exploration. Many series have reported missing the correct diagnosis entirely in their working differential (Roberts and Lifshitz 1982; Mc Murray et al. 1986). Nevertheless, many diagnostic tools are presently under investigation both in the field of medical imaging techniques and in the laboratory medicine.

Imaging Studies

Ultrasonography – US study through a vaginal transducer (TVS) has been shown more effective than pelvic US alone. Some reports (Kol et al. 1990; Kurjak et al. 1992) describe an effective use of TVS in the workup of Fallopian tube cancer, especially if taken into account along with color Doppler evaluation and careful evaluation of tumor markers. The use of TVS and color Doppler present some drawbacks lying in the experience of the operator, the quality of instrumentation, and the dependence of the imaging characteristics on the stage of the disease (Podobnik et al. 1993).

CT and MRI – Even if MRI seems to be superior to CT scan, neither one of these technique can be considered as effective as US (Thurner et al. 1990).

Nuclear scan imaging – Radioimaging studies utilizing labeled MaB or some fragments of them seem to have some relevance in the workup of Fallopian tube cancer. Their sensitivity and specificity may be increased coupling those studies with a correct use of tumor serum markers like CA125. [18]FDG-PET may play a role in the staging process of the disease as well as it does in many other neoplastic conditions (Karlan et al. 1993).

Tumor Markers

CA-125 – High levels, >65 U/mL, are frequently seen in about 50% of all new Fallopian tubes malignancies with a specificity of 98% and a sensitivity of 75% (Tokunaga et al. 1990). As mentioned above, the effectiveness of CA-125 in the work up of Fallopian tube cancer can be enhanced by its coupling with TSV US. CA-125 may also serve as a prognostic indicator and monitor in surgically managed patients. In this respect, it has been proven accountable especially during and after postsurgical chemotherapy treatment, with high specificity, sensitivity, and negative predictive value, with a leading time of 3 months (Gadducci et al. 1993).

CA 19-9 – This marker presents a low sensitivity being not released into the bloodstream and is overtly expressed in poorly differentiated or anaplastic tumors. However, it may play a role in those patients not expressing CA-125 (Sharl et al. 1991).

Differential diagnosis and staging – Differential diagnosis is complex, looking at the very similar aspects of Fallopian tubes cancer and other gynecologic malignancies, specifically those of ovarian origin. Main criteria for differential diagnosis are outlined in Table 1 (Hu et al. 1950).

Even with all the difficulties discussed above, once the presence of a malignant tumor of the Fallopian tube has been ascertained, the disease should be staged according to international classification criteria. Standard FIGO classification of Fallopian tube carcinoma is shown in Table 2.

Fallopian Tube. Table 1 Criteria for diagnosis of primary carcinoma of the Fallopian tube

1. Grossly, the main tumor is in the tube
2. Microscopically, chiefly the mucosa should be involved and should show a papillary pattern
3. If the tubal wall is involved to a great extent, the transition from between benign and malignant tissue should be demonstrable

Pathologic Classification and Prognostic Factors

As well as in the ovary, the most common histopathology found in Fallopian tube malignancies is serous papillary adenocarcinoma, graded as well, moderately and poorly differentiated, instead of the previously used nomenclature of pure papillary, papillary-alveolar, and alveolar-medullary (Hu et al. 1950). Up to one-third of the cases shows a bilateral lesion, thought commonly as a multicentric primary. The gross appearance of the Fallopian tube carcinoma tends to mimic more benign pathologic processes such as hydrosalpinx, pyosalpinx, or hematosalpinx (Anbrokh 1970).

Several prognostic factors have been taken into account when looking at Fallopian tube carcinoma. A statistical significance with a p-value ≤ 0.05 at univariate analysis has been shown in the literature for the following: stage at presentation, age,

Fallopian Tube. Table 2 Staging classification

Stage	T	N	M
1: Growth limited to Fallopian tubes	A: One tube only	–	–
	B: Both tubes, no extra serosa	–	–
	C: Extra serosa or ascites or positive washing	–	–
2: Growth involving one or both tubes with pelvic extension	A: Extended to uterus or ovaries	–	–
	B: Extended to other pelvic sites or tissues	–	–
	C: As A or B plus ascites or positive peritoneal washing	–	–
3: Growth involving one or both tubes, peritoneal implants outside pelvis or positive nodes	A: Gross tumor limited to the true pelvis, negative nodes microscopic seeding of abdominal peritoneum, including liver surface	–	–
	B: Involving one or both tubes, proven implants of abdominal peritoneum <2 cm in diameter, negative nodes	–	–
	C: Abdominal implants >2 cm in diameter and/or positive retroperitoneal or inguinal nodes	+	–
4: Growth involving one or both tubes with distant metastasis, including liver or pleura	Growth involving one or both tubes with distant metastasis, including liver or pleura	±	+

presence of ascites, amount of residual tumor after surgical removal, depth of tubal wall infiltration, vascular space invasion, lymphatic spread, hydrosalpinx like appearance, and, to a lesser degree, serous versus non-serous histology (Baekelandt et al. 2000). Grade of differentiation and the presence of symptoms at diagnosis have not been proven to be of a statistical relevance. Presence of vascular space invasion correlates with both the depth of wall infiltration and the presence of lymphonodal metastasis, whereas the depth of wall infiltration is correlated with stage and postsurgery residual disease. Stromal invasion is associated with a significantly decreased 5-year survival (50–54%) compared with mucosal invasion only (87–100%) (Schiller and Silverberg 1971; Baekelandt et al. 2000).

Treatment

At the present time, a definite therapeutic strategy has not yet found. Several and different approaches have been suggested, but no one seems to prevail over the others. Generally, surgery may be considered the cornerstone of any effective strategy, with the adjuvant support of chemotherapy and radiotherapy, according to the pathologic patterns and prognostic factors.

Surgery – As the base of treatment, extensive surgical resection, and staging, should be carried out through total abdominal hysterectomy, omentectomy, and bilateral salpingectomy, radical pelvic and para-aortic lymphadenectomy, as well as sampling of ascitic fluid or peritoneal washing and peritoneal sampling of diaphragm, bladder, and bowel (Baekelandt et al. 2000; Klein et al. 2000). Great impact has been shown as related to the gross residual disease after surgery, with a cutoff of 2 cm. Patients with favorable prognostic factors at the pathologic examination could be followed up with close observation only. Most of the patients, however, will require to be evaluated for some kind of adjuvant treatment (Baekelandt et al. 2000).

Chemotherapy – Deciphering the literature in search of the most favorable chemotherapy regimens is fraught with difficulties, as no well-designed and large enough randomized studies are available in the literature. The actual tendency is that of considering the utility of treating Fallopian tube carcinomas with the same strategy used in ovarian cancer (Baekelandt et al. 2000; Klein et al. 2000). As well as in other gynecologic malignancies, since the studies done in the 1980s, cisplatin-based combination chemotherapy represents today standard treatment also for Fallopian tube carcinoma as the first-line chemotherapy. The mostly used combinations of cisplatin with adriamycin and cyclophosphamide or Paclitaxel result in an overall response rate accounting for 70–80% (Baekelandt et al. 2000; Harries et al. 2004). Nonresponsive patients may find some degree of relief by the use of second-line chemotherapy, consisting mainly of liposomal doxorubicin, topotecan, and gemcitabine (Markman et al. 2003; Micha et al. 2004).

Radiotherapy – Postoperative radiotherapy has been used routinely up to the 1980s. The ample variability in staging, surgical staging techniques, treatment volume, dose fractionation, and type of radiation used makes difficult to evaluate the past literature. Whole abdomen external beam irradiation or intraperitoneal administration of radioactive colloids (^{32}P, ^{198}Au) seemed to be promising, but there were too few data to scientifically support the point. Better results were associated with higher doses (>50 Gy) and larger volumes including all the areas at risk such as the abdomen and the para-aortic nodes (Mc Murray et al. 1986). No clear-cut answer exists so far over the issue arisen between whole abdominal irradiation versus pelvic only radiotherapy. After the introduction of platinum-derived drugs, radiotherapy has been more and more substituted by chemotherapy even though there is no randomized study available in respect to the superiority of either one of these two

Fallopian Tube. Table 3 Treatment algorithm of primary fallopian tube carcinoma

Stage I	Stage I	Stage II-III-IV	Stage II-III-IV	Stage II-III-IV
	Positive cytology	No residual disease	Bulky residual disease >2 cm	Residual disease in pelvis ($\leq$1 cm)
		Node negative	Node positive	
No further therapy	Intraperitoneal ^{32}P or short-term CDDP or whole abdomen RT	Intraperitoneal ^{32}P or short-term CDDP or pelvic (stage II)/ whole abdomen RT	CDDP containing regimens	CDDP containing regimens followed by whole abdomen RT or whole abdomen RT with pelvic boost

treatment modalities. In general, radiotherapy seems to be more useful in early stages, while chemotherapy should be considered mandatory in more advanced situation (Klein et al. 1994, 2000). A possible future direction for treating patients with more advanced disease could be the exploitation of the cytotoxic activity of both chemotherapy and radiation by using both modalities either sequentially or concurrently (Rawlings et al. 1999). Table 3 reports a possible algorithm for the treatment of Fallopian tube carcinoma.

Future Directions

There is an obvious need for randomized controlled trials to determine the correct and effective management of Fallopian tube carcinomas. However, these trials, because of the rarity of the disease, will require a large national or international cooperative effort. At the moment, one single study by the GOG is running to determine the effectiveness of low dose radiation to the abdomen in combination with docetaxel. An interesting novelty exists also in the field of radiotherapy, where the increased use of IMRT regimen, concurrently or sequentially with chemotherapy when and if indicated, along with the possibility for a better volume definition by the use of functional imaging such as ^{18}FDG-TC/PET, seems to open a wide range of clinical possibilities with a promising perspective of high effectiveness and reasonable efficiency in terms of cost-benefit ratio.

Cross-References

▶ Brachytherapy-GyN

▶ Endometrium

▶ Ovarian Cancer

References

Anbrokh YM (1970) Macroscopic characteristics of cancer of the fallopian tube. Neoplasma 17:557–564

Baekelandt R, Nesbakken AJ, Christensen GB et al (2000) Carcinoma of the fallopian tube. Clinicopathologic study of 151 patients treated at the Norwegian Radium hospital. Cancer 89:2076–2084

Gadducci A, Madrigali A, Ciancia EM et al (1993) The clinical serological pathological and immunocytochemical features of a case of primary carcinoma of the fallopian tube. Eur J Gynaecol Oncol 14:374–379

Hanton E, Malkasian G, Dahlin D et al (1990) Primary carcinoma of the fallopian tube by endovaginal ultrasound. Acta Obstet Gynecol Scand 69:667–668

Harries M, Moss C, Perren T et al (2004) A phase II feasibility study of carboplatin followed by sequential weekly paclitaxel and gemcitabine as first line treatment for ovarian cancer. Br J Cancer 91:627–632

Hu CT, Taymon MZ, Hertig AT (1950) Primary carcinoma of the fallopian tube. Am J Obstet Gynecol 59:58–67

Karlan B, Hoh C, Tse N et al (1993) Whole body positron emission tomography with (Fluorine-18)-2 deoxiglucose can detect metastatic carcinoma of the fallopian tube. Gynecol Oncol 49:383–388

Klein M, Rosen A, Graf A et al (1994) Primary fallopian tube carcinoma: a retrospective survey of 51 cases. Arch Gynecol Obstet 255:141–146

Klein M, Rosen A, Lahousen M et al (2000) The relevance of adjuvant therapy in primary carcinoma of the fallopian tube, stages I and II: irradiation vs chemotherapy. Int J Radiat Oncol Biol Phys 48:1427–1431

Kol S, Gal D, Friedman L et al (1990) Preoperative diagnosis of fallopian tube carcinoma by transvaginal ultrasonography and CA-125. Gynecol Oncol 37: 129–131

Kurjak A, Shulman H, Sosic A et al (1992) Transvaginal ultrasounds: color flow and Doppler wave form of the post menopausal adnexal mass. Obstet Gynecol 80:917–921

Markman M, Glass T, Smith HO et al (2003) Phase II trial of single agent carboplatin followed by dose-intense paclitaxel followed by maintenance paclitaxel therapy in stage IV ovarian, fallopian tube, and peritoneal cancers: a SWOG trial. Gynecol Oncol 88:282–288

Mc Murray EH, Jacobs AJ, Perez CA et al (1986) Carcinoma of the fallopian tube: management and sites of failure. Cancer 58:2070–2075

Micha JP, Goldstein BH, Rettenmeier MA et al (2004) Pilot study of out patients paclitaxel, carboplatin and gemcitabine for advanced stage epithelial ovarian, peritoneal, and fallopian tube cancer. Gynecol Oncol 94:719–724

Nordin A (1994) Primary carcinoma of the fallopian tube: a 20 year literature review. Obstet Gynecol Surv 49:349–561

Phelps H, Chapman K (1974) Role of radiation therapy in treatment of primary carcinoma of uterine tube. Obstet Gynecol 43:669–673

Podobnik M, Singer Z, Ciglar S et al (1993) Preoperative diagnosis of primary fallopian tube carcinoma by transvaginal ultrasound, cytological findings and CA-125. Ultrasound Med Biol 19:687–691

Rawlings G, Bush R, Dembo A et al (1999) Fallopian tube cancer: survival following radiation and chemotherapy. International proceedings, Gynecologic Cancer 3rd biennial meeting

Roberts J, Lifshitz S (1982) Primary adenocarcinoma of the fallopian tube. Gynecol Oncol 13:301–308

Rosenblatt KA, Weiss NS, Schwartz SM (1989) Incidence of malignant fallopian tube tumors. Gynecol Oncol 35:236–239

Schiller HM, Silverberg SG (1971) Staging and prognosis in primary carcinoma of the fallopian tube. Cancer 28:389–395

Sedlis A (1978) Carcinoma of the fallopian tube. Surg Clin North Am 58:121–129

Sharl A, Crombach G, Vurbuchen M et al (1991) Antigen CA19-9 presence in mucosa of nondiseased mullerian duct derivatives and marker for differentiation in their carcinomas. Obstet Gynecol 77:580–585

Thurner S, Older J, Baer S et al (1990) Gadolinium-DOTA enhanced MR imaging of adnexal tumors. J Comput Assist Tomogr 14:939–949

Tokunaga T, Miyazaki K, Matsuyama S et al (1990) Serial measurements of CA-125 in patients with primary carcinoma of the fallopian tube. Gynecol Oncol 36:335–337

Familial Adenomatous Polyposis (FAP)

BRADLEY J. HUTH[1], CLAUS ROEDEL[2]
[1]Department of Radiation Oncology, Philadelphia, PA, USA
[2]Department of Radiotherapy and Radiation Oncology, University Hospital Frankfurt/Main, Frankfurt, Germany

Definition

This is a rare disorder resulting from dysregulation of the APC protein either through direct genomic errors or indirectly through proteins which mediate the function of the APC protein. Classically, FAP displays autosomal dominant inheritance. The disorder has mixed penetrance with 95% patients displaying polyps by age 35 years while some suffer from hundreds of colonic polyps in childhood.

This is an inherited syndrome in which numerous polyps form mainly in the epithelium of the large intestine. While these polyps start out benign, malignant transformation into colorectal cancer occurs when not treated.

Cross-References

▶ Colon Cancer
▶ Rectal Cancer

Fast Neutron Therapy

▶ Neutron Radiotherapy

Fecal Occult Blood Test

Bradley J. Huth
Department of Radiation Oncology,
Philadelphia, PA, USA

Definition

A noninvasive test performed on stool samples to identify microscopic quantities of blood. Multiple modalities are available. The traditional guaiac test has a sensitivity of approximately 30%, which increases to 92% if three separate tests are done over three bowel movements. More sophisticated stool testing has become available including fecal immunochemical tests, fecal porphyrin quantification, and fecal DNA testing. While more sensitive, these tests suffer from high false positive rates.

Cross-References

▶ Colon Cancer
▶ Rectal Cancer

Female Urethra

Stephan Mose
Department of Radiation Oncology,
Schwarzwald-Baar-Klinikum,
Villingen-Schwenningen, Germany

Synonyms

Female urethral cancer; Female urethral carcinoma

Definition/Description

Female urethral cancer is very seldom and occurs in women between 50 and 80 years of age. The tumor is clinically aggressive, mostly diagnosed at a late point of time because of primarily nonspecific symptoms, and associated with a high recurrences rate and a worse prognosis. There are no established therapeutic guidelines due to only few existing data. In general, very small tumors can be cured by surgical excision whereas in circumscribed local carcinomas similar results can be obtained by surgery, brachytherapy alone, combined radiotherapy, and the combination of radiotherapy and surgery. Locally advanced tumors are treated with combined surgery and radiotherapy or radiotherapy alone, balancing bladder-sparing procedures against cure even if the prognosis is worse. The use of combined radiotherapy and chemotherapy in advanced disease is debatable.

Anatomy

The female urethra is 2.5–4.0 cm long and its largest diametral dimension is 6–8 mm. The internal ostium of the urethra is embedded within the lower part of the trigone of the bladder directly above the urogenital diaphragm. This is traversed by the urethra that afterward forms an anterior concavity due to the proximity of the symphysis and then ends in the anterior vaginal wall behind the pubis symphysis.

The female urethra consists of transitional and nonkeratinizing stratified squamous epithelial cells in its proximal one-third and of stratified squamous cells only in its distal part. These membranes are embedded in a thin layer of erectile tissue consisting of small veins and elastic muscle fibers. Together with an external urethral layer of smooth muscles and the voluntary urethral sphincter, these structures provide bladder continence.

The blood supply is derived from the internal pudendal arteries and drains to the correspondent veins. Whereas the lymphatic vessels of the distal urethra drains to the superficial and deep inguinal as well as to the external iliac lymph nodes, the primary drainage of the posterior urethra is to the obturator, presacral, and iliac nodes (Eng 2008).

Epidemiology

The majority of information about this disease is derived from cases accumulated over many decades at major cancer centers because primary carcinoma of the female urethra is uncommon, represents only 0.02% of all cancers diagnosed in women. It accounts for <0.1% of all gynecologic malignancies. Due to recently published population-based tumor registries, the annual age-adjusted incidence is three times lower than that of ▶ male uretheral carcinoma. The tumor mostly (75%) occurs in women between 50 and 80 years of age (average 60 years). In 2% of children diagnosed with Wilms' tumor urethral extension occurs.

Up to now, there is only little information about the pathogenesis of female urethral carcinomas. As it is already known in other lower-tract gynecological carcinomas, ▶ human papilloma virus (HPV) may play a role in the etiology of urethral cancer. Some reports discuss that there is an association with urethral diverticula because in 6% of diverticula invasive carcinomas were found. Furthermore, tumors may be induced by chronic infections and by a dedifferentiation of paraurethral ducts and glands. Patients with transitional cell carcinoma of the bladder are supposed to run a higher risk (10%) of developing urethral cancer (Swartz et al. 2006; Thomas et al. 2008; Ahmed et al. 2010).

Clinical Presentation

Female urethral cancer that mainly represents as squamous, transitional, or adeno cell carcinoma (Table 1) is clinically aggressive. Therefore, most of the patients are diagnosed in a late stage of disease. Furthermore, the first symptoms (30–50%) of urethral cancer are nonspecific (dysuria, itching, irritative, and obstructive symptoms).

Female Urethra. Table 1 Histological types of female urethral cancer and its incidences. Former publications reported a prevalence of squamous cell carcinoma whereas nowadays transitional cell carcinoma is more frequently seen

Squamous cell carcinoma	22–50%	Occurrence in the meatal and distal part of the urethra
Transitional cell carcinoma	15–55%	Occurrence in the proximal urethra
Adeno carcinoma and its subtypes	10–22%	
Melanoma	<1%	
Small cell carcinoma		
Glassy cell carcinoma		
Anaplastic tumor		
Kaposi's sarcoma		
Non-Hodgkin lymphoma		
Metastatic lesions		

Meatus tumors that may be evident by inspection account only for 10–20% of all cases. These tumors are mostly superficial and usually without lymph node involvement. Hematuria (50–60%), urinary retention, overflow incontinence, perineal pain, tumor ulceration, and urethrovaginal and/or vesicovaginal fistulas are often late symptoms in advanced disease. Of these cases, tumors of the proximal part are more often being deeply invasive and tend to spread into the complete urethra. Lymph nodes are described in 13% of distal tumors whereas in proximal carcinomas approximately 30% are found. Bilateral lymph nodes occur in 30% of patients with positive nodes. Careful pelvic examination under anesthesia as well as biopsy is mandatory in all patients.

Differential Diagnosis

As tumors may mimic urinary tract infection and/or benign urethral stricture, these diagnoses have to be excluded. Especially small distal and meatus tumors can resemble a ▶ urethral caruncle or a prolapse of the mucosa throughout the urethral orifice. Furthermore, a urethral diverticulum has to be taken into consideration. Urethral hemangiomas and the rare clear cell "sugar" tumor which is considered to be a type of benign perivascular epitheloid cell tumors were described in case reports.

Imaging Studies

Urethral carcinomas are difficult to detect on imaging studies. Furthermore, the differentiation between various tumor types and benign diseases is hardly possible. Once diagnosed by pelvic examination, biopsy, urethrocystoscopy, and rectoscopy, further staging is needed (see Table 2). Only a few data exist regarding endovaginal ultrasound; concluding results about its value are not reported up to now. CT scanning of the pelvis is limited because of similar densities of urethral carcinoma and bladder wall. In contrast, MRI is accurate in the evaluation of tumor extension (T2-weighted images); however, whereas the negative predictive value is excellent, the tumor extension as well as the extent of lymphadenopathy may be overestimated. Positron emission tomography (PET) has an increasing role in diagnosis and therapy of urologic malignancies; however, considering urethral carcinoma its role is yet not clearly defined.

At the time of diagnosis, 10–15% of patients present with distant metastases especially in liver and lung. Therefore, CT scanning of the abdomen as well as chest X-ray is recommended. Primary metastases in bone

Female Urethra. Table 2 TNM-classification in female urethral cancer

TNM	Stage	
Ta	0a	Noninvasive, polypoid, or verrucous carcinoma
Tis	0is	Carcinoma in situ
T1 N0	I	Invasion of the subepithelial connective tissue
T2 N0	II	Invasion of the periurethral muscle
T3 N0–1 / T1–2 N1	III	Invasion of the anterior vagina or the bladder neck, Metastasis in a single lymph node ≤2 cm in greatest dimension
T4 N0–1 / T1–4 N2 / T1–4 N0–2 M1	IV	Invasion of other adjacent organs, Metastasis in a single lymph node >2 cm or multiple lymph nodes, Distant metastases

and brain are seldom. According to symptomatic lesions, a bone scan and a MRI of the brain are necessary.

Laboratory Studies

All patients should be evaluated by blood chemistry and urine analysis. The evaluation of tumor marker is without value although in adenocarcinoma an initially elevated level of the carbohydrate antigen (CA) 19–9 may be helpful as it is reported in case reports.

Treatment

Up to now, there is no conclusive consensus in the management of this rare tumor. This is due to the small number of patients who were registered and reported summarizing an up to 50 years lasting observation period. Over time, the therapeutic procedures and their technique changed influencing the results as well as the side effects of therapy.

Female Urethra. Table 3 Survival in dependence of prognostic factors

	5-year overall survival	5-year progression-free survival	Median survival
Tu <2 cm	60–80%		
Tu 2–5 cm	37–40%		
Tu >5 cm	7–20%		
Distal tumors	50–60%	69%	
Proximal tumors	20–30%	–	
Tumors of the entire urethra	–	12%	
T1–2	62–80%		60 months
T3–4	27%		43 months

Irrespective of the kind of therapy the 3- and 5-year overall survival is 74% and 30–44%. Local recurrences including lymph node failures occur in 30–50% of patients; these are more often (60%) if only surgery was performed. 30–50% of patients die of distant metastases. The primary histology seems to be less important than expected. However, melanoma of the urethra has a poor prognosis. Lymphoma may be locally cured by irradiation.

Tumor stage, the diagnosis of lymph node metastases and the localization of the tumor are the most important prognostic factors (see Table 3). In proximal urethral carcinomas, cure is seldom possible because of the often advanced stage.

Surgery

In meatal and small distal tumors (Ta, Tis, T1), open excision, electroresection, fulguration, and laser coagulation (Nd-YAG or CO_2) is possible. Larger T1 and T2 tumors need a surgical resection of the distal urethra. If a distal T3–4 tumor is diagnosed, an anterior exenteration and urinary diversion may be discussed; this should be – if a combined radiotherapy is not considered as sole therapy – combined with preoperative radiotherapy.

Lesions of the proximal or entire urethra are usually associated with invasion and high incidence of pelvic lymph node metastases. Therefore, the curative option of (non) exenterative surgery is only kept in tumors <2 cm. Pelvic lymphadenectomy is usually done, whereas inguinal node dissection is only indicated if lymph nodes had been palpable. In selected patients, it may be helpful to remove a part of the pubic symphysis and the inferior pubic rami in order to maximize the surgical margin. Similar results can be achieved with radiotherapy alone or a combination of preoperative radiotherapy and surgery in order to better attain the possibility of a bladder-sparing therapy. In locally advanced tumors, an exenterative surgery (cysto-urethrectomy, anterior vaginal wall resection) and urinary diversion are necessary. To lower the morbidity of surgery and to reduce the incidence of local recurrences preoperative external-beam radiotherapy (45–50 Gy, 1.8–2.0 Gy/day) should be offered to these patients. On the other hand, it has to be primarily discussed whether an organ-sparing procedure is possible abandoning surgery even if the prognosis is worse. In case of local recurrence after radiotherapy, surgical excision should be considered (DiMarco et al. 2004; Eng 2008).

Radiotherapy

The goal of radiotherapy is to maintain both function of the sphincter and the bladder and organ preservation. Therefore, in some reports radiotherapy is presented as treatment of choice with the exception of operable Tis and T1-lesions of the distal urethra. Definitive radiotherapy is recommended in all urethral tumors <70–80 cm^3 with a diameter <4 cm and without infiltration of the bladder. Brachytherapy alone is preferred if the tumor (T1–2) is located in the anterior two-thirds of the urethra while in proximal tumors with/without lymph node infiltration or advanced tumors infiltrating other organs (T3–4) external-beam radiotherapy is performed in combination with a brachytherapy boost. Postoperative radiotherapy may be debatable in case of G3-grading, lymphangiosis, tumor diameter >2 cm, and R0-resection <5 mm. In general, the results of external-beam irradiation alone are worse compared to brachytherapy alone or combined radiation treatment (risk reduction by the factor 4.2). The local tumor control rates (40–75%) are comparable to those of the surgical procedure.

In small meatus or distal located tumors, an interstitial procedure is used placing the needles surrounding the urethral orifice with the help of a sutured template, a Foley catheter within the urethra, and a vaginal tamponade. Some authors prefer a vaginal mold applicator (intraluminal/intracavitary treatment) and needles or guide gutters (interstitial procedure). In principle, CT-based treatment planning is helpful; however, in small tumor transvaginal ultrasound may be better to evaluate the tumor region. The planning target volume includes the tumor (GTV) plus 1(−2) cm safety margin. If brachytherapy is postoperatively performed, the target volume is reduced to the residual tumor region plus safety margins. The dose is expressed to a chosen distance according to the depth of the tumor. The isodose enclosing the target volume is mostly defined as the 85% isodose provided that the needles are located 0.5–1.0 cm lateral to the tumor region. Using LDR brachytherapy (0.4–0.6 Gy/h), 60–70 Gy (definitive treatment) and 20–30 Gy (boost) in 3–5 days are recommended. Using ^{192}Ir HDR brachytherapy, 40–70 Gy or 10–15 Gy is applied (5–10 Gy/week) when afterloading is the sole therapy or is used as a boost in addition to external-beam radiation, respectively.

Applying external therapy in advanced tumors, a three-dimensional treatment planning is obligatory to better reduce therapy-induced side effects and to homogenize the dose distribution. The portals should encompass the extended tumor region and the lymph nodes corresponding to the extension and localization of the tumor. Interestingly, after adjuvant irradiation of lymph nodes, nodal recurrences were seldom reported. The prescribed dose should be 45–50 Gy (1.8–2.0 Gy/day, 5x/week). A boost (10–15 Gy) to affected lymph nodes could be given. The tumor region has to be boosted with brachytherapy to raise the tumor dose up to 70–80 Gy (Milosevic et al. 2000; Gerbaulet 2002; Strnad et al. 2005; Troiano et al. 2009).

Local recurrences after surgery should be treated by combined radiotherapy and surgery whenever possible.

Chemotherapy

Few experiences exist about the influence of chemotherapy in female urethral cancer due to the small number of published patients. In small phase II studies and a few case reports, some encouraging results were reported using the combination of neoadjuvant ifosfamide, paclitaxel, and cisplatin and radiotherapy or concomitant 5-fluorouracil, mitomycin C, and irradiation. The treatment was feasible and toxicity was tolerable. Up to now, conclusions cannot be drawn (Bajorin et al. 2000; Galsky et al. 2007).

Sequelae of Therapy

The incidences of side effects vary in dependence on surgery, radiotherapy, and combined procedures as well in dependence on the treated tumor volume. After 3D-planned modern radiotherapy, acute side effects are relatively common including dry and moist desquamation, urethritis, and dysuria, necessitating antibiotic treatment but they are necessarily not dose limiting. These adverse effects obviously increase if radiotherapy is combined with chemotherapy.

Late sequelae are more important considering quality of life. Irrespective of the mode of treatment, uretheral strictures requiring dilatation or urinary diversion, vaginal stenosis, fistula developing especially in advanced tumors lately because of the tumor itself, necrosis, bowel obstruction, and incontinence were reported in 15–40% of patients. The ability to have sexual relation may be obtained but is often limited by other late effects as well as the woman's self-esteem. Today, the incidence of late effects may be lowered because of optimized therapy.

Cross-References

▶ Carcinoma of the Male Urethra
▶ Clinical Aspects of Brachytherapy (BT)
▶ Kaposi's Sarcoma
▶ Non-Hodgkins Lymphoma
▶ Wilm's Tumor

References

Ahmed K, Dasgupta R, Vats A, Nagpal K, Ashrafian H, Kaj B, Athansiou T, Dasgupta P, Khan MS (2010) Urethral diverticular carcinomas: an overview of current trends in diagnosis and management. Int Urol Nephrol 42:331–341

Bajorin DF, McCaffrey JA, Dodd PM, Hilton S, Mazumdar M, Kelly WK, Herr H, Scher HI, Icasiano E, Higgins G (2000) Ifosfamide, paclitaxel, and cisplatin for patients with advanced transitional cell carcinoma of the urothelial tract: final report of a phase II trial evaluating two dosing schedules. Cancer 88:1671–1678

DiMarco DS, DiMarco CS, Zincke H, Webb MJ, Bass SE, Slezak JM, Lightner DJ (2004) Surgical treatment for local control of female urethra carcinoma. Urol Oncol 22:404–409

Eng TY (2008) Female Urethra. In: Halperin EC, Perez CA, Brady LW (eds) Principles and Practice of Radiation Oncology, 5th edn. Wolters Kluwer/Wiliams and Wilkens, Lippincott/Philadelphia

Galsky MD, Iasonos A, Mironov S, Scattergood J, Donat SM, Bochner BH, Herr HW, Russo P, Boyle MG, Bajorin DF (2007) Prospective trial of ifosfamide, paclitaxel, and cisplatin in patients with advanced non-transitional cell carcinoma of the urothelial tract. Urology 69:255–259

Gerbaulet A (2002) Urethral cancer. In: Gerbaulet A, Pötter R, Materon JJ, Meertens H, van Limbergen E (ed) The GEC ESTRO handbook of brachytherapy, 1st edn. ACCO ESTRO Leuven

Milosevic MF, Warde PR, Banerjee D, Gospodarowicz MK, McLean M, Catton PA, Catton CN (2000) Urethral carcinoma in women: results of treatment with primary radiotherapy. Radiat Oncol 56:29–35

Strnad V, Pötter R, Kovács G (2005) Weibliches Urethrakarzinom. In: Strnad V, Pötter R, Kovács G (eds) Stand und Perspektiven der klinischen Brachytherapie, 1st edn. Science UniMed Bremen, Boston

Swartz MA, Porter MP, Lin DW, Weiss NS (2006) Incidence of primary urethral carcinoma in the United States. Urology 140:1–5

Thomas AA, Rackley RR, Lee U, Goldman HB, Vasavada SP, Hansel DE (2008) Urethral diverticula in 90 female patients: a study with emphasis on neoplastic alterations. J Urol 180:2463–2567

Troiano M, Corsa P, Raguso A, Cossa S, Piombino M, Guglielmi G, Parisi S (2009) Radiation therapy in urinary cancer: state of the art and perspective. Radiol Med 114:70–82

Female Urethral Cancer

▶ Female Urethra

Female Urethral Carcinoma

▶ Female Urethra

Fibrillary Astrocytoma

▶ Spinal Canal Tumor

Fibrohistiocytic Tumors

▶ Soft Tissue Sarcoma

Fibrous Dysplasia

HEDVIG HRICAK[1], OGUZ AKIN[2], HEBERT ALBERTO VARGAS[2]
[1]Department of Radiology, Memorial Sloan-Kettering Cancer Center, New York, NY, USA
[2]Body MRI, Memorial Sloan-Kettering Cancer Center, New York, NY, USA

Definition
Benign skeletal developmental anomaly of the bone-forming mesenchyme that manifests as a defect in osteoblastic differentiation and maturation. This results in lesions that consist of replacement of the medullary bone with fibrous tissue, causing the expansion and weakening of the areas of bone involved.

Cross-References
▶ Imaging in Oncology

Flat Bones

DANIEL J. INDELICATO[1], ROBERT H. SAGERMAN[2]
[1]Department of Radiation Oncology, University of Florida Proton Therapy Institute, University of Florida College of Medicine, Jacksonville, FL, USA
[2]Department of Radiation Oncology, SUNY Upstate Medical University, Syracuse, NY, USA

Definition
Flat bones are made up of a layer of cancellous bone between two thin layers of compact bone. Examples include the cranium, ilium, sternum, rib cage, sacrum, and scapula. Flat bones have marrow, but not a bone marrow cavity. In an adult, most red blood cells are formed in flat bones.

Cross-References
▶ Ewing Sarcoma

Flexible Sigmoidoscopy

▶ Sigmoidoscopy

FLI1 Gene

DANIEL J. INDELICATO[1], ROBERT H. SAGERMAN[2]
[1]Department of Radiation Oncology, University of Florida Proton Therapy Institute, University of Florida College of Medicine, Jacksonville, FL, USA
[2]Department of Radiation Oncology, SUNY Upstate Medical University, Syracuse, NY, USA

Definition
The *FLI1* gene encodes the protein Friend leukemia integration 1 transcription factor (FLI1), also known as proto-oncogene Fli-1 or transcription factor ERGB. In Ewing sarcoma, a chromosomal translocation generates a fusion of the 5′ transactivation domain of EWS with the 3′ Ets domain of Fli-1. The resulting fusion oncoprotein acts as an aberrant transcriptional activator with strong transforming capabilities.

Cross-References
▶ Ewing Sarcoma

Fluoropyrimidines

LYDIA T. KOMARNICKY-KOCHER
Department of Radiation Oncology, College of
Medicine, Drexel University, Philadelphia,
PA, USA

Definition
Family of chemotherapeutic agents used to treat
cancer which function as antimetabolites. Examples include capecitabine, floxuridine, and fluorouracil, temozolamide.

Cross-References
▶ Concurrent Chemoradiation
▶ Induction Chemotherapy
▶ Palliation of Brain and Spinal Cord Metastases
▶ Palliation of Metastatic Disease to the Liver
▶ Primary Intracranial Neoplasms

Forward-Planned Intensity Modulated Radiation Therapy

▶ Forward-Planning

Forward-Planning

ANTHONY E. DRAGUN
Department of Radiation Oncology, James
Graham Brown Cancer Center, University of
Louisville School of Medicine, Louisville,
KY, USA

Synonyms
Collimator-based tissue compensation; Forward-
planned intensity modulated radiation therapy;
Segment weighting

Definition
The use of computer algorithms and three-
dimensional treatment planning software to minimize dosimetric "hot spots" within breast tissue
during the course of whole breast radiation therapy. This technique is used to provide a homogeneous dose throughout the breast from the
base to the apex. Single and multiple institution
analyses have shown decreased acute skin
toxicity and improved late cosmeses in patients
who are treated with this technique as compared
to traditional two-dimensional radiation
techniques.

Cross-References
▶ Early-Stage Breast Cancer
▶ Whole Breast Radiation

Fossa of Rosenmüller

BRANDON J. FISHER[1], LARRY C. DAUGHERTY[2]
[1]Department of Radiation Oncology, College of
Medicine, Drexel University, Philadelphia,
PA, USA
[2]Department of Radiation Oncology,
College of Medicine, Drexel University, Glenside,
PA, USA

Definition
A pharyngeal recess behind the ostium of the
auditory tube; a common site for nasopharyngeal
cancers. At the base of this recess are the
retropharyngeal lymph node(s) also known as
the node of Rouvière.

Cross-References
▶ Hodgkin's Lymphoma
▶ Nasopharynx
▶ Sarcomas of the Head and Neck

Four-Dimensional (4D) Treatment Planning/Respiratory Gating

DAREK MICHALSKI, M. SAIFUL HUQ
Department of Radiation Oncology, University of Pittsburgh Medical Center Cancer Pavilion, Pittsburgh, PA, USA

Definition/Description

For some anatomical regions, conventional three-dimensional (3D) computed tomography (CT) can be replaced by a spatiotemporal data set commonly known as four-dimensional (4D) imaging. This approach affords technology-based solutions for assessing and then correcting for internal organ motion during radiation therapy. This type of intra-fractional motion is addressed by respiratory gating, which synchronizes dose delivery with a preselected signal range associated with the breathing cycle.

Fourth Dimension in Radiation Therapy

New developments in medical imaging have been crucial in qualitative and quantitative advances in radiation therapy. Computed tomography (CT) introduced a three-dimensional (3D) static patient model and afforded 3D conformal radiation therapy and later IMRT treatment delivery. The recognition of the shortcomings of 3D imaging spurred the advent of the time-resolved imaging, which can be perceived as a four-dimensional (4D) version of a given imaging modality. 4D CT as well as 4D positron emission tomography (PET), 4D single photon emission computed tomography (SPECT), and 4D magnetic resonance imaging (MRI) can be used in radiation therapy planning to improve underlying data specificity, sensitivity, and accuracy, and to allow for the shift from population-based to patient-specific parameters. 4D imaging reduces the systematic errors inherent in treatment planning that is based on conventional 3D imaging.

The explicit consideration of the time-dependent characteristics of the patient model and/or dose delivery in radiation therapy is referred to as 4D treatment planning (Keall et al. 2003). The scope and sophistication of the inclusion of temporal effects can vary as not all treatment planning systems have the ability to make use of this vast body of data. Respiratory gating is a method of dose delivery which makes use of clinical 4D treatment planning. Respiratory gating explicitly addresses intra-fractional respiration–induced tumor motion. It can be used for either 3D conformal radiation therapy (3DCRT) or intensity modulation radiation therapy (IMRT).

The quality of medical imaging as with any other probing technique of non-static subjects depends on the time scales of data acquisition and the dynamics of the scanned objects. In terms of the presented methodology, two anatomical regions exhibit conflicting timescales that cause artifacts in 3D imaging and equivalent dose distortions and perturbations during the fractionated radiation therapy. The thorax and the upper abdomen are most susceptible to physiologically induced organ motion. The major cause of motion is due to respiration, but nonnegligible motion is also ascribed to the digestive, cardiac, and muscular systems. Tumors in the lungs as well as in the upper abdomen could exhibit excursions up to 4 cm. It is clear that the conventional approach cannot deal systemically with a patient-specific and an unpredictable magnitude of tumor motion. Slow scans, multiple fast scans, breath-hold scans, or some combination thereof have been used to emulate a 4D data set. However these different strategies are still suboptimal in terms of treatment planning and dose delivery. The artifacts and/or misrepresentation of the anatomical regions of interest in these images prevent the application of protocols aimed at maximizing tumor control with escalated doses to the target and while at the same time minimizing the toxicity to normal structures.

4D CT scans and respiratory gating address these issues in order to enhance the effectiveness of radiation therapy. It is important to note that respiratory gating does not affect or remedy interfractional tumor motion, i.e., the change of tumor location between fractions. This type of tumor location variability can be brought about by physical changes within the patient as well as the psychological state of the patient over the course of treatment. Patients often feel more comfortable after several treatments, which might cause muscular relaxation and a shift in the tumor location. The stomach, bladder, or bowel filling may differ between fractions causing tumor shift. Weight change as well as tumor regression might affect its location as well. Thus if resources permit, when using respiratory gating, it is important to set the patient up using image guidance. The minimization of setup uncertainty is instrumental in decreasing the necessary tumor margins in order to take advantage of respiratory gating based on the 4DCT simulation. The respiratory gating strives to temper the effects of tumor motion during the dose delivery, or equivalently allow for a decrease in the GTV margins thereby ensuring a higher ▶ tumor control probability (TCP) and a lower ▶ normal tissue complication probability (NTCP).

Respiratory Signal

Currently the most common method used to reduce intra-fraction tumor motion is external respiratory gating. It is based on an external surrogate respiratory signal that is generated with an external breathing monitoring device. In contrast, internal respiratory gating uses fluoroscopic information to generate the respiratory signal with or without the radio-opaque fiducial markers implanted in the tumor vicinity. There are various techniques used to produce the external

respiratory motion tracking signal. Spirometers measure air flow or volume displacement (Lu et al. 2005). Strain gauges convert a mechanical strain into an electric signal (Kubo and Hill 1996) (AZ-733V) (Bellows System). These gauges are typically in the form of a belt placed below the diaphragm. Thermometers using either a thermistor or a thermocouple monitor the difference in temperature between inhaled and exhaled air (Kubo and Hill 1996; Wolthaus et al. 2008). The optical Real-Time Position Management Respiratory Gating System (RPM) uses a plastic block with at least two infrared-opaque markers (3 cm apart for quantification). The block is placed half way between the umbilicus and xiphoid. An infrared light source directed at the block allows a charge-coupled device (CCD) camera interfaced with a computer to monitor the vertical movement of the block with respiration. Each of these methods quantifies the amplitude and the period of the breathing cycle. Its utility is based on the assumption of its correlation with tumor motion. The point of concern is the discrepancy and/or variation of phase difference between tumor and respiratory cyclic motion.

There are two ways to realize respiratory gating. The respiratory signal can be described in terms of its phase in the range between 0% and 100%, where the end of inhalation marks the beginning and end of the cycle (phase 0% and 100%), with the end of exhalation falling around phase 50–60%. Usually ten equispaced phases are obtained with 4D scanning. The radiation is administered within a preassigned gating window spanning a certain range of phases. Another way to define the gating window is to use amplitude-based gating. The dose delivery occurs within a preselected range of the respiratory motion amplitude. Figure 1 shows the signal and gating windows for RPM system.

The respiratory signal reproducibility does not automatically imply either tumor motion reproducibility or tumor location reproducibility

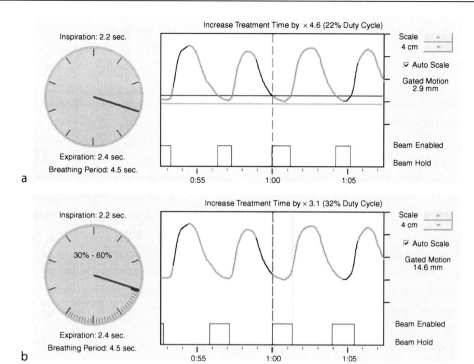

Four-Dimensional (4D) Treatment Planning/Respiratory Gating. Fig. 1 A snapshot of a respiratory signal acquired during 4D CT scanning as replayed by Varian RPM system. (**a**) Shows amplitude gating within the range defined by two horizontal lines superimposed on the signal waveform, the lower step function depicts beam-on signal. (**b**) Shows phase-based respiratory gating with gating window set between phase 30% and 60%. Vertical dashed lines on one of the beam-on signals show the width of the gating window as they cross the respiratory waveform around the end of exhalation. The clockwise motion of the needle on the dial reflects the current breathing phase

with respect to the beam arrangement. Interfractional tumor location shifts occur; these should be determined and the patient appropriately positioned before each fraction using image-guided protocols. Fluoroscopic imaging might also be utilized to confirm the applicability of the initially defined gating window. Ideally one might wish to confirm the congruence of the tumor motion trajectory with the respiratory cycle, especially for phase-based respiratory gating, with another 4D CT scan half way during the treatment course. However, reported studies show that this congruence exists and if the patient breathing pattern is maintained, the shape of the motion trajectories remains the same. The plausible source of

problem, which might invalidate the signal reproducibility and affect the tumor motion trajectory, is the change of respiration from abdominal to chest wall breathing or vice versa between 4D CT simulation and treatment.

4D CT Imaging for Respiratory Gating

Currently, the application of respiratory gating relies mainly on the tumor motion determination obtained with 4D CT. Conceptually, 4D imaging relies on time-resolved data acquisition. A signal associated with respiratory motion allows for temporal correlation of scanned images with a breathing cycle. The signal can be correlated prospectively with scanning effectuated only at given phase or amplitude. Much more efficient is a retrospective correlation for which the scanning and respiratory signals are recorded simultaneously. The post CT scan spatiotemporal binning based on either the amplitude or phase of the breathing track creates 3D CT volumes depicting consecutive stages during the breathing cycle.

Helical and ▶ cine CT scans can be adopted to 4D CT. The phase-based 4D CT helical scan utilizes a very low ▶ pitch for slow couch movement. This enables the CT detectors to obtain axial images of the region over the entire breathing cycle. The projections closest to required phases are binned and reconstructed. For cine CT, at a given couch position, scanning lasts for the average breathing period plus the time required for image reconstruction to ensure that the entire breathing cycle is captured. The images are reconstructed at the given time of scanning and sorted into phases using the respiratory signal recorded during the scan acquisition.

The patient undergoing 4D CT should maintain breath regularity. To help accomplish this, audio and visual coaching is often applied. The audio prompt is set to match the patient's breathing frequency with either "breathe in" and/or "breathe out" commands. The visual prompt that mirrors the respiratory signal amplitude helps the patient maintain the same tidal volume and the functional residual capacity of lungs. The coaching should improve the breathing pattern; however, some patients get confused or frustrated by the procedure, and perform better without any prompts or with minimal audio commands. It is worthwhile to note that coaching does affect the lung mechanics and tumor motion in the sense that coached versus un-coached 4D CT scans can exhibit different tumor positions (Haasbeek et al. 2008). If a 4D CT simulation is carried out with coaching, the treatment must also rely on this technique and vice versa. If the patient seems to be a good candidate for 4DCT, i.e., his or her lung

functionality is not impaired to the degree causing erratic breathing, the tumor motion magnitude and the quality of the 4D CT scan (Yamamoto et al. 2008) determines whether or not respiratory gating can be prescribed.

Tumor Motion Determination

4D CT reconstructs the 3D volumes depicting patient anatomy at various points of the breathing cycle. For tumor motion determination, one of the volumes is used as a reference. Tumor motion magnitude is evaluated with respect to this volume. Currently there are no dedicated tools to carry out the task automatically, although bespoke image registration software can be used to track tumor motion through the breathing cycle (MIMVista) (VelocityAI) (Zhang et al. 2005; Wolthaus et al. 2008). Otherwise tumor motion is determined by measuring the displacement of a preselected anatomical feature which can be identified on all phases on all three DICOM axes. Usually tumors do not deform significantly; the axial, coronal, and sagittal cross sections, including the tumor centroid, are examined in all volumes so that the tumor excursion can be measured from the reference volume. There is always an inherent residual inaccuracy regardless of the method of the tumor displacement determination either due to 4D CT artifacts or image registration. This can be addressed in several ways: (1) using the composite trajectory obtained by averaging the trajectories determined with respect to the different reference volume, (2) by removing the high-frequency components of the discrete inverse Fourier transform of the tumor motion trajectory, or (3) by analyzing the deformation field resulting from image registration (Zhang et al. 2005; Wolthaus et al. 2008). The motion trajectory is comprised of a discrete set of points corresponding to the number of 3D CT volumes in the 4D data set. The motion in between these frames can be derived with a spline interpolation of these discrete points.

A tumor motion threshold of 0.5 cm (Keall et al. 2006) is used to recommend the respiratory gating for patients with the breathing period of at least 3 s.

Respiratory Gating Type and its Parameters

If tumor motion dictates respiratory gating, it must be decided whether the amplitude or phase gating should be prescribed, which segment of the respiratory cycle is most appropriate for the gating window and how big the gating window should be. Tumor motion within the gating window is called residual motion. By selecting a narrow gating window, small residual motion usually can be achieved, but this prolongs the treatment time and decreases the duty cycle. The duty cycle is the ratio of time with beam-on to the entire treatment time. Theoretically one would like to maximize duty cycle and minimize residual motion. By examining the residual motion in prospective gating windows for amplitude and phase respiratory gating, one could determine the optimal window size.

For the majority of patients the breathing cycle is asymmetrical. The exhalation is longer than the inhalation and the end of exhalation is characterized by a certain dwelling time with minimal tumor motion. The end of exhalation is also the most reproducible part of the breathing cycle so it is usually chosen as a reference volume for the motion determination and as a breathing cycle time point reference for anchoring the gating window.

The size of the gating window is determined by a physicist and a physician considering the aforementioned criteria including patient-specific requirements. Our practice has been to limit residual motion to 0.5 cm. This corresponds to the conformal radiation therapy setup accuracy. For special procedures like stereotactic body radiation therapy, the threshold can be decreased to 0.3 cm.

For pulmonary tumors one might consider setting the gating window around the end of inhalation. The rationale for this choice is the possible decrease of lung toxicity due to the increased lung volume during the air intake. However, this intuitively convincing argument does not seem to guarantee the expected gains. A direct treatment plan comparison for gating windows set at the end of exhalation versus the end of inhalation is required to definitely gauge the lung sparing capability of respective plans. The better reproducibility of the end of exhalation compared to the end of inspiration should be considered during the decision process. In addition, the tumor motion at the end of inhalation is usually larger than at the end of exhalation. Thus, due to the magnitude of residual motion, the end of inhalation 3D CT volume is more susceptible to artifacts than its end of exhalation counterpart. This may also weigh-in for the decision process of selecting the gating window and 3D CT volume for treatment planning.

Treatment Planning

The definition of the target using 4D CT must take advantage of information provided by time-resolved CT volumes. Internal target volume (ITV) (ICRU 1999) defines the target object that encompasses the GTV or clinical tumor volume (CTV) during its motion as captured by 4D CT. For respiratory gating, the magnitude of motion is limited to that occurring in gating window. The setup error is added to ITV for planning target volume.

There are a few ways to generate the ITV. The most laborious and apposite to all types of tumors and their locations is manual contouring of GTVs on all CT volumes contained within the gating window. All these CT volumes have the same DICOM coordinates. The DICOM hardware fusion allows for the transfer of the contours to the anchor CT volume. The Boolean union of GTVs from relevant 3D CT frames constitutes the ITV. A variation of this method is contouring only on extreme CT volumes comprising the gating window, but this may not be applicable for cases

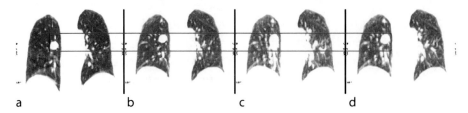

a   b   c   d

Four-Dimensional (4D) Treatment Planning/Respiratory Gating. Fig. 2 The high density differential between the tumor and pulmonary tissue renders the lesion view unambiguously conspicuous with well-defined boundaries in the lung window setting: (**a**) phase 0%, (**b**) phase 50%, (**c**) composite MIP volume built from all phases, and (**d**) composite MIP volume of the gating window created from phases 30% to 60%. The frame facilitates viewing tumor, its locations, and its motion extent

with the residual motion amplitudes comparable with the size of the GTV, or with a motion trajectory exhibiting hysteresis.

As shown in Fig. 2, for well-circumscribed lung tumors with a high ▶ radiodensity as compared with the surrounding pulmonary tissue, the maximum intensity projection (MIP) of CT volumes comprising the gating window may be used as the resultant CT volume for treatment planning. Contouring the tumor on MIP CT data set creates ITV. Tumors in the upper abdomen or in the mediastinum do not exhibit this characteristic and this method cannot be used for ITV generation in these cases. The same can be said about lung tumors with diffuse boundaries. Some treatment centers have used the averaging of CT volumes comprising the gating window. This method reflects the probabilistic nature of ▶ voxel occupancy by the tumor. It does not lend itself directly to the current treatment planning paradigm of definitive characteristics of voxel content. The averaging might also diffuse the tumor boundary resulting in incorrect contouring.

Another method of ITV generation is the use of a single 3D CT frame corresponding to a given reference point during the breathing cycle, e.g., the end of exhalation or inspiration 3D CT volume. The GTV is contoured and margins determined during the motion study that correspond to residual motion within the gating window are added to create ITV.

The critical structures are contoured on CT volumes correlating to the method selected for the ITV creation. Thus intra-fractional tumor motion is factored into the anatomically segmented patient model and the 3D conformal, or intensity modulated radiation therapy plan can be prepared.

Respiratory-Gated Treatment Delivery

Respiratory-gated treatment delivery must comply with all requirements imposed by the patient model and treatment plan, and thus relies on both the 3D and 4D geometry of the patient anatomy. As in conventional treatment, the treatment plan is based on a single static 3D CT patient volume. The 4D dependence is based on a patient model reflecting a specific and definite temporal state of the anatomy. Thus the treatment delivery must be synchronized with a preassigned gating window. As for the 4D image acquisition, the respiratory signal is obtained and the dose delivery is triggered periodically in the gating window. The breathing signal should be acquired with the same device placed at the same position on the patient and with identical breathing coaching as was done for the 4D CT scan. This serves to reproduce the breathing pattern in terms of its periodicity as well as tidal volume. This should guarantee identical respiration-induced tumor kinematics and the correspondence of the patient anatomy during the delivery within the gating window. For amplitude-based gating, visual coaching is more relevant since the breathing period does not affect the breathing signal amplitude. If different breathing signal acquisition systems are used for the 4D imaging and the gated delivery, they should be correlated.

Since gating relies on the tumor location, and vice versa, image-guided patient setup is recommended and in case of ▶ hypofractionation is imperative at every fraction for respiratory-gated treatment delivery, otherwise relevant margins to ITV must be added to accommodate setup errors and daily tumor shifts (Korreman et al. 2008). Fluoroscopic imaging can be used for the verification of the gating window and for its width adjustment if necessary. Therapists should be aware of the complexity of the gated methodology and its procedural subtleties. Therapists should monitor the breathing signal during entire treatment delivery. They should interrupt the treatment in case of significant breathing signal irregularities or in case of shifts of the breathing signal baseline. The treatment should resume after the patient can regain his/her usual breathing pattern. An intrinsic characteristic of the gated delivery is that the beam is on for only a fraction of the breathing cycle. This increased temporal burden may be aided with the increase of the ▶ dose rate.

Cross-References

▶ Image-Guided Radiation Therapy (IGRT): kV Imaging
▶ Image-Guided Radiation Therapy (IGRT): MV Imaging
▶ Intensity Modulated Radiation Therapy (IMRT)
▶ Radiation Oncology Physics

References

Bellows System, Philips Medical Systems, Cleveland
Haasbeek CJA et al (2008) Impact of audio-coaching on the position of lung tumors. Int J Radiat Oncol Biol Phys 71:1118–1123

ICRU (International Commission on Radiation Units and Measurements) (1999) Report 62: prescribing, recording, and reporting photon beam therapy. Supplement to ICRU Report 50. ICRU, Bethesda
Keall PJ et al (2003) Time – the fourth dimension in radiotherapy. Int J Radiat Oncol Biol Phys 57:S8–S9
Keall PJ et al (2006) The management of respiratory motion in radiation oncology report of AAPM Task Group 76. Med Phys 33:3874–3900
Korreman SS et al (2008) Respiratory gated beam delivery cannot facilitate margin reduction, unless combined with respiratory correlated image guidance. Radiother Oncol 86:61–68
Kubo HD, Hill BC (1996) Respiration gated radiotherapy treatment: a technical study Phys Med Biol 41:83–91
Lu W et al (2005) Comparison of spirometry and abdominal height as four-dimensional computed tomography metrics in lung. Med Phys 32:2351–2357
MIMVista, MIM Software Inc., Cleveland
Respiratory Gating System AZ-733V, Anzai Medical Co. Ltd, Tokyo
RPM, Varian Oncology Systems, Palo Alto
VelocityAI, Velocity Medical Solutions, LLC, Atlanta
Wolthaus JWH et al (2008) Comparison of different strategies to use four-dimensional computed tomography in treatment planning for lung cancer patients. Int J Radiat Oncol Biol Phys 70:1229–1238
Yamamoto T et al (2008) Retrospective analysis of artifacts in four-dimensional CT images of 50 abdominal and thoracic radiotherapy patients. Int J Radiat Oncol Biol Phys 74:1250–1258
Zhang T et al (2005) On the automated definition of mobile target volumes from 4D-CT images for stereotactic body radiotherapy. Med Phys 32(11):3493–3502

Fourier Transform

HEDVIG HRICAK[1], OGUZ AKIN[2], HEBERT ALBERTO VARGAS[2]
[1]Department of Radiology, Memorial Sloan-Kettering Cancer Center, New York, NY, USA
[2]Body MRI, Memorial Sloan-Kettering Cancer Center, New York, NY, USA

Definition

Mathematical operation that transforms one complex-valued function of a real variable into another. In such applications as signal processing, the domain of the original function is typically time and is accordingly called the time domain. The domain of the new function is typically called the frequency domain, and the new function itself is called the frequency domain representation of the original function. It describes which frequencies are present in the original function. In effect, the Fourier transform decomposes a function into oscillatory functions.

Cross-References

▶ Imaging in Oncology

Frameless Stereotactic Radiosurgery

BRIAN F. HASSON
Department of Radiation Oncology, Abington Memorial Hospital, Abington, PA, USA
Department of Radiation Oncology, College of Medicine, Drexel University, Philadelphia, PA, USA

Definition

A method or system that is used to monitor a target and its position relative to the coordinate system of a treatment unit. Optical tracking, markers, and digital radiographs are used to determine the position and deviations in positions of the target.

Cross-References

▶ Gamma Knife
▶ Image-Guided Radiation Therapy (IGRT): TomoTherapy
▶ Lung Cancer

▶ Palliation of Brain and Spinal Cord Metastases
▶ Robotic Radiosurgery
▶ Stereotactic Radiosurgery – Cranial

Frey's Syndrome

LINDSAY G. JENSEN, LOREN K. MELL
Center for Advanced Radiotherapy Technologies, Department of Radiation Oncology, San Diego Rebecca and John Moores Cancer Center, University of California, La Jolla, CA, USA

Definition

Sweating from a small area of skin anterior to the ear with exposure to food or thoughts of food.

Cross-References

▶ Salivary Gland Cancer

Frontal Sinus

FILIP T. TROICKI
College of Medicine, Drexel University, Philadelphia, PA, USA

Definition

One of a collection of mucous membrane–lined cavities located within the frontal bone above the orbit.

Cross-References

▶ Nasal Cavity and Paranasal Sinuses

G

Gail

▶ Early-Stage Breast Cancer

Gallbladder Cancer

▶ Liver and Hepatobiliary Tract

Gamma Knife

BRIAN F. HASSON
Department of Radiation Oncology, Abington
Memorial Hospital, Abington, PA, USA
Department of Radiation Oncology, College
of Medicine, Drexel University, Philadelphia,
PA, USA

Definition

A stereotactic radiosurgery unit that incorporates
201 cobalt-60 sources to deliver therapeutic doses
of radiation to a predefined target. The Gamma
Knife was the first high-energy system to be used
for stereotactic radiosurgery.

Cross-References

▶ Radiosurgery
▶ Stereotactic Radiosurgery – Cranial

Ganglioneuroblastoma

BRANDON J. FISHER[1], LARRY C. DAUGHERTY[2]
[1]Department of Radiation Oncology, College
of Medicine, Drexel University, Philadelphia,
PA, USA
[2]Department of Radiation Oncology, College of
Medicine, Drexel University, Glenside,
PA, USA

Definition

A variant of neuroblastoma of intermediate grade
and prognosis.

Cross-References

▶ Neuroblastoma

Ganglioneuroma

BRANDON J. FISHER[1], LARRY C. DAUGHERTY[2]
[1]Department of Radiation Oncology, College
of Medicine, Drexel University, Philadelphia,
PA, USA
[2]Department of Radiation Oncology, College of
Medicine, Drexel University, Glenside, PA, USA

Definition

A benign tumor of the sympathetic nerve fibers
arising from the neural crest cells.

Cross-References

▶ Neuroblastoma

L.W. Brady, T.E. Yaeger (eds.), *Encyclopedia of Radiation Oncology*, DOI 10.1007/978-3-540-85516-3,
© Springer-Verlag Berlin Heidelberg 2013

Gastric Cancer

▶ Stomach Cancer

Gastric Mucosa

FILIP T. TROICKI[1], JAGANMOHAN POLI[2]
[1]College of Medicine, Drexel University, Philadelphia, PA, USA
[2]Department of Radiation Oncology, College of Medicine, Drexel University, Philadelphia, PA, USA

Definition
Stomach lining made up of mucous-secreting cells.

Cross-References
▶ Stomach Cancer

Gastric Tumor

▶ Stomach Cancer

Gastritis

FILIP T. TROICKI[1], JAGANMOHAN POLI[2]
[1]College of Medicine, Drexel University, Philadelphia, PA, USA
[2]Department of Radiation Oncology, College of Medicine, Drexel University, Philadelphia, PA, USA

Definition
Inflammation of the stomach lining, usually causing severe abdominal discomfort.

Cross-References
▶ Stomach Cancer

Gastroenteritis

FILIP T. TROICKI[1], JAGANMOHAN POLI[2]
[1]College of Medicine, Drexel University, Philadelphia, PA, USA
[2]Department of Radiation Oncology, College of Medicine, Drexel University, Philadelphia, PA, USA

Definition
Inflammation of the gastrointestinal tract, involving the stomach and intestines, often causing diarrhea.

Cross-References
▶ Stomach Cancer

Gastroesophageal (GE) Junction

FILIP T. TROICKI[1], JAGANMOHAN POLI[2]
[1]College of Medicine, Drexel University, Philadelphia, PA, USA
[2]Department of Radiation Oncology, College of Medicine, Drexel University, Philadelphia, PA, USA

Definition
The region where the esophagus meets the stomach.

Cross-References
▶ Esophageal Cancer
▶ Stomach Cancer

Gate-Keeper Gene

▶ Tumor Suppressor Gene

Gene Expression Profiling

CLAUDIA E. RÜBE
Department of Radiation Oncology,
Saarland University, Homburg/Saar, Germany

Definition
Measurement of the activity of thousands of genes at once, to create a global picture of cellular functions.

Cross-References
▶ Predictive In vitro Assays in Radiation Oncology

Genomic Instability

SUSAN M. VARNUM, MARIANNE B. SOWA,
WILLIAM F. MORGAN
Biological Sciences Division, Fundamental &
Computational Sciences, Directorate Pacific
Northwest National Laboratory, Richland,
WA, USA

Definition
Characterized by an increased tendency of the genome to acquire mutations when various processes involved in maintaining and replicating the genome are dysfunctional.

Cross-References
▶ Radiation-Induced Genomic Instability and Radiation Sensitivity

Geometry Function

NING J. YUE
The Department of Radiation Oncology, The
Cancer Institute of New Jersey, UMDNJ-Robert
Wood Johnson Medical School, New Brunswick,
NJ, USA

Definition
A quantity accounting for the impacts of spatial radionuclide distribution within the source on the source relative dose distribution, ignoring photon absorption and scattering in the source structure.

Cross-References
▶ Brachytherapy: Low Dose Rate (LDR) Temporary Implants

Germinal Epithelium

JOHANNES CLASSEN
Department of Radiation Oncology,
St. Vincentius-Kliniken Karlsruhe, Karlsruhe,
Germany

Definition
Epithelium of the testis harboring and giving rise to male germ cells.

Cross-References

Glioblastoma Multiforme

Glomus Tumors

CARLOS A. PEREZ, WADE L. THORSTAD
Department of Radiation Oncology, Siteman
Cancer Center, Washington University Medical
Center, St. Louis, MO, USA

Definition

Tumors arising in the regions of the jugular bulb, along the auricular and tympanic branches of the tenth cranial nerve. Typically occurring in the middle ear region but also occurring anywhere along the nerve tracts including the nodose ganglion and carotid body.

Epidemiology

Glomus tumors may be familial: They occur in multiple sites in 10–20% of patients. The mean age at diagnosis has been reported to be 45 years for carotid body tumors and 52 years for glomus tympanicum. These tumors occur three or four times more frequently in women than in men, suggesting a possible estrogen influence (Perez and Thorstad 2008).

Clinical Presentation

Glomus tumors of the middle ear may initially cause earache or discomfort. As they expand, they produce tinnitus, hearing loss, and, in later stages, cranial nerve paralysis resulting from invasion of the base of the skull in 10–15% of patients. If the posterior fossa is involved, symptoms may include occipital headache, ataxia, and paresis of cranial nerves V to VII, IX, and XII;invasion of the jugular foramen causes paralysis of nerves IX to XI.

Chemodectoma of the carotid body usually presents as a painless, slowly growing mass in the upper neck. Occasionally, the mass may be pulsatile and may be associated with thrill or bruit. Very rarely these tumors may be malignant. Metastases occur in 2–5% of cases (Perez and Thorstad 2008).

Diagnostic Workup

In the majority of glomus tympanicum tumors, physical examination demonstrates a red, vascular middle ear mass (Perez and Thorstad 2008). Audiography may demonstrate conductive hearing loss in the ear involved by tumor. Examination of the neck may demonstrate a mass that may be pulsatile or have a bruit or may present with lymph node metastases.

Radiographic studies are invaluable in the diagnosis of these tumors. Plain mastoid radiographs frequently demonstrate clouding of the mastoid air cells, suggesting mastoiditis. Computed tomography (CT) or magnetic resonance (MRI) with contrast has the highest sensitivity and specificity to diagnose this tumor when located in the middle ear or jugular bulb. Recently Astner et al. (2009) reported on the value of PET scanning with Gluc-LysF18-TOCA in the target volume delineation of glomus tumors. Magnification angiography is a sensitive and specific means of detecting glomus tympanicum tumors. Biopsy of glomus tumors may result in severe hemorrhage. Biopsy of an aberrant internal carotid artery can result in major neurologic sequelae or death.

Cytochemical techniques demonstrate increased levels of serotonin, epinephrine, and norepinephrine in normal glomus tissue of the carotid body. Histologic staining techniques, including chromaffin and argentaffin reactions, identify patients with hormonally active tumors. This is important because the glomus tumor may coexist with a pheochromocytoma, which requires special preoperative preparation of the patient.

Staging

The prognosis of these tumors is closely related to the anatomic location and the volume of the lesion, which is reflected in the Glasscock-Jackson classification shown in Table 1. An alternative classification proposed by McCabe and Fletcher is presented in Table 2.

Glomus Tumors. Table 1 Glasscock-Jackson classification of glomus tumors

Glomus tympanicum	
I	Small mass limited to promontory
II	Tumor completely filling middle ear space
III	Tumor filling middle ear and extending into the mastoid
IV	Tumor filling middle ear, extending into the mastoid or through tympanic membrane to fill the external auditory canal; may extend anterior to carotid
Glomus jugulare	
I	Small tumor involving jugular bulb, middle ear, and mastoid
II	Tumor extending under internal auditory canal; may have intracranial canal extension
III	Tumor extending into petrous apex; may have intracranial canal extension
IV	Tumor extending beyond petrous apex into clivus or infratemporal fossa; may have intracranial canal extension

Source: Jackson et al. (1982)

General Management

Surgery is generally selected for treatment of small tumors that can be completely excised. Percutaneous embolization of a low-viscosity silicone polymer has been used frequently as preoperative preparation of the tumor. Preoperative transarterial embolization has proved beneficial but is often limited by vascular anatomy and unfavorable locations.

Surgical treatment of a glomus tumor arising in the jugular bulb often consists of piece-by-piece removal accompanied by significant bleeding. Intraoperative bleeding during surgical removal of head and neck paragangliomas may be a major problem in the management of these highly vascularized tumors.

Local tumor control with surgery alone is about 60%, and it is associated with significant morbidity, particularly cranial nerve injury and bleeding.

Radiation Therapy

Irradiation is frequently used in the treatment of glomus tumors, particularly for those in the tympanicum and jugulare bulb locations. Tumors with destruction of the petrous bone, jugular fossa, or occipital bone or patients with jugular foramen syndrome are more reliably managed with irradiation (Lybeert et al. 1984; Pryzant et al. 1989). Some reports describe successful combinations of surgery with either preoperative or postoperative irradiation (Larner et al. 1992).

Radiation therapy techniques are determined by the location and extent of the tumor (Konefal et al. 1987). In the past, limited, usually bilateral portals were used for localized glomus tumors, whether or not the treatment is combined with surgery.

A three-field arrangement is made with a superior-inferior wedged and lateral open field. Electrons (15–18 MeV) and a lateral portal or combined with ^{60}Co or 4- to 6-MV photon

Glomus Tumors. Table 2 Modification of McCabe and Fletcher classification of chemodectomas

Tumor group	Characteristics
Group I: Tympanic tumors	Absence of bone destruction on x-rays of the mastoid bone and jugular fossa
	Absence of facial nerve weakness
	Intact VIII nerve with conductive deafness only
	Intact jugular foramen nerves (cranial nerves IX, X, and XI)
Group II: Tympanomastoid tumors	X-ray evidence of bone destruction confined to the mastoid bone and not involving the petrous bone
	Normal or paretic VII nerve
	Intact jugular foramen nerves
	No evidence of involvement of the superior bulb of the jugular vein on retrograde venogram
Group III: Petrosal and extrapetrosal tumors	Destruction of the petrous bone, jugular fossa, and/or occipital bone on x-rays
	Positive findings on retrograde jugulography
	Evidence of destruction of the petrous or occipital bones on carotid arteriogram
	Jugular foramen syndrome (paresis of cranial nerves IX, X, or XI)
	Presence of metastasis

Source: Wang et al. (1988)

beams (20–25% of total tumor dose) render a good dose distribution. In patients in whom tumor has spread into the posterior fossa, it was necessary to use parallel-opposed portals with 6–18 MV photon beams. 3D conformal RT or IMRT are highly desirable techniques to treat these tumors, with excellent dose distributions (Fig. 1). Treatment is given at 1.8–2 Gy tumor dose per day with five treatments per week for a total tumor dose of 45–55 Gy in 5 weeks. Table 3 summarizes doses of irradiation recommended by several investigators and the probability of tumor control.

Seventeen patients were treated for glomus tympanicum tumors at Washington University (Konefal et al. 1987). In five patients initial treatment was irradiation alone, and all were tumor free at last follow-up or at death. Seven of eight patients irradiated for surgical recurrence were free of disease 4.5–19 years after irradiation. The remaining four patients were treated preoperatively or postoperatively; only one had recurrence and was salvaged surgically and was tumor free 10 years later. Irradiation doses ranged from 46 to 52 Gy, with 86–100% tumor control with doses over 46 Gy and 50% (2 of 4) with doses below 46 Gy.

Wang and associates (1988) reported on 32 patients with tympanic chemodectomas: 13 treated with surgery alone, 15 with irradiation alone, and 4 with a combination of both modalities. Of the patients treated with irradiation, 84% had initial local tumor control, 77% survived 10 years, and only 11% developed complications. The doses of irradiation used were slightly higher than those reported by others (mean 58.32 Gy). However, no improvement in tumor control was noted with higher doses. Complications occurred in two patients receiving 66 Gy.

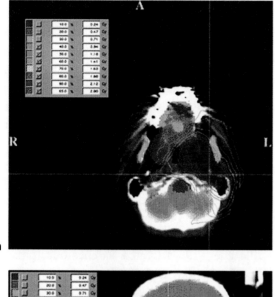

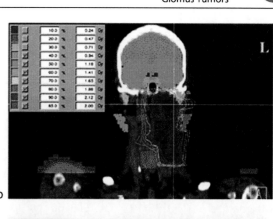

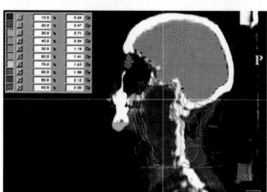

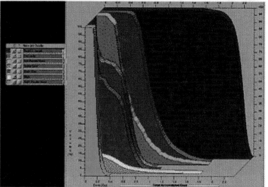

Glomus Tumors. Fig. 1 A 59-year-old female with an unusual malignant left glomus jugulare, who had a metastatic left upper cervical lymph node. She was treated with definitive IMRT (66 Gy in 2 Gy fractions). (**a**) cross, (**b**) coronal, and (**c**) sagittal sections showing dose distributions at primary site and left neck, sparing normal structures (**d**) dose-volume histogram:

Structure	Dose range (Gy)	Mean dose (Gy)
PTV (including left neck)	38–77	70
Brain	0–59	2
Brain stem	6–35	12
Spinal cord	0–32	13

Source: Reproduced with permission from LeVay J, O'Sullivan B, Catton C, et al (1994)

Arthur (1977) observed no recurrences in 24 patients treated with doses of 45–50 Gy; only one failure was observed in a patient receiving 30 Gy in 15 fractions in 21 days. If the tolerances of the brain and brain stem to irradiation are considered, doses of 45–50 Gy (1.8- to 2-Gy fractions) are considered optimal for treatment of these lesions.

Glomus Tumors. Table 3 Local control with radiation therapy for chemodectoma of the temporal bone (glomus tympanicum and jugulare)

Institution	Local control	Nominal dosage schedule
Queen Elizabeth Hospital, Birmingham	19/20[a]	45–50 Gy/ 4–5 weeks
Rotterdamsch Radio-Therapeutisch Instituut, Netherlands	19/19	40–60 Gy/ 4–6 weeks
University of Minnesota	13/14	30–60 Gy/ 3.5–7.5 weeks
University of Virginia	14/17	40–50 Gy/ 4–5 weeks
Princess Margaret Hospital	42/45[b]	35 Gy/ 3 weeks
Total	107/115 (93%)	

[a]One patient listed as a failure was salvaged with further radiation therapy
[b]Two patients listed as failures were salvaged with further treatments
Source: Modified from Wang et al. (1988) and Springate and Weichselbaum (1990)

Powell and associates (1992) reported on 84 patients with chemodectoma of the head and neck, 46 in the glomus jugulare and tympanicum, treated with irradiation alone (45–50 Gy in 25 fractions). Local control of the lesion was 73% at 5 years. Thirty patients were treated with surgery after irradiation with no recurrences (median follow-up of 9 years). Four carotid body and glomus vagale tumors treated with irradiation were locally controlled at 1, 2, 8, and 11 years. In 13 patients treated with surgery alone, the 15-year local control rate was 54%.

Radiation therapy has been used in the treatment of carotid body tumors. Mendenhall and colleagues (1986) treated six chemodectomas of the carotid body and ganglion nodosum in four patients, with doses of 40.8–48.5 Gy using ^{60}Co, 8-MV x-ray beams, or a combination of 8- and 17-MV x-ray beams. Lesions have remained stable in four patients 2–4.5 years after irradiation.

Hinerman and associates (2001) reported on 71 patients with 80 chemodectomas of the temporal body, carotid bone, or glomus vagale treated with radiation therapy alone or subtotal resection and radiation therapy (8 tumors). Fourteen patients had undergone a previous treatment

Glomus Tumors. Table 4 Temporal bone chemodectomas: local control after radiation therapy alone or radiation therapy and surgery

Author	Number of patients	Percent local control	Follow-up (year)
Larner et al.	15	93 (RT alone)	Median, 16.2
Powell et al.	46	90 (RT alone)	Median, 9
Wang et al.	19	84 (RT ± surgery)	5–35
Konefal et al.	23	83 (RT ± surgery)	Mean, 10.5
Pryzant et al.	19	95 (RT ± surgery)	Mean, 11
Cole and Beiler	30	97 (RT alone)	3–27
De Jong et al.	38	89 (RT ± surgery)	Median, 11.5
Hinerman et al.	53	93 (RT ± surgery)	Mean, 15

RT radiation therapy
Source: Hinerman et al. (2001), Wang et al. (1988)

(surgery 11, irradiation 1, or both 2). Fifty-three patients had temporal chemodectomas, 46 of which were classified as glomus jugulare and 9 as glomus tympanicum. Fifty patients were treated with radiation therapy alone and five with subtotal resection followed by postoperative radiation therapy for gross residual tumor. Median dose was 45 Gy with daily fractions of 1.5–2 Gy delivered with cobalt-60, 6 MV, or 8 MV x-ray beams or a combination of different beam energies. Local control was obtained in 43 previously untreated lesions (93%) and in 11 of 12 (92%) previously treated chemodectomas. The results of treatment for temporal bone chemodectoma are summarized in Tables 3 and 4. Complications were rare in these patients.

Cross-References

▶ Primary Intracranial Neoplasms
▶ Sarcomas of the Head and Neck

References

Arthur K (1977) Radiotherapy in chemodectoma of the glomus jugulare. Clin Radiol 28:415–417

Astner ST, Bunduschuh RA, Beer AJ et al (2009) Assessment of tumor volumes in skull base glomus tumors using gluc-lysF^{18}-TOCA positron emission tomography. Int J Radiat Oncol Bio Phys 73:1135–1140

Hinerman RW, Mendenhall WM, Amdur RJ et al (2001) Definitive radiotherapy in the management of chemodectomas arising in the temporal bone, carotid body, and glomus vagale. Head Neck 23:363–371

Jackson CG, Glasscock ME III, Harris PF (1982) Glomus tumors: diagnosis, classification, and management of large lesions. Arch Otolaryngol 108:401–406

Konefal JB, Pilepich MV, Spector GJH et al (1987) Radiation therapy in the treatment of chemodectomas. Laryngoscope 97:1331–1335

Larner JM, Hahn SS, Spaulding CA et al (1992) Glomus jugulare tumors: long-term control by radiation therapy. Cancer 69:1813–1817

LeVay J, O'Sullivan B, Catton C et al (1994) An assessment of prognostic factors in soft tissue sarcoma of the head and neck. Arch Otolaryngol Head Neck Surg 120:981–986

Lybeert MLM, Van Andel JG, Eijkenboom WMH et al (1984) Radiotherapy of paragangliomas. Clin Otolaryngol 9:105–109

Mendenhall WM, Million RR, Parsons JT et al (1986) Chemodectoma of the carotid body and ganglion nodosum treated with radiation therapy. Int J Radiat Oncol Biol Phys 12:2175–2178

Perez CA, Thorstad WL (2008) Unusual non-epithelial tumors of the head and neck. In: Halperin EC, Perez CA, Brady LW (eds) Perez and Brady's principles and practice of radiation oncology, 5th edn. Wolters Kluwer Lippincott Williams & Wilkins, Philadelphia, p 996

Powell S, Peters N, Harmer C (1992) Chemodectoma of the head and neck: results of treatment in 84 patients. Int J Radiat Oncol Biol Phys 22:919–924

Pryzant RM, Chou JL, Easley JD (1989) Twenty year experience with radiation therapy for temporal bone chemodectomas. Int J Radiat Oncol Biol Phys 17:1303–1307

Springate SC, Weichselbaum RR (1990) Radiation or surgery for chemodectoma of the temporal bone: a review of local control and complications. Head Neck 12:303–307

Wang M-L, Hussey DH, Doornbos JF et al (1988) Chemodectoma of the temporal bone: a comparison of surgical and radiotherapeutic results. Int J Radiat Oncol Biol Phys 14:643–648

Gorlin-Gotz Syndrome

▶ Basal Cell Nevus Syndrome

Granulomatous Disease

Jo Ann Chalal
Department of Radiation Oncology, Fox Chase Cancer Center, Philadelphia, PA, USA

Definition

Genetically heterogeneous group of immunodeficiencies causing recurrent bouts of infection due to compromised immune systems.

Cross-References

▶ Multiple Myeloma

Gross Tumor Volume (GTV)

Brandon J. Fisher[1], Larry C. Daugherty[2]
[1]Department of Radiation Oncology, College of Medicine, Drexel University, Philadelphia, PA, USA
[2]Department of Radiation Oncology, College of Medicine, Drexel University, Glenside, PA, USA

Definition

The volume that includes palpable, visible, or demonstrable extent of a tumor. It may consist of the primary tumor, metastatic disease, or lymphadenopathy. The GTV usually represents the part of the malignant growth where the tumor cell density is the largest.

Cross-References

▶ Nasopharynx

Gynecological Tumors

Carsten Nieder
Radiation Oncology Unit, Nordlandssykehuset HF, Bodoe, Norway

Synonyms

TAH-BSO

Definition

Gynecological tumors are a group of pelvic origin malignancies presenting in approximately 11% of females (Dehdusht and Siegal 2011).

Cross-References

▶ Fallopian Tube
▶ Ovary
▶ Total Body Irradiation (TBI)
▶ Uterine Cervix
▶ Vagina

References

Dehdusht and Siegal (2011) Gynecologic tumors, Chapter 11.8, A Journal for Clinicians, Springer, ACS, Atlanta

H

γH2AX Foci Analysis

CLAUDIA E. RÜBE
Department of Radiation Oncology, Saarland
University, Homburg/Saar, Germany

Definition
Histon H2AX is phosporylated rapidly in response to DNA double-strand breaks (DSB), leading to the formation of nuclear foci visualized by immunocytochemical detection of γH2AX. γH2AX analysis is an exquisitely sensitive technique to monitor DSB repair, amenable for use with very low doses.

Cross-References
▶ Predictive In vitro Assays in Radiation Oncology

HAART

BERNADINE R. DONAHUE[1], JAY S. COOPER[2]
[1]Department of Radiation Oncology,
Maimonides Cancer Center, Brooklyn, NY, USA
[2]Maimonides Cancer Center, New York, NY, USA

Definition
Highly active antiretroviral therapy. It primarily consisted of a two-drug nucleoside analogue administered with either a protease inhibitor or a non-nucleoside reverse transcriptase inhibitor. Other classes of drugs employed for treatment of HIV include integrase inhibitors, entry inhibitors, maturation inhibitors, and AntiViral HyperActivation Limiting Therapeutics (AV-HALTs).

Cross-References
▶ cART
▶ Malignant Neoplasms Associated with Acquired Immunodeficiency Syndrome

Hairy Cell Leukemia

CASPIAN OLIAI
Department of Radiation Oncology, College of Medicine, Drexel University, Philadelphia, PA, USA

Definition
An uncommon mature B-cell malignancy that is not included in the four major categories of leukemia. It has a characteristic presentation of pancytopenia, splenomegaly, and circulating "hairy cells" in the bone marrow and hematopoietic organs. The name refers to the cytoplasmic projections resembling hair when seen under the microscope. Comprises up to 2% of all leukemias and highly favors males with a 5:1 male-to-female ratio.

Cross-References
▶ Hodgkin's Lymphoma
▶ Leukemia in General

L.W. Brady, T.E. Yaeger (eds.), *Encyclopedia of Radiation Oncology*, DOI 10.1007/978-3-540-85516-3,
© Springer-Verlag Berlin Heidelberg 2013

Half-Life

YAN YU, LAURA DOYLE
Department of Radiation Oncology, Thomas
Jefferson University Hospital, Philadelphia,
PA, USA

Definition
Length of time for the initial amount of
radioactive material to decrease to half the
original amount.

Cross-References
▶ Brachytherapy: Low Dose Rate (LDR)
Permanent Implants (Prostate)

Hedgehog Pathway Inhibition

RENE RUBIN
Rittenhouse Hematology/Oncology,
Philadelphia, PA, USA

Definition
The hedgehog pathway (adult stem cell regulation) is important for the growth of embryo-
genic and adult cells. Malfunctions may cause
basal cell carcinomas. Vismodegib, an oral medication, appears to modulate the deregulated
pathway and may be used in the treatment
of metastatic or locally advanced basal cell
carcinoma.

Side Effects
- Birth defects (both in men and women)
- Fatigue
- Muscle spasms
- Alopecia
- Diarrhea

Cross-References
▶ Principles of Chemotherapy

Helical CT

DAREK MICHALSKI[1], M. SAIFUL HUQ[2]
[1]Division of Medical Physics, Department of
Radiation Oncology, University of Pittsburgh
Cancer Centers, Pittsburgh,
PA, USA
[2]Department of Radiation Oncology, University
of Pittsburgh Medical Center Cancer Pavilion,
Pittsburgh, PA, USA

Definition
A volume scanning mode in non-planar geometry
with patient being scanned continuously in space
and in time.

Cross-References
▶ Four-Dimensional (4D) Treatment Planning/
Respiratory Gating

Helicobacter (H.) pylori

FILIP T. TROICKI[1], JAGANMOHAN POLI[2]
[1]College of Medicine, Drexel University,
Philadelphia, PA, USA
[2]Department of Radiation Oncology, College of
Medicine, Drexel University, Philadelphia,
PA, USA

Definition
Bacteria shown to cause breakdown of the protective coating of the stomach that can lead to stomach

inflammation (gastritis), stomach ulcers, or even stomach cancer.

Cross-References

▶ Stomach Cancer

Hemangioblastomas

▶ Spinal Canal Tumor

Hemangiopericytomas

CARLOS A. PEREZ, WADE L. THORSTAD
Department of Radiation Oncology, Siteman Cancer Center, Washington University Medical Center, St. Louis, MO, USA

Definition

Rare tumor arising from the perivascular supportive "Pericytes of Zimmerman" that morphologically resemble smooth muscle and believed to provide mechanical support for contractile function of capillaries.

Hemangiopericytomas (HPCs) are rare soft-tissue neoplasms that account for 3–5% of all soft-tissue sarcomas and 1% of all vascular tumors. Some 15–30% of all hemangiopericytomas occur in the head and neck (Perez and Thorstad 2008).

Epidemiology

HPC is an unusual tumor; it occurs in both genders with equal frequency and is found primarily in adults. In the head and neck, the most common sites are the nasal cavity and the paranasal sinuses, followed by the orbital region, the parotid gland, and the neck (Palacios et al. 2005).

Clinical Presentation

Soft-tissue hemangiopericytoma is a firm, painless, slowly expanding mass that is often nodular and well localized (Espat et al. 2002). In the head and neck, the tumor may cause nasal obstruction or epistaxis. Orbital hemangiopericytomas account for 3% of orbital malignancies and most frequently occur with painless proptosis. Hemangiopericytomas may occur intracranially and they carry a high risk of local failure (80%), as well as higher potential for dissemination.

The incidence of metastasis, which depends on the site of origin, can be 50–80%. Late metastases occurring 10 years after diagnosis are not uncommon.

Diagnostic Workup

On plain radiographs, hemangiopericytoma appears as a soft-tissue mass in the nasal cavity or other portions of the head and neck. A defect caused by pressure erosion of the surrounding bones may occur, and calcifications are rare. On arteriography, hemangiopericytoma features include radially arranged or spiderlike branching vessels around and inside the tumor and a long-standing, well-demarcated tumor stain, with high hypervascularity which may be demonstrated with contrast-enhanced CT (Palacios et al. 2005). Intracranially, the diffusely enhancing tumor may closely resemble a meningioma on CT. Both CT and MRI scans are of special value in the delineation of the full extent of the tumor.

General Management

Complete surgical resection, if possible, combined with preoperative embolization of the tumor, is the treatment of choice. More extensive surgery is required in tumors that show features of malignancy. Many patients undergo surgical treatment after embolization of the feeding artery(ies).

For incompletely resected tumors, postoperative radiation therapy is used. The role of chemotherapy in this tumor is not well determined; a few reports have described partial tumor regression in some lesions treated with cytotoxic agents. Doxorubicin (Adriamycin), alone or in combination is the most effective agent for metastatic hemangiopericytoma, producing complete and partial remissions in 50% of cases. Other drugs prescribed when metastasis occurs are cyclophosphamide, dacarbazine, vincristine, and actinomycin-D.

Radiation Therapy

Irradiation alone in the management of hemangiopericytoma is controversial. The main role of irradiation is as an adjuvant after complete excision of the lesion or postoperatively for minimal residual disease (Espat et al. 2002; Mantravadi 1986). The tumor has been considered relatively radioresistant. Tumor doses of 60–65 Gy in 6–7 weeks are required to produce local tumor control in postoperative cases (Perez and Thorstad 2008). The target volume to be irradiated should be wide, to encompass the tumor bed with a margin of at least 5 cm to safely avoid marginal recurrence. Portal arrangement and beam selection are similar to those used in treatment of malignant brain tumors or soft-tissue sarcomas.

Results of Therapy

Spitz and colleagues (1998) published a report on 36 patients with hemangiopericytoma. Median follow-up was 57 months. Twenty-eight patients (78%) underwent complete potentially curative resection. Of the nine patients (32%) who had local recurrences, four had epidural tumors and three had retroperitoneal tumors, but none had extremity tumors. Ten patients (28%) had recurrences at distant sites. Of the 13 patients who experienced a recurrence, 4 had recurrences after a disease-free interval of more than 5 years. The 5-year actuarial survival rate for the entire group of 36 patients was 71%.

Cross-References

▶ Eye and Orbit
▶ Nasal Cavity and Paranasal Sinuses
▶ Salivary Gland Cancer
▶ Sarcomas of the Head and Neck
▶ Sinonasal Cancer

References

Espat NJ, Lewis JJ, Leung D et al (2002) Conventional hemangiopericytoma: modern analysis of outcome. Cancer 95:1746–1751

Mantravadi RVP (1986) Radiation therapy for nonsquamous tumors of the head and neck. Otolaryngol Clin North Am 19:741–754

Palacios E, Restrepo S, Mastrogiovanni L et al (2005) Sinonasal hemangiopericytomas: clinicopathologic and imaging findings. Ear Nose Throat J 84: 99–102

Perez CA, Thorstad WL (2008) Unusual non-epithelial tumors of the head and neck. In: Halperin EC, Perez CA, Brady LW (eds) Perez and Brady's principles and practice of radiation oncology, 5th edn. Wolters Kluwer/Lippincott Williams & Wilkins, Philadelphia, pp 996–1034

Spitz FR, Bouvet M, Pisters PW et al (1998) Hemangiopericytoma: A 20-year single institution experience. Ann Surg Oncol 5:350–55

Hematogenous Spread

Filip T. Troicki[1], Jaganmohan Poli[2]
[1]College of Medicine, Drexel University, Philadelphia, PA, USA
[2]Department of Radiation Oncology, College of Medicine, Drexel University, Philadelphia, PA, USA

Definition

Spread through the blood.

Hematologic Nadir

Lindsay G. Jensen, Brent S. Rose
Arno J. Mundt
Center for Advanced Radiotherapy Technologies,
Department of Radiation Oncology, San Diego
Rebecca and John Moores Cancer Center,
University of California, La Jolla, CA, USA

Definition
The lowest value in a series of peripheral blood
cell count measurements.

Cross-References
▶ Bone Marrow Toxicity in Cancer Treatment

Hematologic System

Lindsay G. Jensen, Brent S. Rose
Arno J. Mundt
Center for Advanced Radiotherapy Technologies,
Department of Radiation Oncology, San Diego
Rebecca and John Moores Cancer Center,
University of California, La Jolla, CA, USA

Definition
The cells, tissues, and organs responsible for the
production and maintenance of blood and blood
cells.

Cross-References
▶ Bone Marrow Toxicity in Cancer Treatment

Hematologically Active Bone Marrow

Lindsay G. Jensen, Brent S. Rose
Arno J. Mundt
Center for Advanced Radiotherapy Technologies,
Department of Radiation Oncology, San Diego
Rebecca and John Moores Cancer Center,
University of California, La Jolla, CA, USA

Definition
Bone marrow that contributes to the development of new blood cells.

Cross-References
▶ Bone Marrow Toxicity in Cancer Treatment

Hematopoiesis

Lindsay G. Jensen[1], Brent S. Rose[1]
Arno J. Mundt[1], Caspian Oliai[2]
[1]Center for Advanced Radiotherapy
Technologies, Department of Radiation
Oncology, San Diego Rebecca and John Moores
Cancer Center, University of California, La Jolla,
CA, USA
[2]Department of Radiation Oncology, College of
Medicine, Drexel University, Philadelphia,
PA, USA

Definition
The formation of blood cellular components.
All blood cell components are derived from
▶ hematopoietic stem cells (HSC) which begin
differentiation while in the bone marrow. HSC

are multipotent and can differentiate into the myeloid lineage: monocytes/macrophages, neutrophils, basophils, eosinophils, erythrocytes, megakaryocytes/platelets, dendritic cells; and the lymphoid lineage: T-cells, B-cells, NK-cells.

Cross-References

▶ Bone Marrow Toxicity in Cancer Treatment
▶ Leukemia in General

Hematopoietic Neoplasms

▶ Leukemia in General

Hematopoietic Stem Cells

LINDSAY G. JENSEN, BRENT S. ROSE, ARNO J. MUNDT
Center for Advanced Radiotherapy Technologies, Department of Radiation Oncology, San Diego Rebecca and John Moores Cancer Center, University of California, La Jolla, CA, USA

Definition

Cells that give rise to lymphoid and myeloid precursor cells which develop into mature blood cells.

Cross-References

▶ Bone Marrow Toxicity in Cancer Treatment

Hepatic Metastasis

▶ Palliation of Metastatic Disease to the Liver

Hepatic Portal System

FILIP T. TROICKI[1], JAGANMOHAN POLI[2]
[1]College of Medicine, Drexel University, Philadelphia, PA, USA
[2]Department of Radiation Oncology, College of Medicine, Drexel University, Philadelphia, PA, USA

Definition

Large collection of veins that drain the gastrointestinal tract which pass through the liver before entering into the heart to be oxygenated.

Hepatocellular Carcinoma

▶ Hepatic Portal System
▶ Liver and Hepatobiliary Tract

Hepatoma

▶ Liver and Hepatobiliary Tract

Her-2

ANTHONY E. DRAGUN
Department of Radiation Oncology, James Graham Brown Cancer Center, University of Louisville School of Medicine, Louisville, KY, USA

Synonyms

ERBB2; Human epidermal growth factor receptor type II; Neu oncogene

Definition

Her-2 is an oncogene amplified in many human breast cancers, resulting in an overexpression of a tyrosine kinase that ultimately enhances tumor growth, invasion, and angiogenesis. Its presence is detected on routine pathologic specimens by immunohistochemitry and/or fluorescent in-situ hybridization (FISH) techniques. Its presence allows a use of novel, targeted systemic agents such as anti Her-2 antibodies (trastuzumab) or small molecular tyrosine kinase inhibitors (lapatinib). These targeted therapies have improved outcomes in the adjuvant and metastatic settings in patients with Her-2-positive breast cancer.

Cross-References

▶ Cancer of the Breast
▶ Early-Stage Breast Cancer
▶ Esophageal Cancer
▶ Locally Advanced and Recurrent Disease
▶ Molecular Markers in Clinical Radiation Oncology
▶ Principles of Chemotherapy
▶ Stage 0 Breast Cancer

Her-2 Inhibitors

RENE RUBIN
Rittenhouse Hematology/Oncology,
Philadelphia, PA, USA

Definition

All Her-2 inhibitors are monoclonal antibodies against her 2-neu human epidermal growth factor receptor Trastuzumab (trade name "Herceptin"). It downregulates the expression of Her-2neu receptors and inhibits the Her-2neu intracellular signaling pathways. Lapatinib blocks Her-1 and Her-2 receptors. TDM-1, which is not yet approved, is Herceptin conjugated to a potent toxin that can be delivered intracellularly without toxicity to non-Her-2-amplified cells. Pertuzumab is another novel Her-2 receptor inhibitor. It inhibits Her-2 dimerization of Her-2 to other "Her-like" receptors. Trastuzumab is currently approved for adjuvant and metastatic breast carcinoma. However, it is effective in Her-2 positive gastric carcinoma and probably all tumors that prove to have Her-2 overexpression. The other drugs are currently under investigation and may be used in metastatic breast carcinoma that has failed other regimens or is indicated for Trastuzumab-resistant tumors.

Side Effects

- Diarrhea
- Rash
- Heart failure

Cross-References

▶ Principles of Chemotherapy

Herbalism

▶ Complementary Medicine

Hereditary Leiomyomatosis Renal Cell Carcinoma

STEPHAN MOSE
Department of Radiation Oncology,
Schwarzwald-Baar-Klinikum,
Villingen-Schwenningen, Germany

Definition

This tumor (FH gene, chromosome 1q42-43) is classified as type 2 papillary renal cell carcinoma associated with leiomyomas of skin or uterus and uterus leiomyosarcomas.

Cross-References
► Kidney
► Uterine Cervix

Hereditary Nonpolyposis Colorectal Cancer (HNPCC)

CHRISTIN A. KNOWLTON[1], MICHELLE KOLTON MACKAY[2], BRADLEY J. HUTH[3], CLAUS ROEDEL[4]
[1]Department of Radiation Oncology, Drexel University, Philadelphia, PA, USA
[2]Department of Radiation Oncology, Marshfield Clinic, Marshfield, WI, USA
[3]Department of Radiation Oncology, Philadelphia, PA, USA
[4]Department of Radiotherapy and Radiation Oncology, University Hospital Frankfurt/Main, Frankfurt, Germany

Synonyms
Lynch syndrome

Definition
Hereditary non-polyposis colorectal cancer (HNPCC) syndrome, also referred to as Lynch syndrome, is an autosomal-dominant, genetically inherited disorder that places patients at a higher incidence of several cancers including colorectal, endometrial, and ovarian cancers. HNPCC syndrome is caused by mutations in one of five DNA mismatch repair genes. The resulting deficiency in repair contributes to the malignant transformation of cells. This is an autosomal dominant genetic condition at high risk of colorectal as well as other cancers including endometrium, ovary, stomach, small intestine, among others. The increased risk for these cancers is due to inherited mutations that impair DNA mismatch repair.

Cross-References
► FAP
► Ovary

Hereditary Papillary Renal Carcinoma

STEPHAN MOSE
Department of Radiation Oncology, Schwarzwald-Baar-Klinikum, Villingen-Schwenningen, Germany

Definition
This tumor (C-Met proto-oncogene, chromosome 7q31-34) is classified as type 1 papillary renal cell carcinoma.

Cross-References
► Kidney

Hereditary Renal Cell Cancer Syndromes

STEPHAN MOSE
Department of Radiation Oncology, Schwarzwald-Baar-Klinikum, Villingen-Schwenningen, Germany

Definition
These syndromes include various autosomal dominant diseases with a different genetic basis and phenotype which are characterized by the possible development and diagnosis of a renal cell carcinoma.

Cross-References
► Kidney

High-Dose Rate (HDR) Brachytherapy

ERIK VAN LIMBERGEN
Department of Radiation Oncology, University Hospital Gasthuisberg, Leuven, Belgium

Definition
The dose is delivered by a stepping source afterloader loaded with 370 GBq Iridium-192 or 74 GBq Cobalt-60 at a dose rate >12 Gy.h^{-1} (>0.2 Gy/min). As in external beam irradiation, enough time is kept in between fractions (>6 h) to allow for full repair. Radiobiological effects are strongly dependent on fraction size, which should be kept low enough in order to avoid exceeding the tolerance dose of irradiated normal tissues. Therefore, the dose is delivered in 1 to several fractions depending on the total dose needed and the body site. Fractions can be delivered to ambulatory patients in many cases.

Cross-References
▶ Clinical Aspects of Brachytherapy (BT)
▶ High-Dose Rate (HDR) Brachytherapy
▶ Low-Dose Rate (LDR) Brachytherapy

High-Risk Neuroblastoma

BRANDON J. FISHER[1], LARRY C. DAUGHERTY[2]
[1]Department of Radiation Oncology, College of Medicine, Drexel University, Philadelphia, PA, USA
[2]Department of Radiation Oncology, College of Medicine, Drexel University, Glenside, PA, USA

Definition
Neuroblastoma in any patient with N-*myc* amplification, patients over the age of 1 year, unfavorable histology, or DNA index of 1 or less.

Cross-References
▶ Neuroblastoma

Histone Deacetylase Inhibitors

RENE RUBIN
Rittenhouse Hematology/Oncology, Philadelphia, PA, USA

Definition
Histone deacetylase inhibitors (Vorinostat) induce cell cycle arrest. They are used in cutaneous T-cell lymphoma (CTCL).

Side Effects
- Nausea
- Myelosuppression
- Fatigue
- QT prolongation
- Hyperglycemia

Cross-References
▶ Principles of Chemotherapy

Histones

TOD W. SPEER
Department of Human Oncology, University of Wisconsin School of Medicine and Public Health, UW Hospital and Clinics, Madison, WI, USA

Definition
Alkaline proteins that are found in eukaryotic cell nuclei and are involved in the packaging and organization of DNA into units termed nucleosomes.

Cross-References
▶ Targeted Radioimmunotherapy

History of Radiation Oncology

HANS-PETER HEILMANN
Director of the Hermann-Holthusen-Institute for Radiotherapy, St. George's Hospital, Hamburg, from 1976 to 2000, Hamburg, Germany

Introduction

"Radiotherapy (radio-oncology), surgery and chemotherapy are the three pillars of successful cancer treatment. Radiotherapy, alone or with surgery, is responsible for nearly half of all cured cancer patients." This statement was made by the "Deutsche Forschungsgemeinschaft" (German Association on Scientific Research) in 1980 and was confirmed by the Alberta Cancer Registry, located in Canada, in 1989.

It has been a long road from the first experiments with newly discovered X-rays in 1895 to the efficacy of radiological cancer treatment today. Bernier et al. (2004) divide the development into four periods and schools: the German school, from 1900 to 1920; the French school, from 1920 to 1940; the British school, from 1940 to 1960; and the United States and European school, from 1970 to present.

Beginnings: 1895–1920

Shortly after the discovery of the "Roentgenstrahlen" (X-rays) by W.C. Röntgen in 1895 (Case 1958), the first observations on the therapeutic effects of this newly discovered radiation were published. In 1897 in Vienna, L. Freund, published a paper detailing his successful treatment of a young girl with a naevus pigmentosus piliferus. In 1896, the first treatment of a breast cancer with ulceration was performed by Emil Grubbe in Chicago. Various other authors published instances of treatment of carcinomas, psoriasis, sarcomas, mycosis fungoides, and leukemia. In 1898, Albers-Schönberg, Hamburg, and others treated the lupus erythematodes successfully with X-rays. During this period, tuberculosis was also treated with X-rays. One female patient who was treated at this time for tuberculosis by Albers-Schönberg at St. George's Hospital, Hamburg, developed a so-called postcricoid carcinoma in the neck region 60 years later. Her original therapy charts were still available at the hospital and she was successfully treated with high-energy X-rays of a betatron (Heilmann 1970).

In 1900 in Stockholm, Thor Stenbeck, cured the first patient with skin cancer with fractionated therapy. In 1902, Pusey from the United States published several cases cured by X-rays, including carcinomas, sarcomas, and breast cancers. In 1903, Cleaves reported the first case of cancer of the cervix cured by X-rays, and Senn irradiated lymph nodes in chronic lymphatic leukemia and the spleen in chronic myelocytic leukemia.

In 1904, Perthes, a surgeon from Tuebingen, Germany, published histological examinations on the effect of X-ray treatment of breast cancer and skin carcinomas. He stated that the tumor had been replaced by connecting tissue. In 1905, Beck discovered the effect of X-rays on hyperthyroidism, and Albers-Schönberg from Hamburg, during the first congress of the "Deutsche Röntgengesellschaft" (German Roentgen Society), demonstrated the cure of a patient with a sarcoma of the skin of the head who was treated and cured by X-rays. The tumor disappeared after 28 treatment visits over a 3-month period.

In 1898, Henry Becquerel discovered natural radioactivity and in Paris, Marie and Pierre Curie, discovered radium. Alpha-, beta-, and gamma-rays were identified in 1900. In 1901 in Paris, Danlos and Bloch treated lupus erythematodes with local application of a sealed radium source. In 1905 in the United States, R. Abbe was the first to use interstitial application of radium needles into tumors.

There were many problems in the beginning of radiotherapy. One was how to bring an efficient radiation dose to the proper depth. In 1904, Perthes and Levy-Dorn invented the cross-fire method, treating the tumor from different directions. In 1906, Pohl for the first time discussed the possibility of rotational therapy. Another problem was how to measure the amount of radiation given to the patient. In 1902, Holzknecht invented the first dosimeter for X-rays, which he called the "chromoradiometer." In the following years other dosimeters were developed by Bordier in France, Hampson et al. in Vienna, Schwarz in Germany, and Kienböck in Austria.

A great technical step forward was made in the United States in 1912 with the development by William Coolidge of the "hot-cathode tube," with a tungsten filament heated by a low-voltage circuit (Buschke 1970). These tubes revolutionized radiology. To diminish the amount of X-rays of low energy causing skin reaction, Pagenstecher and coworkers from Heidelberg, Germany, introduced the filtration of X-rays. Another important observation was made in 1912: Schwarz demonstrated that, with pressure of a tube of an X-ray machine tight to the skin, blood flow was diminished and the radiation reaction of the skin was less severe. This was the first indication of the importance of oxygen in radiation treatment.

Until the 1920s, single-dose treatment was favored in several countries, especially Germany (e.g., by Krönig and Friedrich). In 1914, however, Schwarz, also in Germany, demonstrated the better effect of daily small doses over treatment with a single dose. Unfortunately, this was unknown outside of Germany because of World War I.

In 1906, the "Law of Bergonié und Tribondeau" was published in France. It stated that cells tend to be radiosensitive if they have three properties: a high division rate, a long dividing future, and an unspecialized phenotype. This law had great influence on radiotherapy, but later it became clear that it is not absolutely valid.

In the meantime, the negative effects of the X-rays were becoming obvious. At the 1909 congress of the German Roentgen Society, the sequelae of X-ray treatment were discussed for the first time. Albers-Schönberg, Hamburg, gave a report on the X-ray-induced metastatic cancer of his own hand.

An X-ray machine from 1918 is shown in Fig. 1.

The Second Period: 1920–1940

The limited ability of conventional X-rays to penetrate the tissue spurred multiple efforts to invent new ways of generating radiation. Thus, in 1925 Coolidge introduced a 300-kV tube, and shortly afterward 400-kV generators became available. It was generally agreed that radiation at 500 kV or higher should be designated supervoltage, and in the decade between 1930 and 1940 various supervoltage equipment, varying from 700 to 1,000 kV, was installed in hospitals in the United States and London.

Soon, the importance of the distribution of X-rays in the tissue became clear. Between 1920 and 1925 the first "isodose distribution diagrams" were published by Glasser, Coliez, and Failla.

At the end of the 1920s, R. Wideröe developed the "betatron formula" to construct a circular accelerator. In the United States, France, and Belgium "teleradium therapy" machines, 3–10 g, with a short source-skin distance, were developed. For the first time the build-up effect allowing skin sparing was used. However, these machines were not practical for cancer treatment because of the treatment time of several hours. Telegamma-units became popular after artificial radioactive sources were available in the 1950s. Siemens and Halske, Berlin, presented at the 1922 Congress of the German Roentgen Society an automatic voltage regulation for X-ray tubes, necessary because one of the main technical difficulties of that time was the inconsistency of voltage.

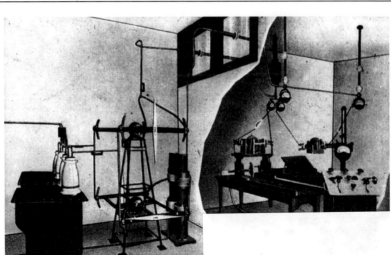

History of Radiation Oncology. Fig. 1 X-ray machine

In addition to technical developments, the main topic of the period was the question of single-dose treatment versus fractionated treatment. As reported, single-dose treatment was favored by many centers until 1920. Then, H. Coutard performed fractionated X-ray treatments at the Paris Radium Institute in 1921 and 1922. He demonstrated his good results and minor sequelae in treating head and neck tumors with fractionated radiotherapy at the American Congress of Roentgenology in 1932. Coutard's meticulous follow-up of his patients is especially notable.

Many institutions began to give up on single dose treatment. Schinz reported good results in 1929–1930 in Zurich with fractionated treatment of tumors of the upper respiratory and gastrointestinal tract. In Hamburg, Holthusen pleaded for fractionated radiotherapy but made clear that the total dose should be elevated, and the gynecological departments of Kiel and Gießen, Germany, used fractionated treatment in cancers of the cervix and the uterus. Thus, in the 1930s, there was consensus in favor of fractionated treatments in

with the radiation dose. The art of radiation therapy consists of finding the optimal dose for cure with only a minimum of side effects.

Technical developments also proceeded. In 1933, the Van de Graaff generator (with 200 kV) was constructed. Also in 1933, the cyclotron, with 5,000 kV, was invented by Lawrence and Livingstone, and in Berlin, Chaoul, at the Charité, developed the method of X-ray treatment with short distance for small volumes (Röntgen-Nahbestrahlung, Fig. 2). The first working betatron was constructed in 1935 in Berlin by M. Steenbeck for Siemens-Schuckert, but it was never manufactured. In 1940, D.W. Kerst, at the University of Illinois in the United States, constructed a betatron based on the 1929 work of Wideröe.

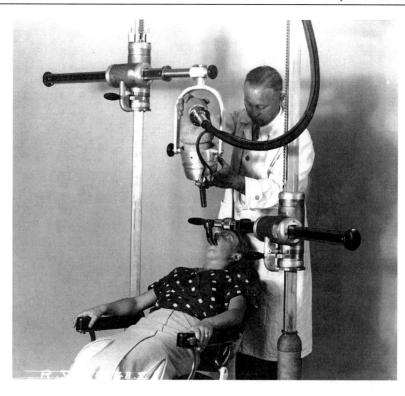

History of Radiation Oncology. Fig. 2 Machine for X-ray treatment with short distance for small volumes (Röntgen-Nahbestrahlung), developed by Chaoul

During this period, technical development in Germany was behind that in the United States because of the political situation. Therefore, rotational treatment techniques were developed and were a popular method for concentrating radiation dose at a target. For example, Du Mesnil de Rochemont published a method of rotational therapy, as did Neumann, Wachsman, and others.

The exact measurement of the X-rays remained a primary problem of radiology. The definition of the "Roentgen" as a unit for radiation measurement was therefore a milestone in the history of radiology. At the 1928 General Assembly of the Second International Congress of Radiology, it was proposed that an international unit of X-radiation be adopted and that it should be called a "roentgen," designated by the small "r" (later "R"). It was based on ionization and was accepted all over the world. In 1937, the definition and standard were altered somewhat to include X-ray and gamma radiation.

Another dosage system for gamma-ray therapy was developed by the English radiologist Paterson and the American-English physicist Parker in 1934.

During this period, various techniques for treating cervical and uterine cancer with radium were developed. In 1917, the "*Stockholm method*" of treating cervical cancer was created by Forssell and Heyman. This method utilizes the uterus and vagina as vehicles for carrying a combination of intrauterine and vaginal radium, selected individually for each patient. It is characterized by short application of high-intensity radium sources repeated two or three times, separated by a 3-week interval.

The "*Paris technique*" (1926), developed by Regaud, uses low-intensity radium treatment over a relatively long period of time, usually for 1 week. Intravaginal sources are placed in a colpostat comprising two impermeable cork cylinders, banded by a metal spring. A central source was used in some patients.

The "*Hamburg technique*" (Anna Hamann and coworkers 1934) uses elements from the Paris and Stockholm techniques for intrauterine application, with a vaginal applicator of the Stockholm-type being used. The applicators are fixed by gauze packing, which allows for distance from the rectum and bladder.

The "*Manchester technique*," originated in 1938 by Tod and Meredith and later modified, uses hard rubber ovoids held apart by a washer or spacer. An intrauterine tandem was associated. The treatment was separated into two fractions over a period of 10 days.

The "*Munich technique*" (Eymer and Ries 1941) uses a fixed combination of intrauterine and vaginal applicators. The vaginal applicator is shaped like a circle, with different sizes allowing for individualization of application.

Later, in 1953, the "*Houston technique*" was developed by Fletcher and Suit. They used a tandem with two ovoids that could be customized to fit the location of the uterus in space. There was no fixation between the ovoids and the uterine tandem. A manual afterloading procedure was developed, and not only radium, but also cesium-137 was used.

For the treatment of carcinomas of the endometrium. Heyman developed in 1936 the "*multicapsule packing technique*" with radium. In 1944, Ries, of Munich, designed "*radium eggs*," and in 1952 in Germany, Becker, Scheer, and Gauwerky used cobalt pearls on a wire instead of radium for the packing method.

In 1923, the Scandinavians Lysholm and Stentstrom used radium needles and tubes for interstitial tumor treatment. These techniques were often used in the 1920s and 1930s. Later, different isotopes and afterloading replaced these methods of interstitial treatment.

A special event took place in 1936. Hans Meyer, a German radiologist, donated the "Roentgen-Ehrenmal," a cenotaph for victims of radiation built at St. George's Hospital, Hamburg, to the German Roentgen Society (Fig. 3). At the time of the first application of X-rays and radium, the risks of these new possibilities were unknown. Therefore, many people were severely injured or died from sequelae of radiation. The names of all known victims of the use of radiation are documented on this monument, with a text in their honor. This monument exists today (Fig. 4) and is visited by doctors, physicists, technicians, and nurses from all over the world. The names on this monument were published in 1937 in the *Book of Honor of Roentgenologists and Radiologists of All Nations* (Holthusen and Meyer 1959). One year earlier, P. Brown edited *American Martyrs to Science through the Roentgen-Rays*. He would later also die from X-ray damage.

Diagnostic radiology and radiotherapy are not immune from political influence, even today. Beginning in 1933 there was massive pressure on medicine by the Nazi regime. At that time, many Jewish radiologists were imprisoned by the Nazis and some Jewish radiologists left Germany. Anna Hamann, originally from Hamburg, became a famous therapeutic radiologist in the United States. A fellowship was named in her honor. The Nazis also passed a law allowing sterilization by X-rays in cases of hereditary diseases. Many therapeutic radiologists objected to this law and were not willing to use radiotherapy for this purpose (Heilmann 1996).

A picture of an X-ray machine from this period is shown in Fig. 5.

The Third Period: 1940–1960

This period is characterized by the development of different machines for megavoltage therapy.

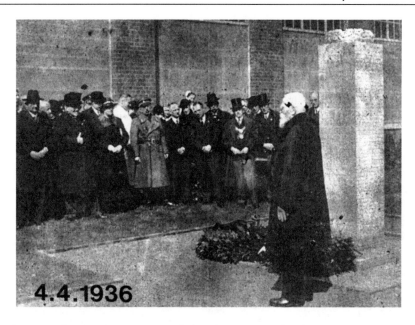

History of Radiation Oncology. Fig. 3 Cenotaph for the victims of radiation (Röntgen-Ehrenmal) in St. George's Hospital, Hamburg, dedication in 1936

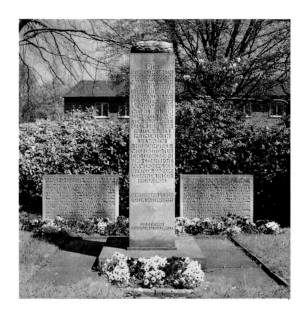

History of Radiation Oncology. Fig. 4 Cenotaph for the victims of radiation (Röntgen-Ehrenmal) in St. George's Hospital, Hamburg, present day

In comparison with conventional X-ray treatment, megavoltage offered the advantage of much higher depth doses, the build-up effect, and the potential to calculate dose distribution by computers. The first dose calculations by computers were reported by Tsien in 1955 and by Richter and Schirrmeister, East Berlin, in 1964.

In 1944, during World War II, the construction of a 6 MeV and 15 MeV betatrons in Erlangen, in association with Siemens, took place. At the end of World War II, the Nazis planned to destroy the betatrons, but the British military government together with German engineers prevented this. In 1947, the first working betatron was realized in Göttingen. This machine is exhibited today at the Smithsonian Institution in Washington, DC. In 1951, the Swiss company Brown, Boveri and Cie (BBC) constructed betatrons with 31 MeV, and Siemens constructed betatrons with more than 40 MeV. Those machines, with 18 MeV (Fig. 6) or more than 30 MeV (Fig. 7), were very popular, especially in Germany, because many radiologists at that time believed in a different biological effectiveness of electrons. Unfortunately, there was a severe accident in 1971 with an 18-MeV betatron at St. George's Hospital in Hamburg.

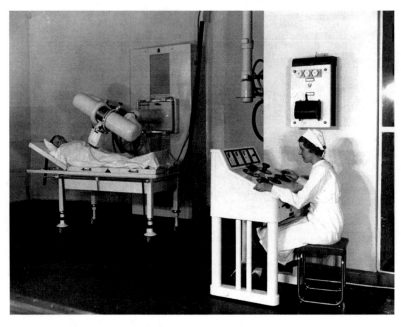

History of Radiation Oncology. Fig. 5 Tuto-Stabilivolt machine for X-ray treatment

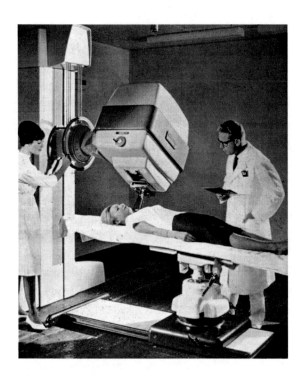

History of Radiation Oncology. Fig. 6 18 MeV betatron manufactured by Siemens

A filter for scattering electrons fell out of the filter support and an unattenuated electron beam hit the patients. Several patients died and there were severe sequelae in the survivors. This accident had a major influence on legal regulations for radiotherapy. In the 1970s, there were about 200 betatrons worldwide, but the production of these machines was halted because of their disadvantages in comparison with linear accelerators.

Another development took place in Great Britain. Before and during the World War II, microwave technology was developed for radar use. Based on this technology, a traveling wave linear accelerator (linac) was described in 1947 by Fry and coworkers and was first installed at the Hammersmith Hospital in 1953. It produced X-rays of 8,000 kV. A 4 MeV linear accelerator was installed in 1953 at Newcastle Hospital. In the United States, a 6 MV accelerator was constructed in 1956 at the Stanford Microwave Laboratory by W.W. Hansen and installed at

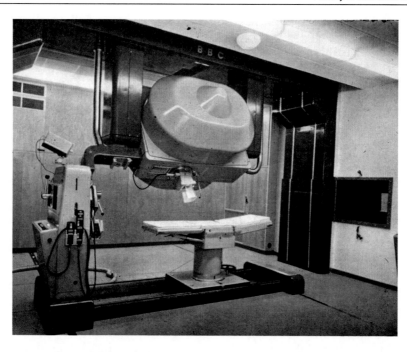

History of Radiation Oncology. Fig. 7 35 MeV betatron manufactured by Brown, Boverie and Cie

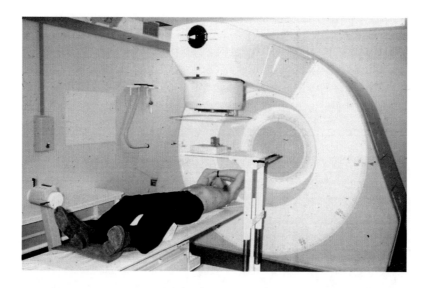

History of Radiation Oncology. Fig. 8 10 MeV linear accelerator manufactured by Philips

Stanford University Hospital. In 1962, the UCLA Medical Center obtained a commercially produced linac. By 1986, there were about 1,000 medical linacs in the United States. In Great Britain, and a short time later all over the world, many linacs were installed. Today, linacs are the machines of choice for medical use of high-energy photons and electrons.

A photograph of a 10-MeV linear accelerator is shown in Fig. 8.

After World War II, it was possible to produce radioactive isotopes artificially by means of nuclear reactors. In 1952, the Canadian Nuclear Society delivered the first 1,000 Ci cobalt-60 sources with gamma energies of 1.17 and 1.33 MeV. The first telecobalt units used a source-skin distance of 60 cm; later on, 80 cm was possible. These machines had a better depth dose than conventional X-ray machines and could use a build-up effect of about 5 mm. Thus, much higher doses to treat tumors were possible. Cobalt units were produced by many manufacturers and became popular (Figs. 9 and 10). In 1968 in Sweden, Leksell constructed the "Gamma Knife" with cobalt sources, the beginning of so-called stereotactic radiosurgery.

Disadvantages of the telecurie machines were the large penumbra due the size of the source, the maximum field size of 30 × 30 cm, need for radiation protection, and the necessity to change the source after about 5 years (cobalt) because of the diminishing activity of the source. Telecesium-137 units (first used at the Oak Ridge Institute of Nuclear Studies in the United States) had still more disadvantages than cobalt units. There have been two severe accidents caused by illegal radioactive waste management: in Brazil in 1987 and in Thailand in 2000. Therefore these machines have been mostly replaced by linear accelerators and today are used only in a few developing countries.

Two other events warrant mention. In 1944, the first publication on intraoperative radiotherapy took place, written by Henschke and Henschke. And in 1952, seeds from gold-198 (Sinclair) were used for interstitial treatment. The seeds were implanted with a pistol-like applicator.

In 1955, some clinics, e.g., St. Thomas Hospital in London, began using hyperbaric oxygen therapy. This was due to the decreasing oxygen levels in a respiring tumor mass through each successive cell layer distal to the lumen of the capillary.

The Fourth Period: 1960 to Present

This period is characterized by, among other things, the development of remote afterloading, stereotactic

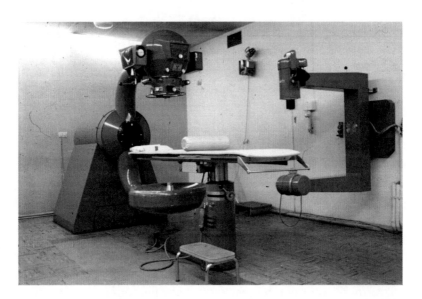

History of Radiation Oncology. Fig. 9 Telecobalt-60 machine with radiation shield manufactured by Canadian Nuclear Society

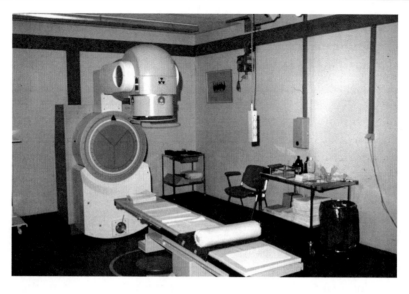

History of Radiation Oncology. Fig. 10 Telecobalt-60 machine with 80 cm source-skin distance manufactured by Philips

radiotherapy ("radiosurgery"), intensity modulated radiotherapy (IMRT), the CyberKnife technique, Hadron treatment, and the combination of radiotherapy and chemotherapy. Because of the sheer number and variety of models of available modern treatment machines, it is not possible to provide illustrations.

During this period, radiotherapy, now called radio-oncology, was separated from diagnostic radiology, even though diagnostic radiology procedures like computer tomography (CT) and magnetic resonance imaging (MRI) became an important element of radiation therapy planning. Scientific societies for radio-oncology were founded, like ASTRO (American Society for Therapeutic Radiology and Oncology, 1958/1966), ESTRO (European Society for Radiotherapy and Oncology, 1980), and numerous national radio-oncology societies. In addition, randomized clinical trials and evidence-based medicine in radiation oncology took place.

In 1953, the ICRU (International Commission on Radiation Units) replaced the "R," the unit of ionization, with the "rad," an abbreviation for "radiation absorbed dose," which was used in medicine until 1985. Since then, the Gy (Gray, named after the British physicist Louis Harold Gray) has been the unit of radiation therapy; 100 rad equal 1 Gy.

Remote afterloading techniques replaced interstitial and intracavitary treatment with radium and cesium and also manual afterloading (Pierquin and Dutreix 1966) with iridium-192 wires. All of these techniques had many disadvantages, above all the exposure of medical personnel to radiation. Therefore, in the 1960s, remote afterloading devices were developed, refined, and used for brachytherapy in Great Britain and later on in the United States. Remote afterloading is an application of the "As Low As Reasonably Achievable" (ALARA) principle in radiation control. Today, a variety of different machines are in use for treatment of gynecological cancers, tumors of the prostate, head and neck, and others. The radioactive nuclides used in remote afterloading are Co-60, Cs-137, and Ir-192. The first two offer longer half-lives but lower specific activities than achieved with Ir-192. Hence, Co-60 and Cs-137 sources are used in low dose rate (LDR), medium dose rate (MDR), or high dose rate (HDR) devices designed for intracavitary treatment with applicators that have larger inner lumens that accommodate the larger diameter (3–4 mm) of Co-60 and Cs-137 sources. Higher activity Ir-192 sources with smaller diameters (about 1–2 mm) are applicable for intraluminal HDR treatments. However, the 73.8-day half-life of Ir-192 necessitates three to four source changes yearly at high cost.

Stereotactic radiotherapy ("radiosurgery") with linear accelerators is an innovation adopted from the technique of Leksell (see above) and is used mainly to treat small lesions with high doses.

Intensity modulated radiotherapy (IMRT) was developed at the University of Wisconsin in 2002 (Welsh and coworkers) and was first clinically used in 2003. It allows molding the dose distribution in the tissue to spare radiosensitive structures and to treat tumors with high doses by nonuniform dose to the target. There are two methods, "dose painting" (in two dimensions) and "dose sculpting" (in three dimensions).

Another technique, the "CyberKnife," was developed in 1990 by J. Adler at Stanford University. Adler had been a coworker of Leksell in Sweden. The CyberKnife technique was published in 1999. A small 6-MeV linac is used in combination with a computer system, two diagnostic X-ray tubes, and digitally reconstructed CT pictures. During the treatment the original pictures are continuously compared with pictures during the treatment, and the linac is adjusted to the situation. Thus, even movements of organs (e.g., lung) during treatment can be compensated for. Since 2002 this machine has also been licensed in Europe.

Standard radiotherapy still uses high-energy photons, mostly from linear accelerators of different energy levels. A variety of treatment facilities with heavy particle irradiation, so-called "Hadron therapy," now also exists. The first neutron therapy of lung tumors was reported by Eichhorn, East Berlin, in 1976. Today, Hadron therapy uses strongly interacting particles, such as neutrons, protons, pions, and ions (alphas, C, Ne). Proton and neutron therapy address deficiencies in photon therapy. Protons have a better dose distribution; neutrons are characterized by better tumor killing. Because of the high costs and the limited indications of this treatment modality, however, there are only a few centers using these facilities.

Another means to increase the effect of radiotherapy with respect to cancer treatment is the combination of chemotherapy and radiotherapy, the so-called chemoradiotherapy. Beginning in the 1960s and 1970s, cisplatin, 5-fluorouracil, mitomycin-C, and other drugs were used. Since the 1980s, significant gains in local tumor control and survival, especially in head and neck tumors and in gastrointestinal tract tumors, have been reported. In addition, hormones are used in combination with radiotherapy, e.g., in mammary carcinoma and prostate cancer.

As with the beginning of radiation therapy, today benign lesions are also treated, including arthritis, inflammation, and other disorders. Details are not given as they are beyond the scope of this essay.

One of the great advantages of radiotherapy, alone or in combination with minimal surgery, is the organ-sparing, nonmutilating treatment of cancer. This was acknowledged by an article for the general public in *Reader's Digest*: "The Invisible Cancer Cure" (Ross 1982).

As demonstrated, technical developments have had an enormous influence on the potential of radiation therapy to treat tumors. However, it is important not to forget that in clinical radiation oncology, the experience and skill of the radio-oncologist, and the accuracy of the team of physicists, technicians, and nurses are the most important factors in treating patients with malignant tumors.

At the time when cobalt-60 was replacing conventional X-ray treatment, a famous American radiologist is reported to have ▓▓▓▓ed which therapy he would prefer in c▓ ▓▓ ▓ cancer: X-rays or cobalt. His reply: he ▓▓ ▓▓ ▓ke to be treated by the better radiologist. This is as true now as it was in the past.

Cross-References

► Brachytherapy
► Intensity Modulated Radiation Therapy (IMRT)
► Linear Accelerators (LINAC)
► Neutron Radiotherapy
► Proton Therapy
► Radiation Detectors
► Robotic Radiosurgery

References

Bernier J, Hall EJ, Giaccia A (2004) Radiation oncology: a century of achievements. Nat Rev Cancer 4:737–747

Buschke F (1970) Radiation therapy: the past, the present, the future. Janeway lecture, 1969. Am J Roentgenol Radium Ther Nucl Med 108(2):236–246

Case JT (1958) History of radiation therapy. Prog Radiat Ther 1:13–41

Deutsche Forschungsgemeinschaft (1980) Bestandsaufnahme Krebsforschung in Deutschland

Eymer H, Ries L (1941) Die Ergebnisse der Strahlenbehandlung der Gebärmutterkrebse an der Münchner Universitäts-Frauenklinik im Jahre 1934. Strahlentherapie 69:12–16

Hamann A, Göbel A, Englmann K (1934) Die Strahlenbehandlung der Gebärmutterkrebse im Allgemeinen Krankenhaus St.Georg in Hamburg (Juni 1929–Dezember 1931). I.Teil Strahlentherapie 50:529–556

Heilmann H-P (1970) Entstehung eines "Postkrikoidkarzinoms" in der Folge mehrfacher Röntgenbestrahlungen der Halsregion wegen Lymphknoten-Tuberkulose. Strahlentherapie 140:388–391

Heilmann H-P (1996) Radiation oncology: historical development in Germany. Int J Radiat Oncol Biol Phys 35:207–217

Holthusen H, Meyer H (1959) Ehrenbuch der Röntgenologen und Radiologen aller Nationen, 2nd edn. Urban & Schwarzenberg, Berlin

Pierquin B, Dutreix A (1966) For a new methodology in curietherapy: the system of Paris (endo- and plesioradiotherapy with non-radioactive preparation). A preliminary note. Ann Radiol (Paris) 9:757–760

Ross W (1982) The invisible cancer cure. The Reader's Digest Association Inc, Pleasantville

HIV-Related Malignancies

Definition

Malignant neoplasms associated with acquired immunodeficiency syndrome.

Cross-References

► Hodgkin's Lymphoma
► HPV
► Sarcoma

HNPCC

► Hereditary Nonpolyposis Colorectal Cancer (HNPCC)

Hodgkin's Lymphoma

THEODORE E. YAEGER
Department Radiation Oncology, Wake Forest University School of Medicine, Winston-Salem NC, USA

Definition

Hodgkin's lymphoma (HL), formerly called Hodgkin's disease, is a distinct classification of lymphoma. HL is first described by Thomas Hodgkin, in 1832, as tumors of absorbant (lymph) glands. It is typically described as a predominately lymphocytic proliferation with histiocytes forming classic Reed-Sternberg cells (see discussion). With the exception of the lymphocytic-predominate Hodgkin's subtype, the proliferated cells often form, at least, a partially nodular pattern. The four basic presentations are categorized below.

Epidemiology

Hodgkin's lymphoma (HL) is a malignancy of unknown pathogenesis. It accounts for less than 1% of all cancers, about 30% of all lymphomas and approximately 0.25% of all cancer deaths annually in the United States. Males predominate slightly and it occurs rarely in less than 10 years of age. The median age at diagnosis is about 26 years of age but there is a well-established bimodal peak based on age. The first peak occurs between an average of 25–30 years while the second peak is seen in the elderly between 75 and 80 years of age. There may be a relationship with the Epstein-Barr virus (EBV) with HL developing 3 months to 13 years following an infection. Also, there is a relationship to infectious mononucleosis as a 2.5-fold increase of HL incidence in patients with a (Hjalgrim et al. 2000) mononucleosis history. There are approximately three cases per 100,000 (10,000 cases per year) in the United States (American Cancer Society (ACS) 2011) with higher rates reported by international registries in developing countries. The highest reported rates are in Hispanics, poor children and young men in countries with a high EBV infection rate. Children have a better prognosis compared to adults and treatment regimens are tailored (Hudson et al. 2007) specific to children. Associations with environmental exposures have not proved conclusive (Greenlee et al. 2001) but cluster incidences have been reported.

Immunology

Hodgkin's lymphoma pathology is a mix of Hodgkin and Reed-Sternberg cells. These are generally derived from germinal B cells (rarely T cells) but have heterogeneous and uncharacterized phenotypes. Gene expression profiles from microarray analyses, molecular studies, and polymerase chain reactions have determined four HL transcription factors. HL lines are clustered despite a B- or T-cell origin with cell lines derived from EBV–activated B cells from diffuse large cell lymphomas. EBV virus can

be detected in 40% of cases (Ambinder and Weiss 2007) of classical HL. Twenty-seven genes, previously unknown, show aberrant expression in Reed-Sternberg (RS) cells. Basically, HL is characterized by clones of malignant cells in a reactive cellular background. They usually constitute less than 1% of the involved tissues. It is a difficult and complex diagnosis with common interobserver disagreements as to a precise diagnosis but to be exact the RS cells must be present. While the presence of the RS cell is necessary for HL, RS cells *alone* are not sufficient for the diagnosis. The primary diagnosis of HL is from the histopathology of a suspected lymph node. RS cells are then identified in a background of reactive cellularity. Still, benign reactive disorders must be eliminated.

Dialogue on Reed-Sternberg cells

Reed-Sternberg (RS) cells are also known as lacunar histiocytes. The name is derived from two researchers, Dorothy Reed Mendenhall (1902) and Carl Sternberg (1898), who provided the first collaborative definitive microscopic description of Hodgkin's "disease." Reed-Sternberg cells are large bilobed or multinucleated nucleus, commonly described as "owl's eyes." They are usually negative for CD20 and CD45 receptors and positive for CD30 and CD15. They can be found in reactive lymphadenopathy such as infectious mononucleosis, carbamazepine-associated lymphadenopathy, and rarely in Non-Hodgkin's lymphoma. The cells have prominent eosinophilic inclusion-like nucleoli and classically are large (15–45 μm) with a background of pale cytoplasm encasing the lobulated nuclei. During fixation the cytoplasm can shrink, leaving an empty space around the nucleus, hence a description as a "lacunar cell." Other RS variants are the L&H or "popcorn" cell with a fluffy, lobulated nucleus containing fine chromatin with small nucleoli and the "mummified" or mononuclear types. These are histopathologic variants of RS cells. In general, the frequency and character of the RS cells are the features contributing to the diagnosis and classification of Hodgkin's Lymphoma.

Diagnosis

Initial evaluation:

When evaluating HL, the initial approach is a thorough history and physical examination.

There are associated HL-related signs and symptoms termed "B" symptoms:

- Unexplained weight loss of greater than 10% in less than 6 months.
- Fevers of 38°C or higher for 3 or more consecutive days.
- Drenching night sweats enough to change clothing.

Patients presenting with "B" symptoms have a poorer prognosis:

- There should be a thorough examination of all lymphoid regions including liver and spleen
- Waldeyer's ring is not commonly involved.

Approximated 80% of patients present with cervical nodes.

Approximately 50% of patients have mediastinal lymphadenopathy and may present with shortness of breath.

Mesenteric involvement occurs in about 5% of patients.

HL typically spreads in an orderly fashion but hematogenous metastases can occur to liver and bone.

HIV/AIDS patients generally demonstrate an atypical, advanced, and aggressive course.

HL commonly presents with enlarged, non-tender, rubbery, movable lymph nodes within usual nodal bearing tissue sites. The liver may be enlarged and nodular. The spleen can be enlarged but is usually non-tender and asymptomatic.

Laboratory tests and imaging studies are outlined below.

Imaging studies:

- Chest X-ray (PA and Lateral views).
- Contrasted, if tolerated, CT scan of chest, abdomen and pelvis.
- FDG-PET or PET/CT total body scan changes the staging in about 20% of patients.

Clinically, the importance of stage is unequivocal for therapy decisions.

Bone scans are not routinely recommended.

Gallium-67 total body scans only if PET/CT not available.

Laparotomy no longer considered a standard diagnostic intervention because most patients will receive systemic chemotherapy (One trial – EORTC 6F – found laparotomy useful in patients receiving radiation alone) (Carde 1993; Diehl 2004).

Contrasted brain CT or MRI brain only for new onset and suspicious CNS symptoms.

Laboratory studies:

- Complete blood count
- Serum chemistry
- Lactate dehydrogenase (LDH)
- Liver/renal function tests
- Erythrocyte sedimentation rate (ESR)
- Alkaline phosphatase
- Beta-microglobulin
- Bone marrow for patients with "B" symptoms
- Fine needle aspiration of suspected nodes and/or masses

Pathology

Requires tissue diagnosis from nodal, extranodal, or cytology specimens.

HL is classified in two main categories and five subtypes.

Classical Hodgkin's lymphoma:
  I. Nodular sclerosis (30% present with "B" symptoms)
  II. Mixed cellularity (typically more advanced stage presentation)
  III. Lymphocyte depleted (rarest presentation and has poorest prognosis)
  IV. Lymphocyte predominate (also known as lymphocyte rich) (most favorable classic HL prognosis)
  V. Nodular lymphocyte predominant (NLPHL) (most favorable HL typically with indolent course) (Halperin 2999)

Staging

The most commonly used staging system is the Ann Arbor anatomically based system with specific prognostic factors (Cancer 1997; Carbone et al. 1971; Wen and LaFave 2008; Hoppe et al. 2006). With the advent of laparoscopy, routine laparotomy is no longer considered a common staging procedure. Laparoscopy can be used in virtually any circumstance to access intracavitary areas when no peripheral site is deemed available.

Stage I:
  Involvement of a single nodal region (I)
  A single extralymphatic site (IE)
Stage II:
  Involvement of two or more nodal sites on the same diaphragm side (II)
  One or more lymph node site with extralymphatic organ on same diaphragm side (IIE)
Stage III:
  Nodes on both sides of diaphragm (III)
  With spleen involvement (IIIS)
  Localized extralymphatic site or organ extension (IIIE)
  IIIE with spleen involvement (IIISE)

Stage IV:
  Diffuse multifocal involvement of extranodal tissues (IV)

Any Stage:

A = no "B" symptoms
B = Fever, weight loss, night sweats
X = Bulky disease

Dialogue on Bulky Disease

Bulky mediastinal disease presentations denotes poorer prognosis and is defined on imaging studies.

Mediastinal mass (MM) greater than 10 cm (Sanford University system, Hughes-Davies 1997)

MM divided by thoracic diameter greater than one-third on PA chest X-ray (EORTC)

MM divided by intrathoracic diameter greater than one-third on PA chest X-ray (GHSG)

Prognostic Factors

Early-stage treated with radiation alone:
Risk factors for relapse following radiation include male, older, mixed cellularity or lymphocyte depletion subtypes, "B" symptoms, bulky mediastinal disease presentations, multiple lymph node involvement, and elevation of erythrocyte sedimentation rate.

Early-stage HL is divided into favorable and unfavorable groups and patients with few poor prognostic factors should be considered for less aggressive treatments. Patients presenting with multiple risk factors should be considered for combined treatment regimens.

Each poor prognostic factor reduces the 5-year freedom from progression by approximately 8%.

Treatment

General management and principles:

Multidrug regimens are the treatment of choice

Dose-intense regimens combined with radiation to bulky presentation sites for locally extensive and/or advanced disease have long-term follow-up with acceptable outcomes.

Radiation, alone, can be an effective therapy intervention for controlling localized to limited regional HL. The volume of presentation to be treated should allow reasonable treatment field sizes.

The current approach is to consider the smallest fields and lowest effective doses.

Chemotherapy with radiotherapy should be delivered sequentially.

Chemotherapy can be used initially to reduce disease volume(s) for radiation.

Chemotherapy is important to use early in disseminated disease presentation.

Favorable HL, stage 1–2A:

Chemotherapy followed by involved-field radiotherapy is the current standard of care.

Doxorubicin, bleomycin, vinblastine, and dacarbazine (ABVD) is the standard for chemotherapy.

Radiation doses are variable, but generally in the lower ranges, e.g., 20–44 Gy, fractionated.

EORTC H9F found a statistical difference between no radiation vs. involved field radiation (IFRT) but not between the doses of 20 Gy versus 36 Gy. Failure after shortened course chemotherapy followed by involved field radiotherapy to an average of 30 Gy is rare.

When a patient refuses or cannot tolerate chemotherapy, radiation alone is a definitive option.

Field arrangement options are described below.

Unfavorable HL, stage 1A–2B:

ABVD-based chemotherapy – or newer regimens – is considered a standard regimen for stage I and II unfavorable HL. The number of cycles is somewhat variable but usually between 4 and 6.

Involved field radiotherapy should be considered to follow chemotherapy. The dose range is generally thought to be between 30 and 36 Gy. Field arrangements should cover the presentation site and contiguous nodal groups. The German Hodgkin Study Group (GHSG) determined that 30 Gy was adequate for prophylaxis.

When radiotherapy is used alone, the National Cancer Center Network (NCCN) recommends a dose range of 30–44 Gy, fractionated. Evenly weighted, opposed fields to involved sites were the general recommended parameters.

Involved field arrangements are usually portions of classic radiation fields (see below)

Treatment of stage III and IV HL:

Systemic treatment is currently the standard choice of care.

Six to eight cycles are planned with restaging at mid-course, typically with a repeat FD-based PET or PET/CT scan, as compared to pretreatment scan, when possible.

Thirty to Forty Gy of IFRT is given for partial responses, sites with bulky disease, or sites greater than 5 cm. This addition of IFRT can convert a partial response to a complete response with similar survival as patients achieving a CR on chemotherapy alone. Thus, routine IFRT is not routinely recommended for chemotherapy-induced complete response.

The use of FDG-based PET scans during or after chemotherapy can assist in determining appropriate candidates for involved field radiotherapy (IFRT).

Rare, nodular lymphocyte-predominant Hodgkin's lymphoma (NLPHL) treatment:

Stage IA:

Can be treated with surgical resection followed by IFRT to 30–36 Gy.

Extended field radiotherapy or combined chemoradiotherapy has no demonstrated a significant additional benefit.

The GHSG is studying the use of anti CD-20 monoclonal antibody therapy.

Stage IIA/B:

Can be treated with chemotherapy followed by IFRT; alternatively with definitive radiation.

Stage IIIA/B, IVA/B:

Are usually treated with chemotherapy, with or without IFRT

Anti CD-20 monoclonal antibody therapy can be considered for poor chemotherapy tolerance or for patients with recurrent and refractory disease presentations.

Treatment of residual, refractory, recurrent disease:

A biopsy should be considered in patients with progression or nonresponse during treatment to confirm the original diagnosis.

Treatment options include, changing standard chemotherapy, high-dose chemotherapy with or without IFRT and with or without autologous stem cell bone marrow transplant.

Restaging includes bone marrow biopsy for all patients considering further aggressive therapy.

Localized failure in original early-stage disease treated by chemotherapy alone is individualized.

Localized failure after lower dose IFRT alone can be retreated to additional radiation doses.

Failure in patients with prior combined chemoradiotherapy, stem cell transplant should be considered. High-dose ablative chemotherapy and transplant can achieve 50% salvage.

A recent prospective series reported an overall survival rate of 83% when recurrences are treated with a combination of total lymphoid radiation, high-dose chemotherapy, and the autologous stem cell transplantation.

Radiation therapy technical specifics:

Involved field radiotherapy (IFRT) is the clinically involved lymph node site.

Regional field radiotherapy (RFRT) is IFRT plus close proximal adjacent nodal sites.

Extended field radiotherapy (EFRT) is RFRT plus distant nodal draining sites.

Diagrams

Mantle EFRT includes the submandibular, cervical, supraclavicular, infraclavicular, axillary, mediastinal subcarinal to the diaphragm crus and hilar node groups. Variations are the minimantle (deletes the fields below the infraclavicular group) and modified mantle that is a truncation laterally, deleting the axillary node basins (Figs. 1 and 2).

Figure 3 inverted "Y" includes the para-aortic, bilateral pelvic, and inguinofemoral node groups. The splenectomy spleen stump or the entire spleen may be included. Subtotal node irradiation (SNI) deletes the pelvic portion of the inverted "Y" with a mantle field. Total nodal radiation (TNI) are all central body nodal groups usually covered with both the mantle and the inverted "Y" fields matched near the diaphragm crus.

Radiation Doses Technical Specifics

Radiation doses are clinically determined by need.

Definitive, is usually defined as "curative" doses with involved areas being treated to 35–44 Gy and uninvolved, associated regions treated with 30–36 Gy.

Adjuvant radiotherapy is usually considered for consolidation after multidrug definitive chemotherapy. In this setting, the original presentation and/or bulky disease should be treated with 30–36 Gy. Also, non-bulky sites can be considered for 20–30 Gy as consolidation.

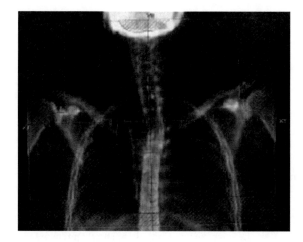

Hodgkin's Lymphoma. Fig. 1 Typical mantle radiation field with shielding of the lungs, humeral heads, larynx, and oral cavity (see text, for detailed description)

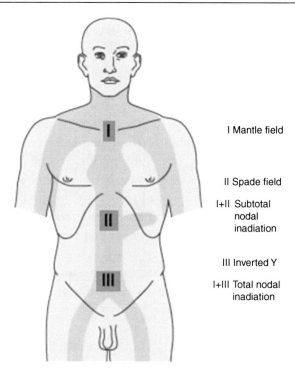

I Mantle field

II Spade field

I+II Subtotal nodal inadiation

III Inverted Y

I+III Total nodal inadiation

Hodgkin's Lymphoma. Fig. 3 Various irradiation fields for lymph nodal coverage in the treatment of Hodgkin's lymphoma or non-Hodgkin's lymphoma (Adapted from the SEER's Training Website http://training.seer.cancer.sov)

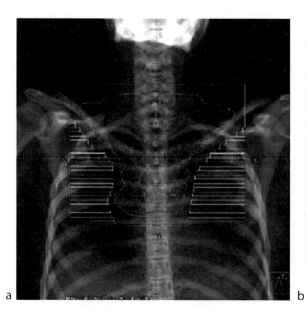

a

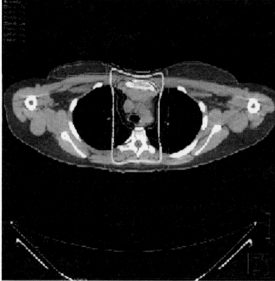

b

Hodgkin's Lymphoma. Fig. 2 Modified Mantle field design and dosimetry

For the relatively rare NLPHL, excision should be followed by localized field to 30 Gy.

Fraction size is somewhat institution dependent but is generally between 1.5 and 2.0 Gy.

Follow-Up

Follow-up is lifelong. Not only are recurrences early but can be late. Additionally, secondary tumors, growth disruptions, hormonal imbalances, early cardiopulmonary disease, infertility, and psychological complications can occur months to years following definitive chemotherapy and radiotherapy.

A typical follow-up schedule is 3 months for a year, 4 months for 2 years, 6 months for 3 years, then annually thereafter.

Specifics include blood counts; thyroid levels; chest X-Rays; CT scans of chest, abdomen, and pelvis; early onset mammograms in female patients; regular cardiac testing for a decade (especially if treated above the diaphragm); annual prophylactic vaccinations as appropriate for active, treated, or no spleen. Specific counseling should be regularly reinforced for psychological support, skin cancer, and cardiovascular risks as well as breast and testicular self-exams (Wen and LaFave 2008).

Current Clinical Trials

Trials for HL are focusing on three major aspects:

1. Decreasing the intensity of therapies in good prognosis patients.
2. Optimizing treatment combinations in patients with early stage but unfavorable prognosis presentations.
3. More intensive treatment programs for advanced stages, resistant tumors, and recurrent disease.

Cross-References

▶ Hodgkin's Lymphoma
▶ Leukemia in General
▶ Lung Cancer
▶ Renal Pelvis and Ureter
▶ Sarcomas of the Head and Neck

References

Ambinder RA, Weiss LM (2007) Association of Epstein-Barr virus with Hodgkin's lymphoma. Lippincott, Philadelphia

American Cancer Society (ACS) Alson cancer statistics, 2011

Cancer (1997) The National Cancer Data Base report on non-Hodgkin's lymphoma. Cancer 80:2311–2320

Carbone PP, Kaplan HS, Musshoff K et al (1971) Report of the committee on Hodgkin's disease staging classification. Cancer Res 31:1860–1861

Greenlee RT, Hill-Harmon MB, Murray T, et al (2001) ACS cancer statistics

Halperin, Perez, Brady, co-editors Principles and practice of radiation oncology, 5th edn, Section III, Chapter 75 as suggested reading

Hjalgrim H, Askling J et al (2000) Risk of Hodgkin's disease and other cancers after infectious mononucleosis. JNCI 92:1522–1528

Hoppe RT, Advani RH, Bierman PJ et al (2006) Hodgkin's disease/lymphoma. Clinical practice guidelines in oncology. J Natl Compr Cancer Netw 4(3):210–230

Hudson M, Korholz D, Donaldson SS (2007) Pediatric Hodgkin's lymphoma. Lippincott, Philadelphia

Wen B-C, LaFave K (2008) Hodgkin's lymphoma, Chapter 28. In: Lu JJ, Brady LW, (eds) Radiation oncology, an evidence-based approach. Springer, Berlin, pp 415–428 (as suggested reading)

Homeopathy

▶ Complementary Medicine

Hormonal Agents

RENE RUBIN
Rittenhouse Hematology/Oncology,
Philadelphia, PA, USA

Definition

Hormonal agents are widely used in curative and palliative treatment of hormone-dependent tumors.

Tamoxifen, toremifene, and raloxifene are all SERM drugs (selective estrogen receptor modulators). They are nonsteroidal antiestrogens with weak estrogenic agonist effects. They bind to the estrogen receptors and inhibit signal transduction. All are used in the treatment of breast carcinoma, except raloxifene which is used to prevent breast carcinoma in high-risk patients.

Anastrozole, letrozole, and exemestane are aromatase inhibitors and are used to treat breast cancer in menopausal patients. They work by inhibiting the conversion of adrenal androgens to estrogen.

Fulvestrant is an estrogen receptor antagonist. It downregulates the expression of the estrogen receptor. It is used in recurrent estrogen receptor positive breast carcinoma.

Goserelin and leuprolide are both luteinizing releasing hormone (LHRH) analogs and are used in prostate carcinoma to prevent gonadal hormone production. In women, it is used to render them menopausal.

Megestrol is a progestational agent used in metastatic breast carcinoma. Currently, it is most commonly used as an appetite stimulant for cancer-induced cachexia.

Estrogen can be used in both prostate carcinoma and in low doses for breast carcinoma.

Aminoglutethimide is a chemical form of adrenalectomy. It is mostly of historical note at this point in time. It must be given with cortisol replacement. It is indicated for both breast and prostate carcinoma.

Bicalutamide, flutamide, and nilutamide are all anti-androgens and are indicated for use in prostate carcinoma. They bind to the androgen receptor. They are indicated in both the adjuvant and metastatic setting for prostate carcinoma.

Estramustine is a conjugate of nitrogen mustard and estradiol. It is indicated in metastatic prostate carcinoma. It works by binding to the androgen receptor.

Abiraterone is newly approved for the treatment of metastatic prostate carcinoma. It inhibits adrenal synthesis of androgens.

Ketoconazole is an antifungal agent. However, when given in high doses it inhibits the production of adrenal steroids and exhibits (marginal) effects on hormone-resistant metastatic prostate cancer.

Side Effects

- Hot flashes
- Vaginal dryness in women
- Erectile dysfunction in men
- Osteoporosis
- Loss of libido
- Elevated lipids (aromatase inhibitors)
- Lowered lipids (SERMS)
- Muscle cramps
- Fluid retention
- Thrombosis

Cross-References

▶ Principles of Chemotherapy

Horner's Syndrome

FENG-MING KONG, JINGBO WANG
Department of Radiation Oncology, Veteran Administration Health Center and University Hospital, University of Michigan, Ann Arbor, MI, USA

Definition

This syndrome is caused by damage to the sympathetic nervous system and presents with a series of ipsilateral signs including ptosis, anhydrosis, miosis, enophthalmos, and loss of ciliospinal reflex.

Cross-References

▶ Lung

HPV

CHRISTIN A. KNOWLTON[1], MICHELLE KOLTON
MACKAY[2], PATRIZIA GUERRIERI[3], PAOLO MONTEMAGGI[3]
[1]Department of Radiation Oncology, Drexel
University, Philadelphia, PA, USA
[2]Department of Radiation Oncology, Marshfield
Clinic, Marshfield, WI, USA
[3]Department of Radiation Oncology, Regional
Cancer Center "M. Ascoli", University of Palermo
Medical School, Palermo, Italy

Synonyms
Human papilloma virus

Definition
The human papilloma virus is a sexually transmitted virus that is known to be causative in
cervical cancer. The two strains of HPV that are
most associated with cervical cancer are HPV 16
and 18, with type 16 being associated with more
than 50% of squamous cell carcinomas of
the cervix. HPV can be assessed with the
Papanicolaou test and found in premalignant
changes. In the United States, two FDA-approved
vaccinations against HPV to prevent cervical
cancer are available.

Cross-References
▶ Sarcomas of the Head and Neck

Human Epidermal Growth Factor Receptor Type II

▶ Her-2

Human Immunodeficiency Virus (HIV)

GERHARD G. GRABENBAUER
Chairman of the Department of Radiation
Oncology, DiaCura Coburg & Klinikum Coburg,
Coburg, Germany

Definition
HIV is a lentivirus which induces the acquired
immunodeficiency syndrome (AIDS). In human,
the disease leads a severe and progressive malfunction
of the immunological system. The course of this life-
threatening disease is characterized by opportunistic
infections and the potential induction of cancer.

Cross-References
▶ Anal Carcinoma
▶ HPV

Human Papilloma Virus

▶ HPV

Human Papilloma Virus (HPV)

STEPHAN MOSE
Department of Radiation Oncology,
Schwarzwald-Baar-Klinikum,
Villingen-Schwenningen, Germany

Synonyms
HPV

Definition
HPV is a papilloma virus of which approximately
130 different types have been identified. High-risk

HPV types are directly associated with the induction of cancer (especially cervical cancer).

Cross-References
▶ Anal Cancer
▶ Female Urethral Cancer
▶ Male Urethral Cancer
▶ Oro-hypopharynx
▶ Penile Cancer
▶ Uterine Cervix

Hybridoma Technique

TOD W. SPEER
Department of Human Oncology, University of Wisconsin School of Medicine and Public Health, UW Hospital and Clinics, Madison, WI, USA

Definition
A technology that produces monoclonal antibodies by fusing antibody-producing B lymphocytes with myeloma cells.

Cross-References
▶ Targeted Radioimmunotherapy

Hydrops Tubae Profluens

PATRIZIA GUERRIERI, PAOLO MONTEMAGGI
Department of Radiation Oncology, Regional Cancer Center "M. Ascoli", University of Palermo Medical School, Palermo, Italy

Definition
A syndrome in which there is a sudden emptying of fluid accumulated in a distended Fallopian tube which causes profuse, watery serosanguinous vaginal discharge with subsequent relief of abdominal discomfort. It may represent in a certain percentage of cases an early sign of a Fallopian tube cancer.

Cross-References
▶ Fallopian Tube

Hyperfractionated Radiotherapy

VOLKER BUDACH[1], CARSTEN NIEDER[2]
[1]Department of Radiotherapy and Radiation Oncology, Charité – University Hospital Berlin, Berlin, Germany
[2]Radiation Oncology Unit, Nordlandssykehuset HF, Bodoe, Norway

Definition
In contrast to conventional fractionation (daily fractions of 1.8–2.0 Gy 5 times per week) a larger number of smaller fractions is administered, e.g., 1.2 Gy twice daily.

Radiotherapy schedules where smaller single doses (fractions) of radiation are given more often than standard radiotherapy (1.8–2 Gy/fraction). In hyperfractionated radiotherapy, individual doses are given more often a day (e.g., twice) than the standard dose of once a day.

Cross-References
▶ Larynx
▶ Lung Cancer
▶ Oro-Hypopharynx
▶ Total Body Irradiation (TBI)

Hypernephroma

▶ Kidney

Hyperthermia

Talha Shaikh[1], Jacqueline Emrich[1],
Lydia T. Komarnicky-Kocher[2]
[1]College of Medicine, Drexel University,
Philadelphia, PA, USA
[2]Department of Radiation Oncology,
College of Medicine, Drexel University,
Philadelphia, PA, USA

Definition

Hyperthermia is a form of cancer therapy which involves the application of heat to tumor cells in order to damage cellular proteins and subsequently cause apoptosis (cell death). This therapy can be used in conjunction with other forms of cancer therapy, particularly radiation therapy, where it can increase the radiosensitivity of cells by inhibiting DNA repair and increasing oxygenation. Although one of the oldest forms of cancer treatments known, it remains a largely underutilized procedure. Recent data has shown success in treating breast, genitourinary, head and neck, and gastrointestinal malignancies.

Background

The concept of using heat to treat tumors is not new. Heat has been used in many cultures as a medical treatment for many diseases. Patients with prolonged infections with erysipelas characterized by high fever and coincidental tumor burden have been noted to have a decrease in the size of the tumor. New York surgeon William B. Coley believed the bacteria causing erysipelas may be responsible for having an effect on cancer and extracted a toxin (Coley's toxin) with which he treated several patients. Coley's work led to a number of studies using local hyperthermia to treat tumors in experimental models. Westermark reported promising results in patients with large carcinomas of the cervix responding to heat. These cases were anecdotal and poorly controlled, but the results were interesting nonetheless.

Twentieth-century worldwide conferences pertaining to hyperthermic oncology have peaked interest in the use of heat to treat malignancies. The first International Congress on Hyperthermic Oncology held in 1975 resulted in worldwide interest with several subsequent trials. Although the field of hyperthermic oncology lost enthusiasm for a time, there appears to be a reemergence of interest and use of hyperthermia to treat malignancies.

Cell Response

The responses of a cancer cell and a normal cell to heat are similar, although it is recognized that individual cells may vary widely in sensitivity to hyperthermia. It is the surrounding architecture which accounts for the difference in outcomes for the two cell types. The physiology of a tumor cell is chaotic with both disorganized vasculature and altered nutrients, theoretically making the tumor more susceptible to hyperthermia due to its inability to dissipate heat. Areas of tumors with decreased blood supply and low pH are particularly sensitive to the cytotoxic effects of hyperthermia as demonstrated by the dramatic response of large, necrotic tumors to heat therapy.

In normal tissue, elevated temperatures cause vasodilation which allows dissipation of heat by the influx of cooler blood. Malignancies vary in that although they have increased blood flow, the poor vasculature impairs cooling of the adjacent surrounding tissue. This factor makes cancerous tissue particularly vulnerable to heat due to the elevated temperatures. In addition, heating a tumor may further alter vasculature and impair cooling. This in effect can alter pH, pO_2, and nutrient status which may also enhance cell killing.

Interestingly, cells respond similarly to heat and x-rays; there is an initial response lag followed by an exponential rate of cell death. Yet the amount of energy needed for cell inactivation is far greater for heat than for x-rays, indicating differences in the cell kill process for each treatment type. The activation energy required for cell kill when using heat as a treatment modality is similar to that necessary to denature a protein. It is widely believed that hyperthermia may actually target nuclear proteins such as those involved in DNA synthesis, although cytoskeleton and membrane components are susceptible as well. Heat therapy causes widespread aggregation of proteins which not only alters DNA replication, but inhibits even routine functions such as glycolysis and the electron transport chain.

The phase of the cell cycle most susceptible to hyperthermia is late synthesis (DNA replication) which is actually the most resistant to x-rays. Unlike x-rays which primarily cause cell death at the time of cell division (mitosis), heated cells typically die by apoptosis. The cell's response to hyperthermia appears in the early response of a tumor to treatment unlike radiotherapy which often produces delayed treatment effects. This may also further indicate the role of combining x-rays and thermotherapy as the effect on cells may be synergistic.

The most important factors governing hyperthermia response include temperature and time of exposure. In vivo tumor cell killing has been best achieved at temperatures between 40°C and 44°C. Most tissue is likely to demonstrate toxic effects at temperatures greater than 44°C with 1 h of exposure. Although acutely intense heat can cause rapid cellular changes, moderate temperature for a prolonged interval is more likely to have long-term implications. In addition, normal tissue is less likely to be damaged with low-level prolonged heat exposure.

The human body is naturally adaptive to its environment and so thermotolerance is a relatively common phenomenon in heat-exposed tissue. Interruption in hyperthermia therapy allows for the alteration of the surrounding milieu, making cells less susceptible to treatment. It has been noted that heat shock proteins coincide with the appearance of thermotolerance and may actually be responsible for the decreased responsiveness following a brief treatment break. These stress proteins are coincidentally also seen after exposure to other toxic substances such as ethanol, heavy metals, and lidocaine. Following a pause in hyperthermia treatment, it may take cells as long as 160 h to revert to normal thermotolerance levels thus limiting treatments to one or two times per week. Studies have not shown a particular difference in response when comparing once weekly or twice weekly treatments.

The CEM 43°CT$_{90}$ measures the cumulative equivalent minutes at 43°C exceeded by 90% of the monitored points within a tumor and is used to determine thermal dose during hyperthermia treatment. This underscores the importance of both temperature and time-dependence in hyperthermia cytotoxicity. Unfortunately, other factors such as acquired thermotolerance and nonuniformity are not accounted for in this measurement.

Methods of Treatment

In vitro experimentation with hyperthermia has been largely successful due to the ability to create easily controlled environments using heated water baths to minimize temperature flux. In clinical practice, uniform heat exposure and constant temperatures are often difficult to maintain.

Hyperthermia treatments can be local, regional, or whole body. Some of the methods of local techniques include shortwave diathermy, ultrasound, microwaves, and interstitial implants. The temperature, regardless of the method used, is dependent on multiple factors including tissue characteristics and blood flow. Local hyperthermia treatment is typically used for superficial tumors which are more likely to be affected by this type of treatment.

Regional hyperthermia often involves traditional methods such as direct heat exposure and warm fluid immersion and may be employed for the treatment of extremities or deep seated tumors. For example, intraperitoneal hyperthermia has been used to improve the delivery of chemotherapy to various deep-seated tumors in the gastrointestinal tract.

Whole-body treatment aims at minimizing energy losses while maximizing energy gains using radiant systems. The temperature is ideally maintained at less than 42°C for 1 h, since higher whole-body temperatures have resulted in greater toxicity. Typically, the procedure involves sedation as well as possible intubation, depending on the facility. Previous methods such as the use of pyrogens, extracorporeal heating, and contact heating have been abandoned due to unacceptable adverse effects.

Unfortunately, although these various techniques have demonstrated some success, there remain problems that need to be addressed. For example, although microwave heat may be appropriate for treating at shallow depths, deep-seated tumors may not be adequately heated. Ultrasound heat may have better heat distribution through a deep-seated tumor but may have distortion of heat patterns due to the presence of bone or air. Other options such as multiphased arrays have shown success by allowing better uniformity of temperature via interstitial methods.

A well-known form of local hyperthermia is radiofrequency ablation (RFA) which involves generating high levels of heat, 50–70°C, by using a high-frequency alternating current. This treatment method involves short exposure of heat powdered by a small RFA probe. Although experience is limited, RFA has been successfully used to ablate nodules particularly in the liver, lung, and kidney. Due to the acute and rapid action of RFA, it typically is not used concurrently with other therapies.

Historically, a large problem with hyperthermia treatment is the difficulty in assessing and maintaining the desired temperature. Recent advances in imaging technology have resulted in improvements in monitoring temperature changes. Ultrasound and magnetic resonance imaging (MRI) have both shown promising results as temperature-dependent parameters have been identified, measured, and calibrated.

Radiotherapy and Hyperthermia

The varying response of cells to x-rays versus heat makes the combination appealing as a potential joint therapy. Cells most susceptible to heat therapy include those that are under hypoxic conditions and are in the S-phase of the cell cycle. Radiotherapy is most effective in conditions with abundant oxygen and during the mitotic phase of the cell cycle. These complementary methods of action make dual treatment attractive.

Theoretically, cells which are out of the "sensitive" phase of the cell cycle and in a hypoxic setting may not respond adequately to x-rays but are likely to be eliminated during heat therapy. Studies have demonstrated that hyperthermia to a temperature of approximately 41°C prior to radiation may promote reoxygenation via increased blood flow which would further make tumor cells more radiosensitive.

Another important means by which these two treatments interact involves the effects of cell repair. Radiotherapy works predominantly by causing breaks in the DNA molecule. Hyperthermia potentiates these effects by interfering with the cellular repair of DNA damage, most likely by denaturing cell proteins. This inability to repair causes both sublethal and lethal damage to the cells.

The thermal enhancement ratio (TER) is defined as the dose of x-rays required to produce a given level of biological damage with and without the application of heat. It is well known that radiotherapy has its greatest thermal enhancement ratio achieved in hypoxic conditions, along with increased temperatures and long exposures. Furthermore, maximum thermal enhancement ratios can be obtained when radiation and hyperthermia are combined. The therapeutic gain factor (TGF) is the ratio of TER in the tumor to the TER in normal tissue. If there is no therapeutic gain for a particular tumor, there is no theoretical advantage for the addition of heat to x-ray treatments.

Trials over the past 20 years have continued to show the effectiveness of hyperthermia as an adjunct to radiation therapy. In particular, superficial tumors such as melanomas and breast cancer recurrences have shown increased responsiveness when hyperthermia is added as a treatment modality. Furthermore, hyperthermia with re-irradiation of the breast has been particularly helpful in recurrent disease.

Although independent treatments, hyperthermia and radiotherapy seem to have additive cytotoxic effects. This may have profound implications in planning therapy. The future of hyperthermia depends largely on current trials assessing its role in conjunction with radiotherapy.

Chemotherapy and Hyperthermia

Similar to the effects of x-rays with hyperthermia, chemotherapy also has several synergistic effects on tumor cells treated with heat therapy. Physiologically, heat results in the vasodilation of blood vessels in order to dissipate heat. This has multiple therapeutic effects. The addition of heat to chemotherapeutic drugs allows for better drug penetration to poorly perfused tumor regions. More importantly, this allows for increased intracellular uptake of chemotherapeutic agents due to blood flow. At the cellular level, this would result in DNA tumor cell damage and death. For example, the addition of heat in patients being treated with bleomycin may further inhibit repair mechanisms and allow for better tumor response.

In vivo experiments have also shown encouraging results with the addition of heat to chemotherapeutic agents. Several drugs have been shown to be potentiated by heat. The combination of these two therapies is thought to counteract drug resistance, avoiding the need for third- and fourth-line therapies. The ideal temperature for treatment remains an important consideration as temperatures above 41°C are believed to be too toxic, while temperatures between 39°C and 40°C appear to be safe and effective.

Unfortunately, although therapeutic gains have been impressive, the toxic effects of combination therapy have been unacceptable. In animal studies, many known adverse effects of chemotherapeutic agents were potentiated. For example, studies with doxorubicin have shown increased risk of heart toxicity while alkylating agents have shown increased damage to the bone marrow. Whole-body hyperthermia has shown evidence of lethal toxicity when combined with chemotherapy. Although a potential future therapy, the combination of chemotherapy and hyperthermia remains largely experimental.

Future Considerations

Hyperthermia remains one of the earliest known treatment modalities for cancer, yet still one of the most underutilized. An important reason for this is the continued difficulty to properly heat/monitor temperatures and therefore treat malignancies. Despite technological advances in the field, improving heating modalities as well as thermometry is of utmost importance in order to achieve better controlled environments during patient treatment.

The continuing development of genomic therapy continues to have implications throughout the medical field. The use of hyperthermia to improve liposomal targeting and accumulation continues to evolve as a future treatment modality. Gene therapy targeting heat shock proteins may allow thermotolerance to be overcome in patients receiving heat therapy.

Combination therapy remains a consideration since hyperthermia alone has produced inadequate responses. Trimodality treatment combining radiation, chemotherapy, and hyperthermia may play an important role in future therapy for cancer patients. Recent studies have demonstrated impressive results in patients treated for breast, rectal, and head and neck tumors.

Although widespread acceptance remains a future goal, the application of hyperthermia treatment and its clinical application remain a topic of debate. With current treatment setups, not all types of tumors can be adequately treated with hyperthermia. Most centers are not adequately equipped with either staff or equipment to treat patients using this modality. Hyperthermia continues to evolve as another possible treatment modality for patients diagnosed with cancer. Trials within the upcoming years will likely dictate its role in oncology.

References

Baronzio GF, Hager ED (eds) (2006) Hyperthermia in cancer treatment: a primer. Springer, New York

Dewhirst MW et al (2005) Re-setting the biologic rationale for thermal therapy. Int J Hyperth 21: 779–790

Gunderson LL, Tepper JE (2007) Clinical radiation oncology. Elsevier Churchill Livingstone, Philadelphia

Hall EJ, Giaccia AJ (2012) Radiobiology for the radiologist. Lippincott Williams & Wilkins, Philadelphia

Hurwitz MD et al (2010) Hyperthermia combined with radiation for the treatment of locally advanced prostate cancer. Cancer 117(3):510–516

Kuban DA et al (2008) Long-term results of the MD Anderson randomized dose escalation trail for prostate cancer. Int J Radiat Oncol Biol Phys 70:67–74

Overgaard J (1989) The current and potential role of hyperthermia in radiotherapy. Int J Radiat Oncol Biol Phys 16:535–549

Perez CA, Brady LW (1992) Principles and practice of radiation oncology. J.B. Lippincott, Philadelphia

Sminia P et al (1994) Effect of hyperthermia on central nervous system: a review. Int J Hyperthermia 10:1–130

Van Der Zee J et al (2002) Heating the patient: a promising approach? Ann Oncol 13:1173–1184

Hypofractionation

DAREK MICHALSKI[1], M. SAIFUL HUQ[2]
[1]Division of Medical Physics, Department of Radiation Oncology, University of Pittsburgh Cancer Centers, Pittsburgh, PA, USA
[2]Department of Radiation Oncology, University of Pittsburgh Medical Center Cancer Pavilion, Pittsburgh, PA, USA

Definition

Radiation therapy based on administering larger dose per fraction but with fewer fractions.

Cross-References

▶ Four-Dimensional (4D) Treatment Planning/Respiratory Gating

Hypogammaglobulinemia

RAMESH RENGAN[1], CHARLES R. THOMAS, JR.[2]
[1]Department of Radiation Oncology, Hospital of the University of Pennsylvania, Philadelphia, PA, USA
[2]Department of Radiation Medicine, Oregon Health Sciences University, Portland, OR, USA

Definition

Present in approximately 5% of patients with thymoma and is characterized by immunodeficiency. Thymectomy does not usually produce a remission in this disorder.

Cross-References

▶ Thymic Neoplasms

Hysteroscopy

CHRISTIN A. KNOWLTON[1], MICHELLE KOLTON MACKAY[2]
[1]Department of Radiation Oncology, Drexel University, Philadelphia, PA, USA
[2]Department of Radiation Oncology, Marshfield Clinic, Marshfield, WI, USA

Definition

A hysteroscope is placed through the cervix to allow for visualization of the uterus. This may be performed as part of the evaluation for abnormal uterine bleeding. A uterine leiomyoma or polyp may be removed by passing an instrument through the hysteroscope. Hysteroscopy may be used for guidance when performing a ▶ dilation and curettage.

Cross-References

▶ Endometrium

H

I

IFRT

▶ Involved Field Radiotherapy

Image-Guided Radiation Therapy (IGRT): kV Imaging

YING XIAO
Radiation Oncology Department, Jefferson
Medical College, Philadelphia, PA, USA

Definition

Image-guided radiation therapy (IGRT) may be broadly defined as a radiation therapy procedure that uses image guidance at various stages of its process: patient data acquisition, treatment planning, treatment simulation, patient setup, and target localization before and during treatment. In the present context, we will use the term IGRT to signify radiotherapy that uses image guidance procedures for target localization before and during treatment. These procedures use imaging technology to identify and correct problems arising from inter- and intrafractional variations in patient setup and anatomy, including shapes and volumes of the treatment target(s), organs at risk, and surrounding normal tissues (Khan 2009). The goal of IGRT is to reduce the geometrical uncertainty in a given treatment fraction by evaluating the patient geometry at the time of treatment and either altering the patient position or adapting the treatment plan with respect to anatomical changes that occur during the radiotherapy treatment course (Korreman et al. 2010).

Background

Image guidance using various imaging modalities has been implemented in radiation therapy for photon, electron, and proton external beam radiation treatments, as well as for brachytherapy in order to reduce the geometrical variations during the course of radiation therapy. These imaging modalities include two-dimensional (2D) x-ray image modalities (2D kV and 2D MV imaging); three-dimensional (3D) x-ray imaging modalities (kilovoltage (kV) helical CT, kV cone-beam CT (kV CBCT), megavoltage (MV) helical CT, MV cone-beam CT); and other imaging modalities, including MRI, ultrasound, PET, etc.

In this entry, the emphasis is on the description of one subset of the image guidance methodologies – kV imaging. They are grouped into 2D, 3D, and four-dimensional (4D) kV image guidance systems. Their basic characteristics, associated image dose, and relevant quality assurance tests will be discussed.

Basic Characteristics

Two-Dimensional Image Guidance
Two-dimensional images, both kV and MV, generated from modern linear accelerators, are produced by two sets of imaging systems: first, a conventional x-ray tube that is mounted, generally orthogonal to the MV radiation gantry, opposes a flat-panel image detector, and second, another flat-panel image detector opposes the

L.W. Brady, T.E. Yaeger (eds.), *Encyclopedia of Radiation Oncology*, DOI 10.1007/978-3-540-85516-3,
© Springer-Verlag Berlin Heidelberg 2013

MV radiation source, the so-called electronic portal imaging device (EPID). The flat-panel image detectors are matrices of 256×256 solid state amorphous silicon (a-Si) photodiodes. The 2D kV images produced by the first imaging system are quite useful in determining the position of the intended target(s) in relation to the bony landmarks and/or radioopaque markers (fiducials) implanted in the target tissues, similar to the functions that can be derived from 2D MV images. In addition, the kV imager can be used in both the radiographic and fluoroscopic modes to check patient setup before each treatment or track the movement of fiducial markers due to respiratory or other involuntary internal motion. The MV imager can provide added online monitoring of the target position during treatment delivery.

Digital Tomosynthesis (DTA)

This intermediate solution lies between 2D fluoroscopy and 3D CBCT (kV or MV), which uses limited gantry rotation with multiple radiographs. The number of degrees spanned by the gantry rotation and acquisition will influence image resolution. The rotational angles are generally between $40°$ and $80°$, which reduce the dose delivered to the patient. The acquisition time is shortened as well, with the major advantage of permitting imaging with just a short breath hold. A $60°$ acquisition requires only 10 s of breath hold which is a realistic level for a typical lung cancer patient to maintain. The images are also of high enough quality to allow the resolution of various soft tissues with good contrast between them. The challenge at the moment for digital tomosynthesis is that the time required for image reconstruction is substantial. However, with the advances in computing technology and the rapid development of image reconstruction algorithms and strategies, it is definitely not an insurmountable obstacle. With the reduction of image dose and image acquisition time for patient comfort and increased feasibility,

and the increase in image quality, this imaging modality holds tremendous potential for future adaptive radiotherapy.

Three-Dimensional Image Guidance

Three-dimensional kV imaging of the patient in treatment position immediately prior to treatment is one of the most common 3D IGRT procedures currently performed in clinical practice. Its main advantage over 3D-in-room MV imaging techniques is the enhanced image contrast for soft tissues with low to moderate imaging doses, owing to the prevalence of photoelectric absorption interactions at low energies. This feature allows for improved alignment of the target volume within the reference frame of the treatment beam. However, as the imaging beam and the treatment beam have different sources, alignment of these two beams is not inherent in these solutions, and has to be established and verified. This requires additional quality control relating to both the dosimetry of the imaging beam and its geometry, which will be covered in a following section. 3D kV imaging is separated into two major categories: kilovoltage fan-beam CT (kV CT) and kilovoltage cone-beam CT (kV CBCT).

Kilovoltage Fan-Beam CT (kV CT)

The use of diagnostic CT in the treatment room is advantageous over planar imaging for the localization and verification of patient positioning due to the availability of the 3D information and the better visibility of soft tissue in the CT scan. With the CT scanner in the treatment room, there is only one couch for the patient. There are two methods of acquiring the CT image for the verification of patient setup: (1) with the treatment table of the actual treatment machine, where the patient on the treatment couch must be moved between the scanner and the treatment unit, or (2) with the CT scanner (and/or the treatment unit) moved to/from the patient. This introduces the various sources of error: the tolerance of the motion of the system itself, the inherent separation of imaging and treatment isocenter, the patient reacting to being moved, and the time taken to move the patient or the equipment.

These CT-on-rails/in-room CT consists of a standard diagnostic CT gantry mounted in the treatment room (Fig. 1, Siemens). This technology requires that the treatment room be sufficiently large to accommodate a CT gantry in addition to the treatment LINAC. One of two possible geometries of these machines may be used; the rotational axes of LINAC and CT gantry can be either parallel or orthogonal to each other. In both cases, the patient is setup on the table before it is moved into the imaging position. Next, CT imaging is performed while the CT gantry slides over and around the static patient couch. After reconstruction of the images, the patient is moved back into the treatment position and the 3D CT images are registered with the original planning CT scan images in order to optimally set up the patient for the day's treatment. The achievable setup accuracy of this technique crucially depends on the geometrical registration of the CT images within the isocentric reference frame of the LINAC. The reference target point defined in the treatment plan can be determined in the CT image by radioopaque markers that were previously fixed either at tattoo marks on the patient's skin or on an immobilization mask. Stereotactic localizers may be used for this purpose.

The main advantage of the CT-on-rails technology is its excellent image quality, which arises from the use of an imaging fan beam (reduced scatter) in combination with highly efficient standard CT detectors. High-contrast CT images of diagnostic quality can be acquired at low additional patient dose for verification of patient setup and target localization as well as adaptive planning using the obtained Hounsfield units for reliable dose calculations.

The primary limitation of the CT-on-rails technology is that by design it cannot be used for the detection of intrafractional patient or organ motion. Another concern is that minor undetectable setup errors might be caused by the required movement of the patient between imaging and treatment. Delineation of the radioopaque markers introduces additional registration errors which are not necessarily negligible. The various steps of the workflow may also limit the throughput efficiency of this method.

Kilovoltage Cone-Beam CT (kV CBCT)

LINAC-Integrated kV CBCT

LINAC-integrated kV CBCT refers to kV imaging equipment, consisting of a diagnostic X-ray source

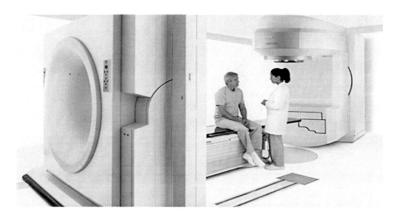

Image-Guided Radiation Therapy (IGRT): kV Imaging. Fig. 1 CT-on-rail, kV CT system, Siemens

and an opposing flat-panel electronic imaging device, mounted on the LINAC gantry. The problem of patient movement between imaging and treatment can be minimized with this gantry-mounted geometry. The technology of LINAC-integrated kV CBCT was first introduced by Jaffray et al. (1999, pp. 773–789) in 1999. In two current commercially available systems, the imaging axis is at a 90° angle to the treatment beam (Fig. 2, Varian Medical Systems, Inc.; Fig. 3, Elekta, Inc.).

The image acquisition of the kV CBCT consists of a number of CT projections (for instance, 330–720), accomplished in either short-scan or full-scan mode in 1 or 2 min, respectively. The achievable image quality is compromised in comparison to diagnostic CT images. The combination of an imaging cone beam with an EPID detection system inevitably leads to intensified scatter artifacts in 3D kV CBCT images. Motion artifacts caused by breathing or peristalsis during the enhanced scanning times can compromise the image quality as well. However, scatter correction methods have been developed to solve the problem of scatter artifacts. Specific calibration and image reconstruction tools warrant sufficient image quality for

a wide range of IGRT procedures at moderate doses. Reproducible mechanical instabilities of the system can be accounted for within the image

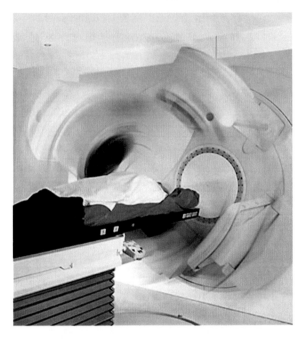

Image-Guided Radiation Therapy (IGRT): kV Imaging. Fig. 3 Linac-integrated kV CBCT system, Elekta

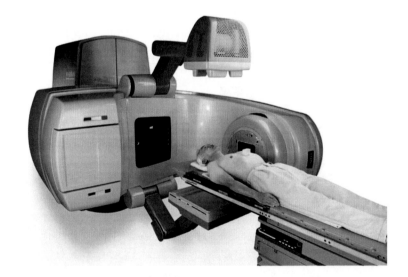

Image-Guided Radiation Therapy (IGRT): kV Imaging. Fig. 2 Linac-integrated kV CBCT system, Varian Medical Systems, Inc

reconstruction through proper calibration processes. Quality assurance measures are needed to guarantee a very precise geometric co-registration of the kV CBCT with the treatment isocenter.

The use of this technique, primarily designed for the correction of interfractional setup errors, is to some extent also suited for the management of intrafraction organ motion using the same equipment. Fluoroscopic imaging and the acquisition of 4D-CBCT scans have been reported (Li et al. 2006; Sonke et al. 2005).

Robotic kV CBCT

For some of the proton treatment facilities, image guidance is performed using in-room robotic cone-beam CT (CBCT) coupled with robotic positioning (Fig. 4, Heidelberg Institute of Technology, Germany). In such a setup, the x-ray imaging generator, detector panel, and patient positioning couch can all be controlled by robotic systems. This setup should ideally offer fast 3D/4D imaging and easy integration with alignment capabilities, as well as the ability to image patients in various positions, with the same ultimate position used for the approved pretreatment images and treatment delivery.

Challenges in establishing such a system include ensuring accurate correlation of the in-room CBCT with the planning CT as well as developing a means of converting Hounsfield numbers to proton stopping power for CBCT. The setup must also offer reproducibility, and the positioning device must not interfere with beam. The issue of intrafraction motion remains a challenge, requiring either 4D tracking or adaptive planning. An appropriate quality assurance regimen for such a system is crucial.

Four-Dimensional Image Guidance: Tracking

Intrafractional tumor motion is managed either by devices to control the motion to a certain extent or by tracking the movement of the tumor with radiation devices. 4D imaging/signal acquisition is required for localizing the target with time. Various systems are used for that purpose, including electromagnetic transponders and detectors, and kV or MV imaging systems. Typical kV systems are described below (Khan 2009).

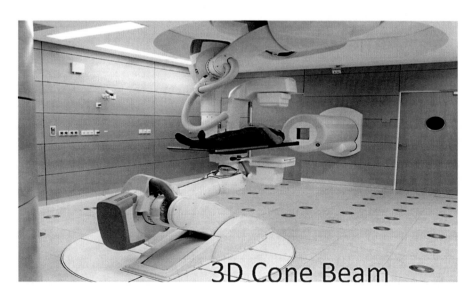

Image-Guided Radiation Therapy (IGRT): kV Imaging. Fig. 4 Robotic controlled CBCT system, HIT proton facility, Heidelberg, Germany

Most commercially available tracking systems use fluoroscopy to detect metal fiducials implanted into the target. Fiducials are continually imaged during irradiation and the treatment beam is turned on or off depending on whether the detected image of the fiducial is within or outside the predefined gating window. Some of these systems are mounted on the accelerator gantry, while others are installed in the treatment room.

Hokkaido University fluoroscopic system is a dual-view fluoroscopy system for tumor tracking (Shirato et al. 2000). The imaging system consists of two diagnostic x-ray tubes that can rotate on a circular track embedded in the floor.

The opposing x-ray detector for each tube rotates synchronously on a track mounted in the ceiling (Fig. 5). During irradiation, the two imaging systems continuously track radioopaque fiducials implanted in the target. The image data from the two fluoroscopic views are combined to construct trajectories of the target motion in three dimensions. Pretreatment imaging is used to define a gating window. During irradiation, the beam is turned on when the image of the fiducial is within the window and turned off when it is outside the window.

ExacTrac/Novalis Body System (Brainlab AG, Germany) (Fig. 6) is a room-mounted system that provides IGRT capabilities for the delivery of

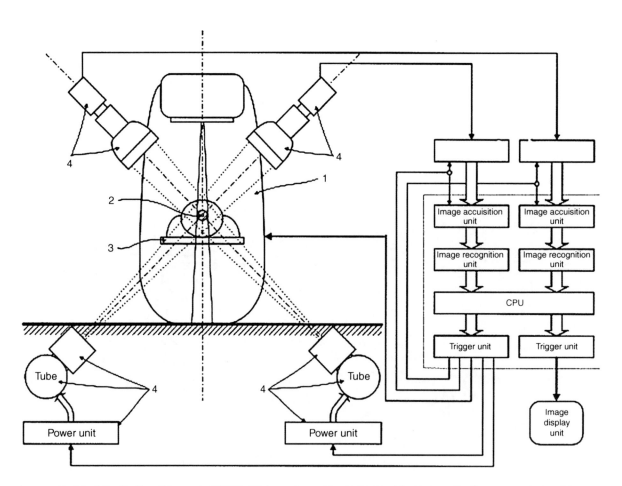

Image-Guided Radiation Therapy (IGRT): kV Imaging. Fig. 5 Hokkaido University fluoroscopic tracking system

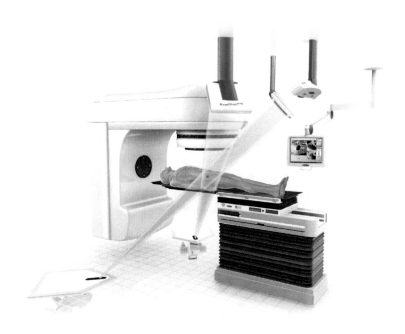

Image-Guided Radiation Therapy (IGRT): kV Imaging. Fig. 6 ExacTrac tracking system

stereotactic radiosurgery or stereotactic radiotherapy. Two real-time tracking systems are used: optical tracking and fluoroscopy-based tracking. In the optical system, IR-reflecting markers are placed on marked spots on the patient's surface or on the immobilization device. Two IR cameras mounted in the ceiling detect the position of the IR markers. Based on the location of the markers, in comparison with the stored reference information, the system automatically steers the treatment couch to match the planned treatment isocenter with the LINAC isocenter. An additional visual feedback of the patient's position is provided by a video camera. Internal target localization and alignment are provided by a stereoscopic x-ray imaging device. This device consists of two x-ray tubes placed in holes in the floor and two opposing a-Si detectors mounted in the ceiling. The system is configured so that the beam axes of both tubes intersect at the LINAC isocenter. The x-ray imaging system is fully integrated into the IR tracking system so that

during treatment delivery, the two systems can work together in monitoring target position. Target alignment is based on implanted fiducials or internal bony landmarks.

The ExacTrac system is capable of providing adaptive gating of the treatment beam given a proper interface to the radiation delivery system, or automatic target alignment using a six-dimensional (6D) robotic couch. The patient positioning parameters are six dimensional: three translations and three rotations about the three orthogonal axes (x, y, z). Evaluation of the intrafraction patient motion is performed with a fusion program that uses internal bony structures visible in the fluoroscopy images to come up with these six parameters.

The CyberKnife (Accuray Inc., Sunnyvale, CA) is an image-guided frameless stereotactic radiosurgery system for treating cranial or extracranial lesions (Fig. 7). It is used for either single-fraction radiosurgery or hypofractionated radiotherapy

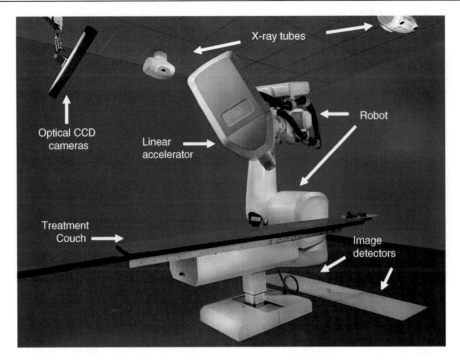

Image-Guided Radiation Therapy (IGRT): kV Imaging. Fig. 7 CyberKnife tracking system

(two to five fractions), with relatively longer delivery time for each fraction. The system consists of an orthogonal pair of x-ray cameras coupled to a small X-band linear accelerator mounted on a robotic arm. Using a higher microwave frequency in the X-band for accelerating electrons reduces the size and weight of the accelerator substantially. As a result, the CyberKnife linear accelerator is small and lightweight (~120 kg), and yet generates a 6-MV x-ray beam. The imaging system in CyberKnife consists of two diagnostic x-ray tubes mounted orthogonally, in the ceiling and two opposing a-Si flat-panel detectors. The system is capable of acquiring and processing multiple images for patient setup as well as for tracking target motion during treatment. The target location is confirmed in relationship to skeletal structure by comparing real-time radiographic images with the reference treatment-planning CT images. The robotic arm has six degrees of freedom and is capable of maneuvering and pointing the linac beam almost anywhere in space. After sensing any target motion, the robotic arm moves the beam to the newly detected target position for alignment.

Image Dose and Quality Assurance

Imaging Dose

The imaging dose associated with these guidance systems depends on the individual system and the particular imaging technique implemented. A comprehensive review of this aspect of the IGRT systems is given in the Task Group 75 report from AAPM (Murphy et al. 2007, pp. 4041–4063). The imaging dose depends on the image acquisition protocols used as well. Typically, the imaging systems come with a number of preprogrammed protocols for image acquisition. These may be specifically intended for imaging of different anatomical regions of the patient by varying the values associated with the different imaging parameters. Also, it may be possible for the user to specify settings not included in a preprogrammed protocol, and to program user-defined protocols. Different settings/protocols will involve different exposures of the patient to imaging dose, and the system will often give an estimate of the dose. The factors for consideration in imaging dose and their relevance are: CTDI doses that are involved for site-specific bony anatomy imaging and soft tissue imaging, the ability to incorporate image dose into treatment planning, dose recording, and QA of imaging dose as estimated from the imaging system.

Quality Assurance (QA) and Calibration

Geometric and dosimetric quality assurance and calibration are important both to ensure correct patient setup and setup verification and to optimize the image quality. For the systems with a separate imaging beam source, that is, kV x-ray systems, it is of great importance to perform and maintain a good alignment and possible compensation of alignment error within the system. For all systems, it is important to avoid unnecessary image distortion and artifacts due to poorly calibrated detector arrays. The imaging systems may come with specialized quality assurance phantoms and guidelines for quality control procedures. While these should be considered a guide to the user, they should not necessarily be considered complete and exhaustive. The factors for consideration in quality assurance and calibration and their relevance are: phantoms for calibration and QA; QA and calibration procedures for image quality, including the CT number relevance and consistency; and QA procedures for geometric alignment and stability.

Cross-References

▶ Electronic Portal Imaging Devices (EPID)
▶ Four-Dimensional (4D) Treatment Planning/ Respiratory Gating
▶ Image-Guided Radiation Therapy (IGRT): MV Imaging

▶ Image-Guided Radiation Therapy (IGRT): TomoTherapy
▶ Robotic Radiosurgery

References

Jaffray D, Drake D, Moreau M et al (1999) A radiographic and tomographic imaging system integrated into a medical linear accelerator for localization of bone and soft-tissue targets. Int J Radiat Oncol Biol Phys 45:773–789
Khan FM (2009) The physics of radiation therapy, 4th edn. Lippincott Williams & Wilkins, Philadelphia
Korreman S, Rasch C, McNair H, Verellen D, Oelfke U, Maingon P, Mijnheer B, Khoo V (2010) The European society of therapeutic radiology and oncology – European institute of radiotherapy (ESTRO–EIR) report on 3D CT-based in-room image guidance systems: A practical and technical review and guide. Radiother Oncol 94(2):129–144
Li T, Xing L, Munro P et al (2006) Four-dimensional cone-beam computed tomography using an on-board imager. Med Phys 33:3825–3833
Murphy MJ, Balter J, Balter S, BenComo JA, Das IJ, Jiang SB, Ma CM, Olivera GH, Rodebaugh RF, Ruchala KJ, Shirato H, Yin FF (2007) The management of imaging dose during image-guided radiotherapy: report of the AAPM task group 75. Med Phys 34:4041–4063
Shirato H et al (2000) Physical aspects of a real-time tumor-tracking system for gated radiotherapy. Int J Radiat Oncol Biol Phys 48:1187–1195
Sonke JJ, Zijp L, Remeijer P, Van Herk M (2005) Respiratory correlated cone beam CT. Med Phys 32:1176–1186

Image-Guided Radiation Therapy (IGRT): MV Imaging

JAY E. REIFF
Department of Radiation Oncology, College of Medicine, Drexel University, Philadelphia, PA, USA

Synonyms

Megavoltage cone beam; Megavoltage cone beam CT; Megavoltage volumetric imaging; MV cone beam

Introduction

Image guidance has become the state of the art for every stage in the process of treating patients with radiation. From patient positioning and target localization through treatment planning and patient/beam alignment, image guidance has allowed physicians to more accurately target and escalate the dose to the affected region(s) while minimizing the dose to the nearby critical structures and adjacent normal, healthy tissue.

The basic premise of image-guided radiation therapy (IGRT) is that soft tissue, key anatomical landmarks, and/or implanted markers can be imaged at the time of treatment. The position of these fiducials is then compared to their expected location based on the initial CT images used for the treatment plan. The patient is then shifted and/or rotated such that the two sets of images are brought into alignment immediately before the treatment commences. Because the target is aligned to its planned location at the time of treatment, the physician is able to reduce the planning margin around the target and spare a larger volume of the adjacent tissue and normal structures from the therapeutic dose being delivered.

Various technologies are used to image the patient while on the treatment table. Those that are most prevalent in radiation oncology centers today include helical TomoTherapy, robotic radiosurgery/radiotherapy, kV imaging, and MV imaging. The detector used in the TomoTherapy unit is a 738 channel xenon-filled ion chamber, the robotic system (CyberKnife) uses cesium iodide scintillators deposited on amorphous silicon photodiodes, and the kV and MV imaging units on traditional linear accelerators use amorphous silicon photodiode panels with an overlying scintillator plate as electronic portal imaging devices (EPID, Fig. 1). As IGRT using helical TomoTherapy, robotic systems, and kV imaging are discussed elsewhere in this Encyclopedia, this entry is limited to IGRT using MV imaging.

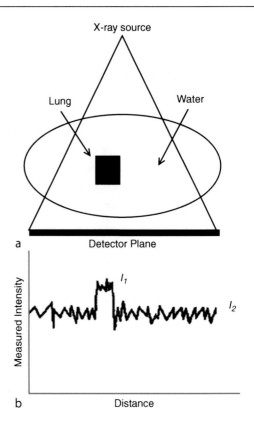

Image-Guided Radiation Therapy (IGRT): MV Imaging. Fig. 1 (**a**) Schematic representing of the definition of contrast in the imaging process. (**b**) Graph depicting the presence of noise in the imaging signal

Megavoltage Imaging

The importance of verifying treatment portals by the use of film has been well documented (Marks et al. 1974, 1976; Rabinowitz et al. 1985) to name just a few. As electronic portal imaging devices (EPIDs) became widely available, many additional studies were performed which demonstrated the utility of these devices, a few of which are referenced here (Ezz et al. 1992; Herman et al. 1994; Van de Steene et al. 1998). Over the last 20 years, many significant improvements have been made to EPIDs in clinical use (▶ Electronic Portal Imaging Devices (EPIDs).

Today these devices can do so much more than just image a treatment portal. Now EPIDs are able to generate a three-dimensional reconstruction of the patient in the treatment position immediately prior to the treatment. In addition to verifying the patient position, these images may be used to track anatomical changes such as tumor growth or regression, monitor the change in tumor location with respect to critical structures due to tumor response or patient weight loss, calculate the dosimetric ramifications based on these changes in order to help the physician decide if a new treatment plan needs to be generated, and assist in planning when a non-CT-compatible object creates artifacts on a diagnostic CT dataset, such as a hip replacement or dental fillings.

MV Cone Beam Image Acquisition

The process begins with the acquisition of data from an MV cone beam CT (MV CBCT). After the patient is set up and aligned in the treatment position, the field size is opened to a square whose dimensions are approximately 27×27 cm. The gantry is set at an angle of $270°$ (right lateral position for a supine, headfirst patient). When the 6 MV beam is turned on, the gantry rotates a total of $200°$ through $0°$ to a final position of $110°$. The accelerator can be preprogrammed to deliver 6, 8, or 10 monitor units (MU) through this $200°$ arc although other values are possible to be input by the user. Typically 6 MU are delivered if the head and neck region is being treated, 8 MU for a thoracic scan, and 10 MU for abdominal and pelvic treatments.

As the gantry is moving, one portal image is acquired per degree of rotation. Thus, a total of 200 megavoltage portal images are used to reconstruct the three-dimensional rendering. Reconstruction begins immediately after the first image is obtained and continues even while subsequent images are being acquired. It takes just under two minutes for the reconstruction to finish.

At this point, the reconstructed three-dimensional rendering may be used to verify and/or modify the patient position, assess the tumor size and location relative to anatomical landmarks, or

be sent to the treatment planning system to assess dosimetric ramifications, or to be fused with a traditional CT scan if that scan contains significant artifacts from non- CT- compatible objects which obscure the anatomical areas needed to be clearly seen by the physician.

Patient Position Verification

Prior to the acquisition of the MV CBCT, the CT scan used for the treatment plan is sent over to the treatment console. Not only are the individual axial slices transferred, the reconstructed sagittal and coronal slices are also transmitted. Additionally, the contoured anatomical structures as well as any dosimetric structures such as the ▶ gross tumor volume (GTV), ▶ clinical target volume (CTV), ▶ internal target volume (ITV), and/or ▶ planning target volume (PTV) associated with the plan (ICRU 1993) are sent to the treatment console; all these structures are clearly demarcated. Isodose lines may be saved as structures and transmitted as well. After the MV CBCT is acquired, this dataset is overlaid with the planning CT dataset. If bony anatomy is being used to register the images as is often the case for skull based, head and neck, and paraspinal tumors, the images are overlaid in all three orthogonal dimensions such that the relevant bony anatomy appears fused, not unlike an image fusion during the treatment planning process. If seeds are being used as a surrogate for the target as in prostate treatments, they become the objects of the fusion. This process may be performed manually by the therapist or automatic registration routines may be employed. If the latter is done, the fusion may still be fine-tuned manually by the therapist. The transparency level of the MV CBCT images may be varied such that both sets of images can be visualized simultaneously and the registration can be validated.

Once the overlay is complete, the system calculates the translation values in the three dimensions (x, y, and z) and if available, the rotation values in the three degrees of freedom (roll, pitch, and yaw) required to obtain the best alignment of the patient with the initial plan. If only translational corrections are being used, the couch may be moved remotely from the treatment console and the treatment may begin.

Tumor Size and Location Verification

Intensity-modulated radiation therapy (IMRT) is often used in the head and neck and thoracic regions to provide a high dose to the target region with a sharp dose gradient to protect adjacent structures. As noted above, the treatment planning CT scan with the associated anatomic and dosimetric contours is sent to the treatment console. As the treatment progresses, any of these dosimetric volumes may shrink and/or suffer a change in position with respect to the bony anatomy or critical structures, thereby possibly requiring a modification of the treatment plan.

MV CBCT is useful in detecting such changes, particularly in the thorax where the higher density tumor is quite obvious in the low-density region of the lung. If, by projecting the initial planning volumes onto the most recent MV CBCT scan, it is determined that the tumor (GTV) has shrunk significantly during the course of treatment, then a revised treatment plan may be necessary in order to treat a smaller volume of healthy lung tissue (Yan et al. 1997; Cheng et al. 2007; Reitz et al. 2007). If this is the case, the recently obtained cone beam CT could be sent back to the treatment planning system and fused with the original planning CT scan so that a new treatment plan using the smaller target volumes may be developed.

Similarly, if a patient who is being treated for a head and neck tumor has suffered significant weight loss, the MV cone beam would indicate the regions of significant tissue loss. It may be that due to the lack of surrounding tissue, the PTV as contoured on the initial CT planning scan has moved closer to a critical structure such as the spinal cord or a parotid gland. This would result

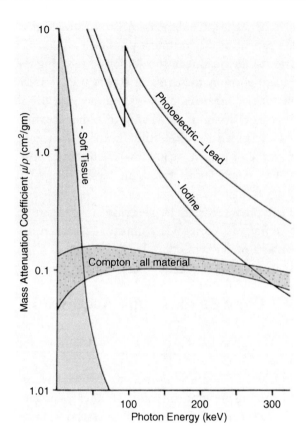

Image-Guided Radiation Therapy (IGRT): MV Imaging. Fig. 2 Compton effect figure

in the critical structure receiving a much higher dose than intended. Projecting the isodose lines of the original plan on the MV CBCT would help in determining the dose that these critical structures are receiving. In these cases the patient might require a complete reevaluation of any immobilization devices that are being used as well as a new planning CT scan in order to generate a revised treatment plan.

Planning with Metallic Objects Within the Patient

Metallic objects such as hip and knee replacements, dental fillings and implants, fiducial markers, and surgical clips often generate artifacts on a conventional kV CT scan. This is an unavoidable radiological consequence of imaging high atomic number objects with x-rays in the diagnostic energy range where the photoelectric effect is dominant. These artifacts, which often appear as white streaks emanating from the metallic object, often obscure anatomic structures that need to be contoured as accurately as possible as part of the treatment planning process.

The image quality of MV images is not affected by these metallic objects due to the nature of the Compton interaction (See ▶ Image-Guided Radiation Therapy (IGRT): TomoTherapy, Fig. 3, p 18) which predominates at megavoltage energies. However, many soft tissue structures as well as most bony landmarks can be visualized on an MV cone beam scan. As a result, MV cone beam images may be sent to the treatment planning system to be fused with the traditional kV CT scan. By adjusting the relative transparencies of the scans, one may contour the relevant structures without interference from the metallic artifacts.

Cross-References

▶ Conformal Therapy: Treatment Planning, Treatment Delivery, and Clinical Results
▶ Electronic Portal Imaging Devices (EPID)
▶ Image-Guided Radiation Therapy (IGRT): kV Imaging
▶ Image-Guided Radiation Therapy (IGRT): TomoTherapy
▶ Intensity Modulated Radiation Therapy (IMRT)
▶ Linear Accelerators (LINAC)
▶ Robotic Radiosurgery

References

Cheng J, Mageras GS, Yorke E, De Arruda F, Sillanpaa J, Rosenzweig KE, Hertanto A, Pham H, Seppi E, Pevsner A, Ling CC, Amols H (2007) Observation of interfractional variations in lung tumor position using respiratory gated and ungated megavoltage cone-beam computed tomography. Int J Radiat Oncol Biol Phys 67(5):1548
Ezz A, Nunro P, Porter AT, Battista J, Jaffray DA, Fenster A, Osborne S (1992) Daily monitoring and correction of radiation field placement using a video-based portal imaging system: a pilot study. Int J Radiat Oncol Biol Phys 22:159
Herman MG, Abrams RA, Mayer RR (1994) Clinical use of on-line portal imaging for daily patient treatment verification. Int J Radiat Oncol Biol Phys 28(4):1017
International Commission of Radiation Units and Measurements (1993) Prescribing, Recording, and Reporting Photon Beam Therapy. ICRU Report 50, Bethesda, MD.
Marks JE, Haus AG, Sutton G, Griem ML (1974) Localization error in the radiotherapy of Hodgkin's disease and malignant lymphoma with extended mantle fields. Cancer 34:83
Marks JE, Haus AG, Sutton G, Griem ML (1976) The value of frequent treatment verification films in reducing localization error in the irradiation of complex fields. Cancer 37:2755
Rabinowitz I, Broomberg J, Goitein M, McCarthy K, Leong J (1985) Accuracy of radiation field alignment in clinical practice. Int J Radiat Oncol Biol Phys 11:1857
Reitz B, Gayou O, Parda DS, Miften M (2007) An adaptive radiotherapy tool for individualizing and verifying treatment margins using MV-CBCT. Int J Radiat Oncol Biol Phys 69(3S):S671
Van de Steene J, Van den Heuvel F, Bel A, Verellen D, De Mey J, Noppen M, De Beukeleer M, Storme G (1998) Electronic portal imaging with on-line correction of setup error in thoracic irradiation: clinical evaluation. Int J Radiat Oncol Biol Phys 40:967
Yan D, Wong J, Vicini F, Michalski J, Pan C, Frazier A, Horwitz E, Martinez A (1997) Adaptive modification of treatment planning to minimize the deleterious effects of treatment setup errors. Int J Radiat Oncol Biol Phys 38(1):197

Image-Guided Radiation Therapy (IGRT): TomoTherapy

Timothy Holmes
Department of Radiation Oncology,
Sinai Hospital, Baltimore, MD, USA

Synonyms

Adaptive radiotherapy; Image-guided radiotherapy; Intensity-modulated radiotherapy

Definition

Helical tomotherapy is a unique form of ▶ intensity-modulated radiotherapy (IMRT) based on a rotating x-ray fan beam. The term "tomotherapy" derives from *tomo*-graphic radio-*therapy*, literally meaning "slice" radiotherapy. Helical tomotherapy treatment delivery is conceptually similar to computerized tomographic (CT) imaging where a three-dimensional image volume is acquired by helical irradiation of the patient using simultaneous source rotation and couch translation. By analogy, a tumor volume can be helically irradiated to achieve a highly ▶ conformal three-dimensional dose distribution by modulating the intensity pattern of the incident x-ray beam profile during rotation. The ▶ intensity modulation is achieved using a pneumatically driven fan-beam multileaf collimator whose leaves achieve near instantaneous leaf transitions between open and closed states.

Background

Helical tomotherapy was initially proposed by Mackie et al., at the University of Wisconsin as a new approach for CT image-guided ▶ intensity-modulated radiotherapy (Mackie et al. 1992). The concept borrowed heavily from the emerging technology of helical computerized tomography where simultaneous source rotation and couch translation were used to perform rapid volumetric diagnostic imaging. A research prototype helical tomotherapy machine was subsequently developed by Dr Mackie's research group and then commercialized as the Hi-ART treatment unit (Fig. 1) by TomoTherapy, Inc., Madison, WI, USA (Mackie 2006). As of this writing, there are approximately 300 systems in use worldwide.

Equipment Description

Figure 2 shows the Hi-ART with gantry covers removed. The major subsystems of the treatment unit are the x-ray source, the CT imaging system, the cooling system, and the treatment couch. The design is based on a CT ring gantry to achieve the high mechanical stability required for accurate, artifact-free CT image reconstruction. The gantry mechanical sag during rotation is approximately 0.1–0.2 mm so no sag corrections are required in the CT reconstruction algorithm. Its isocenter

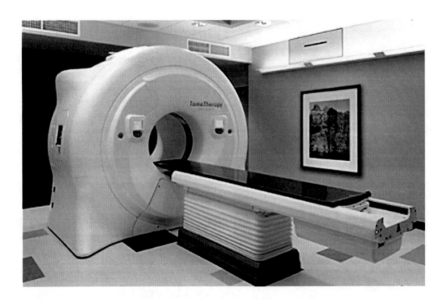

Image-Guided Radiation Therapy (IGRT): TomoTherapy. Fig. 1 The Hi-ART helical tomotherapy CT-guided IMRT system

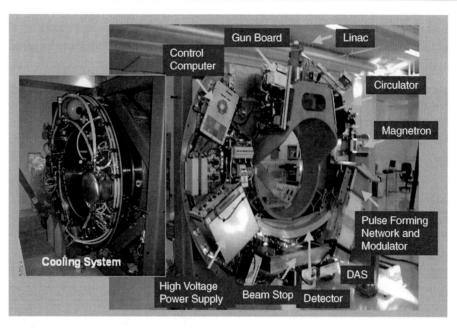

Image-Guided Radiation Therapy (IGRT): TomoTherapy. Fig. 2 The Hi-ART with covers removed showing its major subsystems

specification of 0.2 mm is a factor of 2–10 smaller than that of C-arm gantries (1–2 mm diameter sphere) and is smaller than the pixel size of a reconstructed MVCT image (0.78 mm).

The Hi-ART uses a compact electron linear accelerator (linac) (▶ Linear Accelerators) to generate a 6 MV x-ray beam for treatment and a 3.5 MV x-ray beam for imaging. The linac is a 30 cm long, 6 MV, S-band (nominal 3 GHz) magnetron-powered device with a gridded-gun and a solid-state modulator. An x-ray target is integrated into the body of the linac and is located 85 cm from the gantry rotation axis. There is no beam flattening filter resulting in a high x-ray output for treatment, typically in the range of 8–10 Gy/min at the gantry rotation axis.

The x-ray collimation system consists of a set of moveable primary jaws and the binary multileaf collimator (MLC). The primary jaws have a "clam-shell" design that is used to define discrete beam widths of 5–50 mm in the superior-inferior direction parallel to the MLC leaf motion (Hi-ART systems are typically commissioned with beam widths of 10, 25, and 50 mm). The leakage transmission characteristics of the jaws and MLC are <0.01% and 0.03%, respectively. The 80% to 20% penumbra width of 5 mm corresponds to a gradient of 12%/mm. This gradient corresponds to a dosimetric uncertainty of 2.4% at the edge of the irradiated target due to 0.2 mm mechanical flex of the gantry.

Each binary MLC leaf completely blocks a portion of the x-ray fan beam with a projected shadow of 6.25 mm (nominal) at the gantry rotation axis. The 64 leaves define a 40 cm diameter treatment field-of-view, which combined with the couch travel, enables very large treatment volumes to receive IMRT. Intensity modulation is achieved using pneumatic control of the binary MLC leaves by rapidly (~20 ms) switching the open–closed state of leaves during gantry rotation. The intensity level is proportional to the time a leaf is open, and there are effectively 50 intensity levels that that can be delivered.

The head shielding, including primary collimators, limits the primary leakage to 0.01% of the primary beam, or one tenth the limit (0.1%) used by C-arm radiotherapy treatment units. This added shielding is required since tomotherapy requires a larger number of ▶ monitor units for an IMRT treatment compared to C-arm gantry IMRT methods. Despite this, the whole body dose from tomotherapy is lower than that from C-arm linacs used for fixed-gantry IMRT, due in part to the low leakage transmission of the treatment head and collimation system, and the reduced scatter outside the field due to the lack of a flattening filter (Aoyama et al. 2006). A 13 cm thick lead counterweight is attached to the ring gantry opposite the treatment head that acts as a rotating primary barrier or beam stop.

The treatment couch is a conventional helical CT couch based on a cantilevered (i.e., "cobra") design. Couch positioning accuracy is ±0.5 mm for static positioning and ±1 mm while moving during helical treatment delivery. The precision is 0.1 mm. A carbon fiber couch top (260 cm long by 53 cm wide by 2.2 cm thick) provides rigid patient support and minimal attenuation of the x-ray beam. The maximum longitudinal translation of the couch top is 170 cm. The "modulatable" treatment volume is a cylinder that is approximately 40 cm in diameter and 135 cm long. The couch flex is approximately 0.2 mm over a translation of 3 cm in the region of the head of the table when fully loaded with the weight of a patient.

The Hi-ART system is built upon a single database that integrates all functions of the tomotherapy process. Each patient record in the database contains the patient's treatment plan as well as data generated during each treatment fraction (i.e., MVCT localization images and the treatment "▶ record-and-verification" data). Dedicated workstations are provided for treatment planning and delivery, and are networked to the central dataserver containing the database. The treatment unit operator's workstation combines the functions of CT imaging, image registration, and treatment delivery. In addition, an optional software module (StatRT) is available for this workstation that allows CT-simulation and treatment planning capability for emergent clinical cases where the "sim-and-treat" process can be completed in 20–30 min without moving the patient from the treatment couch.

The ▶ inverse treatment planning system uses a ▶ convolution-superposition dose model for dose calculations (▶ Dose Calculation Algorithms). Inverse treatment planning is typically done using pre-computed 3D "beamlet" dose distributions for individual collimator leaves that directly irradiate the target volume. Most optimization problems require the calculation of thousands of beamlets, consequently a multiprocessor computer system is used to perform the calculations in a reasonable time, typically 7–10 min for intermediate size volumes like a prostate. Once an optimized solution is obtained, a final dose calculation is done that includes the finer details of the MLC leaf thickness and shape, the x-ray output variation as a function of adjacent open leaves, and the latency time to open and close the leaf. Final dose calculations are completed in less than 5 min.

Each 360° gantry rotation is modeled as 51 discrete beams spaced at 7.06° apart – a number chosen to allow a 40 cm diameter target volume to be homogeneously treated with a 2.5 cm completely blocked central avoidance structure. Discretization of the couch travel is determined by the pitch ratio – the ratio of the couch travel distance per rotation to the field width defined at the axis. In helical tomotherapy delivery, the pitch is usually set to be less than ½ to avoid thread-like dose artifacts near the edge of the field. Given a typical pitch of 0.3 for a 25 mm field width, the table motion is modeled by offsetting adjacent beams by 0.147 mm (e.g., 0.3 × 25 mm/51) increments parallel to the direction of table motion.

Plan optimization is performed iteratively by making changes to the incident intensity pattern for all binary MLC leaves that intersect the target, also referred to as the *sinogram* – the name derives from the fact that each point in the target projects back to a sinusoidal path in the intensity pattern. The sinogram describes the opening and closing of the binary MLC leaves as a function of the gantry rotation angle and the translation position of the couch – it is in effect the operational instructions for the Hi-ART treatment delivery. The optimization can be stopped and restarted at any time to review the dose-volume histograms and the dose distribution, and to alter the optimization constraints, without loss of any plan data. Following optimization, the intensity levels are discretized for treatment delivery, with 50 levels chosen to reduce the

uncertainty in the target dose due to intensity discretization to less than 0.1%.

MVCT Imaging

The MVCT x-ray energy is approximately 3.5 MV, therefore the photons interact almost exclusively by Compton interactions producing a linear relationship between CT number and electron density and a higher signal at the MVCT detector than kV x-rays. Consequently, MVCT images do not display image artifacts due to dental fillings or orthopedic implants, making them an attractive alternative to kVCT images for inverse treatment planning when metal is present in treatment volume (Fig. 3).

The MVCT detector is a xenon-filled gas detector with tungsten septa separating

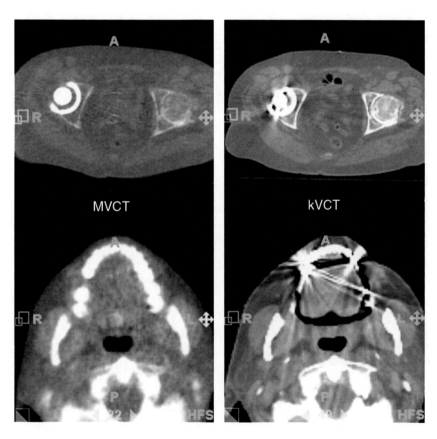

Image-Guided Radiation Therapy (IGRT): TomoTherapy. Fig. 3 Two examples showing the impact of implanted metal on MVCT and kVCT images

ionization cavities. The detector resolution at the rotation axis is about 0.6 mm in the transverse direction and equal to the MVCT beam width (4 mm) in the longitudinal direction. The size of the electron beam on the target is about 1 mm so that the high contrast resolution is about 1.2–1.6 mm. The MVCT images have soft tissue contrast of 2–3% at a dose of 1–2 cGy, which is sufficient for radiotherapy localization (Fig. 4).

The gantry rotation period for MVCT imaging is 10 s compared to rotation periods of 20–60 s for an IMRT treatment delivery. Approximately 800 transmission images are measured per rotation, sufficient to reconstruct two axial images. Helical pitches of 1, 1.5, and 2 are available for MVCT imaging allowing a typical tumor of 8–10 cm length to be imaged in as little as 2 min. Image reconstruction is carried out in parallel with data acquisition so there is little delay following data acquisition for the MVCT images to be analyzed. Automatic registration of the MVCT images to the planning CT images is based on a mutual information algorithm and takes

10–20 s, although manual registration is also possible. The registration quality can be evaluated using a checkerboard tool and overlays of the anatomical and isodose contours. The Hi-ART can automatically adjust translation and roll offsets; pitch and yaw adjustments must be handled using a tertiary positioning device with angle readouts.

Clinical Application

Most treatment procedures are completed within 15–20 min; patient setup and image guidance require less than 10 min and treatment delivery can be completed within 3–10 min depending on the length of the target volume and the prescribed dose. Recent research into a fully dynamic jaw delivery has demonstrated the potential to reduce overall treatment time by 40–50% including a reduction in out-of-field dose occurring in the superior-inferior direction.

Overall treatment delivery time T is a function of target length (L), beam width (W), prescribed dose D, average dose rate at the target R, and the user-defined modulation factor M (ratio of the maximum leaf open time to the average leaf opening time):

$$T = MD(L + W)/WR \sim (M/W) \times \text{constant}$$

Treatment time can be shortened by reducing the intensity modulation or by increasing the beam width. Modulation factors of 2–3 are commonly used as higher values do not significantly improve plan quality but increase overall treatment time. The choice of beam width (1.0, 2.5, or 5.0 cm) can significantly alter the overall treatment time. For example, a 7 cm long prostate volume can be treated in approximately 3–5 min using a 2.5 cm beam width, or 12–20 min with a 1 cm beam width without noticeable improvement in dose conformance. Regardless of the overall length of the treatment volume, it should be recognized that a slab of tissue defined by the beam width will receive a conventional fractionation

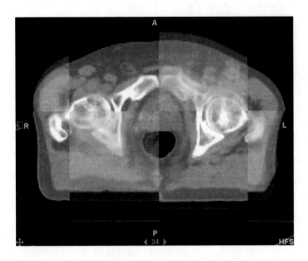

Image-Guided Radiation Therapy (IGRT): TomoTherapy. Fig. 4 Example of MVCT image localization of a prostate. The MVCT is shown as a transparent blue-scale checkerboard overlay on the original planning CT data

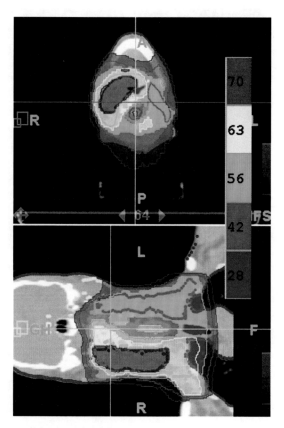

Image-Guided Radiation Therapy (IGRT): TomoTherapy. Fig. 5 Axial and coronal images of a head and neck case showing high (*red*), intermediate (*yellow*) and low (*green*) risk target regions simultaneously treated to 70 Gy, 63 Gy and 56 Gy, respectively

dose of 1.8–2.0 Gy within 1–2 min due to the slice-based delivery. Consequently, the average dose rate in the tumor is typically 1–2 Gy/min minimizing the impact of cell repair during the treatment delivery.

Helical tomotherapy has been successfully applied to image-guided IMRT throughout the body for curative and palliative cases. Treatment volumes range from small metastatic lesions in the brain and lung to intermediate-sized tumors such as prostate and head and neck tumors to the extreme case of total bone irradiation with organ avoidance for bone marrow transplantation (Schultheiss et al. 2007). In most curative situations, the rationale for using CT-guided IMRT is to deliver a high tumorcidal dose (60–80 Gy) while minimizing dose to adjacent structures. Helical tomotherapy has proven very useful for head and neck irradiation where it is common to concurrently "dose paint" the high-, intermediate-, and low-risk regions to different dose levels as shown in the example of Fig. 5.

Dosimetry Quality Assurance

All patient treatment plans must be verified by dosimetry measurement prior to the first treatment delivery, a process referred to as Dosimetry Quality Assurance, or DQA. Applying the patient's treatment plan parameters to CT images of a DQA test phantom creates a DQA verification test plan. The DQA test phantom is then irradiated with dosimeters inside it (e.g., film plus ion chambers or an ion chamber/diode array) after first localizing it on the treatment couch using MVCT. The measured data is then imported into the planning system and compared to the computed dose in at the same location as the measured data. Comparison methods include 1D dose profiles, 2D isodose distributions, and a 2D "gamma distribution" that represents how well a pixel in the measured dose image agrees in magnitude and spatial position to a neighborhood of pixels in the calculated dose image (Low et al. 1998). A DQA plan verification example is shown in Fig. 6.

Machine Quality Assurance

Helical tomotherapy QA includes both static and dynamic quality assurance tests (Fenwick et al. 2004). Static QA tests are carried out on the non-rotating beam and are similar to tests performed on a conventional C-arm linac (x-ray output, beam geometry, collimation system alignment, laser alignment, etc.) Since treatments are delivered using dynamic motions of the couch, gantry, and MLC, a suite of dynamic tests must also be performed to test the machine's performance under conditions

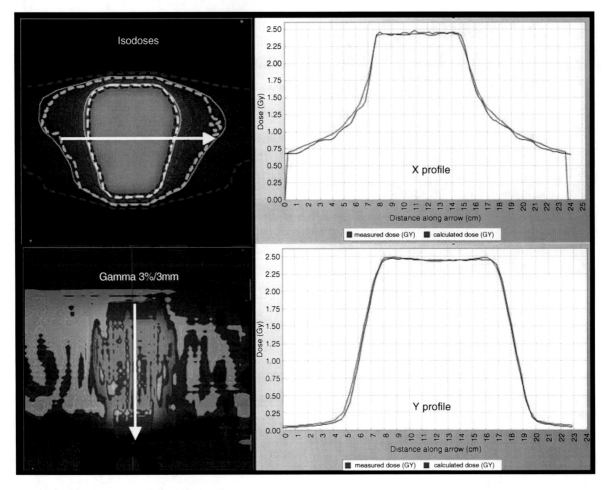

Image-Guided Radiation Therapy (IGRT): TomoTherapy. Fig. 6 Example of DQA verification for a prostate case showing isodose, profile and gamma distribution comparisons

similar to clinical use. These tests include gantry rotation speed, couch speed, and MLC leaf transitions. These can be tested separately or in combination. For example, Balog et al. have described a dynamic quality assurance procedure that measures constancy of dynamic output, x-ray energy, couch–gantry speed synchronization, couch offset, moveable laser calibration, MVCT localization imaging, and image quality parameters (high and low contrast resolutions, CT number constancy) in a single imaging and delivery procedure (Balog et al. 2006). TomoTherapy, Inc. provides an optional

quality assurance software tool called TQA that implements many of these static and dynamic tests.

Adaptive Radiotherapy

The availability of daily MVCT images of the patient provides the means of evaluating the impact of ongoing changes in patient anatomy due to weight loss and tumor shrinkage on the delivered dose. Specifically, daily dose estimates are computed using these images, the results then added to obtain the cumulative dose using

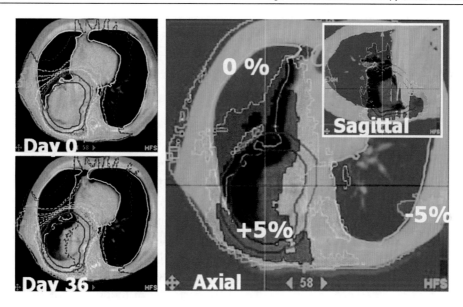

Image-Guided Radiation Therapy (IGRT): TomoTherapy. Fig. 7 An adaptive-planning example showing the impact of lung tumor shrinkage on treated dose. Here, the treated dose was approximately 5% higher than the treatment plan with the dose increase largely in the region of tumor shrinkage

deformable registration. Differences between the cumulative dose and the planned dose can be determined and decisions made to adapt future treatments to compensate for these errors (Tome' et al. 2007). An adaptive-planning tool is provided with the Hi-ART system to assess the effect of patient weight loss and tumor shrinkage on the treated dose. An example of the use of this tool to assess lung tumor shrinkage during the course of a 1-month treatment is shown in Fig. 7.

Cross-References

▶ Conformal Therapy: Treatment Planning, Treatment Delivery, and Clinical Results
▶ Image-Guided Radiation Therapy (IGRT): kV Imaging
▶ Image-Guided Radiation Therapy (IGRT): MV Imaging
▶ Imaging in Oncology
▶ Intensity-Modulated Proton Therapy (IMPT)
▶ Linear Accelerators (LINAC)
▶ Oro-Hypopharynx
▶ Palliation of Brain and Spinal Cord Metastases
▶ Prostate
▶ Radiation Detectors
▶ Radiation Oncology Physics
▶ Robotic Radiosurgery
▶ Stereotactic Radiosurgery – Cranial
▶ Stereotactic Radiosurgery: Extracranial
▶ Total Body Irradiation (TBI)

References

Aoyama H, Westerly DC et al (2006) Integral radiation dose to normal structures with conformal external beam radiation. Int J Radiat Oncol Biol Phys 64(3):962–967

Balog J, Holmes T, Vaden R (2006) Helical tomotherapy dynamic quality assurance. Med Phys 33(10):3939–3950

Fenwick JD, Tomo WA et al (2004) Quality assurance of a helical tomotherapy unit. Phys Med Biol 49(13): 2933–2953

Low DA, Harms WB et al (1998) A technique for the quantitative evaluation of dose distributions. Med Phys 25(5):656–661

Mackie TR (2006) History of tomotherapy. Phys Med Biol 51(13):R427–R453

Mackie TR, Holmes T et al (1992) Tomotherapy: a new concept for the delivery of dynamic conformal radiotherapy. Med Phys 20:1709–1719

Schultheiss TE, Wong J et al (2007) Image-guided total marrow and total lymphatic irradiation using helical tomotherapy. Int J Radiat Oncol Biol Phys 67(4):1259–1267

Tome' WA, Jaradat HA, Nelson IA, Ritter MA, Mehta MP (2007) Helical tomotherapy: image guidance and adaptive dose guidance. In: Meyer JL (ed) IMRT, IGRT, SBRT – Advances in the treatment planning and delivery of radiotherapy. Front Radiat Ther Oncol 40:162–168

Image-Guided Radiotherapy (IGRT)

TIMOTHY HOLMES
Department of Radiation Oncology, Sinai Hospital, Baltimore, MD, USA

Definition

Radiotherapy methods that use imaging methods to localize the tumor prior to and during treatment to improve accuracy of dose delivery to the tumor. Common imaging methods include pretreatment localization using CT, ultrasound, planar X-ray imaging, or tracking of implanted electromagnetic markers. Tumor tracking is also commonly carried out by planar X-ray imaging of implanted markers or by real-time tracking of electromagnetic markers.

Cross-References

▶ Image-Guided Radiation Therapy (IGRT): TomoTherapy

▶ Image-Guided Radiation Therapy (IGRT): kV Imaging

▶ Image-Guided Radiation Therapy (IGRT): MV Imaging

▶ Image-Guided Radiotherapy (IGRT)

▶ Robotic Radiosurgery

Imaging in Oncology

HEBERT ALBERTO VARGAS[1], OGUZ AKIN[1], HEDVIG HRICAK[2]
[1]Body MRI, Memorial Sloan-Kettering Cancer Center, New York, NY, USA
[2]Department of Radiology, Memorial Sloan-Kettering Cancer Center, New York, NY, USA

Introduction

The field of medical imaging includes a wide variety of techniques that allow direct visualization of anatomy and provide insights into physiologic, metabolic, and pathological processes within the human body. Imaging plays a role in all aspects of oncology, from primary cancer diagnosis (including screening) to cancer staging, treatment planning, treatment response assessment, and long-term follow-up. Technical advances in recent decades have broadly expanded the number of imaging modalities used in routine clinical practice in oncology and have allowed structural information to be combined with functional information regarding tumor biology and metabolism. Furthermore, significant developments in ▶ molecular imaging are opening new horizons in preclinical cancer detection and personalized, targeted cancer therapy. Each imaging modality has specific advantages and limitations with regard to each cancer type and site. Therefore, it is important – though often challenging – to choose the modality most likely to answer the pertinent clinical questions in an individual patient, so as to maximize efficacy and avoid unnecessary diagnostic and therapeutic delays.

Imaging Modalities

X-Ray-Based Modalities

Plain Radiography

Synonyms: Conventional radiography; Plain film radiography; Radiography; Roentgenography; Simple x-rays

Basic Principle: An x-ray beam (a form of ► electromagnetic radiation) is attenuated as it passes through a tissue, to a degree that is proportional to the thickness, density, and composition of that tissue. Air causes minimal attenuation of the x-ray beam, so air-filled structures (such as lungs and bowel) appear lucent (black) on plain radiography. At the other extreme, dense materials (such as calcium in bones, metals in prosthesis) extensively attenuate x-ray beams and appear opaque (white) on radiography.

Current Role in Oncology: Mammography, which forms the mainstay for screening in breast cancer, uses low-dose x-rays and multiple projections to detect abnormal findings in the breast (Fig. 1). In other areas of oncology, plain radiography has largely been replaced by more advanced techniques, though it is still often used as a first-line examination. In skeletal pathology, it is helpful for characterizing bone lesions (e.g., fractures, calcified matrix, and ► periosteal reaction) (Fig. 2), particularly when rapid assessment is needed in the context of trauma. Also, bone radiographs are commonly evaluated together with findings from other modalities (such as bone scintigraphy or MRI) to prevent misdiagnosis of various osseous abnormalities (such as ► stress fracture or ► fibrous dysplasia). Chest and abdominal radiography are in steady decline, as, ultimately, further imaging (mostly computed tomography (CT)) is needed for

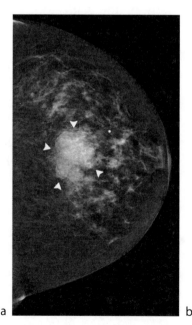 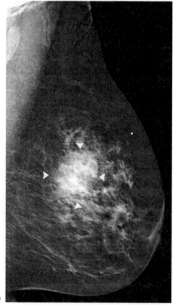

a   b

Imaging in Oncology. Fig. 1 Cranio-caudal (**a**) and mediolateral oblique (**b**) views from a screening mammogram in a 65-year-old woman showing a mass in the left breast (*arrowheads*)

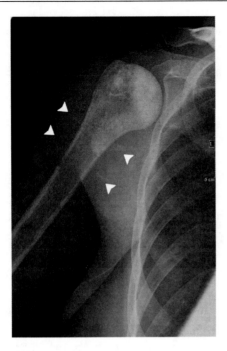

Imaging in Oncology. Fig. 2 Plain radiograph shows an osteosarcoma of the right proximal humerus with ill-defined margins and a permeative pattern. Soft tissue calcification is also present (*arrowheads*)

clarifying radiographic findings. However, they may be useful in some acute circumstances, such as ▶ pneumothorax or ▶ pneumoperitoneum.

Advantages: Quick, inexpensive, and widely available.

Limitations: Most soft tissues attenuate x-ray beam to a similar degree, resulting in the markedly limited ability of radiography to distinguish soft tissue abnormalities (such as liver metastases from normal liver tissue).

Advanced Applications

- *Dual-energy radiography*: Allows two images of the same object, one created with a low-energy spectrum and another created with a high-energy spectrum of the x-ray source, to be combined. Potential uses include evaluating the calcium content of a pulmonary nodule to assess the likelihood that it is malignant.

Computed Tomography (CT)

Synonyms: ▶ Computed axial tomography (CAT)

Basic Principle: The basic physics principle is the same as for plain radiography and is based on the attenuation of x-ray beams as they pass through tissues. In CT, however, an x-ray-producing source and x-ray detector(s) are positioned opposite each other within a gantry which rotates continuously around the patient. As a result, x-ray beams are directed toward the patient from multiple angles, and a large amount of data is generated regarding the attenuation of each x-ray beam. Computer algorithms are then applied to produce a detailed representation of a "slice" of the human body, typically in the axial plane, based on the differences in x-ray attenuation by different organs.

Current Role in Oncology: CT is helpful in evaluating body parts composed of various tissue densities such as air (lung, bowel), fat, soft tissue, and bone. In many types of cancers, CT can accurately show the extent of local and distant spread of tumor. Change in tumor size is the basis of the standard guidelines for assessing response to therapy (Miller et al. 1981; Eisenhauer et al. 2009) and is most commonly measured on CT. Ultrafast acquisitions allow three-dimensional reconstruction of blood-filled structures (CT angiography) or fluid-filled structures (CT urography) (Fig. 3). CT can also be used to guide interventional procedures, such as biopsy and drainage, and to facilitate the targeting of radiation treatment. Finally, CT is also useful in diagnosing complications of cancer and cancer therapy, such as ▶ pulmonary embolism, postoperative collections, and ▶ opportunistic infections.

Advantages: Cost-effective and widely available. With the current technology, high-quality images of multiple body parts can be acquired in seconds.

Limitations: Both plain radiography and CT involve ionizing radiation, but the dose delivered to the patient with CT is higher. Overutilization

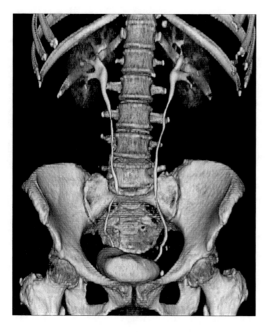

Imaging in Oncology. Fig. 3 Three-dimensional reconstruction from a computed tomography (*CT*) urogram allowing visualization of the pelvicalyceal systems, ureters, and bladder

of CT is a recognized problem in some health care settings and is an issue under increasing scrutiny. Also, the iodinated intravenous contrast materials often used with CT can cause adverse reactions, which are usually mild (e.g., mild transient pruritus or skin rashes) but occasionally severe (e.g., renal failure or death).

Advanced Applications

- *Virtual endoscopy*: The large volume of data obtained with current CT technology can be used to produce multiplanar 2D, 3D and endoluminal views of different structures. The most studied of these techniques is CT colonography, which in a recent revision of the American Cancer Society (ACS) guidelines for colorectal cancer screening was included as one of the screening options for average-risk individuals (Levin et al. 2008).

Other applications of these techniques, such as CT bronchoscopy, are currently under evaluation.

- *Dual-source CT*: Two x-ray tubes work in parallel at different energy levels. This technology can be used to automatically differentiate various tissue types in one scan.
- *Functional CT*: Advanced computational analysis allows quantitative assessment of tissue perfusion, blood volume and capillary permeability "in vivo." Currently, the main limitation of this technique is the high radiation dose delivered. In the future, further developments in the ability to lower radiation dose may allow functional CT to become a valuable tool for obtaining physiological information to assist with diagnosis, staging, and therapy monitoring for patients with cancer.

Ultrasound (US)

Synonyms: Echography (echocardiography refers to ultrasound of the heart); Sonography

Basic Principle: This modality exploits the physical properties of sound waves to generate "real-time" images of the human anatomy. The properties of US are similar to those of audible sound, except that the frequency of audible sound is between 0.01 and 0.02 MHz while the frequency of medical US is typically in the range of 3–12 MHz. A US transducer in contact with a body surface emits an US pulse, which is transmitted into the body, then reflects off anatomical structures and returns to the transducer. The time from emission to reception is used to calculate the depth of a structure and its "brightness" or echogenicity on gray-scale images (B-mode US). US can also be used to detect the change in frequency of a moving sound wave, which is the basis for Doppler ultrasound, commonly used to image vascular structures.

Current Role in Oncology: In cancer patients, US is most commonly used to image superficial

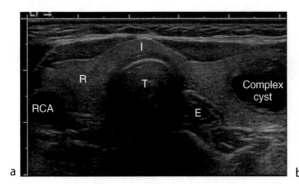
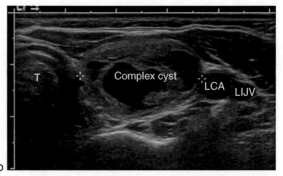

a   b

Imaging in Oncology. Fig. 4 (**a, b**) Thyroid ultrasound demonstrates a mixed-echogenicity complex cystic lesion in the left lobe of the thyroid. *I* thyroid isthmus, *R* right lobe of thyroid, *T* trachea, *E* esophagus, *RCA* right carotid artery, *LCA* left carotid artery, *LIJV* left internal jugular vein

structures (e.g., thyroid, breast, testes) (Fig. 4), the thorax (pleural or pericardial effusions, chest wall masses), the abdomen (especially liver, biliary system, and kidneys), pelvic genitourinary organs, and the vascular system. In addition, US can be used to guide interventional radiology procedures such as biopsy, tumor ablation, and drainage.

Advantages: No ionizing radiation is involved, and there are no proven harmful effects to humans at the frequencies used in diagnostic US. Also, "real-time" images are produced, and modern equipment is extremely portable (some devices are the size of a conventional hand-held or laptop computer) and relatively inexpensive.

Limitations: US waves cannot propagate through air and dense tissue (calcium), therefore the presence of air-containing or calcified structures (such as bowel gas, lungs, and bones) hinders the evaluation of the adjacent anatomy. Also, US is more operator-dependent and less reproducible than other imaging modalities.

Advanced Applications

- *Contrast-enhanced ultrasound*: Small (1–7 μm) gas-filled agents usually referred to as "micro bubbles" are injected intravenously. They can then be visualized on real-time

ultrasound, as they do not diffuse out of the circulation and thus behave as blood-pool markers. They can also be coated with surface ligands to target and provide useful information about tumor microvasculature.

- *Ultrasound elastography*: Exploits the differences in tissue strain produced by freehand compression. Using elastography, the operator is able to discriminate hard from soft tissue regions, with stiffness values marked in different colors and shown in real-time images. Elastography is being investigated as a novel tool for cancer detection, based on the hypothesis that the consistency of solid tumors differs from that of adjacent normal tissues.

Magnetic Resonance Imaging (MRI)

Synonyms: ▶ Nuclear magnetic resonance (NMR)

Basic Principle: When nuclei composed of an odd number of protons and neutrons are placed in a magnetic field (usually measured in units of Tesla) and excited by the addition of radiofrequency pulses, they momentarily gain energy. When the radiofrequency pulses are turned off, the nuclei return to their resting state and emit the previously absorbed energy. Complex mathematical algorithms

(▶ Fourier transform) are then performed to convert the data generated from these changes in energy levels into images. The magnitude of the emitted signal and the time it takes for the nuclei to return to the resting state is dependent upon certain intrinsic properties of the nuclei, including the nuclear spin density (or proton density), longitudinal (T1) relaxation time, and transverse (T2) relaxation time. The most commonly imaged nucleus is hydrogen (^{1}H).

Current Role in Oncology: MRI plays an important role in the assessment of multiple cancers (Figs. 5–6). A detailed discussion of specific scenarios where MRI is indicated rather than other imaging modalities and vice versa is beyond the scope of this chapter, but a few points are worth mentioning. First, the lack of ionizing radiation from MRI makes this modality preferable for use in patients who may be more susceptible to the harmful effects of ionizing radiation, such as children and patients who require repeated examinations. Also, MRI technology is rapidly evolving. The spatial resolution of some modern MRI sequences is similar to that of CT; in addition, unlike CT, where contrast between tissues is based solely on the difference in their x-ray attenuation, many MRI parameters can be manipulated to change the tissue contrast of an image. Ultimately, the decision of whether to image with MRI or another modality depends on many factors, perhaps, most importantly, the clinical question that needs to be answered.

Advantages: No ionizing radiation, excellent soft tissue resolution, allows multiparametric

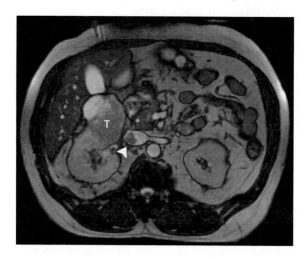

Imaging in Oncology. Fig. 6 Steady-state free precession (*SSFP*) magnetic resonance imaging (*MRI*) shows a right renal tumor (*T*) with extension into the inferior vena cava (*arrowhead*)

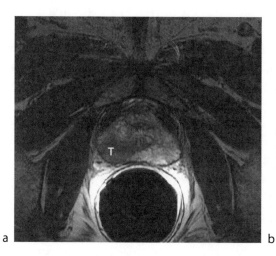

a

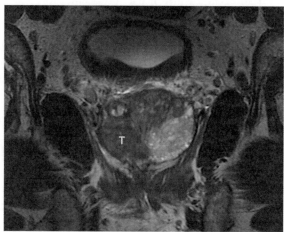

b

Imaging in Oncology. Fig. 5 Axial (**a**) and coronal (**b**) T2-weighted magnetic resonance (*MR*) images of the prostate showing a right peripheral zone tumor (*T*)

assessment (with perfusion, diffusion-weighted, and spectroscopic imaging).

Disadvantages: More expensive, not as widely available as other imaging modalities. Gadolinium-based contrast agents used in MRI have recently been implicated in a very rare form of severe toxicity called nephrogenic systemic fibrosis.

Advanced Applications

- *Functional MRI (fMRI)*: Based on the different paramagnetic properties of oxy- and deoxy-hemoglobin and on changes in blood flow, fMRI can evaluate regions of the brain that are activated by specific tasks (such as hand-tactile stimulation or hand motor activity). This functional data can be superimposed on anatomical images, thus providing helpful information for pre-treatment planning in neuro-oncology, particularly regarding the avoidance of critical areas and minimizing the loss of essential functions.

- *MR Spectroscopy (MRS)*: This technique exploits the phenomenon of "chemical shift," or small changes in resonant frequency due to molecular structure, for the purpose of in vivo detection of multiple metabolites within tissues (including citrate, choline, lactate, and creatine). Variations in the presence and concentration of such metabolites form the basis for differentiating cancerous from non-cancerous tissues using this technique, which has been predominantly studied in the brain and prostate.

- *Diffusion-weighted MRI (DW-MRI)*: Based on the variability of the rate of water movement ("diffusion") in different biological tissues. Diffusion within tumors is restricted relative to that in normal tissue. By obtaining multiple images with different diffusion "weighting" factors, it is possible to calculate the apparent diffusion coefficient (ADC), a measure of the distance water molecules have traveled. The ADC values are calculated for all pixels of the image and displayed as a parametric map.

- *Dynamic contrast-enhanced (DCE) MRI*: Also known as "perfusion" MRI, this technique uses fast MRI sequences to repeatedly image the passage of a gadolinium-based intravenous contrast agent through a volume of interest. The basic principle is that the MRI signal will change relative to the amount of contrast material present at any given time. This is used to assess tissue microcirculation, with cancers often demonstrating early nodular enhancement before the rest of the parenchyma and early contrast washout.

Nuclear Medicine Imaging Modalities

Basic Principle: Radioactive tracers (which emit gamma rays) are injected into the body and then their physiological and pathological distribution is recorded using a ▶ radioactivity detector system. Several such detectors exist, including the gamma camera, which produces two-dimensional images, and ▶ single photon emission computed tomography (SPECT) and ▶ positron emission tomography (PET), which provide three-dimensional information.

Current Role in Oncology: The most commonly used nuclear medicine study is the bone scintigram (Fig. 7). The radiotracer used, 99^{m}Technicium-Methyl diphosphonate (Tc-99m-MDP), is injected intravenously. Some of the tracer is excreted through the kidneys, but some also accumulates in the skeleton, predominantly in regions of increased osteoblastic activity. An image of the distribution of the radiotracer uptake is taken with a gamma camera a few hours after injection. The presence of a tumor or other damage to the bone shows up as a "hot-spot" superimposed on a background of normal bone uptake. A similar principle is also applied in nuclear cardiology, where the uptake or distribution of a radiotracer can be used to calculate physiologic parameters such as the ventricular ejection fraction or to detect areas of myocardial ischemia. Lymphoscintigraphy

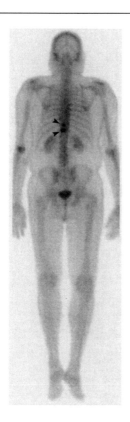

Imaging in Oncology. Fig. 7 Bone scintigraphy shows two areas of increased uptake in the spine (*arrowheads*) in keeping with bone metastases in a patient with prostate cancer

is also used to detect spread from a primary tumor site to a regional "sentinel" lymph node at an early stage of metastasis.

Advantages: Provides "functional" information to complement anatomical information from other modalities. The most commonly used radiotracers are safe and relatively inexpensive.

Limitations: Gamma rays are also a form of ionizing radiation. Some radiotracers have a very short half-life and are not widely available. Examinations are time-consuming.

Hybrid Modalities → PET/CT

Basic Principle: Combines detailed anatomical information from CT with information from PET on the spatial distribution of a radiolabeled, biologically relevant molecule. A common feature of many tumors is accelerated glycolysis. As a result, the radiolabeled glucose analog ^{18}F-2-fluoro-D-deoxy-glucose, or ^{18}F-FDG, has been widely used to quantitatively image the biochemistry of glucose utilization by tumors.

Current Role in Oncology: The advantages of having both PET and CT in a single device have resulted in rapid dissemination of this relatively new technology. Although certain issues such as equipment specifications, image acquisition protocols, supervision, interpretation, professional qualifications, and safety still need to be standardized, the American College of Radiology Practice Guidelines (American College of Radiology 2007) list many potential uses for FDG PET/CT in oncology, including evaluating an abnormality detected by another imaging method to determine the level of metabolism and the likelihood of malignancy, and searching for an unknown primary tumor when metastatic disease is discovered as the first manifestation of cancer. However, it should be noted that PET/CT does not work equally well for all tumors, and a continuing review of the literature is essential to monitor the most effective applications of this technique.

Advantages: Depicts tissue function and biochemistry in a high-resolution, anatomic context. Fused images are easier to interpret than images from PET and CT performed separately (Fig. 8).

Limitations: Both PET and CT involve ionizing radiation. Not as widely available as other imaging modalities. Radiotracers used have a short half-life.

Advanced Applications

FDG is not the only agent used in PET/CT. A vast array of radiotracers can be used to image many key molecules and molecularly based events with this technique, including carbon-11, fluorine-18, oxygen-15, and nitrogen-13.

Future Directions: Molecular Imaging

Molecular imaging is not a new phenomenon; it has been practiced indirectly for decades, using

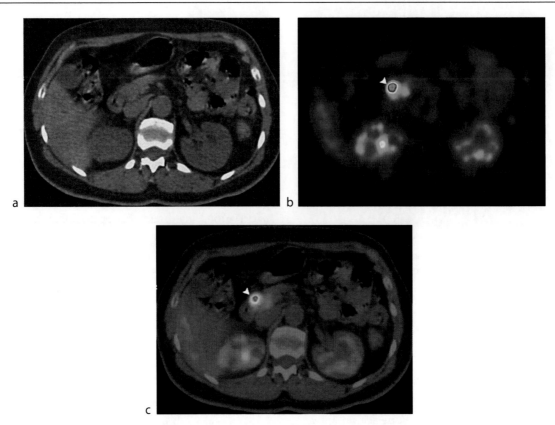

Imaging in Oncology. Fig. 8 Axial unenhanced computed tomography (*CT*) image of the abdomen (**a**) does not show any significant abnormality. Positron emission tomography (*PET*) study in the corresponding location (**b**) shows a hypermetabolic focus (*arrowhead*); however, anatomical correlation is difficult. Fused PET and CT image (**c**) demonstrate that the focus of high uptake is localized in the head of the pancreas. The patient had a confirmed pancreatic malignant tumor

nuclear medicine techniques (e.g., indium-111 – octreotide receptor imaging of carcinoid tumors and iodine-131 imaging of the thyroid) and other imaging techniques. However, interest in molecular imaging as a tool for oncology has surged in recent years, as improvements in the understanding of cancer biology, coupled with advanced techniques for imaging metabolic and biochemical pathways, have allowed implementation of the concept of "personalized" medicine. Molecular imaging research themes include cancer biology (gene expression imaging, cancer phenotype imaging), drug discovery based on antibody and small molecules (including treatment selection and response assessment), and cellular tracers (cancer immunology, stem cell physiology, and physiology of metastases). Potential future clinical uses of molecular imaging include treatment response assessment through evaluation of changes in metabolism and cellular proliferation, which are known to precede changes in tumor size.

Cross-References

▶ Image-Guided Radiotherapy (IGRT)
▶ Molecular Markers in Clinical Radiation Oncology
▶ Nuclear Medicine

References

American College of Radiology (2007) ACR practice guidelines for performing FDG-PET/CT in oncology. Available at: http://www.acr.org/Secondary-MainMenuCategories/quality_safety/guidelines/nuc_med.aspx. Accessed April 30, 2010

Eisenhauer E, Therasse P, Bogaerts J et al (2009) New response evaluation criteria in solid tumours: revised RECIST guideline (version 1.1). Eur J Cancer 45:228–247

Levin B, Lieberman D, McFarland B et al (2008) Screening and surveillance for the early detection of colorectal cancer and adenomatous polyps: a joint guideline from the American Cancer Society, the US Multi-Society Task Force on Colorectal Cancer, and the American College of Radiology. CA Cancer J Clin 58:130–160

Miller A, Hoogstraten B, Staquet M et al (1981) Reporting results of cancer treatment. Cancer 47:207–214

Immediate-Delayed Reconstruction

▶ Post Mastectomy Reconstruction

Immunohistochemically Positive Lymph Node

▶ Microscopic Lymph Node Disease

Immunoreactivity

TOD W. SPEER
Department of Human Oncology, University of Wisconsin School of Medicine and Public Health, UW Hospital and Clinics, Madison, WI, USA

Definition

The ability of a targeting construct to maintain a high level of affinity after it has been conjugated to a radionuclide.

Cross-References

▶ Targeted Radioimmunotherapy

In Situ Carcinoma

DAVID E. WAZER
Radiation Oncology Department, Tufts Medical Center, Tufts University School of Medicine, Boston, MA, USA
Radiation Oncology Department, Rhode Island Hospital, Brown University School of Medicine, Providence, RI, USA

Definition

A proliferation of malignant-appearing cells without evidence of invasion through the epithelial basement membrane; variants arising from the breast include LCIS, Paget's disease, or DCIS.

Cross-References

▶ Cancer of the Breast Tis

In Vivo Verification

IRIS RUSU
Department of Radiation Oncology, Loyola University Medical Center, Maywood, IL, USA

Definition

Employs external dosimeters to monitor the dose received during treatment at different locations on the patient body.

Cross-References

▶ Total Body Irradiation (TBI)

Induction Chemotherapy

VOLKER BUDACH
Department of Radiotherapy and Radiation
Oncology, Charité – University Hospital Berlin,
Berlin, Germany

Definition

The use of chemotherapy delivered prior to the
radiation course (e.g., in three cycles every
3 weeks). Typical agents used for squamous cell
cancer of the head and neck region are a triple of
taxane, cis-platinum, 5-FU (TPF).

Cross-References

▶ Larynx
▶ Oro-Hypopharynx

Inflammation

SUSAN M. VARNUM, MARIANNE B. SOWA,
WILLIAM F. MORGAN
Biological Sciences Division, Fundamental &
Computational Sciences, Directorate Pacific
Northwest National Laboratory, Richland,
WA, USA

Definition

A protective tissue response to irritation,
injury, or infection. The process includes
increased blood flow and activation of defense
mechanisms.

Cross-References

▶ Radiation-Induced Genomic Instability and
Radiation Sensitivity

Intensity Modulated Radiation Therapy: Beam Modulation

ALBERT S. DENITTIS
Lankenau Institute for Medical Research,
Lankenau Hospital, Wynnewood, PA, USA

Definition

Using computer software to develop a treatment
plan based on prescription dose-volume constraints of target and normal tissues defined by
the user which produces optimal intensity modulated profiles. The generated plans can account
for convexity and concavity in target volume,
thus sparing normal tissue.

Cross-References

▶ Cancer of the Pancreas
▶ Esophageal Cancer
▶ Sarcomas of the Head and Neck
▶ Stage 0 Breast Cancer
▶ Prostate

Intensity Modulated Radiation Therapy (IMRT)

ROBERT A. PRICE, JR.
Department of Radiation Oncology, Fox Chase
Cancer Center, Philadelphia, PA, USA

Definition

In this work IMRT will be defined as varying the
energy fluence, and subsequent dose, across
a radiation therapy treatment field. The intersection
of the nonuniform dose distributions from multiple
treatment fields allows for a higher degree of
dose conformity around the intended target and

increased normal structure sparing as compared to conventional, three-dimensional conformal radiation therapy (3D CRT) techniques.

The IMRT Process

IMRT has become a mature treatment modality benefitting many patients requiring radiotherapy. The fundamental theories involved with almost every aspect of this technique are numerous and complex and are beyond the scope of this work. To this end the following sections describe the routine clinical processes associated with IMRT.

Figure 1 represents a flow diagram, the individual components of which will be described in greater detail throughout this chapter.

Patient Selection

IMRT can be significantly more labor intensive for the entire treatment team as compared to conventional methods. Physicians must delineate both abnormal and normal structures on the treatment planning imaging studies to allow for optimization. Even though inverse planning is typically used it is still an iterative process.

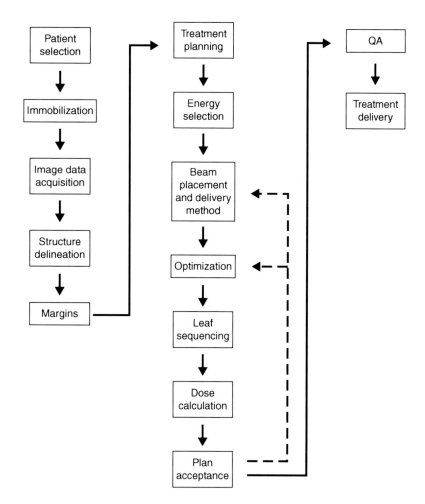

Intensity Modulated Radiation Therapy (IMRT). Fig. 1 This diagram illustrates the typical clinical flow of tasks related to the IMRT process. *Dotted lines* indicate routine components that are addressed in an iterative fashion until plan acceptance is achieved

The dosimetrist may need to generate and evaluate multiple plans in order to meet the physician's acceptance criteria. The physicist may need to assist in the planning process, assure accuracy of the dose distribution in the patient, as well as assure treatment delivery accuracy through the quality assurance (QA) process. The very nature of IMRT, treating a volume with multiple beams each made up of multiple segments, results in significant mechanical wear on the linear accelerator. Additionally, this type of treatment delivery inherently takes more time than conventional delivery meaning that the patient may have to lie on the treatment couch, immobile, for an increased amount of time. All of the aforementioned reasons support the concept of appropriate patient selection for IMRT planning and delivery. If the resultant dose distribution from conventional methods encompassing the surrounding normal tissues will not cause additional adverse effects, IMRT may not be warranted.

While IMRT has been used for treatment in practically every anatomical site to date, the most prevalent uses are probably for treatment of prostate and head and neck cancers. In the treatment of prostate cancer, it is generally not possible to adequately treat the prostate and associated margin to the high doses considered standard while limiting the adjacent critical structures, primarily the rectum, to acceptable dose levels using 3D CRT techniques. The physician must invariably choose between inadequately covering the target with the intended dose or accepting higher doses to the rectum and the potential adverse effects. Through IMRT planning and delivery, these compromises are made to a much more limited degree given that ideally the target would receive full dose and the critical structure(s) would receive none. In the case of head and neck cancers, there are a multitude of critical structures that may be spared dosimetrically through the use of IMRT. For example, in the treatment of nasopharyngeal cancer, one must limit the dose to the spinal cord, brain stem, and brain. This is typically done with 3D CRT through a series of opposed lateral fields designed to limit dose to these structures through avoidance by decreasing the field size at various dose levels (cone downs). Depending on the shape of the target and the proximity to the critical structures, the physician is often faced with making the aforementioned choices between target coverage and critical structure sparing. For other head and neck sites, the parotid glands are typically exposed to doses that severely limit or inhibit altogether their function with this technique due to the through-and-through type of dose distributions that result. With IMRT, we are again able to shape the dose distribution to more adequately cover the target while sparing the critical structures.

Immobilization

It is intuitive that patient motion defeats the purpose of generating dose distributions with the degree of conformality achievable with IMRT delivery. Immobilization devices can be used to expedite the setup and alignment process, aid the patient in remaining as immobile as possible following setup, and suppress motion due to respiration. Furthermore, devices that are indexable with the treatment couch offer increased reproducibility and allow for the implementation of couch shift tolerances that may aid in the quality control process. An overview of commonly used patient positioning systems is given by Balter (2005) and includes styrofoam casts, evacuated bean bags, thermoplastic materials, as well as dental molds and bite blocks. These systems are used in a patient-specific manner to aid in reproducibility of setup for treatment of practically every body site. It is important to note that these systems need to be employed prior to simulation and throughout patient treatment.

Image Data Acquisition

Great care must be taken to acquire image data with the patient in the treatment position including all immobilization devices where possible. When fusing data sets from different modalities (e.g., MR to CT), an understanding of structure location as a function of the time of data acquisition is necessary. It is most often the case that the CT data set will be used as the base for treatment planning due to our understanding of the relationship between Hounsfield numbers and electron density and the application of heterogeneity corrections. Image artifacts typically caused by high-Z materials should be masked and assigned the appropriate values to prevent potential errors in dose calculation.

Target/Normal Structure Delineation (Contouring)

Structure delineation may represent the single largest increase in time for the radiation oncologist when compared with conventional radiotherapy techniques. Inverse planning, inherent to the majority of IMRT planning, requires volumetric structures to be identified in order for the optimization algorithm to work. If a structure has not been delineated it does not exist from the point of view of the optimizer. The physician must possess an increased knowledge of cross-sectional anatomy in order to define tumor as well as normal structures. While this knowledge may have appeared adequate with 3D CRT techniques, outcomes may have been attributed to irradiating larger volumes based on these techniques (e.g., opposed laterals for H&N treatment). Insufficient or inaccurate contouring and structure definition may result in potential underdosing with the degree of target conformality achievable with IMRT.

Daily Localization/Immobilization Uncertainties (PTV/PRVs) and IGRT

In an effort to account for uncertainties in daily setup and localization, margins are routinely added to both the target (Planning Target Volume or PTV) and critical structures (Planning Organ at Risk Volume or PRV) during the treatment planning process. The absolute sizes of these margins should be based on the evaluation of measured

results for each uncertainty and are ideally treatment center dependent. Caution should be exercised if the physician is to delineate PTVs in order to avoid sensitive structures. The overlap of a properly generated PTV with a critical structure may represent a potential space for the target to occupy with respect to the aforementioned uncertainties. An understanding of the changing (or fixed) spatial relationship between a target and critical structure may be crucial. Artificially limiting this space may result in the target being underdosed. A more appropriate method may be to allow the overlap but to control the dose in this region with separate optimization objectives and/or constraints. This will yield more meaningful results when comparing dose distributions with patient outcome. Ideally, the physical size of these margins should not change regardless if 3D CRT or IMRT is utilized. However, great care must be exercised by the physician if the expected response is based on non-IMRT treatments targeting an anatomical region with minimal or no target delineation. In this scenario, beam penumbra may be the only uncertainty taken into account. Given the 3D nature of IMRT and the use of optimization algorithms, the target(s) and critical structures must be delineated. The physician must assure that he/she understands any differences between these two targeting methods to assure similar disease response.

In order to potentially minimize the aforementioned uncertainties and safely take advantage of the high degree of conformality afforded with IMRT, pretreatment image guidance is often utilized. Image guidance methods allow the patient to be positioned in a manner consistent with planning data acquisition and subsequently move the target and critical structures into the appropriate spatial positions of the planned dose distribution. This process may also allow for a reduction in the size of the margins used for both target(s) and critical structures. For a more complete explanation of these modalities, the reader is referred to IGRT sections of this encyclopedia.

Treatment Planning

Energy Selection

In keeping with the concept of maximizing dose to abnormal tissue and minimizing dose to normal tissue, as well as ongoing questions concerning integral dose, care should be exercised in selecting IMRT beam energy. However, the addition of neutron dose should be considered for energies greater than 10 MV. In regions of the body where it has been the convention to treat with 6 MV (e.g., head and neck), this energy should continue to be utilized to maintain the link with our response data. If it is necessary for a PTV to come within 5 mm of the skin surface it may be prudent to add bolus material to assure appropriate buildup. This bolus should be placed prior to acquisition of the CT planning data to insure that accurate placement and any imperfections are taken into account during planning. If this is not done, there is potential for the optimizer to assign increased dose to the buildup region in order to meet the assigned input parameters. Additionally, the dose in the surface region of a treatment plan may be highly inaccurate due to many factors including calculation matrix voxel size, tangential beam placement, etc., and may lead to unexpected, adverse effects.

Beam Placement/Orientation

IMRT does not allow us to change the physics of a photon beam. It is not possible to arrive at a conformal dose distribution through a parallel-opposed beam orientation. In general, choosing orientations that do not include opposing beams will increase target conformity since entrance and exit doses are not being summated. Figure 2 illustrates this principle. One should not abandon what we have learned from 3D CRT planning. If a critical structure can be geometrically avoided it may be prudent to do so. However, since one rarely needs to assign a critical structure a zero dose limit, it is often helpful in cases with complex geometries to have a beam traverse a critical structure; the optimizer will aid in limiting the dose accordingly and while perhaps not intuitive, may result in a more optimal plan. In all cases, it is imperative that patient-specific treatment planning be performed.

Optimization

The term "optimization" as it pertains to IMRT typically refers to the computational process of determining the "best" combination of physical parameters such as number of beamlets, the shape of the combination of beamlets, individual beamlet weights, etc. The treatment planner influences this process through the use of input parameters such as beam orientation and energy as well as dose-volume relationships for both targets and organs at risk. These input parameters are utilized to minimize or maximize an objective or cost function to determine a compromise between what is desired and what is physically achievable given the complexity of the problem. Should the resultant plan be determined to be unacceptable, changes to the input parameters are typically made and the process is reinitiated in an iterative fashion. The degree of "optimality" is determined by the radiation oncologist with reference to his/her patient's needs by evaluating specific, predetermined dose-volume histogram (DVH) and isodose distribution endpoints. Since by definition there can be no "degrees of optimality," no plan is ever truly optimal. Paraphrasing Webb (2001), "the term 'optimum' should strictly be reserved for the one probably unachievable plan which leads to unity TCP with zero NTCP," with TCP meaning tumor control probability and NTCP meaning normal tissue complication probability. It should be noted that, although not as common, biological indices can also be used as input parameters for optimization. One example is the equivalent uniform dose (EUD) defined as the uniform dose that would result in the same biological effect as the

Intensity Modulated Radiation Therapy (IMRT). Fig. 2 A simplistic illustration of a parallel-opposed (AP/PA) dose distribution is presented on the *left*. Doses higher than the prescription of 60 Gy are located outside the target and conformality is nonexistent. The three-field example on the *right* (AP, LPO, RPO) maintains the highest doses within the target and conformality is greatly improved

actual nonuniform dose distribution for a specific organ. For a more complete explanation of optimization, the reader is referred to the aforementioned reference.

Leaf Sequencing

The primary variable in the optimization process is the individual beam's intensity maps. Each beam is typically divided into beam elements or bixels that range in size from 5×5 mm^2 to 10×10 mm^2 and it is the intensity or fluence of each of the bixels that is actually optimized. However, these intensity maps must be converted into something deliverable with a linear accelerator. The intensity maps are converted into a series of shapes defined by the multileaf collimator (MLC) with each individual shape referred to as a segment (Bortfeld 2003). The individual segments are sequenced and delivered according to one of the methods to be described later.

Dose Calculation

As explained by Dong (2003), some planning systems separate the optimization process into two distinct steps. The first endeavors to find the ideal intensity patterns that satisfy the objective function while the second converts the ideal intensity patterns into deliverable MLC sequences. If the MLC characteristics were not taken into account in the first step there can be significant deviation between the optimal and final (deliverable) treatment plan. While this process may appear to be more expedient it may add additional iterations into the planning process. Furthermore, in the opinion of this author, it adds to the degree of difficulty in determining the "best" plan by placing an additional interpretive step between assessing the effects of the input parameters on the final plan. With the improvement in calculation speed of today's computers, perhaps all vendors will migrate toward combining the aforementioned optimization processes and provide the planner with a deliverable dose distribution following each iteration.

The need for the use of heterogeneity corrections is still controversial. At the time of this writing, there are still RTOG protocols being written prohibiting their use. Low (2005) points out that the dose delivered by the small, complex portals used with IMRT may be significantly altered in the presence of heterogeneities due to the change in electron transport. He cautions the user to conduct experimental validations in "patientlike" geometries prior to incorporating heterogeneity corrections. This author is in total agreement and would suggest that these validations be part of the IMRT commissioning process. It seems intuitive that our understanding of the relationship between dose and response will be improved with an accurate knowledge of delivered dose distributions.

Plan Analysis (Acceptance Criteria)

As previously mentioned, IMRT, even with inverse planning, remains an iterative process. Rarely does one arrive at the "best" plan on the first try and even if a suitable plan is achieved it may still be possible to improve upon it. It is advantageous for each center to develop acceptance criteria to be used during treatment plan analysis. These criteria allow the dosimetrist/physicist to know when to stop planning and consult the radiation oncologist. Additionally, these criteria promote the concept of similar treatments between patients and aid in outcome analysis. Acceptance criteria are usually DVH based and include target coverage limits and homogeneity as well as dose volume relationships for normal structures. These limits should be based on randomized clinical trial outcomes whenever possible. Since no spatial information is available in a DVH, it is also prudent to develop acceptance criteria based on isodose distributions. An example of both DVH and isodose acceptance criteria for prostate cancer IMRT is given by Price (2005). These acceptance criteria include 95% of the prostate PTV (PTV_{95}) receiving at least 100% of the prescription dose. Rectal constraints must be met such that no more than 17% of the rectum receives ≥ 65 Gy (R_{65}) and no more than 35% receives ≥ 40 Gy (R_{40}). Spatial constraints indicate that the 50% isodose line should fall within the rectal contour on any individual CT slice and

the 90% isodose line should not exceed ½ the diameter of the rectal contour on any slice. Bladder constraints are such that no more than 25% of the bladder receives >65 Gy (B_{65}) and no more than 50% receives >40 Gy (B_{40}). Additional criteria include no more than 10% of either femoral head receiving 50 Gy.

To aid in demonstrating the use of these acceptance criteria, a simple comparative study was made for a patient with clinical stage T1C N0 M0 adenocarcinoma of the prostate. The goal is to treat the prostate and proximal seminal vesicles to 80 Gy in 40 fractions. A treatment plan was generated using a simple 10 MV, four-field box technique using 8 mm PTV to MLC margins. This margin was selected to account for beam penumbra and allow the overall normalization scheme between the 3D CRT and IMRT plans to be somewhat consistent. The IMRT plan consisted of an eight-field, 10 MV beam orientation using the step-and-shoot delivery method. The resulting plans are illustrated in Fig. 3 in both the transverse and sagittal planes. It is clear that IMRT results in a much more conformal isodose distribution with respect to the high dose, 80 Gy region (magenta line) as well as the lower dose spread. The aforementioned isodose criteria can be seen to be acceptable for the IMRT plan by viewing the sagittal plane while the criteria are not met in the 3D CRT plan.

A DVH comparison was made between the two plans and is illustrated in Fig. 4. The IMRT plan was superior with respect to all criteria evaluated as follows: R_{65} (12.6%, 42.2%), R_{40} (24.0%, 83.0%), B_{65} (18.7%, 32.8%), B_{40} (44.7%, 70.6%), Rt FH (1.7%, 15.3%), Lt FH (0%, 23.0%) for IMRT and 3D CRT, respectively.

Acceptance criteria should be developed for each site treated with IMRT. One must exercise caution when combining acceptance criteria from different institutions and assure that an appropriate understanding of how they were arrived at is achieved. Careful analysis of the aforementioned

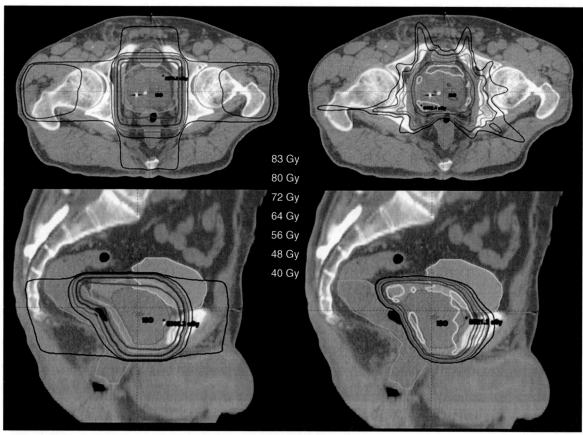

83 Gy
80 Gy
72 Gy
64 Gy
56 Gy
48 Gy
40 Gy

Intensity Modulated Radiation Therapy (IMRT). Fig. 3 3D CRT, four-field axial dose distribution (*upper left panel*) and sagittal distribution (*lower left panel*) compared with eight-field IMRT axial dose distribution (*upper right panel*) and sagittal distribution (*lower right panel*). Isodose lines given are 83 Gy, 80 Gy, 72 Gy, 64 Gy, 56 Gy, 48 Gy, and 40 Gy. The PTV and prostate are also illustrated

information will increase the efficacy of an IMRT program.

Treatment Delivery

Step-and-Shoot
This delivery mode is characterized by the use of static gantry and MLC positions. While the radiation beam is "ON" the gantry position remains fixed. Additionally, MLC configuration changes occur only when the beam is "OFF." Physical compensator-based IMRT would fall into this category since the gantry is in a fixed position when the beam is "ON."

Dynamic Multileaf Collimation (DMLC)
This delivery mode is characterized by the use of static gantry and dynamic or moving MLC positions. While the radiation beam is "ON" the gantry position remains fixed. However, the MLC configuration changes during irradiation.

Arc-Based or Rotational IMRT
This delivery mode is characterized by the use of moving gantry and MLC positions. While the radiation beam is "ON" the gantry position as well as the MLC configuration is changing. It is possible to deliver dose throughout gantry rotation of an entire

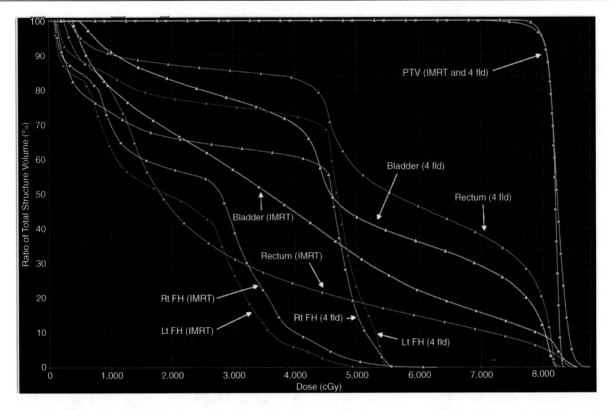

Intensity Modulated Radiation Therapy (IMRT). Fig. 4 DVH comparison between a 3D CRT, four-field box and an eight-field, IMRT prostate plan

360° or multiples thereof or through subsets (Arcs) or combinations of the aforementioned. Depending on the MLC employed, incremental movement of the treatment couch may or may not be necessary as well. Arc-based therapies are gaining popularity due in large part to their faster delivery times. It is advisable for centers anticipating implementing this delivery technique to compare plan quality (acceptance criteria) with plans generated for their routine fixed gantry IMRT delivery method. In addition, endpoints such as energy deposition in the low dose areas, integral dose, and machine head leakage (evaluated as a function of monitor units) should be compared between modalities. Caution should be exercised when selecting a more expedient delivery method at the expense of plan quality. A reasonable

approach may be to assure that the arc-based plans are at least dosimetrically equivalent to the routine IMRT plans and allow for a faster delivery time. It is preferable to achieve improvements in both plan quality and delivery time.

Quality Assurance (QA)

QA for IMRT encompasses everything from planning system commissioning to accuracy of treatment delivery with the majority of the subjects in between being beyond the scope of this chapter. Therefore, within the confines of this work we will concentrate on patient-specific QA as it pertains to delivery accuracy. Typically, once an acceptable IMRT treatment plan has been formulated, the delivery parameters (gantry angles, leaf sequences, MU, etc.) are used to generate a forward planned

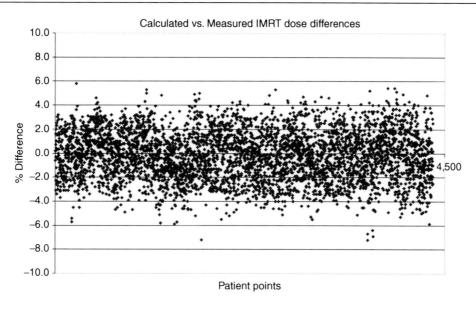

Intensity Modulated Radiation Therapy (IMRT). Fig. 5 Comparison of measurement vs. calculated dose values for a single point in the high-dose, low-gradient region for the first 4,350 IMRT patients treated at Fox Chase Cancer Center. Agreement rates of 36.9%, 65.3%, 86.8%, and 96.7% were observed for ranges of ±1%, ±2%, ±3%, and ±4%, respectively

dose distribution on a homogeneous virtual phantom. The physical phantom (from which the virtual phantom was created) is then irradiated under the same conditions as patient treatment. This physical phantom will contain measuring devices such as ionization chambers, film, diode arrays, or ionization chamber arrays. The data collected can be formatted into absolute dose values as well as spatial dose distributions. These values and distributions are then compared with data obtained from the virtual phantom within the treatment planning system. Limits to the agreement between dose values and spatial distributions are applied during analysis to determine plan delivery acceptability. Exceeding these limits should trigger further investigation and hopefully assist the physicist in determining the cause(s) of the disagreement. As an example, Fig. 5 illustrates comparisons between measured and absolute doses. Given that these points were selected in a high-dose, low-gradient region, a ±3% window was selected. Values

obtained outside these limits trigger repeat or additional measurements and/or further investigation to explain the deviation. When using 2D or 3D detection devices (e.g., film, ionization chamber arrays), limits can be set based on the percent difference between or distance to agreement for isodose lines allowing for the inclusion of spatial dose distribution analysis. It should be noted that the phantom testing method evaluates delivery accuracy only as the phantom geometry and composition differ significantly from that of the patient. However, within the accuracy of the dose calculation algorithm in the presence of heterogeneities, one can infer that if the measured data agree with the calculated data on the virtual phantom, delivery to the patient will be accurate as well.

References

Balter J (2005) Immobilization and localization. In: Mundt AJ, Roeske JC (eds) Intensity modulated radiation therapy, a clinical perspective. BC Decker, Lewiston

Bortfeld T (2003) Physical optimization. In: Palta JR, Mackie TR (eds) Intensity-modulated radiation therapy: the state of the art. Medical Physics Publishing, Madison, pp 51–75

Dong L (2003) Intensity-modulated radiation therapy physics and quality assurance. In: Chao KSC (ed) Practical essentials of intensity modulated radiation therapy. Lippincott Williams & Wilkins, Philadelphia

Low (2005) Physics of intensity modulated radiation therapy for head and neck cancer. In: Chao KSC, Ozyigit G (eds) Intensity modulated radiation therapy for head and neck cancer. Lippincott Williams & Wilkins, Philadelphia

Price RA Jr (2005) Intact prostate cancer: case study. In: Mundt AJ, Roeske JC (eds) Intensity modulated radiation therapy, a clinical perspective. BC Decker, Lewiston

Webb S (2001) Intensity-modulated radiation therapy. Institute of Physics Publishing, London

Intensity-Modulated Proton Therapy (IMPT)

DANIEL YEUNG[1], JATINDER PALTA[2]
[1]Department of Radiation Oncology, Univeristy of Florida Proton Therapy Institute, Jacksonville, FL, USA
[2]Department of Radiation Oncology, University of Florida Health Science Center, Gainesville, FL, USA

Definition

A technique that allows for three-dimensional dose conformity to a target volume using protons through pencil-beam scanning with dynamic control and optimization of the beam energy and intensity throughout the scan.

Cross-References

▶ Proton Therapy

Intention to Treat

EDWARD J. GRACELY
Department of Epidemiology and Biostatistics, College of Medicine, Drexel University, Philadelphia, PA, USA

Definition

A conservative method of handling data from subjects in a randomized trial who do not receive the intended treatment.

Cross-References

▶ Statistics and Clinical Trials

Intermediate-Risk Neuroblastoma

BRANDON J. FISHER[1], LARRY C. DAUGHERTY[2]
[1]Department of Radiation Oncology, College of Medicine, Drexel University, Philadelphia, PA, USA
[2]Department of Radiation Oncology, College of Medicine, Drexel University, Glenside, PA, USA

Definition

Stage 3 and 4 patients with nonamplification of N-*myc*, favorable histology, younger than 1 year of age.

Cross-References

▶ Neuroblastoma

Internal Organs

▶ Visceral Organs (also Viscera or Internal Organs)

Internal Target Volume (ITV)

Jay E. Reiff
Department of Radiation Oncology, College of
Medicine, Drexel University, Philadelphia,
PA, USA

Definition
Internal target volume (ITV) consists of an internal margin added to the CTV to compensate for internal physiologic movement and variations in size, shape, and position of the CTV.

Cross-References
▶ Image-Guided Radiation Therapy (IGRT): MV Imaging

International Breast Cancer Intervention Survey (IBIS) Models

▶ Breast Cancer Risk Models

Interstitial Implant

Yan Yu, Laura Doyle
Department of Radiation Oncology, Thomas
Jefferson University Hospital, Philadelphia,
PA, USA

Definition
Brachytherapy technique that involves inserting radioactive material directly into the tumor or surrounding tissue. This technique may involve a permanent or temporary implant.

Cross-References
▶ Brachytherapy
▶ Low-Dose Rate (LDR) Brachytherapy
▶ Permanent Implants

Interstitial Brachytherapy

Erik van Limbergen
Department of Radiation Oncology, University
Hospital Gasthuisberg, Leuven, Belgium

Definition
The sources or source carriers are implanted in the clinical target volume: different possibilities are seeds or needles of various length and thickness, or plastic tubes, or needles of varying diameter and rigidity. These techniques are used for breast cancer, prostate, head and neck, anal canal, interstitial pelvic for vaginal and cervical cancer, bladder, pediatrics and soft tissue sarcoma.

Cross-References
▶ Clinical Aspects of Brachytherapy (BT)
▶ High-Dose Rate (HDR) Brachytherapy
▶ Low-Dose Rate (LDR) Brachytherapy

Interstitial High Dose Rate (HDR) Brachytherapy

Patrizia Guerrieri, Paolo Montemaggi
Department of Radiation Oncology, Regional
Cancer Center "M. Ascoli", University of Palermo
Medical School, Palermo, Italy

Definition
This is a brachytherapy technique in which the dose rate is higher than 300 cGy/min; at the present time this

is frequently used to replace LDR techniques. Brachytherapy is carried out by using a ^{192}Ir miniaturized source held in a safe, which would step out, through the inserted needles according to the planned dosimetry, to deliver the dose usually in a hypo-fractionated fashion. Generally, it is used as a boost dose after completion of an external beam course to the pelvis.

Cross-References

▶ Brachytherapy
▶ Vulvar Carcinoma

Interstitial Low Dose Rate (LDR) Brachytherapy

PATRIZIA GUERRIERI, PAOLO MONTEMAGGI
Department of Radiation Oncology, Regional Cancer Center "M. Ascoli", University of Palermo Medical School, Palermo, Italy

Definition

LDR standard treatment schemes delivering a dose of 70–80 Gy in 6–8 days at a dose rate of 50–100 cGy/h are considered a possible conservative treatment for particular early stage vulvar cancers through the insertion of needles or pins loaded with ^{226}Ra substitutes isotopes, mostly ^{192}Ir. Smaller doses, ranging from 25 to 35 Gy, are frequently used through shorter application times for the post-surgical treatment to prevent local relapse risk of more advanced cancers after completion of an external beam radiation therapy course of 45–50 Gy at standard fractionation.

Cross-References

▶ Vulvar Carcinoma

Intestinal Cancer

▶ Colon Cancer

Intracavitary Brachytherapy

CHRISTIN A. KNOWLTON[1], MICHELLE KOLTON MACKAY[2], ERIK VAN LIMBERGEN[3]
[1]Department of Radiation Oncology, Drexel University, Philadelphia, PA, USA
[2]Department of Radiation Oncology, Marshfield Clinic, Marshfield, WI, USA
[3]Department of Radiation Oncology, University Hospital Gasthuisberg, Leuven, Belgium

Definition

Brachytherapy, derived from the Greek term for "close" therapy, refers to placing a radiation source in or close to the tumor region. Intracavitary means the placement of the brachytherapy delivery device in a body cavity, such as in the vagina for endometrial cancer, as opposed to directly into tissue. With endometrial cancer, brachytherapy is often used to treat the vaginal cuff in postoperative patients to allow a higher dose to this region with limited side effects.

Brachytherapy sources are contained by dedicated applicators designed for cervical, endometrial, and vaginal as well as nasopharyngeal cancers. Nowadays they are made of carbon, plastic (MRI compatible), or metal (MRI compatible when made of Titanium): Standardized: Fletcher type with intrauterine catheter and two vaginal catheters with ovoids, Stockholm type with intrauterine tube and endovaginal ring, or individualized Pierquin-Chassagne type individualized molds.

Cross-References

▶ Brachytherapy: High Dose Rate (HDR) Implants
▶ Clinical Aspects of Brachytherapy (BT)
▶ Endometrium
▶ High-Dose Rate (HDR) Brachytherapy
▶ Low-Dose Rate (LDR) Brachytherapy

Intracavitary High-Dose-Rate (HDR) Brachytherapy

Patrizia Guerrieri, Paolo Montemaggi
Department of Radiation Oncology, Regional Cancer Center "M. Ascoli", University of Palermo Medical School, Palermo, Italy

Definition

It is a brachytherapy technique, at the present time used to replace LDR technique, in which the dose rate is higher than 300 cGy/min. The brachytherapy is carried out by using a ^{192}Ir miniaturized source, held in a safe, which would step out, through the inserted device according to the planned dosimetry, to deliver the dose usually in a hypo-fractionated fashion. More frequently, therapeutic schemes have been designed using hyperfractionated BID (bis in die) schedules. Generally it is used as a boost dose after completion of an external beam course to the pelvis. Techniques and instruments are the same as those used to treat cervical cancers.

Cross-References

▶ Vagina

Intracavitary Low-Dose-Rate (LDR) Brachytherapy

Patrizia Guerrieri, Paolo Montemaggi
Department of Radiation Oncology, Regional Cancer Center "M. Ascoli", University of Palermo Medical School, Palermo, Italy

Definition

LDR standard treatment schemes delivering a dose of 60 Gy in 6–7 days at a dose rate of 40–60 cGy/h are considered a reference schedule for the exclusive treatment of early stage cervical cancer through the intracervical insertion of brachytherapy applicators loaded with ^{226}Ra substitutes isotopes, mostly ^{137}Cs. Smaller doses, ranging from 25 to 35 Gy, are commonly used through shorter application times for the treatment of more advanced gynecological cancer after completion of an external beam radiation therapy to the pelvis. Analogue concepts can be used when a vaginal involvement is present and/or to treat extensive vaginal lesions by the use of specifically designed cylinders, coupled or not with the classic intracervical tandem.

Cross-References

▶ Vagina

Intramedullary Spinal Cord Compression (Also Intramedullary Spinal Cord Metastases)

James H. Brashears, III
Radiation Oncologist, Venice, FL, USA

Synonyms

Intramedullary spinal cord metastases

Definition

Direct involvement of the spinal cord with metastatic disease by hematogenous dissemination. It is most associated with lung cancer and is usually a harbinger of advanced, disseminated disease. Shortly after diagnosis, massive neurologic compromise usually results followed by death in short order.

Cross-References

▶ Palliation of Brain and Spinal Cord Metastases

Intramedullary Spinal Cord Metastases

▶ Intramedullary Spinal Cord Compression (Also Intramedullary Spinal Cord Metastases)

Intraoperative Brachytherapy

FELIPE A. CALVO
Department of Oncology, Hospital General
Universitario Gregorio Maranon, Madrid, Spain

Definition
Surgically guided placement of radioactive sources into the anatomic region defined by the surgical procedure.

Cross-References
▶ Intraoperative Irradiation
▶ Intraoperative Radiation Therapy (IORT)

Intraoperative Electron Radiation Therapy (IOERT)

FELIPE A. CALVO
Department of Oncology, Hospital General
Universitario Gregorio Maranon, Madrid, Spain

Definition
Direct delivery of a linear accelerator-generated electron beam to a surgically exposed tumor or tumor bed.

Cross-References
▶ Intraoperative Irradiation

Intraoperative Electrons

▶ Intraoperative Radiation Therapy (IORT)

Intraoperative High-Dose-Rate Brachytherapy

FELIPE A. CALVO
Department of Oncology, Hospital General
Universitario Gregorio Maranon, Madrid, Spain

Definition
Intraoperative high-dose-rate brachytherapy: Intra-surgical placement of catheters to guide radioactive isotopes with high-dose-rate delivery characteristics.

Cross-References
▶ Intraoperative Irradiation

Intraoperative Irradiation

FELIPE A. CALVO[1], MANUEL GONZÁLEZ-DOMINGO[2],
SERGEY USYCHKIN[3]
[1]Department of Oncology, Hospital General
Universitario Gregorio Maranon, Madrid, Spain
[2]Department of Radiation Oncology, Oncology
Institute, Viña del Mar, Chile
[3]Department of Radiation Oncology, Instituto
Madrileño de Oncologia, Madrid, Spain

Definition
Intraoperative radiotherapy (IORT) is a therapeutic modality that incorporates a high-dose single fraction of radiation directly to the tumor or tumor bed at the time of surgery. The radiation dose may be delivered as a boost or as

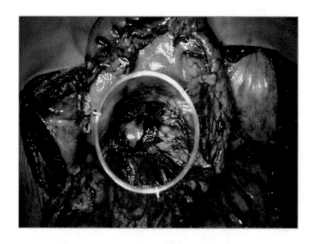

Intraoperative Irradiation. Fig. 1
Pre-pancreatectomy assessment of the surgical field encompassed by an 8 cm diameter applicator (15° beveled angle) with exclusion from the radiation beam normal uninvolved upper abdominal organs and tissues by mechanical displacement (stomach, transverse colon, liver, and small intestine) and the non-resected tumor inside the applicator

the only radiation therapy component. The radiation is often administered in an unresectable or partially resected tumor or in the post-resected surgical field. An advantage of this technique is that it allows for the displacement and protection of normal tissues from the radiation beam (Fig. 1).

Purpose

Patients for whom intraoperative radiation therapy (IORT) may be a viable radiation treatment regimen are those who are expected to undergo surgical cancer resection with a high risk of local recurrence, and/or those who have nearby critical organs whose normal tissue dose tolerance may be exceeded by using standard external beam radiation therapy. Other indications for IORT are early stage cancers which are amenable to being treated with the IORT component alone (breast cancer, pediatric tumors).

Two methods of IORT treatment are external intraoperative electron radiotherapy and intraoperative high-dose-rate brachytherapy. External IORT (IOERT) using an electron beam can be performed with a conventional linear accelerator (Fig. 2) or a miniature, mobile accelerator which is movable from one operating room to another. Its advantages compared to IORT with brachytherapy are the shorter treatment time, the possibility of using different electron beam energies with different depth dose and isodose distribution characteristics, and that it requires minimal shielding of treatment room. The dose is generally prescribed to the depth of the 90% isodose (Fig. 3).

IORT using brachytherapy with a high-dose-rate remote afterloader (HDR-IORT) is given using either special applicators or via direct catheter implantation (Fig. 4). The advantages of brachytherapy IORT over IOERT include better adaptation of the dose to curved surfaces, the accessibility of narrow cavities to brachytherapy catheters compared to IOERT cones, irradiation of very limited volumes, and the possibility of irradiating the skin and subcutaneous tissue. A common dose prescription policy is 1 cm from the plane of the catheters or 0.5 cm from the surface of the applicator.

In either case, IORT is often given in conjunction with external beam radiotherapy as an intraoperative boost. This reduces the risk of marginal recurrences and increases the total dose of radiotherapy given to the GTV with the radiobiological advantages of fractionated irradiation.

Principles

The basic aim of IORT is to improve the therapeutic index of radiotherapy by increasing the dose gradient between the tumor and the surrounding normal tissues. When administered as an exclusive irradiation (IORT alone), it maximizes the biological effective dose, with

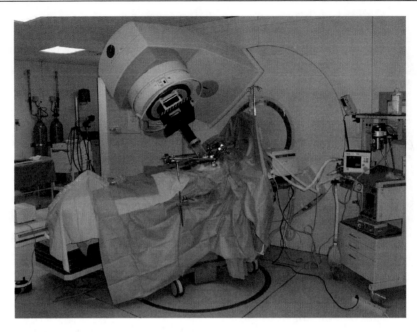

Intraoperative Irradiation. Fig. 2 IORT procedure with a conventional linear accelerator. General vision of the treatment room: gantry angulation, electron applicator, and patient under surgical and anesthetic monitoring

a bioequivalence between two and three times higher than using conventional fractionation.

Considering the linear-quadratic model and assuming an α/β of 3 for late responding normal tissues and an α/β of 10 for tumor tissues, the bioequivalence established is:

- 12 Gy of single fraction IORT = 25–30 Gy of conventional fractionation
- 15 Gy of single fraction IORT = 30–37.5 Gy of conventional fractionation
- 20 Gy of single fraction IORT = 40–50 Gy of conventional fractionation

Advantages of IORT

Following the principles of radiobiology, IORT has the advantage of reducing the risk of tumor repopulation after surgical treatment. The tumor control probability decreases with increasing the initial number of residual malignant cells. Administering a large dose of radiation at the time of surgery not only decreases the repopulation of malignant cells during the interval between surgery and conventional radiation therapy but also between fractions of conventional treatment. This serves to improve the radiobiological benefit.

Another advantage of IORT is that it acts on well vascularized tissues with optimal aerobic metabolism due to the vasodilation associated with increased vascular flow-induced anesthesia, and ventilation with pure oxygen during surgery. However, the beneficial effect of reoxygenation between fractions could be lost when using hypofractionated radiation schemes on hypoxic cells.

Disadvantages of IORT

IORT eliminates the potential benefits of fractionation with regard to cancer cell cycle redistribution. Moreover, its main drawback appears as adverse effects on normal tissues due to their poor long-term tolerance of very high doses

Dose Volume Histogram

Intraoperative Irradiation. **Fig. 3** Treatment planning system for IOERT (radiance). Example of 2D and 3D dosimetric distribution and surgical navigation in a case with para-aortic recurrence

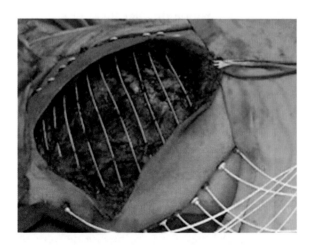

Intraoperative Irradiation. **Fig. 4** Perioperative brachytherapy with catheters implanted in the surgical bed of a soft tissue sarcoma

when IORT is used as the only mode of radiotherapy (i.e., no subsequent external beam treatments). Due to emergence of late side effects, starting at doses of 15–17 Gy, it is recommended not to exceed a dose of 20 Gy in anatomic structures at risk for neurotoxicity and/or vascular damage.

Indications

IORT with electron beams is the preferred technique for treating unresected or partially resected tumors, or tumor bed regions in which the prescribed dose to the target needs to cover a nonuniform depth across the intended treatment volume. Applicator systems may be either hard-docking or non-docking to the accelerator gantry (alignment among applicator components is mandatory to assure appropriate dose distribution). Although most of the electron applicators are circular, elliptical and rectangular applicators can also be used when dictated by the size and shape of the target volume. The use of electron beams offers a wide range of treatment depths (from 0.5 to 5.5 cm). Flat bottom cones are used to deliver the dose when the cone can be centered directly over the target. When the cone cannot be centered directly over the target due to physical constraints, beveled cones may be used. The effect of the beveled bottom is to skew the isodose distribution asymmetrically to the open side of the cone. The price to pay is a slightly lower coverage in depth compared to the same size flat bottom cone. Miniaturized, portable linear accelerators are commercially available (Mobetron, Novac 7, Liac). The portability permits moving the linear accelerator from one operating room to another.

High-dose-rate (HDR) brachytherapy is used for targets with either planar or curve surface characteristics. HDR brachytherapy is most often used for sites that have microscopically close margins or a minimum of post-resected residual disease. The technical and dosimetric differences between the different IORT delivery systems are summarized in Table 1. Low energy X-ray beams are being implemented for its IORT use with the INTRABEAM system and widely used in early breast cancer.

Today, IORT is used predominantly for treating breast cancer, certain digestive tract tumors (pancreas, rectum, and stomach), sarcomas, head and neck, and selected pediatric neoplasms and isolated cancer recurrences. The cosmetic advantages and the possibility of shortening the total treatment time while performing dose escalation coupled with promising local control data, make IORT an excellent adjuvant therapy in these sites. Table 2 presents IORT clinical results consolidated from multiple studies

Intraoperative Irradiation. Table 1 Potential differences between electron and high-dose-rate brachytherapy intraoperative irradiation systems

Parameters	IOERT	HDR-IORT
Actual treatment time	2–4 min	5–30 min
Total procedure time	30–45 min	45–120 min
Treatment sites	Accessible locations	All areas with depth at risk ≤0.5 cm from the surface of applicator
Surface dose	Lower (75–93%)	Higher (150–200%)
Dose at depth (2 cm)	Higher (70–100%)	Lower (30%)
Dosimetric homogeneity (surface to depth)	≤10% variation	≥100% variation

and publications. It provides a comprehensive analysis of results of over 5,500 patients reported by expert institutions over the last 20 years. The data show high local control rates (over 80%) with the combination of IORT boost (10–20 Gy) and a full external-beam fractionated irradiation component (45–50 Gy). The data is remarkable as well in terms of local control (over 50%) of unresected or macroscopic residual cancer, when a high integral dose of radiation is delivered. Survival results are tempered by the systemic progression of disease in most tumor sites with adverse prognostic features, or in the case of recurrent disease where the risk of systemic micrometastatic disease is fairly high.

Modern IORT is considered an excellent alternative technique for the precise delivery of radiotherapy. It provides a component of the total required radiation dose without compromising advances in surgery (it is feasible at the time of

Intraoperative Irradiation. Table 2 International results presented at the International Society of Intraoperative Radiation Therapy Conference (ISIORT) 2008 in locally advanced human cancer of different histology, tumor site, and stage/status

Tumor	References	Stage/Status	No. of patients	Local control (%)	Survival (%)
Breast (single)	González et al. (2008), Gunderson et al. (1999, 2008, 2011)	pT1-2, pN0-1	542	94–100	100
Breast (boost)	Haddock et al. (2008), Hu et al. (2002, 2008), Karasawa et al. (2008)	pT1-2,pN0-1	1,757	99–100	86–100
Rectal	Kinsella et al. (1985), Cividalli et al. (2005), Kopp et al. (2008)	p/cT3-4; cN+	998	88–95	65–68
Sarcomas	De la Mata et al. (2008), Drognitz et al. (2008), Krempien et al. (2008), Lesti et al. (2008), Majewski et al. (2008), Merrick et al. (2003)	Primary/ recurrence	821	71–100	50–79
Pancreatic	Fernández Lizarbe et al. (2008), Mussari et al. (2008), Oreccia and Veronesi (2005), Petersen et al. (2008), Piroth et al. (2008)	pT3-4 unresectable/ resected	421	23–95	17–47
Gastric	Garrán et al. (2008a, b, Polowski et al. (2008), Radziszewski et al. (2008)	p/cT2-3,cNx	162	84–96	25–62
Head and neck	Roeder et al. (2008), Rutten et al. (2008), Sedlmayer et al. (2008), Flaquer et al. (2008)	pT3, Nx primary/ recurrent	126	61–100	44–70
Pelvic recurrences	Gomez-Espí et al. (2008), Sindelar et al. (1994, 1999), Skoropad et al. (2008), Valentini et al. (2008)	Localized	697	61–71	25–30

laparoscopic resection) or systemic treatment (minimal bone marrow toxicity).

Clinical models particularly suitable for single-dose IORT are early breast and prostate cancer and post-neoadjuvant responding pediatric cancers. A contemporary tendency in clinical radiation oncology is to use hypofractionation with limited target volumes. This new paradigm provides an excellent opportunity to test the possibilities of IORT. Single-dose IORT not only tests this hypothesis, but it is extremely efficient in limiting the total treatment time for a patient as it combines surgery and radiotherapy into a single procedure.

Contraindication

The majority of late side effects are known from experimental studies in large animals, mostly dogs, carried out in the 1980s. In general, although of great scientific interest, the results in animal models are not completely extrapolated to results in humans. These effects as well as those of other treatments such as chemotherapy or the influence of wide excision of tissues and organs have not been able to be reproduced in humans.

In addition to information provided by these studies, the experience from using IORT in practice has allowed a better understanding of the late toxicity expected with this technique. Side effects, in addition to being dose-dependent, are related to other parameters such as the other cancer treatments given (chemotherapy, etc.), the volume of irradiation, the length of the tubular structures contained in the irradiated volume, and the ability to move or protect the healthy organs at risk.

The main dose-limiting normal tissue structure is the peripheral nerve, where the risk of serious late toxicity is 35% at 5 years if the dose exceeds tolerance. With doses of 10–15 Gy, axonal destruction and perineural increase of connective tissue become apparent. After 20 Gy, the risks of hyalinization of the capillary thrombosis and bleeding are multiplied. It is therefore recommended not to exceed a dose of 16 Gy when the treatment volume includes a significant length of a peripheral nerve.

Another dose-limiting structure is the ureter. Its involvement is more common if there was a dissection of the vascular tunic. A dose of 12.5 Gy can produce up to two-thirds of stenotic complications. However, unlike the peripheral nerve, the ureter can be moved away from the IORT treatment field.

The possibility of vascular damage, present in clinical IORT, leads to progressive ischemia by intimal proliferation of the microvasculature, which also may be obliterated at the same dose level starting at 20 Gy. With doses of 40 Gy, there is a fibrosis of the intima with hyaline necrosis of the middle layer.

It is important to mention that while an increased risk of radiation-induced tumors has been described in animal models, it has not been identified in long-term survivors treated with IORT.

Future

Many multidisciplinary collaborations are currently studying the expanded use of IORT. Topics included in these groups include the development of miniature technology, treatment planning and surgical navigation, and the use of IORT during laparoscopic surgery. Translational research with immunohistochemical and cytogenetic studies of both irradiated and nonirradiated normal tissue samples is being carried out by several working groups using well-defined prospective clinical models.

Cross-References

▶ Brachytherapy
▶ Electron Dosimetry and Treatment
▶ High-Dose Rate (HDR) Brachytherapy
▶ Intraoperative Irradiation
▶ Renal Pelvis and Ureter
▶ Total Body Irradiation (TBI)
▶ Whole Breast Radiation

References

Alvarez A, Calvo FA, Lozano MA et al (2008a) Recurrence of soft tissue sarcoma treated with IORT: topography, timing, and inmunohistochemical molecular profile. Rev Cancer (Madrid) 22:51

Alvarez A, Calvo FA, García-Sabrido JL et al (2008b) Long term results of intraoperative electron beam radiotherapy for retroperitoneal soft tissue sarcomas. Rev Cancer (Madrid) 22:53

Arcangeli G, Arcangeli S, Giordano C et al (2008) Intraoperative (IORT) vs. standard radiotherapy (EBRT) in breast cancer: an update of an ongoing Italian multicenter, randomized study. Rev Cancer (Madrid) 22:12–13

Azinovic I, Calvo FA, Puebla F, Aristu J, Martínez-Monge R (2001) Long-term normal tissue effects of intraoperative electron radiation therapy (IOERT): late sequelae, tumor recurrence, and second malignancies. Int J Radiat Oncol Biol Phys 49:597–604

Beddar AS, Biggs PJ, Chang S et al (2006a) Intraoperative radiation therapy using mobile electron linear accelerators: report of AAPM Radiation Therapy Committee Task Group No. 72. Med Phys 33:1476–1489

Beddar AS, Krishnan S, Briere TM et al (2006b) The optimization of dose delivery for intraoperative high-dose-rate radiation therapy using curved HAM applicators. Radiother Oncol 78:207–212

Calín A, Calvo FA, De Torres M et al (2008) Pancreatic cancer resection with or without intraoperative electrons plus chemoradiation: an update of a contemporary institutional experience (1995–2008). Rev Cancer (Madrid) 22:31

Callister MD, Beauchamp CP, Fitch TR et al (2008) Preoperative radiation and IOERT for soft-tissue sarcomas of the extremities and trunk. Rev Cancer (Madrid) 22:54

Calvo FA, Meiriño R, Gunderson LL, Willet CG (2004) Intraoperative radiation therapy. In: Perez CA, Bradys LW, Halperin EC, Schimdt-Ullrich RK (eds) Principles and practice of radiation oncology, 4th edn. Lippincott Williams and Wilkins, Philadelphia, pp 428–456

Calvo FA, Meiriño RM, Orecchia R (2006) Intraoperative radiation therapy. First part: rationale and techniques. Crit Rev Oncol Hematol 59:106–115

Calvo FA, Rodríguez M, Jiménez LM, Díaz-Zorita B, Infante JM, López-Baena JA et al (2008a) Intraoperative electron irradiation (IOERT) during laparoscopic radical surgery: a technical innovative development. Rev Cancer (Madrid) 22:3–4

Calvo FA, Sánchez S, Flaquer A et al (2008b) Multiorgan resection and intraoperative irradiation in recurrent pelvic cancer: long-term results. Rev Cancer (Madrid) 22:47

Ciabattoni A, Mirri MA, Checcaglini F et al (2008a) Italian report on IORT as anticipated boost in I and II stage breast cancer. Rev Cancer (Madrid) 22:14

Ciabattoni A, Cosentino LM, Belardi A et al (2008b) IORT in advanced rectal cancer: long term outcomes and toxicity in 66 patients treated at S.Filippo Neri Hospital. Rev Cancer (Madrid) 22:44

Ciérvide R, Gómez-Iturriaga A, Gastañaga M et al (2008) Surgery, preoperative high-dose rate brachytherapy and external radiation in soft tissue sarcomas of the extremities and the superficial trunk. Rev Cancer (Madrid) 22:54

Cividalli A, Creton G, Ceciarelli F, Strigari L, Danesi D, Benassi M (2005) Influence of time interval between surgery and radiotherapy on tumor regrowth. J Exp Clin Cancer Res 24:109–116

De la Mata MD, Carballo N, Delapuente F et al (2008) Recurrent gynecologic cancer treated with radical surgical resection and combined HDR-IORT: institutional experience. Rev Cancer (Madrid) 22:49

Drognitz O, Henne K, Saum R et al (2008) Intraoperative radiotherapy for patients with gastric cancer, long term results. Rev Cancer (Madrid) 22:24

Fernández Lizarbe E, Montero A, Hernanz R et al (2008) Intraoperative radiation therapy (IORT) for the treatment of sarcomas of extremities and retroperitoneo. Rev Cancer (Madrid) 22:55

Flaquer A, Calvo FA, González C et al (2008) Esophageal and gastric cancer treated with IOERT containing adjuvant treatment. Rev Cancer (Madrid) 22:24–25

Garrán C, Pagola M, Ciérvide R et al (2008a) Surgery, perioperative high-dose rate brachytherapy and paclitaxel/cisplatin-based postoperative chemotherapy in locally advanced head and neck cancer. Rev Cancer (Madrid) 22:22–23

Garrán C, Gómez-Iturriaga A, Pagola M et al (2008b) Perioperative high dose rate brachytherapy (PHDRB) in the management of locally recurrent gynaecological tumors (LRGT). Rev Cancer (Madrid) 22:49–50

Gomez-Espí M, Calvo FA, González C et al (2008) Timing and intensity of neoadjuvant treatment in rectal cancer: results of pre (Plus IOERT) vs. post (No IOERT) chemoradiation. Rev Cancer (Madrid) 22:45

González C, Calvo FA, García R et al (2008) IOERT pediatric cancer patients: omission of external beam irradiation under individualized patients consideration does not compromise local control. Rev Cancer (Madrid) 22:35

Gunderson LL, Wilett CG, Harrison LB, Calvo FA (1999) Intraoperative irradiation. Techniques and results. Humana Press, Totowa

Gunderson LL, Moss AA, Callister MG et al (2008) Preoperative chemoradiation and IOERT for unresectable or borderline resectable pancreas cancer. Rev Cancer (Madrid) 22:32

Gunderson LL, Willet CG, Calvo FA, Harrison LB (2011) Intraoperative irradiation, 2nd edn. Springer, Heidelberg

Haddock MG, Miller RC, Nelson H et al (2008) Intraoperative electron irradiation for locally recurrent colorectal cancer. Rev Cancer (Madrid) 22:49–50

Hu KS, Enker WE, Harrison LB (2002) High-dose-rate intraoperative irradiation: current status and future directions. Semin Radiat Oncol 12:62–80

Hu K, Ng J, Shah N et al (2008) High dose-rate intraoperative radiation therapy for the treatment of head and neck cancer. Rev Cancer (Madrid) 22:23

Karasawa K, Sunamura M, Okamoto A et al (2008) Efficacy of novel hypoxic cell sensitiser doranidazole combined with intraoperative radiotherapy in the treatment of locally advanced pancreatic cancer. Rev Cancer (Madrid) 22:33

Kinsella TJ, Sindelar WF, DeLuca AM et al (1985) Tolerance of peripheral nerve to intraoperative radiotherapy (IORT): clinical and experimental studies. Int J Radiat Oncol Biol Phys 11:1579–1585

Kopp M, Deutschmann H, Kopp P et al (2008) IOERT in advanced anterior skull base tumors: the results of 30 patients over a 6 year period. Rev Cancer (Madrid) 22:23

Krempien R, Roedeer F, Buchler MW et al (2008) Intraoperative Radiation Therapy (IORT) for primary and recurrent extremity soft tissue sarcoma: first results of a pooled analysis. Rev Cancer (Madrid) 22:56

Lesti G, Ciampaglia F, Tidona V (2008) Breast conserving surgery with intraoperative radiotherapy in single dose of 21 Gy 5 year follow-up. Rev Cancer (Madrid) 22:17

Majewski W, Wydmanski J, Kaniewska-Dorsz Z et al (2008) Early results of targeted intraoperative radiation therapy (TARGIT) as a boost in breast conserving treatment. Rev Cancer (Madrid) 22:17–18

Merrick HW, Gunderson LL, Calvo FA (2003) Future directions in intraoperative radiation therapy. Surg Oncol Clin N Am 12:1099–1105

Mussari S, Cionini L, Fatigante L et al (2008) IORT with electrons in breast carcinoma. Experience of two radiotherapy Italian centers. Rev Cancer (Madrid) 22:19

Oreccia R, Veronesi U (2005) Intraoperative electrons. Semen Radiat Oncol 15:76–83

Petersen IA, Haddock MG, Stafford SL et al (2008) Use of intraoperative radiation therapy in retroperitoneal sarcomas: update of the Mayo Clinic Rochester experience. Rev Cancer (Madrid) 22:57

Piroth MD, Heindrichs U, Gagel B et al (2008) Intraoperative radiotherapy in breast cancer. Experiences with the mobile linear accelerator NOVAC7 from physicians, physicists and patients point of view. Rev Cancer (Madrid) 22:20–21

Polowski WP, Jankiewicz M, Romanek J et al (2008) Breast and axillary lymph node sparing surgery with targeted intraoperative radiotherapy and sentinel node biopsy for early breast carcinoma. Rev Cancer (Madrid) 22:21

Radziszewski J, Lyczek J, Gierej P et al (2008) Intraoperative brachytherapy in pelvic recurrences and locally advanced rectal cancer. a preliminary report. Rev Cancer (Madrid) 22:51

Roeder F, Timke C, Krauter U et al (2008) Combination of neoadjuvant radiochemotherapy, surgery and intraoperative radiotherapy in patients with locally advanced pancreatic cancer. Rev Cancer (Madrid) 22:34

Rutten HJ, Valentini V, Krempien R et al (2008) Treatment of locally advanced rectal cancer by intraoperative electron beam radiotherapy containing multimodality treatment, results of a European pooled analysis. Rev Cancer (Madrid) 22:45

Sedlmayer F, Fastner G, Merz F et al (2008) Isiort pooled analysis on linac-based IORT as boost strategy during breast conserving therapy. Rev Cancer (Madrid) 22:21–22

Sindelar WF, Tepper JE, Kinsella TJ et al (1994) Late effects of intraoperative radiation therapy on retroperitoneal tissues, intestine, and bile duct in a large animal model. Int J Radiat Oncol Biol Phys 29:781–788

Sindelar WF, Johnstone PAS, Hoekstra HJ et al (1999) Normal tissue tolerance to intraoperative irradiation: The National Cancer Institute experimental studies. In: Gunderson LL, Willett CG, Harrison LB, Calvo FA (eds) Intraoperative irradiation: techniques and results. Human Press, Totowa, pp 131–146

Skoropad V, Berdov B, Evdokimov L et al (2008) Intraoperative radiotherapy for gastric and colon cancer: Obninsk Radiological Center 15-Years experience. Rev Cancer (Madrid) 22:26–27

Valentini V, D'Agostino G, Mattiucci GC et al (2008) IORT in pancreatic cancer: a joint analysis on 270 patients. Rev Cancer (Madrid) 22:34–35

Vaidya JS, Joseph DJ, Tobias JS (2010) Targeted intraoperative radiotherapy versus whole breast radiotherapy for breast cancer (TARGIT-A trial): an international, prospective, randomised, non-inferiority phase 3 trial. Lancet 376(9735):91–102

Willet CG, Czito BG, Tyler DS (2007) Intraoperative radiation therapy. J Clin Oncol 25:971–977

Intraoperative Radiation Therapy (IORT)

ANTHONY E. DRAGUN
Department of Radiation Oncology, James Graham Brown Cancer Center, University of Louisville School of Medicine, Louisville, KY, USA

Synonyms

Intraoperative brachytherapy; Intraoperative electrons

Definition

A technique of accelerated partial breast irradiation using a single fraction of electrons (3–9 MeV), photons (50 kVp), or high-dose rate brachytherapy to deliver approximately 18–21 Gy to the tumor bed at the time of lumpectomy. Initial experience with these techniques has shown great promise with acceptable toxicity and cosmetic outcome. Currently, early results of randomized trials comparing efficacy to whole breast radiation therapy show favorable results in selected patients.

Cross-References

▶ Accelerated Partial Breast Irradiation
▶ Early-Stage Breast Cancer
▶ Intraoperative Irradiation

Intraperitoneal Chemotherapy

CHRISTIN A. KNOWLTON[1], MICHELLE KOLTON MACKAY[2]
[1]Department of Radiation Oncology, Drexel University, Philadelphia, PA, USA
[2]Department of Radiation Oncology, Marshfield Clinic, Marshfield, WI, USA

Synonyms

IP chemotherapy

Definition

Intraperitoneal chemotherapy is administered through a thin catheter that is surgically implanted directly into the peritoneal cavity. Common agents used for IP chemotherapy include cisplatin and paclitaxel. This treatment is most often considered in patients with stage II and III disease. Advantages to IP chemotherapy include higher drug concentrations and longer drug half-lives in the peritoneal cavity.

Cross-References

▶ Ovary
▶ Principles of Chemotherapy

Intraperitoneal Phosphorus-32 (32-P)

PATRIZIA GUERRIERI, PAOLO MONTEMAGGI
Department of Radiation Oncology, Regional Cancer Center "M. Ascoli", University of Palermo Medical School, Palermo, Italy

Definition

A Beta particle–emitting radiopharmaceutical used as ^{32}P-chromic phosphate for intraperitoneal instillations in ovarian or Fallopian tube cancer patients at risk for relapse in the intraperitoneal space.

Cross-References

▶ Carcinoma of the Fallopian Tube

Intrinsic Radiosensitivity

CLAUDIA E. RÜBE
Department of Radiation Oncology, Saarland University, Homburg/Saar, Germany

Definition

Inherent cellular radiosensitivity.

Cross-References

▶ Predictive In vitro Assays in Radiation Oncology

Inverse Treatment Planning

TIMOTHY HOLMES
Department of Radiation Oncology, Sinai Hospital, Baltimore, MD, USA

Definition

The complexity of IMRT treatments require that an automated method of treatment planning using optimization algorithms be used to compute the large number of parameters that make up an IMRT plan (i.e., the positions of mechanical components as a function of elapsed treatment time). The term "inverse" treatment planning refers to the simple idea of inverting the "optimal" dose distribution to obtain the intensity modulated beams that produce the dose distribution.

Cross-References

▶ Image Guided Radiation Therapy (IMRT) - Helical TomoTherapy

Involved Field Radiotherapy

FENG-MING KONG, JINGBO WANG
Department of Radiation Oncology, Veteran Administration Health Center and University Hospital, University of Michigan, Ann Arbor, MI, USA

Synonyms

IFRT

Definition

Involved field radiotherapy is only targeted to the regions involved by tumor and the prophylactic irradiation to the nodal regions is not planned.

Cross-References

▶ Lung

Ion Chamber

YAN YU, LAURA DOYLE
Department of Radiation Oncology, Thomas Jefferson University Hospital, Philadelphia, PA, USA

Definition

Instrument for obtaining exposure measurements. Uses applied voltage across electrodes to collect charge produced by radiation interactions within an air volume inside the instrument. Current is proportional to exposure rate, which is usually displayed in units of mR/h.

Cross-References

▶ Brachytherapy: Low Dose Rate (LDR) Permanent Implants (Prostate)

IP Chemotherapy

▶ Intraperitoneal Chemotherapy

Irish Node

FILIP T. TROICKI[1], JAGANMOHAN POLI[2]
[1]College of Medicine, Drexel University, Philadelphia, PA, USA
[2]Department of Radiation Oncology, College of Medicine, Drexel University, Philadelphia, PA, USA

Definition

Enlarged axillary node, often associated with advanced gastric cancer.

Cross-References

▶ Stomach Cancer

Isolated Tumor Cells

▶ Microscopic Lymph Node Disease

Isotypes

Tod W. Speer
Department of Human Oncology, University of
Wisconsin School of Medicine and Public Health,
UW Hospital and Clinics, Madison,
WI, USA

Definition

The specific type or class of antibody that is based
upon the makeup of the amino acid sequence and
configuration of the heavy chain. In mammals,
there are five different isotypes: IgA, IgD, IgE,
IgG, and IgM.

J

Jun Gene Expression

THEODORE E. YAEGER
Department Radiation Oncology, Wake Forest
University School of Medicine, Winston-Salem,
NC, USA

Synonyms
Radiation induced gene expression

Definition
A proto-oncogene mediated by a protein kinase
and by reactive oxygen intermediates. It is an early
response to radiation exposure that modifies
gene expression as a heterodimer that expresses
transcription AP-1. The transcription is a central
regulator of cell proliferation, differentiation and
cell death.

Cross-References
► Genomic Instability
► Short-Term and Long-Term Health Risk of
Nuclear Power Plant Accident

References
Kufe D, Weichselbaum R (2003) Radiation therapy: activation for gene transcription and the development of
genetic radiotherapy-therapeutic strategies in oncology. Cancer Biol Ther 2:326–329

Juvenile Granulosa Cell Tumors

THEODORE E. YAEGER
Department Radiation Oncology, Wake Forest
University School of Medicine, Winston-Salem,
NC, USA

Synonyms
Pediatric ovarian cancer

Discussion
Similar to the adult female presentation these are
rare mostly unilateral ovarian tumors that typically behave in a benign presentation. They present in prepubertal females and up to the age of 30
years are considered "juvenile." They may secrete
estrogens forcing prepubertal girls to demonstrate isosexual precious puberty seen before age
8–10 years. The sexual manifestations are somewhat dramatic however the most common sign is
that of an abdominal mass. Bilateralism occurs in
only about 5% of cases. Since most are early stage
the overall prognosis is good except for post surgical recurrences and the unfortunate neglected
cases with advanced stage. Radiotherapy can be
palliative but surgical intervention is typical.

Cross-References
► Ovarian Cancer
► Pediatric Ovarian Cancer

L.W. Brady, T.E. Yaeger (eds.), *Encyclopedia of Radiation Oncology*, DOI 10.1007/978-3-540-85516-3,
© Springer-Verlag Berlin Heidelberg 2013

References

Young RH et al (1984) Juvenile granulosa cell tumor of the ovary. A clinicopathologic analysis of 125 cases. Am J Surg Path 8:575–596

Juvenile Nasopharyngeal Angiofibroma

THEODORE E. YAEGER
Department Radiation Oncology, Wake Forest University School of Medicine, Winston-Salem, NC, USA

Definition

A malignant vascular tumor arising from the posterior or posterolateral wall of the nasopharynx. It can extend into the surrounding sinuses, orbits and infratemporal fossae. It often presents signs of an intraorbital tumor, epistaxis, cranial nerve deficits and/or facial (cheek) swelling. Patient often have a history of familial adenomatous Polyposis associated with a gene mutation. Radiation therapy is useful for post-operative therapy for incomplete resections (a failure rate about 60%), as adjuvant therapy, or as sole treatment for recurrences or in locally advanced presentations. Modern IMRT is recommended with doses approaching but not exceeding 36 Gy.

Cross-References

▶ Pediatric Ovarian Cancer
▶ Sarcomas of the Head and Neck

References

Kuppersmith RB et al (2000) The use of intensity modulated radiotherapy for the treatment of extensive and recurrent juvenile angiofibroma. Int J Pediatr Otorhinolarygol 52:261–268

Juvenile Secretory Breast Carcinoma

THEODORE E. YAEGER
Department Radiation Oncology, Wake Forest University School of Medicine, Winston-Salem, NC, USA

Definition

Childhood breast carcinoma.

Discussion

A rare pediatric tumor characterized by abundant mucin and mucopolysaccharid containing material by pathology analysis of the specimen. Hormone receptors are usually not identified. Local surgical resection of the tumor is consider adequate in most cases as adjuvant radiation for this age group of 3–15 years of age is considered a risk for secondary malignancy.

Cross-References

▶ Pediatric Ovarian Cancer
▶ Stage 0 Breast Cancer

References

Eskelinen M et al (1990) Carcinoma of the breast in children. Z Kinderchir 45:52–55

Juxtaspinal Cord Tumors

THEODORE E. YAEGER
Department Radiation Oncology, Wake Forest University School of Medicine, Winston-Salem, NC, USA

Definition

Tumors presenting adjacent to the spinal cord demonstrating invasion or adherence to the vertebral body, spinal cord or peripheral nerve roots. Typically a sarcomatous origin tumor but can be a complex metastasis. Advanced radiotherapy techniques to "wrap" the cord are required for adequate dose delivery. Intensity Modulated delivery of photons or protons also require accurate and reproducible patient immobilization techniques.

Cross-References
▶ Palliation of Bone Metastases
▶ Pancoast Syndrome
▶ Proton Therapy

References

Weber DC et al (2004) A treatment planning comparison of intensity modulated photon and proton therapy for paraspinous sarcomas. IJROBP 58:1596–1606

K

Kantianism

THEODORE E. YAEGER
Department Radiation Oncology, Wake Forest
University School of Medicine, Winston-Salem,
NC, USA

Synonyms
Denotology

Definition
Consistent standards of behavior at all times
regardless of consequences. It contrasts with Util-
itarianism which is based on the best positive (or
least negative) outcome for the greatest benefit to
the greatest numbers of beneficiaries.

Kaposi's Sarcoma

THEODORE E. YAEGER
Department Radiation Oncology, Wake Forest
University School of Medicine, Winston-Salem,
NC, USA

Synonyms
Skin cancer

Definition
A vascular tumor, predominantly in the skin,
characterized by purplish lesions on the skin and
mucosal surfaces. It is a highly vascular tumor
produced by angiogenic growth factors affecting
the supportive network of the stromal supportive
cells and extracellular matrix. The lesions can be
macular, plaque-like, or nodular. It can be associated with lymphadenopathy or lymphedema
and may cause pain, bleeding or disfigurement.
Common presentations are in the lower extremities, genitalia, inguinal regions and facial areas.
Visceral Kaposi's Sarcoma typically involves the
aero-digestive tracts, in particular, oropharynx
and pulmonary lesions can lead to airway
obstruction and death.

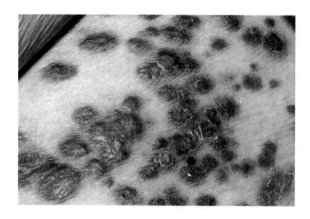

Cross-References
▶ Human Immunodeficiency Virus (HIV)
▶ Malignant Neoplasms Associated with
Acquired Immunodeficiency Syndrome

L.W. Brady, T.E. Yaeger (eds.), *Encyclopedia of Radiation Oncology*, DOI 10.1007/978-3-540-85516-3,
© Springer-Verlag Berlin Heidelberg 2013

Keloid

THEODORE E. YAEGER
Department Radiation Oncology, Wake Forest
University School of Medicine, Winston-Salem,
NC, USA

Synonym
Benign skin tumors

Definition
Excessive skin proliferation about scars after superficial injuries but can be spontaneous. They differ from hypertrophic scars in that the proliferation is infiltrative and can cause local pain especially when associated with inflammatory reactions. Common presentations involve skin with high tension such as the earlobes or sternum.

Cross-References
▶ Radiotherapy of Nonmalignant Diseases

Kidney

STEPHAN MOSE
Department of Radiation Oncology,
Schwarzwald-Baar-Klinikum,
Villingen-Schwenningen, Germany

Synonyms
Hypernephroma; Kidney cancer; Renal cell carcinoma; Urinary tract

Definition/Description
Renal cell carcinoma accounts for 2–3% of malignant diseases. Recent years have led to an improved understanding of this tumor, which is not one entity but rather a collection of different types of tumors with distinct genetic characteristics and histological features. In 2–3% of patients, ▶ hereditary renal cell cancer syndromes are diagnosed. In acquired tumors, risk factors are nicotine abuse, obesity, hypertension, end-stage-renal failure (dialysis), and acquired renal cystic disease. Partial nephrectomy and radical nephrectomy are the treatment of choice in localized and advanced disease, respectively. Adjuvant therapies are investigational. Whereas the impact of immunotherapy is still a matter of debate, targeted therapies are successfully included in the treatment of metastases.

Anatomy
The kidneys are a paired bean-shaped, vertically placed organ (length 11–12 cm) mainly consisting of blood vessels and epithelial collecting duct systems. The kidneys are surrounded by a tough fibrous capsule, perinephric fat – including the adrenal glands on top of each kidney – and the renal fascia (Gerota's fascia) retroperitoneally located between the eleventh rib and the transverse process of the third lumbar vertebral body. Both organs are breath-dependently mobile (3–4 cm) and paralleled to the lateral border of the psoas muscle. Adjacent organs to the kidney are the diaphragm (superiorly), the liver to the right kidney, the spleen to the left kidney (each posteriorly and laterally), and the duodenum (right), the stomach and pancreas (left), and the small bowels and the colon (medially and anteriorly). Because of its proximity to the liver, the right kidney typically lies slightly more inferior than the left one. The renal parenchyma is divided into the superficial renal cortex and the deep renal medulla. These structures contain the blood plasma filtrating and urine producing formations (renal lobes, pyramids, corpuscles, tubules, collecting ducts, minor and major calyces) draining the urine into the renal pelvis. This is

a part of the renal hilum where the renal artery as a direct branch of the abdominal aorta is located as well as the renal veins and lymph vessels, which on the right side predominantly drain to the paracaval and interaortocaval lymph nodes and on the left side drain to the paraaortic lymph nodes.

Epidemiology

Renal cell carcinomas account for 2–3% of all cancers in adults. The worldwide incidence is about 209,000 new cases per year. Most patients are 60 years of age (average) although recently the largest increase of tumor incidence is found in older patients. The tumor is more often diagnosed in men compared to women (1.5–2:1). In 1.5%, the tumor occurs bilaterally. However, simultaneous disease is rare and the metachronous occurrence is higher in young patients. Established risk factors are long-term nicotine abuse, obesity, hypertension, end-stage-renal failure (dialysis), and acquired renal cystic disease. Other potential environmental causes (exposure to asbestos, cadmium, thorium, trichloroethylene, abuse of phenacetin-containing analgetics) have been associated, but not convincingly linked to carcinogenesis in renal cell cancer. Two to three percent of tumors are familial; several autosomal dominant ▶ hereditary renal cell cancer syndromes (von Hippel–Lindau syndrome, hereditary papillary renal cell carcinoma, ▶ hereditary leiomyomatosis renal cell carcinoma, ▶ Birt–Hogg–Dubé syndrome, ▶ tuberous sclerosis) are known. These tumors are more often multifocally and bilaterally located. They occur more often in younger patients than sporadic tumors suggesting the strong genetic predisposition (Rini et al. 2009).

Clinical Presentation

At initial diagnosis, approximately 60–70% of tumors are confined to the kidney (Table 1) (Fig. 1). In 5–10% an invasion of the renal vein and the vena cava occurs, respectively. Ten to twenty-seven percent of tumors are lymph node positive, 16–30% of patients are diagnosed with simultaneous metastases (lung: 55–75%, soft tissue: 36%, bone: 20–30%, liver: 18–30%, skin: 8%, brain: 5–8%), and 1–3% present with solitary metastases. Compared to women, men present with larger tumors, a higher incidence of lymph nodes and metastases. The classical symptom triad of macrohematuria, abdominal mass, and pain is seldom (5–10%) and – if diagnosed – an advice for a probably advanced stage. Most patients suffer from microhematuria (50%). In 15–40% of patients, paraneoplastic syndromes (e.g., anemia, hypertension, cachexia, fever, hypercalcaemia, erythrocytosis, and neuropathia) are described. A well known presentation is a paraneoplastic liver dysfunction of cholestasis called 'Stauffer Syndrome'. Likewise, these systemic symptoms may refer to advanced disease Stauffer syndrome (Michalski 2008; Rini et al. 2009).

Renal cell carcinomas are derived from various parts of the renal parenchyma and are partially characterized by a distinct molecular signature reflecting their morphological, biological, and behavioral differences (Table 2). Primary renal sarcomas and renal lymphomas are very rare.

Furthermore, it is worldwide known that the Fuhrman nuclear grading has a prognostic value. It is based on three reproducible factors: nuclear size (10, 15, 20, >20 µg), nuclear irregularity (round and uniform, slightly irregular, moderately irregular, and multilobular nuclei) and the evidence of nucleoli (absent, visible at high power, visible at low power, and large with heavy chromatin clumps).

Differential Diagnosis

In imaging studies, 20% of diagnosed tumors are benign masses; therefore, each finding has to be evaluated carefully. Angiomyolipomas can be differentiated from malign disease because of their

Kidney. Table 1 TNM classification and staging. The TNM classification is still a matter of scientific debate because small tumors <4 cm – although the incidence increases – are not yet considered. Regarding their impact on prognosis in pT3–4 tumors, the following criteria are still controversially discussed: invasion of the perirenal fat, adrenal gland invasion ± venous involvement, infiltration of renal sinus fat, level of venous involvement, and invasion of the urinary collecting system. Furthermore, it is questionable if the differentiation between N1 and N2 as well as the selective reflection of the number and localization of distant metastases should be integrated into the classification (Moch et al. 2009)

TNM	
T1a	Tumor ≤4 cm and confined to kidney
T1b	Tumor >4 cm and ≤7 cm, confined to kidney
T2	Tumor >7 cm and confined to kidney
T3a	Invasion of the adrenal gland or perinephric fat but not beyond Gerota's fascia
T3b	Extension into renal vein (or its segmental branches) or vena cava below diaphragm
T3c	Extension into vena cava above the diaphragm or invasion of the wall of vena cava
T4	Invasion beyond Gerota's fascia
N0	No regional lymph node metastases
N1	Metastasis in one regional lymph node
N2	Metastases in more than one regional inguinal lymph node
M0	No distant metastases
M1	Distant metastases
Staging	
Stage I	T1 N0 M0
Stage II	T2 N0 M0
Stage III	T1–2 N1 M0
	T3 N0-1 M0
Stage IV	T4 N0-1 M0
	any T N2 M0
	any T any N M1

typical patches of dense fat, which are unusual in renal cancer. Furthermore, hematoma, abscesses, renal infarction, cysts and renal metastases of another malignancy have to be excluded. In case of hematuria, all inflammatory and malign diseases of the urinary tract system should be considered.

Imaging Studies

Today most renal carcinomas (up to 75%) are incidentally diagnosed by routinely performed imaging (ultrasonography, computed tomography) for unrelated abdominal symptoms. Ultrasonography is ideally completed and optimized by contrast agent to differentiate between cysts,

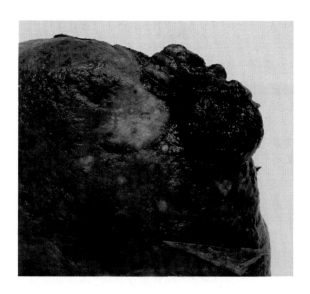

Kidney. Fig. 1 Renal cell carcinoma (with courtesy of A.Lampel, MD, Professor and Head of Department of Urology and Paediatric Urology, Schwarzwald-Baar-Klinikum Villingen-Schwenningen, Germany)

solid tumors and an abscess. In experienced hands, a tumor invasion into the renal vein or the vena cava can be evaluated by duplex sonography. Further diagnostic work-up includes an abdominal computed tomography (CT), which is equivalent to a magnetic resonance tomography (MRT) considering the local extension of the mostly solid carcinoma, the invasion of the renal collecting system and pelvis, the invasion into vessels and the lymph node staging (sensitivity and specificity 80–90%) (Figs. 2 and 3). Whereas the MRT enables to better differentiate a malign tumor from complex cysts, the CT has its advantage in the visualization of calcifications. Therefore, in some patients both modalities have to be performed at the time of primary diagnosis and/or preoperative staging. Likewise, both are established during therapy monitoring. In special mostly preoperative cases, a computerized angiography is added. Furthermore, CT, MRT as well as bone scan are needed to evaluate or exclude metastases (thorax, liver, bone, brain) during – if clinically indicated – initially staging and during follow-up of metastasized patients.

Although several advances in positron emission tomography (PET) with/without computerized tomography (PET/CT) had been made in recent years, there is no role of PET and PET/CT for primary diagnosis because of the renal excretion of the tracer. However, PET may be helpful to diagnose metastasized disease or to reevaluate treatment in patients with visceral, lymph node, and/or bone metastases (Bouchelouche & Oehr 2008; Graser et al. 2009).

Laboratory Studies

Blood count, blood chemistry, and urine analysis do not account for further diagnostic evaluation; however, they are needed for preparation of further therapy. An increase of alkaline phosphatase may be an advice for bone metastases. The pathological finding of secreted proteins (parathyroidlike hormone, erythropoietin, renin, gonadotropins, placental lactogen, prolactin, enteroglucagon, insulinlike hormone, adrenocorticotropic hormone, prostaglandine) demonstrates the association of renal cell carcinoma with various paraneoplastic syndromes. Serum tumor markers are not known.

Therefore, in renal cell carcinoma, biopsy is still argumentative although it is not routinely performed considering the reported incidence of in-transit metastases, the usual radiological accuracy, and the ease of removal of renal masses. However, recently reported, still experimental data about molecular tumor analysis (i.e., fluorescence-in-situ-hybridization, FISH-test), necessitating biopsy before surgery, has gained more investigational interest, because these tests may allow selective treatment decisions regarding the distinct molecular behavior of the individual cancer. Furthermore, this is due to the higher incidence of early diagnosed tumors where the

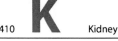
Kidney. Table 2 Histological subtypes, their incidence and mostly seen chromosomal aberrations, and further characteristics

Subtype	Incidence (in%)	Chromosomal aberrations	Further characteristics
Clear cell	70–80	– Depletion of 3p segments – Gain of 5q, 7 – Loss of 6q, 8p, 9p, 14q	– Mutation of the VHL gene in 60–70% of sporadic renal cell carcinoma – In 5% sarcomatoid pattern (worse prognosis) – More often in women
Papillary	10–15	– Trisomy or tetrasomy of 7 and 17 – Gain of 3, 12, 16, 20 – Loss of chromosome Y	– Type I (low-grade nuclei) with better prognosis than type II (high-grade nuclei) – In 5% sarcomatoid pattern – More often in men
Chromophobe	3–5	– Combined loss of 1, 2, 6, 10, 13, 17, 21	– Prognosis probably better than in clear cell carcinoma
Collecting duct (ductus bellini)	<1		– Mostly locally advanced with lymph node metastases at diagnosis (worse prognosis)
Medullary	<1		– Occurring almost in patients with sickle-cell trait (worse prognosis)
Multilocular-cystic	<1		– Characterized by multiple cysts – No local/distant failure reported
Unclassified	<5		– Consists of various tumor cell components without identifiable differentiation
TFE3-fusion-tumor	<1%	– Various translocation of region Xp11.2	– More often in children and young adults
Mucinous tubular and spindle cell	<1%	– Gain of 7, 11, 16, 17 – Combined loss 1, 4, 6, 8, 13, 14	– Probably good prognosis – May resemble sarcomatoid tumors
Papillary adenoma	<1%	– Combined trisomy of 7 and 17 – Loss of chromosome Y	– Putative precursor of papillary renal cell carcinoma
Oncocytoma (benign)	<5%	– Loss of 1p, 14q and Y – Balanced translocation between 11q13 and another chromosome	– Good prognosis

physician must differentiate benign from malignant disease and suggest surgery with/without organ sparing or optionally active surveillance (Rini et al. 2009).

Treatment

In renal cell carcinoma, prognosis strongly depends on the time of diagnosis. In incidentally diagnosed tumors, being often smaller, and in

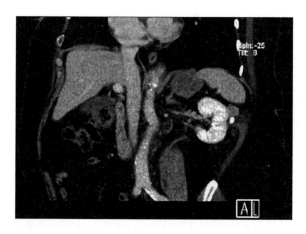

Kidney. Fig. 2 Peripheral renal cell carcinoma (computed tomography) (with courtesy of A. Lampel, MD, Professor and Head of Department of Urology and Paediatric Urology, Schwarzwald-Baar-Klinikum Villingen-Schwenningen, Germany)

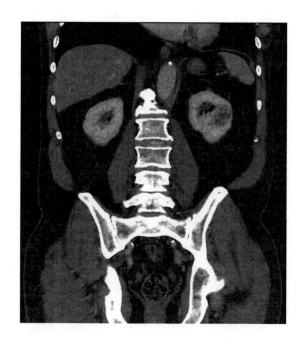

Kidney. Fig. 3 Central renal cell carcinoma (computed tomography) (with courtesy of A. Lampel, MD, Professor and Head of Department of Urology and Paediatric Urology, Schwarzwald-Baar-Klinikum Villingen-Schwenningen, Germany)

elective indication regarding surgery, the 5-year overall survival is 80–100% compared to those which are diagnosed because of abdominal symptoms, risk of renal failure, and therefore imperative indication (40–70%). In addition, this reflects the important role of the extension of the tumor. Also, the lymph node status is relevant regarding prognosis; the 5-year overall survival in node negative and positive patients is 60–80% and 10–20%, respectively. In those 20–40% of patients who will develop metastases, the 5-year overall survival is <10% (median survival 6–8 months). Bone and liver metastases are associated with a worse prognosis compared to lung metastases. Most of local and distant failure occurs within 3 (85%) and 5 (93%) years after surgery. Furthermore, prognosis depends on the histological subtype (see Table 2).

Although studies revealed a worse median overall survival in men, gender has no assured impact on the cancer-specific survival. However, increasing age may be related to worse outcome in patients with tumors 4–7 cm hypothesizing that there may be an influence of age and hormonal status on tumor aggressiveness.

Prognostic algorithm models using perioperative risk stratification are widely used. The model developed at the Memorial Sloan-Kettering Cancer Center (MSKCC-Score) considers five variables as risk factors for short term survival in advanced tumors (Table 3). Up to now, all models are not yet reliable enough to be completely implemented into therapeutic strategies. Due to the improved understanding of molecular mechanism in renal cell carcinoma, it is hoped that individualized therapeutic and prognostic assessment will be improved by the use of molecular biomarkers combined with clinical parameters (Aron et al. 2008; Scoll et al. 2009; Rini et al. 2009).

Surgery

Surgery is the treatment of choice in renal cell carcinoma achieving, regardless of tumor and

Kidney. Table 3 Risk stratification in advanced renal cell carcinoma (MSKCC-Score)

Risk factors	– Low Karnofsky performance status (<80) – Elevated lactate dehydrogenase (1.5 fold) – Low serum hemoglobin (< normal value) – Elevated "corrected" serum calcium (>10 mg/dl) – Time from initial tumor diagnosis to recurrence and start of treatment <12 months
Risk group	**Median survival**
Favorable: no risk factors	30 months
Intermediate: 1–2 risk factors	14 months
Poor: 3–5 risk factors	6 months

nodal staging, postoperative 5- and 10-year tumor-specific survival rates of 74% and 67%, respectively. Although there are no randomized studies considering the best surgical procedure in localized tumors, it is accepted that nephron-sparing surgery is gold standard in tumors ≤4 cm (T1a) and should be performed whenever technically possible. (Large cohort trials demonstrated that partial and radical nephrectomy yielded the same oncological outcome and that even radical nephrectomy is associated with a higher overall mortality whereas partial nephrectomy protects from loss of renal function and the deleterious effects of renal insufficiency independently of a normal contralateral kidney function combined with less use of analgetics and a shorter convalescence). The incidence of local recurrences is 0–10%; the 5- and 10-year overall survival rates are 92–98% and 90–96%, respectively. Benign tumors will be finally diagnosed in 17–25% of patients. Complications (e.g., bleeding with consecutive reoperation, urine fistula, renal failure due to ischemia) are reported in <20%. Comparable data are obtained in patients in whom a laparoscopic partial nephrectomy was performed. However, there are no randomized trials and the incidence of complications is higher (<25%); therefore, this procedure needs further evaluation. In experienced hands and – from a technical point of view – in favorable localized tumors, partial nephrectomy may be also possible in larger carcinomas that are confined to the kidney. But it has to be taken under consideration that higher tumor stage is related to unfavorable grading and a higher incidence of multifocality.

Other minimally invasive procedures (cryoablation, radiofrequency ablation, and high intensity focused ultrasound) have gained more interest in recent years. However, there are some technical limitations and randomized trials as well as long-time follow-up are still lacking, although in the USA radiofrequency ablation ± selective embolization is an equally approved therapy for T1a tumors. Depending upon the tumor diameter, 71–97% of patients are locally controlled; a 5-year overall survival of 93–98% is reported (Rini et al. 2009; Zini et al. 2009).

In (elderly) patients with relevant comorbidities, a high risk considering surgical intervention and a small tumor, active surveillance may be justified due to long-term follow-up data demonstrating that those tumors slowly grow and only 1% of tumors metastasize. Tumors <1 cm and <2 cm are found to be benign diseases in 46% and 30%, respectively (Crispen et al. 2009).

In T2–4 tumors radical nephrectomy with occasionally on block resection of adjacent organs and venous thrombectomy is necessary obtaining cure in 40–60% of patients. An adrenalectomy is indicated only in highly selected cases where involvement is suspected due to preoperative imaging and/or risk factors (i.e., multifocality, upper pole location and large tumor, venous thrombosis).

If preoperative staging is well done, micrometastases are found in only 4% of dissected lymph nodes. Therefore, a routine indication for lymph node dissection is not given; a survival benefit could not be shown in a randomized trial. Consequently, only selected cases with aggressive tumors may benefit from this procedure concerning the reduction of tumor burden and taking into consideration that in most of these patients, prognosis is limited by the development of distant metastases. Lymph node dissection may probably experience more importance if, for example, adjuvant target therapies will be proven to be successful (Blohm et al. 2009).

In metastasized disease and large renal tumor burden, nephrectomy is selectively indicated. In 0.8% spontaneous remission of metastases have been described following nephrectomy. Solitary metastases may be comparably considered for metastasectomy; in a favorable setting (i.e., complete respectability, long interval between primary diagnosis and development of metastases) 5-year survival rates of 24–30% are reported (Rini et al. 2009).

Radiotherapy

The motivation to include radiotherapy into the treatment of renal cell carcinoma is to preoperatively shrink the tumor to improve operability, or postoperatively to decrease the incidence of local recurrences. But radiotherapy has been historically regarded as ineffective in this disease, because up to now in clinical trials, which had been rarely performed, a beneficial effect on overall survival of (neo)adjuvant radiotherapy could not be demonstrated. An improvement in disease-free survival was solely obtained in incompletely resected pT3–4 tumors as well as in lymph node negative pT3 tumors where the local recurrences rate could be decreased from 16–37% to 9–11%. In pT1–2 tumors, radiotherapy is redundant because of the low risk of local recurrence whereas it is unnecessary in pT3b-c and pT4 tumors because of the high and – considering the prognosis – relevant risk of distant metastases.

If radiotherapy is to be implemented in renal cancer therapy, this should be done with the help of three-dimensional treatment planning. Intensity-modulated radiotherapy may be theoretically helpful in preventing side effects (nausea, vomiting, diarrhea, bowel dysfunction, decrease of liver function). However, the formerly reported high incidence of radiotherapy-induced severe side effects is definitively lowered by the application of modern treatment techniques (risk <5%). The applied dose (preoperative 45 Gy, postoperative 45–50 Gy, 1.8–2.0 Gy 5x/week) should encompass the renal bed, the renal and paraaortic lymph nodes as well as the scar because of the reported risk of in-transit metastases. If a boost is given, this should be ideally defined by clips (Michalski 2008; Troiano et al. 2009).

Recent experimental data demonstrate that a reduction or inhibition of transcription factors downstream of the interferon-signaling pathway (i.e., signal transducer and activator of transcription 1 = STAT 1) leads to radiosensitization in renal cancer cell lines hypothesizing that induced changes of this pathway could overcome radioresistance and enhance the effect of irradiation (Hui et al. 2009). Interestingly, reports about successful definitive carbon ion radiation therapy and about intraoperative radiotherapy in local recurrent diseases demonstrate the potential of new radiotherapy techniques in single cases. Furthermore, there are interesting data about hypofractionated extracranial stereotactic radiotherapy (40–48 Gy in 3–5 fractions) in

Kidney. Table 4 ESMO-Algorithm for systemic treatment of metastasized renal cell carcinoma

Histology	Risk group (MSKCC)	Standard treatment	Optional therapy
Clear cell carcinoma First line	Good/intermediate	Sunitinib or alternatively bevacizumab plus IFN α	High-dose IL-2 (in patients with good performance status only)
	Poor	Temsirolimus or alternatively sorafenib	
Second line	Cytokine refractory patients TKI-refractory patients	Sorafenib Everolimus	Sunitinib
Nonclear cell histology			Temsirolimus Sunitinib Sorafenib

primary and metastatic cases achieving partial and complete local responses in 90–98% suggesting an effect of fractionation on renal cell carcinoma.

Palliative radiotherapy yields good pain reduction (70–80%) and symptomatic neurological control (55–76%) in bone and multiple (>3) brain metastases, respectively. As alternative to surgery, (hypofractionated) radiosurgery obtains a local control in 64–96% of solitary brain metastases, so that in the most of selected patients the extracranial progress of renal cancer is life limiting.

Chemotherapy, Immunotherapy, and Targeted Therapy

Despite radical surgery, progression-free survival decreases in tumors >4 cm (65–80%) giving the rationale to adjuvant treatment. However, to date, adjuvant systemic therapy is investigational. Renal cell cancer is resistant to adjuvant and palliative chemotherapy; only gemcitabine and doxorubicine obtained small activity (<15%) in metastasized disease. In adjuvant phase-III-trials neither Interferon (IFN) α, Interleukin-2 (IL-2), nor combined therapy (IFN α, IL-2, 5-Fluorouracil) have shown any improvement regarding progression-free survival and overall survival after nephrectomy of advanced tumors (i.e., ≥pT2 or ≥pN1). Moreover, relevant side effects were reported. The randomized data regarding heat shock protein vaccine demonstrated no benefit and those data on the proving tumor cell lysate vaccine while initially not convincing, need to be scrutinized. Actually, important postoperative trials are ongoing studying the effect of multikinase inhibitors (sunitinib, sorafenib) and the effect of the monoclonal antibody G250 on tumors >4 cm (Rini et al. 2009).

In metastasized disease, systemic therapy changed dramatically within the last years due to the recent promising data achieved by targeted therapy, which is based on molecular mechanism:

- Sunitinib (tyrosine kinase inhibitor, TKI) and sorafenib (multikinase inhibitor) with activity against vascular endothelial growth factor (VEGF) and platelet-derived growth factor (PDGF)

- Bevazizumab (anti-angiogenic monoclonal antibody) targeting VEGF itself
- Everolimus and temsirolimus (mTOR-kinase inhibitors) inhibit the mammalian target of rapamycin pathway, which is responsible for regulation of cell growth and death

Due to recently reported data of randomized studies and integrating the MSKCC-score, an algorithm for systemic treatment of metastasized renal cell carcinoma was presented by the ESMO (European Society for Medical Oncology) (Table 4) taken under consideration that most of the studies have included tumors with clear cell histology (de Reijke et al. 2009). In first-line therapy, a median overall and progression-free survival of 18–26 months and 5–11 months was achieved in good and intermediate risk groups, respectively, whereas in the poor risk group the corresponding data were 11 and 6 months. Partial remissions in 9–31% and stable disease in 46–74% of treated patients are reported. The role of IL-2 is still controversial; however, ongoing trials with these and other new agents will demonstrate if there will be a role for cytokines.

Cross-References

▶ Pain Management
▶ Paraneoplastic Syndromes
▶ Wilm's Tumor

References

Aron M, Nguyen MN, Stein RJ, Gill IS (2008) Impact of gender in renal cell carcinoma: an analysis of the SEER database. Eur Urol 54:133–142

Blom JHN, van Poppel H, Maréchal JM, Jacqmin D, Schröder FH, de Prijck L, Sylvester R, EORTC Genitourinary Tract Cancer Group (2009) Radical nephrectomy with and without lymph-node dissection: final results of European Organization for Research and Treatment of Cancer (EORTC) randomized phase III trial 30881. Eur Urol 55:28–34

Bouchelouche K, Oehr P (2008) Positron emission tomography and positron emission tomography/

computerized tomography of urological malignancies: an update review. J Urol 179:34–45

Crispen PL, Viterbo R, Boorjian SA, Greenberg RE, Chenn DYT, Uzzo RG (2009) Natural history, growth kinetics, and outcome of untreated clinically localized renal tumors under active surveillance. Cancer 115:2844–2852

Graser A, Zech CJ, Stief CG, Reiser MF, Staehler M (2009) Bildgebung des Nierenzellkarzinoms – Imaging renal cell carcinoma. Urologe 48:427–438

Hui Z, Tretiakova M, Thang Z, Li Y, Wang X, Zhu JX, Gao Y, Mai W, Furge K, Qian C, Amato R, Butler B, Teh BT, Teh BS (2009) Radiosensitization by inhibiting STAT1 in renal cell carcinoma. Int J Radiat Oncol Biol Phys 73:288–295

Michalski J (2008) Kidney, renal pelvis, and ureter. In: Halperin EC, Perez CA, Brady LW (eds) Principles and practice of radiation oncology, 5th edn. Kluwer/Lippincott, Philadelphia

Moch H, Artibani W, Delahunt B, Ficarra V, Knuechel R, Montorsi F, Patard JJ, Stief CG, Sulser T, Wild PJ (2009) Reassessing the current UICC/AJCC TNM staging for renal cell carcinoma. Eur Urol 56:636–643

de Reijke TM, Bellmunt J, van Poppel H, Marreaud S, Aapro M (2009) EORTC-GU group expert opinion on metastatic renal cell cancer. Eur J Cancer 45:765–773

Rini BI, Campbell SC, Escudier B (2009) Renal cell carcinoma. Lancet 373:1119–1132

Scoll BJ, Wong YN, Egleston BL, Kunkle DA, Saad IR, Uzzo RG (2009) Age, tumor size and relative survival of patients with localized renal cell carcinoma: a surveillance, epidemiology and end results analysis. J Urol 181:506–511

Troiano M, Corsa P, Raguso A, Cossa S, Piombino M, Guglielmi G, Parisi S (2009) Radiation therapy in urinary cancer: state of the art and perspective. Radiol Med 114:70–82

Zini L, Perrotte P, Capitanio U, Jeldres C, Shariat SF, Antebi E, Saad F, Patard JJ, Montorsi F, Karakiewicz PI (2009) Radical versus partial nephrectomy – effect on overall and noncancer mortality. Cancer 115:1465–1471

Kidney Cancer

▶ Kidney
▶ Renal Cell Carcinoma
▶ Wilm's Tumor

Klinefelter's Syndrome

RAMESH RENGAN[1], CHARLES R. THOMAS, JR.[2]
[1]Department of Radiation Oncology, Hospital of
the University of Pennsylvania, Philadelphia, PA,
USA
[2]Department of Radiation Medicine, Oregon
Health Sciences University, Portland, OR, USA

Definition

This is a syndrome in which males have an extra
X chromosome (XXY). This is the most common
sex chromosome disorder. Males are characterized by small testicles and infertility.

Cross-References

► Mediastinal Germ Cell Tumor

L

Labeled MaB (Labeled Monoclonal Antibodies)

PATRIZIA GUERRIERI, PAOLO MONTEMAGGI
Department of Radiation Oncology, Regional
Cancer Center "M. Ascoli", University of Palermo
Medical School, Palermo, Italy

Definition

Monoclonal antibodies genetically engineered into
mammalian or yeast cells or immunologically built
in the laboratories by using animal (usually mice)
immunological reactions against human antigens
from various diseases. The ones against Fallopian
tube or ovary cells components, usually an epitope
on the CA-125 containing mucin protein, are used
for the diagnosis and follow-up of the respective
cancers by labeling them with radioactive tracers.
In recent clinical trials, they are being labeled with
radiopharmaceuticals such as radioactive Iodine-
131 and intraperitoneally administered for therapy
of small-volume stage III ovarian cancer.

Cross-References

► Carcinoma of the Fallopian Tube
► Chemotherapy
► Non-Hodgkins Lymphoma
► Radioimmunotherapy (RIT)
► Targeted Radioimmunotherapy

Laboratory Biology

► Clinical Research and the Practice of Evidence-
Based Medicine in Radiation Oncology

Larynx

VOLKER BUDACH, CARMEN STROMBERGER
Department of Radiotherapy and Radiation
Oncology, Charité - University Hospital Berlin,
Berlin, Germany

Description

Most patients suffering from larynx cancer want
to preserve their organ function. Therefore, treatment of laryngeal cancer is not only aimed at
cancer cure but also at the preservation of voice
and swallowing function, both factors of utmost
importance. Nowadays, improved surgical and
radiotherapeutic techniques often combined
with chemotherapy provide great potential for
a functional ► larynx preservation even for
patients with locally advanced disease. Surgery,
laser surgery, or radiotherapy offers comparable
cure rates (80–90%) for early stage cancer (T1/
T2a N0) in terms of local control (Rosier et al.
1998). Radiotherapy was reported to lead to
significantly better voice and speech quality.
This is the reason for radiotherapy being the
favored treatment modality for invasive tumors.
For locally advanced cancers a combined treatment approach for organ preservation is provided
by ► concurrent chemoradiation or induction
sequential chemoradiation (ICT). If organ
preservation is not feasible due to tumor site
and tumor extension, total laryngectomy combined with postoperative chemo-(radio)-therapy
is favored. Before starting any treatment, all
patients must be discussed in an interdisciplinary

L.W. Brady, T.E. Yaeger (eds.), *Encyclopedia of Radiation Oncology*, DOI 10.1007/978-3-540-85516-3,
© Springer-Verlag Berlin Heidelberg 2013

tumor board, whose decision should be executed to attain an optimized treatment outcome. The TNM staging system can be found in Table 1.

Etiology and Epidemiology

▶ Tumors of the larynx are the most common cancers of the head and neck region (42%) with a male predominance of m:f = 5:1. Consumption of tobacco, alcohol and betel nuts, and deficiencies of vitamin B12 or iron are associated risk factors. Laryngeal cancer is only weakly associated with a latent infection of the human papilloma virus (HPV) type 16 or 18 compared with pharyngeal tumors (Hobbs et al. 2006). However, as in other subsites of head and neck cancer, HPV positivity is a favorable prognostic factor and predicts good radiation response with and without chemotherapy.

Anatomy

The larynx has three subsites, the supraglottic region (suprahyoidal and infrahyoidal epiglottis, aryepiglottic folds, arytenoids, and false cord), the glottis region (true vocal cords with the anterior and posterior commissures), and the subglottic region from the lower boundary (≈5 mm) of the true vocal cord to the inferior area of the cricoid cartilage. The sensible and motoric nerval innervation of the larynx is provided by the recurrent vagal and the upper laryngeal nerve. Branches of the external carotid artery (A. pharyngea ascendens, A. thyroidea superior and inferior) provide the blood flow to the larynx. The lymph node drainage is typically to the levels II–IV (supraglottic region) and for the infraglottic subsite additionally to the pre-tracheal lymph node level. Early stage, T1/T2 glottic tumors seldom have a lymphogenic spread.

Clinical Presentation

Clinical signs of laryngeal cancer are site and stage dependent. Persistent and increasing dysfunction of the voice and/or hoarseness are frequently the first symptoms for tumors of the glottic region.

Supraglottic tumors often present with a more or less unspecific sore throat, dysphagia, or otalgia. For tumors of the epiglottis there are no specific early symptoms. Dyspnea is predominantly seen in tumors of the subglottic subsite.

Diagnostics

- Medical history
- Physical examination including tumor consistence and mobility, and cervical lymph node status
- Inspection
- Flexible endoscopy/laryngoscopy for tumor localization and extension
- Panendoscopy with biopsy, to detect synchronous secondary malignancies in the pharyngeal or esophageal region
- Bronchoscopy if clinically indicated
- Contrast media–enhanced CT (potential cartilage invasion) or MRI of the head and neck region (tumor dimensions) prior to biopsy
- Ultrasound of the cervical lymph node regions
- Ultrasound of the abdomen
- CT or X-ray of the chest
- Optional: PET-CT scanning for locally advanced stages
- Preventive dental care with potential tooth extraction at least 10 days prior to radiotherapy
- Speech and swallowing evaluation
- HPV status

Differential Diagnosis

Ninety-five percent of laryngeal tumors and almost all of the glottic tumors are squamous cell carcinomas (SCC). Other histologic types are rare (≈5%) and include adenocarcinoma, mucoepidermoid, adenoid cystic, small cell carcinoma, non-Hodgkin lymphomas, and sarcomas. Small cell carcinomas occur most frequently in the supraglottic region and behave similarly as small cell lung cancer.

Larynx. Table 1 UICC, TNM Staging System (7th Edition, 2010)

Stage 0	Tis	N0	M0
Stage I	T1	N0	M0
Stage II	T2	N0	M0
Stage III	T1, T2	N1	M0
	T3	N0, N1	M0
Stage IVA	T1, T2, T3	N2	M0
	T4a	N0, N1, N2	M0
Stage IVB	T4b	any N	M0
	any T	N3	M0
Stage IVC	any T	any N	M1

Supraglottic Tumor (T)

T1: Tumor limited to one subsite of supraglottis with normal vocal cord mobility

T2: Tumor invades mucosa of more than one adjacent subsite of supraglottis or glottis or region outside the supraglottis, without fixation of the larynx

T3: Tumor limited to larynx with vocal cord fixation and/or invades any of the following: postcricoid area, pre-epiglottic tissues, para-glottic space, minimal invasion of thyroid cartilage

T4a: Tumor invades through the thyroid cartilage, trachea, and/or extends into soft tissues of the neck, deep muscle of tongue, thyroid/esophagus

T4b: Tumor invades through the paravertebral space, mediastinum, or internal carotid artery

Glottic Tumor (T)

T1: Tumor limited to vocal cord(s) with normal mobility

T1a: Tumor limited to one vocal cord

T1b: Tumor involves both vocal cords

T2: Tumor extends to supraglottis and/or subglottis, impaired vocal cord mobility

T3: Tumor limited to the larynx with vocal cord fixation

T4a: Tumor invades through the thyroid cartilage, trachea, and/or extends into soft tissues of the neck, deep muscle of tongue, thyroid/esophagus

T4b: Tumor invades through the paravertebral space, mediastinum, or internal carotid artery

Subglottic Tumor (T)

T1: Tumor limited to the subglottis

T2: Tumor extends to vocal cord(s) with normal or impaired mobility

T3: Tumor limited to larynx with vocal cord fixation

T4a: Tumor invades through the thyroid cartilage, trachea, and/or extends into soft tissues of the neck, deep muscle of tongue, thyroid/esophagus

T4b: Tumor invades through the paravertebral space, mediastinum, or internal carotid artery

Regional Lymph Nodes (N)

N0: No regional lymph node metastasis

N1: Metastasis in a single ipsilateral lymph node, <3 cm in greatest dimension

N2a: Metastasis in a single ipsilateral lymph node >3–6 cm in greatest dimension

N2b: Metastasis in multiple ipsilateral lymph nodes, ≤6 cm in greatest dimension

N2c: Metastasis in bilateral or contralateral lymph nodes, ≤6 cm in greatest dimension

N3: Metastasis in a lymph node >6 cm in greatest dimension

Distant Metastasis (M)

M0: No distant metastasis

M1: Distant metastasis

Therapy

As mentioned above the aim for the treatment for laryngeal cancer is cure and also speech and swallowing preservation. Surgery and/or radiotherapy supplemented by chemotherapy depending on risk factors involved are the main treatment options for a potential cure. Treatment is always stage dependent. Surgical options are limited surgery (stripping or laser), cordectomy, vertical partial laryngectomy or total laryngectomy with permanent tracheostoma and reconstruction of the pharynx. Vaporization of the respective tumor tissue by using lasers offers no chances for a histologic workup and is therefore not the treatment of choice in these cases. A micro-dissection for a Cis (carcinoma in situ) should be favored.

Based on a pivotal phase III clinical trial concurrent chemoradiation has become the worldwide standard of care for locally advanced SCC of the larynx (Forstiere et al. 2003). ICT with a triplet of cis-platinum, 5-fluorouracil, and docetaxel (TPF) has been investigated in the last years and is superior to the doublet of cis-platinum and 5-fluorouracil alone with a loss of compliance for subsequent radiotherapy. ▶ Induction chemotherapy in patients with laryngeal cancer showed an organ preservation rate of 80%.

Adjuvant chemoradiation is established as treatment of choice for high-risk patients only. Extracapsular extension (ECE) and/or microscopically involved surgical margins are the only independent risk factors that could be established by multivariate analyses. For palliative treatment chemotherapy is used exclusively. All treatment decisions have to be taken before the start of treatment by an interdisciplinary tumor board.

Surgery

Early stage glottic tumors can be resected and cured by limited and function-preserving surgery. For glottic Tis, limited surgery can be carried out by endoscopic removal (stripping or laser) or preferably by micro-dissection to allow a histological workup for exclusion of micro-invasive or invasive carcinomas. Glottic T1/T2a N0 can be resected with chordectomy or partial laryngectomy (T2b with limited cord movement).

Glottic T3-primaries (fixation of the vocal cord) require total laryngectomy in most cases. T4 glottic tumors with extra-laryngeal spread or invasion of the cartilage require total laryngectomy with a permanent tracheostoma and reconstruction of the pharynx. For T4 tumors, generally adjuvant radiotherapy is required independent of a cervical lymph node involvement.

Supraglottic T1-2 tumors are treated with a partial supraglottic laryngectomy with or without a selective neck dissection. For involved lymph nodes with an ipsilateral modified radical neck dissection supraglottic T3 tumors need a total laryngectomy with a permanent tracheostoma with an ipsilateral or bilateral modified radical neck dissection (N0-1) and for N2-3 with a bilateral neck dissection. For resectable T4 supraglottic tumors, a total laryngectomy with a permanent tracheostoma and reconstruction of the pharynx supplemented by an ipsilateral or bilateral neck dissection (N0-1) and for N2-3 by bilateral neck dissection is necessary followed by adjuvant chemoradiation.

Subglottic tumors are rare and prognostic unfavorable. Surgical treatment often includes a total laryngectomy with or without thyroidectomy followed by adjuvant chemoradiation. The neck dissection should include also the paratracheal lymph node region.

Radical neck dissection removes levels II–V, the sternocleidomastoid muscle, the omohyoid muscle, the internal and external jugular veins, the N. accessorius (XI) and the submandibular glands. Modified neck dissection leaves one or more of the following structures in situ: the sternocleidomastoid muscle, the internal jugular vein, or the XI nerve. Selective neck dissection does not remove one or more lymph node levels from I–V. The lateral neck dissection removes levels II–IV.

Salvage surgery can be added to the treatment for persistent bulky or residual lymph nodes or tumors >12 weeks following definitive chemoradiation or in the case of local or regional recurrence.

Radiotherapy

Modern radiotherapy is based on multi-section imaging techniques to derive 3-D target volumes, which are used for the treatment planning (▶ Oro-Hypopharynx). Radiation therapy for laryngeal tumors is delivered by linear accelerator–based external beam radiotherapy. Brachytherapy has no role in the treatment of laryngeal tumors. Early stage tumors can be cured and larynx function can be preserved by radiotherapy alone (TD 66–70 Gy). T1 and T2 N0 tumors of the glottic larynx can be treated by small volume radiotherapy of the larynx due to the low risk of nodal spread. IMRT or rapid arc is not recommended for the treatment of glottic T1/T2 N0 tumors; opposed lateral fields should be used to optimally spare normal tissue. T1/T2 N0 supraglottic tumors need treatment of the primary (TD 66–70 Gy) with lymph node level II–III (TD 50–54 Gy) due to an increased risk of microscopic nodal involvement.

Adjuvant radiotherapy is always based on preoperative imaging and is indicated for intermediate risk patients such as multiple or large involved lymph nodes (≥N2a) and ≥T3 (dose prescription: TD 50–60 Gy). Adjuvant chemoradiation with cis-platinum ± 5-fluorouracil is indicated in high-risk situations (ECE and/or microscopically involved surgical margins; dose prescription: TD 64–66 Gy).

Standard treatment for locally advanced tumors (T3-T4 N0 N+) of the larynx is concurrent chemoradiation with cis-platinum conventionally fractionated (SD: 2 Gy, TD 70 Gy) (Forastiere et al. 2003), hyperfractionated (TD 72 Gy), or using ICT followed by radiotherapy for organ preservation. Locally advanced tumors of the larynx always need treatment of the macroscopic tumor and nodes (TD 70–72 Gy) with adjuvant radiation therapy of the lymph node level II–V (TD 50–60 Gy). For subglottic tumors the radiotherapy should include the paratracheal lymph node level.

Modern high-precision radiotherapy does not only rely on highly complex radiation techniques like ▶ intensity modulated radiotherapy (IMRT, Fig. 1) but also on regular positioning controls of the patients during fractionated radiation therapy (▶ Oro-Hypopharynx).

Chemotherapy

Cis-platinum ± 5-fluorouracil is the most common agent used for concurrent chemoradiation. ICT is carried out using cis-platinum-based agents, 5-fluorouracil, and docetaxel followed by (chemo) radiotherapy.

First-line palliative chemotherapy for recurrent or metastatic squamous-cell carcinoma of the head and neck uses platinum-based agents, 5-fluorouracil, and cetuximab.

Targeted Therapies

The monoclonal antibody, cetuximab, blocks extracellular the epidermal growth receptor and the signaling to activate tyrosinkinase and the cell proliferation. For patients with locally advanced head and neck tumors, cetuximab plus radiotherapy significantly improves overall survival at 5 years compared with radiotherapy alone; the improvement is less pronounced in patients with laryngeal cancer.

Side Effects

Surgery

Perioperative complications include hemorrhage, bleeding, infections, prolonged wound healing, edema, and airway obstruction. Postoperative complications of surgery include stenosis, fistula, chondritis, and aspiration with consecutive pneumonia. ▶ Late reactions include hoarseness, voice

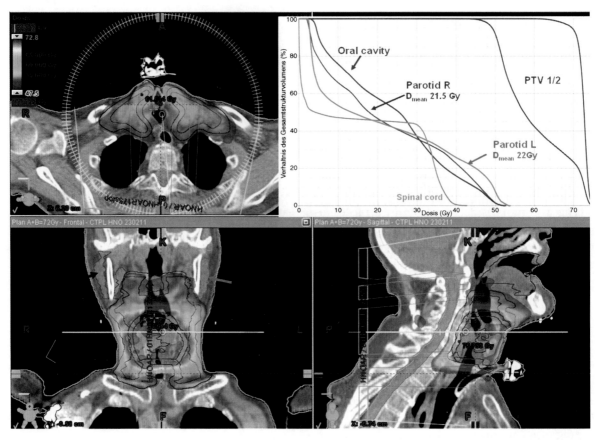

Larynx. Fig. 1 Example for dose distribution and DVH for a patient with a SCC of the larynx; cT4, cN0, M0; definitive chemoradiation (Rapid Arc® technique); dose prescription: SD of 2 Gy to a TD 60 Gy (PTV 2) and SD of 2 Gy to a TD of 72 Gy (PTV 1) with sparing of the right and left parotid gland

and speech as well as swallowing dysfunctions. A permanent tracheostoma requires an electronic voice box to communicate.

Radiotherapy

Early side effects include different degrees of dermatitis, mucositis, dysphagia, taste alteration, weight loss, hoarseness, edema of the larynx, chondritis, and sticky saliva. Late toxicity of radiotherapy (>90 days) includes fibrosis of the soft tissue, hyperpigmentation, teleangiectasia, submental edema, edema of the larynx, xerostomia, and rarely radionecrosis, osteoradionecrosis, or chondritis. Swallowing and voice and speech function can be impaired.

Chemotherapy and Targeted Therapy

Complications are drug dependent. Hematologic (anemia, neutropenia, thrombocytopenia), gastrointestinal side effects (nausea and vomiting), mucositis, and transient infertility are most common. Cis-platinum is known to affect the nephrologic function and has the potential to alter hearing permanently. Neurologic impairment (hand-foot syndrome) or allergic reactions have been reported with the use of drugs such as taxanes. Allergic reactions to anaphylactic shock, skin rash (acne-like), and hair and nail alterations can be associated with the use of cetuximab.

Prognosis

Early stage glottic (T1-T2a) tumors can be cured in the majority of all cases (80–90%) using any single treatment modality (surgery, laser surgery or radiotherapy) with similar results in terms of local control. Nevertheless, radiation therapy is significantly correlated with better long-term speech and voice quality qualifying the treatment modality as the preferred one. Subglottic tumors are rare and prognostic unfavorable. The prognosis is generally hampered by higher disease stages and positive resection margins (R1, R2) and ECE. The disease-free survival is negatively influenced by a positive nodal status. A latent HPV infection is a positive prognostic factor. ► Hyperfractionated radiotherapy but not acceleration provides a survival benefit. No benefit was observed with adjuvant chemotherapy. However, ICT as a predictive marker of tumor response for later chemoradiation was convincing, irrespective that a survival benefit when compared with concurrent chemoradiation was not observed.

Cross-References

► Oro-Hypopharynx
► Targeted Radioimmunotherapy

References

Forastiere AA, Goepfert H, Maor M et al (2003) Concurrent chemotherapy and radiotherapy for organ preservation in advanced laryngeal cancer. N Engl J Med 349:2091–2098

Fung K, Lyden TH, Lee J et al (2005) Voice and swallowing outcomes of an organ-preservation trial for advanced laryngeal cancer. Int J Radiat Oncol Biol Phys 63:1395–1399

Giro C, Hoffmann T, Budach W (2009) Kehlkopf. In: Bamberg M, Molls M, Sacks H (eds) Radioonkologie Klinik, 2nd edn. W. Zuckschwerdt, München/New York

Hansen EK, Schechter NR (2007) Cancer of the larynx and hypopharynx. In: Hansen EK, Roach M III (eds) Handbook of evidence-based radiation oncology, 1st edn. Springer, New York

Hobbs CG, Sterne JA, Bailey M et al (2006) Human papilloma virus and head and neck cancer: a systematic review and meta-analysis. Clin Otolaryngol 31:259–266

Levendag P, Al-Mamgani TD (2009) Contouring in head & neck cancer. Elsevier, Munich

Rosier JF, Grégoire V, Counoy H et al (1998) Comparison of external radiotherapy, laser microsurgery and partial laryngectomy for the treatment of T1N0M0 glottic carcinomas: a retrospective evaluation. Radiother Oncol 48:175–183

Larynx Preservation

VOLKER BUDACH
Department of Radiotherapy and Radiation Oncology, Charité - University Hospital Berlin, Berlin, Germany

Definition

Treatment strategy for laryngeal cancer to preserve the larynx itself or its function.

Cross-References

► Larynx

Larynx Tumor

VOLKER BUDACH
Department of Radiotherapy and Radiation Oncology, Charité - University Hospital Berlin, Berlin, Germany

Definition

Benign or malignant neoplasm or formation of cells in any area of the larynx as part of the respiratory track.

Cross-References

► Larynx

Late Radiation Toxicity

ANTHONY E. DRAGUN
Department of Radiation Oncology, James
Graham Brown Cancer Center, University of
Louisville School of Medicine, Louisville,
KY, USA

Definition

This refers to a group of side effects that occur in the months and years after treatment with radiation therapy. Breast fibrosis, which may have a negative impact on long-term cosmetic outcome, is described in 10–15% of cases. Breast pain is not unusual, but is more difficult to quantify, but rarely requires medical therapy. Seroma, which is an accumulation of fluid within the lumpectomy cavity, may contribute to pain or discomfort and has been described in up to 25–30% of patients, although the need for intervention is rare. Most seromas resolve spontaneously over a period of months. Lymphedema of the ipsilateral breast and/or upper extremity was more common in the past, when axillary dissections were performed in all patients. Cardiac, pulmonary, and chest wall injury have been described in the historical literature but are rare in the modern age of treatment of early-stage breast cancer, due to improvements in surgical technique, more accurate radiation therapy used and the less-frequent use of elective nodal irradiation.

Cross-References

► Early-Stage Breast Cancer
► Lymphedema
► Radiation Pneumonitis

Late Reactions

VOLKER BUDACH
Department of Radiotherapy and Radiation
Oncology, Charité - University Hospital Berlin,
Berlin, Germany

Definition

Reaction of the healthy tissue >90 days after end of radiotherapy treatment. The type and severity of late reaction is related to the body region treated, the applied radiation dose, the radiation technique (e.g., IMRT with sparing of organs at risk), and the individual predisposition of the patient. Late side effects can be long term or permanent.

Cross-References

► Larynx
► Oro-Hypopharynx

Leiomyosarcoma

FILIP T. TROICKI[1], JAGANMOHAN POLI[2]
[1]College of Medicine, Drexel University,
Philadelphia, PA, USA
[2]Department of Radiation Oncology, College of
Medicine, Drexel University, Philadelphia,
PA, USA

Definition

Tumor of the smooth muscle.

Cross-References

▶ Stomach Cancer

Leptomeningeal Spinal Cord Compression (Also Leptomeningeal Spinal Cord Metastases)

James H. Brashears, III
Radiation Oncologist, Venice, FL, USA

Synonyms

Leptomeningeal spinal cord metastases

Definition

Diffuse involvement of tumor cells to the spinal cord or subarachnoid fluid. The soft tissue of the brain is also usually invaded and lumbar puncture may show the presence of tumor cells. It is frequently seen with breast cancer and portends a bleak prognosis. While rare, leptomeningeal metastases are increasingly diagnosed and treatment often includes intraventricular chemotherapy.

Cross-References

▶ Palliation of Brain and Spinal Cord Metastases

Leptomeningeal Spinal Cord Metastases

▶ Leptomeningeal Spinal Cord Compression (Also Leptomeningeal Spinal Cord Metastases)

LET

George E. Laramore, Jay J. Liao, Jason K. Rockhill
Department of Radiation Oncology, University of Washington Medical Center, Seattle, WA, USA

Definition

▶ Linear energy transfer. The amount of energy a particle or quantum of ionizing radiation deposits along its path, typically measured in kiloelectron volts per micron (keV/μm). Fast neutrons are high LET particles with energy deposition in the range of 20–100 keV/μm, whereas megavoltage photons are low LET radiation with energy deposition in the range of 0.2–2 keV/μm.

Cross-References

▶ Neutron Radiotherapy

Lethal Midline Granuloma

Carlos A. Perez, Wade L. Thorstad
Department of Radiation Oncology, Siteman Cancer Center, Washington University Medical Center, St. Louis, MO, USA

Definition

Lethal midline granuloma (LMG) or midline malignant polymorphic reticulosis is characterized by progressive, unrelenting ulceration and necrosis of the midline facial tissues.

LMG is associated with Epstein-Barr virus. Despite considerable controversy, three clinicopathologic entities remain identified: Wegener's granulomatosis, LMG, and polymorphic reticulosis

(PMR). A review of the literature suggests that cases described as idiopathic midline destructive disease and PMR are an evolutionary spectrum from almost benign to fatal malignant lymphoma. Wegener's granulomatosis is an epithelioid necrotizing granulomatosis with vasculitis of small vessels. Systemic involvement of the kidneys and lungs is common.

PMR is an unusual disorder, characterized by atypical mixed lymphoid infiltration of the submucosa with necrosis, sometimes extending to bone or cartilage. PMR has been considered a lymphoproliferative disorder; most, if not all, cases are peripheral T-cell lymphomas. Several authorities believe that PMR and systemic lymphomatoid granulomatosis are the same disease with the latter predominantly involving the lungs.

Idiopathic LMG describes a localized disorder not characterized by visceral lesions but by destruction of the midfacial area, which, if left untreated, is uniformly fatal. Despite specific clinicopathologic features, the distinction between LMG and PMR is often difficult; although controversial, they may represent two phases of the same disease, with LMG remaining histologically benign or evolving into PMR.

LMG occurs more frequently in men. Ages range from 21 to 64 years; almost half of the patients are in their 50s at presentation. Most patients have involvement of the nasal cavity (including destruction of the septum) and the paranasal sinuses (particularly maxillary antrum). The primary lesion may extend into the orbits, the oral cavity (palate, gingiva), and even the pharynx.

Clinical Features and Diagnostic Workup

Clinical manifestations include progressive nasal discharge, obstruction, foul odor emanating from the nose, and, in later stages, pain in the nasal cavity, paranasal areas, and even in the orbits.

Examination discloses ulceration and necrosis in the nasal cavity, perforation or destruction of nasal septum and turbinates, and even ulceration of the nose. Edema of the face and eyelids may be noted, and the bridge of the nose may be sunken.

CT is invaluable in demonstrating the full extent of the tumor, including bone or cartilage destruction. MRI is also helpful because it could distinguish fluid retained within the paranasal sinuses from solid masses and tumor from granulation tissue; it is of little value for detecting bone lysis.

General Management and Radiation Therapy Techniques

When treatment of these patients is planned, it is extremely important to exclude the diagnosis of Wegener's granulomatosis, a benign process that is commonly treated with antimicrobial agents, steroids, and systemic chemotherapy. Bonafide LMG does not respond to steroids; the treatment of choice is radiation therapy.

Target volume should encompass all areas of involvement, including adjacent areas at risk (i.e., for a lesion of the maxillary antrum it will include the antrum as well as all of the paranasal sinuses) with a 2- to 3-cm margin. Because marginal failures are a significant problem, wide margins are necessary for treatment of these patients.

Irradiation techniques are similar to those described for tumors of the paranasal sinuses, nasal cavity, or nasopharynx. Several investigators have described complete responses with doses of 30–50 Gy; most patients are treated with 35–45 Gy in 3–4.5 weeks (Fauci et al. 1982). We recommend 45–50 Gy in 4.5–5.5 weeks in 1.8- to 2-Gy daily fractions.

Results of Therapy

Because of the rarity of this tumor, experience is limited. Fauci and colleagues (1982) reported on ten patients with extensive midline granuloma treated with irradiation. In seven patients receiving 40–50 Gy local control of disease was 77%; two patients had local recurrences, one outside the initially irradiated volume.

The Mayo Clinic reported the most extensive experience in treatment of PMR or LMG with irradiation doses of 40–42 Gy. Of 20 patients irradiated for localized upper airway PMR, 13 were alive and well for an average of 9.5 years.

A retrospective study found that a minimum dose of 42 Gy was necessary to achieve long-term local control. Systemic failure occurred in 25% of their patients initially presenting with limited disease. The salvage of these patients required effective combination chemotherapy, usually containing doxorubicin, cyclophosphamide, vincristine, and prednisone (CHOP) or other combinations, including CHOP or nitrogen mustard, vincristine, procarbazine, and prednisone (MOPP) in some patients.

Fauci and coworkers (1982) published a prospective study of 15 patients with systemic lymphomatoid granulomatosis. Of 13 patients treated with cyclophosphamide and prednisone, seven sustained complete remission (mean duration of remission, 5.2 ± 0.6 years). Six deaths were associated with biopsy-proven lymphoma; one was caused by a lymphoma-like illness unproven by biopsy. None of these patients received radiation therapy.

Cross-References

▶ Hodgkin's Lymphoma
▶ Lung Cancer
▶ Rectal Cancer
▶ Sarcomas of the Head and Neck

References

Fauci AS, Hayes BF, Costa J et al (1982) Lymphomatoid granulomatosis: prospective clinical and therapeutic experience over 10 years. N Engl J Med 306: 68–74

Leukemia Cutis

CASPIAN OLIAI
Department of Radiation Oncology, College of Medicine, Drexel University, Philadelphia, PA, USA

Definition

The infiltration of malignant leukemic cells into the skin resulting in clinically identifiable cutaneous lesions. This condition may be contrasted with leukemids, which are skin lesions that occur with leukemia, but which are not related to leukemic cell infiltration.

Cross-References

▶ Leukemia in General

Leukemia in General

CASPIAN OLIAI
Department of Radiation Oncology, College of Medicine, Drexel University, Philadelphia, PA, USA

Synonyms

Acute lymphocytic leukemia (ALL); Acute myelogenous leukemia (AML); Chronic lymphocytic leukemia; Chronic myelogenous leukemia; Hematopoietic neoplasms; Lymphoblastic neoplasms

Definition

Leukemia: A progressive malignant disease of the blood-forming organs characterized by aberrant development and distorted proliferation of leukocytes at some point in ▶ hematopoiesis. It is classified as acute or chronic based on the degree of malignant cell maturity, and as either myeloid or lymphoid in origin. The vast majority of leukemias fall under this classification, and these will be the focus of this chapter. Of note, ▶ hairy cell leukemia and T-cell prolymphocytic leukemia are usually considered to be outside of this classification scheme.

Acute Lymphoblastic Leukemia (ALL): A neoplasm composed of immature B or T-cells, referred to as lymphoblasts. The lymphoid neoplasms are separated based upon cell maturity and further grouped by B- or T-cell origin. The precursor B-cell type arise in the bone marrow and may spread to the peripheral blood. The precursor T-cell type arise within the thymus or bone marrow. These can be further divided into either lymphoblastic lymphoma or lymphoblastic leukemia. Clinically, a case is defined as lymphoma if there is a mass lesion in the mediastinum or elsewhere and <25% blasts in the bone marrow. It is classified as leukemia if there are ≥25% bone marrow blasts, with or without a mass. Nevertheless, these can be considered the same disease since both conditions eventually develop characteristics of one another.

Acute Myeloid Leukemia (AML): A group of hematopoietic neoplasms involving cells committed to the myeloid line of cellular development. It is characterized by a clonal proliferation of myeloid precursors with reduced capacity to differentiate into more mature cellular elements. More specifically, AML is defined as >20% myeloid blasts in the bone marrow/peripheral blood, or the presence of particular genetic aberrations, regardless of the blast count.

> **World Health Organization (WHO) subdivides AML into:**
> ● AML with genetic aberrations
> ● AML with myelodysplastic syndrome-like features
> ● AML, therapy related
> ● AML not otherwise specified

The French-American-British (FAB) system is based upon the degree of differentiation and lineage. It may not be as useful as the WHO classification, but can help when associating cytogenetic abnormalities to particular subtypes:

> **French-American-British System**
> ● M0 – minimally differentiated acute myeloblastic leukemia
> ● M1 – acute myeloblastic leukemia, without maturation
> ● M2 – acute myeloblastic leukemia, with granulocytic maturation
> ● M3 – acute promyelocytic leukemia
> ● M4 – acute myelomonocytic leukemia
> ● M4eo – myelomonocytic with bone marrow eosinophilia
> ● M5a – acute monoblastic leukemia
> ● M5b – acute monocytic leukemia
> ● M6 – acute erythroid leukemias
> ● M7 – acute megaloblastic leukemia
> ● M8 – acute basophilic leukemia

Chronic Myeloid Leukemia (CML): A ▶ myeloproliferative disease (MPD) characterized by over-proliferation of the granulocytic lineage at any stage of maturation. It is always associated with the presence of a BCR-ABL fusion gene, which is usually created by a reciprocal translocation that results in the formation of the Philadelphia chromosome t(9;22).

Chronic Lymphocytic Leukemia (CLL): A neoplasm of mature lymphocytes in which there is accumulation of functionally incompetent monoclonal cells. The absolute B-lymphocyte count in the peripheral blood is ≥5,000/μL. B-cell origin is seen in 95% of cases. CLL is considered to be identical to ▶ small lymphocytic lymphoma, a slowly progressing type of ▶ non-Hodgkin lymphoma (NHL). They both represent different areas of the spectrum within the same disease.

Background

The American Cancer Society estimated incidence of leukemia in 2010 was 43,050 new cases, with

21,840 estimated deaths. Leukemia is estimated to comprise 3% of new US cancer cases, and 4% of the total US cancer deaths in 2010. Leukemia is the most common cancer among children 14 years and younger, comprising approximately 30% of all childhood cancers. Leukemia also accounts for the most cancer deaths in children.

Radiotherapy was used to treat leukemia more frequently in the past and has been largely supplanted by CNS-penetrating chemotherapeutics and small molecule-targeted pharmaceuticals. In 2010, radiotherapy is administered in relatively small percentage of leukemia cases. Common indications for radiotherapy in leukemic patients include total body irradiation as myeloablative preparation for hematopoietic stem cell transplant, CNS prophylaxis, testicular relapse, and palliative splenic/chloroma irradiation. Despite the limited role of radiotherapy, leukemia is a major topic that all healthcare professionals working in the field of radiation oncology should include in their fund of knowledge. This chapter will briefly discuss the chemotherapeutics used to treat the leukemias in addition to radiotherapy.

Etiology

ALL: Heterogeneous in that it can arise from any lymphoid developmental stage. Transformation from a normal functioning cell into a single malignant cell is the first step followed by monoclonal proliferation and dissemination. A sole etiology has yet to be determined. Most cases are not associated with risk factors; however, some do exist. These include previous cancer treatment, exposure to high levels of radiation (nuclear reactor accident, atomic bomb), immunodeficiency, and viral infection. The genetic aspect of the disease is exemplified by the association between AML and Down syndrome, in addition to affected first-degree relatives.

AML: Derived from bone marrow progenitors that are restricted to developing into granulocytes, erythrocytes, monocytes, or megakaryocytes. It is the consequence of a series of genetic changes including translocations, inversions, or deletions. The most common cytogenetic abnormalities are:

$$M2 - t(8; 21)(q22; q22)$$

$$M3 - t(15; 17)(q22; 11 - 12)$$

$$M4eo - inv(16)(p13; q22)$$

$$M4, 5 - t(11q23; v)$$

Malignant blood diseases such as ▶ myelodysplastic syndrome (MDS) and the myeloproliferative diseases can transform into AML. In addition, benign blood diseases like paroxysmal nocturnal hemoglobinuria show an association. Increased risk is also seen in alkylating agents, anthracyclins, high levels of radiation exposure, and in working conditions of early twentieth century radiologists prior to modern safety practices. The genetic aspect of the disease is exemplified by the association between AML and Down syndrome, in addition to affected first-degree relatives.

CML: Arises from the fusion of two genes: BCR on chromosome 22 and ABL1 on chromosome 9, resulting in the BCR-ABL fusion gene. This usually results from a reciprocal translocation, t(9;22)(q34;q11), that gives rise to the Philadelphia chromosome (Ph+). The fusion protein functions as a tyrosine kinase, resulting in leukemic transformation. This is present in over 90% of individuals with CML. The only known risk factors are male gender, older age, and radiation exposure.

CLL: The etiology is unclear; however, several risk factors are thought to exist. They include age >50 years, male gender, Caucasian race, family history of CLL or other hematopoietic neoplasms, and exposure to herbicides and insecticides like Agent Orange used during the Vietnam war.

Clinical Presentation

The signs and symptoms typical of most leukemias are related to cellular expansion in the bone marrow causing anemia, neutropenia, and thrombocytopenia. They include fatigue, weight loss, bone pain, pallor, ecchymoses, petechiae, dyspnea, dizziness, heart palpitations, and recurrent infections.

ALL: Patients may experience B-symptoms: fever >38°C, drenching night sweats, and unintentional weight loss ≥10% of total body weight within 6 months.

Precursor B-cell ALL invades the CNS frequently creating an increase in intracranial pressure which disrupts the meninges. Focal neurological deficits may result. Adults may experience lymphadenopathy (LAD) and hepatosplenomegaly. Mass lesions occur and usually are found in lymph nodes, skin, testicles, and the CNS.

Precursor T-cell ALL typically presents with a mediastinal mass or LAD. The former may lead to complications including pleural/pericardial effusion, ▶ superior vena cava syndrome, or obstruction. Other characteristics specific to the T-cell type include more frequent B-symptoms, advanced disease upon diagnosis, increased serum LDH, and a low incidence of extranodal disease.

AML: Fever may be present from two sources: (1) the process of leukemia itself, usually seen in the M3 type and (2) infection due to neutropenia, which is more common. CNS symptoms of headache, visual changes, and cranial nerve deficits may occur, usually in those with M4/5 disease. A significant percentage of these subtypes also manifest leukemic skin infiltration. The lack of LAD and hepatosplenomegaly is a key, which helps distinguish AML from ALL upon physical exam. A small percentage may experience arthritis or arthralgias.

▶ Chloroma may be found in patients with AML. If a chloroma occurs simultaneously with bone marrow involvement, it is found in the skin or gingiva. In the absence of bone marrow involvement, chloroma sites include bone, lymph nodes, ovary, and uterus.

CML: Individuals are frequently asymptomatic at diagnosis, in which case the disease is found upon routine blood work. Once symptomatic, the disease shows the typical signs/symptoms of leukemia in addition to excessive sweating, splenomegaly, and abdominal fullness. Extramedullary involvement may include skin, lymph nodes, and soft tissue. WBC counts can reach levels above 100,000/µL and platelet counts of 600,000/µL.

The clinical course is biphasic or triphasic: (1) chronic phase, present at diagnosis in the vast majority of cases; (2) accelerated phase, in which neutrophil differentiation becomes impaired and leukocyte proliferation becomes difficult to suppress; and (3) blast crisis, resembling acute leukemia in which blast cells proliferate uncontrollably. Blast crisis is defined as ≥20% blasts in the peripheral blood or ≥30% blasts in the marrow, presence of chloroma, or large regions of blast clusters upon bone marrow biopsy. This phase typically occurs 3–5 years after the diagnosis of CML and 1.5 years after the onset of the accelerated phase.

CLL: Patients are usually asymptomatic upon diagnosis or may present with painless cervical LAD. Hepatic and splenic enlargement is also common. A small percentage of patients experience B-symptoms. The most common non-lymphatic organ involvement is the skin, which is a condition known as ▶ leukemia cutis, usually involving the face. Hypersensitivity to insect bites is a feature in some cases of CLL. There is an association with autoimmune hemolytic anemias, pure red blood cell aplasia, and membranoproliferative glomerulonephritis. The majority of patients present with WBC count levels >100,000/µL. Blood levels of LDH and β2-microglobulin are also frequently elevated.

A unique characteristic of CLL is its propensity to transform into other lymphoproliferative conditions usually occurring as the final phase of disease. The most common resulting disorders include prolymphocytic leukemia, ▶ Richter transformation, ▶ Hodgkin lymphoma, and ▶ multiple myeloma.

Diagnostics

ALL: Diagnosis is dependent upon bone marrow aspirate/biopsy, as well as samples from involved extranodal sites. Subsequently, these samples are evaluated by flow cytometry, cytogenetic studies, and histology. Blood smears are also needed to identify blast cells.

The blast cell surface is positive for terminal deoxytransferase (TDT) and commonly expresses the CALLA antigen. Blast cells are usually PAS-stain positive and myeloperoxidase negative. Precursor B- and T-cell ALL are indistinguishable upon blood smear. B-cell type is identified by presence of surface markers CD19, 20, 22, and 79a. T-cell type is distinguished by CD3.

AML: The WHO classification specifies that bone marrow aspirate or peripheral blood analysis must show ≥20% blasts of the myeloid lineage (FAB system uses a ≥30% cutoff). AML can also be diagnosed without meeting the above criterion in the presence of one of the following cytogenetic abnormalities: t(8;21), inv(16), t(15;17), or the presence of chloroma. In addition, the malignant cells must be confirmed as from the myeloid lineage by presence of Auer rods or positive staining for myeloperoxidase.

CML: Peripheral blood smear and bone marrow aspirate are the most revealing early steps in diagnosis. CML demonstrates leukocytosis with WBC counts around 100,000/μL. The WBC differential includes all levels of neutrophilic maturity, the most abundant being myelocytes and segmented neutrophils. Although present, blast cells comprise a very low percentage of total WBCs. A high myelocyte-to-metamyelocyte ratio is characteristic of CML. Basophilia and eosinophilia are also frequently seen.

The most common method to classify phase is based on percentage of blast cells. Accelerated phase has a blast range from 10% to 19%, which may progress to blast crisis defined as ≥20% blasts.

Tests must be done to identify the Philadelphia chromosome (Ph+), BCR-ABL1 fusion gene or its mRNA product. This can be achieved by karyotyping, FISH analysis, or RT-PCR. Over 90% of patients are Ph+, but the diagnosis can still be made without it; however, evidence of the fusion gene is necessary in Ph− individuals.

CLL: Complete blood count (CBC) with a differential, peripheral blood smear, and flow cytometry are all necessary tests in the workup of these patients. They must show an absolute B-cell count ≥5,000/μL in the peripheral blood with a mature phenotype. Flow cytometry must show monoclonal markers which include the B-cell markers CD19, 20, 23, the T-cell antigen CD5, and very low levels of SmIg with either κ or λ light chains.

Differential Diagnosis

ALL: AML, small cell lung cancer, rhabdomyosarcoma, aplastic anemia, idiopathic thrombocytopenic purpura.

AML: ALL, myelodysplastic syndrome, biphenotypic leukemia, CML blast crisis, myelofibrosis, vitamin B12 deficiency.

CML: Leukemoid reaction, juvenile myelomonocytic leukemia, chronic myelomonocytic leukemia, "Atypical CML," chronic eosinophilic leukemia, chronic neutrophilic leukemia, essential thrombocytosis, Ph+ ALL.

CLL: Leukemoid reaction, small lymphocytic leukemia, monoclonal B-cell lymphocytosis, prolymphocytic leukemia, follicular lymphoma, mantle cell lymphoma.

Prognosis

The American Cancer Society reports that the overall trend in 5-year survival for those diagnosed with leukemia has improved from 35% in the mid 1970s to 54% in the present day.

ALL: Overall survival rates for ALL improved greatly in the past decades now reaching 75–85%. Risk stratification is important to direct treatment, which uses the following factors: age, WBC count at diagnosis, cytogenetics, immunological subtype, and time to cytoreduction. The strongest predictors of survival are age at diagnosis and cytogenetics. Precursor T-cell ALL and mature B-cell ALL have a poorer prognosis than precursor B-cell ALL. Age <1 year and adulthood are poor prognostic factors. The MLL gene (11q23) and Ph+ suggests less favorable outcome due to their occurrence in adult disease. More favorable prognostic factors include hyperploidy (>50 chromosomes) which is usually accompanied by t(12;21) and are found in childhood disease (Rubnitz and Look 2000) (Table 1).

AML: The strongest predictors of short-term expected survival are age at diagnosis and performance status, most likely due to the association of comorbidities. The strongest predictors of treatment failure are cytogenetic characteristics. Favorable chromosomal features include: t(8;21), inv(16), t(15;17). In clinical trials, cure rates have been <40% but actual rates may not reach that level due to more elderly being affected than participating in studies. The M3 subtype has an excellent prognosis of >90% when treated with retinoic acid (Table 2).

CML: The strongest predictor of outcome is phase at diagnosis. Accelerated phase and blast crisis have much poorer prognosis than those with chronic phase. Many years of disease control can be achieved by treating those in the chronic phase. Of high significance is the BCR-ABL T315I mutation, since these patients are resistant to tyrosine kinase inhibitors. A common scoring system to predict outcome is the Euro scale. It predicts poorer prognosis with increased age, blast count, platelet count, percent basophils, and spleen size. Patients with a higher score are less likely to achieve complete remission. However, once achieved, all patients have a good prognosis. In general, patients on tyrosine kinase inhibitors can achieve 5-year survival of approximately 90% (Druker et al. 2006).

CLL: The natural history is variable, with a median survival of 10 years in asymptomatic patients (range 2–20 years). The Rai staging system is commonly used for prognostic outlook (Table 3).

Other factors of useful value include lymphocyte doubling time and cytogenetic abnormalities.

Leukemia in General. Table 1 ALL risk groups

Risk group	Features
Low	Hyperploidy
	Trisomy 4,10,17
	t(12;22)
Standard	WBC <50,000/μL
	Age 1 to less than 10 years
High	T-cell ALL
	Age >10 years or
	WBC >50,000/μL
	t(1;19)
Very high	Age <1 year
	t(9;22)
	t(4;11)
	MLL gene
	Induction failure

Leukemia in General. Table 2 AML prognostic features

Unfavorable features
Age >55 years
WBC count ≥30,000/μL
ECOG performance status ≥3
Myelodysplastic Syndrome, etc.
AML, therapy related type
t(6;9), 11q23 abnormalities excluding t(9;11)
CD34-positive
MDR1-positive
BAALC over-expression

Leukemia in General. Table 3 Rai staging and survival without therapy

Risk group	Stage	Clinical features	Survival (mo)
Low	0	Lymphocytosis	150
Intermediate	I	LAD	101
	II	Organomegaly	71
High	III	Anemia	19
	IV	Thrombocytopenia	~

Early-staged patients with short doubling time (<12 months) may develop more rapid disease progression. Other markers associated with poorer prognosis include β2-microglobulin and CD38.

Therapy

Treatment is specific for each disease and risk group, but can be generally divided into the following components in those with acute disease: (1) remission induction, (2) CNS prophylaxis, (3) intensification and/or consolidation, and (4) maintenance therapy.

ALL: Remission induction seeks to achieve complete response which is considered no evidence of leukemia in the bone marrow, CNS, or extramedullary sites. This is achieved when bone marrow has <5% lymphoblasts, has normal appearing cellularity, normal peripheral CBC, and normal CSF counts. Induction therapy for children typically includes vincristine, L-asparginase, and dexamethasone. Addition of anthracycline in high-risk patients can result in remission rates up to 95%. Subsequently, patients who achieve complete response are administered intensification with high-dose methotrexate (MTX), *ara-C*, or L-asparaginase. Similarly to induction, addition of anthracycline has been shown to benefit high-risk patients during intensification (Rivera et al. 1991). This is followed by maintenance therapy of intermittent low-dose MTX and daily 6-mercaptopurine. Evidence exists for an additional round of intensification after completion of maintenance therapy for high-risk patients (Roberts and Seropian 2008).

In comparison, adult treatment has some variation and is successfully treated with high-dose MTX, cyclophosphamide, and *ara-C*. Combining these agents with vincristine, L-asparaginase, doxorubicin, and steroids attain remission rates of up to 85%.

Prior to the 1980s, cranial irradiation of 24 Gy was used to prophylactically treat children with ALL. However, late sequela was shown to include cognitive deficits, hypopituitarism, growth retardation, leukoencephalopathy, and secondary malignancy. This evidence shifted the standard away from cranial RT to newer high-dose chemotherapeutic agents which are able to penetrate the blood-brain barrier more effectively than past chemotherapy. Triple intrathecal (MTX, *ara-C*, hydrocortisone) and systemic chemotherapy adequately prevents CNS disease in standard-risk children. In addition, the risk-to-benefit ratio justifies CNS prophylaxis in high-risk patients or those with CNS-3 disease. High-risk features include patient age <1 year or >10 years, WBC count >50,000, T-cell ALL phenotype, or Ph+ ALL. Several protocols exist and most established dosing schemes use 1.8-Gy fractions, but some 1.6 and 2.0-Gy fractions have been reported. Commonly accepted indications are shown in Table 4 (Schrappe et al. 1998). In 2010, a long-term study has suggested that reducing the dose from 18 Gy to 12 Gy does not compromise efficacy in T-cell ALL or any high-risk patients treated with high-dose intrathecal MTX (Möricke et al. 2010).

The technique used in cranial radiation is parallel-opposed lateral fields which encompass the cranial meninges and areas where the CNS can be infiltrated. These mainly include the subarachnoid space within the cranial vault. The inferior boundary is at the first or second cervical

Leukemia in General. Table 4 CNS prophylactic therapy

Therapy	Risk	CNS-type
Chemo alone	Standard	CNS 1,2
12 Gy	High	CNS 1,2
18 Gy	Standard, High	CNS 3

CNS 1, negative cytology (no blasts); CNS 2, +blasts, <5 WBC/μL; CNS 3, +blasts, ≥5 WBC/μL

vertebra. A 'flashing technique' is frequently used over the scalp. The cribriform plate and the cranial nerves as they exit the superior orbital fissure are also targeted. Particular attention to the posterior globe of the orbit has been recommended due to the propensity of the retina as a site for relapse (Marcus 2007).

Testicular relapse is a sign that systemic and/or CNS relapse will likely follow. However, this occurs in <5% of modern cases that have been treated with intensive chemotherapy. Testicular RT is associated with sterility. Thus, prophylactic testicular RT protocols have not been widely used. In the case that testicular relapse does occur, local RT and systemic therapy are indicated, achieving EFS rates up to 65% (Wofford et al. 1992). Dose schemes include 24–26 Gy in 2.0-Gy fractions. Bilateral RT is preferred since clinical involvement of one testicle is associated with a likelihood of contralateral occult disease and subsequent contralateral relapse. The 'frog-leg' position is typically used with the penile shaft lifted and secured to the abdomen (Marcus 2007).

Allogeneic hematopoietic stem cell transplantation (HSCT) may be used in high-risk patients who relapse or those who fail induction therapy. Conditioning regimens prior to transplant seek to prevent graft rejection and destroy malignant cells. This is typically accomplished by chemotherapy (usually cyclophosphamide) with or without ▶ total body irradiation (TBI) (Roberts and Seropian 2008).

AML: Induction therapy includes *ara-C* plus an anthracycline with or without etoposide, dexamethasone, and/or thioguanine. Intensification is achieved with high-dose *ara-C* which enhances the efficacy of the treatment regimen. CNS prophylaxis is not as well defined as in ALL. Nonetheless, intrathecal *ara-C* and MTX have shown to significantly reduce CNS relapse rate. Those who benefit the most from intrathecal therapy are children with M4/5 subtype or those with exceedingly high peripheral blasts. RT may be used to treat extramedullary disease that causes acute symptoms like cord compression or visual changes, but has no role otherwise. M3 disease is treated with all-*trans* retinoic acid making it one of the most effectively treated subtypes (Roberts and Seropian 2008). Allogeneic HSCT may be considered for adults with poor prognostic features following remission therapy, and offers the highest survival advantage for children with AML (Cassileth et al. 1998). Therefore, TBI is the most common radiation strategy for AML.

CML: In the early twentieth century, CML was treated with radiotherapy to the abdomen, which was later replaced by chemotherapeutic regimens. Recently, these have been replaced by the highly efficacious drug, Imatinib, which specifically inhibits the BCR-ABL tyrosine kinase. Newer generation tyrosine kinase inhibitors (TKI) have been developed which include Nilotinib and Dasatinib. TKI do not offer cure, but are able to achieve long-term disease control in the majority of patients. Therefore, they have become the treatment of choice for almost all newly diagnosed patients in the chronic or accelerated phase. Nilotinib or Dasatinib may be used in patients in chronic or accelerated phase refractory to Imatinib. Only Dasatinib may be used for blast crisis refractory to Imatinib. The potential for cure is possible by allogeneic HSCT which uses TBI. It is indicated in younger patients with stable disease who have a suitable donor, those with blast crisis, and those intolerant or refractory to Imatinib (Gale et al. 1998).

Accelerated phase and blast crisis is relatively difficult to control. Patients in these phases who initially respond to TKI usually relapse. Subsequently, they may undergo an additional round with a TKI and/or HSCT. Palliative radiotherapy is indicated during accelerated phase or blast crisis when enlargement of the spleen becomes painful or when chloroma manifest. Dosing schemes for these conditions range from 10 to 20 Gy.

CLL: Delayed treatment does not affect overall survival; therefore, not all CLL patients need to be treated upon diagnosis. Asymptomatic individuals with early disease have a median survival >10 years and many oncologists choose close observation over treatment. Symptomatic patients or those with progressive disease have a median survival without treatment of 1.5–3 years, which is increased to 5 years following treatment. In the past, single-agent chlorambucil had been used. Recently, combination regimens in these patients may include alkylating agents, purine analogs, and monoclonal antibodies. Specific agents in each group have yet to become established as the standard of care and therapy should be tailored to the individual. However, early results demonstrate the high potential for the combination of fludarabine, cyclophosphamide, and rituximab (Keating et al. 2005). The role for intensification and maintenance therapy has not been established. The role for allogeneic HSCT has not been established either and is currently being tested in younger CLL patients <55 years of age.

The role for radiotherapy is limited to palliative treatment. CLL patients with painful splenomegaly or nonsurgical candidates who experience cytopenia associated with splenomegaly may receive targeted radiation. Reported doses vary from 4 to 10 Gy in 1-Gy fractions (Weinmann et al. 2001). Radiotherapy is also indicated for unresponsive disease manifesting with adenopathy or non-lymphoid organ involvement.

Epidemiology

Epidemiology of individual leukemia type is seen in Table 5.

ALL: ALL is the most common form of leukemia in children.

Precursor B-ALL occurs most frequently in childhood, but may present in adults. If present in adulthood, the median age at diagnosis is 39 years. It has a slight male predominance, with Hispanics having the highest incidence, and is three times more common in whites than African-Americans.

Precursor T-ALL has a more narrow age distribution manifesting in late childhood through young adulthood. It accounts for 25% of childhood ALL and 25% of adult ALL. It is twice more common in males than females.

AML: The most deadly form of leukemia. AML accounts for 80% of acute leukemias in adults, in which the median age at diagnosis in adults is 65 years. It is less common in children, accounting for 10% of acute leukemias in those under 10 years of age. AML has a slight male predominance.

Leukemia in General. Table 5 American Cancer Society 2010, estimated rates

	Incidence	% of new leukemic cases	Annual deaths	% of annual leukemic deaths
ALL	5,330	12%	1,420	6%
AML	12,330	28%	8,950	41%
CML	4,870	11%	440	2%
CLL	14,990	35%	4,390	20%

CML: The prevalence is increasing in developed nations due to the dramatic effect of specific tyrosine kinase inhibitors on survival. The typical age at diagnosis is 50–60 years. There is a slight male predominance.

CLL: Typically diagnosed in the elderly with a median age of 70 years, but the disease may manifest in adults during their 30s. Caucasians have a higher incidence than African-Americans or Asian Pacific Islanders. There is a slight male predominance. Richter transformation has been reported to occur in up to 10% of patients with CLL.

Cross-References

▶ Hodgkin's Lymphoma
▶ Non-Hodgkins Lymphoma
▶ Total Body Irradiation (TBI)

References

Cassileth PA, Harrington DP, Appelbaum FR et al (1998) Chemotherapy compared with autologous or allogeneic bone marrow transplantation in the management of AML in the first remission. N Engl J Med 339:1649–1656

Druker BJ, Guilhot F, O'Brien SG et al (2006) Five-year follow-up of patients receiving imatinib for chronic myeloid leukemia. N Engl J Med 355(23): 2408–2417

Gale RP, Hehlmann R, Zhang MJ et al (1998) Survival with bone marrow transplantation versus hydroxyurea or interferon for CML. The German CML Study Group. Blood 91:1810–1819

Keating MJ, O'Brien S, Albitar M et al (2005) Early results of a chemoimmunotherapy regimen of fludarabine, cyclophosphamide, and rituximab as initial therapy for CLL. J Clin Oncol 23: 4079–4088

Marcus KJ (2007) Pediatric leukemias and lymphomas. In: Gunderson LL, Tepper TE (eds) Clinical radiation oncology, 2nd edn. Churchill Livingstone, Philadelphia

Möricke A, Zimmermann M, Reiter A (2010) Long-term results of five consecutive trials in childhood acute lymphoblastic leukemia performed by the ALL-BFM study group from 1981 to 2000. Leukemia 24(2): 265–284

Rivera GK, Raimondi SC, Hancock ML et al (1991) Improved outcome in childhood ALL with reinforced early treatment and rotational combination chemotherapy. Lancet 337:61–66

Roberts KB, Seropian S (2008) Leukemia. In: Halperin EC, Perez CA, Brady LW (eds) Principles and practice of radiation oncology, 5th edn. Wolters Kluwer/Lippincott Wiliams & Wilkens, Philadelphia

Rubnitz JE, Look AT (2000) Pathobiology of acute lymphoblastic leukemia. In: Hoffman R (ed) Hematology: basic principles and practice, 3rd edn. Churchill Livingston, New York

Schrappe M, Reiter A, Henze G et al (1998) Prevention of CNS recurrence in childhood ALL: results with reduced radiotherapy combined with CNS-directed chemotherapy in four consecutive ALL-BFM trials. Klin Pädiatr 210(4):192–199

Weinmann M, Becker G, Einsele H et al (2001) Clinical indications and biological mechanisms of splenic irradiation in chronic leukaemias and myeloproliferative disorders. Radiother Oncol 58(3): 235–246

Wofford MM, Smith SD, Shuster JJ et al (1992) Treatment of overt or late testicular relapse in children with ALL: a Pediatric Oncology Group Study. J Clin Oncol 11:271–278

L'Hermitte's Sign

Tony S. Quang[1], Linna Li[2]
[1]Department of Radiation Oncology, VA Puget Sound Health Care System University of Washington Medical Center, Seattle, WA, USA
[2]Radiation Oncology, Fox Chase Cancer Center, Philadelphia, PA, USA

Definition

Shock-like sensations radiating to the hands and feet when the neck is flexed.

Cross-References

▶ Oro-Hypopharynx
▶ Spinal Canal Tumor

Li-Fraumeni Syndrome

JOHN P. LAMOND[1], STEPHAN MOSE[2], TONY S. QUANG[3]
[1]Department of Radiation Oncology, Temple University, Crozer-Chester Medical Center, Upland, PA, USA
[2]Department of Radiation Oncology, Schwarzwald-Baar-Klinikum, Villingen-Schwenningen, Germany
[3]Department of Radiation Oncology, VA Puget Sound Health Care System, University of Washington Medical Center, Seattle, WA, USA

Definition

Rare mutation to the p53 tumor suppressor gene. The syndrome increases the risk of breast cancer, brain tumors, acute leukemia, soft tissue sarcoma, bone sarcoma, and adrenal cortical carcinoma.

This syndrome includes the diagnosis of following cancers: breast cancer, soft tissue and bone sarcoma, brain tumors, and ACC.

Cross-References

▶ Breast Cancer: Locally Advanced and Recurrent Disease, Postmastectomy Radiation and Systemic Therapies
▶ Carcinoma of the Adrenal Gland
▶ Early-Stage Breast Cancer
▶ Primary Intracranial Neoplasms
▶ Soft Tissue Sarcoma

Linear Accelerators (LINAC)

TIMOTHY C. ZHU, KEN K.-H. WANG
Department of Radiation Oncology, University of Pennsylvania Medical Center, Philadelphia, PA, USA

Introduction

Medical electron linear accelerators (LINACs) are commonly used to produce megavoltage photon and electron beams for radiation therapy. Most modern linear accelerators are also equipped with sophisticated imaging devices for MV and/or kV portal imaging, and cone-beam computer tomography (CBCT). The primary accelerating structure in a conventional linear accelerator is the waveguide which accelerates electrons to megavoltage energies. The x-ray beams are generated by the Bremsstrahlung process, that is, hitting the electron beams on a high-Z target. There are auxiliary systems which produce electrons, modulate the radiation pulse width, and power the waveguide. Additional systems are used to steer the beam via a series of focusing and steering magnets, shape the beam using the primary and secondary collimators, change the intensity distribution using flattening filters and wedges, and quantify the beam output using a monitor chamber. This chapter provides an introduction on the basic components of an electron linear accelerator. A brief discussion on the future direction of medical linear accelerators is also included.

Commercial Medical Linear Accelerators

There are three major linear accelerator vendors in the USA: Elekta, Siemens, and Varian (in alphabetic order). All of them are capable of producing multiple electron and photon beams of various energies for radiation treatments. Some of the specifics of each type of LINAC are described here.

Elekta

The Elekta linear accelerators include the SL series, Synergy, and Infinity. An Electa Synergy is shown in Fig. 1a. A modern Elekta accelerator is made of a magnetron, circulator, accelerating waveguide, bending magnet, and collimating jaws. The upper secondary collimator jaws in an Elekta accelerator is replaced by a multileaf collimator (MLC). The basic characteristics of the components of an Elekta accelerator are listed in Table 1.

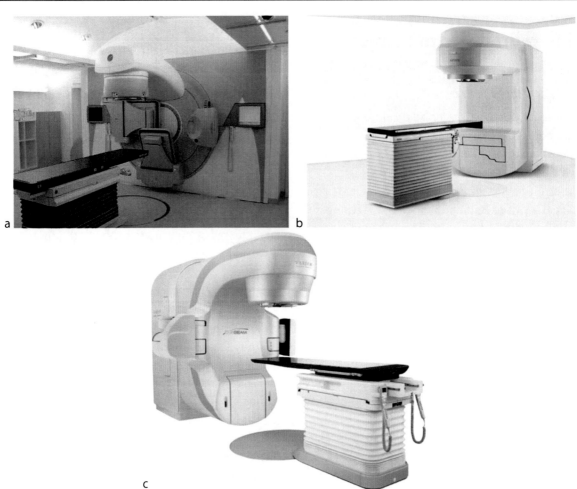

Linear Accelerators (LINAC). Fig. 1 Images of modern electron linear accelerators from (**a**) Elekta, Synergy (**b**) Siemens, Artiste, and (**c**) Varian TrueBeam (Courtesy of respective companies Elekta, Siemens, and Varian)

Siemens

The Siemens linear accelerators have undergone many evolutions. Its model lines include MXE, MD, KD2, Primus, Oncor, and Artiste. The last three are the current model lineup. A Siemens Artiste is shown in Fig. 1b. A modern Siemens accelerator is made of a klystron, circulator, accelerating waveguide, bending magnet, and collimating jaws. The lower secondary collimator jaws in a Siemens accelerator is replaced by a multileaf collimator (MLC). The basic characteristics of the components of a Siemens accelerator are listed in Table 1.

Varian

The Varian linear accelerators include Clinac (6/100, 600C, 1800, 2100CD, 2300ix), Trilogy, and the Truebeam. A Varian TrueBeam is shown in Fig. 1c. A modern Varian accelerator is made of a klystron, circulator, accelerating waveguide, bending magnet, and collimating jaws. The MLC is attached to the existing secondary collimator jaws and thus acts as a tertiary collimator. One unique feature of the Varian accelerator is its grid gun, which allows the radiation beam to be turned on and off instantly. The basic characteristics of the components of a Varian accelerator are listed in Table 1.

Linear Accelerators (LINAC). Table 1 Comparison of commercial medical linear accelerators

Accelerator items	Siemens	Varian	Elekta
Pulse repetition freq. (PRF)	Low energy: 400 Hz	Low energy: 360 Hz	Low energy: 400 Hz
	High energy: 200 Hz	High energy: 180 Hz	High energy: 200 Hz
RF power generators	Klystron	Klystron	Magnetron
Accelerating waveguide type	Standing wave	Standing wave	Traveling wave
Max. RF power levels	Low energy: 5 MW	Low energy: 7 MW	Low energy: 2.5 MW
	High energy: 10 MW	High energy: 12 MW	High energy: 5 MW
MLC types	Replacement of lower jaws	Attachment in addition to jaws	Replacement of upper jaws
MLC leave pairs	58, 80, 160	52, 80, 120	80, 160
Wedge types	Virtual wedge	Enhanced dynamic wedge	Omni physical wedge
Focusing magnet type	270 bending magnet	270 bending magnet	90 Slalom bending magnet
Available energies	2–3 photons: 4–23 MV	2–5 photons: 4–23 MV	2–3 photons: 4–25 MV
	6 electrons: 4–23 MeV	6 electrons: 4–23 MeV	6 electrons: 4–25 MeV

Electron Accelerator Waveguide

The waveguide is an evacuated metallic structure and is the most essential part of linear accelerators. It is where the electrons are accelerated to the desired energy. These electrons may be used directly or may produce an x-ray beam by impinging them upon a metal target. By sending high-power microwaves using a klystron or magnetron into the accelerator waveguide, the microwave fields induce an electric current within the guide wall, and the current generates an electric field. If electrons are introduced into one end of the guide, the electric field will exert a force on the electrons and accelerate them.

The length of waveguide can be as short as 30 cm for a 4-MeV accelerator or as long as 1–3 m in order to produce higher electron energies (Karzmark and Morton 1997; Greene and Williams 1997). In addition to the rigid mechanical specifications, conductivity is an important factor which determines the stability and accuracy of a waveguide. To achieve the high electrical conductivity at microwave frequencies, the accelerating guide is usually made of copper, resulting in minimal microwave power loss. The high vacuum (10^{-6} Torr) maintained inside the waveguide is to prevent electron loss and arcing by interacting with air particles (Metcalfe et al. 2007).

A single waveguide cavity, which is a completely hollow structure, is not suitable for accelerating electrons because the microwaves are transmitted much faster than the injected electrons. Hence, the advancing microwave fields are slowed by introducing into the waveguide a series of disks (irises) with a hole in the center of each one. The guide is therefore divided into a series of cavities. These cavities distribute microwave power between adjacent cavities and produce an appropriate electric field pattern for accelerating the electrons (Podgorsak 2005). Two types, traveling and standing waveguides, are most

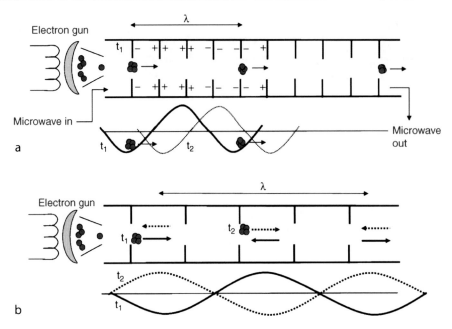

Linear Accelerators (LINAC). Fig. 2 (**a**) Simplified layout of a traveling waveguide. Electron bunches are shown as *red spots*. The electric field distributions at time t_1 (*solid*) and t_2 (*dash*) along the waveguide are displayed beneath the guide layout. The electric field propagates from left to right end. Three electron bunches are shown in the waveguide. The *arrow* indicates the direction of electric field exerting on these electron bunches at time t_1. The corresponding electric polarity distributed on the cavity wall at time t_1 is also shown. (**b**) Simplified layout of a standing waveguide. The electric field distribution at time t_1 (*solid*) and t_2 (*dash*) are shown beneath the waveguide layout. The *solid* and *dash arrows* shown in the waveguide cavities are the negative electric field direction at t_1 and t_2, respectively

commonly used in medical linear accelerators, and their principles of operation are briefly explained below.

Traveling Waveguide (TW)

A picture of a person surfing on the crest of an ocean wave may provide a simple analogy for understanding the electron advancing in a traveling waveguide. As the wave propagates forward, the surfer is carried along with the wave. If now we transfer the water sport to the traveling waveguide, the surfer is analogous to the electrons and the water wave corresponds to the electric field induced by the input microwaves. The electrons pass through the waveguide due to the propagating electric field.

A simplified layout of a traveling waveguide is shown in Fig. 2a. An electron gun sends electrons into the waveguide. The high-power microwaves are introduced into the waveguide by microwave generators. The emitted electrons are formed as "bunch" in a buncher cavity before entering the main accelerating waveguide, as shown in Fig. 2a (Karzmark et al. 1993). As the microwave travels within the guide, it induces an advancing electric field pattern which accelerates the electron bunches. There are three independent electron bunches shown in Fig. 2a in different cavities within the waveguide at time point t_1. The corresponding electric field propagating within the waveguide at time point t_1 (solid line) is illustrated beneath the waveguide layout.

At time t_1, the electron bunch at the beginning of waveguide is affected by an electric force accelerating it toward right. One wavelength spans four cavities in length, and only one out of four cavities accelerates the electron bunches at a given moment. At time t_2, the electric field advances toward right (dash line shown in Fig. 2a), and at the same time, the electron bunch traveling from the first cavity will reach the second cavity, and be accelerated again. The accelerated electrons eventually reach the speed of light. The input high-power microwaves are either absorbed without any reflection in the output end or exit the waveguide and hit a resistive load (Fig. 2a).

Standing Waveguide (SW)

The essential difference between the traveling and standing waveguide is that the wave is reflected in the standing waveguide instead of exiting the waveguide. In the standing wave structure, both ends of the waveguide are terminated with a conducting disc to reflect the microwave. The forward going wave and the reflected wave interfere with each other and result in a standing wave (Fig. 2b). Figure 2b shows a simplified standing waveguide, and the electron bunches propagating inside. The corresponding standing wave electric field at time t_1 (solid) and t_2 (dash) are shown beneath the waveguide drawing. The electric field oscillates up and down within the guide but does not propagate. The electron bunch is first accelerated by the electric field (solid line) in the cavity on the left end of the waveguide at time t_1. At time t_2, the bunch reaches the third cavity relative to

the first one, and the bunch is accelerated again by the standing wave (dash line). Following the illustration of Fig. 2b, there are some cavities without an electric field contribution. These cavities can be moved to the side of waveguide, in order to reduce the dimension of waveguide and optimize the electric field pattern.

Operational and Auxiliary Systems

The other operational components of linear accelerators are the pulse modulator, microwave generators (klystron and magnetrons), and electron gun. Only a general picture of these components is explained here, Further technique details can be found in Karzmark et al. (1993), Slater, J. C. (1948), and Greene and Williams (1997).

The Modulator

The pulsed modulator supports the high-voltage DC pulse required by the injection system which consists of the electron gun and the microwave source, either a magnetron or a klystron. The operation of a linear accelerator requires a fairly large amount of electrical power to successfully accelerate the electrons. This power is pulsed in order to accelerate the electrons in bursts. The pulse modulator and the microwave sources are used to accomplish this. The primary function of the modulator is to supply negative high voltage pulses to the cathode of the microwave source, and apply the same DC pulse to electron gun. A block diagram of a modulator is shown in Fig. 3. The three-phase full-wave rectifier with solid state diodes delivers about 10 kV to the

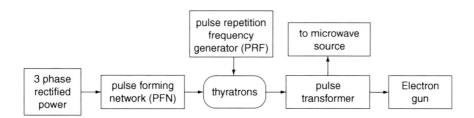

Linear Accelerators (LINAC). Fig. 3 Block diagram of modulator (Modified from Metcalfe et al. 2007)

pulse forming network (PFN). The PFN modulates this into pulses. The PFN is a capacitor and inductor circuit, serving a twofold purpose; it stores the required energy in order to produce the pulse, and it subsequently discharges this energy into the pulse transformer. The thyratron is essentially a switching tube. When the hydrogen-filled thyratron is fired, it will discharge the PFN, and the resulting current pulse will pass through the primary windings of pulse transformer (Greene and Williams 1997). The low-voltage of the transformer is connected to ground and the high-voltage end is connected to the cathode of the microwave generator. The frequency of the thyratron on-and-off switching is controlled by the pulse repetition frequency generator (PRF). In the other words, ultimately the dose rate from the accelerating waveguide is regulated by PRF.

Klystrons and Magnetrons

Modern linear accelerators generally employ either a klystron or a magnetron to generate high-power microwaves to accelerate the electrons traveling in the accelerating waveguide. During World War II, high-power microwave generators working at short wavelengths (such as 10 cm) were urgently needed to increase the spatial resolution of radar systems. In 1940, John Randall and Harry Boot at the University of Birmingham improved the output power of cavity-like magnetrons to 1 MW and increased the frequency stability. This breakthrough largely broadened the application of magnetrons. The klystron was invented by the brothers Russell and Sigurd Varian at the Stanford University. Similar to magnetrons, the klystron amplifier underwent a significant evolution during World War II, and has become one of most popular devices to amplify microwaves on a multimegawatt power scale.

The difference between klystrons and magnetrons is that the klystron is essentially an amplifier with a low-power microwave input, while the magnetron is a self-oscillator, thus producing microwaves in response to a DC input. Klystrons are usually used to power high-energy LINACs; magnetrons are generally used for lower energy accelerators. The microwave frequency employed by medical accelerator is 3,000 MHz in S Band (1.6–5.2 GHz). The reason that the S Band frequency is chosen is because the wavelength is on the order of 10 cm, which is an appropriate length such that the accelerator components can be reasonably designed and manufactured. The S Band magnetron and klystron output is usually 2 and 5 MV peak power, respectively, for a medical LINAC. The operational life is about 10,000 h for klystrons compared to 2,000 h for magnetrons (Karzmark et al. 1993). Operationally, magnetrons are temperature dependent while klystrons are not. Klystrons are large and cannot be mounted on the gantry, while the smaller magnetrons are gantry-mounted. This can cause slight frequency changes from magnetrons as a function of gantry angle. Compared to magnetrons, the klystrons are more stable, but also more expensive and more complicated. Details of the working principles for klystrons and magnetrons are explained below.

Klystron

The klystron is an evacuated vacuum tube used to produce high-energy microwaves. A good analogy to describe the klystron is a pipe organ. When air is sent throughout the organ, the air induces the vibration of the organ's tubes. This vibration makes the tubes emit sound waves at a specific frequency. Different pipe structures make the sound waves travel at different frequencies; therefore, we can hear various notes. In klystrons, instead of air, bunches of electrons propagate through the klystron vacuum tube. The cavity of the tube is resonant with the propagating electron bunches. Therefore, the kinetic energy of the electron bunches is transferred to the output microwaves in an electromagnetic energy form.

Figure 4 shows the cross section of an elementary two-cavity klystron. The electrons are first boiled off the cathode by heating the filament. The cathode/electron gun end is submerged in an oil-filled tank which provides necessary electrical insulation. Low-power microwaves are sent into the first cavity, the so-called buncher cavity. The microwaves then set up an alternating electric field. The negative electric field accelerates the electrons, and the positive field decelerates them. These accelerations and decelerations modulate the electron propagating velocity and separate the electrons into "bunches." The process of varying the electron velocity is known as velocity modulation. The second cavity, the so-called catcher cavity, has the resonant frequency of the electron bunches. After the electron bunches pass through a field-free space in the drift tube, they arrive at the catcher cavity (Fig. 4) and induce charges on the ends of the cavity, thereby generating a retarding electric field. The arriving electrons suffer deceleration. By the principle of conservation of energy, much of the kinetic energy of electrons is converted into intense electric fields, creating the high-power microwaves which are used to accelerate the electrons down the accelerator

waveguide. The rest of the electron energy that is not converted into microwave energy is dissipated as heat in the beam collector in the end of klystron (Fig. 4). The heat is removed by the water cooling system.

Magnetron

A magnetron is a device that converts high-voltage DC electrical power into microwave power (Fig. 5). One obvious difference between the magnetron and the klystron is that the magnetron employs a circular geometry whereas the klystron uses a linear geometry (Comparing Fig. 4 vs Fig. 5).

Figure 5 is a schematic diagram of a cylindrical cathode which is heated by inner filaments connected to both ends of cathode. The coaxial anode is surrounding the cathode, located close to the magnetron wall. An axial magnetic field perpendicular to the cross plane of magnetron is supplied by a large permanent magnet. After the electrons are boiled out from the cathode surface, a pulsed DC voltage is applied between the cathode and anode so that the electrons will travel radially in the opposite direction of the electric field E_{dc}, in the absence of the magnetic field (Fig. 5). The axial magnetic field exerts a magnetic force (Lorentz force) on these traveling electrons, which is perpendicular to their initially radial

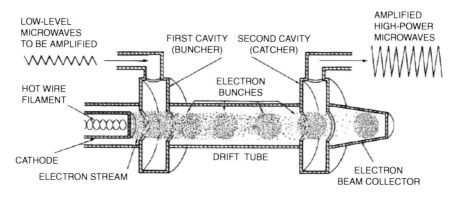

Linear Accelerators (LINAC). Fig. 4 Cross-sectional view of a two-cavity klystron (From Karzmark and Morton 1997)

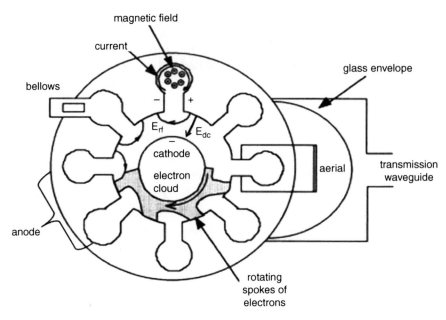

Linear Accelerators (LINAC). Fig. 5 A cross-sectional view of a magnetron. Electrons generated by the cathode move in a coiled path due to the influence of E_{dc}, E_{rf}, and the magnetic field. An output aerial is inserted into one of the cavities to transfer the microwaves from the magnetron to the waveguide (From Metcalfe et al. 2007)

motion, and thus the electrons tend to be swept around in a circular path. When the electrons approach the ring anode, they induce an additional charge distribution and a radio frequency (microwave) electric field E_{rf} (Fig. 5). In a manner similar to that in the catcher cavity of the klystron, the E_{rf} fields act to remove the energy from those moving electrons, and the reduction of kinetic energy will be transferred as the high-frequency microwave energy. In the process, approximately 60% of the kinetic energy of the electrons can be converted into the microwave energy. An output aerial is inserted into one of the cavities to transfer the microwave power from the magnetron to the waveguide (Fig. 5).

Automatic Frequency Control Circuit (AFC)

The temperature of the various components of the linear accelerator tends to increase while the machine is running. In particular, a 1°C temperature rise in the accelerator waveguide can sufficiently change the resonant frequency by 60 kHz (Hendee et al. 2005). In addition to temperature, the resonant frequency of accelerator structures varies with the input power level, the beam loading, and other mechanical and electrical perturbations of the accelerating cavities. This makes a feedback system necessary in order to adjust the accelerator components, such as the klystron and magnetron, so that the resonant frequency is generated accurately. Modern microwave sources, such as klystrons and magnetrons, are equipped with motor-driven tuners controlled by a circuit which senses and compensates for any change of frequency. This kind of circuit is called an automatic frequency control circuit (AFC).

Electron Gun

An electron gun provides the source of electrons injected into the waveguide. There are two types of electron guns used in medical linear accelerators, the diode type and the triode type. Both of these contain a heated filament cathode, a focus electrode, and an anode. The triode type incorporates an additional grid. A photograph of a removable triode gun from a high-energy linear accelerator is shown in Fig. 6. A heater boils electrons out from a spherically shaped cathode. The cathode is held at a static negative potential with respect to the grounded anode; the typical range for this is between 0 and −30 kV. The emitted electrons are accelerated toward the anode and are focused into a pencil beam by a cone-shaped focusing electrode.

The current of electrons produced by a given cathode–anode voltage heavily depends on the cathode–anode spacing and the cathode diameter (Karzmark et al. 1993). In order to vary the current without varying the cathode–anode voltage, a control grid is incorporated between the cathode and anode, forming the triode type gun

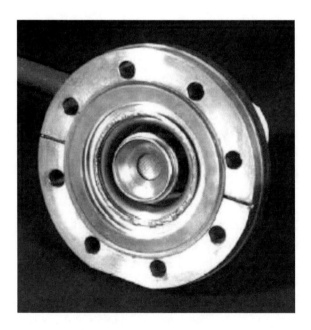

Linear Accelerators (LINAC). Fig. 6 Removable electron triode gun from a high-energy linac, Varian Clinac-18 (From Podgorsak 2005)

(Fig. 6). This gun grid controls the flow of electrons from the cathode to anode by applying voltage pulses to the gun. Typical amplitudes of −150 to −180 V are applied to the grid to control the gun current (Metcalfe et al. 2007). The more positive the voltage applied by the grid, the higher the resulting gun current will be. If the full −150 V is applied to the grid, the electrons are prevented from passing through the anode. To inject electrons simultaneously with the high-power microwaves into the accelerator waveguide, the voltage pulses applied to the grid must be synchronized with the pulses applied to the microwave generator.

Beam Delivery Systems

Bending and Focus Magnet Assembly

After the electrons are accelerated through the waveguide, they are focused and bent to the desired direction using magnets. The magnet bends a charged particle beam circularly if the magnetic field is perpendicular to the direction of the beam velocity. Except for some single low-energy accelerators (e.g., Varian 600C), which direct the electrons to the target without the use of a bending magnet, most modern LINACs steer the electron beam using magnetic coils. Two pairs of magnetic coils are usually placed near the entrance (far end) of the waveguide to bend the direction of electron beam radially and transversely. These are called directional bending magnetic coils. Two additional pairs of magnetic coils are placed near the exit of the waveguide. These are called positional bending magnetic coils. In addition, most modern accelerators focus the electron beam achromatically to a very small spot through a series of focusing magnets that bends electron beam either 270° or 90° (Fig. 7).

An energy selection slit (Fig. 7a) can be inserted between the first and second electromagnets to minimize the spread of electron energies

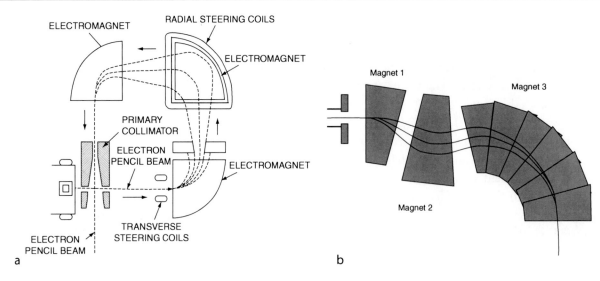

Linear Accelerators (LINAC). Fig. 7 Achromatic focusing magnets bend the electron beam either (**a**) 270° or (**b**) 90°. They maintain the focal spot size regardless the energy of the incident electron beams, and thus is called an achromatic focusing magnet (Figures modified from Karzmark et al. (1993) and Smith (1999))

hitting the focal spot. The placement and design of the three magnets is such that after passing through the three magnets, all the electrons will focus on the same spot. The 270° focusing magnet is usually used in the Varian and Siemens accelerators while the 90° focusing magnet is usually used in the Elekta accelerators.

Target and Flattening Filter

To generate a Bremsstrahlung x-ray beam, a thick transmission target is usually used. The target is made of high-Z materials to increase the efficiency of the Bremsstrahlung yield (Khan 2003). The thickness of the target is sufficient to stop all incident electrons. Each manufacturer chooses a proprietary design geometry for the target to keep the target cool during x-ray production. A flattening filter is usually inserted in the beam path to flatten the profile of the resulting radiation beam. The flattening filter for photon beams is often made of aluminum, steel, copper, and/or tungsten, and its thickness is often energy dependent. The flattening filter has cylindrical symmetry to produce a uniform beam. Recently,

manufacturers have begun to produce accelerators which produce unflattened beams. These beams do not pass through a flattening filter. The dose rate produced by these beams is much higher than that produced by the typical flattened beam.

For electron beams, a dual scattering foil system is often used to produce monoenergetic electron beams, where the first scattering foil produces a broad electron beam and the second scattering foil flattens the resulting electron beam. Details of flattening filter designs can be found elsewhere (Metcalfe et al. 2007; Karzmark et al. 1993).

Switching between Electron and X-Ray Modes

Most modern linear accelerators are dual modality; they allow for both electron and photon beams to be used. When switching between electron and x-ray mode, several changes occur in the various components of the accelerator. Firstly, the electron beam intensity emanating from the waveguide for the x-ray mode is about 1,000 times larger than that when the machine is in electron mode. In the x-ray mode, a thick target is inserted to produce Bremsstrahlung photons and stop all the incident electrons; in electron mode, the target is removed from the beam path. Second, a carousel will rotate to different positions to replace the flattening filter used by the photon beams with the dual scattering foils suitable for the electron beams. For some accelerators (Siemens), different monitor chambers are used for electron and x-ray beams due to the fact that a thick metal coating is added to the back of the photon monitor chamber to reduce monitor backscattering effects. Lastly, in addition to the existing movable collimators in the head of the accelerator, an additional applicator should be used when treating with an electron beam so that the final electron beam collimation can be placed close to the patient surface in order to reduce the width of the electron penumbra.

Monitor Chamber

The monitor chamber is often made of multiple layers of parallel plate ionization chambers (Metcalfe et al. 2007). Within each layer, multiple chambers are used to monitor the beam flatness and symmetry in both the radial and transverse directions. Primary and secondary monitor chamber readings are used to determine the dosage (or monitor unit) and will stop the radiation when the appropriate level has been delivered. Additionally, these chambers act as a safety guard which will turn off the radiation beam if the beam flatness or symmetry drifts out of machine specification. In addition, there is a timer which is correlated to the dose rate that will shut off the radiation beam should the monitor chambers fail to do so.

Collimation (Primary Collimator, Secondary Collimator Jaws, Block)

The beam collimator system is used to define and shape the radiation field. Typically, it is composed of the cone-shaped primary collimator and the secondary movable collimator jaws that form a rectangular field. The primary collimator typically forms a 50 cm diameter circle at the isocenter (usually 100 cm from the source). The secondary collimators are often made of two pairs of divergence focused tungsten blocks in the X (usually outer jaws) and Y (usually inner jaws) directions. The collimator jaws in modern accelerators are either replaced or supplemented by multileaf collimators (MLC) that can be shaped to tumor size and can be dynamically adjusted for intensity modulated radiotherapy (IMRT). Additional patient-specific lead or Cerrobend blocks can be added on a block tray to provide additional shielding. The leakage radiation through the primary and secondary collimators is usually less than 0.1% of the primary radiation. The radiation transmission through the external blocks and MLC are usually larger, but are typically in the 1–2% range unless they passes through the gaps between MLC leaves (tongue and groove effect) or the inherent opening when the MLC leaves are fully closed as a 1 mm gap typically exists between MLC leaf pairs to avoid collision.

Multileaf Collimator (MLC)

One of the major developments that allows intensity-modulated radiation therapy (IMRT) is the multileaf collimator. The MLC is available for LINACs from all the major vendors although the physical design of the MLC between manufacturers is very different. In addition to the variation in leaf design between the vendors, the number of leaves comprising the MLC varies between the vendors as well (see Table 1). MLC leaves are made of a tungsten alloy and are typically single focused leaves with rounded leaf ends, that is, the leading edge of each leaf has a rounded edge. The leaves travel perpendicular to the direction of the beam and conform to the divergence of the beam emanating from the source (Boyer et al. 2001). Because of the difference in MLC

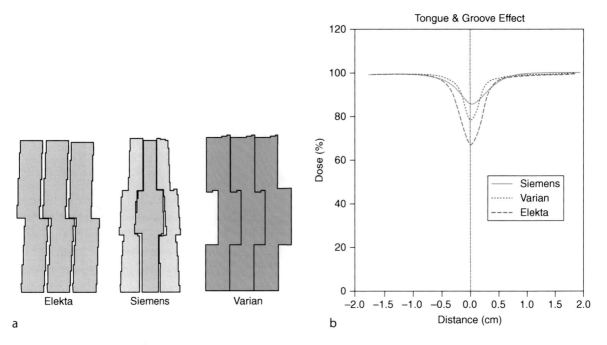

Elekta   Siemens   Varian

a   b

Linear Accelerators (LINAC). Fig. 8 (**a**) Schematics of the tongue and groove end of various leaves from different manufacturer (**b**) the corresponding leakages due to the tongue and groove effect (Data taken from Huq et al. 2002)

design (Elekta MLC replaces the upper collimator jaws, Siemens MLC replaces the lower collimator jaws, and Varian MLC is an attachment), the dosimetric properties of the different MLCs are quite different. The MLC tongue and groove effect is due to radiation leaking through the thinner parts of the leaves as well as between the leaf edges (Fig. 8a) (Huq et al. 2002). Huq et al. have compared the radiation leakage among different MLC types for 6 MV photon beams (Fig. 8b) (Huq et al. 2002). This leakage can vary by up to 17% between machines from the different manufacturers.

Wedges

Wedge-shape filters are used to produce "tilted" dose distributions (Fig. 9). Once they have been characterized, they may be used as missing tissue compensators and/or dose compensators. Wedges may be classified as physical, soft, or

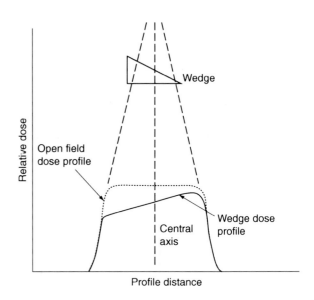

Linear Accelerators (LINAC). Fig. 9 A conceptual figure of relative dose/profile change relative to the open field after a wedge was inserted into the treatment head

universal (Das et al. 2008). Physical wedges, or so called removable wedges, are individually designed metal wedges which are used to produce a defined skewed (i.e., nonuniform) dose distribution at a specific depth. The physical wedge can be inserted into treatment head externally or internally. The effect of the uncertainty in positioning the wedge in the exact location needed for reproducing the "tilted" dose distribution is greater for the internally positioned wedge than the external wedge. This is because the internal wedge is much closer to the target, and therefore a small error in positioning may result in a large error in the isodose distribution. Instead of inserting a physical wedge into the treatment head, soft wedge mimics the tilting isodose line by moving only one collimator jaw, usually a Y-jaw, while keeping the other Y-jaw stationary during beam on time. Two major linear accelerator vendors in the USA implement soft wedges; enhanced dynamic wedge (EDW) is used by Varian, and virtual wedge (VW) is used by Siemens. The EDW operates by varying jaw speed and dose rate, while the VW only varies the jaw speed; the dose rate is based on a built-in analytical function, which depends on the required effective wedge angle (Boyer et al. 2001). The omni universal wedge, used in Elekta accelerators, is a built-in 60° motorized physical wedge, which when combined with an open field enables users to achieve any desired effective wedge angle up to 60°.

Future Electron Linear Accelerators

The modern linear accelerator based on waveguide technique typically requires approximately 1 m to generate the required energy. The recent development of laser wakefield acceleration (LWA) has made it possible to accelerate electron beams to the same energy within a few millimeters, thus making it possible to establish table-top medical accelerators (Kainz et al. 2004). A recent experiment has demonstrated the feasibility for intraoperative radiation therapy (Gamucci et al. 2008). Even though the current LWA method has not produced a clinically stable beam with features similar to today's linear accelerators, it is certainly feasible to expect production of these machines within the next 5–10 years.

Cross-References

▶ Conformal Therapy: Treatment Planning, Treatment Delivery, and Clinical Results
▶ Electron Dosimetry and Treatment
▶ Electronic Portal Imaging Devices (EPID)
▶ History of Radiation Oncology
▶ Image-Guided Radiation Therapy (IGRT): kV Imaging
▶ Image-Guided Radiation Therapy (IGRT): TomoTherapy
▶ Image-Guided Radiation Therapy (IGRT): MV Imaging
▶ Intensity-Modulated Proton Therapy (IMPT)
▶ Radiation Detectors
▶ Radiation Oncology Physics
▶ Radiation Therapy Shielding
▶ Robotic Radiosurgery
▶ Stereotactic Radiosurgery – Cranial

References

Boyer A, Biggs P, Galvin J, Klein E, LoSasso T, Low D, Mah K, Yu C (2001) Basic applications of multileaf collimators, Report of Task Group No. 50, AAPM Report No. 72. Medical Physics, Madison

Das IJ et al (2008) Accelerator beam data commissioning equipment and procedures: report of the TG-106 of the Therapy Physics Committee of the AAPM. Med Phys 35(9):4186–4215

Gamucci AA et al (2008) Electron acceleration in laser-plasma interaction at moderate intensity and perspectives of application. Phys Rev Lett 101:105002

Greene D, Williams PC (1997) Linear accelerators for radiation therapy, 2nd edn. Taylor & Francis Group, New York

Hendee WR, Ibbott GS, Hendee EG (2005) Radiation therapy physics, 3rd edn. Wiley, Hoboken

Huq MS, Das IJ, Steinberg T, Galvin JM (2002) A dosimetric comparison of various multileaf collimators. Phys Med Biol 47:N159–N170

Kainz KK et al (2004) Dose properties of a laser accelerated electron beam and prospects for clinical application. Med Phys 31:2053–2067

Karzmark CJ, Morton RJ (eds) (1997) A primer on theory and operation of linear accelerators in radiation therapy, 2nd edn. Medical Physics, Madison

Karzmark CJ, Nunan CS, Tanabe E (1993) Medical electron accelerators, 1st edn. McGraw-Hill, New York

Khan FM (2003) The physics of radiation therapy, 3rd edn. Lippincott Williams & Wilkins, Philadelphia

Metcalfe PE, Kron T, Hoban P (eds) (2007) The physics of radiotherapy X-rays and electrons, 1st edn. Medical Physics, Madison

Podgorsak EB (ed) (2005) Radiation oncology physics: a handbook for teachers and students. International Atomic Energy Agency, Vienna

Slater JC (1948) The design of linear accelerators. Rev Mod Phys 20:473–518

Smith FA (1999) A primer in applied radiation physics. World Scientific, London

Linear Energy of Transfer (LET)

Tod W. Speer
Department of Human Oncology, University of Wisconsin School of Medicine and Public Health, UW Hospital and Clinics, Madison, WI, USA

Definition

The energy (keV) deposited in a medium over a defined track length (μm). Thus, the International Commission on Radiological Units (ICRU) defines LET as follows:

$$LET = dE/dl$$

where dE is the average energy transferred to the medium by a charged particle of certain energy over distance dl.

Cross-References

▶ Targeted Radioimmunotherapy

Liposomal Doxorubicin

Patrizia Guerrieri, Paolo Montemaggi
Department of Radiation Oncology, Regional Cancer Center "M. Ascoli", University of Palermo Medical School, Palermo, Italy

Definition

Doxorubicin hydrochloride liposome is a form of doxorubicin hydrochloride contained inside liposomes (very tiny particles of fat). This form may work better than other forms of doxorubicin hydrochloride and have fewer side effects. Also, because its effects last longer in the body, it does not need to be given as often. Liposomal doxorubicin seems to have substantial activity against ovarian and Fallopian tube cancer refractory to platinum and paclitaxel.

Cross-References

▶ Carcinoma of the Fallopian Tube

Liver and Hepatobiliary Tract

Rachelle Lanciano
Department of Radiation Oncology, Philadelphia Cyberknife Center, Delaware County Memorial Hospital, Drexel Hill, PA, USA

Synonyms

Ampullary carcinoma; Bile duct cancer; Cholangiocarcinoma; Gallbladder cancer; Hepatocellular carcinoma; Hepatoma

Definition/Description

Carcinoma of the hepatobiliary tract includes a diverse group of malignancies extending from the ampulla of Vater (ampullary carcinoma) through the biliary system (cholangiocarcinoma) to the liver (hepatocellular carcinoma).

It was estimated that 24,120 patients will present with primary hepatocellular carcinoma or intrahepatic cholangiocarcinoma with 18,910 deaths in the USA in 2010, while 9,760 patients will present with gallbladder or extrahepatic cholangiocarcinoma with 3,320 deaths. With the exception of true ampullary cancers, cancers of the hepatobiliary tract tend to be unresectable at presentation. They are usually associated with poor survival unless detected at an early stage. Etiologic factors such as hepatitis of any strain, chronic infection, and cirrhosis play an important role in pathogenesis for hepatocellular carcinoma. Surgery remains the mainstay of treatment for cancers in this region from Whipple procedures for ampullary and distal bile duct carcinomas to liver resection and transplant for proximal bile duct carcinoma or primary liver tumors. Radiotherapy plays an important role in combination with chemotherapy for postoperative treatment. Radiation can also be used for unresectable tumors, medically inoperable patients, or palliation of symptoms.

Anatomy

Periampullary tumors arise in the vicinity of the ampulla of Vater and can originate from the pancreas, duodenum, distal common bile duct, or the ampulla of Vater itself (primary ampullary carcinoma). The ampulla of Vater begins distal to the confluence of the distal common bile and pancreatic ducts and ends at the papilla on the medial aspect of the second portion of the duodenum (Fig. 1).

Cholangiocarcinoma is a cancer of the bile duct and is classified as distal (extrahepatic), perihilar, or intrahepatic based on the position of the cancer relative to the bifurcation of the right and left hepatic ducts. Bile duct tumors that involve the common hepatic duct bifurcation are referred to as Klatskin tumors (Fig. 2). The gallbladder and the cystic duct originate from the perihilar portion of the bile duct. The liver is separated into the right and left lobes with eight functional subsections including two in the right posterior, two in the right anterior, two in the left medial, and two in the left lateral sections (Fig. 3).

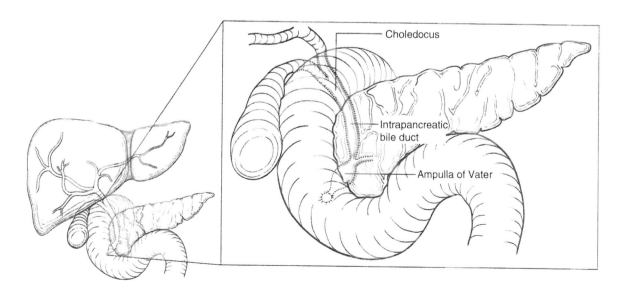

Liver and Hepatobiliary Tract. Fig. 1 Liver and hepatobiliary tract

Epidemiology

Primary ampullary tumors are rare and account for only 6% of tumors that arise in the periampullary region. The risk of ampullary tumors is markedly increased among patients with hereditary polyposis syndromes which present at a younger age than sporadic tumors. The most common subtype of ampullary adenocarcinoma is intestinal followed by pancreatobiliary which are thought to arise from ampullary adenomas. True ampullary cancers have a better prognosis compared with other periampullary cancers such as pancreatic or bile duct cancer, consistent with its presumed intestinal origin.

In the USA, approximately 5,000 cases of cholangiocarcinoma and 6,000 cases of gallbladder cancer were diagnosed in 2006. Perihilar tumors account for 60% of all cholangiocarcinomas while 30% are distal extrahepatic and the remainder are intrahepatic. The incidence of intrahepatic cholangiocarcinoma has been increasing while extrahepatic cholangiocarcinoma has been decreasing. Major risk factors for cholangiocarcinoma are primary sclerosing cholangitis (an inflammatory disorder of the biliary tree that leads to fibrosis and stricture of the bile ducts associated with ulcerative colitis) and biliary cysts (congenital cystic dilation of the bile ducts).

Gallbladder cancer is the most common cancer in the biliary tract with the majority found incidentally in patients undergoing gallbladder surgery for cholelithiasis. Gallbladder cancer is associated with chronic gallbladder inflammation such as found with gallstones, chronic infection with *Salmonella*, *Helicobacter*, or congenital abnormalities such as biliary cysts or abnormal pancreaticobiliary duct junction.

Pathologic precursors to cholangiocarcinoma include biliary intraepithelial neoplasia and intraductal papillary neoplasm similar to pancreas cancer. Pathologic precursors to gallbladder cancer are similar to other GI tract adenocarcinomas which progress from dysplasia, to carcinoma in situ and then invasive cancer. The majority of cholangiocarcinomas and gall bladder cancers are adenocarcinomas with the rest squamous cell cancer.

Hepatocellular carcinoma is the third leading cause of cancer-related deaths in the world and the ninth leading cause of cancer deaths in the USA with 80% of cases due to chronic hepatitis B and C infection frequently occurring in the setting of chronic liver disease and cirrhosis. Rare metabolic disorders such as hemochromatosis, porphyria cutanea tarda, alpha-1 antitrypsin deficiency, Wilson's disease, and inflammatory conditions such as primary biliary cirrhosis and the sequela of nonalcoholic fatty liver disease increase the risk of hepatocellular carcinoma.

Clinical Presentation

Cancers of the ampullary region, gall bladder, and bile ducts frequently present with painless jaundice, clay colored stools, dark urine, less commonly weight loss, anemia, or abdominal pain. Primary hepatocellular carcinoma presents with symptoms late in the course of disease such as ascites, encephalopathy, jaundice, variceal bleeding, or decompensation of previously controlled cirrhosis. Patients with hepatocellular carcinoma occasionally develop paraneoplastic syndromes with erythrocytosis, hypercalcemia, hypoglycemia and diarrhea or cutaneous manifestations of the disease.

Diagnostic Workup and Staging

Ultrasound of the liver and biliary tree and CT scan of the abdomen and pelvis are the standard initial diagnostic tests when a hepatobiliary malignancy is suspected. Tumor markers can be helpful which include CA 19-9 and CEA for ampullary and biliary tumors and AFP for hepatocellular carcinoma. The preferred drainage procedure for jaundice is endoscopic retrograde cholangiopancreatography (ERCP) since visualization of the ductal system is

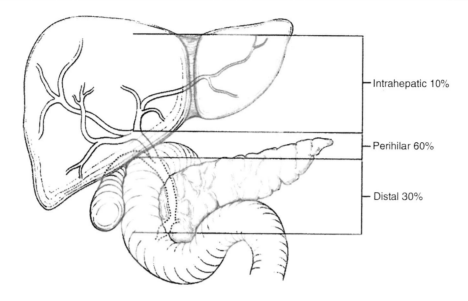

Liver and Hepatobiliary Tract. Fig. 2 Ampullary cancer

possible with biopsy and stent placement. Endoscopic ultrasound is useful to stage the depth of tumor penetration and to assess nodal metastases which can be sampled pathologically.

AJCC stage for ampullary cancers accounts for invasion into the duodenal wall, pancreas, or adjacent organs including peripancreatic soft tissues (T stage) and nodal metastases (N stage) (Fig. 4).

AJCC stage for cholangiocarcinoma is reported separately for intrahepatic, perihilar, and distal cholangiocarcinoma. Intrahepatic cholangiocarcinoma stage accounts for vascular invasion, presence of multiple tumors, perforation of the visceral peritoneum, or direct extension to extrahepatic structures (T stage) and nodal metastases (N stage). Perihilar cholangiocarcinoma stage accounts for invasion of liver, hepatic artery, portal vein (T stage), and nodal metastases (N stage). Distal cholangiocarcinoma stage accounts for extension outside the duct to pancreas, duodenum, gallbladder, or involvement of celiac axis/superior mesenteric artery (T stage)

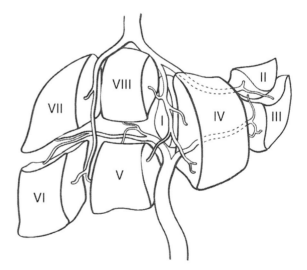

Liver and Hepatobiliary Tract. Fig. 3 Cholangiocarcinoma

and nodal metastases (N stage) (Figs. 5–7). Gallbladder cancer stage accounts for increasing depth of muscular invasion and extension to portal vein, hepatic artery or extrahepatic organs or

Primary Tumor (T)

TX	Primary tumor cannot be assessed
T0	No evidence of primary tumor
Tis	Carcinoma in situ
T1	Tumor limited to ampulla of Vater or sphincter of Oddi
T2	Tumor invades duodenal wall
T3	Tumor invades pancreas
T4	Tumor invades peripancreatic soft tissues or other adjacent organs or structures other than pancreas

Regional Lymph Nodes (N)

NX	Regional lymph nodes cannot be assessed
N0	No regional lymph node metastasis
N1	Regional lymph node metastasis

Distant Metastasis (M)

M0	No distant metastasis
M1	Distant metastasis

ANATOMIC STAGE/PROGNOSTIC GROUPS

Stage 0	Tis	N0	M0
Stage IA	T1	N0	M0
Stage IB	T2	N0	M0
Stage IIA	T3	N0	M0
Stage IIB	T1	N1	M0
	T2	N1	M0
	T3	N1	M0
Stage III	T4	Any N	M0
Stage IV	Any T	Any N	M1

Liver and Hepatobiliary Tract. Fig. 4 AJCC staging for ampullary cancers

Primary Tumor (T)

TX	Primary tumor cannot be assessed
T0	No evidence of primary tumor
Tis	Carcinoma in situ (intraductal tumor)
T1	Solitary tumor without vascular invasion
T2a	Solitary tumor with vascular invasion
T2b	Multiple tumors, with or without vascular invasion
T3	Tumor perforating the visceral peritoneum or involving the local extra hepatic structures by direct invasion
T4	Tumor with periductal invasion

Regional Lymph Nodes (N)

NX	Regional lymph nodes cannot be assessed
N0	No regional lymph node metastasis
N1	Regional lymph node metastasis present

Distant Metastasis (M)

M0	No distant metastasis
M1	Distant metastasis present

ANATOMIC STAGE/PROGNOSTIC GROUPS

Stage 0	Tis	N0	M0
Stage I	T1	N0	M0
Stage II	T2	N0	M0
Stage III	T3	N0	M0
Stage IVA	T4	N0	M0
	Any T	N1	M0
Stage IVB	Any T	Any N	M1

Liver and Hepatobiliary Tract. Fig. 5 AJCC staging for intrahepatic cholangiocarcinoma

structures (T stage), and nodal metastases (N stage) (Fig. 8).

Many clinical staging systems have been used for hepatocellular carcinoma; however, the CLIP system (Cancer of the Liver Italian Program) is preferred which combines tumor-related features (extent of disease in liver, serum AFP levels, and presence or absence of portal vein thrombosis) with an index of the severity of cirrhosis (Child-Pugh stage) (Table 1). Median survival for CLIP stages 0,1,2,3,4,5, and 6 treated with nonsurgical therapy for hepatocellular carcinoma were 31, 27, 13, 8, 2, and 2 months, respectively. Secondary

AJCC staging is recommended for patients undergoing surgery (liver transplantation and resection) with 5-year survival of 55%, 37%, and 16% for stage I, II, and III, respectively (Fig. 9).

Treatment

Ampullary Cancer/ Cholangiocarcinoma/Gall Bladder Cancer

Surgery for cancers of the hepatobiliary tract is the preferred initial treatment approach with radiation and chemotherapy reserved postoperatively for patients with a high risk of local-regional recurrence or inoperable disease.

Primary Tumor (T)

TX Primary tumor cannot be assessed
T0 No evidence of primary tumor
Tis Carcinoma in situ
T1 Tumor confined to the bile duct, with extension up to the muscle layer or fibrous tissue
T2a Tumor invades beyond the wall of the bile duct to surrounding adipose tissue
T2b Tumor invades adjacent hepatic parenchyma
T3 Tumor invades unilateral branches of the portal vein or hepatic artery
T4 Tumor invades main portal vein or its branches bilaterally; or the common hepatic artery; or the second-order biliary radicals bilaterally; or unilateral second-order biliary radicals with contralateral portal vein or hepatic artery involvement

Regional Lymph Nodes (N)

NX Regional lymph nodes cannot be assessed
N0 No regional lymph node metastasis
N1 Regional lymph node metastasis (including nodes along the cystic duct, common bile duct, hepatic artery, and portal vein)
N2 Metastasis to periaortic, pericaval, superior mesenteric artery, and/or celiac artery lymph nodes

Distant Metastasis (M)

M0 No distant metastasis
M1 Distant metastasis

ANATOMIC STAGE/PROGNOSTIC GROUPS

Stage 0	Tis	N0	M0
Stage I	T1	N0	M0
Stage II	T2a-b	N0	M0
Stage IIIA	T3	N0	M0
Stage IIIB	T1-3	N1	M0
Stage IVA	T4	N0-1	M0
Stage IVB	Any T	N2	M0
	Any T	Any N	M1

Liver and Hepatobiliary Tract. Fig. 6 AJCC staging for perihilar cholangiocarcinoma

Pancreaticoduodenectomy (Whipple operation) is the standard surgical approach for ampullary cancer and distal cholangiocarcinoma. Poor prognostic factors following surgery for ampullary cancer include high-grade histology, positive surgical margins, as well as increasing T stage and nodal involvement. Five-year survival in a series of over 1,300 patients with ampullary cancer from the

Primary Tumor (T)

TX Primary tumor cannot be assessed
T0 No evidence of primary tumor
Tis Carcinoma in situ
T1 Tumor confined to the bile duct histologically
T2 Tumor invades beyond the wall of the bile duct
T3 Tumor invades the gallbladder, pancreas, duodenum, or other adjacent organs without involvement of the celiac axis, or the superior mesenteric artery
T4 Tumor involves the celiac axis, or the superior mesenteric artery

Regional Lymph Nodes (N)

NX Regional lymph nodes cannot be assessed
N0 No regional lymph node metastasis
N1 Regional lymph node metastasis

Distant Metastasis (M)

M0 No distant metastasis
M1 Distant metastasis

ANATOMIC STAGE/PROGNOSTIC GROUPS

Stage 0	Tis	N0	M0
Stage IA	T1	N0	M0
Stage IB	T2	N0	M0
Stage IIA	T3	N0	M0
Stage IIB	T1	N1	M0
	T2	N1	M0
	T3	N1	M0
Stage III	T4	Any N	M0
Stage IV	Any T	Any N	M1

Liver and Hepatobiliary Tract. Fig. 7 AJCC staging for distal cholangiocarcinoma

SEER registry between 1988 and 2003 reveals overall survival for stage I patients of 57–60%, stage II of 22–30%, stage III of 27%, and stage IV of 0%. Nodal metastases decreased survival by 50% from 48% to 21% at 5 years. Patterns of recurrence suggest half of recurrences occur local-regionally; therefore, patients with highest risk of local recurrence could be offered postoperative radiation with chemotherapy. Unfortunately, two randomized trials of chemotherapy alone versus chemoradiation failed to show a benefit for radiation over surgery and chemotherapy for ampullary cancers that were included in periampullary/pancreas cancer trials.

Primary Tumor (T)

TX   Primary tumor cannot be assessed

T0   No evidence of primary tumor

Tis Carcinoma in situ

T1   Tumor invades lamina propria or muscular layer
     (Figure 20.3)

T1a Tumor invades lamina propria

T1b Tumor invades muscular layer

T2   Tumor invades perimuscular connective tissue; no
     extension beyond serosa or into liver (Figure 20.4)

T3   Tumor perforates the serosa (visceral peritoneum)
     and/or directly invades the liver and/or one other
     adjacent organ or structure, such as the stomach,
     duodenum, colon, pancreas, omentum, or extra-
     hepatic bile ducts

T4   Tumor invades main portal vein or hepatic artery
     or invades two or more extrahepatic organs or
     structures

Regional Lymph Nodes (N)

NX   Regional lymph nodes cannot be assessed

N0   No regional lymph node metastasis

N1   Metastases to nodes along the cystic duct, common
     bile duct, hepatic artery, and/or portal vein

N2   Metastases to periaortic, pericaval, superior
     mesenteric artery, and/or celiac artery lymph nodes

Distant Metastasis (M)

M0   No distant metastasis

M1   Distant metastasis

ANATOMIC STAGE/PROGNOSTIC GROUPS

Stage 0	Tis	N0	M0
Stage I	T1	N0	M0
Stage II	T2	N0	M0
Stage IIIA	T3	N0	M0
Stage IIIB	T1-3	N1	M0
Stage IVA	T4	N0-1	M0
Stage IVB	Any T	N2	M0
	Any T	Any N	M1

Liver and Hepatobiliary Tract. Fig. 8 AJCC staging for gallbladder cancer

In the USA, however, ampullary cancers are treated postoperatively like pancreas cancer with common regimens including 50.4 Gy involved field radiation with concurrent infusional 5FU and adjuvant gemcitabine chemotherapy.

Distal cholangiocarcinoma requires pancreaticoduodenectomy (Whipple) while intrahepatic cholangiocarcinoma requires liver resection if curative resection is possible. Distal cholangiocarcinoma has the highest resectability rate (90%) with proximal (intrahepatic and perihilar) the lowest (55–60%). Criteria for resectability include absence of pancreatic and celiac nodal metastases, absence of liver metastases or extrahepatic adjacent organ invasion, and absence of portal vein or main hepatic artery invasion.

Prognostic factors among patients who undergo curative resection for cholangiocarcinoma include location of cancer, presence of vascular invasion and stage with the more proximal and lower stage cancers having higher resection rates and 5-year survival. For extrahepatic bile duct cancer, nodal metastasis decreases 5-year survival from 38% with negative nodes to 10% with positive nodes. Margin status after curative resection affects 5-year survival from 19–47% with negative margins to 0–12% with positive margins. Preoperative portal vein embolization may be used to induce lobar hypertrophy in patients who have a predicted postoperative liver remnant volume of less than 25% to achieve negative surgical margins. Selective use of portal lymphadenectomy generally for more proximal cancers of the bile duct may be used to increase surgical margins and for staging. Five-year survival rates with intrahepatic cholangiocarcinoma range from 74% for T1 to 48% for T2a, 18% for T2b, and 7% for N1 disease.

Adjuvant chemotherapy and radiation is recommended for patients with microscopic or macroscopic residual disease following resection as per NCCN guidelines with reported increase in local control and possibly survival. Chemotherapy and radiation is also recommended for the 50–90% of patients with unresectable cholangiocarcinoma for palliation of symptoms including pain, pruritus, jaundice, and improvement in quality of life. Radiation techniques include external beam conformal radiation therapy (CRT), intensity-modulated radiation therapy (IMRT), brachytherapy, and stereotactic radiosurgery (SRS). The type of radiation used

Liver and Hepatobiliary Tract. Table 1 Clinical staging for hepatocellular carcinoma; Cancer of the Liver Italian Program system

Table 57.2	GRADING SYSTEM FOR CIRRHOSIS: THE CHILD-PUGH SCORE				
Score	Bilirubin (mg/dL)	Albumin (g/dL)	Prothrombin Time (sec)	Hepatic Encephalopathy (grade)	Ascites
1	<2	>3.5	<4	None	None
2	2–3	2.8–3.5	4–6	1–2	Mild (detectable)
3	>3	<2.8	>6	3–4	Severe (tense)

Child class: A, 5 to 6; B, 7 to 9; C, >9.

Modified Child-Pugh classification of the severity of liver disease according to the degree of ascites, the plasma concentrations of bilirubin and albumin, the prothrombin time, and the degree of encephalopathy

can be tailored to expertise of oncologist and the site of the bile duct cancer with SRS being most appropriate for intrahepatic bile duct cancers, where literature exists for primary liver tumors, intrahepatic cholangiocarcinoma, and liver metastases, while standard external beam techniques (CRT and IMRT) +/− brachytherapy reserved for more distal presentations. Generally, 50.4 Gy is delivered with concurrent chemotherapy in the postoperative setting directed to the tumor bed and regional lymph nodes with CRT or IMRT techniques.

Locally advanced and unresectable disease should receive higher doses of radiation for local control if possible within normal tissue constraints such as liver or bowel tolerance. Other local treatments for palliation have been used including radiofrequency ablation (RFA), transarterial chemoembolization (TACE), radioembolization with yttrium-90-tagged microspheres, and photodynamic therapy. Chemotherapy also is useful for palliation including 5FU, cisplatin, or gemcitiabine as single or multiagent regimens.

Gallbladder cancer is often found incidentally for benign gallbladder disease after cholecystectomy. These patients may undergo a second curative procedure including resection of at least 2 cm of liver in the gallbladder bed (generally segments IVB and V) and dissection of the regional lymph nodes from the hepatoduodenal ligament except for patients with T1a cancer. Reexploration will reveal residual tumor in 40–76% of cases. In medically high-risk patients who cannot tolerate further surgery, chemotherapy and radiation postoperatively can decrease local failure and improve survival. The SEER database of 4,180 patients with gallbladder cancer revealed older age, male sex, nonpapillary histology, and no adjuvant radiation were significant predictors of worse survival in multivariate analysis. Patients in this series with >T2, node positive gallbladder cancer derived the most benefit from radiation. Usually 5FU-based chemotherapy is given with radiation to the tumor bed and regional lymph nodes with doses of 50.4 Gy. Five-year survival rates from National Cancer Data Base for gallbladder cancer are 50% stage I, 29% stage II, 8% stage IIIA, 7% stage IIIB, 3% stage IVA, and 2% stage IVB. Locally advanced and unresectable gallbladder cancer is usually treated with a combination of radiation and chemotherapy. Radiation techniques may include CRT and IMRT external beam with SRS boost or SRS alone if appropriate. Chemotherapy can induce objective response rates of 50–60% and commonly used regimens include gemcitabine +/− cisplatin, capecitabine, or oxaliplatin-based regimens. The Southwest Oncology Group phase II trial is accruing patients with resected extrahepatic

Primary Tumor (T)	
TX	Primary tumor cannot be assessed
T0	No evidence of primary tumor
T1	Solitary tumor without vascular invasion
T2	Solitary tumor with vascular invasion or multiple tumors none more than 5 cm
T3a	Multiple tumors more than 5 cm
T3b	Single tumor or multiple tumors of any size involving a major branch of the portal vein or hepatic vein
T4	Tumor(s) with direct invasion of adjacent organs other than the gallbladder or with perforation of visceral peritoneum

Regional Lymph Nodes (N)	
NX	Regional lymph nodes cannot be assessed
N0	No regional lymph node metastasis
N1	Regional lymph node metastasis

Distant Metastasis (M)	
M0	No distant metastasis
M1	Distant metastasis

ANATOMIC STAGE/PROGNOSTIC GROUPS

Stage I	T1	N0	M0
Stage II	T2	N0	M0
Stage IIIA	T3a	N0	M0
Stage IIIB	T3b	N0	M0
Stage IIIC	T4	N0	M0
Stage IVA	Any T	N1	M0
Stage IVB	Any T	Any N	M1

Liver and Hepatobiliary Tract. Fig. 9 Secondary AJCC staging for hepatocellular carcinoma

bile duct or gallbladder cancer with T2-4 and/or N1 and/or positive margins following resection to adjuvant treatment with capecitabine/gemcitabine chemotherapy followed by capecitabine with concurrent radiation.

Hepatocellular Carcinoma

Surgery is possible for only about 5% of patients presenting with hepatocellular carcinoma because of invasion of a major portal or hepatic vein, direct invasion of organs other than the gallbladder, perforation of the visceral peritoneum, nodal or distant metastases, or because of comorbid medical issues, primarily cirrhosis or the complications of the disease. Assessment of hepatic reserve and extent of liver cirrhosis are key selection factors with surgery generally reserved for patients with no cirrhosis or Child-Pugh A. Liver transplantation is an option for unresectable patients who have a solitary hepatocellular carcinoma less than 5 cm or up to three separate lesions not larger than 3 cm, no evidence of gross vascular invasion, and no regional nodal or distant metastases. Long-term relapse-free survival of 40% or better and 5-year survival rates of 50–90% are possible in selected patients following resection or transplantation.

Although a diagnosis of hepatocellular carcinoma increases the priority score for donor organs, there can be a significant wait for transplantation. A variety of local treatments have been used as a bridge to transplant or for unresectable disease, such as radiofrequency ablation (RFA), transarterial chemoembolization (TACE), external beam conformal radiation therapy (CRT), intensity-modulated radiation therapy (IMRT), stereotactic radiosurgery (SRS), proton beam radiation therapy, and radioembolization. External beam CRT/IMRT and SRS can achieve local control rates of 60–95% at 1–2 years with fractionation schemes of 66 Gy in 33 fractions or 30–45 Gy in 3–5 fractions, respectively, for limited tumors in patients with relatively good liver function (Child-Pugh A,B). Sometimes TACE is combined with radiation. An international phase III trial is currently open to compare repeat application of TACE versus SRS (36-45 Gy/3fx) for inoperable recurrent hepatocellular carcinoma ≤7.5 cm following initial treatment with TACE. Volume constraints include >800 cc. Uninvolved liver should receive <12 Gy. All patients require fiducial placement for respiratory tracking and usually 3-mm margins are applied to the gross tumor volume which should receive the full dose.

Patients with disease spread outside the liver are considered for systemic therapy. Sorafenib has been shown to improve survival over supportive care alone in patients with advanced hepatocellular carcinoma.

Cross-References

► Nuclear Medicine
► Palliation of Metastatic Disease to the Liver
► Primary Cancer of The Duodenum
► Principles of Chemotherapy
► Stereotactic Radiosurgery: Extracranial

References

Abdalla E, Stuart K (2011) Overview of treatment approaches for hepatocellular carcinoma
American Joint Commission on Cancer (AJCC) (2010) AJCC cancer staging manual, 7th edn. Springer, New York (Chap 18–23, pg 191–240)
Anderson C, Stuart K (2011) Treatment of localized cholangiocarcinoma: surgical management and adjuvant therapy
Anderson C, Stuart K (2011) Treatment options for locally advanced cholangiocarcinoma
Curley S, Stuart K, Schwartz J, Carithers R (2011) Nonsurgical therapies for localized hepatocellular carcinoma: transarterial embolization, radiotherapy, radioembolization, radiofrequency ablation, percutaneous ethanol injection, thermal ablation and cryoablation
Curley S, Barnett C, Abdalla E (2011) Staging and prognostic factors in hepatocellular carcinoma. www.uptodate.com
International Randomized study of transarterial chemoembolization (TACE) vs. cyberknife radiosurgery for recurrent hepatocellular carcinoma. Principle Investigator: Albert Koong MD Stanford University, Sponsor: Accuray International, IRB approval 2/8/2011
Lowe R, Afdhal N, Anderson C (2011) Epidemiology, patholgenesis and classification of cholangiocarcinoma
Lowe R, Afdhal N, Anderson C (2011) Clinical manifestations and diagnosis of cholangiocarcinoma
Martin J, Moser A, Lora M (2011) Ampullary carcinoma: epidemiology, clinical manifestations, diagnosis and staging
Mehrotra B (2011) Gallbladder cancer: epidemiology, risk factors, clinical features, and diagnosis
Mehrotra B (2011) Treatment of advanced, unresectable gallbladder cancer
National Comprehensive Cancer Network (2011) Practice guidelines in oncology. Version 1. Hepatobiliary cancers. www.nccn.org
Ryan D, Mamon H, Fernandez-del Castillo C (2011) Ampullary carcinoma: treatment and prognosis
Schwartz J, Carithers R (2011) Epidemiology and etiologic associations of hepatocellular carcinoma
Schwartz J, Carithers R (2011) Clinical features and diagnosis of primary hepatocellular carcinoma
Swanson R, Mehrotra B (2011) Gallbladder cancer: treatment of localized, potentially resectable disease

Lobular Carcinoma In Situ (LCIS)

David E. Wazer
Radiation Oncology Department, Tufts Medical Center, Tufts University School of Medicine, Boston, MA, USA
Radiation Oncology Department, Rhode Island Hospital, Brown University School of Medicine, Providence, RI, USA

Definition

Non-infiltrating lobular proliferation of loosely cohesive carcinoma cells filling the acinar space.

Cross-References

► Cancer of the Breast Tis
► Stage 0 Breast Cancer

Low-Dose Rate (LDR) Brachytherapy

Ning J. Yue[1], Erik van Limbergen[2], Cheng B. Saw[3]
[1]The Department of Radiation Oncology, The Cancer Institute of New Jersey, UMDNJ-Robert Wood Johnson Medical School, New Brunswick, NJ, USA
[2]Department of Radiation Oncology, University Hospital Gasthuisberg, Leuven, Belgium
[3]Division of Radiation Oncology, Penn State Hershey Cancer Institute, Hershey, PA, USA

Definition

The sources commonly used for LDR are cesium-137 (LDR afterloaders), or iridium-192 as LDR wires. The dose is delivered at 0.4–2 Gy h^{-1} (10 Gy/day). Irradiation is continuous and can take depending on the dose 1–6 days. Patients have to be hospitalized in rooms that fulfill the requirements of radioprotection legislation. Since the dose rate is low, repair of sublethal damage is possible during irradiation. LDR is therefore considered as having a wider therapeutic ratio to spare normal tissues while treating cancer cells.

Cross-References

▶ Brachytherapy: High Dose Rate (HDR) Implants
▶ Clinical Aspects of Brachytherapy (BT)
▶ High-Dose Rate (HDR) Brachytherapy
▶ Low-Dose Rate (LDR) Brachytherapy

Low-Risk Neuroblastoma

BRANDON J. FISHER[1], LARRY C. DAUGHERTY[2]
[1]Department of Radiation Oncology, College of Medicine, Drexel University, Philadelphia, PA, USA
[2]Department of Radiation Oncology, College of Medicine, Drexel University, Glenside, PA, USA

Definition
Young patients with favorable histology, non-amplification of N-*myc*, and DNA index >1.

Cross-References
▶ Ganglioneuroma
▶ Ganglioneuroblastoma
▶ N-myc
▶ Neural Crest Cells
▶ Neuroblastoma
▶ Round Blue-Cell Tumors
▶ Shimada Pathologic Classification System
▶ Wilm's Tumor

Luminal Subtypes

▶ Breast Cancer Risk Models
▶ Stage 0 Breast Cancer

Lumpectomy/Segmental Mastectomy

DAVID E. WAZER
Radiation Oncology Department, Tufts Medical Center, Tufts University School of Medicine, Boston, MA, USA
Radiation Oncology Department, Rhode Island Hospital, Brown University School of Medicine, Providence, RI, USA

Definition
The removal of breast disease with the goal of complete excision with negative surgical margins while conserving the breast.

Cross-References
▶ Cancer of the Breast Tis
▶ Early Stage Breast Cancer

Lung

JINGBO WANG, FENG-MING KONG
Department of Radiation Oncology, Veteran Administration Health Center and University Hospital, University of Michigan, Ann Arbor, MI, USA

Synonyms
Bronchopulmonary carcinoma; Carcinoma of lungs

Definition/Description

Bronchopulmonary carcinoma refers to the malignancy that derives from epithelial cells within the lungs and bronchus and is usually simply termed as lung cancer.

Background

Lung cancer is the most common malignancy worldwide as well as the leading cause of cancer deaths, with a 5-year survival rate of only 15.9% (Jemal et al. 2009). Smoking is the greatest risk factor for lung cancer. More than 85% of lung cancer deaths are related to tobacco abuse. Exposed nonsmokers (passive smoking) have a 24% higher risk to develop lung cancer than unexposed never-smokers (Hackshaw et al. 1997).

Histology

Lung cancer is generally divided into non-small-cell lung cancer (NSCLC) and small-cell lung cancer (SCLC) based on biological behavior, therapeutic strategy, and prognosis. NSCLC accounts for approximately 85% of all lung cancer cases in the United States with a broad spectrum of histological types. Adenocarcinoma has surpassed squamous cell carcinoma and becomes the predominant histological subtype of lung cancer since the mid-1980s.

Clinical Presentation

Common signs and symptoms of lung cancer can be sorted into four categories according to their mechanisms: (1) those resulting from local tumor growth and intrathoracic spread, such as dyspnea, wheezing, coughing, chest pain, hemoptysis, hoarseness, dysphagia, or corresponding syndromes such as superior vena cava syndrome (▶ SVCS), ▶ Horner's syndrome, and ▶ Pancoast's Syndrome; (2) those due to distant metastases, such as bone pain caused by bone involvement and headache, nausea, vomiting, or seizure, resulting from brain spread; (3) ▶ paraneoplastic syndromes; and (4) nonspecific symptoms and signs such as fever, anorexia, anemia, fatigue, weakness, and weight loss.

Imaging Studies

Chest X-ray is the simplest and most traditional method for pulmonary tumor detection. Chest CT (IV contrast CT in particular) is the most prevalent and effective approach for defining mediastinal status and the suspicious nodule in lung. At present, CT remains the dominant role in lung cancer diagnosis, staging as well as response evaluation. A minimum diameter of 10 mm or more on a CT image is the most commonly used criterion for defining malignant nodes. ▶ PET has been widely used for defining pulmonary malignancies, staging, treatment planning, and monitoring treatment response in NSCLC. The sensitivity and specificity of PET for the mediastinal evaluation were 91% and 86%, respectively. The corresponding values of CT were 75% and 66%. The sensitivity and specificity of PET for detecting distant metastases alone were 82% and 93%, respectively (Pieterman et al. 2000). The main drawback of PET is poor quality in anatomical information. Integrated PET-CT can obtain a better diagnostic and staging accuracy than either modality alone and is the preferred approach for NSCLC evaluation (Lardinois et al. 2003). In terms of the predicting capability, the diagnostic accuracy and sensitivity were 79% and 64%, and the corresponding values for the conventional-staging group were 60% and 32%, respectively. The use of PET for preoperative staging of NSCLC may reduce both the total number and the number of futile thoracotomies but did not affect the overall mortality (Fischer et al. 2009). The use of chest MRI for the initial evaluation of lung cancer is less frequent but may be valuable in evaluating superior sulcus lesions abutting the spine, brachial plexus, or subclavian vessels. Brain MRI should be performed for those with more advanced disease (II and III) if aggressive combined-modality therapy is being considered. Brain MRI is also recommended as a preferred staging evaluation for SCLC.

Pathological Diagnosis

The gold standard for lung cancer diagnosis is histological evidence. Biopsy can be performed by bronchial endoscopy, CT-guided transthoracic percutaneous fine-needle aspiration (FNA), endoscopic ultrasound-guided FNA (EUS-FNA), or endobronchial ultrasound-guided transbronchial needle aspiration (EBUS-TBNA). Currently, mediastinoscopy is still considered as the best approach for assessing mediastinal lymph node involvement. The average sensitivity of mediastinoscopy is approximately 80% and the average false negative rate is around 10%. Video mediastinoscopy is likely to further improve diagnostic performance, with the sensitivity of 90% and false negative rate of 7% (Detterbeck et al. 2007).

Treatment

Lung cancer is a disease with extremely poor 5-year survival of only 15.9% (Jemal et al. 2009). Surgery, radiation therapy, chemotherapy, and the emerging targeted therapy are the main modalities used to treat lung cancer patients.

Treatment for NSCLC

Surgery

An overall evaluation, including complete history acquisition, physical examination, performance status, comorbidity assessment, imaging studies, blood test, and pulmonary function test should be performed before surgery to determine medical fitness for surgery. The surgical-approach selection depends on the extent of tumor and individual tolerance. Anatomic pulmonary resection (lobectomy, bilobectomy, or pneumonectomy) remains to be standard care for patients with resectable NSCLC, and lobectomy is used most frequently if complete resection can be achieved. Lymph nodal dissection or sampling is required as a component of radical surgical resection.

Radiation Therapy

Over 60% of patients with NSCLC require radiotherapy at least once during the course of the disease. Radiation therapy (RT) can be used alone or mostly combined with chemotherapy as (1) a neoadjuvant or adjuvant therapy for patients with surgical resection, (2) a definitive therapy for those with unresectable or inoperable NSCLC, (3) a palliative treatment for patients with incurable NSCLC.

Simulation initiates the preparation for radiation therapy, which can be implemented under conventional simulator, CT, MRI, or PET-CT. CT simulation is considered the preferred option and IV contrast should be used whenever possible for better target definition, and respiratory motion should be managed. Due to the aforementioned superiority of PET-CT over CT, it is recommended as the preferred method in cases with significant atelectasis or those who cannot have IV contrast.

External-beam radiation therapy, including three-dimensional conformal radiation therapy (▶ 3D-CRT), ▶ intensity modulated radiation therapy (IMRT), and ▶ stereotactic radiosurgery: extracranial are frequently used for radiation therapy of lung cancer. At present, 3DCRT is the most widely used irradiation technique. It is yet unclear whether IMRT can offer significant improvements over 3DCRT. IMRT seems to have limited extra value for patients without node metastases, but is beneficial in node-positive cases (Grills et al. 2003). Recent evidence suggests SBRT could offer benefit over 3DCRT in both survival and local control for patients with peripheral stage I NSCLC (Grutters et al. 2010). ICRU Report 62 offers the primary principle for consideration of lung cancer treatment volume: The gross tumor volume (GTV) should include the primary tumor and involved regional lymph nodes as identified on the planning scan and other examinations. The clinical target volume (CTV) should account for uncertainties in microscopic tumor spread. The planning volume (PTV) should include the CTV plus an external expansion considering geometric and other uncertainties. Considering respiratory motion, internal target volume (ITV) is specifically defined as an expansion of CTV with margins of target motion. Standard target definition for mediastinal lymph nodes has not yet been determined. The role of ENI (elective nodal irradiation) is controversial. To allow high-dose radiation without causing severe toxicity from concurrent chemoradiation, involved field radiotherapy (IFRT) is a common practice, with a failure rate outside the PTV of only about 6% (Kong et al. 2005; Rosenzweig et al. 2007; Senan et al. 2004).

RT dose for definitive radiotherapy alone or sequential chemoradiation therapy in patients with NSCLC is 60–74 Gy at 2 Gy per fraction. Concurrent chemoradiotherapy requires a moderate dose and 60–70 Gy with conventional fraction may be preferable. Escalated dose has potential to attain better overall survival and local control, provided normal tissue toxicity is within constraint (Kong et al. 2005). PORT (postoperative radiation therapy) dose is determined on the margin status. At the present time, conventional fraction to 50 Gy is recommended to individuals with negative margins, and definitive dose should be delivered if there is gross residual tumor (Douillard et al. 2008). Common-dose strategies of SBRT in patients with stage I include 30–34 Gy once, 15–20 Gy × 3 fractions, 12–12.5 Gy × 4 fractions, or 10–11 Gy × 5 fractions (Timmerman et al. 2007). As soon as an adequate biologic equivalent dose is given, various fractionation regimens offer a similar tumor control outcome. RTOG 0915 is comparing the effect of 34 Gy in one single fraction with 12.5 Gy x 4 fractions.

Radiation-related toxicity is a series of normal tissue damage associated with complicated interaction among multiple factors such as irradiation location and dosimetric factors. Nonspecific side effects such as skin irritation, fatigue, or nausea can be observed in most patients. Thoracic radiation specific side effects include pulmonary toxicity, esophagitis, or cardiac toxicity. Hair loss is common in patients who undergo brain irradiation.

Chemotherapy

Chemotherapy plays an important role in patients with NSCLC. Chemotherapy can be used as: (1) a neoadjuvant or adjuvant therapy for patients treated with surgical resection, (2) a part of combined therapy for inoperable or unresectable NSCLC, and (3) a palliative therapy for metastatic disease.

Neoadjuvant chemotherapy before surgical resection improves survival in stage IIIA NSCLC. Adjuvant chemotherapy with cisplatin-based regimen provides a 5.4% benefit in 5-year survival to patients in stage II and III resected NSCLC (Pignon et al. 2008) and is thus considered to be standard of care (Ardizzoni et al. 2007).

The role of chemotherapy in stage III NSCLC will be summarized later under chemoradiation. For patients with metastatic NSCLC, chemotherapy offers modest improvement in overall survival (Group NM-AC 2008) and quality of life. Platinum-based combined regimens are most commonly used currently and display superiority to single drug.

Chemoradiation Therapy

Chemoradiation therapy (CRT) plays an important role in the multimodality treatment for NSCLC. Basically, this strategy can be divided into sequential and concurrent CRT according to the sequence of two therapy procedures.

Chemoradiation therapy is mostly used for patients with unresectable locally advanced disease (IIIA and IIIB). Compared to sequential pattern, concurrent CRT offers a significant absolute survival benefit of 4.5% at 5 years primarily because of better locoregional control (Aupérin et al. 2010; Belderbos et al. 2007; Fournel et al. 2005; Furuse et al. 1999; Zatloukal et al. 2004). Although concurrent CRT is associated with higher incidence of radiation esophagitis, the adverse event is acceptable and manageable. At present, concurrent CRT is the standard therapy for locally advanced unresectable NSCLC. Cisplatin-etoposide, cisplatin-vinblastine, and carboplatin-paclitaxel are commonly used chemotherapy regimens. Radiation dose can be 60–70 Gy by 2 Gy per fraction if the tolerances of adjacent normal structures are met.

For patients with resectable tumors located in the superior sulcus, neoadjuvant current chemoradiation therapy followed by surgical resection and adjuvant chemotherapy is recommended, presenting a 5-year survival rate of 44% for all patients and 54% for those achieving pathologic complete response (Rusch et al. 2007). Postoperative chemoradiation therapy can be performed as an option for patients with positive margin.

For patients with pN2 nodal disease after complete resection, postoperative radiation therapy (PORT) following adjuvant chemotherapy showed promising survival benefit (Douillard et al. 2008; Lally et al. 2006). Further confirmation in prospectively designed randomized studies are warranted to confirm the role of PORT in completely resected pN2 NSCLC.

Targeted Therapy

In recent years, molecular-targeted therapy aimed at cell receptors, signal transduction, cell cycles, or angiogenesis has been developed for cancer treatment.

Gefitinib is a tyrosine kinase inhibitor targeting the tyrosine kinase domain of the epidermal growth factor receptor (EGFR). Asian female non-smokers with adenocarcinoma (bronchioloalveolar carcinoma in particular) and EGFR gene somatic mutations, specifically the deletion mutation in exon19 and a single-point mutation in exon 21, appear to have great potential to obtain survival advantage from this drug (Lynch et al. 2004). As compared with the chemotherapy of carboplatin-paclitaxel, gifitinib significantly prolonged the progression free survival, increased the objective response rate, and improved the quality of life in these selected patients (Mok et al. 2009).

Erlotinib, another tyrosine kinase inhibitor, also provided longer survival for patients with NSCLC after first-line or second-line chemotherapy (Shepherd et al. 2005). It has been approved by the FDA as a second-line therapy for patients with locally advanced or metastatic NSCLC who had progression after one or two previous chemotherapy regimens. It has also been approved as a maintenance therapy for patients with locally advanced or metastatic NSCLC after 4 cycles of platinum-based first-line chemotherapy.

Bevacizumab is a FDA-approved angiogenesis inhibitor used in patients with unresectable, locally advanced, recurrent, or metastatic non-squamous NSCLC, preferably combined with paclitaxel and carboplatin (Sandler et al. 2006).

Treatment for SCLC

Small-cell lung cancer is distinguished from NSCLC by its more aggressive biological behavior. Without any treatment, patients with SCLC have shorter life expectancy than NSCLC. Most patients of SCLC present hematogenous metastases, while only about one third of patients have diseases confined to the chest. Thus, a distinct strategy is utilized for the treatment of SCLC.

Surgery may be considered in patients with T1 N0 disease, and these patients may achieve complete resection and acquire survival benefit from surgery (de Antonio et al. 2006).

Chemotherapy is an essential component of treatment for patients with SCLC and should be administered to all patients without poor performance status. Cisplatin-etoposide is the standard regimen, with carboplatin-irinotecan as the surrogate if the former is contraindicated or poorly tolerated (Lara et al. 2009).

The addition of thoracic radiation therapy improves overall survival for patients with limited SCLC resulting in a 5% increase of 3-year survival as compared with chemotherapy alone (Pignon et al. 1992).

Concurrent chemoradiotherapy is recommended as the preferred sequence for limited SCLC. Furthermore, early initiation of radiotherapy (started at cycle 1 or 2 chemotherapy) presents small but significant survival benefit compared with late concurrent or sequential radiotherapy (Fried et al. 2004). Irradiation dose of 1.5 Gy, twice per day, to a total dose of 45 Gy is the preferred option provided patients have excellent performance status and good baseline pulmonary function (Turrisi et al. 1999); otherwise, 1.8–2.0 Gy once daily to 60–70 Gy should be delivered.

Over 50% of SCLC patients will develop brain metastases during the course of the disease. Prophylactic cranial irradiation (PCI) can reduce incidence of cerebral metastases and increase overall survival for patients with SCLC regardless of initial stage for both limited and extensive stage diseases (Aupérin et al. 1999; Slotman et al. 2007). At the present time, PCI is recommended for patients with either limited or extensive SCLC who achieve a complete or partial response from chemoradiation or chemotherapy. The preferred dose for this is 25 Gy in 10 fractions (Le Péchoux et al. 2009).

Cross-References

▶ Carcinoid Tumor
▶ Four-Dimensional (4D) Treatment Planning/Respiratory Gating
▶ Intensity Modulated Radiation Therapy (IMRT)
▶ Ganglioneuroma
▶ Paraneoplastic Syndromes
▶ Stereotactic Radiosurgery: Extracranial

References

Ardizzoni A, Boni L, Tiseo M et al (2007) Cisplatin- versus carboplatin-based chemotherapy in first-line treatment of advanced non-small-cell lung cancer: an individual patient data meta-analysis. J Natl Cancer Inst 99:847–857

Aupérin A, Arriagada R, Pignon J et al (1999) Prophylactic cranial irradiation for patients with small-cell lung cancer in complete remission. Prophylactic Cranial Irradiation Overview Collaborative Group. N Engl J Med 341:476–484

Aupérin A, Le Péchoux C, Rolland E et al (2010) Meta-analysis of concomitant versus sequential radiochemotherapy in locally advanced non-small-cell lung cancer. J Clin Oncol 28:2181–2190

Belderbos J, Uitterhoeve L, van Zandwijk N et al (2007) Randomised trial of sequential versus concurrent chemo-radiotherapy in patients with inoperable non-small cell lung cancer (EORTC 08972–22973). Eur J Cancer 43:114–121

de Antonio D, Alfageme F, Gámez P et al (2006) Results of surgery in small cell carcinoma of the lung. Lung Cancer 52:299–304

Detterbeck FC, Jantz MA, Wallace M et al (2007) Invasive mediastinal staging of lung cancer: ACCP evidence-based clinical practice guidelines, 2nd edn. Chest 132:202S–220S

Douillard J, Rosell R, De Lena M et al (2008) Impact of postoperative radiation therapy on survival in patients with complete resection and stage I, II, or IIIA non-small-cell lung cancer treated with adjuvant chemotherapy: the adjuvant Navelbine International Trialist Association (ANITA) Randomized trial. Int J Radiat Oncol Biol Phys 72:695–701

Fischer B, Lassen U, Mortensen J et al (2009) Preoperative staging of lung cancer with combined PET-CT. N Engl J Med 361:32–39

Fournel P, Robinet G, Thomas P et al (2005) Randomized phase III trial of sequential chemoradiotherapy compared with concurrent chemoradiotherapy in locally advanced non-small-cell lung cancer: Groupe Lyon-Saint-Etienne d'Oncologie Thoracique-Groupe Français de Pneumo-Cancérologie NPC 95–01 Study. J Clin Oncol 23:5910–5917

Fried D, Morris D, Poole C et al (2004) Systematic review evaluating the timing of thoracic radiation therapy in combined modality therapy for limited-stage small-cell lung cancer. J Clin Oncol 22:4837–4845

Furuse K, Fukuoka M, Kawahara M et al (1999) Phase III study of concurrent versus sequential thoracic radiotherapy in combination with mitomycin, vindesine, and cisplatin in unresectable stage III non-small-cell lung cancer. J Clin Oncol 17:2692–2699

Grills IS, Yan D, Martinez AA et al (2003) Potential for reduced toxicity and dose escalation in the treatment of inoperable non-small-cell lung cancer: a comparison of intensity-modulated radiation therapy (IMRT),

3D conformal radiation, and elective nodal irradiation. Int J Radiat Oncol Biol Phys 57:875–890

Group NM-AC (2008) Chemotherapy in addition to supportive care improves survival in advanced non-small-cell lung cancer: a systematic review and meta-analysis of individual patient data from 16 randomized controlled trials. J Clin Oncol 26:4617–4625

Grutters J, Kessels A, Pijls-Johannesma M et al (2010) Comparison of the effectiveness of radiotherapy with photons, protons and carbon-ions for non-small cell lung cancer: a meta-analysis. Radiother Oncol 95:32–40

Hackshaw A, Law M, Wald N (1997) The accumulated evidence on lung cancer and environmental tobacco smoke. BMJ 315:980–988

Jemal A, Siegel R, Ward E et al (2009) Cancer statistics, 2009. CA Cancer J Clin 59:225–249

Kong F-M, Ten Haken RK, Schipper MJ et al (2005) High-dose radiation improved local tumor control and overall survival in patients with inoperable/unresectable non-small-cell lung cancer: long-term results of a radiation dose escalation study. Int J Radiat Oncol Biol Phys 63:324–333

Lally B, Zelterman D, Colasanto J et al (2006) Postoperative radiotherapy for stage II or III non-small-cell lung cancer using the surveillance, epidemiology, and end results database. J Clin Oncol 24:2998–3006

Lara PJ, Natale R, Crowley J et al (2009) Phase III trial of irinotecan/cisplatin compared with etoposide/cisplatin in extensive-stage small-cell lung cancer: clinical and pharmacogenomic results from SWOG S0124. J Clin Oncol 27:2530–2535

Lardinois D, Weder W, Hany T et al (2003) Staging of non-small-cell lung cancer with integrated positron-emission tomography and computed tomography. N Engl J Med 348:2500–2507

Le Péchoux C, Dunant A, Senan S et al (2009) Standard-dose versus higher-dose prophylactic cranial irradiation (PCI) in patients with limited-stage small-cell lung cancer in complete remission after chemotherapy and thoracic radiotherapy (PCI 99–01, EORTC 22003–08004, RTOG 0212, and IFCT 99–01): a randomised clinical trial. Lancet Oncol 10:467–474

Lynch T, Bell D, Sordella R et al (2004) Activating mutations in the epidermal growth factor receptor underlying responsiveness of non-small-cell lung cancer to gefitinib. N Engl J Med 350:2129–2139

Mok T, Wu Y, Thongprasert S et al (2009) Gefitinib or carboplatin-paclitaxel in pulmonary adenocarcinoma. N Engl J Med 361:947–957

Pieterman R, van Putten J, Meuzelaar J et al (2000) Preoperative staging of non-small-cell lung cancer with positron-emission tomography. N Engl J Med 343:254–261

Pignon J, Arriagada R, Ihde D et al (1992) A meta-analysis of thoracic radiotherapy for small-cell lung cancer. N Engl J Med 327:1618–1624

Pignon JP, Tribodet H, Scagliotti GV et al (2008) Lung adjuvant cisplatin evaluation: a pooled analysis by the LACE Collaborative Group. In J Clin Oncol 26:3552–3559

Rosenzweig K, Sura S, Jackson A et al (2007) Involved-field radiation therapy for inoperable non small-cell lung cancer. J Clin Oncol 25:5557–5561

Rusch V, Giroux D, Kraut M et al (2007) Induction chemoradiation and surgical resection for superior sulcus non-small-cell lung carcinomas: long-term results of Southwest Oncology Group Trial 9416 (Intergroup Trial 0160). J Clin Oncol 25:313–318

Sandler A, Gray R, Perry M et al (2006) Paclitaxel-carboplatin alone or with bevacizumab for non-small-cell lung cancer. N Engl J Med 355:2542–2550

Senan S, Chapet O, Lagerwaard F et al (2004) Defining target volumes for non-small cell lung carcinoma. Semin Radiat Oncol 14:308–314

Shepherd F, Rodrigues Pereira J, Ciuleanu T et al (2005) Erlotinib in previously treated non-small-cell lung cancer. N Engl J Med 353:123–132

Slotman B, Faivre-Finn C, Kramer G et al (2007) Prophylactic cranial irradiation in extensive small-cell lung cancer. N Engl J Med 357:664–672

Timmerman R, Park C, Kavanagh B (2007) The North American experience with stereotactic body radiation therapy in non-small cell lung cancer. J Thorac Oncol 2:S101–S112

Turrisi Ar, Kim K, Blum R et al (1999) Twice-daily compared with once-daily thoracic radiotherapy in limited small-cell lung cancer treated concurrently with cisplatin and etoposide. N Engl J Med 340:265–271

Zatloukal P, Petruzelka L, Zemanova M et al (2004) Concurrent versus sequential chemoradiotherapy with cisplatin and vinorelbine in locally advanced non-small cell lung cancer: a randomized study. Lung Cancer 46:87–98

Lung Shielding

Iris Rusu

Department of Radiation Oncology, Loyola University Medical Center, Maywood, IL, USA

Definition

Shielding blocks employed to reduce the dose to the lung; used only for part of the treatment after a certain dose is reached.

Cross-References

▶ Total Body Irradiation (TBI)

Lymph Node Regions in Head and Neck

BRANDON J. FISHER[1], LARRY C. DAUGHERTY[2]
[1]Department of Radiation Oncology, College of Medicine, Drexel University, Philadelphia, PA, USA
[2]Department of Radiation Oncology, College of Medicine, Drexel University, Glenside, PA, USA

Definition

Level I – Submental and submandibular

Level II – Internal jugular chain, extends from the base of the skull to the bottom of the hyoid bone

Level III – Internal jugular chain between the bottom of the hyoid bone and the bottom of the cricoids; lies anteriorly to the back of the sternocleidomastoid muscle

Level IV – Internal jugular chain, extends from the bottom of the cricoid to the level of the clavicles

Level V – Spinal accessory chain, corresponds to nodes in the posterior triangle

Level VI– Upper visceral nodes, anterior to the thyroid region

Cross-References

▶ Nasopharynx

Lymphedema

ANTHONY E. DRAGUN
Department of Radiation Oncology,
James Graham Brown Cancer Center, University of Louisville School of Medicine, Louisville, KY, USA

Definition

This refers to chronic, painful swelling and restricted mobility of the ipsilateral upper extremity following breast cancer treatment. It is important to distinguish progressive lymphedema symptoms from a disease recurrence in the axilla or supraclavicular fossa. The overall risk of clinically significant lymphedema after breast and axillary surgery is approximately 5–15%. Risk mainly depends on the extent of axillary surgery (complete dissection vs. sentinel lymph node biopsy). The use of axillary irradiation (especially with more antiquated radiotherapy techniques), may increase this risk slightly. Early detection of lymphedema and intervention with complex decongestive physiotherapy is beneficial. Liposuction has also been used in severe cases.

Cross-References

▶ Stage 0 Breast Cancer

Lymphoblastic Neoplasms

▶ Leukemia in General

Lynch Syndrome

▶ Hereditary Nonpolyposis Colorectal Cancer (HNPCC)

M

MACIS

Nisha R. Patel, Michael L. Wong
Department of Radiation Oncology,
College of Medicine, Drexel University,
Philadelphia, PA, USA

Definition
Scoring schema used to calculate a prognostic score with variables such as metastasis, age, primary tumor size, extrathyroidal invasion, and completeness of surgical resection for papillary thyroid cancer.

Cross-References
▶ Thyroid Cancer

Male Breast Cancer

Anthony E. Dragun
Department of Radiation Oncology,
James Graham Brown Cancer Center, University of Louisville School of Medicine, Louisville, KY, USA

Definition
Male breast cancer accounts for less than 1% of all breast cancers in the United States and less than 0.5% of all cancers diagnosed in men. Risk factors include familial genetic breast cancers (BRCA1/2), hyperestrogenic states, and gynecomastia. The majority of men with breast cancer present with a palpable lump, and approximately two-thirds have greater than stage I disease at diagnosis. The principles of diagnostic workup, staging, and management are the same as that for female breast cancer. Mastectomy is usually the operation of choice and indications for post mastectomy radiotherapy are the same as those for women. For early-stage disease, the overall prognosis is similar to that of female breast cancer. Prognosis is worse for men with locally advanced breast cancer or metastatic disease at diagnosis.

Cross-References
▶ Stage 0 Breast Cancer

Male Urethra

Stephan Mose
Department of Radiation Oncology,
Schwarzwald-Baar-Klinikum,
Villingen-Schwenningen, Germany

Synonyms
Carcinoma of the male urethra; Male urethral cancer

Definition/Description
Urethral cancer of the male is an extremely rare disease mostly diagnosed at an advanced tumor stage in patients who are often older than

60 years. The pathogenesis is not clearly defined (history of urethral strictures, sexual transmitted diseases, coincidence with bladder cancer, and HPV infection). Due to the seldom occurrence, there is no standardized therapy. Superficial tumors, which have the best outcome, as well as those of the penile urethra may be treated by transurethral procedures (electroresection and laser), brachytherapy, and partial or complete penectomy. In locally advanced tumors and especially in posterior carcinoma of the bulbomembraneous and prostatic urethra single modalities even if radically performed are inadequate. In small, recently published series, promising results are obtained by simultaneously applied radiochemotherapy with or without salvage surgery.

Anatomy

The male urethra is a mucous membrane embedded in connective tissue, elastic fibers, and smooth muscles. With a length of 20–25 cm and an extension from the bladder neck to the external urethral meatus, the male urethra is divided into three parts. The posterior urethra passes through the prostate (prostatic urethra: length 3–3.5 cm, average diameter 1 cm) and the urogenital diaphragm (membraneous urethra) with the voluntary bladder sphincter. The anterior part passing through the corpus spongiosum is defined as bulbous urethra with its slightly dilated portion from the urogenital diaphragm to the penoscrotal junction and the penile or pendulous urethra that ends in the boat-shaped fossa navicularis and the external ostium within the glans penis. The corpus spongiosum itself lies between the two corpora cavernosa and close to adjacent structures (pubic symphysis, perineum, and scrotum).

While the prostatic urethra contains transitional epithelium only, this gradually changes during its passage through the urogenital diaphragm into pseudostratified columnar epithelium which is also seen in the bulbous urethra.

The more distal part of the anterior urethra is covered by stratified columnar epithelium.

The blood supply is derived from the internal pudendal arteries (A. urethralis) and drains to the correspondent veins. The anterior urethra preferentially drains into the superficial and deep inguinal lymph nodes, whereas the bulbomembranous and the prostatic portion empty themselves into the external iliac, obturator, internal iliac, and presacral nodes.

Epidemiology

Male urethral carcinomas are extremely rare (US population: incidence 4.3 per million), causing the lack of conclusive data. It seems that the disease is twice as high in African-Americans as in whites. The tumor is found in men >60 years of age although approximately 10% are diagnosed in men who are younger than 40 years.

The pathogenesis is rather unknown. Obviously, men with bladder cancer can be expected to coincidentally have or to develop at a later point of time urethral cancer with transitional cell histology. There may be a correlation to chronic irritations, infection with ▶ human papilloma virus (HPV), and sexually transmitted diseases. Urethral trauma and urethral polyps may seldom play a role in tumorgenesis. Furthermore, a history of urethral strictures could be relevant as a high prevalence of cancer is seen in the bulbomembraneous portion where urethral strictures are more common (Swartz et al. 2006).

Clinical Presentation

At the time of diagnosis, most of the patients are symptomatic. These symptoms mostly are not pathognomonic often mimicking benign diseases (infections, obstructive symptoms, and incontinence). However, in 43–72% a stricture is seen; in 17–20% and 11–20% pain and hematuria are reported, respectively. Urethral fistulas, abscess formations, purulent discharge, and necrosis are diagnosed in advanced tumors. A tumor mass is

Male Urethra. Table 1 TNM-classification in male urethral cancer

TNM	Stage	
Ta	0a	Noninvasive, papillary, polypoid, or verrucous carcinoma
Tis	0is	Carcinoma in situ
T1 N0	I	Invasion of the subepithelial connective tissue
T2 N0	II	Invasion of the corpus spongiosum or prostate
T3 N0–1	III	Invasion of the corpus cavernosum or beyond prostate capsule or the bladder neck,
T1–2 N1		Metastasis in a single lymph node ≤2 cm in greatest dimension
T4 N0–1	IV	Invasion of other adjacent organs,
T1–4 N2		Metastasis in a single lymph node >2 cm or multiple lymph nodes
T1–4 N0–2 M1		Distant metastases

palpable in 28–33%. Up to 80% of patients present with T3–4 cancer emphasizing the local tumor growth, while less than 15% demonstrate metastases (especially lung metastases) at the time of initial diagnosis; most of those metastasized tumors are transitional cell carcinomas of the prostatic urethra. Lymph nodes occur in 20–34% nearly almost representing metastatic disease (see Table 1).

Forty to fifty percent of tumors are diagnosed within the anterior urethra, whereas 50–60% of them are found within the posterior portion. More than 50% are undifferentiated tumors (G3). Whereas in former publications there was a prevalence of squamous cell carcinoma, this has changed in recent reports demonstrating a higher incidence of transitional cell carcinomas. This may be partially due to the reported and probably underestimated coincidence of bladder cancer and urethral carcinoma in the prostatic urethra. It has to be argued that a transitional cell carcinoma of the prostatic urethra without simultaneous bladder cancer is diagnosed as urethral cancer whereas in case of simultaneous bladder cancer this urethral involvement is staged as a carcinoma of the bladder. Adenocarcinomas are diagnosed in 2–16%. Other histologic types are

very seldom (epidermoid carcinoma, melanoma, rhabdomyosarcoma, anaplastic carcinomsarcoma, small-cell carcinoma, carcinoid tumors, and non-Hodgkin's lymphoma). Due to the location of the tumor the histology varies: 90% of carcinoma of the prostatic urethra are of transitional cell type, whereas tumors of the penile urethra are primarily squamous cell carcinoma. A transurethral or needle biopsy has to be performed to assure the tumor diagnosis (Mansur 2008).

Differential Diagnosis

Because most of the reported symptoms are nonspecific, benign diseases have to be excluded. This is related to any kind of infections with or without possible complications (urethrocutaneous fistula, abscess, and necrosis), diverticula, and benign strictures. The incidence of a ▶ urethral inverted papilloma is seldom reported; however, the symptoms may mimic a carcinoma.

Imaging Studies

In addition to the physical examination of the external genitalia, rectum, perineum, and palpation of the inguinal lymph nodes, both urethrocytoscopy and rectoscopy add to the findings. Retrograde urethrography is accepted as an initial method to evaluate the urethra although it may be replaced by ultrasound, CT, and MRI. Local staging is completed by CT scanning of the abdomen and pelvis with regard to the tumor invasion into adjacent structures, to the lymph nodes, and the upper urinary tract. The MRI allows the precise definition of the tumor volume and its locoregional extension and is being increasingly used for both staging and follow-up.

To complete the staging, a chest radiography and/or a computer tomography of the lung are necessary; a bone scan should be done as clinically indicated. Up to now, conclusions considering the value of PET (positron emission tomography) scanning cannot be drawn (Kawashima et al. 2004).

Laboratory Studies

Laboratory studies include the complete blood count, basic liver and kidney tests, as well as urine analysis, although none of these tests are diagnostic with regard to urethral cancer. However, they may give an advice about possible infections and organ function in face of further therapies. Tumor markers are not known.

Treatment

Because of the rare incidence of male urethral carcinoma and the consequential lack of secure statistical data, there are no final conclusions regarding therapy. Reported data are often case reports and single center experiences collecting patients over up to 30 years. However, especially in advanced cases, single modality therapies are obviously inadequate, achieving a dismal outcome; after surgery alone the 5-year disease-free survival is 22–38% and 0–15% in tumors of the anterior and posterior urethra respectively; after radiotherapy alone 0–12% were obtained.

Furthermore, therapy varies with staging and location of the tumor. Superficial tumors have a better prognosis (5-year overall survival <83%) independent of location compared to infiltrating tumors (5-year overall survival <45%), which more often tend to develop nodal and distant metastases. Otherwise, in carcinoma of the anterior urethra the 5-year overall survival is 69%, whereas it is 26% in posterior tumors. This holds true in surgically treated patients whereas the localization of the tumor is supposed to be not significantly relevant in radiochemotherapy. Furthermore, the subtype of the common histological diagnoses does not seem to be as important whereas in tumors with rare histological types the outcome in anaplastic carcinomas is poor. However, melanoma may be treated by a combination of surgery, radiotherapy, and chemotherapy; patients with localized lymphoma may be cured by radiotherapy alone.

Surgery

Surgery is the primary therapy in male urethral cancer. The extent of surgery depends on the location and the tumor stage. In those seldom tumors involving the mucosa only (stage Tis, Ta) transurethral endoscopic resection may be performed (electroresection, fulguration, Nd-YAG, and carbon dioxide laser). In superficial lesions of the anterior urethra, partial urethrectomy with the preservation of the penile corpora may be possible, which has to be balanced against the risk of local relapse and/or early dissemination.

Well-selected infiltrating lesions of the fossa navicularis or otherwise distally located small tumors can be cured by amputation of the glans penis or partial penectomy with a 2 cm-margin. A total penectomy should be done if the tumor infiltrates more than the proximal half of the penile urethra. In T1–2 tumors, local recurrences after amputation are seldom described. The prophylactic inguinal lymphonodectomy is not recommended.

In tumors of the bulbomembraneous or prostatic urethra, cystoprostatectomy, en bloc penectomy, and resection of the inferior pubic rami are recommended. In bulky disease, the lower portion of the pubic symphysis may be dissected as well to increase the surgical margins. Also, in posterior urethral carcinoma pelvic lymph nodes should be removed because of the higher incidence of positive nodes and the potential, though limited possibility, of cure, whereas inguinal node resection is performed only if affected nodes are palpable. Because of the high recurrences rate in advanced tumors, preoperative radio(chemo)therapy may be discussed.

The 5-year overall survival after surgery alone is 40–45% with local control rates of approximately 50%. Improved survival was reported in patients with anterior lesions (69%) compared to those with posterior tumors (6–26%) (Dalbagni et al. 1998; Mansur 2008).

Radiotherapy

Although tumor control has been reported especially in superficial anterior lesions alone or in combination with surgery in advanced carcinomas, the role of radiotherapy in male urethral carcinoma is not well defined due to small data.

In very superficial (<5 mm depth) penile urethral carcinoma, an intraluminal brachytherapy implant may be indicated where an afterloading-catheter is introduced into the urethra. The complete penile urethra as well as a safety margin of 5–10 mm may be considered as planning target volume; after surgical endourethral resection, this volume should be reduced to residual disease. An interstitial implant is used in larger penile lesions; after introduction of a Foley catheter hypodermic needles are implanted perpendicular to the axis of the organ and arranged above and below the urethra. Then radioactive wires are loaded. The procedure is comparable to that in brachytherapy of penile cancer; for dosimetry, the rules of the Paris system are used. In selected superficial anterior tumors, a survival rate of 67% was achieved with brachytherapy alone which is comparable to surgical results; in more localized tumors treated by a combination of surgery and brachytherapy, the survival rate was 55%.

If external radiotherapy is performed in larger, mainly posterior tumors the planning target volume should encompass the genital region from the perineum to the upper part of the sacrum including the inguinal and pelvic external/internal iliac lymph nodes. Three-dimensional planning is mandatory; intensity-modulated radiotherapy may be effective in reducing side effects. The recommended dose is 45–50 Gy (1.8–2.0 Gy/day, 5×/week). In definitive radiotherapy, a boost is given with 10–15 Gy, although the results of radiotherapy alone are disappointing. Interestingly, in small series with preoperative radiotherapy local control rates of 83% and a survival rate of 42% were obtained.

In analogy to anal cancer, its comparable histology and association to HPV 16, its similar embryological development, and the pattern of nodal spread it was supposed that the combination of external radiotherapy (tumor and lymph nodes: 45–50 Gy, boost: 10–15 Gy) and effective chemotherapy with mitomycin-c and 5-fluorouracil could achieve encouraging results in male urethral cancer provided that modern techniques are used. In fact, there are some recently published data supporting this standardized procedure with complete responses in 83% and a mean survival of 34 months (5-year overall survival: 60%, 5-year disease-free survival 54%) offering the possibility of organ preservation. In one-third of patients, recurrences were documented (75% local, 25% distant). Interestingly, nonresponder after salvage surgery died within 1 year leading to the presumption that surgery is unable to achieve a complete remission in those aggressive tumors refractory to multimodality therapy. In contrast, in patients responding to chemoradiotherapy salvage surgery provided better survival rates. It is remarkable that these results were obtained in patients with locally advanced tumors with or without lymph node metastases. Furthermore, localization of the tumor, evidence of lymph node metastases, and grading do not seem to predict response and prognosis although the number of published patients is too small to draw final conclusions (Gerbaulet 2002; Cohen et al. 2008; Mansur 2008; Troiano et al. 2009).

Chemotherapy

There is no indication to use chemotherapy alone in primary male urethral carcinoma. Promising data exist when chemotherapy is combined with simultaneous radiotherapy (see above). In metastasized disease, chemotherapy provides a palliative effect; cisplatin, 5-fluorouracil, and mitomycin-c are recommended in squamous cell carcinoma, whereas methotrexate, vinblastine, doxorubicin, and cisplatin may be used in transitional cell carcinoma. In general, the experience is small due to the rarity of this disease.

Sequelae of Therapy

Independent on the modality used (surgery, radiotherapy) the incidence of urethral strictures, urethral fistulas, and urinary incontinence due to the damage of the bladder sphincter are often reported (0–40%) necessitating balloon dilation and/or complex urethral reconstruction. Because organ preservation is not almost possible or, even if it was possible, in most patients sexual function may be impaired or cannot be preserved.

After radical surgery, bowel obstruction, infections, and dysfunction of the conduits for urinary diversion are reported. Reversible acute side effects of radiotherapy that are more pronounced if chemotherapy is simultaneously given include dry and moist desquamation, erythema, and swelling of subcutaneous tissue. Ulceration, necrosis of skin, and lymphedema are seldom after modern radiation treatment; if lymphedema develop a lymphatic spread of tumor is most likely.

Cross-References

▶ Anal Carcinoma
▶ Bladder Cancer
▶ Clinical Aspects of Brachytherapy (BT)
▶ Female Urethral Carcinoma
▶ Penile Cancer

References

Cohen MS, Triaca V, Billmeyer B, Hanley RS, Girshovich L, Shuster T, Oberfield RA, Zinman L (2008) Coordinated chemoradiation therapy with genital preservation for the treatment of primary invasive carcinoma of the male urethra. J Urol 179:536–541

Dalbagni G, Zhang ZF, Lacombe L, Herr HW (1998) Male urethral carcinoma: analysis of treatment outcome. Urology 53:1126–1132

Gerbaulet A (2002) Urethral cancer. In: Gerbaulet A, Pötter R, Materon JJ, Meertens H, van Limbergen E (eds) The GEC ESTRO handbook of brachytherapy, 1st edn. ACCO ESTRO, Leuven

Kawashima A, Sandler CM, Wasserman NF, LeRoy AJ, King BF Jr, Goldman SM (2004) Imaging of urethral disease: a pictorial review. Radiographics 24(Suppl 1):195–216

Mansur DB (2008) Penis and male urethra. In: Halperin EC, Perez CA, Brady LW (eds) Principles and practice of radiation oncology, 5th edn. Wolters Kluwer/Lippincott Wiliams and Wilkens, Philadelphia

Swartz MA, Porter MP, Lin DW, Weiss NS (2006) Incidence of primary urethral carcinoma in the United States. Urology 140:1–5

Troiano M, Corsa P, Raguso A, Cossa S, Piombino M, Guglielmi G, Parisi S (2009) Radiation therapy in urinary cancer: state of the art and perspective. Radiol Med 114:70–82

Male Urethral Cancer

▶ Male Urethra

Malignant Lesion of the Nasopharynx

▶ Nasopharynx

Malignant Melanoma

▶ Melanoma

Malignant Mesothelioma

▶ Pleural Mesothelioma

Malignant Myeloma

▶ Plasma Cell Myeloma

Malignant Neoplasms Associated with Acquired Immunodeficiency Syndrome

BERNADINE R. DONAHUE[1], JAY S. COOPER[2]
[1]Department of Radiation Oncology,
Maimonides Cancer Center, Brooklyn, NY, USA
[2]Maimonides Cancer Center, New York, NY, USA

Synonyms
AIDS-related malignancies; HIV-related malignancies

Definition/Description
HIV-related malignancies are those tumors whose incidence is preferentially increased by prior infection of the host by the human immunodeficiency virus. The incidence and characteristics of malignancies associated with HIV infection have changed over time (Engels et al. 2006a). Early in the epidemic, three types of malignancies occurred at a sufficiently increased incidence in the setting of HIV infection that they qualified as AIDS-defining conditions: Kaposi's sarcoma (KS), non-Hodgkin's lymphoma (NHL), and carcinoma of the uterine cervix. Although not considered AIDS-defining illnesses, anal carcinoma, Hodgkin's disease, and some unusual pediatric-age malignancies also appeared to be more common than expected in the HIV-infected population. More recently, other malignancies, particularly lung, head and neck, and liver cancers appear to have arisen at a somewhat increased frequency in the setting of HIV (Engels et al. 2006b; Patel et al. 2008).

HIV Infection and Combined Antiretroviral Therapy
Over 24 million people have died of AIDS since 1981. Highly active antiretroviral therapy (▶ HAART) was introduced in 1996 and primarily consisted of a two drug nucleoside analog administered with either a protease inhibitor or a non-nucleoside reverse transcriptase inhibitor; other classes of drugs now employed for treatment of HIV include integrase inhibitors, entry inhibitors, maturation inhibitors, and antiviral hyperactivation limiting therapeutics. HAART had a dramatic effect on the prognosis of HIV-infected individuals. In parts of the world where this combination antiretroviral therapy became readily available, the number of opportunistic infections and the number of deaths from AIDS were dramatically reduced. The identification of subtypes of HIV and the specific chemokine receptors to which they bind, provide future hope of further improving the outcome of patients infected with HIV. Unfortunately, the death rate from AIDS remains high in resource-constrained areas of the world where AIDS transmission is unchecked and where medical care and drugs often are lacking. In 2009 alone, an estimated 2.7 million persons contracted HIV and two million people died from AIDS (http://www.data.unaids.org/en/KnowledgeCenter/HIVData/Epidemiology/2009 2010).

Although the survival of HIV-infected individuals unquestionably has improved as a direct consequence of treatment with immunomodulatory agents, the effect of such therapies on HIV-related malignancies has been mixed (Clifford et al. 2005). The incidence of NHL and Kaposi's sarcoma has declined substantially, and hopefully the incidence of cervical cancer will dramatically decline as a result of increasingly widespread vaccination against HPV, but there has been no major change in the incidence of other malignancies. Furthermore, it (not surprisingly) appears that HIV infection does not decrease the incidence of other cancers, and the non-AIDS-related cancers that become increasingly common as humans age will be seen in greater numbers in HIV-infected populations as they age (Herida et al. 2003; Bower et al. 2006; Bedimo et al. 2009; Powles et al. 2008; Silverberg and Abrams 2009).

In general, for persons who are infected by HIV, "standard" stage-directed therapies for each malignancy are required for control of the malignancy (Donahue and Cooper 2008; Spano et al. 2008). However, such "standard" treatments may need to be attenuated based on the immunologic status, the viral load, coexisting opportunistic infections and comorbidities in any given individual. A major remaining challenge in the management of persons with cancer and HIV is how most appropriately to integrate antiretroviral therapy into cancer treatment regimens. Whether such therapy should be delivered concomitantly with, or just after, particular chemotherapy regimens is still debated. Laboratory data suggests that certain protease inhibitors may increase radiosensitivity, however, this has not been borne out in the clinic. Nevertheless, the myelosuppressive nature of some of the antiretrovirals should raise some concern in the face of aggressive chemotherapy and/or when radiation therapy is delivered to large volumes of bone marrow. Similarly the neurotoxicity of other antiretrovirals may need to be considered when radiation therapy includes the CNS (Housri et al. 2010).

The epidemiology, the clinical presentation, the diagnostic evaluation, the treatment, and the prognosis of each of the HIV-associated malignancies in adults are presented below. For additional details regarding the delivery of radiation, the sections addressing the specific neoplasm in this encyclopedia should be consulted. Lung, head and neck, and liver cancers have been included in this section because of the suggestive available data; however, other malignancies which are being identified in the aging HIV population include skin cancers, breast cancer, prostate cancer, colorectal cancer, and testicular tumors.

AIDS-Defining Malignancies

Systemic Non-Hodgkin's Lymphoma

Epidemiology

▶ Non-Hodgkin's lymphoma (NHL) in HIV-infected persons was one of the first malignancies designated by the CDC as an AIDS-defining illness. Its incidence has been shown to correlate with the duration of immunosuppression, CD4 count 1 year prior to the diagnosis of NHL, and B-cell stimulation. The observed fall in the incidence of NHL with the introduction of HAART was most likely secondary to an overall decrease in the proportion of patients who had low CD4 counts.

Clinical Presentation

The most common presentations of HIV-associated systemic NHL are rapidly developing adenopathy and/or constitutional "B" symptoms (fevers, unexplained weight loss, night sweats). The majority of patients will present with advanced-stage disease and symptoms. Diagnosis generally is obtained from the histologic examination of a clinically suspicious peripheral lymph node. The most common histologic subtypes are high-grade B-cell lymphoma and Burkitt's lymphoma; however, intermediate-grade (diffuse large cell type) lymphomas are often seen as well. Additionally, during the height of the AIDS era, a previously unrecognized form of lymphoma, called primary effusion or body cavity lymphoma, was identified in HIV-infected patients. It appears to be associated with Human Herpesvirus 8 (HHV-8) and is characterized by body cavity lymphomatous effusions in the absence of widespread lymphadenopathy. Survival from this entity was worse than for other types of NHL, on the order of 2–5 months even with aggressive therapy.

Diagnostic Evaluation

As patients who have HIV-NHL frequently have extranodal involvement, staging evaluation should include chest, abdomen, and pelvic computerized tomograms; bone marrow biopsy; and CSF analysis.

Treatment

Early in the AIDS epidemic it was recognized that treatment of HIV-NHL lymphoma with high-dose chemotherapy regimens designed to cure non-AIDS-related lymphomas was not well tolerated and resulted in substantial toxicity, as well as high rates of infectious complications. As a result, attenuated doses of cytotoxic chemotherapy or standard-dose chemotherapy plus cytokine support were introduced. However, with the availability of HAART, it became feasible to employ standard chemotherapy regimens, and a major question now is whether HAART should be administered in conjunction with, or after, chemotherapy. In general, it is recommended that zidovudine be avoided because of its myelosuppressive effects. The current paradigm is to treat HIV-infected persons in the same aggressive fashion as noninfected persons; however, the prognosis remains worse and the toxicity is higher.

Chemotherapy

Early studies reported complete remission rates of approximately 50%, but median survivals of only 6–7 months and 1-year survivals of approximately 25%. Further study helped to define regimens with high efficacy with acceptable toxicity such as CDE (cyclophosphamide, doxorubicin, and etoposide)

and EPOCH (etoposide, prednisone, vincristine, cyclophosphamide, and doxorubicin). The advent of rituximab, an anti-CD20 antibody, which has improved in survival for patients with non-HIV-associated NHL, may improve the outcome in HIV-NHL. Trials incorporating rituximab have shown complete response rates of approximately 60–75%, and 2 year overall survivals of 55–75% (Spano et al. 2008). However, data has been somewhat contradictory about the safety of this approach because of potential infectious complications. Early trials showed increased rates of infections with the addition of rituximab; however, more recent trials including Aids Malignancy Consortium 034 reported no increased risk of severe toxicity (Levine et al. 2008). In countries challenged by the lack of HAART, regimens employing dose-modified oral chemotherapy have been developed which appear to result in outcomes comparable to the pre-HAART experience in the USA.

CNS prophylaxis with intrathecal chemotherapy was frequently used routinely in the setting of high grade NHL and HIV infection, particularly in patients with extranodal disease. However, the risk of CNS involvement appears to be higher in Epstein-Barr Virus (EBV)-positive persons and it may be that prophylaxis can be reserved for a selected subset of patients with EBV-infected tumors.

Radiotherapy

The role of radiotherapy in the treatment of HIV-NHL has not been evaluated methodically. Radiation therapy probably should be considered for the same indications it is considered in immunocompetent individuals; however, it is not clear whether treatment modifications are indicated in the setting of HIV-NHL because of concerns of HIV-related radiosensitization.

Radiation therapy clearly can provide palliative therapy for patients who develop lymphomatous meningitis. The majority of these patients have far-advanced AIDS and although this approach has been shown to result in a 60–70% clinical and/or cytological response, median time to progression is generally only 2–2.5 months.

Prognosis

Median survival for patients who have HIV-NHL more than doubled, from approximately 4 to 9 months, after the introduction of HAART. Currently, one half to three fourths of patients with HIV-NHL survive 2 years. The International Prognostic Index (IPI), a model designed to predict the outcome of NHL, generally is a reliable prognostic indicator of outcome for patients who have HIV-NHL. However, the degree of immunodeficiency imparted by HIV, as measured by surrogates such as CD4 level and HIV plasma RNA, also plays an important role in the outcome of patients who have HIV-NHL.

Primary CNS Lymphoma

Epidemiology

At the height of the AIDS epidemic, the incidence of primary CNS lymphoma (PCNSL) in persons who had AIDS was more than 3,000 times higher than in the general population. PCNSL was most commonly seen when the CD4 count dropped below 50 cells/mm^3. HAART dramatically decreased the incidence of HIV-PCNSL (from 8.4 per 1,000 person-years pre-HAART to 1.1 once HAART was available), although it is still seen in geographic regions where combined antiretroviral therapy (▶ cART) is not available.

Clinical Presentation

In most patients who have HIV-associated PCNSL, the diagnosis is suggested by the onset of headaches or a change in mental status. Nearly one third have motor or sensory abnormalities, but PCNSL may present as other symptoms that result from an intracranial mass such as seizures, visual changes, vomiting, etc. PCNSL in individuals with AIDS is more likely to be multifocal as compared to PCNSL in immunocompetent persons. The vast majority of cases are EBV-positive.

Diagnostic Evaluation

The clinical and radiographic findings of PCNSL are often indistinguishable from other pathologic processes (primarily toxoplasmosis) that also tend to occur in HIV-infected patients. The typical radiographic appearance is multiple contrast-enhancing lesions, frequently in a periventricular location. Early in the AIDS era patients often were treated empirically for toxoplasmosis and, if this treatment did not result in clinical improvement, empiric treatment for presumed PCNSL was delivered. Outcomes with this approach were poor; however, as survival from AIDS improved with HAART, biopsy for definitive diagnosis became customary. Pathology specimens usually show high-grade, diffuse large B-cell tumors, often of the immunoblastic subtype; low-grade lymphomas are very rarely seen. If biopsy cannot be performed, there should be a high suspicion of PCNSL in the proper clinical setting of low CD4, negative toxoplasmosis titers, appropriate radiographic findings, and the identification of EBV DNA by PCR of the CSF.

The standardized guidelines for the baseline evaluation and response assessment of PCNSL established by the International PCNSL Collaborative Group should be employed in patients who are able to be treated with definitive intent. These include initial staging with gadolinium–enhanced MRI, lumbar puncture for CSF cytology (unless medically contraindicated), detailed ophthalmological examination, CT scans of the chest, abdomen, and pelvis, bone marrow biopsy with aspirate, and consideration of testicular ultrasound.

Treatment

Chemotherapy

When possible, methotrexate-based chemotherapy should be considered for patients who have

HIV-PCNSL. High-dose methotrexate-based chemotherapy with leukovorin rescue is now the standard of care for immunocompetent patients who have PCNSL and results in median survivals ≥3 years. However, many HIV-infected patients, who are sufficiently immunosuppressed to develop PCNSL, may be unable to tolerate methotrexate. Drugs such as temozolomide and rituximab, which are being explored in the setting of PCNSL in immunocompetent patients, have not been tested to any degree in persons with HIV-PCNSL.

Radiotherapy

The role of radiotherapy alone in the treatment of PCNSL is palliative although it usually produces clinical and radiographic evidence of tumor response. Various fractionation schedules ranging from a short palliative-intent course of 3,000 cGy in ten fractions over 2 weeks to a more protracted course of 5,000 cGy, delivered in 180–200 cGy per fraction over 5–6 weeks, have been employed. However, mean overall survival with radiation therapy has been in the range of 2–5 months. HAART may have an impact on this poor outcome. The irradiated volume typically includes the cranial meninges and posterior orbits.

The practice of withholding RT or of employing "low-dose" consolidative cranial RT (i.e., 2,340 cGy) after a complete response to chemotherapy has been adopted for immunocompetent patients with PCNSL, and although this approach seems appealing for patients who are infected by HIV, it has not been fully evaluated in the setting of combined antiretroviral therapy.

Prognosis

HAART has decreased the incidence of HIV-PCNSL; however, its effect on the outcome of the disease remains uncertain (Kreisl et al. 2008). In general, the results of treatment of HIV-PCNSL uniformly are poor and the strategy of up-front chemotherapy that has proven successful in immunocompetent patients has not

been closely replicated in the setting of AIDS. The majority of series predate the use of HAART, and the precise influence of aggressive antiretroviral treatment on outcome remains unclear, although there is some hope that HAART has improved outcome (Skiest and Crosby 2003). There are anecdotal reports of regression of PCNSL with the institution of HAART and case reports of survival ≥2 years (Aboulafia and Puswella 2007). Recent intriguing data from Japan reports a survival rate of 64% at 3 years in a cohort of irradiated patients who were receiving HAART. Patients who received (or, perhaps more accurately, who were able to receive) doses ≥3,000 cGy fared better than those receiving lower doses. Unfortunately, one third of persons who lived >12 months manifested leukoencephalopathy (Nagai et al. 2010).

Given the virtually uniform finding of EBV in HIV-PCNSL, treatment directed at both HIV and EBV has been explored. Combinations of zidovudine, ganciclovir, and interleukin-2 have been piloted (AIDS Malignancy Consortium trial 019). The incidence of myelosuppression with this regimen is high, and this remains an experimental approach (Aboulafia et al. 2006). For the subgroup of AIDS patients who have CD4 >200, no concurrent opportunistic infections, and who can tolerate aggressive therapy consisting of either methotrexate and/or whole brain radiotherapy, median survival appears to be on the order of 10–18 months.

Cervical Cancer

Epidemiology

Uterine cervix carcinoma in the presence of HIV infection was accepted by the CDC as an AIDS-defining illness in 1993. It was the sixth most common initial AIDS-defining illness in women and the most common AIDS-related malignancy. Cervical dysplasia, the precursor to invasive disease, was found in nearly 50% of HIV-infected women.

However, it was never entirely clear whether there was a substantially higher incidence of invasive disease. Invasive cervical cancer does not appear to have as strong a relationship to immune function as other HIV associated malignancies and, in fact, it can be argued that since the introduction of HAART, there is little evidence to support the continued status of cervical cancer as an AIDS-defining illness. Even in Africa where constrained resources have limited the availability of HAART and the incidence of HIV infection in women continues to rise, an increased incidence of invasive cervical carcinoma has not been documented.

As in immunocompetent women, there is a strong association between human papilloma virus (HPV) infection and risk for cervical epithelial abnormalities (Chaturvedi et al. 2009). As compared with HIV-seronegative women, HIV-infected women have a higher rate of persistent infection with HPV-16 or HPV-18, the viral types which are most strongly associated with cervical carcinoma. Women who are coinfected with HIV and HPV are at particular risk of developing intermediate and high grade dysplasia and the frequency and severity of dysplasia appear to correlate inversely with CD4 counts. Data suggest that the introduction of HAART may reduce HPV infection and squamous intraepithelial neoplasms in HIV-positive women (Minkoff et al. 2010).

Clinical Presentation

HIV-infected women often present with advanced-stage disease and, as observed in Africa, frequently at a younger age than their noninfected counterparts. In addition to vaginal bleeding and dyspareunia, patients may present complaining of abdominal or back pain, weight loss, or palpable cervical adenopathy.

Diagnostic Evaluation

Routine gynecological evaluation, including PAP smears (and colposcopy when warranted), is the most successful means of detecting the dysplastic and in situ lesions (CIN) that are precursors to invasive lesions. In the setting of advanced invasive cancer, EUA, cystoscopy and sigmoidoscopy, and full body CT scans are indicated.

Treatment

Surgery

HIV-infected women treated with laser/cone or cryotherapy for CIN have an increased risk of major bleeding or infection as compared with uninfected patients. The small proportion of patients who have early-stage, non-bulky disease are well treated in a fashion similar to non-HIV-infected women, that is, with radical hysterectomy and pelvic lymph node dissection.

Chemotherapy-Enhanced Radiotherapy

The stage of disease should guide treatment and patients who have advanced local-regional disease should be treated in the same fashion as their non-HIV-infected counterparts if permitted by their immune status and overall medical condition (see the section on cervical cancer in this encyclopedia for the standard of care for each stage of cervical cancer). The current standard of care for advanced cervical cancer is a combination of concurrent radiation therapy and cisplatin-based chemotherapy. There is little data to demonstrate the routine feasibility and/or efficacy of this approach in the setting of AIDS; however, as RT alone historically resulted in poor outcome in patients who had HIV-associated cervical cancer (50% with no or minimal response to treatment and uniform rapid progression disease), advanced cervical cancers in women who do not have a specific contraindication to chemotherapy should be treated with chemotherapy-enhanced external-beam radiotherapy and an intracavitary brachytherapy boost.

Radiotherapy Alone

Radiation therapy alone is appropriate only for patients who are too ill for chemotherapy and, in such circumstances, is not innocuous. When RT alone has been used to treat cervical cancer in HIV-infected women the rates of acute toxicity, particularly GU, GI, and cutaneous toxicity, have been higher than would otherwise be expected (Gichangi et al. 2006). However, palliative radiation therapy (or chemotherapy) may be used to reduce symptoms such as pain and bleeding.

Prognosis

The exact outcome of cervical carcinoma in HIV-infected patients who are treated with "standard" chemoradiation is unclear. Unfortunately, as is true of other malignancies, cervical carcinoma appears to be more aggressive in the HIV-infected population than in the immunocompetent population. Thus the key to improving outcome is prevention and, when that is not possible, early diagnosis of cervical abnormalities. Recombinant vaccines targeting HPV-16 and HPV-18, and close surveillance, including PAP smears and colposcopy, currently are the best weapons against HIV-cervical cancer. Prospective data from the Women's Interagency Human Immunodeficiency Virus Study has confirmed that with close monitoring, that is, PAP smears every 6 months, and appropriate intervention, the incidence of invasive cervical cancer among women who were infected by HIV was not higher than in other women (Massad et al. 2009).

Kaposi's Sarcoma

▶ Kaposi's sarcoma (KS) is a mesenchymal neoplasm whose histologic diagnosis requires the identification of both spindle cell (the malignant component) and vascular elements within the lesion (Mitsuyasu et al. 2010).

Epidemiology

AIDS-Kaposi's sarcoma (arises from the interplay of two viruses: the Human Immunodeficiency Virus (HIV) and the HHV-8 (also known as KS-associated herpesvirus (KSHV)). The HHV-8 virus has been detected in AIDS-related, endemic (the common African form), and classic (occurring in elderly men of Eastern European or Mediterranean ancestry) Kaposi's sarcoma; however, AIDS-KS is unique in that it appears to require coinfection with both HIV and HHV-8. HIV produces the immunosuppression that facilitates HHV-8 induction of KS and likely fosters its widespread growth pattern.

Clinical Presentation

AIDS-KS can be seen on virtually any skin or mucosal surface and initially is typically light to moderate purple in color. Over time it tends to darken. The lesions can be macular, plaque-like, or nodular, with or without associated adenopathy and/or lymphedema. Unlike classic KS, which nearly always initially presents as an asymptomatic singular lesion or a cluster on the skin, at or near the ankles, at presentation AIDS-KS lesions can be either single or numerous, can occur on virtually any skin or mucosal surface and may cause pain, bleeding, and/or disfigurement. Oropharyngeal lesions can result in life-threatening airway obstruction and pulmonary involvement can result in life-threatening respiratory compromise. Visceral KS often involves the aerodigestive tract and can cause bleeding or obstruction. As infiltration of lymph nodes and lymphatics occurs, progressive edema can result, particularly with involvement of the lower extremity.

Diagnostic Evaluation

In deference to the potential widespread involvement by KS, inspection of all skin and visible mucosal surfaces is required; endoscopic evaluation of the gastrointestinal tract also is appropriate for any patient who has GI symptoms. When KS is not confined to the ankle region and/or is detected in a relatively young person, a workup for HIV should be obtained: complete physical examination, blood count and chemistries including CD4 lymphocyte count and viral load, chest x-ray, tuberculin test, anergy screen, and screen for sexually transmitted diseases. Biopsy confirmation of skin lesions prior to the initiation of therapy is generally appropriate, but biopsy of visceral lesions may be contraindicated because of the risk of hemorrhage. The characteristic endoscopic and radiographic findings of GI Kaposi's should suffice when the rest of the clinical picture is concordant.

Treatment

Where available, the best treatment of AIDS-KS is its prevention with combined antiretroviral therapy designed to suppress HIV. However, even after lesions form, combined therapy can induce durable regression in approximately 60% of patients.

Chemotherapy

For widely disseminated disease that fails to respond to combined antiretroviral therapy, a variety of regimens can be chosen based on the urgency of symptom relief, the overall condition of the patient and the specific comorbidities present. The combination of Adriamycin (doxorubicin), bleomycin, and vincristine (ABV), the initial "gold standard" of therapy has largely been replaced by liposomal encapsulated daunorubicin and doxorubicin because they have at least comparable activity with a more favorable toxicity profiles. The liposomal drugs are generally now used as first-line therapy with response rates of 25% and a median duration of 4 months. Paclitaxel also has been approved for treatment; toxicity is mild except for myelosuppression and response rates of approximately 60% (nearly all partial responses) with a 10 month median duration have been reported. Consequently, Paclitaxel has become a common second or third line drug (following the liposomally encapsulated agents), by virtue of its activity and acceptable toxicity.

Radiotherapy

Radiation therapy can provide effective palliation of pain, bleeding, or edema. Typically, small fields that include only the distressing lesion and a small margin are treated. A wide variety of doses produce regression of disease; however, greater doses are associated with a higher response rates, a lower incidence of residual pigmentation and a longer duration of tumor control. A total of 3,000 cGy delivered in 10 fractions over 2 weeks produces response in more than 90% of lesions and approximately 70% respond completely. However, for patients who have far-advanced AIDS (where a briefer duration of palliation will suffice and the appearance of the lesion is not as important), a dose of 800 cGy in one fraction often is preferable. Similarly, palliation of the pain associated with swollen extremities can be obtained with a single fraction of 800 cGy.

Prognosis

At present it is not possible to predict which lesions will behave in a more chronic versus aggressive fashion. As a general tendency, patients who have very few helper T-cells, prior opportunistic infections and/or constitutional symptoms (fevers, night sweats, weight loss) have a worse prognosis. Pulmonary lesions also tend to herald a poor prognosis. In contrast, with combined antiretroviral therapy, cutaneous KS poses far less risk today than at the beginning of the AIDS era. In fact, they largely have stopped needing to be treated by radiotherapy.

Non-AIDS Defining Malignancies

As we enter the third decade of the AIDS epidemic, it has become increasingly evident that the underlying immunosuppression that is the hallmark of AIDS will influence the incidence and manifestations of diseases which are not specifically related to infection with HIV. Furthermore, as HIV infection becomes more treatable and the population living with AIDS ages, it is becoming clear that HIV-infected individuals are at higher risk for the development of non-AIDS-defining malignancies, and may present with more advanced disease. Generally, stage-for-stage, the diagnostic evaluation of these cancers in persons infected by HIV is similar to those without HIV infection. However, the epidemiology and, where data is available, the influence of HIV on the treatment and the prognoses of these non-AIDS defining malignancies is unique.

Anal Cancer

HIV infection was implicated as an independent risk for ▶ anal carcinoma in the 1990s with its incidence reported to be approximately 100-fold greater in the HIV-infected population as compared to the noninfected population. However, studies of homosexual men in New York City and San Francisco showed a greater increase in the incidence of anal cancer in HIV-seronegative men than in HIV-seropositive men. It is clear that anal carcinomas appear to be related to sexually transmitted HPV (with anal intercourse being a risk factor) and HIV-infected homosexual men have increased serum HPV DNA as compared with HIV-seronegative homosexual men. How combined antiretroviral therapy has influenced the incidence is still being defined, but recent data from large European cohorts evaluating the incidence of non-AIDS-defining cancers showed an elevated incidence of anal cancer during the pre-HAART era (1983–1995), the "early HAART" era (1996–2001), and the "established HAART" era (2002–2007) with similar standardized incidence ratios in all three periods (Powles et al. 2008). Thus, at present, it appears that HAART does not diminish the excess risk of anal cancer in the HIV positive population.

Early stage lesions may present as an incidental finding during excision of condylomata or hemorrhoids, or may be identified when patients present with anal fissures. However, the majority of patients who have HIV-anal carcinoma present with advanced disease and signs and symptoms may include perianal/rectal pain, tenesmus, bleeding, mucous drainage or palpable inguinal adenopathy. Evaluation and work-up includes DRE, inguinal node evaluation with biopsy or FNA of suspicious nodes, anoscopy, gynecological exam in women, body CTs, and consideration of a PET scan.

In patients who have small, low-grade, early-stage lesions without any evidence of nodal involvement, local excision with wide margins *may* be acceptable if the sphincter function is preserved. Generally, if treatment is to be definitive, chemoradiation is the treatment of choice, the standard being radiation therapy and concurrent 5-FU/Mitomycin-c. This treatment should be offered to HIV-infected patients with appropriately staged anal carcinoma if possible. However, patients who have advanced HIV have the potential for severe myelosuppression and hemolytic uremic syndrome and the decision to eliminate mitomycin-c or substitute cisplatinum (which in immunocompetent patients is associated with higher rates of colostomy), and/or treat with reduced volume pelvic fields, should be made on an individual basis. Although treatment breaks are associated with a higher incidence of recurrence, radiation therapy administered in conjunction with chemotherapy for anal cancer frequently results in marked moist desquamation, necessitating temporary interruption of therapy. Initial series utilizing chemoradiation in the setting of HIV-anal cancer reported that patients with HIV infection manifested more toxicity than non-HIV-infected persons and required longer breaks for severe skin reactions and chemotherapy dose reductions because of neutropenia. However, recent series have shown that with modern management, including IMRT and growth factor support, hematologic toxicity in HIV patient was similar to immunocompetent patients. Because CD4 counts may decrease and viral load increase after combined modality treatment monitoring of these immunologic parameters is warranted (Barriger et al. 2009; Fraunholz et al. 2009; Salama et al. 2007; Seo et al. 2009).

In the pre-HAART era, HIV-anal carcinoma appeared to be associated with a shorter survival and a higher incidence of local failure than non-HIV-anal cancer. It appears that after the introduction of HAART, the outcome for persons who have HIV-anal cancer has improved with recent series showing local control rates of 60–65% and overall 2 year survival rates of 70–75%, which is similar to rates in the non-HIV population. Newer strategies employing targeted agents, such as in an AIDS Malignancy Consortium phase II study, which is evaluating cetuximab in addition to 5-FU/cisplatin with radiation, may improve the outcome of HIV-associated anal carcinoma (http://clinicaltrials. gov/ct2/show/NCT00324415 2010).

Given the similar etiology of anal and cervical carcinoma, it makes sense that the key to improving outcome will be prevention and early diagnosis of anal mucosal abnormalities. Rigorous surveillance for anal intraepithelial neoplasia with cytology and anoscopy in the population at risk is warranted and there is hope that widespread vaccination for HPV would be a major public health advance against anal cancer.

Hodgkin's Lymphoma

The relative risk of developing ▶ Hodgkin's lymphoma in the setting of HIV infection is increased as compared with the general population (Biggar et al. 2006). The exact magnitude of the increase has been difficult to calculate, but a study of 302,824 HIV-infected (including AIDS) patients between the ages of 15 and 69 years showed a relative risk of 11.5 of developing Hodgkin's lymphoma in HIV-infected individuals (Frisch et al. 2001). The incidence of this disease in the HIV-infected population substantially *increased* after the introduction of HAART as documented by recent data from large European cohort clearly

showing a rising standardized incidence ratio from 1983 through 2007, and with multivariate analysis showing that HAART was associated with an increased risk of disease (Powles et al. 2008).

The explanation for the rise after combined antiretroviral therapy became widely available is unclear; however, one intriguing explanation involves the relationship between Reed Sternberg cells and CD4 cells (Levine 2006). The risk of Hodgkin's lymphoma appears to peak when HAART reconstitutes the immune system and CD4 cells reach levels of 150–190 cells/mm^3. It is postulated that Reed Sternberg cells produce growth factors that increase the influx of CD4 cells, which in turn provide signals that cause the proliferation of Reed Sternberg cells. If CD4 cells stimulate the growth of Reed Sternberg cells, it would stand to reason that as HAART improves the CD4 cell count, more of these cells are available to stimulate growth of the cell associated with Hodgkin's lymphoma.

Hodgkin's lymphoma in patients who are HIV infected tends to be advanced (bone marrow involvement is seen in 50% of patients) and is usually accompanied by B symptoms. Importantly, it can be associated with very unusual manifestations, such as presentation with a gastric or intracranial mass. In addition to the usual prognostic factors for Hodgkin's lymphoma, low CD4 count and preexisting AIDS confer a worse prognosis.

In the past, only 50% of patients had a complete response following combination chemotherapy and 2-year survival was on the order of 45%. However, more recent data suggests that the outcome may be improving in the setting of HAART and combination chemotherapy (regimens typically employed for the treatment of Hodgkin lymphoma such as ABVD). The use of the Stanford V regimen with concurrent HAART resulted in a complete response rate of 81%, although nearly one third of patients required reduction in drug doses because of toxicity (Spina et al. 2002). Radiation therapy should be considered for the same indications it is considered in non-HIV-associated Hodgkin's lymphoma; however, little data on its use and tolerance in this setting exists.

Lung Cancer

Studies reporting an increased incidence of ▶ lung cancer in persons with HIV infection may be somewhat confounded by the fact that there is a higher incidence of smoking in the HIV population (Cadranel et al. 2006). Nevertheless, multiple epidemiologic studies have shown standardized incidence ratios of 2:3 for lung cancer. The presentation of lung cancer in this population is marked by young age at presentation (38–50 years) and 75–100% of patients have advanced disease at diagnosis. The most common subtype is adenocarcinoma. It is unclear as to whether combined antiretroviral therapy improves the outcome of these patients. Case reports have documented increased toxicity (particularly esophageal) in patients with HIV irradiated for lung cancer, however, larger series do not necessarily report increased toxicity (although doses of >6,000 cGy usually were not employed) (Housri et al. 2010). How to incorporate antiretroviral drug regimens into lung cancer treatment regimens remains undefined. In general, an attempt should be made to deliver "standard" treatment based on the stage of the disease with the caveat that the treatment approach may need to be modified based on the patient's immunological status, viral load, and coexisting opportunistic infections.

Head and Neck Tumors

Given the increased smoking rate and HPV infection rate observed in persons who are infected by HIV, it should not be surprising to see an increased incidence of both smoking and HPV-related squamous cell head and neck tumors in HIV-infected persons. North American data provides some evidence that since the beginning of the HAART era, there is an increased incidence of head and neck cancers in persons with HIV infection. And, a recent report of a large European cohort of HIV-infected persons documented a trend in increasing incidence from the pre-HAART era through the present, but this did not reach statistical incidence. To date, there have been only a few case reports describing the treatment of head and neck malignancies in patients infected by HIV; they do not suggest the same increased mucosal sensitivity as is seen in patients with HIV-KS.

Liver Cancer

Increased levels of hepatitis B and C coinfections in the HIV population may explain the higher standardized incidence ratios reported in both North American and European data sets, although the data is conflicting as to whether the incidence is higher for persons receiving combined antiretroviral therapy. The French have published on the feasibility of liver transplant for cirrhosis in persons with hepatitis and HIV (Tateo et al. 2009) but data on the treatment of ▶ hepatocellular carcinoma in the setting of HIV is lacking.

Cross-References

▶ Anal Carcinoma
▶ Hodgkin's Lymphoma
▶ Larynx
▶ Liver and Hepatobiliary Tract
▶ Lung
▶ Non-Hodgkins Lymphoma
▶ Skin Cancer
▶ Uterine Cervix

References

Aboulafia DM, Puswella AL (2007) Highly active antiretroviral therapy as the sole treatment for AIDS-related primary central nervous system lymphoma: a case report with implications for treatment. AIDS Patient Care STDs 21(12):900–907

Aboulafia DM, Ratner L, Miles SA, Harrington WJ (2006) Jr. AIDS Associated Malignancies Clinical Trials

Consortium. Antiviral and immunomodulatory treatment for AIDS-related primary central nervous system lymphoma: AIDS Malignancies Consortium pilot study 019. Clin Lymphoma Myeloma 6:399–402

Barriger RB, Calley C, Cárdenes HR (2009) Treatment of anal carcinoma in immune-compromised patients. Clin Transl Oncol 11(9):609–614

Bedimo RJ, McGinnis KA, Dunlap M et al (2009) Incidence of non-AIDS-defining malignancies in HIV-infected versus noninfected patients in the HAART era: impact of immunosuppression. J Acquir Immune Defic Syndr 52(2):203–208

Biggar RJ, Jaffe ES, Goedart JJ et al (2006) Hodgkin lymphoma and immunodeficiency in persons with HIV/AIDS. Blood 108:3786–3791

Bower M, Palmieri C, Dhillon T (2006) AIDS-related malignancies: changing epidemiology and the impact of highly active antiretroviral therapy. Curr Opin Infect Dis 19(1):14–19

Cadranel J, Garfield D, Lavole A et al (2006) Lung cancer in HIV infected patients: facts, questions and challenges. Thorax 61:1000–1008

Chaturvedi AK, Madeleine MM, Biggar RJ, Engels EA (2009) Risk of human papillomavirus-associated cancers among persons with AIDS. J Natl Cancer Inst 101(16):1120–1130

Clifford GM, Polesol J, Rickenbach M et al (2005) Cancer in the Swiss HIV cohort study: association with immunodeficiency, smoking, and highly active antiretroviral therapy. J Natl Cancer Inst 97:425–432

Donahue B, Cooper JS (2008) Malignant neoplasms associated with the Acquired Immunodeficiency Syndrome (AIDS), chapter 31. In: Perez C, Brady L (eds) Principles and practice of radiation oncology, 5th edn. Lippincott Williams & Wilkins, Philadelphia

Engels EA, Pfeiffer RM, Goedert JJ et al (2006a) Trends in cancer risk among people with AIDS in the United States 1980–2002. AIDS 20:1645–1654

Engels EA, Brock MV, Chen J et al (2006b) Elevated incidence of lung cancer among HIV-infected individuals. J Clin Oncol 24:1383–1388

Fraunholz I, Weiss C, Eberlein K et al (2009) Concurrent chemoradiotherapy with 5-fluorouracil and mitomycin-C for invasive anal carcinoma in human immunodeficiency virus-positive patients receiving highly active antiretroviral therapy. Int J Radiat Oncol Biol Phys 76(5):1425–1432

Frisch M, Biggar RJ, Engels EA et al (2001) Association of cancer with AIDS-related immunosuppression in adults. JAMA 285:1736–1745

Gichangi P, Bwayo J, Estimable B et al (2006) HIV impact on acute morbidity and pelvic tumor control following radiotherapy for cervical cancer. Gynecol Oncol 100:405–411

Herida M, Mary-Krause M, Kaphan R et al (2003) Incidence of non-AIDS-defining cancers before and during the highly active antiretroviral therapy era in a cohort of human immunodeficiency virus-infected patients. J Clin Oncol 21:3447–3453

Housri N, Yarchoan R, Kaushal A (2010) Radiotherapy for patients with the human immunodeficiency virus: are special precautions necessary? Cancer 116:273–283

http://www.data.unaids.org/en/KnowledgeCenter/HIVData/Epidemiology/2009. Accessed 26 May 2010

http://clinicaltrials.gov/ct2/show/NCT00324415. Accessed 26 May 2010

Kreisl TN, Panageas KS, Elkin EB et al (2008) Treatment patterns and prognosis in patients with human immunodeficiency virus and primary central system lymphoma. Leuk Lymphoma 49(9):1710–1716

Levine AM (2006) Hodgkin lymphoma: to the HAART of the matter. Blood 108:3630

Levine AM, Lee J, Kaplan L et al (2008) Efficacy and toxicity of concurrent rituximab plus infusional EPOCH in HIV-associated lymphoma: AIDS Malignancy Consortium Trial 034. J Clin Oncol 26:460s (suppl;abst 8527)

Massad LS, Seaberg EC, Watts DH et al (2009) Long-term incidence of cervical cancer in women with human immunodeficiency virus. Cancer 115(3):524–530

Minkoff H, Zhong Y, Burk RD et al (2010) Influence of adherent and effective antiretroviral therapy use on human papillomavirus infection and squamous intraepithelial lesions in human immunodeficiency virus-positive women. J Infect Dis 201(5):681–690

Mitsuyasu RT, Cooper JS (2010) AIDS-related malignancies, chapter 24. In: Pazdur R, Wagman LD, Camphausen KA, Hoskins WJ (eds) Cancer management: a multidisciplinary approach, 20th edn. CMPMedica, Norwalk, CT

Nagai H, Odawara T, Ajisawa A et al (2010) Whole brain radiation alone produces favourable outcomes for AIDS-related primary central nervous system lymphoma in the HAART era. Eur J Haematol 84(6):499–505

Patel P, Hanson DL, Sullivan PS et al (2008) Incidence of types of cancer among HIV-infected persons compared with the general population in the United States, 1992–2003. Ann Intern Med 148:728–736

Powles T, Robinson D, Stebbing J et al (2008) Highly active antiretroviral therapy and the incidence of non-AIDS-defining cancers in people with HIV infection. J Clin Oncol 27:884–890

Salama JK, Mell LK, Schomas DA et al (2007) Concurrent chemotherapy and intensity-modulated radiation therapy for anal canal cancer patients: a multicenter experience. J Clin Oncol 25(29):4581–4586

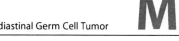

Seo Y, Kinsella MT, Reynolds HL et al (2009) Outcomes of chemoradiotherapy with 5-fluorouracil and mitomycin-c for anal cancer in immunocompetent versus immunodeficient patients. Int J Radiat Oncol Biol Phys 75(1):143–149

Silverberg MJ, Abrams DI (2009) Do antiretrovirals reduce the risk of non-AIDS-defining malignancies? Curr Opin HIV AIDS 4(1):42–51

Skiest DJ, Crosby C (2003) Survival is prolonged by highly active antiretroviral therapy in AIDS patients with primary central nervous system lymphoma. AIDS 17:1787–1793

Spano J-P, Costagliola D, Katlama C et al (2008) AIDS-related malignancies: state of the art and therapeutic challenges. J Clin Oncol 26(29):4834–4842

Spina M, Gabarre J, Rossi G et al (2002) Stanford V regimen and concomitant HAART in 59 patients with Hodgkin disease and HIV infection. Blood 100: 1984–1988

Tateo M, Roque-Afonso AM, Antonini TM et al (2009) Long-term follow-up of liver transplanted HIV/hepatitis B virus coinfected patients: perfect control of hepatitis B virus replication and absence of mitochondrial toxicity. AIDS 23:1069–1076

Management or Treatment of Osseous Disease

▶ Palliation of Bone Metastases

Maxillary Sinus

FILIP T. TROICKI
College of Medicine, Drexel University, Philadelphia, PA, USA

Definition
One of a pair of mucous membrane–lined cavities in the maxilla.

Cross-References
▶ Nasal Cavity and Paranasal Sinuses

Maximum Intensity Projection (MIP) CT Volume

DAREK MICHALSKI[1], M. SAIFUL HUQ[2]
[1]Division of Medical Physics, Department of Radiation Oncology, University of Pittsburgh Cancer Centers, Pittsburgh, PA, USA
[2]Department of Radiation Oncology, University of Pittsburgh Medical Center Cancer Pavilion, Pittsburgh, PA, USA

Definition
A composite CT volume with voxel values equal to maximal voxel value of the equivalent voxels from a given series of other 3D CT volumes.

Cross-References
▶ Four-Dimensional (4D) Treatment Planning/ Respiratory Gating

Mediastinal Germ Cell Tumor

RAMESH RENGAN[1], CHARLES R. THOMAS, JR.[2]
[1]Department of Radiation Oncology, Hospital of the University of Pennsylvania, Philadelphia, PA, USA
[2]Department of Radiation Medicine, Oregon Health Sciences University, Portland, OR, USA

Synonyms
Extragonadal germ cell tumor

Definition/Description
The most common site for germ cell tumors to arise is within the gonadal tissue. However, a small percentage of germ cell tumors arise in extragonadal sites. The most common site for an extragonadal

germ cell tumor is the anterior mediastinum. These tumors account for approximately 10% of all primary mediastinal neoplasms. These tumors are usually divided into benign (∼70% of all tumors) and malignant (∼30% of all tumors) categories (Chetaille et al. 2010). Mature teratomas and teratomas with a minority (<50%) immature component are considered benign. Dysgerminomas (seminomas) and non-seminomatous germ cell tumors are considered malignant. The majority of benign tumors are asymptomatic at the time of diagnosis. The majority of malignant germ cell tumors are symptomatic at diagnosis with patients usually presenting with chest pain and dyspnea. The treatment of mediastinal germ cell tumors is heavily dependent upon histology. Surgical resection is the mainstay of therapy for benign tumors with chemotherapy +/− radiotherapy being the optimal treatment for malignant tumors.

Anatomy

The mediastinum occupies the central portion of the thoracic cavity. It is bounded by the lungs and parietal pleura within the pleural cavities laterally, the thoracic inlet superiorly, the diaphragm inferiorly, the sternum and attached thoracic musculature anteriorly, and by the thoracic vertebrae and associated ribs posteriorly. The mediastinum can be divided into three clinically relevant compartments: anterior, middle, and posterior. The anterior mediastinum lies posterior to the sternum and anterior to the pericardium and great vessels, extends from the thoracic inlet to the diaphragm, and contains the thymus gland, lymph nodes, and, rarely, ectopic thyroid and parathyroid glands. The middle mediastinum is defined as the space occupied by the heart, pericardium, proximal great vessels, and central airways, including both phrenic nerves and lymph nodes. The posterior mediastinum is bounded by the heart and great vessels anteriorly, the thoracic inlet superiorly, the diaphragm inferiorly, and the

chest wall of the back posteriorly, and includes the paravertebral gutters, esophagus, descending aorta, sympathetic chains and vagus nerves, azygous vein, thoracic duct, and lymph nodes.

Epidemiology

The majority (70%) of mediastinal germ cell tumors are benign and consist of either pure mature teratomas or teratomas with a minority immature component. Benign tumors do not exhibit any male or female predominance. In contrast, malignant tumors (30% of all tumors) are most commonly seen in men (∼90%). Patients usually present in the third decade of life, however, these tumors can present up to age 60. Germ cell tumors also account for 3% of all pediatric tumors with the vast majority (∼80%) being benign teratomas. Approximately 20% of pediatric germ cell tumors are malignant. However, only 4% of pediatric germ cell tumors arise in the mediastinum. (Billmire 2006) Germ cell tumors account for approximately 10–15% of all mediastinal tumors in adults. There is an increased incidence of mediastinal non-seminomatous germ cell tumors in ▶ Klinefelter's syndrome (KS) patients, with up to 20% of patients with non-seminomatous germ cell tumors having a diagnosis of KS.

Clinical Presentation

The majority of benign tumors present as an incidental finding as identified on routine thoracic imaging. In contrast, the majority of malignant mediastinal germ cell tumors are symptomatic at presentation – usually with signs of mediastinal compression, including chest pain, dyspnea, and cough.

Differential Diagnosis

The differential diagnosis for an anterior mediastinal mass includes thymoma, lymphoma, tumors of the thyroid gland and parathyroid glands, and mesenchymal tumors such as a fibroma or leiyomysosarcoma.

Imaging Studies

A contrast-enhanced computed tomographic scan of the chest is the diagnostic test of choice. Magnetic resonance imaging can also be used. It has the advantage of multiplanar imaging and is superior to computed tomography in identifying vessel invasion. Additionally, imaging can be used with greater latitude in the setting of renal insufficiency or allergy to iodinated contrast dye. There is no formal AJCC staging system for mediastinal germ cell tumors. The role of FDG-PET is the diagnosis and assessment of response to therapy is under active investigation. FDG-PET may have an application in identification of mediastinal nodal involvement and this modality may also aid in confirmation of recurrence when tumor markers are elevated (De Giorgi et al. 2005).

Laboratory Studies

Complete blood count and serum chemistries should be ordered as they may be abnormal in associated syndromes. Serum tumor markers, including alpha-fetoprotein (AFP), beta human chorionic gonadotropin (β-HCG), and lactate dehydrogenase (LDH) are secreted by many germ cell tumors. Additionally, a hormone profile including thyroid hormone and parathyroid hormone may help identify tumors of the thyroid and parathyroid glands. Adrenocorticotropic hormone may be elevated in carcinoid tumors.

Treatment

Teratoma

The standard therapeutic approach for a mature teratoma is complete surgical resection. Local recurrence is rare after complete resection. There is no established role for either chemotherapy or radiation in the management of a mature teratoma. Complete surgical resection is also the treatment of choice for an immature teratoma. However, neoadjuvant chemotherapy may be employed in younger patients or to facilitate surgical resection. The likelihood of response is heavily dependent upon the extent of the immature component of the tumor.

Dysgerminoma (Seminomas)

There are a variety of potentially curative approaches for the treatment of pure seminomas including definitive radiotherapy to 40–50 Gy. (Hainsworth and Greco 1992) Recently, chemotherapy has been shown to have significant efficacy in mediastinal germ cell tumors. The usual approach is to utilize a cisplatin-based regimen. (Kesler and Einhorn 2009) The majority of patients will have a residual mediastinal mass after chemotherapy; however, this usually represents a scirrhous reaction in the mediastinal bed. There is some evidence to suggest that larger masses (>3 cm in diameter) may have an increased likelihood of residual disease and therefore should be monitored carefully for progression. Radiation without confirmation of viable residual tumor is not recommended (Schultz et al. 1989).

Nonseminomatous Germ Cell Tumors (NSGCT)

The NSGCTs include choriocarcinoma, embyonal carcinomas, endodermal sinus tumors, and teratomas. These can exist both in pure form and as mixed histology. The standard treatment approach is with a cisplatin-based regimen (Kesler and Einhorn 2009). Approximately 50% of patients will achieve long-term cure with this approach. In contrast to dysgerminomas, patients with a residual mediastinal mass after chemotherapy should be referred for complete surgical resection. Patients who have persistent elevation of serum markers after chemotherapy should be considered for salvage chemotherapy or high dose chemotherapy with stem cell transplant (Sirohi and Huddart 2005).

M

Prognosis

Teratoma

The prognosis for mature teratoma is excellent with complete surgical extirpation. Immature teratomas are exceedingly rare; however, complete surgical resection and chemotherapy are associated with increased survival.

Seminoma

In the absence of metastases, the prognosis for dysgerminomas is excellent with 5-year survival approaching 90%. In the presence of non-pulmonary visceral metastases, 5-year survivorship drops to 72% (IGCCG 1997).

Nonseminomatous Germ Cell Tumors (NSGCT)

The prognosis for NSGCT is generally poorer than for dysgerminoma. 5-year survival with chemotherapy and complete surgical excision in patients without evidence of visceral metastasis is 60–70%. In contrast, the median survival in patients with visceral metastases is on 22 months (Ganjoo, Rieger et al. 2000).

Pediatric Mediastinal Germ Cell Tumors

The overall survival for these tumors in the POG/CCG series of 22 patients was 71% (Billmire et al. 2001).

Cross-References

▶ Lung
▶ Testes
▶ Thymic Neoplasms

References

Billmire DF (2006) Malignant germ cell tumors in childhood. Semin Pediatr Surg 15(1):30–36

Billmire D, Vinocur C et al (2001) Malignant mediastinal germ cell tumors: an intergroup study. J Pediatr Surg 36(1):18–24

Chetaille B, Massard G et al (2010) Mediastinal germ cell tumors: anatomopathology, classification, teratomas and malignant tumors. Rev Pneumol Clin 66(1):63–70

De Giorgi U, Pupi A et al (2005) FDG-PET in the management of germ cell tumor. Ann Oncol 16(4):iv90–iv94

Ganjoo KN, Rieger KM et al (2000) Results of modern therapy for patients with mediastinal nonseminomatous germ cell tumors. Cancer 88(5):1051–1056

Hainsworth JD, Greco FA (1992) Extragonadal germ cell tumors and unrecognized germ cell tumors. Semin Oncol 19(2):119–127

IGCCG, I. G. C. C. C. G (1997) International Germ Cell Consensus Classification: a prognostic factor-based staging system for metastatic germ cell cancers. International Germ Cell Cancer Collaborative Group. J Clin Oncol 15(2):594–603

Kesler KA, Einhorn LH (2009) Multimodality treatment of germ cell tumors of the mediastinum. Thorac Surg Clin 19(1):63–69

Schultz SM, Einhorn LH et al (1989) Management of postchemotherapy residual mass in patients with advanced seminoma: Indiana University experience. J Clin Oncol 7(10):1497–1503

Sirohi B, Huddart R (2005) The management of poor-prognosis, non-seminomatous germ-cell tumours. Clin Oncol (R Coll Radiol) 17(7):543–552

Mediastinal Thymic Neoplasms

▶ Thymic Neoplasms

Medical Physics

JAY E. REIFF
Department of Radiation Oncology, College of Medicine, Drexel University, Philadelphia, PA, USA

Definition

The branch of physics associated with the practice of medicine which includes radiological physics, therapeutic radiological physics, diagnostic imaging physics, medical nuclear physics, and medical health physics.

Cross-References

▶ Radiation Oncology Physics

Medium-Dose Rate (MDR)

ERIK VAN LIMBERGEN
Department of Radiation Oncology, University Hospital Gasthuisberg, Leuven, Belgium

Definition

The dose is delivered at 2–12 Gy/h $(+/-10$ Gy/h) usually by cesium-137 sources in depending on the dose in 1–3 fractions. Because of the higher dose rate, total dose has to be lowered as compared to LDR treatments. Hospitalization in a brachytherapy ward is necessary.

Cross-References

▶ High-Dose Rate (HDR) Brachytherapy
▶ Low-Dose Rate (LDR) Brachytherapy
▶ Clinical Aspects of Brachytherapy (BT)

Megavoltage Cone Beam

▶ Image-Guided Radiation Therapy (IGRT): MV Imaging

Megavoltage Cone Beam CT

▶ Image-Guided Radiation Therapy (IGRT): MV Imaging

Megavoltage Volumetric Imaging

▶ Image-Guided Radiation Therapy (IGRT): MV Imaging

Melanoma

LYDIA T. KOMARNICKY-KOCHER[1], FIORI ALITE[2]
[1]Department of Radiation Oncology, College of Medicine, Drexel University, Philadelphia, PA, USA
[2]College of Medicine, Drexel University, Philadelphia, PA, USA

Synonyms

Cutaneous melanoma; Malignant melanoma

Definition/Description

Melanoma represents a malignant tumor of melanocytes, which are embryological derivatives of neural crest tissue. Therefore, melanoma can occur from any site of neural crest migration, but most often arises from the skin. When the fetus develops, these cells migrate to areas of skin, meninges, mucous membranes, upper esophagus, and eyes. The most common area of malignant potential is the skin where melanocytes reside at the dermal–epidermal junction. Melanoma of the skin, or cutaneous melanoma, comprises only 4% of skin malignancies, but is responsible for the majority of skin cancer mortality. Melanoma has exhibited a dramatic increase in incidence since the 1930s, which is thought to be secondary to increased surveillance and changes in diagnostic criteria. At the same time, there has been a dramatic decrease in mortality with the cumulative 5 year survival increasing to 91% in 2005 from 81% in the 1980s, mostly attributed to heightened awareness and early detection. Melanoma tends to arise more frequently in white adults with peek incidence in the 40s and 50s, more frequently occurring in the head, neck, and trunk region in men, and more commonly in the extremities in women. These findings highlight the central role that ultraviolet radiation exposure from the sun plays in the development of the disease. The transformation of melanocytes to melanoma involves a complex set of molecular events and a stepwise progression through dysplasia, hyperplasia, invasion, and metastasis. Melanoma can arise from preexisting nevi or directly from normal melanocytes. Although patients with multiple nevi are at increased risk for the development of melanoma and that nevi can undergo malignant degeneration, it is thought that the presence of multiple nevi signifies a predisposition to melanoma and that most develop as new lesions in unblemished skin from normal melanocytes. Melanoma first involves the regional draining lymph nodes, and is notorious for distant metastasis at which point the disease is often intractable and 5 year survival drops to only 14%. ▶ Sentinel lymph node involvement has emerged as the most important prognostic factor for recurrence and survival. Depth of invasion (*vertical thickness*) is highly predictive of dissemination, with 20% of lesions greater than 2 mm in depth demonstrating positive sentinel lymph node involvement. The treatment of localized melanoma centers around surgical excision with adequate margins. Although often underutilized, radiation therapy is indicated in the adjuvant setting after surgical resection for high-risk lesions, to treat regional nodes in patients with high-risk features, as palliative treatment for metastatic disease, and rarely as definitive therapy for primary lesions.

Epidemiology

There are approximately 68,000 new cases of melanoma every year and 8,700 deaths, with less than 10% of cases developing from non-cutaneous sites. The incidence of melanoma is increasing more rapidly than any other malignancy. Currently, 1 in 64 women will develop melanoma and 1 in 42 men will be diagnosed with melanoma of the skin during their lifetime. The highest incidence per capita worldwide is in Australia, with the highest incidence in persons of Western European descent. In nonwhite populations, there is a higher frequency of melanoma developing in subungal, plantar, palmar, and mucosal areas. Ocular and nonacral melanomas are more likely in white than nonwhite populations. The increased incidence in melanomas has mainly been seen in white populations.

Prevention and Screening

The US Preventive Services Task Force review of evidence for routine screening for cutaneous melanoma in asymptomatic patients in the primary care clinical setting using a total-skin examination for early detection found that there was insufficient evidence to recommend for or against screening. More selective patient screening based on risk factors may be more effective, however, currently, there is no validated risk assessment scale with which to screen patients for melanoma. Furthermore, although lesions detected by a physician are significantly thinner than those detected by a patient or spouse, and physicians are encouraged to take advantage of the physical examination to screen for skin cancer, studies have not shown a decrease in mortality. An emphasis on minimizing ultraviolet radiation exposure from the sun on the skin is important in helping prevent the development of melanoma. Recently, a meta-analysis found no association between sunscreen use and decreased incidence of melanoma, possibly related to incorrect use or a false sense of security that sunscreen provides, resulting in increased exposure activities (Halfand et al. 2004). The strongest evidence in helping prevent melanoma points to increasing efforts of reducing intermittent sunburns in childhood, best accomplished by avoiding midday sun exposure, and wearing copious protective clothing. Prevention efforts must place the focus on reducing skin exposure to the sun, as opposed to increasing sunscreen use.

Etiology

Risk for developing melanoma exhibits a genetic or acquired sensitivity to ultraviolet radiation coupled with excessive environmental exposure to the sun. The strongest risk factors are family history of melanoma, benign or atypical nevi, or previous history of melanoma. Immunosuppression, sun sensitivity, light skin, history of severe sunburns in childhood, and polyvinyl chloride all increase risk. Familial forms of melanoma are associated with gene mutations of tumor suppressor factors cyclin-dependent kinase-4 (CDK4), cyclin-dependent kinase inhibitor 2A (CDKN2A), and p16 in as many as 45–50% of cases.

Demographic characteristics of those who develop melanoma support an association between ultraviolet irradiation and the development of melanoma. ultraviolet-C radiation is typically absorbed by the ozone layer, but ultraviolet-B radiation (290–320 nm) is associated with sunburn and triggering tanning by the induction of melanin production. It is the form of radiation most strongly associated with the development of melanoma. For example, human skin grafted on mice develops nevi and melanoma under UVB radiation exposure. The role of ultraviolet-A (320–400 nm) irradiation in melanoma etiology is more controversial and this form of radiation is associated more with chronic sun damage skin changes. Previous radiation therapy also increases the risk for development of melanoma as well as other skin cancers. This is especially relevant in patients who have been treated with a combination of chemotherapy and radiation therapy, as well as younger patients treated for testicular cancers or lymphomas.

The malignant transformation from normal melanocytes to metastatic melanoma occurs through a stepwise histological progression. Atypical melanocytes arise in either a preexisting nevus or de novo in unblemished skin, yet they very rarely progress to melanoma. The development of atypical melanocytic hyperplasia at the dermal–epidermal junction or the development of nests of atypical melanocytes in the epidermis marks a further step toward malignant transformation. As this process progresses, an early melanoma can be diagnosed and growth is marked by radial extension. The radial growth phase (RGP) of a cutaneous melanoma can include either melanoma in situ or superficial invasion as far as the papillary dermis. It can be years before the radial growth phase converts to a vertical growth phase (VGP), which is marked by extension into the dermis and beyond. The radial growth phase has very low metastatic potential, estimated at 0–5%, but the development of the vertical growth phase represents progression toward metastatic transformation due to acquisition of subsequent mutations leading to clonal changes in the cells of the RGP. Lesions exhibiting vertical growth are at increased risk for nodal involvement and distant metastases.

Pathology

The pathogenesis of malignant melanoma consists of progression through two distinct growth phases. Initially, radial growth represents melanoma spreading horizontally within the epidermis and superficial papillary dermis, and cells lack metastatic potential during this phase. During the latter stages of the natural history of melanoma, vertical growth occurs when cells invade perpendicularly from the skin into the deeper layers of the dermis as an evolving mass, while gaining metastatic potential.

Cytologically, melanoma cells appear larger than normal melanocytes and can exhibit epithelioid, spindle cell, or nonspecific appearance which places them in a cytologic gray zone. Immunohistochemical staining is often required to distinguish melanoma cells which often contain S-100, HMB-45, and MART-1 antigens. The histologic subtypes of melanoma correlate chronologically with the different growth phases.

- Superficial spreading melanoma represents 70% of melanomas and exhibits primarily a radial growth pattern with low (5%) risk of metastasis, only progressing to vertical growth late in the disease. Development of vertical growth correlates with a more aggressive and rapidly growing tumor, imparting a 35–80% risk of metastasis. Most commonly occurring between the ages of 40 and 60 they are usually flat, pigmented lesions with an epithelioid microscopic pattern. It is associated with intermittent sun exposure, often occurs in the trunk and extremities, and can develop from precursor nevi.
- Nodular melanoma comprises 30% of lesions, and they are often highly pigmented or amelanotic, and often develop de novo. They display only vertical growth, which is heralded by the distinctive nodular appearance. There is a 2:1 male predominance, and lesions are often found on the trunk or head and neck.
- Lentigo maligna melanoma represents 4% of cases and is a disease of the elderly, often involving the face and dorsum of the hands. It has the most benign progression pattern and does not arise from precursor nevi.
- Acral lentiginous melanoma accounts for 2–8% of lesions, and is the most common type in nonwhite patients. It often occurs in the palms, soles, or subungal areas. It is most common by the 60s and rapidly metastasizes.
- Desmoplastic melanoma is a rare variant, found to be deeply invasive and have a high local recurrence rate. Lesions exhibit prominent neutropism, are very locally aggressive, but often lack lymphatic or distant spread. Desmoplastic melanoma is also more likely to lack the common histochemical staining pattern of the other subtypes (Fig. 1).

TYPE	SITE
Superficial spreading melanoma	Trunk/Extremities
Nodular melanoma	Trunk/Head and Neck
Lentigo Maligna	Face/Dorsum of the Hands
Acral Lentiginous	Melanoma Palms/Soles/Sub-Ungual
Desmoplastic	Melanoma Skin/Peripheral Nerves

Melanoma. Fig. 1 Histologic subtypes of cutaneous melanoma by most likely site of presentation

Prognostic Factors

Depth of invasion, first described by Breslow, serves as the best predictor of distant metastases. The Breslow thickness is measured from the granular layer of the epidermis, and has been incorporated in the current staging system. Clark levels do not add much prognostic value except in thin melanomas where Clark level IV and V lesions impart a higher risk of metastases. Ulceration of the primary lesion, a high mitotic rate (>6 mitoses per square millimeter), as well as nodular type of melanoma are all considered poor prognostic indicators. Anatomic site, gender, and age are all prognostic with lesions of the trunk, male gender, and older age groups imparting a poorer prognosis. Prognosis for early lesions is good, but only 15.9% of patients with metastatic disease survive 5 years.

Clinical Presentation

Melanoma most often presents as a pigmented skin lesion, sometimes developing from preexisting benign nevi. Although patients with multiple nevi are at increased risk for the development of melanoma and those nevi can undergo malignant degeneration, it is thought that the presence of multiple nevi signifies a predisposition to melanoma and that most develop as new lesions in unblemished skin. Melanoma of the skin is rarely symptomatic in its early stages, although itching, ulceration, bleeding, and pain can sometimes be associated with late lesions. Clinical manifestations most consistent with melanoma include changes in a pigmented skin lesion with time, such as change in color (hyper- or hypo-pigmentation), shape, growth in size (>6 mm), or development of ulceration. This paradigm termed the "ugly duckling approach," requires that physicians consider lesions suspicious for biopsy when they look or feel different from the patient's other coexisting or nearby nevi.

Differential Diagnosis

Several similarly appearing benign or malignant lesions can develop on the skin. Melanoma must often be distinguished from ▶ atypical (dysplastic) nevi which are benign. Blue nevi, solar lentigo, and seborrheic keratosis, as well as vascular lesions are all benign skin manifestations resembling melanoma. Other skin malignancies such as basal cell carcinoma, squamous cell carcinoma, Merkel cell carcinoma, and cutaneous lymphoma may be difficult to distinguish from melanoma. Lentigo maligna (Hutchinson's freckle) is melanoma in situ that can be present for years without malignant progression, but often resembles melanoma on the clinical examination.

Workup

Evaluation of a patient for newly diagnosed melanoma begins with a detailed history and physical examination with a focus on eliciting risk factors, sun exposure, and family history of melanoma. A complete survey of the skin should be performed, the lesion should be palpated to delineate the extent of non-superficial tumor, and examination should focus on determining the presence of ulceration, satellite lesions, or regional lymph node involvement. For head and face lesions, a detailed cranial nerve examination is critical.

▶ Surface microscopy (dermoscopy, epiluminescence microscopy) has gained acceptance as a tool for aiding in the diagnosis of cutaneous melanoma. The skin is covered with oil, and a handheld instrument magnifies that skin at least ten times. Pseudopods, radial streaming, blue/grey veil, and peripheral black dots have been identified

as factors suggestive of melanoma and can aid physicians in the decision making process.

All suspicious lesions should be biopsied, optimally with an excisional biopsy with 1–3 mm margins. Orientation of the excision should be planned with definitive treatment in mind, and wider margins should be avoided since they can disrupt the lymphovascular architecture which must be intact should a sentinel lymph node biopsy be indicated.

Staging for melanoma has evolved through the Clark, Breslow, and now the TNM staging systems. Clark levels describe the extent of anatomical invasion of the melanoma through the histological layers of the skin. Breslow classification system stratifies tumors based on distance of vertical invasion or tumor thickness (Tables 1 and 2).

Melanoma. Table 1 Breslow thickness has been found to be prognostic and has been incorporated in the AJCC and NCCN staging guidelines

Clark levels		Breslow thickness (mm)	Approximate 5 year survival (%)
I	Melanoma confined to the epidermis (melanoma in situ)	<1	95–100
II	Invasion into the papillary dermis	1–2	80–96
III	Invasion to the junction of the papillary and reticular dermis	2.1–4	60–75
IV	Invasion into the reticular dermis	>4	50
V	Invasion into the subcutaneous fat http://en.wikipedia.org/wiki/Breslow%27s_depth-cite_note-weedon-5		

Melanoma. Table 2 TNM Staging

Stage 0	Melanoma in situ
Stage IA	<1 mm without ulceration
Stage IB	<1 mm with ulceration or 1–2 mm without ulceration
Stage IIA	1–2 mm with ulceration or 2–4 mm without ulceration
Stage IIB	2–4 mm with ulceration or >4 mm without ulceration
Stage IIC	>4 mm with ulceration
Stage IIIA	Any depth without ulceration with 1–3 nodes positive for micrometastases
Stage IIIB	Any depth with ulceration with 1–3 nodes positive for micrometastases or any depth without ulceration with 1–3 nodes positive for macrometastases or in-transit mets/satellite(s) *without* metastatic node(s)
Stage IIIC	Any depth with ulceration with 1–3 nodes positive for macrometastases or in-transit mets/satellite(s) *without* metastatic node(s) or any depth with four or more metastatic nodes, matted nodes, or in-transit mets/satellite(s) *with* metastatic node(s)
Stage IV	Distant metastasis

Source: Adapted from AJCC Staging Manual 7th edition (2010)

Treatment

Surgery is indicated in almost all patients for primary melanoma excision. Metastatic disease may also lend itself to surgical excision when it presents with solitary masses of the subcutaneous tissue, lung, nonregional lymph nodes, or the brain. This is particularly pertinent in patients with long time intervals between a primary lesion and development of metastasis, a feature classically associated with melanoma. Elective lymph node resection has lost favor in the literature, with sentinel lymph node biopsy followed

Melanoma. Table 3 Recommended surgical margins by tumor thickness

Tumor thickness	Recommended clinical margins
In situ	0.5 cm
≤1 mm	1 cm
1.01–2 mm	1–2 cm
2.01–4 mm	2 cm
>4 mm	2 cm

by lymphadenectomy being recommended in patients with at least a 15% risk of occult lymph node involvement. Incomplete excision, tumors with high-risk features, nodal involvement, and metastasis necessitate the use of chemotherapy and radiation in an adjuvant setting.

Surgery

Wide excision is the primary treatment for melanoma. Achieving adequate margins is an important predictor of local recurrence. Several prospective randomized trials have helped shape criteria for surgical margins. The National Comprehensive Cancer Network currently recommends the surgical margins mentioned in Table 3.

For patients undergoing wide local excision for lesions between 1 and 3.5 cm, sentinel lymph node biopsy status was found to be the most prognostic for disease-specific survival, although there was no association with decreased local recurrence, or melanoma-specific survival. Patients with lesions less than 1 mm in thickness rarely have occult nodal disease; therefore, sentinel lymph node biopsy is not recommended unless high-risk features are present pathologically, such as ulceration or Clark level IV to V. For patients with lesions that are more than 1 mm in thickness, risk of occult nodal involvement climbs to 15–35% and sentinel lymph node staging should be performed in order to better formulate the prognosis and determine if adjuvant therapy is indicated. Patients with melanomas of head and neck, mucous membranes/anorectal region, and fingers and toes require special considerations since obtaining optimal margins is often difficult or not feasible. Melanomas of the head and neck often do not lend themselves to complete optimal surgical excision due to anatomical and cosmetic constraints, especially those near the eye. In such circumstances, the largest margins possible should be obtained and closed with an advancement flap, skin graft, or limited rotation flap. The head and neck region is also a common site of desmoplastic melanoma, whose often amelanotic gross appearance and difficult to demarcate histological appearance makes obtaining adequate surgical resection margins increasingly difficult. If efforts at obtaining adequate margins fail in desmoplastic melanoma, adjuvant radiation therapy to the resected region with 2–3 cm margins should be considered. Mucosal melanomas of the head and neck, anorectal region, and female genital tract are often diagnosed late and represent much deeper lesions associated with higher rates of local recurrence and nodal involvement. These lesions often require wide local excisions, with anorectal melanomas often requiring an abdominaperineal resection and incorporation of adjuvant radiation therapy. Special considerations must be made in vulvovaginal melanomas when attempting wide local excision in order to preserve sexual and urinary function. Subungal melanomas of the fingers and toes are managed by amputation at the interphalangeal joint of the toe or at the distal interphalangeal joint of the finger. More proximal melanomas of the fingers and toes often require amputation, except for small, thin proximal lesions where wide local excision with skin grafting may be attempted.

Chemotherapy

Immune modulation is an important mechanism employed by the various forms of systemic treatment of melanoma. Patients recognized to be at increased risk for recurrence or distant metastasis may be candidates for adjuvant systemic treatment. High-dose interferon alpha-2b improves relapse-free survival by as much as 30% and is currently indicated in lesions thicker than 4 mm or in cases of nodal involvement (Stages IIB, IIC, and III). Given the unfavorable toxicity profile of interferon alpha-2b, including acute constitutional symptoms, chronic fatigue, headache, nausea, weight loss, myelosuppression, and depression, it is important to consider performance status and life expectancy when choosing it for systemic treatment. Incorporating interleukin-2 and conventional chemotherapy consisting of cisplatin, vinblastine, dacarbazine (CVD) to interferon alpha-2b, termed biochemotherapy, has been shown to have superior progression-free survival to chemotherapy alone. Various tumor-specific vaccines targeting specific gangliosides in the melanoma cell membranes or unique melanoma-expressed antigens are currently under investigation.

Radiotherapy

Radiotherapy remains an underutilized modality in melanomas of the skin, estimated to be incorporated in treatment in less than half of indicated cases.

For in situ disease (Lentigo Maligna) that often presents on the face and is not amenable to surgery due to cosmetic considerations, there is evidence that external beam radiation can be used to prevent tumor growth and progression. At 15 month median follow-up, 42 patients treated with high-dose superficial radiation for lentigo maligna showed no local recurrences. Radiation is a safe and effective means of management and may be considered as definitive therapy for in situ lesions not amenable to surgery.

Large lentigo maligna melanoma lesions of the face often do not lend themselves to surgical excision. Excellent local control was achieved in 20/22 patients using superficial radiation of 100 Gy in 10 Gy fractions over 2 weeks

(Schmid-Wendtner et al. 2000). Surgery was employed in this setting to excise only the nodular portion of the lesion. Excellent cosmesis was achieved, with only hyperpigmentation being reported in the treatment field but no fibrosis.

The most significant application of radiation therapy in the management of cutaneous melanoma is in the adjuvant setting. Although adequate surgical excision imparts less than a 5% chance of local recurrence, several factors carry increased local recurrence risk at the primary site from 14% to 48%. Head and neck location, lesions greater 4 mm in thickness, positive surgical margins, ulceration, presence of satellite lesions, and the desmoplastic melanoma histologic variant are all indications for adjuvant radiation therapy to the primary tumor bed due to increased recurrence risk.

Therapeutic lymph node dissection is associated with 85% control of nodal disease, however, several factors increase the risk of local nodal recurrence. Extracapsular extension, multiple (4+) nodal involvement, lymph node size ≥ 3 cm, cervical nodal location and recurrent nodal disease after initial dissection all increase recurrence risk 30–50%. In a large series of 466 patients with at least one of the high-risk features mentioned above, adjuvant radiation therapy consisting of 30 Gy in five fractions delivered twice weekly showed excellent regional control of 89% at 5 years (Ballo et al. 2006). When considering addition of adjuvant radiation therapy to regional lymph nodes, potential benefit should always be balanced against expected toxicity, as well as the independent risk of distant failure. It may be that the same risk factors which are predictive of local nodal failure, may portend a similar risk for distant metastatic failure, diminishing the utility of nodal irradiation. This may be why sentinel lymph node biopsy, although predictive of survival and provides prognostic information, has not been shown to improve survival. The most significant added toxicity of nodal irradiation is lymphedema. A higher threshold for irradiation should be employed when the draining basin involves the axillary or inguinal lymph nodes since lymphedema has been associated in as high as 20% and 27% of cases, respectively. Therefore, the MD Anderson Cancer Center (MDACC) treatment algorithm recommends that irradiation to these sites be limited to those patients that exhibit two or more of the high-risk features (Table 4).

The target volume for radiation treatment technique includes the primary site with a 2–4 cm margin, with additional lymph nodal target volumes inclusions depending on primary site. Conventional fractionation schemes with dose recommendations similar to squamous cell carcinoma or basal cell carcinoma can be employed, namely, 2–3 Gy fractions to a cumulative dose of 45–55 Gy. Although there is no specific data to support a commonly held belief that melanoma is radioresistant, radiobiological studies suggest that melanoma cell lines have dose–response characteristics favoring hypofractionation. Recent data comparing hypofractionated radiation therapy for high-risk diseases consisting of 30 Gy in 5 fractions versus conventional fractionation of 60 Gy in 30 fractions showed no difference in local control or overall survival (Chang et al. 2006). Toxicity considerations associated with the

Melanoma. Table 4 High-risk features of the primary lesion and nodal involvement used to determine indications for adjuvant radiation therapy

Primary	Nodes
Head and neck lesion	Cervical nodal involvement
>4 mm thickness	>4 Nodes involved
Positive surgical margins	Extracapsular extension
Ulceration	Lymph node size ≥3 cm
Satellite lesions	Recurrent nodal disease
Desmoplastic melanoma	

hypofractionated scheme seen in a minority of patients include osteoradionecrosis of temporal bone or radiation-induced plexopathies. The Trans Tasman Radiation Oncology Group (TROG Study 96.06) is the only large phase II adjuvant postoperative radiation trial, where 234 patients were treated with lymph node dissection followed by 48 Gy in 20 fractions over 4 weeks. The regional in-field recurrence rate was 6.8% and distant relapse of 62.8% was reported. The 5 year overall survival was 35%, and the 5 year local control was 91%. Significant axillary and inguinal lymphedema was seen in 9% and 19% of patients, respectively.

Stage IV melanoma harbors a very poor prognosis, with a median survival between 6 and 10 months, and a 5-year survival of less than 5%. Development of unresectable locoregional disease such as dermal, subcutaneous, lymph node metastases, or distant metastasis such as brain metastases, or painful bony lesions is often managed by palliative radiotherapy. The general goal of palliative radiotherapy is to deliver a relatively large dose of radiation expediently in order to achieve a significant symptomatic response. A hypofractionated regimen of five to six fractions of 6 Gy given twice weekly can be employed for skin nodules or local lymphatic involvement. For axillary and inguinal adenopathy a standard fractionation regimen may be more appropriate to prevent lymphedema. Whole brain radiotherapy is effective at palliating symptoms from brain metastasis. WBRT given at 35 Gy in 14 fractions has also been shown to improve median survival and time to recurrence when employed postoperatively after resection of solitary brain metastasis. Stereotactic radiosurgery is an alternative to resection when lesions are less than 3 cm, when dealing with multiple lesions (<6), when lesions are surgically inaccessible, or patients are poor surgical candidates. Pain from bony metastasis can be alleviated in up to 80% of patients with regimens of 20 Gy in five fractions or 30 Gy in ten fractions delivered in 2 weeks. When facing the risk of cord compression, it is imperative that patients be evaluated for neurosurgical debulking followed by standard fractionated radiotherapy usually delivered in ten fractions to 30 Gy.

Cross-References

► Basal Cell Nevus Syndrome
► Clark Level
► External Beam Radiation Therapy
► Eye and Orbit
► Merkel Cell Carcinoma (MCC)
► Neutron Radiotherapy
► Palliation of Bone Metastases
► Skin Cancer
► Squamous Cell Carcinoma

References

Altekruse SF, Kosary CL, Krapcho M et al. (2010) *SEER Cancer Statistics Review, 1975–2007*, National Cancer Institute. Bethesda, MD, http://seer.cancer.gov/csr/1975_2007/, based on November 2009 SEER data submission, posted to the SEER web site, 2010

Ballo MT, Ross MI, Cormier JN et al (2006) Combined modality therapy for patients with regional nodal metastases from melanoma. Int J Radiat Oncol Biol Phys 64:106–113

Boyle P, Levin B (eds) (2008) Melanoma. In: World cancer report 2008. International Agency for Research on Cancer, Lyon, France

Burmeister BH, Mark Smithers B, Burmeister E et al (2006) A prospective phase II study of adjuvant postoperative radiation therapy following nodal surgery in malignant melanoma — Trans Tasman Radiation Oncology Group (TROG) Study 96.06. Radiother Oncol 81:136–142

Chang DT, Amdur RJ, Morris CG et al (2006) Adjuvant radiotherapy for cutaneous melanoma: comparing hypofractionation to conventional fractionation. Int J Radiat Oncol Biol Phys 66(4):1051–1055

Helfand M, Krages KP (2010) Counseling to prevent skin cancer: a summary of the evidence for the U.S. Preventive Services Task Force. Agency for Healthcare Research and Quality, 2003, Rockville, MD http://www.ahrq.gov/clinic/3rduspstf/skcacoun/skcounsum.htm. Accessed 2 Nov 2010

Miller AJ, Mihm MC (2006) Review: melanoma, mechanism of disease. N Engl J Med 355:51–65

National Comprehensive Cancer Network (2010) NCCN clinical practice guidelines in oncology: Melanoma, V.I.2010. Available at: http://www.nccn.org/professionals/physician_gls/PDF/melanoma.pdf Accessed 15 August 2010

Rager EL, Bridgeford EP, Ollila DW (2005) Cutaneous melanoma: update on prevention, screening, diagnosis, and treatment. Am Fam Physician 72(2):269–276

Schmid-Wendtner MH, Brunner B, Konz B (2000) Fractionated radiotherapy of lentigo maligna and lentigo maligna melanoma in 64 patients. J Am Acad Dermatol 43:447–482

Slingluff CL, Flaherty K, Rosenberg SA, Read PW (2008) Cutaneous melanoma. In: DeVita VT, Hellman S, Rosenberg SA (eds) Cancer: principles and practice of oncology, 2nd edn. Wolters Kluwer, Lippincott Williams & Wilkins, Philadelphia

Solan MJ, Brady LW (2008) Skin cancer. In: Halperin EC, Perez CA, Brady LW (eds) Principles and practice of radiation oncology, 5th edn. Wolters Kluwer, Lippincott Williams & Wilkins, Philadelphia

Tsao H, Atkins M, Sober A (2004) Review: management of cutaneous melanoma. N Engl J Med 351:998–1012

MEN2a

NISHA R. PATEL, MICHAEL L. WONG
Department of Radiation Oncology,
College of Medicine, Drexel University,
Philadelphia, PA, USA

Definition
Multiple endocrine neoplasia is a familial syndrome characterized by medullary neoplasm associated with the development of primary hyperparathyroidism and pheochromocytoma.

Cross-References
▶ Thyroid Cancer

MEN2b

NISHA R. PATEL, MICHAEL L. WONG
Department of Radiation Oncology,
College of Medicine, Drexel University,
Philadelphia, PA, USA

Definition
Multiple endocrine neoplasia is a familial syndrome characterized by medullary neoplasm associated with pheochromocytoma, marfanoid habitus, and mucosal neuromas.

Cross-References
▶ Thyroid Cancer

Meningioma

Definition
Benign or malignant tumor arising from the lining of the brain or spinal cord and rarely extracranial.

Cross-References
▶ Extracranial Meningioma
▶ Primary Intracranial Neoplasms
▶ Spinal Canal Tumor

Merkel Cell Carcinoma (MCC)

BRANDON J. FISHER
Department of Radiation Oncology,
College of Medicine, Drexel University,
Philadelphia, PA, USA

Synonyms
Neuroendocrine carcinoma of the skin

Definition
MCC, also known as neuroendocrine carcinoma of the skin, is a rare tumor with roughly 500 cases per year in the United States. These tumors tend to be aggressive with a high frequency of local and distant metastases. MCC is usually present in the sixth decade of life and involves sun-exposed areas of the skin. It has three subtypes: trabecular, intermediate, and small cell. Treatment involves

surgical excision with a 2–3-cm margin followed by adjuvant radiation therapy. MCC tends to be sensitive to radiation. Volumes should include the primary tumor, surgical bed, scar, and draining lymphatics. Radiation dosing is similar to that for other skin cancers.

Cross-References

▶ Skin Cancer

Mick Applicator

Yan Yu, Laura Doyle
Department of Radiation Oncology, Thomas Jefferson University Hospital, Philadelphia, PA, USA

Definition

Device used to implant radioactive seeds in permanent LDR prostate implant. Seeds are loaded in a cartridge and ejected individually into the prostate.

Cross-References

▶ Brachytherapy: Low Dose Rate (LDR) Permanent Implants (Prostate)

Microarray Analysis

Anthony E. Dragun
Department of Radiation Oncology, James Graham Brown Cancer Center, University of Louisville School of Medicine, Louisville, KY, USA

Synonyms
Oncotype DX

Definition

A reverse-transcription-polymerase chain reaction (RT-PCR) analysis of paraffin-fixed tissue yielding a twenty-one gene panel combined with a mathematical algorithm to derive a "recurrence score," which is extrapolated to predict an individual patient's risk of recurrence of and survival from a diagnosis of breast cancer. This test has been validated on NSABP-derived tissue banks. It is most useful to guide treatment for patients who are estrogen receptor and progesterone receptor positive, lymph node negative, early-stage breast cancer patients. Its use is mainly to define the utility of adjuvant cytotoxic chemotherapy.

Cross-References

▶ Early-Stage Breast Cancer

Microenvironment

Lindsay G. Jensen, Brent S. Rose, Arno J. Mundt
Center for Advanced Radiotherapy Technologies, Department of Radiation Oncology, San Diego Rebecca and John Moores Cancer Center, University of California, La Jolla, CA, USA

Definition

Network of cells, extracellular matrix, and vasculature within the bone marrow that support hematopoiesis.

Cross-References

▶ Bone Marrow Toxicity in Cancer Treatment

Microsatellite Instability

BRADLEY J. HUTH[1], CHRISTIN A. KNOWLTON[2],
MICHELLE KOLTON MACKAY[3]
[1]Department of Radiation Oncology,
Philadelphia, PA, USA
[2]Department of Radiation Oncology,
Drexel University, Philadelphia, PA, USA
[3]Department of Radiation Oncology, Marshfield
Clinic, Marshfield, WI, USA

Synonyms
MSI

Definition
Microsatellites are short repeated sequences of DNA. Multiple sequences of microsatellites result in long stretches of uniform DNA which cause instability of the strand. The resulting microsatellite instability is found frequently in colon, ovarian, and uterine cancers. Its presence raises the suspicion of hereditary syndromes but may also confer an improved prognosis.

Cross-References
▶ Colon Cancer
▶ Endometrium
▶ Rectal Cancer

Microscopic Lymph Node Disease

ANTHONY E. DRAGUN
Department of Radiation Oncology, James Graham Brown Cancer Center, University of Louisville School of Medicine, Louisville, KY, USA

Synonyms
Immunohistochemically positive lymph node; Isolated tumor cells

Definition
This refers to the low-volume, microscopic lymph node disease that is occasionally detected by detailed pathologic analysis that is a supplement to routine H and E staining after sentinel lymph node biopsy. Although these patients are most often managed in a similar fashion to patients with N0 disease, current controversy exists over the routine use of full axillary dissection and/or systemic cytotoxic chemotherapy in such patients.

Cross-References
▶ Early-Stage Breast Cancer

Mixed Beam Radiation

GEORGE E. LARAMORE, JAY J. LIAO, JASON K. ROCKHILL
Department of Radiation Oncology, University of Washington Medical Center, Seattle, WA, USA

Definition
This refers to a treatment fractionation schema utilizing both neutron and conventional photon/electron radiotherapy rather than just fast neutrons alone.

Cross-References
▶ Electron Dosimetry and Treatment
▶ Neutron Radiotherapy

MLC

GEORGE E. LARAMORE, JAY J. LIAO, JASON K. ROCKHILL
Department of Radiation Oncology, University of Washington Medical Center, Seattle, WA, USA

Definition
A device which uses independently controlled leaves to shape the radiation beam, allowing for more precise control of the delivered dose.

Cross-References

► IMRT (Intensity Modulated Radiotherapy)
► Linear Accelerators (LINAC)
► Neutron Radiotherapy

Modified Radical Hysterectomy

CHRISTIN A. KNOWLTON[1], MICHELLE KOLTON MACKAY[2]
[1]Department of Radiation Oncology,
Drexel University, Philadelphia, PA, USA
[2]Department of Radiation Oncology, Marshfield
Clinic, Marshfield, WI, USA

Synonyms

Class II hysterectomy

Definition

A modified radical hysterectomy is the surgical removal of the uterus, the cervix, the upper 1–2 cm of the vagina, and the parametrial tissues surrounding these organs medial to the ureters. Pelvic lymphadenectomy and para-aortic lymph node sampling are often included with this procedure.

Cross-References

► Uterine Cervix

Modified Radical Mastectomy

DAVID E. WAZER
Radiation Oncology Department, Tufts Medical
Center, Tufts University School of Medicine,
Boston, MA, USA
Radiation Oncology Department, Rhode Island
Hospital, Brown University School of Medicine,
Providence, RI, USA

Definition

An axillary nodal dissection, levels I and II, in addition to the removal of the entire breast tissue, from the clavicle to the rectus abdominus muscle, between the sternal edge of the latissimus dorsi muscle, including the removal of the fascia of the pectoralis major muscle.

Cross-References

► Cancer of the Breast Tis
► Stage 0 Breast Cancer

Modulation Transfer Function (MTF)

JOHN W. WONG
Department of Radiation Oncology and
Molecular Radiation Sciences, Johns Hopkins
University, Baltimore, MD, USA

Definition

The ratio of the information recorded by a detector system to the total amount of information available.

Cross-References

► Electronic Portal Imaging Devices (EPID)

Mohs Micrographic Surgery

BRANDON J. FISHER
Department of Radiation Oncology,
College of Medicine, Drexel University,
Philadelphia, PA, USA

Definition

Originally developed by Dr. Frederic Mohs, Mohs microsurgery is used to decrease the cosmetic morbidity of skin cancer surgery. The surgical procedure allows for maximal skin sparing through a process of fixation and mapping of the surgical margins with multiple frozen sections to obtain microscopically clear margins. This technique is preferred for deeply invasive tumors; diffuse laterally spreading tumors; perineural invasion or any tumor on the face; and recurrent tumors. Mohs surgery is used primarily for basal cell carcinomas and squamous cell carcinomas.

Cross-References

▶ Skin Cancer

Molecular Imaging

HEDVIG HRICAK[1], OGUZ AKIN[2], HEBERT ALBERTO VARGAS[2]
[1]Department of Radiology, Memorial Sloan-Kettering Cancer Center, New York, NY, USA
[2]Body MRI, Memorial Sloan-Kettering Cancer Center, New York, NY, USA

Definition

Visualization, characterization, and measurement of biological processes at the molecular and cellular levels in humans and other living systems. Molecular imaging typically includes two- or three-dimensional imaging as well as quantification over time. The techniques used include radiotracer imaging/nuclear medicine, MRI, MR spectroscopy, optical imaging, ultrasound, and others.

Cross-References

▶ Imaging in Oncology

Molecular Markers in Clinical Radiation Oncology

BRUCE G. HAFFTY
Department of Radiation Oncology, UMDNJ-Robert Wood Johnson Medical School, Cancer Institute of New Jersey, New Brunswick, NJ, USA

Introduction and Overview

Radiation therapy is a potent DNA damaging agent and one of the most powerful tools in the management of cancer (Haffty and Wilson 2009). The use of therapeutic doses of radiation as a primary treatment modality or in combination with surgery and/or chemotherapy results in high response rates and excellent local-regional control across a broad spectrum of malignancies. Despite the use of near tolerance doses of radiation, however, a significant number of patients will experience relapse within the radiation field (Suit 1996). Therefore, identification of factors that help to predict local-regional failure after radiation remains an active area of investigation. Conventional clinical and pathologic factors, including patient age, sex, race, TNM stage, histologic subtype, tumor grade, differentiation, and margin status have been extensively evaluated as prognostic risk factors for both local and systemic relapse. While these conventional factors have been helpful in identifying risk and guiding clinical decision making for both local and systemic management, there is clearly a need to identify additional prognostic markers, which can aid in refining our treatment strategies and improve treatment outcomes (Gorski et al. 1998; Smith et al. 2000; Haffty 2002; Haffty and Glazer 2003; Haffty and Wilson 2009).

Substantial research efforts have been focused on genetic and molecular factors related to metastatic disease and overall survival, and many of these factors have been integrated into routine clinical management (Folkman 1985; Brennan and Sidransky 1996; Agrup et al. 2000; Linderholm et al. 2000b; Perou et al. 2000; Perez et al. 2002; Harris et al. 2004; Romond et al. 2005; Harris et al. 2006). While molecular and genetic markers have not been fully integrated into local-regional management, there is a rapidly growing body of literature focused on molecular and genetic factors associated with radiation resistance and risk of local-regional failure (Elkhuizen et al. 1999; Linderholm et al. 1999; Haffty and Glazer 2003; Nuyten et al. 2006; Freedman et al. 2009; Goyal et al. 2009).

There are several reasons to explore the area of molecular markers as they relate to radiation resistance and local-regional failure. First, such factors can be used to identify which patients are at risk for failure using standard therapy, and ultimately to modify that therapy with dose escalation, concurrent chemotherapy, or targeted therapies. In addition to employing markers simply as prognostic factors to guide in clinical decision making, molecular markers provide a unique and exciting opportunity as potential targets for therapeutic intervention (Harari and Huang 2002; Romond et al. 2005). If overexpression of a given marker is associated with radiation resistance, targeting this marker with antibodies, or using other therapeutic modalities to downregulate or upregulate expression of the marker, may improve radiation sensitivity and ultimately improve local control and may result in cure. This strategy has already entered the clinical arena and proven effective in targeting EGFR in head and neck cancers, and an ongoing NSABP trial is evaluating targeted therapy to HER2/neu in patients receiving radiation for DCIS to improve local-regional control (Harari and Huang 2002).

As with any biologic model, it should be emphasized that the interpretation and potential use of molecular markers is complex, and there are often conflicting and seemingly contradictory data. A given molecular marker may not have prognostic significance for radiation failure for a specific disease site, but may be a powerful predictor in subsets of those patients, or may be a factor when evaluated in combination with another marker. As an example, COX-2 expression has been shown to correlate with outcomes in breast cancers which express estrogen receptor, but does not correlate strongly in patients with ER-negative disease (Haffty et al. 2008). In this regard there have been recent studies demonstrating the prognostic utility of profiles of expression of multiple molecular markers including a 21 gene expression profile, a 70 gene expression profile, and other profiles such as a hypoxic marker profile or wound healing profiles (Cheng et al. 2006; Nuyten et al. 2006; Mamounas et al. 2010).

In addition to molecular/genetic profiling of tumors in an effort to improve outcomes and individualize therapeutic strategies, genetic profiling of the host is being increasingly evaluated as a prognostic tool to evaluate both tumor response and normal tissue response (Haffty et al. 2002; Iannuzzi et al. 2002; Ho et al. 2006; Pierce et al. 2006). The mapping of the human genome has afforded unique opportunities to understand and evaluate the impact of treating cancers associated with relatively rare disease-associated genetic mutations such as BRCA1/BRCA2, ▶ Li-Fraumeni, and ATM. In addition, recent studies have focused on treatment outcomes associated with relatively common variants and polymorphisms in a broad spectrum of genes. For example, a common polymorphism in tamoxifen metabolism, CYP2D6, has been associated with poor response to tamoxifen and is being used by some oncologists in the selection of hormonal therapy options (Schroth et al. 2009). Polymorphisms in a number of genes associated with DNA repair and radiation response, such as 53BP1, TGF-Beta, MDM2, BCL-2, and others, are being investigated as prognostic factors for normal tissue reactions and response to radiation (Hirata et al. 2009; Lehnerdt et al. 2009; Yuan et al. 2009).

In this review, we will attempt to summarize recent advances and the available literature evaluating molecular and genetic markers as they relate to radiation sensitivity of solid tumors. We will focus on the area of molecular markers in the primary tumors. The rapidly evolving literature evaluating genetic mutations in the host, as they relate to radiation response and sensitivity, represents a broad and rapidly growing area of investigation. However, the focus of this review will be limited to expression of molecular markers in the primary tumor, as they relate to radiation sensitivity and local control of disease. We have attempted to highlight a portion of molecular markers that have potential clinical significance with respect to radiation sensitivity and local control. Novel markers continue to be rapidly identified and it is clearly not possible in this review to include all the available literature. For the majority of markers, we have attempted to provide some of the basic biology and laboratory evidence demonstrating how the marker relates to radiation response, and have provided some of the available correlative clinical studies employing these markers as prognostic tools.

Epidermal Growth Factor Receptor

The epidermal growth factor receptor (EGFR) is a transmembrane protein of the ErbB family of tyrosine kinase receptors, and it has been demonstrated that signaling through EGFR stimulates the cell cycle pathways that control cell proliferation. EGFR inhibitors generally result in growth arrest and/or anti-proliferation (Nicholson et al. 2001; Harari and Huang 2002). It is presumed that the success of EGFR with radiation is in part attributable to the combination of EGFR G1 cell cycle arrest and the G2 cell cycle arrest of radiation (Harari and Huang 2002). In addition, EGFR inhibitors enhance radiation-induced

apoptosis and inhibit radiation-induced damage repair (Huang et al. 2001).

Epidermal growth factor receptor is expressed in a wide variety of cancers. While there are several studies demonstrating expression of EGFR correlates with poor overall and disease-free survival, there are several studies correlating EGFR expression with local failure in irradiated patients (Grandis et al. 1998; Almadori et al. 1999; Grandis et al. 2000; Kwok and Sutherland 1991; Harari and Huang 2001, 2002). Taken together, these studies suggest an association between EGFR expression, radiation resistance, and local relapse in patients treated with radiation therapy.

Given the laboratory and clinical data correlating EGFR expression with radiation response, and the availability of antibodies directed at EGFR which can affect the signaling pathways and theoretically alter radiosensitivity, laboratory and clinical efforts have focused on employing antibodies to EGFR, concurrently with radiation in an effort to improve response. Numerous laboratory studies to date have demonstrated significantly enhanced antitumor activity in cell lines treated with a combination of radiation therapy and antibody to EGFR. Ultimately this led to a landmark phase III trial of radiation alone compared to radiation with antibody to EGFR (Cetuximab). The median duration of locoregional control was 24.4 months among patients treated with cetuximab plus radiotherapy and 14.9 months among those given radiotherapy alone (hazard ratio = 0.68, $p = 0.0005$). In addition, the median overall survival was 49 months among patients treated with combined therapy and 29.3 months among those treated with radiotherapy alone (hazard ratio for death, 0.74; $p = 0.03$) (Bonner et al. 2000, 2006, 2010). This is one of the first and most significant studies to demonstrate the effectiveness of molecular targeted therapy in combination with radiation therapy where the targeted therapy significantly prolonged progression-free and overall survival. This strategy of identifying molecular markers associated with radiation resistance, attempting to regulate these markers and ultimately using these markers as a direct target for therapeutic intervention to achieve a therapeutic gain, highlights the exciting potential of molecular markers as they relate to radiation oncology.

HER2/Neu

Another member of the tyrosine kinase family, erbB-2 or HER2/neu, has been extensively studied in breast cancer (Romond et al. 2005). Although initial studies evaluating its prognostic significance were conflicting, recent data clearly demonstrate poorer survival rates and poorer response rates to specific chemotherapeutic agents in those patients whose primary breast tumors overexpress HER2/neu. Development of antibodies to HER2/neu has had a significant impact on clinical management. Patients with metastatic disease who overexpress HER2/neu benefit significantly from antibody therapy alone or antibody to HER2/neu in combination with cytotoxic chemotherapy, and anti-HER2/neu therapy, have been shown to improve outcomes when used in the adjuvant setting in patients with early stage and advanced breast cancers which are HER2/neu positive (Romond et al. 2005).

Data regarding HER2/neu and radiation sensitivity are less prevalent, but there appear to be both laboratory and clinical data suggesting that patients who overexpress HER2/neu do not respond as well as others (Haffty et al. 1996; Haffty et al. 2004; Freedman et al. 2009). In cell culture experiments, Pietras et al. reported increased radioresistance in cells overexpressing HER2/neu. Furthermore they demonstrated that therapy with antibody to HER2/neu enhanced radiation sensitivity. Stackhouse demonstrated that cells transfected with anti-erbB2 single chain antibody were radiosensitized

(Stackhouse et al. 1998). These and other laboratory studies indicate that overexpression of HER2/neu, as with overexpression of EGFR, may be associated with relative radioresistance.

There are several clinical studies supporting the laboratory studies that suggest that HER2/neu overexpression may be associated with relative radiation resistance. In a pilot case-control study of conservatively managed breast cancer patients, Haffty et al. observed that patients who sustained a local relapse were more likely to overexpress HER2/neu (Haffty et al. 1996). A similar trend was noted in conservatively treated patients in a study by Elkhuizen et al. although the difference did not reach statistical significance (Elkhuizen et al. 1999). More recently, in a cohort of patients treated with radiation for post-mastectomy chest wall relapses, Haffty et al. observed a higher rate of chest wall progression in patients overexpressing HER2/neu (Haffty et al. 2004). In a series of patients with locally advanced breast cancer treated with chemotherapy and radiation, Formenti et al. noted that low HER2/neu gene expression was associated with a better response to therapy (Formenti et al. 2002). Several other studies have also recently demonstrated higher local relapse rates in HER2/neu expressing tumors (Nguyen et al. 2008; Freedman et al. 2009). There are, however, several conflicting studies showing no correlation between radiation response/local relapse and HER2/neu expression (Pierce et al. 1994; Elkhuizen et al. 1999). Most of the studies evaluating HER2/neu, however, have utilized immunohistochemical staining. Recently, fluorescent in situ hybridization (FISH) evaluation of gene amplification has evolved as a more accurate and clinically meaningful measure of HER2/neu status (Perez et al. 2002). It is anticipated that future studies evaluating the prognostic significance of HER2/neu and radiation sensitivity will employ both immunohistochemical as well as FISH analysis. Of note, however, is that a majority of HER2/neu positive breast cancers are currently receiving adjuvant Trastuzumab, which theoretically should improve radiation sensitivity and is likely to improve local-regional relapse rates in HER2/neu positive cancers (Romond et al. 2005).

In this regard, the NSABP recently launched a study using anti-HER2/neu therapy as an adjunct to radiation in patients with DCIS. DCIS patients where HER2/neu is overexpressed generally have higher grade tumors and may be at increased risk of local relapse. In this recently launched NSABP study, patients with DCIS whose tumors overexpress HER2/neu by FISH will be treated with conventional whole breast irradiation and randomized to no other treatment or anti-HER2/neu therapy (trastuzumab) for two cycles during the course of radiation. This is one of the first studies in breast cancer where targeted molecular therapy will be used in combination with radiation to potentially improve local control.

P53

The P53 tumor suppressor protein plays a critical role in the cell cycle transition, DNA repair, and apoptosis (Lane 1992; Levine 1997; Bouvard et al. 2000; Agarwal et al. 2001; Alsner et al. 2001; Edstrom et al. 2001; Koelbl et al. 2001). Normal, wild type P53 is necessary to activate apoptosis and the role of P53 is therefore pivotal in assessing the response of tumors to ionizing radiation and chemotherapy. Growth arrest in wild type P53 is dependent on transcriptional activation of P21, which ultimately inhibits cyclin complexes and arrests cells in the G1 to S-phase transition. Through activation of BAX, a pro-apoptotic gene, and downregulation of BCL-2, an anti-apoptotic gene, P53 plays an essential role in apoptosis (Lowe et al. 1993; Wilson et al. 1995; Silvestrini et al. 1996; Xie et al. 1999). It follows that cellular response to radiation may be dependent on a normally functioning P53 protein. The complex role of P53, however, can result in opposing forces with respect to response to ionizing radiation. It has been suggested that this may be due to the fact that any decrease in apoptosis seen in P53-deficient cells may be offset by a defect in DNA repair (Mineta et al. 1998; Xia and Powell 2002).

Tumor cells with mutations in the P53 gene generally show accumulation and overexpression of the P53 protein. However, there is often discordance between mutation status of the P53 gene, and evaluation of the protein levels (i.e., expression of the protein does not always correlate with underlying mutations, and underlying P53 mutations may not always result in overexpression of the protein) (Mineta et al. 1998; Xia and Powell 2002). This factor, along with the complicated role of P53 in cell cycle regulation, apoptosis, and DNA repair, has resulted in confusing and conflicting data regarding P53 and response to radiation. Depending on the methodology in assessing P53, experimental conditions, and the status of other genetic and molecular factors within the cellular model, expression of P53 has been associated with increase radiation sensitivity, decreased radiation sensitivity, or no effect (Mineta et al. 1998; Elkhuizen et al. 1999; Overgaard et al. 2000; Turner et al. 2000; Alsner et al. 2001; Xia and Powell 2002).

Numerous translational clinical research studies have assessed the prognostic significance of P53 with respect to local control and response to radiation therapy. Given the complexities noted above, along with heterogeneity between and within the clinical data sets evaluated, the studies to date have been inconsistent and conflicting. There have been, however, numerous studies suggesting that P53 may be a significant factor in predicting response to radiation. In order to overcome the difficulties associated with discordant results between protein expression and gene mutations, Alsner et al. used denaturing gradient gel electrophoresis to assess the P53 gene mutation status in a cohort of patients with squamous cell carcinoma of the head and neck (Alsner et al. 2001). In patients treated with radiation therapy, P-53 gene mutations were associated with poor local control and disease-free survival. Koch et al. also demonstrated poorer local control in patients with P53 mutations with a relative risk of 2.4 compared to tumors with wild type P53 (Koch et al. 1996). Several of these studies report that mutation status, but not necessarily protein expression, correlates with local relapse and radiation response. Given the mixed results of P53 protein expression as a prognostic factor in head and neck cancer, the value of P53 protein expression alone as a prognostic factor remains questionable. In a study in early stage larynx cancer, Rewari et al. reported that the combination of P53 expression and the BRCA2 interactive protein BCCIP was found to have prognostic significance for local relapse (Rewari et al. 2009).

P53 protein expression has also been evaluated as a prognostic factor for local control and radiation response in breast cancer. In a case-control study of locally recurrent breast cancer patients and a matched group of locally controlled patients, Turner et al. observed a higher rate of overexpression of P53 in the locally recurrent cohort (Turner et al. 2000). A similar study reported by Elkhuizen et al., however, failed to show a correlation between P53 expression and local control in conservatively managed breast cancer patients (Elkhuizen et al. 1999). Silvestrini et al. also did not show a correlation with local relapse following conservative surgery and radiation. They did report, however, that nonirradiated conservatively managed patients had a higher rate of local relapse with overexpression of P53 (Silvestrini et al. 1993, 1996). Finally, in a large cohort of mastectomized patients, Zellars et al. reported higher rates of local relapse with and without postoperative radiation in those patients overexpressing P53 (Zellars et al. 2000).

There have been numerous studies in other sites, including cervix, lung, prostate, colo-rectum, and brain, which demonstrate both positive and negative results using P53 expression as a prognostic factor for radiation sensitivity and local control with therapeutic doses of radiation. It is apparent that the data with respect to P53 overexpression based on immunohistochemical staining remain conflicting. Given the differences in techniques between studies, patient heterogeneity, relatively small patient populations, discordance between protein expression and gene status, along with the complex role of P53 in cell cycle regulation, repair, and apoptosis, the conflicting results are not surprising. Clearly, further studies are warranted, that evaluate P53 status at both the protein and gene level, and that evaluate co-expression of P53 with other markers, to determine the potential clinical utility of P53 status in assessing radiation response. Since P53 does play such a potential pivotal role in cellular response, and can potentially be used as a target for therapeutic intervention, clarifying its role as a prognostic factor and as a target to improve radiation sensitivity is a worthy avenue of investigation.

BCL-2 and Apoptotic Markers

Overexpression of genes that suppress apoptosis or down regulation of pro-apoptotic genes can theoretically result in radioresistant phenotypes. The protein product of the BCL-2 oncogene promotes cell survival by suppressing apoptosis. BAX, a related homologue of the BCL-2 protein has been shown to form heterodimers with BCL-2, thereby antagonizing its function and promoting apoptosis (Reed 1998). Therefore, the combination of overexpression of BCL-2 and low expression of BAX are theoretically associated with decreased apoptotic response to radiation and increased radiation resistance. Conversely, elevated BAX and low BCL-2 protein levels should be associated with increased apoptotic response and higher sensitivity to radiation. Several studies have evaluated these related proto-oncogenes as a function of clinical response to radiation. In a series of 41 patients undergoing external beam radiation for prostate cancer, Mackey et al. demonstrated that patients with higher BCL-2/bax ratios were at increased risk of failing radiation (Mackey et al. 1998). In carcinoma of the cervix treated with definitive radiotherapy, Harima et al. reported that BCL-2 and bax prior to therapy did not correlate with response to therapy, but increased bax expression after 10.8 Gy correlated with good response and increase BCL-2 expression after 10.8 Gy correlated with poor response (Harima et al. 2000).

In a recent study of conservatively treated breast cancer patients, Yang et al. demonstrated that BCL-2 expression correlated with higher local relapse rates (Yang et al. 2009). As with the other markers, larger, more homogenous patient populations using standardized techniques are required prior to routinely using these markers in clinical decision making. This area of BCL-2 as a molecular marker may become increasingly clinically relevant as there are now commercially available agents targeting BCL-2 that are currently in Phase I/II human trials for patients with metastatic disease. Use of these agents in combination with radiation therapy may result in increased response and local-regional control rates, as has been shown with antibodies directed at EGFR.

Angiogenic Factors

Molecular markers related to tumor neovascularization have been evaluated as a possible predictor of disease-free survival, overall survival, and response to therapy. The most commonly evaluated angiogenic markers include the microvessel density and vascular endothelial growth factor. Several laboratory and translational clinical studies have evaluated angiogenic molecular markers as they relate to radiation sensitivity. Although there are many growth factors (VEGF) involved in the angiogenic process, vascular endothelial growth factor has been identified as the most dominant protein that mediates endothelial cell growth. In a series of experiments employing cell lines transformed to overexpress VEGF, Gupta et al. demonstrated that VEGF enhanced endothelial cell survival and VEGF-positive xenografts were more resistant to cytotoxic effects of ionizing radiation while treatment with anti-VEGF antibody enhanced radiation sensitivity (Gupta et al. 2002a, b). Gorski et al. demonstrated that blockade of the VEGF stress response enhanced the antitumor effects of radiation (Gorski et al. 1998). These studies, as well as others, provide strong laboratory evidence that overexpression of VEGF is associated with radiation resistance, and that reversal of radiation resistance may be achieved through specific targeting of the VEGF pathway.

There are several clinical studies that support VEGF as a predictive factor for radiation resistance. In a series of early stage laryngeal carcinomas treated with radiation therapy, Homer et al. noted increased expression of VEGF in tumor specimens compared to normal tissue (Homer et al. 2001). However, they did not observe a difference in expression of VEGF between radiosensitive and radioresistant tumors. In a series of squamous cell carcinomas of the oral cavity and oropharynx, treated with surgery and postoperative radiation, Smith et al. noted an increased relative risk of local relapse (RR = 3.08) associated with VEGF-positive tumors (Smith et al. 2000). In a meta-analysis of over 1,000 patients in 12 studies where angiogenic markers were evaluated in head and neck cancers, Kyzas et al. reported a 1.88-fold increase in 2-year mortality with overexpression of VEGF (Kyzas et al. 2005).

In node-negative breast cancer patients treated with radiotherapy alone, Linderholm et al. noted that expression of VEGF correlated with relapse-free and overall survival (Linderholm et al. 2000a). Although they showed no specific correlation with local relapse alone, they hypothesized that VEGF expression may define a radioresistant phenotype. Although there are conflicting data, these studies support a potential role for VEGF as a prognostic factor and as a potential target for therapeutic intervention to enhance tumor radiocurability.

COX-2

Cyclooxygenase-2 is induced by a variety of factors and has been shown to be linked to carcinogenesis, tumor growth, and metastatic spread (Denkert et al. 2004). The cytokine inducible enzyme has been shown to be upregulated in inflammatory conditions, metabolizes protaglandins, suppresses apoptosis, and promotes tumor invasion and angiogenesis (Costa et al. 2002; Brueggemeier et al. 2003). Recent laboratory investigations have shown that inhibitors of COX-2 can result in enhanced radiation sensitivity (Milas 2001; Bundred and Barnes 2005). This coupled with studies demonstrating that overexpression of COX-2 may be related to radiation resistance make this marker particularly appealing. Theoretically, the relatively nontoxic use of COX-2 inhibitors or nonsteroidal anti-inflammatory drugs used in combination with radiation may help to overcome the relative radioresistance of tumors overexpressing COX-2. Studies by Milas et al. and Kishi et al. clearly demonstrated enhancement of tumor response to gamma radiation by inhibiting the cyclooxygenase-2. Clinical translational studies in carcinoma of the cervix demonstrated that overexpression of COX-2 is associated with decreased responsiveness to radiation and local relapse within the irradiated

volume (Kishi et al. 2000; Milas 2001, 2003; Bundred and Barnes 2005). Overexpression of COX-2 was reported by Gaffney et al. to be correlated with poorer overall and disease-free survival in a cohort of cervical carcinoma patients treated with definitive radiation therapy (Gaffney et al. 2001a, b). In a related study, Kim et al. demonstrated overexpression of COX-2 to be associated with a higher incidence of central and lymph node failure (Kim et al. 2002). In a study of early stage breast cancer patients treated with conservative surgery and radiation, Haffty et al. demonstrated a higher rate of local and distant relapse in COX-2 expressing tumors (Haffty et al. 2008). However, the significance was limited to estrogen receptor positive disease, a finding also noted by others (Spizzo et al. 2003). This may be related to the fact that overexpression of COX-2 drives an increase in aromatase levels that may negatively impact on hormone sensitive tumors (Spizzo et al. 2003; Bundred and Barnes 2005).

These pilot studies, although small, demonstrate the potential prognostic use of COX-2 expression with respect to radiation. If the use of commonly available COX-2 inhibitors can be combined with radiation in tumors that are known to overexpress COX-2, it is feasible that a therapeutic gain can be realized with relatively low cost and toxicity. This is currently an active area of investigation.

Cell Kinetic/Proliferative Markers

Proliferation markers that have been evaluated as predictors of radiation response include Ki-67, proliferating cell nuclear antigen, p105, thymidine labeling index, S-phase fraction, and potential doubling time. We will not extensively review this topic and the reader is referred to numerous reports and reviews of these proliferative markers as predictors of radiation response in the literature (Begg 1995, 1999; Bradford 1999). There are conflicting reports regarding the majority of proliferative markers with respect to radiation sensitivity and local control with radiation therapy. The conflicting reports are likely a reflection of a number of competing and conflicting factors including patient heterogeneity, tumor heterogeneity, changes in proliferative indices induced by radiation, differences in techniques, and relatively small sample sizes. Currently, the weight of evidence suggests that although proliferative markers may be of prognostic value in predicting radiation response in subsets of patients, given the inconsistencies and conflicting data to date, one cannot reliably use these markers for clinical decision making at this time.

Gene Profiling of Tumors

Recent advances in technology allow for evaluation of the expression of multiple genes in a given tumor simultaneously. While the initial research in this arena was limited to fresh-frozen tissue specimens, currently paraffin embedded specimens can be processed for gene expression profiling (Perou et al. 2000; Esteva et al. 2002; Paik et al. 2004; Sorlie 2004; Mamounas et al. 2010). There has been a broad spectrum of studies evaluating gene profiles as potential prognostic tools in local-regional management. A few of these will be highlighted here.

Cheng et al. evaluated 97 post-mastectomy patients (67 without a local-regional relapse and 30 with a local-regional relapse) who all were treated by mastectomy without radiation. Using a 258 gene profile assay they were able to define a high risk and low risk group (Cheng et al. 2006). They also demonstrated that the 258 gene profile could be reduced to a 34 gene profile without loss of prognostic value. In patients treated with mastectomy with one to three positive nodes, those with a poor prognostic signature had a high risk of local relapse (12 of 19), in comparison to only 1 of 34 relapses in the favorable prognostic signature group. Validation of this study in a larger cohort is eagerly awaited.

Nuyton et al. showed in a cohort of patients treated with BCS+RT that a wound profiling signature was prognostic of local relapse (Nuyten et al. 2006). This profile demonstrated prognostic value in a training set, and was validated in a second validation cohort. Again, confirmation in a larger cohort is needed to assess its potential clinical utility.

Mamounas et al. recently demonstrated using a 21 gene profile assay (Oncotype DX) that a high recurrence score correlated with local relapse in early stage node-negative ER positive breast cancer patients (Mamounas et al. 2010). In another study of nearly 3,000 breast cancers, using a panel of five markers (ER, PR, HER2, Cytokeratin, and Ki-67), Voduc et al. reported a higher rate of local relapse following mastectomy among basal-like tumors, and a higher rate of local relapse following breast conserving surgery in HER2-enriched tumors (Voduc et al. 2010). These and other studies will require further validation prior to routine clinical use.

Summary

In summary, the application of molecular and genetic markers in clinical radiation oncology as prognostic factors and as potential targets for therapeutic intervention continues to evolve rapidly. There is tremendous potential for employing molecular and genetic markers as prognostic factors, as they relate to local-regional control of disease and response to radiation. Although we have covered a broad scope of the relevant literature, there are many studies that may have been overlooked, and many important ongoing investigations with promise for the future. Despite the rapid expansion of data and ongoing studies, efforts evaluating molecular markers as they relate to radiation oncology and local-regional control of disease lag far behind molecular strategies in combination with chemotherapy for systemic control of disease. This relatively under-explored area of molecular strategies for clinical decision making and to improve radiocurability creates an exciting opportunity for investigation, and more importantly has potential for impacting on clinical care and improving patient outcome.

Cross-References

▶ Breast Cancer: Locally Advanced and Recurrent Disease, Postmastectomy Radiation and Systemic Therapies
▶ Cancer of the Breast Tis
▶ Early-Stage Breast Cancer
▶ Larynx
▶ Lung
▶ Nasopharynx
▶ Oro-Hypopharynx
▶ Prostate
▶ Uterine Cervix

References

Agarwal ML, Ramana CV, Hamilton M, Taylor WR, DePrimo SE, Bean LJ, Agarwal A, Agarwal MK, Wolfman A, Stark GR (2001) Regulation of p53 expression by the RAS-MAP kinase pathway. Oncogene 20:2527–2536

Agrup M, Stal O, Olsen K, Wingren S (2000) C-erbB-2 overexpression and survival in early onset breast cancer. Breast Cancer Res Treat 63:23–29

Almadori G, Cadoni G, Galli J, Ferrandina G, Scambia G, Exarchakos G, Paludetti G, Ottaviani F (1999) Epidermal growth factor receptor expression in primary laryngeal cancer: an independent prognostic factor of neck node relapse. Int J Cancer 84:188–191

Alsner J, Hoyer M, Sorensen SB, Overgaard J (2001) Interaction between potential doubling time and TP53 mutation: predicting radiotherapy outcome in squamous cell carcinoma of the head and neck. Int J Radiat Oncol Biol Phys 49:519–525

Begg AC (1995) The clinical status of Tpot as a predictor? Or why no tempest in the Tpot! Int J Radiat Oncol Biol Phys 32:1539–1541

Bonner JA, Raisch KP, Trummell HQ, Robert F, Meredith RF, Spencer SA, Buchsbaum DJ, Saleh MN, Stackhouse MA, LoBuglio AF, Peters GE, Carroll WR, Waksal HW (2000) J Clin Oncol 18:47S–53S

Bonner JA, Harari PM, Giralt J, Azarnia N, Shin DM, Cohen RB, Jones CU, Sur R, Raben D, Jassem J, Ove R, Kies MS, Baselga J, Youssoufian H, Amellal N, Rowinsky EK, Ang KK (2006) N Engl J Med 354:567–578

Bonner JA, Harari PM, Giralt J, Cohen RB, Jones CU, Sur RK, Raben D, Baselga J, Spencer SA, Zhu J, Youssoufian H, Rowinsky EK, Ang KK (2010) Radiotherapy plus cetuximab for loco-regionally advanced head and neck cancer: 5-year survival data from a phase 3 randomised trial, and relation between cetuximab-induced rash and survival. Lancet Oncol 11:21–28

Cheng SH, Horng CF, West M, Huang E, Pittman J, Tsou MH, Dressman H, Chen CM, Tsai SY, Jian JJ, Liu MC, Nevins JR, Huang AT (2006) Genomic prediction of locoregional recurrence after mastectomy in breast cancer. J Clin Oncol 24:4594–4602

Costa C, Soares R, Reis-Filho JS, Leitao D, Amendoeira I, Schmitt FC (2002) Cyclo-oxygenase 2 expression is associated with angiogenesis and lymph node metastasis in human breast cancer. J Clin Pathol 55:429–434

Denkert C, Winzer KJ, Hauptmann S (2004) Prognostic impact of cyclooxygenase-2 in breast cancer. Clin Breast Cancer 4:428–433

Edstrom S, Cvetkovska E, Westin T, Young C (2001) Overexpression of p53-related proteins predicts rapid growth rate of head and neck cancer. Laryngoscope 111:124–130

Elkhuizen PH, Voogd AC, van den Broek LC, Tan IT, van Houwelingen HC, Leer JW, van de Vijver MJ (1999) Risk factors for local recurrence after breast-conserving therapy for invasive carcinoma: a case-control study of histological factors and alterations in oncogene expression. Int J Radiat Oncol Biol Phys 45:73–83

Esteva FJ, Sahin AA, Cristofanilli M, Arun B, Hortobagyi GN (2002) Molecular prognostic factors for breast cancer metastasis and survival. Semin Radiat Oncol 12:319–328

Formenti SC, Spicer D, Skinner K, Cohen D, Groshen S, Bettini A, Naritoku W, Press M, Salonga D, Tsao-Wei D, Danenberg K, Danenberg P (2002) Low HER2/neu gene expression is associated with pathological response to concurrent paclitaxel and radiation therapy in locally advanced breast cancer. Int J Radiat Oncol Biol Phys 52:397–405

Freedman GM, Anderson PR, Li T, Nicolaou N (2009) Locoregional recurrence of triple-negative breast cancer after breast-conserving surgery and radiation. Cancer 115:946–951

Gaffney DK, Holden J, Davis M, Zempolich K, Murphy KJ, Dodson M (2001a) Elevated cyclooxygenase-2 expression correlates with diminished survival in carcinoma of the cervix treated with radiotherapy. Int J Radiat Oncol Biol Phys 49:1213–1217

Gaffney DK, Holden J, Zempolich K, Murphy KJ, Dicker AP, Dodson M (2001b) Am J Clin Oncol 24:443–446

Goyal S, Parikh RR, Green C, Schiff D, Moran MS, Yang Q, Haffty BG (2009) Int J Radiat Oncol Biol Phys 75(5):1304–1308

Grandis JR, Melhem MF, Gooding WE, Day R, Holst VA, Wagener MM, Drenning SD, Tweardy DJ (1998) J Natl Cancer Inst 90:824–832

Grandis JR, Zeng Q, Drenning SD (2000) Laryngoscope 110:868–874

Gupta VK, Jaskowiak NT, Beckett MA, Mauceri HJ, Grunstein J, Johnson RS, Calvin DA, Nodzenski E, Pejovic M, Kufe DW, Posner MC, Weichselbaum RR (2002a) Cancer J 8:47–54

Gupta VK, Park JO, Jaskowiak NT, Mauceri HJ, Seetharam S, Weichselbaum RR, Posner MC (2002b) Ann Surg Oncol 9:500–504

Harari PM, Huang SM (2002) Semin Radiat Oncol 12:21–26

Harima Y, Nagata K, Harima K, Oka A, Ostapenko VV, Shikata N, Ohnishi T, Tanaka Y (2000) Cancer 88:132–138

Harris J, Lippman M, Morrow M, Osborne C (2004) Diseases of the breast. Lippincott Williams & Wilkins, Philadelphia

Ho AY, Atencio DP, Peters S, Stock RG, Formenti SC, Cesaretti JA, Green S, Haffty B, Drumea K, Leitzin L, Kuten A, Azria D, Ozsahin M, Overgaard J, Andreassen CN, Trop CS, Park J, Rosenstein BS (2006) Int J Radiat Oncol Biol Phys 65:646–655

Homer JJ, Greenman J, Stafford ND (2001) Clin Otolaryngol 26:498–504

Iannuzzi CM, Atencio DP, Green S, Stock RG, Rosenstein BS (2002) Int J Radiat Oncol Biol Phys 52:606–613

Kim YB, Kim GE, Cho NH, Pyo HR, Shim SJ, Chang SK, Park HC, Suh CO, Park TK, Kim BS (2002) Cancer 95:531–539

Kishi K, Petersen S, Petersen C, Hunter N, Mason K, Masferrer JL, Tofilon PJ, Milas L (2000) Cancer Res 60:1326–1331

Koch WM, Brennan JA, Zahurak M, Goodman SN, Westra WH, Schwab D, Yoo GH, Lee DJ, Forastiere AA, Sidransky D (1996) J Natl Cancer Inst 88:1580–1586

Koelbl O, Rosenwald A, Haberl M, Muller J, Reuther J, Flentje M (2001) Int J Radiat Oncol Biol Phys 49:147–154

Kwok TT, Sutherland RM (1991) Br J Cancer 64:251–254

Lehnerdt GF, Franz P, Bankfalvi A, Grehl S, Kelava A, Nuckel H, Lang S, Schmid KW, Siffert W, Bachmann HS (2009) Ann Oncol 20:1094–1099

Linderholm B, Tavelin B, Grankvist K, Henriksson R (1999) Br J Cancer 81:727–732

Linderholm B, Grankvist K, Wilking N, Johansson M, Tavelin B, Henriksson R (2000a) J Clin Oncol 18:1423–1431

Linderholm B, Lindh B, Tavelin B, Grankvist K, Henriksson R (2000b) Int J Cancer 89:51–62

Mackey TJ, Borkowski A, Amin P, Jacobs SC, Kyprianou N (1998) Urology 52:1085–1090

Mamounas EP, Tang G, Fisher B, Paik S, Shak S, Costantino JP, Watson D, Geyer CE Jr, Wickerham DL, Wolmark N (2010) Association between the 21-gene recurrence score assay and risk of locoregional recurrence in node-negative, estrogen receptor-positive breast cancer: results from NSABP B-14 and NSABP B-20. J Clin Oncol 28(10):1677–1683

Milas L (2001) Semin Radiat Oncol 11:290–299

Milas L (2003) Am J Clin Oncol 26:S66–S69

Mineta H, Borg A, Dictor M, Wahlberg P, Akervall J, Wennerberg J (1998) Br J Cancer 78:1084–1090

Nguyen PL, Taghian AG, Katz MS, Niemierko A, Abi Raad RF, Boon WL, Bellon JR, Wong JS, Smith BL, Harris JR (2008) J Clin Oncol 26:2373–2378

Nicholson RI, Gee JM, Harper ME (2001) Eur J Cancer 37(suppl 4):S9–S15

Paik S, Shak S, Tang G, Kim C, Baker J, Cronin M, Baehner FL, Walker MG, Watson D, Park T, Hiller W, Fisher ER, Wickerham DL, Bryant J, Wolmark N (2004) N Engl J Med 351:2817–2826

Pierce LJ, Merino MJ, D'Angelo T, Barker EA, Gilbert L, Cowan KH, Steinberg SM, Glatstein E (1994) Int J Radiat Oncol Biol Phys 28:395–403

Pierce LJ, Levin AM, Rebbeck TR, Ben-David MA, Friedman E, Solin LJ, Harris EE, Gaffney DK, Haffty BG, Dawson LA, Narod SA, Olivotto IA, Eisen A, Whelan TJ, Olopade OI, Isaacs C, Merajver SD, Wong JS, Garber JE, Weber BL (2006) J Clin Oncol 24:2437–2443

Reed JC (1998) Oncogene 17:3225–3236

Rewari A, Lu H, Parikh R, Yang Q, Shen Z, Haffty BG (2009) Radiother Oncol 90:183–188

Romond EH, Perez EA, Bryant J, Suman VJ, Geyer CE Jr, Davidson NE, Tan-Chiu E, Martino S, Paik S, Kaufman PA, Swain SM, Pisansky TM, Fehrenbacher L, Kutteh LA, Vogel VG, Visscher DW, Yothers G, Jenkins RB, Brown AM, Dakhil SR, Mamounas EP, Lingle WL, Klein PM, Ingle JN, Wolmark N (2005) N Engl J Med 353:1673–1684

Schroth W, Goetz MP, Hamann U, Fasching PA, Schmidt M, Winter S, Fritz P, Simon W, Suman VJ, Ames MM, Safgren SL, Kuffel MJ, Ulmer HU, Bolander J, Strick R, Beckmann MW, Koelbl H, Weinshilboum RM, Ingle JN, Eichelbaum M, Schwab M, Brauch H (2009) JAMA 302:1429–1436

Silvestrini R, Benini E, Daidone MG, Veneroni S, Boracchi P, Cappelletti V, Di Fronzo G, Veronesi U (1993) J Natl Cancer Inst 85:965–970

Silvestrini R, Benini E, Veneroni S, Daidone MG, Tomasic G, Squicciarini P, Salvadori B (1996) J Clin Oncol 14:1604–1610

Smith BD, Smith GL, Carter D, Sasaki CT, Haffty BG (2000) J Clin Oncol 18:2046–2052

Sorlie T (2004) Eur J Cancer 40:2667–2675

Spizzo G, Gastl G, Wolf D, Gunsilius E, Steurer M, Fong D, Amberger A, Margreiter R, Obrist P (2003) Br J Cancer 88:574–578

Stackhouse MA, Buchsbaum DJ, Grizzle WE, Bright SJ, Olsen CC, Kancharla S, Mayo MS, Curiel DT (1998) Int J Radiat Oncol Biol Phys 42:817–822

Suit H (1996) Front Radiat Ther Oncol 29:17–23

Turner BC, Gumbs AA, Carbone CJ, Carter D, Glazer PM, Haffty BG (2000) Cancer 88:1091–1098

Voduc KD, Cheang MC, Tyldesley S, Gelmon K, Nielsen TO, Kennecke H (2010) Breast cancer subtypes and the risk of local and regional relapse. J Clin Oncol 28(10): 1684–1691

Wilson GD, Richman PI, Dische S, Saunders MI, Robinson B, Daley FM, Ross DA (1995) Br J Cancer 71:1248–1252

Xia F, Powell SN (2002) Semin Radiat Oncol 12:296–304

Xie X, Clausen OP, De Angelis P, Boysen M (1999) Cancer 86:913–920

Yang Q, Moran MS, Haffty BG (2009) Breast Cancer Res Treat 115:343–348

Yuan X, Liao Z, Liu Z, Wang LE, Tucker SL, Mao L, Wang XS, Martel M, Komaki R, Cox JD, Milas L, Wei Q (2009) J Clin Oncol 27:3370–3378

Zellars RC, Hilsenbeck SG, Clark GM, Allred DC, Herman TS, Chamness GC, Elledge RM (2000) J Clin Oncol 18:1906–1913

Molecular Targeting

CLAUDIA E. RÜBE
Department of Radiation Oncology, Saarland University, Homburg/Saar, Germany

Definition

To design drugs that specifically attack the molecular pathways that cause malignant disease, without disrupting the normal functions in other cells and tissues.

Cross-References

▶ Predictive In vitro Assays in Radiation Oncology

Monitor Unit

TIMOTHY HOLMES[1], CHARLIE MA[2], LU WANG[2]
[1]Department of Radiation Oncology, Sinai Hospital, Baltimore, MD, USA
[2]Department of Radiation Oncology, Fox Chase Cancer Center, Philadelphia, PA, USA

Definition

Monitor unit – A measure of radiation "beam-on" time used for medical linear accelerators. By convention, one monitor unit equals 1 cGy of absorbed dose in water under specific calibration conditions for the medical linac.

Cross-References

▶ Dose Calculation Algorithms
▶ Image-Guided Radiation Therapy (IGRT): TomoTherapy
▶ Image-Guided Radiotherapy (IGRT)

M

Monoclonal Antibodies

RENE RUBIN
Rittenhouse Hematology/Oncology, Philadelphia, PA, USA

Definition

Alemtuzumab is a monoclonal antibody to CD52 which is used in chronic lymphocytic leukemia.

Brentuximab vedotin is a monoclonal antibody to CD30 (microtubule inhibitor) and approved for relapsed Hodgkin's disease and anaplastic large cell lymphoma.

Gemtuzumab/ozogamicin is a monoclonal antibody to CD33 conjugated to calicheamicin and used in relapsed acute myelogenous leukemia and myelodysplastic syndrome.

Ibritumomab is a CD20 monoclonal antibody radiolabeled to yttrium. It is used in CD20-positive B-cell malignancies.

Ipilimumab is a newly approved monoclonal antibody for use in melanoma. It binds to cytotoxic T lymphocyte associated antigen 4 and causes an immune response by blocking the activity of CTLA 4 and causes T-cell activation and proliferation. The substance is also being studied in prostate carcinoma.

Rituximab is a monoclonal antibody to CD20-positive lymphocytes. It is used in combination with other chemotherapeutic drugs to treat B-cell malignancies that are CD20 positive (chronic lymphocytic leukemia, non-Hodgkin's disease) and as maintenance. Furthermore, it is also used in the treatment of autoimmune diseases.

Tositumomab is a CD20 monoclonal antibody attached to radioactive iodine. It is indicated in B-cell malignancies.

Side Effects

- Allergy (rituximab, brentuximab vedotin)
- Fever
- Immunosuppression (rituximab)
- Hepatotoxicity/veno-occlusive liver disease
- Abdominal pain (brentuximab vedotin)
- Bloating, constipation, diarrhea (ipilimumab)
- Myelosuppression/thrombocytopenia
- Pulmonary edema
- Tumor lysis syndrome
- Arrythmia (brentuximab vedotin)
- Hypotension
- Urinary retention (ipilimumab)

Cross-References

▶ Non-Hodgkin's Lymphoma
▶ Principles of Chemotherapy

Morbus Bowen

Stephan Mose[1], Gerhard G. Grabenbauer[2]
[1]Department of Radiation Oncology, Schwarzwald-Baar-Klinikum, Villingen-Schwenningen, Germany
[2]Chairman of the Department of Radiation Oncology, DiaCura Coburg & Klinikum Coburg, Coburg, Germany

Definition

Bowen's disease is an intraepidermal carcinoma in situ which may merge into a squamous cell carcinoma. It presents as circumscribed erythematous sometimes scaly and crusted plaque with irregular borders. This disease may affect any site of the skin surface or on mucosal surfaces.

Cross-References

▶ Anal Carcinoma
▶ Penile Cancer
▶ Skin Cancer

MSI

▶ Microsatellite Instability

mTOR Inhibitors

Rene Rubin
Rittenhouse Hematology/Oncology, Philadelphia, PA, USA

Definition

The mammalian target of rapamycin is a protein kinase that regulates cell growth, proliferation, and motility. It is integrated with insulin-like receptors. The mTOR pathway is dysregulated in certain cancers. The mTOR-inhibitors everolimus (oral) and temsirolimus (I.V.) are approved for renal cell carcinoma. Furthermore, everolimus is used in pancreatic neuroendocrine carcinomas and astrocytoma. Rapamycin is used to prevent transplant rejection.

Side Effects
- Allergy
- Rash
- Myelosuppression
- Hyperglycemia
- Hyperlipidemia
- Interstitial lung disease
- Nausea
- Liver enzyme dysfunction

Cross-References
▶ Principles of Chemotherapy

MTT Assay

CLAUDIA E. RÜBE
Department of Radiation Oncology,
Saarland University, Homburg/Saar, Germany

Definition
Allows to estimate cell survival based upon the capacity of living cells to reduce a tetrazolium compound to a colored product that can be measured spectrophotometrically.

Cross-References
▶ Predictive In vitro Assays in Radiation Oncology

Mucoepidermoid Carcinoma

LINDSAY G. JENSEN, LOREN K. MELL
Center for Advanced Radiotherapy Technologies,
Department of Radiation Oncology, San Diego
Rebecca and John Moores Cancer Center,
University of California, La Jolla, CA, USA

Definition
Most common malignant tumor of the parotid gland. Graded as low, intermediate, or high grade. Higher grades are associated with poorer prognosis (Carlson and Ord 2009).

Cross-References
▶ Salivary Gland Cancer

Mucosa-Associated Lymphoid Tissue (MALT)

FILIP T. TROICKI[1], JAGANMOHAN POLI[2]
[1]College of Medicine, Drexel University,
Philadelphia, PA, USA
[2]Department of Radiation Oncology, College of
Medicine, Drexel University, Philadelphia,
PA, USA

Definition
Concentration of lymphatic tissue (containing B cells, T cells, macrophages, plasma cells) that exist within various sites of the body, including the gastrointestinal tract.

Cross-References
▶ Stomach Cancer

Mucosal Melanomas

THEODORE E. YAEGER
Department Radiation Oncology, Wake Forest
University School of Medicine, Winston-Salem
NC, USA

Definition

Primary melanoma of the head and neck region occurring in mucosal surfaces typically in the fifth to seventh decades of life with an equal male-to-female ratio.

Primary mucosal melanomas of the head and neck regions comprise less than 10% of melanoma cases in the United States up to 25% of presentations in Japan (Umeda et al. 1988; Batsakis et al. 1982). They are very rare in the first two decades of life and are fairly split evenly between the upper respiratory tract and the pharynx or oral cavity. Presentations in the nasal cavity/paranasal sinuses are even rarer, compromising less than 1% of melanomas. The hard palate in the oral cavity is the most common site of occurrences and is typically preceded by a pigmented area lasting over 1 year in duration. (Buchner and Hansen 1987) The upper then lower gingival are next in presentations.

Suspicious masses appearing in otherwise normal appearing mucosal should be considered for "excisional" surgical removal since approximate 25–30% of mucosal melanomas can be amelanotic. (Hoki et al. 1985) The differentiation for a metastatic melanoma can usually be determined by the presence of normal tissue between the subepidermal tumor and the basal layer of melanocytes. Also, the location of metastatic melanoma sites is different from primary mucosal melanomas in that the former is usually located in the tongue, larynx, and tonsil areas and typically are represented as discrete nodular masses rather than more flatter and superficial growths. Also, metastases can be associated with known melanoma primary sites.

The prognosis for mucosal melanomas is far worse than cutaneous counterparts (Trapp et al. 1987) with invasion greater than 0.5–0.7 mm as a particularly poor prognostic predictor. Interestingly, lymph node involvement does not contribute to poorer prognosis as in cutaneous types; so, elective lymph node dissections are not helpful even though somewhere between 30–60% of patients may develop latent nodal metastases (Kingdom and Kaplan 1995).

Therapy has taken two distinct approaches. Some researchers recommend surgical excision with microscopically negative margins, then apply postoperative radiotherapy attempting to prolong disease-free intervals. In this situation, about 85% will still have a local recurrence and about 50% will develop either neck metastases, distant metastases, or both (Kingdom and Kaplan 1995). Another approach is to use primary radiotherapy to the biopsied site saving radical excisional surgery for local failure. This approach is more applicable to nasal cavity/paranasal mucosal melanomas and produces similar survival rates of about 24% over 5 years of follow-up. Laryngeal primary mucosal melanomas have the worst prognosis with only about a 13% 5-year survival. Novel biotherapy interventions are considered for all (Harwood and Larson 1982).

Cross-References

▶ Esophageal Cancer
▶ Lung
▶ Melanoma
▶ Nasal Cavity and Paranasal Sinuses
▶ Nasopharynx
▶ Oro-Hypopharynx
▶ Skin Cancer

References

Batsakis JG et al (1982) The pathology of head and neck tumors: mucosal melanomas. Head and Neck Surgery 4:404–418

Buchner A, Hansen LS (1987) Pigmented nevi of the oral mucosa: a clinicopathologic study of 36 new cases and a review of 155 cases from the literature. Analysis of 191 cases. Oral Surgery 63:676–682

Harwood AR, Larson VG (1982) Radiation therapy for melanomas of the head and neck. Head Neck Surg 4:468–474

Hoki K et al (1985) Malignant melanoma in the maxillary sinus: a case successfully treated with radiotherapy. Auris Nasus Larynx (Tokyo) 12:81–87

Kingdom TT, Kaplan MJ (1995) Mucosal melanoma of the nasal cavity and paranasal sinuses. Head Neck 17: 184–189

Trapp TK et al (1987) Melanoma of the nasal and paranasal sinus mucosa. Arch Otolaryngol Head and Neck Surgery113:1086–1089

Umeda M et al (1988) Heterogeneity of primary malignant melanomas in oral mucosa: an analysis of 43 cases in Japan. Pathology 20:234–241

Multicentric Disease

DAVID E. WAZER
Radiation Oncology Department, Tufts Medical Center, Tufts University School of Medicine, Boston, MA, USA
Radiation Oncology Department, Rhode Island Hospital, Brown University School of Medicine, Providence, RI, USA

Definition

At least two areas of discontinuous disease within the breast that are separated by more than 4 cm signifying the inability to remove known disease in one lumpectomy specimen. Multicentric disease is a contraindication to breast conservation therapy.

Cross-References

► Breast Cancer Locally Advanced
► Cancer of the Breast Tis

Multifocal Disease

DAVID E. WAZER
Radiation Oncology Department, Tufts Medical Center, Tufts University School of Medicine, Boston, MA, USA
Radiation Oncology Department, Rhode Island Hospital, Brown University School of Medicine, Providence, RI, USA

Definition

At least two areas of discontinuous disease that are within 4 cm of one another and removable within one lumpectomy specimen. Multifocality is not a contraindication to breast conservation therapy.

Cross-References

► Breast Cancer Locally Advanced
► Cancer of the Breast Tis

Multimodality Treatment

Definition

A treatment regimen that utilizes more than one approach/technique to treat a disease state.

Cross-References

► Bladder
► Multimodality Treatment/Combined Modality Treatment

Multimodality Treatment/ Combined Modality Treatment

CHRISTIAN WEISS, CLAUS ROEDEL
Department of Radiotherapy and Radiation Oncology, University Hospital Frankfurt/Main, Frankfurt, Germany

Definition
Combination of several therapies to improve efficacy without increasing toxicity (in bladder cancer with the aim of organ preservation).

Cross-References
- ▶ Anal Carcinoma
- ▶ Bladder
- ▶ Bladder Cancer
- ▶ Clinical Aspects of Brachytherapy (BT)
- ▶ Esophageal Cancer
- ▶ Intensity Modulated Radiation Therapy
- ▶ Larynx
- ▶ Nasopharynx
- ▶ Oro-Hypopharynx
- ▶ Rectal Cancer
- ▶ Soft Tissue Sarcoma
- ▶ Stomach Cancer
- ▶ Uterine Cervix
- ▶ Vagina

Multiple Basal Cell Carcinoma Syndrome

- ▶ Basal Cell Nevus Syndrome

Multiple Endocrine Neoplasia Type I

STEPHAN MOSE
Department of Radiation Oncology, Schwarzwald-Baar-Klinikum, Villingen-Schwenningen, Germany

Definition
Parathyroid, pituitary and pancreatic neuroendocine tumors, adrenal adenomas, and ACC.

Cross-References
- ▶ Carcinoma of the Adrenal Gland

Multiple Endocrine Neoplasia Type II

STEPHAN MOSE
Department of Radiation Oncology, Schwarzwald-Baar-Klinikum, Villingen-Schwenningen, Germany

Definition
This syndrome is divided into type II A (MEN II A) which is defined by the diagnoses of a pheochromocytoma, a medullary thyroid carcinoma, and a parathyroid hyperplasia, and type II B (MEN II B) which includes a pheochromocytoma, a medullary thyroid carcinoma, and mucosal neuromas. Furthermore, type II B is associated with a marfonoid habitus.

Cross-References
- ▶ Carcinoma of the Adrenal Gland

Multiple Myeloma

Caspian Oliai
Department of Radiation Oncology,
College of Medicine, Drexel University,
Philadelphia, PA, USA

Definition
Collections of abnormal plasma cells in bones where they cause lytic lesions, and in the bone marrow where they interfere with hematopoiesis. Most cases feature the production of a paraprotein, an abnormal antibody that can cause ► kidney problems and interferes with the production of normal antibodies leading to immunodeficiency. The constellation of increased serum calcium, anemia, bone pain, and kidney failure suggests multiple myeloma.

Cross-References
► Leukemia in General

MV Cone Beam

► Image-Guided Radiation Therapy (IGRT): MV Imaging

Myasthenia Gravis

Ramesh Rengan[1], Charles R. Thomas, Jr.[2]
[1]Department of Radiation Oncology, Hospital of the University of Pennsylvania, Philadelphia, PA, USA
[2]Department of Radiation Medicine, Oregon Health Sciences University, Portland, OR, USA

Definition
A disorder of neuromuscular transmission secondary to antibody production against the postsynaptic nicotinic acetylcholine receptor. The syndrome is initially characterized by ocular weakness and eventually progresses to generalized weakness in the majority of patients.

Cross-References
► Thymic Neoplasms

Mycosis Fungoides

Curt Heese
Department of Radiation Oncology, Eastern Regional Cancer Treatment Centers of America, Philadelphia, PA, USA

Synonyms
Alibert-Bazin syndrome or granuloma fungoides

Definition
Mycosis fungoides, also known as Alibert-Bazin syndrome or granuloma fungoides, is the most common form of ► cutaneous T-cell lymphoma. It generally affects the skin, but may progress internally over time.

Cross-References
► Cutaneous T-Cell Lymphoma
► Total Skin Electron Therapy (TSET)

M

Myelodysplastic Syndrome (MDS)

Caspian Oliai
Department of Radiation Oncology,
College of Medicine, Drexel University,
Philadelphia, PA, USA

Definition
A chronic disease of ineffective production of myeloid blood cells with gradually worsening

cytopenias due to progressive bone marrow failure. Approximately one-third of patients will progress to AML within months to a few years.

Cross-References
▶ Leukemia in General

Myeloma

▶ Plasma Cell Myeloma

Myelopathy

JAMES H. BRASHEARS, III
Radiation Oncologist, Venice, FL, USA

Definition
Disease of the spinal cord. For radiation-related toxicity, severe myelopathy (RTOG $\geq$ Grade 2) ranges from severe Lhermitte's syndrome to chronically progressive radiation myelitis that ends in permanent paralysis.

Cross-References
▶ Palliation of Bone Metastases

Myeloproliferative Disease (MPD)

CASPIAN OLIAI
Department of Radiation Oncology,
College of Medicine, Drexel University,
Philadelphia, PA, USA

Definition
A group of diseases of the bone marrow creating excess cellular proliferation in the marrow. This group of disease includes: CML, polycythemia vera, essential thrombocytosis, and myelofibrosis. They may evolve into ▶ myelodysplastic syndrome or AML. However, MPD has a better prognosis than these two conditions.

Cross-References
▶ Leukemia in General

Myometrium

CHRISTIN A. KNOWLTON[1], MICHELLE KOLTON MACKAY[2]
[1]Department of Radiation Oncology, Drexel University, Philadelphia, PA, USA
[2]Department of Radiation Oncology, Marshfield Clinic, Marshfield, WI, USA

Definition
The myometrium is the middle layer of the uterine wall, between the endometrium (the inner lining) and the perimetrium/serosa (the outer layer). The myometrium is composed primarily of smooth muscle cells. The extent of invasion of endometrial cancer into the myometrium is key for determining stage of the cancer and appropriate treatment.

Cross-References
▶ Endometrium

Myxopapillary Ependymomas

▶ Spinal Canal Tumor

N

Nasal Cavity

FILIP T. TROICKI
College of Medicine, Drexel University,
Philadelphia, PA, USA

Definition

Nasal cavity is a cavity inside the head, extending from the face to the pharynx posteriorly and from the floor of the skull to the roof of the mouth inferiorly.

Cross-References

▶ Nasal Cavity and Paranasal Sinuses

Nasal Cavity and Paranasal Sinuses

FILIP T. TROICKI
College of Medicine, Drexel University,
Philadelphia, PA, USA

Synonyms

Sinonasal cancer

Definition

▶ Nasal cavity and ▶ paranasal sinuses include the ▶ nasal vestibule, nasal cavity, ethmoid sinuses, maxillary sinuses, the ▶ sphenoid sinus, and the frontal sinuses.

Background

Nasal cavity and paranasal sinus tumors are exceedingly rare, comprising less than 1% of all malignant neoplasms. The incidence of these tumors is highest in Japan and South Africa and is four times more likely to occur in men than women. Cancers of the ▶ maxillary sinus make up approximately one half of all sinonasal carcinomas. Occupational exposure is believed to contribute to the development of these tumors because they are seen more commonly in carpenters and sawmill and nickel workers.

The nasal vestibule is lined with skin and as a result most frequently gives rise to squamous cell cancers. Other cancers found in the area include basal cell carcinoma, sebaceous carcinoma, ▶ melanoma, and ▶ non-Hodgkin's lymphoma (NHL). Nasal vestibule carcinomas can spread by direct invasion of the upper lip, gingivolabial sulcus, premaxilla, or nasal cavity and can lead to septal perforation. These tumors tend not to spread hematologically but rather follow ipsilateral facial (buccinator and mandibular) as well as submandibular lymph nodes.

The nasal cavity includes a transition from skin to mucous membrane as well as the bony septum that divides the nasal cavity. Like the cancers of the nasal vestibule, the majority (85–90%) of cancers of the nasal cavity are ▶ squamous cell carcinomas with approximately 10–15% being adenocarcinomas, adenoid cystic carcinomas, and mucoepidermoid carcinomas. The tumors of the nasal cavity can extend into the surrounding spaces. Some of the areas of tumor extension from the nasal cavity include superiorly the orbit and the anterior cranial fossa; laterally, the maxillary antrum,

L.W. Brady, T.E. Yaeger (eds.), *Encyclopedia of Radiation Oncology*, DOI 10.1007/978-3-540-85516-3,
© Springer-Verlag Berlin Heidelberg 2013

ethmoid cells, orbit, pterygopalatine fossa, and ▶ nasopharynx; inferiorly, the palate and maxillary antrum. Although lymphatic spread of tumors arising in the nasal cavity is not common, it is certainly possible, especially to the retropharyngeal and cervical lymph nodes. The adenoid cystic carcinomas, which are known to spread along the trigeminal nerve, are an exception.

Maxillary sinus tumors are the most common of the nasal cavity and paranasal sinus tumors, comprising approximately 70% of the paranasal cancers. The ethmoid and maxillary sinuses are lined by bony structures and contain mostly empty space through which tumors can invade. Tumors that originate in the maxillary sinus can extend to the ethmoid sinuses, nasal cavity, palate, orbit, alveolar process, gingivobuccal sulcus, andpterygoid, infratemporal, and pterygopalatine fossa, as well as to the base of skull and to adjacent soft tissues and muscles. Treatment of any invading tumor in this area is difficult because of the proximity to critical structures such as the brain stem and ocular structures. Due to the limited lymphatic and vascular supply to the sinuses, for the most part, only the aggressive tumors such as squamous cell and poorly differentiated carcinomas metastasize. By the same token, lymphadenopathy is a rare occurrence in patients with tumors of the sinuses but may be present in ipsilateral subdigastric and submandibular lymph nodes.

Initial Evaluation

A thorough history and physical examination are the mainstays of finding tumors of the nasal cavity and paranasal sinuses. The skin should be inspected for lesions; sinuses and lymph nodes should be palpated; a thorough eye examination should be done to look for proptosis and visual field deficits. An otoscopic examination of the nasal cavity is paramount and may warrant further inspection with an endoscope and a biopsy.

Cancers of the nasal vestibule are easy to spot but can be mistaken for noncancerous lesions and as a result can be ignored by the patient as well as by the practitioner. A thorough skin examination is warranted, and biopsies should be obtained even from patients with asymptomatic plaques or nodules.

Tumors of the nasal cavity may also be brought to the attention of the physician by patients who notice a mass protruding from the nose. Patients may complain of headaches, nasal congestion, chronic unilateral discharge, or nosebleeds. Large lesions may cause proptosis, diplopia, eye pain, epiphora, facial or nasal swelling, or even anosmia.

Unlike tumors of the nasal vestibule and nasal cavity, tumors of the sinuses are usually not seen on a physical examination until they are large enough to cause an effect on surrounding structures. Patients with ▶ ethmoid sinus cancers can present with facial pain, headaches, and sinus pressure. They can also complain of nasal discharge and bleeding, nasal obstruction, excessive tearing, diplopia, and proptosis. Due to the location and structure of the maxillary sinuses, patients with these cancers are usually diagnosed at an advanced stage of the disease. Like patients with ethmoid sinus tumors, these patients can present with facial numbness or pain, facial swelling, nasal obstruction, intermittent bleeding, proptosis, and diplopia. In addition, patients can also complain of an ill-fitting denture or present with an alveolar or palatal mass.

The results of a complete blood count and chemistry panel should also be considered to look for a low hemoglobin count that may suggest a bleed and for other abnormalities in laboratory values that may suggest distant metastases. Images of the head and neck region should be taken in anyone suspected of having a nasal cavity or paranasal sinus tumor. Detailed magnetic resonance imaging (MRI) and computed tomographic (CT) scans of the nose and sinuses should be obtained and evaluated for masses, lymph node enlargement, and cortical bone destruction.

Differential Diagnosis

Benign skin lesions, nasal polyps, osteomas, chondromas, schwannomas, neurofibromas, ossifying fibromas, cementomas, odontogenic tumors, papillomas, meningiomas, hemangiomas, hemangiopericytomas, lymphomas, sarcomas, Wegener's granulomatosis, extramedullary plasmacytomas, squamous cell carcinomas, adenoid cystic carcinomas, adenocarcinomas, olfactory neuroblastomas, sarcomas, and melanomas.

Imaging Studies

In addition to a thorough history and physical examination, a proper radiographic evaluation is imperative for any patient suspected of having a nasal cavity or paranasal tumor. MRI and CT are the main imaging modalities that should be used together. MRI is best for differentiating solid masses from secretions and for detecting direct intracranial, perineural, and leptomeningeal spread. A CT image of the head, on the other hand, can show bone destruction that may be missed on an MRI scan.

Laboratory Studies

Complete blood count and serum chemistries can screen for occult metastases if abnormal.

Treatment

Surgery with or without radiation is the mainstay of treatment for nasal cavity and paranasal carcinomas because surgical excision and postoperative radiation yield high rates of local control (>95%) and 5-year overall survival (>90%). Given the excellent results obtained with surgery and irradiation, chemotherapy is not often used in cancers of the nasal cavity and paranasal sinuses. Chemotherapy can be used in a neoadjuvant setting to shrink the tumor as can a radiosensitizing agent when given concomitant with radiation. In fact, some evidence indicates that concomitant chemoradiation improves local control in patients with inoperable tumors.

In patients with persistent or recurrent lesions, salvage radiation or surgery is possible, especially in those who did not receive combined modality treatment. The main limitation to reirradiation, however, is the maximum allowable dose to neural structures surrounding the tumor site.

Regardless of the treatment modality, patients with nasal cavity and paranasal sinus tumors should be reevaluated with a CT or MRI scan 3 months after treatment. Patients should be seen every 4 months for the first 3 years, every 6 months for the next 2 years, and then annually thereafter.

Nasal Vestibule

Location is an important factor in the treatment of nasal cavity and paranasal sinus tumors. Although surgical resection of a nasal vestibule carcinoma yields higher control rates, radiation therapy is often used to give patients improved cosmesis. Both external-beam irradiation using orthovoltage x-rays or electrons to a total dose of 60–66 Gy and/or ▶ low dose rate brachytherapy using ^{192}Ir wire implants can be used to treat small tumors of the nasal vestibule (T1 and T2 lesions). In patients with large, invasive tumors, surgical excision with pre- or postoperative radiation is recommended. Well-differentiated tumors that are ≤1.5 cm in size can be irradiated with a 1–2-cm margin, whereas larger or more aggressive tumors usually require a 2–3-cm margin. The latter also require radiation using photons to bilateral facial, submandibular, and subdigastric nodes even in cases where no palpable lymphadenopathy is present. In patients who have pathological involvement of any lymph nodes, the lower neck should be included in the radiation field. The most common fractionation schedule in a postoperative setting includes 50 Gy in 25 fractions to the tumor plus any lymph nodes, followed by an additional 6 Gy in 3 fractions to the surgical bed, followed by a final cone-down of an additional 4 Gy in 2 fractions to the negative margin versus 10 Gy in 5 fractions to the positive-margin presurgical tumor bed. In cases where ▶ low-dose rate brachytherapy is used, the patient should be treated with doses between 60 and 65 Gy using ^{192}Ir wire implants for 5–7 days. A combination of external-beam radiation and a high-dose rate brachytherapy boost can be used effectively according to the following fractionation schedule: 50 Gy delivered in 25 fractions using external-beam radiation, followed by 18 Gy delivered in 6 fractions over 3 days using ▶ high-dose rate brachytherapy.

Cure rates for cancers of the nasal vestibule using external-beam radiation or brachytherapy are as high as 95–100% for tumors smaller than 2 cm and 70–80% for tumors larger than 2 cm. Overall local control for radiotherapy as well as surgery is greater than 90% and is dependant primarily on tumor size (<2 cm vs. >2 cm) and site of lesion (external skin vs. vestibule).

Nasal Cavity

Similarly to the tumors of the nasal vestibule, tumors of the nasal cavity can be treated either with surgery or radiation, depending on the size and location of the lesion. For example, large, posterior tumors are usually resected, whereas small, anterior-inferior tumors are treated with radiation. Locally advanced lesions (stages II–IVa) should undergo resection with or without postoperative radiation. Nasal cavity tumors within the first 4 cm of the nasal apex can be safely treated with electrons, as long as a 1-cm margin is included in the treatment area. Any tumor within the nasal cavity that is beyond the reach of the electron beam should be treated with intensity-modulated radiotherapy (IMRT) to spare dosing critical structures in the area. Three-dimensional (3D) conformal radiotherapy can be used in place of IMRT provided that the ethmoid sinuses are not involved. In this case, either anterior oblique wedge-pair photon fields or opposed-lateral fields can be used when treating tumors located in the anterior and posterior nasal cavities, respectively. The fractionation schedule for postoperative 3-D conformal radiotherapy includes 50 Gy to elective tissue, followed by additional 6 Gy to the operative bed, finally followed by an optional boost of 4 Gy to positive surgical margins. In addition to external-beam options, single-plane implant brachytherapy can also be used to treat anterior tumors of the nasal cavity as long as radiation covers a 2-cm tumor margin. Like the low-dose brachytherapy fractionation schedule for cancers of the nasal vestibule, the schedule for treating the nasal cavity should be 60–65 Gy over 5–7 days.

Tumors confined to the nasal cavity (Kadish stage A) have local control exceeding 90% when treated with surgery or radiation alone. Kadish stage B (confined to the nasal cavity and one or more paranasal sinuses) and stage C tumors (extending beyond the nasal cavity and paranasal sinuses) usually require surgery followed by radiation to the tumor bed without nodal radiation. Overall local control for all nasal cavity tumors is between 60% and 80% with a 5-year survival rate between 28% for undifferentiated tumors and over 60% for esthesioneuroblastomas or adenocarcinomas.

Ethmoid and Maxillary Sinuses

Most tumors of the ethmoid sinus also require surgery followed by postoperative irradiation. Like the treatment of nasal cavity tumors, postoperative radiation to the ethmoid sinus carcinomas should use IMRT and include the cribiform plate in the clinical tumor volume. Carcinomas of the maxillary sinuses, on the other hand, are treated differently based on the stage of the tumor. Patients presenting with T1-2 maxillary sinus carcinomas can often undergo surgery alone, whereas patients with more advanced tumors require radiation with or without surgery, depending on resectability. Due to the location of the tumor, most patients with maxillary tumors present with a locally advanced stage. These cases are usually treated with surgery followed by IMRT radiotherapy. The prechemotherapy gross tumor volume plus 1–1.5-cm margin should receive between 66 and 70 Gy. If 3D conformal radiation is used postoperatively, the target volume treated to 56 Gy should include a margin of 1–2 cm around the surgical bed. A boost up to 66 Gy should be given to the tumor bed plus the positive margins, areas of ▶ perineural invasion, and any other high-risk regions. When the initial radiation field extends to the optic nerve and chiasm, a field adjustment must be made to spare those critical structures after 50–54 Gy. Although patients with squamous or poorly differentiated cancers can receive radiation to the cervical as well as submandibular and subdigastric lymph nodes, any positive cervical lymph nodes require neck irradiation to 50 Gy regardless of histological appearance.

The combination of surgery and radiation provides the best local control (up to 75%) and 5-year overall survival rate (up to 60% using conventional RT and up to 80% using IMRT) for patients with maxillary sinus tumors.

Cross-References
▶ Brachytherapy: High Dose Rate (HDR) Implants
▶ Eye and Orbit
▶ Intensity-Modulated Proton Therapy (IMPT)
▶ Low-Dose Rate (LDR) Brachytherapy
▶ Nasopharynx
▶ Oro-Hypopharynx
▶ Principles of Surgical Oncology
▶ Unusual Nonepithelial Tumors of the Head and Neck

References
Ahamad A, Ang KK (2008) Nasal cavity and paranasal sinuuses, chapter 39. In: Halperin EC, Perez CA, Brady LW (eds) Principles and practice of radiation oncology, 5th edn. Lippincott Williams & Wilkins, Philadelphia, p 861

Gunderson LL, Tepper JE (2007) Clinical radiation oncology, 2nd edn. Elsevier Churchill Livingstone, Edinburgh

Hansen EK, Roach M III (eds) (2006) Handbook of evidence-based radiation oncology. Springer, New York

Levitt SH, Purdy JA, Perez CA, Vijayakumar S (eds) (2006) Technical basis of radiation therapy, 4th rev edn. Springer, Berlin/Heidelberg

Nasal Vestibule

FILIP T. TROICKI
College of Medicine, Drexel University, Philadelphia, PA, USA

Definition
Nasal vestibule is the most anterior and hollow part of the nasal cavity.

Cross-References
▶ Nasal Cavity and Paranasal Sinuses

N

Nasopharyngeal Angiofibroma

CARLOS A. PEREZ, WADE L. THORSTAD
Department of Radiation Oncology, Siteman Cancer Center, Washington University Medical Center, St. Louis, MO, USA

Definition
A rare tumor of children and young adults usually arising in the roof of the pterygoid process from the posterior wall of the sphenoid cavity where there is a junction of the palatine bone and "Ala of Vomer."

Epidemiology
Juvenile nasopharyngeal angiofibroma (JNPA) comprises less than 0.05% of head and neck tumors. It is found more frequently in young

pubertal boys; it has been shown to contain androgen receptors. Patient age at presentation ranges from 9 to 30 years, with a median of 15 years. Females comprise less than 4% of the total cases (Cummings et al. 1984).

The tumor is believed to originate from the posterolateral wall of the nasal cavity where the sphenoidal process of the palatine bone meets the horizontal ala of the vomer and the roof of the pterygoid process because it is always involved. Other investigators agree, because involution of tumor after irradiation usually occurs in this direction.

Clinical Presentation and Pathology

The most common complaints are nasal obstruction or epistaxis, followed by nasal voice or discharge, cheek swelling, proptosis, diplopia, hearing loss, and headaches. Nasopharyngeal angiofibroma may initially extend into the nasal fossae and maxillary antrum and push the soft palate downward, then through the pterygopalatine fossa and superoanteriorly through the inferior orbital fissure or laterally through the pterygomaxillary fissure to the cheek and temporal regions.

Diagnostic Workup

After clinical history and physical examination, CT scans with and without contrast should be obtained. The pattern of enhancement in this highly vascular tumor is diagnostic, and many investigators believe carotid angiograms are unnecessary after CT diagnosis of the lesion, unless embolizations, which are also controversial, are contemplated.

CT scans are especially helpful in regions involving thin bony structures (paranasal sinuses, orbits), where CT performs better than MRI. In the nasopharynx and parapharyngeal space, MRI is superior to CT. Obtaining tumor volumetric data with spiral CT or MRI facilitates 3D treatment planning (Perez and Thorstad 2008).

If intracranial extension is noted and radiation therapy is contemplated, no further studies are indicated. If the lesion is extracranial and surgery is indicated, bilateral carotid angiograms will identify the feeding vessels and delineate the boundaries of the tumor.

Biopsies are not indicated in all patients because of the potential for severe hemorrhage, unless the clinical picture (sex, age, location, and behavior of the lesion) is not consistent with JNPA because some lesions have proven to be sarcomas or chronic sinusitis.

Staging

Two staging schemes have been proposed: (1) The system of Chandler and colleagues (Table 1). (2) A radiographic staging system was proposed by Sessions and associates (Sessions et al. 1981): Stage Ia is limited to the nasopharynx and posterior nares; stage Ib extends to the paranasal sinuses; stages IIa, b, and c extend to other extracranial locations; and stage III is intracranial.

General Management

In patients with extracranial tumors, surgery is the treatment of choice and yields near-zero mortality or any long-term morbidity. Tumor remnants in symptom-free patients should be kept under surveillance by repeated CT scanning, since

Nasopharyngeal Angiofibroma. Table 1 Staging of nasopharyngeal angiofibromas

Stage I	Confined to the nasopharynx
Stage II	Extension to nasal cavity and/or sphenoid sinus
Stage III	Extension to one or more: antrum, ethmoid, pterygomaxillary and infratemporal fossae, orbit, and/or cheek
Stage IV	Intracranial extension

Source: Chandler et al. (1984)

involution may occur. Recurrent symptoms may be treated by radiation therapy rather than by extended surgery or combined procedures.

When there is intracranial tumor extension (seen in about 20% of patients), the risk of surgically related death increases. Most of these patients are best treated with irradiation (Cummings et al. 1984).

Some investigators recommend preoperative intra-arterial tumor vessel embolization at the time of diagnostic bilateral carotid angiography, claiming a decrease in operative bleeding. Salvage with embolizations of polyvinyl alcohol has been described. Others have reported anecdotal evidence of partial regression with the use of estrogens, believed to be the result of feedback inhibition of the pituitary's production of gonadotropin-releasing hormone.

Radiation Therapy

Photon irradiation should be used for these patients, and target volume must be individualized to cover the tumor completely with a margin (1–2 cm). Standard treatment portals are similar to those used in carcinoma of the nasopharynx (without irradiating the cervical lymph nodes) or carcinoma of the paranasal sinuses when these structures or the nasal cavity is involved. Opposing lateral portals are suitable in most patients, with larger fields and compensators used for tumors extending into the nose. More extensive disease requires three-field or wedge-pair arrangements. 3D CRT or IMRT can yield excellent dose distributions, particularly when there is nasopharyngeal or intracranial tumor extension. In all cases, the eyes are protected as much as possible. The recommended tumor dose ranges from 30 Gy in 15 fractions in 3 weeks to 50 Gy in 24–28 fractions in 5 weeks (Cummings et al. 1984). A conventional setup uses 6- to 18-MV photons to treat the lesion with parallel-opposed fields to 50 Gy (2-Gy fractions).

The advantages of IMRT for the treatment of extensive and/or recurrent JNPA have been described (Kuppersmith et al. 2000). Tumor doses varied from 35 to 45 Gy in 1.8–2 Gy fractions.

Results of Therapy

Jones and associates (1986) reported the results of 40 patients with JNPA treated with surgery alone. With a mean follow-up of 17 months (6–36 months), the control rates according to the Sessions staging system were as follows: 100% (stages I and IIa), 83% (stage IIb), 80% (stage IIc), and 50% (stage III). All failures were controlled with irradiation ($n = 18$ patients), embolization ($n = 8$), or surgical resection ($n = 8$). These findings are consistent with other series reporting initial surgical control of 86% with an ultimate control rate of 96%.

Cummings, Blend, and colleagues (1984) treated 42 patients primarily with irradiation and 13 for postsurgical failures; all except six had biopsy. Nine had stage IV disease according to Chandler's staging system. Dose was 30–35 Gy in 14–16 fractions over a 3-week period. Follow-up ranged from 3 to 26 years. The control rate was 80% and was equivalent for all dose ranges. Local control was 89% and 74%, respectively, when three fields versus two fields were used. When the field size was more than 6×6 cm, the control rate was 83% versus 55% for smaller portals, indicating the importance of accurately determining the target volume, including any potential tumor extension. Of 11 recurrences, 8 were controlled by a second course of irradiation and 3 by surgery. Tumor regression usually occurs slowly after either irradiation or chemotherapy; therefore, the presence of tumor up to 2 years after treatment is not an invariable sign of failure unless it is symptomatic or progressing.

Malignant degeneration in JNPA undergoing radiation therapy has been occasionally reported (Cummings et al. 1984).

Cross-References

- ▶ Nasal Cavity and Paranasal Sinuses
- ▶ Nasopharynx
- ▶ Sarcomas of the Head and Neck

References

Chandler JR, Goulding R, Moskowitz L et al (1984) Nasopharyngeal angiofibromas: staging and management. Ann Otol Rhinol Laryngol 93:322

Cummings BJ, Blend R, Fitzpatrick P et al (1984) Primary radiation therapy for juvenile nasopharyngeal angiofibroma. Laryngoscope 94:1599–1604

Jones GC, DeSanto LW, Bremer JW et al (1986) Juvenile angiofibromas. Arch Otolarygol Head Neck Surg 112:1191–1193

Kuppersmith RB, The BS, Donovan DT et al (2000) The use of intensity modulated radiotherapy for the treatment of extensive and recurrent juvenile angiofibroma. Int J Pediatr Otorhinolaryngol 52:261–268

Perez CA, Thorstad WL (2008) Unusual non-epithelial tumors of the head and neck. In: Halperin EC, Perez CA, Brady LW (eds) Perez and Brady's principles and practice of radiation oncology, 5th edn. Wolters Kluwer/Lippincott Williams & Wilkins, Philadelphia, p 996

Sessions RB, Bryan RN, Naclerio RM et al (1981) Radiographic staging of juvenile angiofibroma. Head Neck Surg 3:279–83

Nasopharynx

Brandon J. Fisher[1], Larry C. Daugherty[2]

[1]Department of Radiation Oncology, College of Medicine, Drexel University, Philadelphia, PA, USA

[2]Department of Radiation Oncology, College of Medicine, Drexel University, Glenside, PA, USA

Synonyms

Malignant lesion of the nasopharynx; Neoplasm of the rhinopharynx; Neoplasms of the nasopharynx

Definition/Description

Nasopharyngeal carcinoma (NPC) includes all malignant lesions arising from the nasopharyngeal mucosa.

The nasopharynx is a cuboidal-shaped cavity that begins at the posterior choana and slopes posteriorly along the airway to the level of the soft palate. It communicates anteriorly with the nasal cavity and inferiorly into the oropharynx. The roof and the posterior wall are formed by the sphenoid sinus, the clivus, and the first cervical vertebra. The floor is the superior surface of the soft palate. The eustachian tube opens into the lateral wall of the nasopharynx. The posterior portion of the eustachian tube is a cartilaginous protrusion called the ▶ torus tubarius. Posterior to the torus is a recess called the ▶ fossa of Rosenmüller.

The most common malignant lesion of the nasopharynx is squamous cell carcinoma, accounting for more than 70% of cases. Lymphomas account for roughly 20% and the remaining may be seromucinous minor salivary gland tumors.

Background

Nasopharyngeal carcinoma shows distinct racial and geographical distributions, with higher incidence among Chinese men. Chinese people who have migrated to Western countries show progressively lower risk. The age of onset typically follows a bimodal distribution: The first peak occurs at 15–25 and the second peak at 50–59 years of age. The age distribution is similar in both genders. The incidence rates in men are typically two- to threefold of those in women.

Epidemiological observations reveal multiple causes that include both genetic predisposition and environmental factors. An association has been made between the presence of ▶ Epstein–Barr virus (EBV) and the development of NPC. EBV DNA or RNA has been found in tumor cells of people with NPC, indicating that the virus may play an oncogenic role in the carcinogenesis. NPC has been linked to exposures to carcinogens in traditional southern Chinese food (nitrosamines). Cigarette smoking, previous irradiation, and occupational exposures to dust, smoke, and chemical fumes have also been implicated;

however, no direct link to any of these irritants has been identified.

The lymphatics of the nasopharynx (▶ lymph node regions in the head and neck) follow various pathways including the parapharyngeal lymph node region, the retropharyngeal node (*node of Rouvière*), and the jugular lymph node chain to involve the jugulodigastric and deep jugular nodes. Finally, lymphatic pathways may also drain into the spinal accessory chain, the uppermost node lying beneath the sternomastoid muscle at the tip of the mastoid process.

A number of foramina and fissures located in the base of the skull provide routes along which a NPC can extend and invade intracranially and can involve various cranial nerves. Because the foramen lacerum and the foramen ovale have a close anatomic relationship with the cavernous sinus, NPC invasion into this region can involve cranial nerves III–VI. Cranial nerve involvement is a sign of more advanced disease.

Initial Evaluation

Diagnosis and evaluation of NPC should begin with a thorough history and physical examination. Special attention should be paid to specific disease-related signs and symptoms (Table 1).

Nasopharynx. Table 1 Symptoms and physical signs of nasopharyngeal carcinoma at presentation (Brady 2008)

Symptom/sign	Incidence %
Neck mass	80
Nasal discharge, bleeding, obstruction	>37
Aural: tinnitus, hearing loss, pain, discharge	41
Headache	40
Cranial nerve palsy	23
Sore throat	16

The clinical presentation of NPC is highly dependent on the location and size of these lesions. The most common presenting symptom is a painless enlargement of upper neck nodes. Nodal metastases are found in 75–90% of cases of squamous cell carcinoma at the time of initial presentation. About 20% of patients have signs of ▶ cranial nerve palsy at diagnosis. Nerves V and VI are most commonly involved.

An initial work-up should include endoscopic examination of the nasal cavities and the entire pharynx, thorough testing of all cranial nerves, and assessment of neck node involvement. Imaging is mandatory for complete evaluation and is critical in the staging process.

Differential Diagnosis

Angiofibroma, tuberculosis, lymphoma, chordoma.

Imaging Studies

Imaging studies are essential for accurately defining the tumor extent as well as for defining the presence of regional nodal involvement. Computed tomography (CT) and magnetic resonance imaging (MRI) are the most valuable imaging methods. MRI is the study of choice because of its superior sensitivity compared to CT imaging. MRI is able to better define and delineate neoplastic lesions from surrounding structures, including the base of the skull and cervical vertebrae and surrounding tissue. A CT scan is, however, more sensitive in detecting early bone invasion. CT with axial and coronal reconstructions with contrast is accepted as an alternative and is most commonly used. CT may be better suited for depicting metastases to the cervical nodes.

A chest radiograph is indicated to rule out pulmonary metastases and often requires further imaging of the thorax. CT is often required if the result from the chest radiograph is equivocal. A comprehensive search for distant metastases is indicated for patients with advanced

N

locoregional disease (particularly N3) and those with suspicious clinical or laboratory abnormalities. Positron emission tomographic (18-FDG PET) imaging has proved superior to conventional work-up (using chest radiograph, isotope bone scan, and abdominal ultrasonograph) in detection of distant metastases and is often essential for radiation planning. PET coupled with CT is the modality of choice, if available. If nuclear medicine techniques are not used, liver ultrasound and bone scan are recommended for patients with more advanced disease.

Laboratory Studies

Initial laboratory tests should include a complete blood count, a basic blood chemistry panel, a liver function test, and renal function tests. EBV serologic tests should also be performed. Ig-A antiviral capsule antigen and Ig-G anti-early antigen are often recommended. High pretreatment titers were associated with advanced stages and poor prognosis. Circulating cell-free DNA of EBV is a useful prognostic marker. More clinical data are necessary to determine the consistency and reliability of this test before it can be recommended for routine use.

Other biological factors that might have prognostic significance include E-cadherin and β-catenin, c-erbB2, p53, nm23-HI, interleukin-10, and vascular endothelial growth factor. However, clinical data on their usefulness are limited, and further substantiation is needed.

Histological confirmation is mandatory for the diagnosis of NPC. Tissue samples can be obtained from the primary tumor with endoscopic biopsy or fine-needle aspiration of an enlarged neck node.

Staging System

An accurate staging system is crucial not only for predicting the prognosis but also for guiding treatment strategies for different risk groups and facilitating the exchange of experiences between oncology centers (Table 2). Staging is based on

Nasopharynx. Table 2 Diagnostic and staging work-up for nasopharyngeal carcinoma (Brady 2008)

General
History and physical examination
Palpation of neck node
Testing of cranial nerve
Signs of distant metastases
Endoscopic examination
Nasopharyngoscopy and biopsies and panendoscopy Laboratory studies
Laboratory studies
Complete blood studies
Liver function studies
Radiographic studies
Assessment of locoregional extent
Magnetic resonance imaging
Computed tomography
Chest radiograph
Additional metastatic work-up
Positron-emission tomography
Computed tomography of thorax and upper abdomen, ultrasound of liver, bone scan (acceptable alternative)

the system used by the American Joint Committee on Cancer and International Union Against Cancer (Table 3).

Treatment

Due to the deep-seated location of the nasopharynx and its proximity to critical structures, radical surgical resection is difficult and typically not recommended. The role of surgery is limited to obtaining a biopsy for histological confirmation and salvage for persistent or recurrent disease.

Treatment strategy should be tailored to the specific pattern of growth and stage for different risk groups. The current recommendation is to treat patients with stage I disease with radiation

Nasopharynx. Table 3 Staging criteria of The American Joint Committee on Cancer, 7th edition (Edge et al. 2010. With permission)

Stage	Staging criteria		
T category			
TX	Primary tumor cannot be assessed		
T0	No evidence of primary tumor		
Tis	Carcinoma in situ		
T1	Tumor confined to the nasopharynx or tumor extends to the oropharynx and/or nasal cavity without parapharyngeal extension		
T2	Tumor with parapharyngeal extension		
T3	Tumor involves bony structures of skull base and/or paranasal sinuses		
T4	Tumor with intracranial extension and/or involvement of cranial nerves, hypopharynx, orbit, or with extension to the infratemporal fossa or masticator space		
N category			
NX	Regional lymph nodes cannot be assessed		
N0	No regional lymph node metastasis		
N1	Unilateral metastasis in cervical lymph node(s), ≤6 cm in greatest dimension, above the supraclavicular fossa and/or unilateral or bilateral retropharyngeal lymph nodes ≤6 cm in greatest dimension		
N2	Bilateral metastasis in lymph node(s), ≤6 cm in greatest dimension, above the supraclavicular fossa		
N3	Metastasis in lymph node(s)		
	N3a >6 cm in dimension		
	N3b Extension to the supraclavicular fossa		
M category			
MX	Distant metastasis cannot be assessed		
M0	No distant metastasis		
M1	Distant metastasis		
Stage grouping			
0	Tis	N0	M0
I	T1	N0	M0
II	T1	N1	M0
	T2	N0	M0
	T2	N1	M0

Nasopharynx. Table 3 (continued)

Stage	Staging criteria		
III	T1	N2	M0
	T2	N2	M0
	T3	N0	M0
	T3	N1	M0
	T3	N2	M0
Stage IVA	T4	N0	M0
	T4	N1	M0
	T4	N2	M0
Stage IVB	Any T	N3	M0
Stage IVC	Any T	Any N	M1

therapy with or without chemotherapy and those with stages II, III, and IVA, and B disease with concurrent chemoradiation therapy followed by adjuvant chemotherapy. Neck dissection is reserved for persistent or recurrent neck nodes.

Radiation Therapy

All patients should have a dental evaluation and dietary and nutritional consultation prior to commencement of radiation therapy. A feeding tube is often needed to maintain nutrition during treatments. Patients should be advised to abstain from smoking and drinking alcohol. The patient is put in a supine position with the head extended. A customized thermoplastic mask covering the head to shoulder region is made to immobilize the patient. Computerized planning for intensity-modulated radiation therapy (IMRT) is recommended. Fusion of diagnostic MRI and/or PET with planning CT is useful and highly recommended for more accurate delineation of tumor targets and critical structures.

Dose

Local tumor control is improved in patients who received more than 67 Gy to the tumor target.

The prescription generally recommended for NPC is a total dose to the gross tumor of about 70 Gy during 7 weeks and 50–60 Gy for elective treatment of potential risk sites. Various Radiation Therapy Oncology Group protocols exist to give guidance for dosing and treatment regimens. IMRT is recommended. Different investigators are exploring various methods and dose fractionation schemes for IMRT. Most of the patients treated in these series also received additional chemotherapy and/or enhanced radiation therapy with boosts (Table 4).

Tumor Target Volumes

The ▶ gross tumor volume (GTV) includes the primary nasopharyngeal tumor and grossly involved lymph nodes as shown by clinical, endoscopic, and radiologic examinations. If the patient has induction chemotherapy, it is recommended that the targets be based on the prechemotherapy extent.

The ▶ clinical target volume (CTV) includes the GTV, microscopic infiltration, and anatomic structures at risk. Elective irradiation of bilateral cervical lymphatics is recommended in N0 patients. The level I nodes can be spared for patients with N0 disease but should include the bilateral

Nasopharynx. Table 4 Dose constraints for intensity-modulated radiation therapy for nasopharyngeal carcinoma (Brady 2008)

Critical organ at risk	First criteria: ideal	Second criteria: acceptable
Brain stem	Point < 54 Gy	1% volume < 60 Gy
Spinal cord	Point < 45 Gy	1 mL volume < 50 Gy
Optic chiasm	Point < 54 Gy	1% volume < 60 Gy
Optic nerve	Point < 54 Gy	1% volume < 60 Gy
Temporal lobes	Point < 65 Gy & 1% volume < 60 Gy	1% volume < 65 Gy
Pituitary gland	Point < 60 Gy	1% volume < 65 Gy
Mandible/TMJ	1% volume < 70 Gy	1% volume < 75 Gy
Lens	Point < 6 Gy	1% volume < 10 Gy
Eyeball	Point < 50 Gy	Mean < 35 Gy
Parotid glands	Mean < 26 Gy (at least 1 gland)	50% volume < 30 Gy (1 gland)
Cochlea	Mean < 50 Gy	–
Tongue	1% volume < 70 Gy	Mean dose < 55 Gy
Larynx	Mean < 30 Gy	Mean < 45 Gy

▶ retropharyngeal nodes, levels II, III, IV, and V nodal regions. Definition of CTV differs with the various protocols; for example, one protocol describes three different CTVs. A CTV aimed at 70 Gy (CTV70) includes the GTV with a 5- to 10-mm margin (if possible) and the whole nasopharynx. A CTV aimed at 60 Gy (CTV60) covers high-risk local structures (including the parapharyngeal spaces, posterior third of nasal cavities and maxillary sinuses, pterygoid processes, base of skull, lower half of sphenoid sinus, anterior half of the clivus, and petrous tips), and lymphatic regions, II, III, and some of V. A CTV aimed at 50 Gy (CTV50) covers the remaining levels IV–V.

The ▶ planning target volume (PTV) includes the CTV with a margin for setup variation, typically ranging from 2 to 5 mm.

Chemotherapy

The chemotherapeutic agent used concurrently with radiotherapy is cisplatin followed by adjuvant cisplatin and fluorouracil (5-FU).

Effective systemic therapy is needed for patients with advanced locoregional disease because of the predilection for hematogenous spread and the need for further improvement of local control. For patients with more advanced and aggressive stage IV locoregional disease infiltrating neighboring neurologic structures, a more aggressive approach combining induction-concurrent radiotherapy cisplatin and 5-FU or just chemotherapy alone may be necessary.

Cross-References

▶ Nasal Cavity and Paranasal Sinuses

References

Al-Sarraf M et al (1998) Chemoradiotherapy versus radiotherapy in patients with advanced nasopharyngeal cancer: Phase III randomized Intergroup study 0099. J Clin Oncol 16:1310–1317

Baert AL (2008) Encyclopedia of diagnostic imaging, vol 2. Springer, Berlin/Heidelberg

Brady LW, Lu JJ (eds) (2008) Radiation oncology, an evidence-based approach. Springer, Berlin

Brady LW et al (eds) (2008) Principles and practice of radiation oncology, 5th edn. Lippincott, Williams & Wilkins, Philadelphia

Edge SB et al (eds) (2010) Cancer staging handbook, 7th edn. Springer, New York

Hansen EK, Roach M III (eds) (2007) Handbook of evidence-based radiation oncology. Springer, New York

Naturopathy

▶ Complementary Medicine

Neoadjuvant Chemotherapy

FILIP T. TROICKI[1], JAGANMOHAN POLI[2]
[1]College of Medicine, Drexel University, Philadelphia, PA, USA
[2]Department of Radiation Oncology, College of Medicine, Drexel University, Philadelphia, PA, USA

Definition
Initial use of chemotherapy in patients with advanced stages of cancer presentation in order to decrease the tumor burden prior to treatment by other modalities.

Cross-References
▶ Breast Cancer
▶ Esophagus Cancer
▶ Head and Neck Cancer
▶ Lung Cancer
▶ Ovarian Cancer
▶ Stomach Cancer

Neoplasm of the Rhinopharynx

▶ Nasopharynx

Neoplasms of the Nasopharynx

▶ Nasopharynx

Nephroblastoma

LARRY C. DAUGHERTY[1], BRANDON J. FISHER[2]
[1]Department of Radiation Oncology, College of Medicine, Drexel University, Glenside, PA, USA
[2]Department of Radiation Oncology, College of Medicine, Drexel University, Philadelphia, PA, USA

Definition
Synonymous with Wilm's tumor, the most common malignant tumor of the kidney in children.

Cross-References
▶ Wilm's Tumor

Nerve Sheath Tumor

▶ Spinal Canal Tumor

Nerve-Sparing Retroperitoneal Lymph Node Dissection

JOHANNES CLASSEN
Department of Radiation Oncology, St. Vincentius-Kliniken Karlsruhe, Karlsruhe, Germany

Definition
Surgical procedure trying to spare in part retroperitoneal nerves from dissection in order to limit side effects of surgery, namely difficulties in ejaculation.

Cross-References

► Testes

Neu Oncogene

► Her-2

Neural Crest Cells

Brandon J. Fisher[1], Larry C. Daugherty[2]
[1]Department of Radiation Oncology, College of Medicine, Drexel University, Philadelphia, PA, USA
[2]Department of Radiation Oncology, College of Medicine, Drexel University, Glenside, PA, USA

Definition

Migratory embryonic cells derived from the ectoderm.

Cross-References

► Neuroblastoma

Neuroblastoma

Larry C. Daugherty[1], Brandon J. Fisher[2]
[1]Department of Radiation Oncology, College of Medicine, Drexel University, Glenside, PA, USA
[2]Department of Radiation Oncology, College of Medicine, Drexel University, Philadelphia, PA, USA

Synonyms

Extraskeletal small cell tumors

Definition/Description

Neuroblastoma is the third most common childhood cancer (behind leukemia and CNS neoplasms), accounting for approximately 10% of pediatric malignancies (Smith et al. 1999). Neuroblastoma is the most common extracranial solid malignancy of childhood and the most common malignancy diagnosed in infants – accounting for 50% of all cases. The incidence is approximately nine cases per one million children, or approximately 650 cases annually in the USA each year. The median age at diagnosis is 17 months (Brodeur and Maris 2002).

Neuroblastoma is a pediatric tumor which arises from embryonic ► neural crest cells. Because of the natural migratory process of these cells, neuroblastoma can arise in any portion of the sympathetic nervous system including the adrenal glands (40%), abdominal ganglia (25%), thoracic ganglia (15%), cervical ganglia (5%), and pelvic ganglia (5%) (Wolden 2007).

Neuroblastoma is an oddity among tumors. Most (60%) are metastatic at presentation. However, unlike other metastatic tumors, neuroblastoma has "favorable" metastatic sites which are considered curable: liver and skin. Unfavorable metastatic sites include bone marrow and the bones of the skull (such as the orbits) (Brodeur and Maris 2002).

Neuroblastoma is associated with paraneoplastic syndromes such as vasoactive intestinal polypeptide secretion and opsoclonus-myoclonus-ataxia syndrome which can complicate both diagnosis and treatment.

Background

During embryonic development, all human fetuses develop cell clusters in the adrenal glands between 17 and 20 weeks gestation. These cells regress spontaneously by birth or early infancy in the vast majority of cases. Very rarely, there appears to be some disruption in this process and tumors persist and develop into what we call neuroblastoma (Ikeda et al. 1981).

A cause for neuroblastoma has not been elicited and no link has been established between neuroblastoma and exposure to carcinogens such as radiation, chemicals, or pharmaceuticals. A small fraction of neuroblastomas are considered familial and associated with germline mutation. These patients tend to have more extensive, bilateral disease and typically present at an earlier age than their somatically mutated counterparts.

Initial Evaluation

The clinical presentation of neuroblastoma is variable with age. Children younger than 1 year are more likely to have local or regional disease at diagnosis. Physical examination on these children with abdominal tumors as the sole site of disease will present with increased abdominal girth, abdominal pain, and gastrointestinal disturbance. Conversely, children older than 1 year are much more likely to have disseminated disease at presentation and will complain of bone pain, fever, and weight loss. Clinicians should also be aware of opsomyoclonus, a paraneoplastic syndrome which presents with myoclonic jerking and random eye movements.

Evaluation of regional lymphatics is important. Neuroblastoma can involve the para-aortic chain and (uncommonly) the left supraclavicular fossa (Virchow's node). Lung and brain metastases are possible, but rare at initial presentation. However, with increasing improvements in systemic therapy, many high-risk patients will at some point in their clinical course have distant spread to the lungs or central nervous system. Clinicians should routinely evaluate these organ systems in high-risk children.

In addition, two bilateral posterior iliac crest bone marrow aspirates and biopsies are required for staging purposes. One positive biopsy is sufficient to document involvement of the bone marrow.

Increased sympathetic tone from catecholamine release can cause hypertension, flushing, and tachycardia. Urine should be collected and examined for catecholamines and their metabolites, such as norepinephrine, vanillylmandelic acid (VMA), homovanillic acid (HVA), and 3-methoxy-4-hydroxyphenylglycol (MHPG) (LaBrosse et al. 1976).

Staging

The issue of staging has evolved over the decades and several staging systems have historically been used, including the Children's Cancer Group (CCG) staging system as well as the Pediatric Oncology Group system. However, these systems have been replaced by the International Neuroblastoma Staging System (INSS), which is the currently accepted standard staging system (Brodeur et al. 1993).

INSS Stage 1 patients have localized disease, which has been completely excised surgically. Patients can have microscopic residual disease, but negative ipsilateral lymph nodes. However, lymph nodes directly adherent to the primary tumor are allowed to be positive.

INSS Stage 2 is divided into 2A and 2B. Patients with 2A disease have local disease with gross residual tumor after surgery and negative ipsilateral lymph nodes. The distinguishing feature of 2B disease is the positivity of ipsilateral nonadherent lymph nodes.

INSS Stage 3 disease crosses midline (defined as the vertebral column). Regional lymph nodes can be positive or negative. Conversely, Stage 3 disease can consist of a unilateral tumor (i.e., does not cross midline) with positive contralateral lymph nodes.

INSS Stage 4 disease is an interesting and unique class of patients among cancer staging. Stage 4 disease is divided into unfavorable patients with distant metastases to unfavorable sites (lymph nodes, bone, bone marrow, skin, and liver) or the much more favorable 4S category, which consists of a localized primary tumor with dissemination to skin, liver, and/or bone marrow in infants less than 1 year of age. Stage 4S patients tend to behave more like early stage disease and typically respond very favorably to treatment (Brodeur et al. 1993).

Apart from INSS staging, risk stratification based on histology and other prognostic features is extremely important in neuroblastoma. Histologic examination is of the utmost importance in this disease and histologic features dramatically impact prognosis.

Given the complex milieu of prognostic features, the Shimada system was developed as a uniform means of classifying patients into favorable versus unfavorable categories. The Shimada system recognizes age, histologic pattern (nodular versus diffuse), amount of Schwann cell stroma in the tumor, and mitotic-karyorrhectic index (MKI) as prognostic features. Based on these four features, patients can be classified as either favorable or unfavorable (Wolden 2007).

Differential Diagnosis

Neuroblastoma is classified as one of the many small, round, blue-cell tumors of childhood. The remaining eight small ▶ round blue-cell tumors can best be recalled using the pneumonic "Lemon Powder" (LEMN PWDR):

L – Leukemia, Acute
E – Ewing's Sarcoma
M – Mesothelioma, small cell
N – Neuroblastoma
P – Primitive neuroectodermal tumor
W – Wilm's Tumor
D – Desmoplastic small round blue-cell tumor
R – Rhabdomyosarcoma

Pathologic staining as well as clinical clues will assist the clinician with the appropriate diagnosis of a small, round, blue-cell tumor.

Neuroblastoma itself represents a spectrum of disease with different histologic subtypes of the disease reflecting the spectrum of maturation and increasing differentiation from ▶ ganglioneuroma to ▶ ganglioneuroblastoma to neuroblastoma (Fig. 1). Ganglioneuromas are typically benign. Ganglioneuroblastomas are histologically similar to both ganglioneuroma and neuroblastoma with

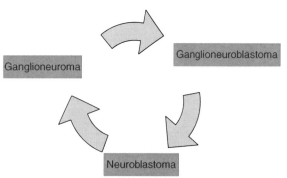

Neuroblastoma. Fig. 1 Histologic spectrum of neuroblastoma including ganglioneuroma (benign), ganglioneuroblastoma (features of both ganglioneuroma and ganglioneuroblastoma), and neuroblastoma

an intermediate behavior which can be either quite aggressive or more benign. Neuroblastoma represents the most aggressive end of the spectrum (Wolden 2007).

Imaging Studies

Workup generally begins with plain radiography of the abdomen which may reveal a large tumor with calcifications – a feature present in 85% of tumors. Further characterization of the tumor and regional lymphatics should be accomplished with computerized tomography (CT) or magnetic resonance imaging (MRI). These studies are helpful to clinically stage a patient and can be used to determine resectability. Neuroblastoma commonly metastasizes to the liver, so this organ should be paid its due respect in evaluating abdominal imaging studies (Golding et al. 1984; Fletcher et al. 1985).

Bone metastases are also common in neuroblastoma. The disease has a proclivity to involve the base of skull – giving rise to the classic "raccoon eyes," or periorbital ecchymosis. Studies which may be helpful in assessing skeletal spread include metaiodobenzylguanidine (MIBG) scan, bone scan, and/or fluorodeoxyglucose positron emission tomography (FDG PET) scan (Voute et al. 1985).

Laboratory Studies

In addition to routine laboratory tests such as CBC and serum chemistries, molecular and genetic testing is helpful in determining both treatment and prognosis in children diagnosed with neuroblastoma (Wolden 2007).

Molecular alterations of neuroblastoma have been well described and are of particular importance for the prognosis of children with this disease. The two most widely described genetic mutations are the deletion of the short arm of chromosome 1 (1p) and ▶ N-*myc* amplification. Either of these genetic events portends a worse prognosis and is typically described in more advanced disease.

Chromosomal ploidy, also known as DNA index (DI) is an additional prognostic marker of importance, particularly in children 18 months of age and younger. Pseudodiploid and near-diploid tumors have nuclear DNA content which approximates normal but usually have structural chromosomal abnormalities, including N-*myc* amplification. Hyperdiploid and near-triploid tumors usually do not have N-*myc* amplification or chromosome 1p deletion and have a more favorable prognosis (Matthay 1997).

Treatment

Risk stratification (based on stage and the ▶ Shimada Pathologic Classification System) is of utmost importance when approaching treatment for patients with neuroblastoma. Treatment typically consists of a multimodality, team-based approach. Many patients will require surgery, chemotherapy, and radiotherapy. New experimental treatments, including radioimmunotherapy, are also being investigated. Below is outlined the treatment considerations for patients of low-, intermediate-, and high-risk status. Additionally, treatment of recurrent disease will be discussed. The reader is referred to Fig. 2 for an at-a-glance view of treatment recommendations for low-, intermediate-, and high-risk disease.

Low Risk

Low risk neuroblastoma is typically treated with surgery alone. Even patients with subtotal resection can be cured in the vast majority of cases. No benefit has been demonstrated for adjuvant chemotherapy or radiotherapy in addressing gross residual disease, and these modalities are typically reserved for progressive or recurrent disease. Radiation, when indicated, is typically to a dose of 21 Gy (Perez et al. 2000).

High risk features, such as N-*myc* amplification, are rare in low-risk patients. When present, N-*myc* amplification in this subgroup does not confer a worsened prognosis (Cohn et al. 1995).

Patients with stage 4S are considered low risk, despite having disseminated disease at presentation. Distant metastases often regress spontaneously in this subgroup and overall survival is excellent (Nickerson et al. 2000). However, it is important to be able to recognize rapidly progressive stage 4S disease because these patients can require prompt radiotherapeutic intervention when lung or liver metastases cause respiratory distress or bowel ischemia, respectively. In such situations, low-dose radiotherapy has proven successful. A patient with severe hepatomegaly can be treated to a dose of 4.5 Gy in three fractions with rapid relief of symptoms (Wolden 2007). This is a situation in which the risk of treatment is minimal due to the low dose, and the reward maximal with palliation of symptoms which can be fatal. The astute radiation oncologist would be wise to intervene rapidly in any pediatric patient with neuroblastoma who complains of dyspnea or severe abdominal pain.

Intermediate Risk

Intermediate risk patients, as determined by the Shimada Pathologic Classification System as well as stage, require multimodality treatment including surgical resection and 4–8 months of chemotherapy. The timing of chemotherapy in relation to surgery depends entirely on the respectability

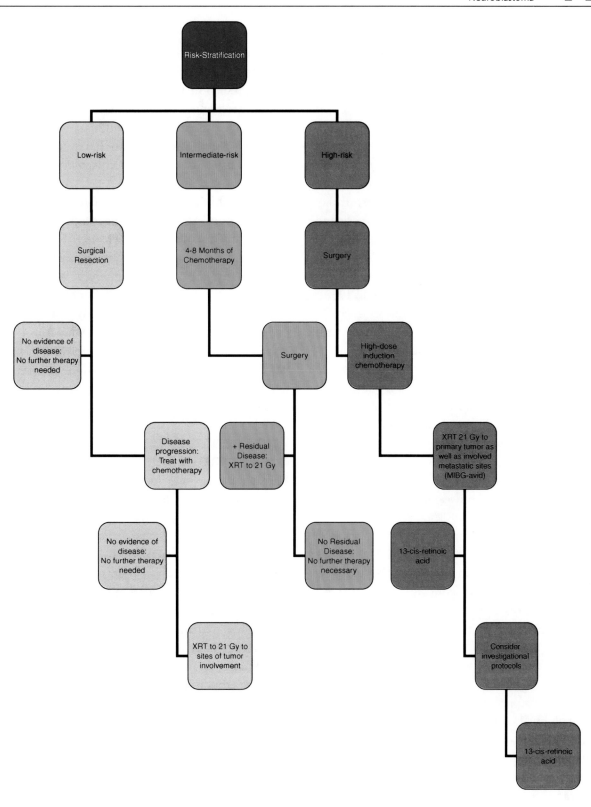

Neuroblastoma. Fig. 2 Treatment algorithm by risk-stratified groups

of the tumor. Oftentimes, surgery is delayed until after chemotherapy, allowing a less extensive operation.

Evidence for radiotherapy is based on older data with outdated techniques. Extrapolation of this data to the modern era proves difficult. Patients with intermediate-risk stage 2 disease can be successfully treated with surgery and chemotherapy, forgoing radiotherapy. Patients with stage 3 intermediate-risk disease have historically been treated with radiotherapy after surgery and chemotherapy. However, changes in the staging system over time blur the previously distinct categories of which stage- and risk-stratified patient will benefit from radiation (Matthay et al. 1989).

In the most recent COG study (#A3961) intermediate-risk patients were treated with surgery and chemotherapy consisting of cyclophosphamide, doxorubicin, carboplatin, and etopiside. In this protocol, radiation is indicated only for persistent disease after chemotherapy or in patients with disease progression. With this study as a guideline, stage 3 intermediate-risk patients, with favorable biology, likely do not require radiation unless treatment with surgery and chemotherapy proves ineffective (Wolden 2007).

High Risk

Despite advances in therapy over the past few decades, prognosis is poor for patients with high-risk disease. However, prognosis is age-dependent, with children diagnosed at an earlier age (less than 1 year) outperforming those diagnosed at a later age (over 1 year).

The Chidren's Cancer Group (CCG) conducted a phase III clinical trial, which demonstrated the benefit of high-dose chemotherapy, radiotherapy, and autologous bone marrow transplantation in these patients. Administration of 13-*cis*-retinoic acid upon completion of chemotherapy has also shown a dramatic benefit (Matthay et al. 1999).

Given the results of the CCG trial, children with high-risk disease today are managed with high-dose induction chemotherapy followed by surgical resection. Consideration is given to adjuvant consolidative myeloablation and stem cell rescue. Subsequently, residual disease is targeted with radiotherapy. Response to therapy portends a better prognosis than patients who do not respond.

The Children's Oncology Group recommends a dose of 21 Gy to the primary tumor and any metastatic sites which are MIBG-avid on the pre-transplant scan. The ideal timing of radiotherapy appears to be after myeloablative chemotherapy, when the total volume of disease to be treated is minimal. Total body irradiation (TBI) has historically been used with a good response prior to transplantation. However, TBI has been replaced at most institutions with systemic myeloablative therapy (Haas-Kogan et al. 2003).

Treatment of Recurrent Disease and Palliative Considerations

Therapeutic options for disease recurrence or refractory disease include chemotherapy or novel therapies such as radionuclides or immunotherapy. Radiation therapy also plays a central role in disease palliation. With improvement in systemic therapy, many patients are living long enough to experience discomfort or functional impairment from disease progression or metastasis. In these patients, external beam radiotherapy can provide effective palliation. There are many dose/fractionation schemes which have been successfully employed – most of which are quite similar to radiation schemes employed in adults suffering from metastatic disease requiring palliation (Wolden 2007).

Radiation Therapy Volume

The irradiated volume will depend on the region being treated. However, as most tumors are intra-abdominal, there are a few governing principles which should guide the individuals assigned to plan the prescribed course of radiotherapy.

Neuroblastoma commonly recurs in the para-aortic chain, so these nodal structures should be included in the radiation field (Wolden et al. 2000). In covering the para-aortics, it is important to remember to encompass entire vertebral bodies to reduce the risk of long-term scoliosis (Wolden 2007).

Given the often large fields employed, most patients are treated with simple anterior and posterior beams. However, intensity modulated radiation therapy may occasionally be helpful to spare critical organs such as the kidney or spinal cord (Wolden 2007).

Oftentimes anesthesia will be required in order to ensure that very young children remain still and the treatment is appropriately and accurately delivered.

Cross-References

▶ Palliation of Bone Metastases
▶ Palliation of Metastatic Disease to the Liver
▶ Total Body Irradiation (TBI)
▶ Wilm's Tumor

References

Brodeur G, Maris J (2002) Neuroblastoma. Principles and practice of pediatric oncology, 4th edn. Lippincott Williams and Wilkins, Philadelphia, pp 895–937

Brodeur GM, Pritchard J, Berthold F et al (1993) Revisions in the international criteria neuroblastoma diagnosis, staging and response to treatment. J Clin Oncol 11:1466

Cohn SL, Look AT, Joshi VV et al (1995) Lack of correlation of N-*myc* gene amplification with prognosis in localized neuroblastoma: a Pediatric Oncology Group study. Cancer Res 55:721–726

Fletcher BD, Kopiwoda SY, Strandjord SE et al (1985) Abdominal neuroblastoma: magnetic resonance imaging and tissue characterization. Radiology 155:699

Golding SJ, McElwain TJ, Husband JE (1984) The role of computed tomography in the management of children with advanced neuroblastoma. Br J Radiol 57:661

Haas-Kogan DA, Swift PS, Selch M et al (2003) Impact of radiotherapy for high-risk neuroblastoma: a Children's Cancer Group study. Int J Radiat Oncol Biol Phys 56:28–39

Ikeda Y, Lister J, Bouton JM, Buyukpamukcu M (1981) Congenital neuroblastoma, neuroblastoma in situ, and the normal fetal development of the adrenal. J Pediatr Surg 16:636

LaBrosse EH, Comay E, Bohuan C et al (1976) Catecholamine metabolism in neuroblastoma. J Natl Cancer Inst 57:633–643

Matthay KK (1997) Neuroblastoma: biology and therapy. Oncology 11:1857–1866

Matthay KK, Sather HN, Seeger RC et al (1989) Excellent outcome of stage II neuroblastoma is independent of residual disease and radiation therapy. J Clin Oncol 7:236–244

Matthay KK, Villablanca JG, Seeger RC et al (1999) Treatment of high-risk neuroblastoma with intensive chemotherapy, radiotherapy, autologous bone marrow transplantation, and 13-cis-retinoic acid. Children's Cancer Group. N Engl J Med 341:1165–1173

Nickerson HJ, Matthay KK, Seeger RC et al (2000) Favorable biology and outcome of stage IV-S neuroblastoma with supportive care or minimal therapy: a Children's Cancer Group Study. J Clin Oncol 18:477–486

Perez CA, Matthay KK, Atkinson JB et al (2000) Biologic variables in the outcome of stages I and II neuroblastoma treated with surgery as primary therapy: a Children's Cancer Group Study. J Clin Oncol 18:18–26

Smith M, Ries L, Gurney J (1999) Cancer incidence and survival among children and adolescents: United States SEER program 1975–1995, National Cancer Institute, SEER program, Bethesda

Voute PA, Hoefnagel C, Marcuse HR et al (1985) Detection of neuroblastoma with [I-13]meta-iodobenzylguanidine. Prog Clin Biol Res 175:389–398

Wolden SL (2007) Neuroblastoma. In: Clinical radiation oncology, 2nd edn. Elsevier/Churchill Livingstone, Philadelphia, pp 1637–1643

Wolden SL, Gollamudi SV, Kushner BH et al (2000) Local control with multi-modality therapy for stage 4 neuroblastoma. Int J Radiat Oncol Biol Phys 47:985–992

Neuroendocrine Carcinoma of the Skin

▶ Merkel Cell Carcinoma (MCC)

Neurofibromatosis Type 1

JOHN P. LAMOND
Department of Radiation Oncology,
Temple University, Crozer-Chester Medical
Center, Upland, PA, USA

Definition

Genetic syndrome associated with skin pigmented lesions, multiple neurofibromas, and schwannomas. Formerly called von Recklinghausen disease.

Cross-References

▶ Soft Tissue Sarcoma

Neutron

GEORGE E. LARAMORE, JAY J. LIAO,
JASON K. ROCKHILL
Department of Radiation Oncology, University of
Washington Medical Center, Seattle, WA, USA

Definition

The neutron is a subatomic particle that is a constituent of all atomic nuclei except for ^{1}H. It is approximately 1,839 times more massive than an electron. As a neutral particle, it does not interact directly with the atomic electrons but rather with the atomic nuclei of the material through which it passes. The knock-off protons and nuclear fragments produced in these interactions produce dense ionization events along their path, which give rise to the unique radiobiological properties of neutrons.

Cross-References

▶ Neutron Radiotherapy
▶ X-Ray

Neutron Radiotherapy

JAY J. LIAO, GEORGE E. LARAMORE, JASON K. ROCKHILL
Department of Radiation Oncology, University of
Washington Medical Center, Seattle, WA, USA

Synonyms

Fast neutron therapy

Definition

▶ Neutron radiotherapy refers to the clinical application of ionizing radiation using fast neutrons. It falls under the broader category of hadron radiotherapy, which also includes protons and carbon ions. The underlying radiobiological properties of neutron radiotherapy compared to standard photon/electron treatment have led to clinical studies for a wide range of tumors. Based on this experience, neutron radiotherapy has been demonstrated to be advantageous primarily in the treatment of specific tumors that are relatively radioresistant, including malignant salivary gland tumors, soft tissue sarcomas, and melanoma.

Background

Historical Perspective

The neutron was first discovered by Sir James Chadwick in 1932 while studying certain nuclear reactions. Clinical trials in cancer patients were initiated several years later by Dr. Robert Stone at the Lawrence Berkeley Laboratory ▶ cyclotron in Berkeley, California. At that time, the understanding of the relationship between neutron doses and clinical effects was still immature. As a result, many patients developed significant radiation complications due to inadvertent overdoses. This discouraging early experience as well as the beginning of World War II led to discontinuation of further neutron therapy investigation for nearly 20 years.

In the 1970s, investigators at Hammersmith Hospital in London, with a better understanding of neutron radiobiology, resumed neutron clinical trials using the Medical Research Council (MRC) cyclotron. The initial studies were performed mainly in patients with advanced head and neck cancers because the neutrons generated by this relatively low-energy cyclotron made treatment of only superficial tumors feasible. Encouraging local control outcomes with acceptable side effects were reported. This ushered in a period of clinical investigation across many tumor sites, and neutron radiotherapy was ultimately utilized in 39 different centers in North America, Europe, Asia, and Africa. Larger cyclotrons capable of generating high-energy neutrons in the range of 20–50 MeV as well as the increased flexibility of facilities with rotating gantries and more advanced beam shaping made it possible to treat a wider array of tumors.

For many tumor types the results of these clinical trials failed to demonstrate a significant advantage compared to widely available photon-based therapy. Neutron radiotherapy was clearly not the panacea that was hoped for, and the early widespread clinical interest waned. Nevertheless, neutrons have consistently demonstrated improved outcomes in select clinical applications, mainly in relatively radioresistant tumors such as salivary gland tumors, soft tissue sarcomas, and melanoma. There remain five operating fast neutron radiotherapy centers throughout the world, including two in the United States, which offer this specialized therapy to select patients who continue to benefit from the unique advantages of this treatment.

Physics and Radiobiology

Neutrons are produced using a cyclotron or a particle ▶ linear accelerator which accelerates positively charged protons or deuterons to several million electron volts (eV). These high-energy particles then impact a beryllium target generating a neutron distribution that is approximately spherically symmetric. Shaped collimators are used to produce the clinical beams. Typical neutron energy ranges are 20–70 MeV. Many early neutron facilities were actually modified high-energy physics research installations. The development of dedicated hospital-based systems, isocentrically mounted gantries, multileaf collimator (▶ MLC) beam shaping, and neutrons in the 50 MeV range made it possible to generate beams with depth dose characteristics similar to 6 MV linear accelerator x-ray units and to deliver more conformal treatment plans.

The potential advantages of neutron therapy are based on several important radiobiological concepts (Hall and Giaccia 2006). Neutrons are classified as a form of high linear energy transfer (▶ LET) radiation, which also includes carbon and heavier ions. LET is the rate of energy loss along the pathway of an ionizing particle, usually expressed in keV/μm. Neutrons are densely ionizing radiation, meaning that they create a dense column of ionization in their path and therefore more double strand DNA breaks and other non-repairable damage. High LET is usually considered to be in the range of 20–100 keV/μm. In contrast, x-rays as well as gamma rays and electrons are more sparsely ionizing in the range of 0.2–2 keV/μm and therefore considered to be low LET. As LET increases, the relative biologic effectiveness of a particular radiation type also increases up to a certain point. RBE is the ratio of physical doses between two different types of radiations required to produce the same biological endpoint. Typically, the comparison is made to 250 kV_p x-ray radiation. The specific RBE depends upon the specific tissue and endpoint chosen. The higher RBE associated with high LET forms of radiation such as neutrons results in greater tumor cell killing compared to x-rays. For instance, the RBE of neutrons for malignant salivary tumors is 8.0, while the neutron RBE for most normal tissue late effects is 3.0–3.5 and for late central nervous system effects 4.0–4.5. As a result, neutrons show a therapeutic gain for a number of tumor types, especially relatively slow-growing tumors and radioresistant tumors that typically do not respond well to low LET radiation.

Another potential advantage of neutrons relates to oxygenation. Many tumors harbor subvolumes of hypoxic cells. The mechanism of action of tumor cell killing by x-ray therapy is predominantly indirect damage to DNA mediated by free radicals. This depends on the presence of oxygen for maximal effect, which acts as a stabilizer of free radical damage. It has been observed that hypoxic tumors both in the lab and in the clinic demonstrate decreased sensitivity to x-ray therapy. This is quantified by the oxygen enhancement ratio (▶ OER), which is the ratio of doses to achieve the same biologic effect in hypoxic versus aerated cells. X-ray- or gamma-ray-based therapies are characterized by an OER in the range of 2.5–3.0. In contrast, fast neutron therapy causes more direct damage to critical cellular targets and has an OER in the range of 1.5–2.0. Therefore, neutrons may be more effective in treating hypoxic tumors.

High LET radiotherapy is associated with a reduced shoulder in the cell survival curve, which is nearly log-linear in contrast to low LET radiotherapy. This is explained in part by reduced potential for both sublethal and potentially lethal DNA damage repair with high LET therapy such as neutrons. Finally, radiosensitivity typically varies across the different parts of the cell cycle with greater radiosensitivity observed in M and late G1/early S phase. This effect is more evident in photon therapy and may be a source of radioresistance in an asynchronously dividing cell population. High LET radiation is less dependent on these cell cycle effects and therefore may be more effective than photons in tumors with long cell cycle times.

Treatment Techniques

Fast Neutron Therapy

The neutron radiotherapy planning process is similar to conventional photon-based treatment. Patients undergo a simulation procedure, usually with a treatment planning CT scan and custom immobilization, which depends on the particular site being treated. For instance, patients with head and neck tumors are typically immobilized with a thermoplastic mask, occipital mold, shoulder restraints, and occasionally a dental stent or bite block. Depending on the clinical situation, treatment planning MRI or FDG-PET scans may be obtained for image registration and fusion.

Target and organ at risk volumes are then delineated. Three-dimensional conformal treatment planning based on these contours is performed followed by evaluation of the dose distributions and dose–volume histograms. Compared to photon therapy, several differences are notable. Neutron dose distributions have a broader penumbra as well as a different shape in the build-up region, which depends on the specific neutron energy and beam path. Neutron interactions with tissue generate a cascade of photons, neutrons, and charged particles that must be taken into account when calculating doses.

Given the higher neutron RBE, the total physical dose for a course of neutron therapy is about 1/3 of the physical dose for a typical photon therapy course. Doses range from 18 to 20 ▶ nGy (Neutron Gray) delivered in daily fractions of 1.15–1.20 nGy over about 4 weeks. Dose limits to organs at risk are well-established and based on neutron RBE in various normal tissues as well as clinical experience. The expected acute and late effects from neutron therapy are similar to effects observed with conventional photon therapy but may be more exacerbated. The delivered dose is designed to achieve a similar rate of normal tissue late effects as a course of photon therapy.

Mixed Beam

Mixed beam approaches combining neutron therapy with conventional photon or electron therapy have been utilized. In the past, a number of approaches employed neutron therapy alternating with or used as a boost after photon therapy. In current practice, the application of mixed beam approaches typically relate to specific dosimetric concerns. The most common scenario is the addition of electron therapy to supplement a neutron therapy plan in areas of relative neutron underdose superficially. This may be necessary due to limitations imposed by adjacent normal tissue constraints. For instance, electrons may be used to boost a superficial component of a periorbital or paranasal sinus tumor after tolerance doses to adjacent optic structures are reached with neutrons. Electrons are also commonly used to boost the posterior neck lymph nodes after spinal cord tolerance is reached with neutrons. More recently, newer approaches have been pioneered, which combine neutron therapy with Gamma Knife® stereotactic radiosurgery boost in patients with tumor invasion into the base of skull.

Clinical Applications

Early clinical investigations studied a wide variety of tumor types including head and neck squamous cell cancers, salivary gland tumors, lung cancer, cervical cancer, prostate cancer, sarcomas, and melanoma (Laramore et al. 2008). Approximately 30,000 patients have been treated with neutron therapy as a component of their care. We highlight below some important clinical studies of fast neutron radiotherapy.

Salivary Gland Tumors

Neutron therapy has been used most widely in the management of salivary gland tumors, where the therapeutic advantage of neutron therapy has been most clearly demonstrated (Laramore et al. 1993a; Huber et al. 2001; Douglas et al. 2003).

Given the neutron RBE of approximately 8 for salivary tumors and 3.0–3.5 for most normal tissues, there is a significant therapeutic gain factor on the order of 2.3–2.6. Therefore, a typical fractionated course of 18–20 nGy translates into 60–70 Gy-equivalent with respect to normal tissues and approximately 160 Gy-equivalent with respect to the tumor.

Single institution studies supported the efficacy of neutrons in this setting with acceptable toxicity. This led to a prospective randomized trial (RTOG-MRC), which confirmed a significant improvement in locoregional control with neutrons compared to photon therapy, in a population of patients primarily with locally advanced disease. Although no clear survival advantage was apparent in this trial, patterns of failure shifted such that a greater proportion of patients with locally advanced disease treated with neutrons achieved long-term control of locoregional disease but succumbed eventually to distant metastases.

A number of single institutions including the University of Washington and the German Cancer Research Center have reported long-term experiences of primary neutron therapy for locally advanced malignant salivary gland tumors. Overall long-term locoregional control is around 60–75%. This represents a dramatic improvement over the historically poor rates of locoregional control around 25% with conventional approaches for this cohort of patients. Negative prognostic factors for local control include tumors >4 cm, lack of surgical resection, and the presence of skull-base invasion. The poor outcomes of patients with base of skull invasion relate to the proximity of critical structures (temporal lobes, optic chiasm, optic nerves), which limit the delivery of full neutron doses. Improved locoregional control without an apparent increase in complications has recently been reported with a strategy of neutron therapy followed by Gamma Knife® boost to the skull base (Douglas et al. 2008). However, patients with locally advanced salivary gland tumors continue to be plagued by a high rate of eventual distant metastases ranging from 30% to 50%. On the other hand, patients treated adjuvantly for microscopic disease only, who comprise a much smaller proportion of patients treated with neutrons, fare extremely well with locoregional control achieved in approximately 90% of cases.

The aforementioned studies include a wide range of salivary gland histologies including adenoid cystic carcinoma, mucoepidermoid carcinoma, acinic cell carcinoma, adenocarcinoma, and squamous cell carcinoma of both major and minor salivary gland origin. Neutron radiotherapy has also been used to treat high-risk, recurrent pleomorphic adenomas of the major salivary glands. Excellent long-term locoregional control has been achieved around 76% for gross disease and 100% for microscopic disease. Finally, neutrons have also been used in the selective retreatment of unresectable gross recurrent salivary gland tumors, usually after prior photon radiotherapy. The local control rates are approximately 50% in this cohort of patients with limited therapeutic options. There is expected increased late morbidity including soft tissue fibrosis, osteoradionecrosis, trismus, etc. However, significant palliation is achieved in many patients.

Prostate Cancer

Some radiobiological work suggests that prostate cancer has a relatively low α/β ratio in the range of 1.5–3.0, which would predict for a potential advantage in favor of high LET radiotherapy. The reported early clinical experience in locally advanced prostate cancer in fact supports this hypothesis with apparent improvement in locoregional control with neutrons compared to photons. Two early randomized clinical trials comparing neutrons (either alone or mixed beam) with photons in locally advanced prostate cancer were conducted by the RTOG and NTCWG (Laramore et al. 1993b; Russell et al. 1994). A locoregional control advantage on the order of 10–20% absolute increase in favor of neutrons was observed. However, increased rectal and bowel toxicity with neutrons was noted in several series, which lessened enthusiasm for neutrons in prostate cancer. Acceptable complication rates have actually been observed at institutions where MLC beam shaping allows for appropriate rectal shielding.

Sarcoma

Sarcomas are traditionally considered to be relatively radioresistant, except in the setting of microscopic disease following surgical resection. Retrospective data comparing neutrons to photons in the setting of inoperable gross disease suggests a benefit in favor of neutrons with local control rates around 50% compared to 20–30% for photons. The largest clinical report of neutron therapy for sarcomas reviewed the European experience in 11 centers of over 1,000 patients and demonstrated local control around 90% for microscopic disease and 47% for unresectable disease (Schwarz et al. 1998).

Melanoma

Melanoma is a tumor that would be expected to benefit from high LET radiotherapy. The reported clinical experience with neutrons is actually quite limited. However, neutrons have been used in the treatment of primary, recurrent, and metastatic melanoma of both cutaneous and sinonasal mucosal origin, especially in the setting of gross disease. The response rates are quite high with some patients achieving complete clinical regression of gross disease. Local control with neutrons in the setting of gross disease is achieved in 50–70% of patients and compares favorably to outcomes with photon therapy. Many patients have control of local disease until time of death. Neutron therapy can be considered for the primary treatment or palliation of gross disease in melanoma, especially in the setting of inoperable disease.

Head and Neck Squamous Cell Carcinoma (HNSCC)

The results of neutron radiotherapy for the more common HNSCC have not been as impressive as the results in salivary gland tumors. Two important randomized controlled trials have been reported in patients with locally advanced disease. An RTOG trial compared conventional photons with a mixed beam approach (neutron/photon), and an NTCWG trial compared photons with neutrons (Griffin et al. 1989; Maor et al. 1995). Both trials found no significant benefit in terms of locoregional control or survival for the neutron-treated patients. There was a trend toward improved regional control in favor of neutrons in patients with clinically positive nodes, although more late complications were observed. Therefore, neutrons are not routinely indicated in the management of HNSCC but may have a role in patients with massive cervical lymphadenopathy in certain scenarios.

Central Nervous System (CNS)

Neutron therapy has been used to treat primary gliomas and some anaplastic meningiomas. In the 1980s, the University of Washington ran several trials looking at treatment response of high-grade gliomas to fast neutrons or mixtures of neutrons and photons. Survival times were not improved when compared to standard photon irradiation and in some cases worse. Remarkably, autopsy studies showed tumor sterilization but also significant normal tissue toxicity including widespread, coagulation necrosis (Laramore et al. 1978; Catterall et al. 1980). Due to this treatment toxicity, neutron radiotherapy is no longer being used for high-grade brain tumors.

Summary

Neutron radiotherapy is a specialized form of high LET radiotherapy which offers several radiobiological advantages compared to conventional photon therapy including high RBE for a number of tumor types, decreased oxygen dependence, decreased sublethal and potentially lethal damage repair, and decreased cell cycle dependence. Clinical investigation in a wide range of tumor sites has demonstrated that neutrons are not universally beneficial, but do appear to benefit a small but important niche of patients with relatively radioresistant tumors that are difficult to manage with other therapeutic options.

Cross-References

► Melanoma
► Prostate
► Proton Therapy
► Salivary Gland Cancer
► Soft Tissue Sarcoma
► X-Ray

References

Catterall M, Bloom JG, Ash DV et al (1980) Fast neutrons compared with megavoltage x-rays in the treatment of patients with supratentorial glioblastoma: a controlled pilot study. Int J Radiat Oncol Biol Phys 6:261–266

Douglas JG, Koh WJ, Austin-Seymour M et al (2003) Treatment of salivary gland neoplasms with fast neutron radiotherapy. Arch Otolaryngol Head Neck Surg 129:944–948

Douglas JG, Goodkin R, Laramore GE (2008) Gamma knife stereotactic radiosurgery for salivary gland neoplasms with base of skull invasion following neutron radiotherapy. Head Neck 30:492–496

Griffin TW, Pajak TF, Maor MH et al (1989) Mixed neutron/photon irradiation of unresectable squamous cell carcinomas of the head and neck: the final report of a randomized cooperative trial. Int J Radiat Oncol Biol Phys 17:959–965

Hall EJ, Giaccia AJ (2006) Radiobiology for the radiologist, 6th edn. Lippencott, Williams & Wilkins, Philadelphia

Huber PE, Debus J, Latz D et al (2001) Radiotherapy for advanced adenoid cystic carcinoma: neutrons, photons or mixed beam? Radiother Oncol 59:161–167

Laramore GE, Griffin TW, Gerdes AJ et al (1978) Fast neutron and mixed (neutron/photon) beam teletherapy for grades III and IV astrocytomas. Cancer 42:96–103

Laramore GE, Krall JM, Griffin TW et al (1993a) Neutron versus photon irradiation for unresectable salivary gland tumors: final report of an RTOG-MRC randomized clinical trial. Radiation therapy oncology group, medical research council. Int J Radiat Oncol Biol Phys 27:235–240

Laramore GE, Krall JM, Thomas FJ et al (1993b) Fast neutron radiotherapy for locally advanced prostate cancer. Final report of radiation therapy oncology group randomized clinical trial. Am J Clin Oncol 16:164–167

Laramore GE, Phillips MH, DeLaney TP (2008) Particle beam radiotherapy. In: Halperin EC, Perez CA, Brady LW (eds) Perez and Brady's principles and practice of radiation oncology, 5th edn. Wolters Kluwer/Lippincott Williams & Wilkins, Philadelphia

Maor MH, Errington RD, Caplan RJ et al (1995) Fast-neutron therapy in advanced head and neck cancer: a collaborative international randomized trial. Int J Radiat Oncol Biol Phys 32:599–604

Russell KJ, Caplan RJ, Laramore GE et al (1994) Photon versus fast neutron external beam radiotherapy in the treatment of locally advanced prostate cancer: results of a randomized prospective trial. Int J Radiat Oncol Biol Phys 28:47–54

Schwarz R, Krull A, Lessel A et al (1998) European results of neutron therapy in soft tissue sarcomas. Recent Results Cancer Res 150:100–112

Neutropenia

LINDSAY G. JENSEN, BRENT S. ROSE,
ARNO J. MUNDT
Center for Advanced Radiotherapy Technologies,
Department of Radiation Oncology, San Diego
Rebecca and John Moores Cancer Center,
University of California, La Jolla, CA, USA

Definition
Decreased peripheral neutrophil count, typically <1,500 per microliter.

Cross-References
▶ Bone Marrow Toxicity in Cancer Treatment

Nevoid Basal Cell Carcinoma Syndrome

▶ Basal Cell Nevus Syndrome

Nevus with Architectural Disorder

▶ Atypical (Dysplastic) Nevi

nGy

GEORGE E. LARAMORE, JAY J. LIAO, JASON K. ROCKHILL
Department of Radiation Oncology, University of Washington Medical Center, Seattle, WA, USA

Definition
nGy or Gy_n is defined as the physical absorbed dose from the neutron beam. By convention, it also includes the dose from γ-rays produced by neutron interactions with atomic nuclei.

Cross-References
▶ Neutron Radiotherapy

N-myc

BRANDON J. FISHER[1], LARRY C. DAUGHERTY[2]
[1]Department of Radiation Oncology, College of Medicine, Drexel University, Philadelphia, PA, USA
[2]Department of Radiation Oncology, College of Medicine, Drexel University, Glenside, PA, USA

Definition
N-myc is a genetic alteration seen in unfavorable cases of neuroblastoma.

Cross-References
▶ Neuroblastoma

Nomogram

YAN YU, LAURA DOYLE
Department of Radiation Oncology, Thomas Jefferson University Hospital, Philadelphia, PA, USA

Definition
Lookup table used for calculating the amount of activity needed for a brachytherapy implant based on volume and prescription dose.

Cross-References
▶ Brachytherapy: Low Dose Rate (LDR) Permanent Implants (Prostate)

Nonconventional Medicine

▶ Alternative Medicine
▶ Nontraditional Medicine

Non-Hodgkins Lymphoma

THEODORE E. YAEGER
Department Radiation Oncology, Wake Forest University School of Medicine, Winston-Salem, NC, USA

Definition
Non-Hodgkin's Lymphoma is a group of many different types of lymphomas which takes into account the cell of origin, whether it is classified as indolent or aggressive, and stage at presentation with or without systemic symptoms.

Introduction
Non-Hodgkin's Lymphoma, the fifth most common malignancy in the United States, is generally considered a systemic disease process in 80–85% of patients. The majority are a B-cell origin with a wide variety of clinical phenotypes (Armitage and Weisenberger 1998). A multidisciplinary approach for appropriate management is appropriate for most cases.

Chemotherapy is the mainstay of treatment in the majority of symptomatic presentations. When lymphomas possess the CD20 cell membrane receptor immunotherapy (Rituximab – Rituxan) is often added to chemotherapy either concurrently or sequentially. External beam radiation therapy is a useful primary treatment modality for limited, localized, and slower growing disease. Radiation therapy is also an important consideration for most catastrophic symptomatic presentations. Catastrophic symptoms (superior vena cava obstruction, spinal cord compression, pulmonary obstruction, severe pain, etc.) can often be an urgent treatment situation and radiotherapy would be crucial to alleviating life-threatening or crippling presentations.

Radiolabeled immunotherapy (^{131}I tositumomab – Bexxar or ^{90}Y ibritumamab – Zevalin) is becoming an important treatment option for consolidative treatment after initial chemoimmunotherapy or for recurrent/persistent disease after chemotherapy and/or non-radiolabeled immunotreatments (Cheson 2001, 2003).

Diagnosis, Staging and Prognosis

Diagnosis

Initial Evaluation
Diagnosis and evaluation of Non-Hodgkin's lymphoma (NHL) usually starts with a complete history and physical. Special attention should be focused upon externally palpable nodal sites, liver, spleen, skin, and oral cavity. NHL commonly

presents as an enlarged, non-tender, rubbery, moveable lymph node within a typical node bearing area, an enlarged nodular liver, enlarged non-tender spleen, or enlarged non-ulcerated tonsil.

Attention should be paid to a described history that reveals exposure to toxic chemicals – solvents, benzene compounds, and tobacco use/exposure, and non-specific symptoms such as night sweating, unexplained weight loss, shortness of breath, hemoptysis, pruritis, recent onset alcohol beverage intolerance, and unusual fatigue.

A thorough physical examination should include epitrochlear, axillary, supraclavicular node areas, and Waldeyer's ring as commonly involved areas.

Laboratory Tests

Initial lab tests should include complete blood count and chemistries including liver function, alkaline phosphatase, lactate dehydrogenase, sedimentation rate, imaging studies, and a bone marrow biopsy.

Imaging Studies

Diagnostic imaging studies are required to appropriately evaluate and stage NHL. A chest X-Ray and CT of chest, abdomen, and pelvis are the minimum. Recently positron emission tomography (PET) in combination with a concurrent CT scan has become an approved study for baseline systemic staging and for restaging when failure is suspected. Follow-up diagnostic quality CT scans can then be performed on suspected sites of nodal or organ involvement. Departing from past experience, laparotomy is no longer considered a standard of care and is rarely beneficial. If needed a laparoscopy may be performed for biopsy when no peripheral site is available. In the absence of neurologic symptoms a CT or MRI of the brain is not routinely needed. Similarly, the bone scan and gallium scans have been replaced by the PET scan.

Pathology

Tissue for pathologic confirmation is critical to determine the type, histopathology, and cell receptor status for treatment determination. Typically fine needle aspiration of a suspected lymph node, soft tissue nodule/organ mass, cytologic spin of an effusion or a bone marrow biopsy will yield enough cells to analyze. The Revised European-American classification now recognizes three major subtypes of lymphomas: B-cell, T-cell, and Hodgkin's disease. The main classification is based on cell cytology rather than architecture including the recognition of a widely variable morphologic grades and clinical aggressiveness. The most common North American lymphomas are the low-grade follicular, small cleaved cell type, and the intermediate grade diffuse large cell lymphoma. Mycosis fungoides, extramedullary plasmacytomas, mantle cell, and mucosa-associated lymphoid tissue (MALT) cell lymphomas are rarer subtype falling into the miscellaneous category. Burkitt's cell lymphoma is associated with a particular MYC translocation and over expression (Gospodarowicz and Wasserman 1998). CD-20 receptor analysis has become crucial to determine as newer biologic agents utilized this receptor therapeutically (Fisher et al. 2005) (Table 1).

MALT lymphomas are considered to be low-grade B-cell tumors. They usually arise in the stomach, thyroid, salivary glands, breasts, and bladder. An indolent, localized course is anticipated and they can be treated with localized therapies. In particular, stomach MALT tumors can be associated with a helicobacter infestation and once treated with antibiotics the lymphoma can resolve, as well. Mantle cell lymphomas generally occur in older adults and are typically a systemic presentation, with a median survival of only 3–5 years, regardless of treatment. Likewise T-cell lymphomas, are usually systemic at outset, are more common in Asian heritage with a typical aggressive clinical course. They are potentially

Non-Hodgkins Lymphoma. Table 1

Low grade	Small lymphocytic
	Follicular, small cleaved cell
	Follicular, mixed small cleaved, and large cells
Intermediate grade	Follicular, predominately large cell
	Diffuse, small cleaved cell
	Diffuse, mixed small, and large cell
	Diffuse, large cell
High grade	Large cell immunoblastic
	Lymphoblastic
	Small, non-cleaved cell

curable, but some are entirely resistant to any existing therapy. Skin involvement is also quite common with anaplastic large cell lymphoma that contains the CD30 receptor. The course is generally aggressive. Angiocentric lymphomas, characterized by angiocentric and angioinvasive presentations have been described as lethal midline granuloma, nasal T-cell lymphoma, and lymphomatoid granulomatosis.

Staging

The Ann Arbor staging classification is still widely used:

Stage I
    Involvement of a single lymph node region
Stage II
    Involve of two or more regions on the same side of the diaphragm
    Localized involvement of one extra lymphatic organ and one lymph node region both on the same side of the diaphragm
Stage III
    Involvement of lymph node regions on both sides of the diaphragm (III)
    Associated involvement of the spleen (IIIs) or a extralymphatic site (IIIe) or site or both (IIIes)

Stage IV
    Diffuse or disseminated involvement of one or more organs or tissues with or without lymph node involvement

In the Ann Arbor classification, Waldeyer's ring, thymus, spleen, appendix, and Peyer's patches of the small intestine are considered lymphatic tissue and not stage "e" involvement. Some clinicians consider them as separate entities.

Prognostic Factors

Stage is important but there are many other factors that can influence the outcome of patients with NHL.

Ten-year cause-specific survival for patients with stage I, II, III, and IV follicular cell type are 68%, 56%, 42%, and 18%, respectively (Gospodarowicz et al. 1984).

Five significant good prognosis factors that affect overall survival have been identified:

Age less than 60 years
Normal serum LDH
ECOG performance status 0
Early stage (I and II)
Only one extranodal site

Patients with two or more risk factors, bone marrow, major organ, CNS, or GI tract involvement have about a 50% chance of a 5-year survival. Generally, very elder patients have a worse prognosis.

Female gender has a better prognosis when low-grade lymphoma is diagnosed.

B-symptoms (sweating, pruritis, weight loss), especially when associated with elevated LDH have the risks of bulky tumors and advanced disease.

Tumor presenting as a bulky lesion of greater than 5 cm has a higher local relapse rate.

Tumors greater than 10 cm, larger than one third of the chest diameter, palpable abdominal masses, and/or the combination of pelvic and paraaortic node involvement are poorer prognostic factors for stage III and IV disease (International Non-Hodgkin's Lymphoma Prognostic Factors Project 2003).

The total number of involved sites is an independent prognostic factor for patients treated with multiagent chemotherapy, immunotherapy, and radiotherapy.

Almost 50% of patients with stage I and II disease have extranodal site involvement.

For Asian origin, elevated serum calcium is an adverse factor.

Primary brain lymphomas that produce high CSF protein is an adverse factor.

Overexpression of Ki-67 is an impendent poor prognostic factor.

Treatment Options

General

The primary treatment modalities used to treat NHL are chemotherapy, immunotherapy, radiation therapy, and combination chemoradiotherapy techniques (Habermann et al. 2006).

Also, radiation can be given as radiolabeled immunotherapy (Dillman 2002) (Table 2).

The initial decision for curative patients is between the use of local treatment, systemic treatments, and local plus systemic treatments. The choice must recognize the potential for local control and inherit risks of occult systemic disease, and the availability of curable therapies. Observation with delayed treatment for symptoms is an appropriate choice for low grades, marginal treatment capability, and the very elderly patients.

The role of surgery is usually limited to obtaining tissue for diagnosis or orthopedic stabilization, insertion of vascular access, and CNS shunts.

Planned combined chemotherapy and radiotherapy for advance or bulky disease usually employs the chemotherapy/chemoimmunotherapy first to reduce the tumor size allowing tumor response assessment and smaller radiotherapy fields for consolidation.

Management by Stage

Stage I and Stage II Low Grade

Stage I and II follicular lymphoma patients treated with radiation alone have an excellent survival risk. The overall survival rate at 5 years is 80–100%. There is no clear evidence that extended field treatment offers any survival advantage (Chen et al. 1979).

Low-grade lymphomas are generally more responsive to radiotherapy. Doses of 20–35 Gy over 10–20 fractions have produced control rates approaching 95%.

Most centers will prescribe doses between 30 and 40 Gy, fractionated, for curative intent.

Non-Hodgkins Lymphoma. Table 2

Common modern interventions	Carmustine (BCNU)
	Cyclophosmide
	Cytarabine
	Doxorubicin
	Etoposide
	Fludarabine
	Ibritumomab tiuxetan (Zevalin)
	Melphalan
	Prednisone
	Rituximab (Rituxan)
	Tositumomab/I-131 tositumomab (Bexxar)
	Vincristine

Non-Hodgkins Lymphoma. Table 3
Recommended systemic therapies for low-grade lymphoma

First-line	Chlorambucil
	Cyclophosphamide
	Rituximab
	CHOP +/− Rituximab
	CVP +/− Rituximab
	Fludarabine +/− Rituximab
	FND +/− Rituximab
	Radioimmunotherapy
	CHOP plus Rituximab +/− radioimmunotherapy
Second-line	Rituximab
	Chemoimmunotherapy
	Radioimmunotherapy
	Autologous transplant +/− Rituximab
	Allogenic transplant
Novel interventions	Radioimmunotherapy
	Bortezomib
	Bendamustine
	Lenalidomide (Kahl 2007)

CHOP cyclophosphamide, doxirubicin, vincristine, prednisone
CVP cyclophosphamide, vincristine, prednisone
FND fludarabine, mitoxantrone, dexamethasone

Stage III and IV Low Grade

Stage III low-grade lymphomas have an excellent 5 and 10 year survival with conservative management in asymptomatic patients.

Treatment can also be deferred until symptoms develop but this usually infers more aggressive management at that time. Initially small field radiation can be applied for symptom relief. When symptoms are not imminently threatening

Non-Hodgkins Lymphoma. Table 4 The principles of modern thought about the application of radiotherapy

Stage I and II	III and IV
Low grades, indolent	
Recommended: involved field radiation	Recommended: observe and defer for asymptomatic small bulk disease
Radiation with immunotherapy chemotherapy or both	Other treatment options: Symptomatic or bulky disease: combined chemotherapy with or without immunotherapy
Chemotherapy alone	
Immunotherapy alone	Other treatment options
Combined modality therapy	
Observation and deferred treatment	Asymptomatic or small bulk disease: single agent chemotherapy or wide field radiation
Intermediate and high-grade lymphomas	
Recommended: Doxorubicin based chemotherapy	Recommended: Doxorubicin based chemotherapy
Involved field radiotherapy	Adjuvant or prophylactic radiation to selected high-risk sites
Immunotherapy	Transplantation with chemotherapy or chemoimmunotherapy
Radioimmunotherapy	Craniospinal axis radiation in selected cases
	Immunotherapy, radioimmunotherapy

Non-Hodgkins Lymphoma. Table 5 Primary extranodal lymphomas, general principles

Gastric lymphoma	Most common primary extranodal lymphoma
	Helicobacter pylori is lined to MALT lymphoma
	Clinical trials nearing completion comparing surgery plus chemotherapy versus chemotherapy and radiation
	Surgery alone does not alter overall or relapse-free survival (d'Amore et al. 1994)
Intestinal lymphoma	Surgical resection is standard
	Postoperative chemotherapy should be considered
	Radiation may palliate bulky disease, possibly preoperatively
Oropharynx, salivary, thyroid lymphomas	Combined modality therapy including chemotherapy and involved field radiotherapy produce high rates of local control
	Salivary and thyroid may be part of the MALT lymphoma spectrum
Orbital lymphoma	Symptoms include ptosis, chemosis, epiphora, visual field disruptions
	Retrobulbar lesions can produce proptosis and decreased ocular movements
	Unilateral and bilateral lesions have similar outcomes
	Low-dose radiation with lens sparing techniques is favored
	Typical radiation dose is 20–30 Gy for low to intermediate grades
	Doxirubicin-based chemotherapy followed by up to 35 Gy for higher grades
Breast lymphomas	High-grade breast presentations tend to be bilateral, associated with pregnancy (younger women) and may quickly disseminate to the central nervous system
	Breast preservation is possible in most cases with 40–50 Gy commonly used
	Intermediate and high grade should be treated with multimodality therapy
	CNS prophylaxis should be considered, especially in high grade with bulky or bilateral presentation
Testicular lymphoma	Most common testicular tumor in men over age 60
	25–50% of men over age 50
	Intermediate to high-grade diffuse large cell type is most common. Doxirubicin-based chemotherapy produces about 90% control rates
	The role of radiotherapy is palliative for bulky, painful lesions
	Radiotherapy can also be used initially, treating bilaterally including pelvic and paraaortic nodes
	CNS prophylaxis should be considered

Non-Hodgkins Lymphoma. Table 5 (continued)

Bone lymphoma	Long bones are the most common presentation
	Primary bone presentation should be treated with chemotherapy and reserving whole bone radiotherapy for consolidation
	Combined modality therapies have achieved relapse-free rates of about 70% at 5 years
	The role of immunotherapy is investigational
	MRI is an important tool to evaluate the extent of disease for planning purposes
Primary central nervous system lymphoma	About 60% of patients present with cerebral soft tissue disease
	A smaller subset present with meningeal, cord, or ocular disease
	Radiation fields should include the whole brain plus an extension to C2, inferiorly. Doses are usually between 40 and 50 Gy
	Concurrent chemotherapy does not improve outcome over radiotherapy alone and is not currently routinely recommended (O'Neill et al. 1995)
	HIV-associated CNS lymphoma is associated with poorer prognosis and is resistant to even aggressive chemoradiotherapy
Cutaneous lymphomas	Primary cutaneous lymphomas are divided into three subsets: low grade presenting as mycosis fungoides/Sezary syndrome – 65%, large T-cell lymphomas as pleomorphic, immunoblastic or anaplastic – 10%, and cutaneous B-cell lymphomas – 25% (Chao et al. 2001)
	Both initial radiation therapy, including total body electron therapy and chemotherapy produce a good initial response (Rijlarrsdam and Willemze 1994)
	Rapid extra-cutaneous dissemination is common in T-cell types
	Infection with *Borrelia burgdorferi* is associated with B-cell types
	B-cell type response to chemoimmunotherapy is investigational (Schaefer-Cutillo et al. 2007)

then single agent chemotherapy or upfront radioimmunotherapy can be considered as an alternate to external beam radiation (Kaminski et al. 2005a).

Intensive, multiagent chemotherapy is associated with a high rate of response but also with a continuous risk of relapse and long-term bone marrow suppression.

Although prolonged survival is expected, there are few actual cures (Table 3).

Stage I and II Intermediate Grade

Radiation therapy alone is curative in 40–50% of patients (Horwich et al. 1988).

Extranodal presentations without poor prognostic factors that can complete a combined modality therapy course can have an 80–90% 5-year survival.

When combined therapy is used, patients have an excellent local control with doses between 30 and 35 Gy given at 1.75–3.0 per fraction.

Patients achieving a complete response to CHOP chemotherapy then undergo involved field radiotherapy and have superior local control rates to CHOP alone and a trend for improved overall survival in two major trials; ECOG and SWOG.

For patients without bulky disease, a short course of CHOP chemotherapy followed by involved radiotherapy is a currently acceptable course of action (Miller et al. 1996).

For bulky presentations, long course chemotherapy followed by radiotherapy to bulky residual or unfavorable extranodal sites (bone, extradural, etc.) may be favored.

Radiolabeled immunotherapy (Bexxar, Zevalin) is also an approach to treat bulky residual masses. The reported response rates are excellent (Kaminski et al. 2005b) but these modalities require specialized equipment and training and are not often widely available.

Stage III and IV Intermediate and High Grade

In advanced stage disease, chemotherapy is generally the mainstay of treatment. CHOP and/or CHOP with immunotherapy for CD20 positive tumors is considered standard (Zelenetz et al. 2002). More aggressive drug combinations have not proven to be more beneficial; however, bone marrow transplantation may achieve a response (Friedberg et al. 1999).

Radiation can be applied to symptomatic areas, mostly for palliative intent.

Stage III and IV NHL Overall

The role of radiotherapy in advanced stage aggressive NHL presentations is poorly defined and mostly palliative.

The presence of residual mass at a bulky site does not always represent active disease. PET follow-up scans have been helpful to define activity to guide radiation (Tables 4, 5).

Cross-References

► Hodgkin's Lymphoma
► Leukemia in General
► Multiple Myeloma
► Sarcomas of the Head and Neck

References

Armitage RO, Weisenberger DD (1998) Non-Hodgkin's lymphoma classification project. J Clin Oncol 16:2780–2795

Chao KS, Perez CA, Brady LW (2001) Non-Hodgkin's lymphoma. In: Chao KS, Perez CA, Brady LW (eds) Radiation oncology management decisions, 2nd edn. Lippincott Williams & Wilkins, Philadelphia/London, pp 589–599

Chen MG et al (1979) Results of radiotherapy in control of Stage I and II non-Hodgkin's lymphoma. Cancer 43:1245–1254

Cheson BD (2001) Some like it hot! J Clin Oncol 19:3908–3911

Cheson BD (2003) Radioimmunotherapy of non-Hodgkin lymphoma. Blood 101:391–398

d'Amore F et al (1994) Non-Hodgkin's lymphoma of the gastrointestinal tract: a population based analysis of incidence, geographical distribution, clinical pathological presentation features and prognosis. J Clin Oncol 12:1673–1684

Dillman RO (2002) Radiolabeled anti-CD20 monoclonal antibodies for the treatment of B-cell lymphomas. J Clin Oncol 20:3545–3557

Fisher RI et al (2005) New treatment options have changed the survival of patients with follicular lymphoma. J Clin Oncol 23:8447–8452

Friedberg JW et al (1999) Autologous bone marrow transplantation after histologic transformation of indolent B-cell malignancies. Biol Blood Marrow Transplant 5:262–268

Gospodarowicz MK, Wasserman TH (1998) Non-Hodgkin's lymphoma. In: Perez CA et al (eds) Principle and practice of radiation oncology, 3rd edn. Lippincott Williams & Wilkins, Philadelphia, pp 1987–2011

Gospodarowicz MK, Bush RS, Brown TC et al (1984) Prognostic factors in nodular lymphomas. Int J Radiat Oncol Biol Phys 10:489–497

Habermann TM, Weller EA et al (2006) Rituximab-CHOP versus CHOP alone or with maintenance Rituximab in older patients with diffuse large B-cell lymphoma. J Clin Oncol 24:3121–3127

Horwich A et al (1988) The management of early stage aggressive non-Hodgkin's lymphoma. Hematol Oncol 6:291–298

International Non-Hodgkin's Lymphoma Prognostic Factors Project (2003) N Engl J Med 329:987–994

Kahl B (2007) Current standards and future directions in treatment of follicular lymphoma. Community Oncol 4:5–10

Kaminski MS et al (2005a) I-131 tositumomab therapy as initial treatment for follicular lymphomas. N Engl J Med 352:441–449

Kaminski MS et al (2005b) Re-treatment with I-131 tositumomab in patients with non-Hodgkin's lymphoma who had previously responded to I-131 tositumomab. J Clin Oncol 23:7985–7993

Miller TP et al (1996) Three cycles of CHOP plus radiotherapy is superior to eight cycles of CHOP alone for localized intermediate and high-grade non-Hodgkin's lymphoma: a Southwest Oncology Group Study. Proc Am Soc Clin Oncol 15:401a

O'Neill LB et al (1995) Primary nervous system non-Hodgkin's lymphoma: survival advantages with combined initial therapy? Int J Radiat Oncol Biol Phys 33:663–673

Rijlarrsdam JU, Willemze R (1994) Primary cutaneous B-cell lymphomas. Leuk Lymphoma 14:213–218

Schaefer-Cutillo J et al (2007) Novel concepts in radioimmunotherapy for non-Hodgkin's lymphoma. Oncology 21:203–212

Zelenetz AD et al (2002) Patients with transformed low grade lymphoma attain durable responses following outpatient radioimmunotherapy with tositumomab and I-131 tositumomab. Blood 100:357a

Noninvasive Breast Cancer

▶ Cancer of the Breast Tis

Nonmalignant Disease

▶ Radiotherapy of Nonmalignant Diseases

Nonmelanoma Skin Cancer

▶ Skin Cancer

Non-targeted Effects of Ionizing Radiation

SUSAN M. VARNUM, MARIANNE B. SOWA,
WILLIAM F. MORGAN
Biological Sciences Division, Fundamental & Computational Sciences, Directorate Pacific Northwest National Laboratory, Richland, WA, USA

Definition

An all embracing concept that describes responses in nonirradiated cells (hence the term non-targeted) after receiving signals from an irradiated cell (i.e., a targeted cell). These non-targeted effects include, but are not limited to, bystander effects and radiation-induced genomic instability.

Cross-References

▶ Radiation-Induced Genomic Instability and Radiation Sensitivity

Nontraditional Medicine

JAMES H. BRASHEARS, III
Radiation Oncologist, Venice, FL, USA

Synonyms

Alternative medicine; Nonconventional medicine

Definition

Also alternative, complementary, nonconventional, or complementary and alternative medicine (CAM). The knowledge, research, and practice of medicine other than that typically taught in Western medical schools, not based on the natural sciences or not consistently shown effectual in randomized, controlled trials typically used to evaluate biomedicine. CAM comprises a broad range of diagnostic and therapeutic techniques including acupuncture, aromatherapy, herbalism, biofeedback, homeopathy, meditation, yoga, Ayurveda, and chiropractry. Some draw a difference between complementary medicine, which is used in conjunction with biomedicine and alternative (or nontraditional) medicine that is used in place of biomedicine.

Cross-References
▶ Pain Management

Normal Tissue Complication Probability (NTCP)

DAREK MICHALSKI[1], M. SAIFUL HUQ[2],
BRIAN F. HASSON[3,4]
[1]Division of Medical Physics, Department of Radiation Oncology, University of Pittsburgh Cancer Centers, Pittsburgh, PA, USA
[2]Department of Radiation Oncology, University of Pittsburgh Medical Center Cancer Pavilion, Pittsburgh, PA, USA
[3]Department of Radiation Oncology, Abington Memorial Hospital, Abington, PA, USA
[4]Department of Radiation Oncology, College of Medicine, Drexel University, Philadelphia, PA, USA

Definition
The probability that a given dose of radiation will cause an organ or structure to experience complications considering the specific biological cells of the organ or structure. The NTCP is used in treatment planning as a tool to differentiate among treatment plans.

A dose-dependent mathematical model to gauge the probability of dose-induced complications in noncancerous tissue.

Cross-References
▶ Four-Dimensional (4D) Treatment Planning/Respiratory Gating
▶ Stereotactic Radiosurgery – Cranial

Nuclear Energy Accidents

▶ Short-Term and Long-Term Health Risk of Nuclear Power Plant Accident

Nuclear Medicine

THEODORE E. YAEGER[1], LUTHER W. BRADY[2],
CHERIE YAEGER[1]
[1]Department Radiation Oncology, Wake Forest University School of Medicine, Winston-Salem, NC, USA
[2]Department of Radiation Oncology, College of Medicine, Drexel University, Philadelphia, PA, USA

Definition
A medical specialty involving the use of radioactive substances for the diagnosis and treatment of diseases based on cellular function and physiology. It utilizes radiation emitting from the body for diagnosis or calculated therapeutic radiation delivered internally to targeted organs.

The first radionuclide to gain clinical application was radium produced by the Curies in December of 1898. It was rapidly recognized that this radionuclide had major significant biologic effects not only in normal tissues but also in tumor tissues. It was introduced into clinical practice in the form of needles or capsules. Data accumulated rapidly that this radionuclide had a significant and important role in the treatment of patients with cancer.

However, from a nuclear medicine point of view, it was not until radioactive iodine was produced by a technique of neutron bombardment of stable iodine that the field of nuclear medicine was born in the mid 1930s.

In 1934, Hertz et al. produced iodine-131 demonstrating that the thyroid gland had an affinity for the radioactive iodine. This set the stage for the development of various technologies to assess the physiologic characteristics of the thyroid and its function (Table 1). It was also in the mid 1930s that Erf et al. at the University of California, Berkeley, produced the phosphorus radionuclide (radioactive P-32) to assess hematologic dynamics.

In the late 1930s, early 1940s, Hamilton et al. studied radioactive iodine in the evaluation of the human thyroid gland. Iodine-131 was produced by the cyclotron at the University of California, Berkeley. It was possible to measure the uptake of radioactive iodine in excised specimens of human thyroid glands after tracer doses were given preoperatively. Subsequently, they demonstrated that the distribution of the radioactive iodine-131 could be measured in the thyroid gland by external detectors in humans.

In 1942, a group from Columbia University demonstrated the first case of metastatic thyroid carcinoma to show uptake with radioactive iodine. The utilization of this radionuclide in the treatment of hyperthyroidism was demonstrated about the same time. In May 1943, the group at Columbia also demonstrated uptake in metastatic lesions from the thyroid gland. Subsequently, Cidlin et al. demonstrated that metastatic carcinoma of the thyroid could be successfully treated with radioactive iodine when the lesions concentrated the radionuclide.

The evolution of events subsequent to these demonstrations confirmed the utilization of this radionuclide as an active treatment technology for hyperthyroidism as well as functioning carcinoma of the thyroid. This technology now

Nuclear Medicine. Table 1 Radiopharmaceutical affinity for various tumors

Gallium-67 Citrate
Hodgkin's disease
Non-Hodgkin's lymphoma (especially high grade)
Hepatoma
Bronchogenic carcinoma
Melanoma
Seminoma
Rhabdomyosarcoma
Thallium-201 Chloride
Gliomas (high-grade)
Thyroid carcinoma
Benign tumors (usually fade over 2 h)
Osteosarcoma
Lymphoma (especially low grade)
Kaposi's sarcoma (gallium-negative)
Technetium-99^m Sestamibi
Cancer metastases
Breast cancer
Parathyroid adenomas
Gliomas
Lymphoma
Thyroid
Indium-111 Pentertreotide
APUD cell tumors
Pancreatic islet cell
Pituitary adenoma
Pheochromocytoma
Neuroblastoma
Paragangliomas
Carcinoid
Gastrinoma
Medullary carcinoma of thyroid
Small-cell lung cancer

Nuclear Medicine. Table 1 (continued)

Indium-111 Pentertreotide
Meningioma
Fluorine-18 Fluorodeoxyglucose
Most tumors
Head and neck cancer
Esophageal cancer
Non-small-cell lung cancer
Melanoma
Lymphoma
Colorectal cancer
Breast cancer
Iodine-123 or 131 Soduim iodide
Thyroid cancer
Iodine-123 or 131 Metaiodobenzylguanidine
Pheochromocytoma
Neuroblastoma
Paraganglioma
Monoclonal antibodies
Lymphoma

represents the standard in the management of patients with both hyperthyroidism and primary and secondary malignant tumors of the thyroid gland that are demonstrated to localize the material.

Radioactive iodine is the central focus in more than 98% of the workup of patients in diagnosis of thyroid disease.

Today, thyroid studies constitute a significant portion of the activity in the field of nuclear medicine. The original emphasis on the utilization of iodine-131 has now been replaced by the 24 h thyroid uptake test using iodine-123. Concomitant with this early development of the clinical applications of the radioisotopes of iodine as well as P-32 there was significant improvement in the technology of nuclear detection and quantification equipment.

Initially, the equipment was developed to do hand counting with plots that involved the drawing of small circles for less activity and larger circles for more activity. Even though this was very primitive, it allowed for adequate and appropriate evolution of technologies for dose counting. In the 1950s came the rapid development of not only single probes for assessment of thyroid function but also the development of rectilinear scanners. This subsequently lead to the emergence of more sophisticated equipment including gamma cameras with improved sensitivity for better detection capabilities, better collimators for improved precision and localization, and more rapid turnaround in studies being done allowing more access for patients.

In the contemporary laboratory, the emphasis now is on the high technology with regards to external counting techniques for diagnostic purposes with very sophisticated cameras for total body or more limited body imaging technology.

Along with the development in the techniques for radionuclide detection was a major emphasis on the development of radionuclides for imaging purposes. The major emphasis at the moment is on technetium-99 generators but also others which can be used for multiple radionuclide studies. The emphasis is also on the utilization of iodine-123 for a short assay of thyroid function and iodine-131 for therapeutic purposes for hyperthyroidism and treatment of patients with cancer of the thyroid. Xenon-133 has been used actively in the evaluation of pulmonary function and with technetium DPTA significant ability to diagnose early pulmonary emboli.

From a therapeutic point of view, radionuclides have been actively explored for therapeutic purposes.

Early on, radioactive gold-198 was used for the control of malignant pleural effusions and malignant peritoneal effusions now replaced by the utilization of colloidal chromic phosphate P-32. In spite of the efficacy of these technologies in the treatment of malignant effusions, they are not used very actively in clinical practice.

Iodine-131 has been actively utilized and reported for the utilization of hyperthyroidism within the context of proper dose administration, the side effect of hypothyroidism can be avoided. The assessment of the patient with thyroid cancer often indicates that the tumor is functioning not only in the primary site but also in secondary sites, and radioactive iodine-131 is useful in the management of those patients with primary local disease as well as disseminated disease.

Bone scanning has emerged to be a significant and important diagnostic tool in the assessment of patients with malignant disease. It is regularly used in the assessment of patients for the potential of early diagnosis of metastatic bone disease. The bone scanning agent is labeled as technetium. However, samarium-153 and strontium-89 have been used in the therapeutic management of patients with metastatic disease to the bone. More recently, from a therapeutic point of view, Bexxar (Tositumomab) labeled with iodine-131 and zevalin (Ibritumomab tiuxetan) labeled with yttrium-90 or indium-111 have been used in the treatment of patients with B-cell non-Hodgkin's lymphomas with very successful results. Around 2005, the Food and Drug Administration approved yttrium-90 delivered transarterially for liver-directed primary cancer and metastases. Yttrium-90 is impregnated within glass or resin microspheres and become point sources that deliver focused areas of radiation in peritumoral and intratumoral perivasculature. This unique capability makes it suitable to selectively deliver very high radiation doses to liver tumors while radiation exposure to normal hepatic parenchyma remains within tolerable limits. There are two absolute contraindications to sphere therapy: exaggerated hepatopulmonary shunting and arterial reflux into the gastroduodenal regions.

Relative contraindications are portal venous thrombosis and baseline decreased hepatocellular reserve. Another use for indium-111 is attaching it to a somatostatin analogue, commonly called an Octreotide scan, which is useful in the diagnosis and follow-up to therapy of true carcinoid tumors, other similar tumors, and sarcoidosis.

With the development of monoclonal antibodies, the research work done by Kohler and Milstein indicated that a human tumor cell could be wedded to a mouse leukemic cell. Then, as long as that hybrid cell was transmitted from one immunologic deficient mouse to another, antibodies against that tumor cell would be produced. This was explored extensively by the group at Wistar Institute, and a wide variety of monoclonal antibodies have been produced. Presently, the most commonly *applied* antibodies (assembled utilizing theuropic cloning procedures) are the colon receptor 17-1A and the anti-epidermal growth factor receptor, monoclonal antibody CA-425. The latter has found receptors in high-grade glioma of the brain, breast, head and neck malignancies, etc. Ongoing research is very fertile in this area with a myriad of active antibodies being regularly discovered. It is leading to a new branch of cancer therapy.

For a specific example, CA-425 has been explored extensively in the treatment of patients with primary brain tumors. Very early it was found that the antibody therapy was weak as a sole therapeutic agent but it could be enhanced in its activity with leukophoresis and cellular incubation with the antibody. It would then be given to the patient or labeled with iodine-125 as the intended therapeutic agent, then given to the patient with the various human tumor types as above.

In essence, the efficacy of radionuclides in the treatment of human cancer has been, and still is being, explored. It has proven to extensively support therapeutic interventions not only in the above-mentioned tumors but also in many types of cancers and tumor cell lines/types.

The field of nuclear medicine now is a broad array of practical and potential applications from a diagnostic as well as therapeutic point of view. The advent of new scanning devices, the utilization of computers, the discovery of cell receptors, and the analysis of the genetic code have considerably expanded the potential primary nuclear-based assessment and treatment of the patient with malignancy.

Cross-References
▶ Carcinoma of the Adrenal Gland
▶ Colon Cancer
▶ Hodgkin's Lymphoma
▶ Imaging in Oncology
▶ Liver and Hepatobiliary Tract
▶ Lung
▶ Non-Hodgkins Lymphoma
▶ Palliation of Bone Metastases
▶ Palliation of Metastatic Disease to the Liver
▶ Primary Intracranial Neoplasms
▶ Thyroid Cancer

References
Freeman LM, Blaufox MD (eds) (1979) Seminars in nuclear medicine, vol IX, no 3. Grune & Stratton, New York
Freeman LM, Blaufox MD (eds) (2010) Seminars in nuclear medicine, vol 40, no 2. Elsevier New York
Mettler FA, Guiberteau MJ (eds) (2006) Essentials of nuclear medicine imaging, 5th edn. Saunders Elsevier, Philadelphia

Nuclear Reactor Cores

JOHN P. CHRISTODOULEAS
The Perelman Cancer Center, Department of Radiation Oncology, University of Pennsylvania Hospital, Philadelphia, PA, USA

Definition
Nuclear reactor cores are the part of the power plant that contain the radioactive fuel and materials to control the fission of the fuel.

Cross-References
▶ Short-Term and Long-Term Health Risk of Nuclear Power Plant Accident

Null Hypothesis

EDWARD J. GRACELY
Department of Epidemiology and Biostatistics, College of Medicine, Drexel University, Philadelphia, PA, USA

Definition
The statistical hypothesis that serves as the starting point for data analysis and usually asserts the absence of an effect or a difference.

Cross-References
▶ Statistics and Clinical Trials

O

OER

George E. Laramore, Jay J. Liao, Jason K. Rockhill
Department of Radiation Oncology,
University of Washington Medical Center,
Seattle, WA, USA

Definition
A ratio of the physical radiation doses required to produce a given endpoint such as the percentage of cell killing between hypoxic conditions and normoxic conditions. This is LET-dependent and for low LET radiation is in the range of 2.5–3.0 compared with 1.5–2.0 for fast neutrons.

Cross-References
▶ Neutron Radiotherapy

Oligoastrocytoma

▶ Primary Intracranial Neoplasms

Oligodendroglioma

▶ Primary Intracranial Neoplasms

Oligodendrogliomas

▶ Spinal Canal Tumor

Omentum

Filip T. Troicki[1], Jaganmohan Poli[2]
[1]College of Medicine, Drexel University,
Philadelphia, PA, USA
[2]Department of Radiation Oncology,
College of Medicine, Drexel University,
Philadelphia, PA, USA

Definition
Large layer of fatty tissue connected to the stomach and the intestines.

Cross-References
▶ Colon Cancer
▶ Ovarian Cancer
▶ Stomach Cancer

Oncogene

▶ Proto-oncogene

Oncotype DX

▶ Microarray Analysis

L.W. Brady, T.E. Yaeger (eds.), *Encyclopedia of Radiation Oncology*, DOI 10.1007/978-3-540-85516-3,
© Springer-Verlag Berlin Heidelberg 2013

Oophorectomy

CHRISTIN A. KNOWLTON[1], MICHELLE KOLTON MACKAY[2]
[1]Department of Radiation Oncology, Drexel University, Philadelphia, PA, USA
[2]Department of Radiation Oncology, Marshfield Clinic, Marshfield, WI, USA

Definition
The surgical removal of an ovary or ovaries. This procedure can be done alone but is most frequently performed with a hysterectomy and salpingectomy in cases of ovarian cancer. Because the ovaries produce the majority of the body's hormones including estrogen, removal of the ovaries is linked to development of menopausal signs and symptoms such as hot flashes, vaginal dryness, depression, heart disease, osteoporosis, and decreased libido.

Cross-References
▶ Ovary

Opportunistic Infections

HEDVIG HRICAK[1], OGUZ AKIN[2], HEBERT ALBERTO VARGAS[2]
[1]Department of Radiology, Memorial Sloan-Kettering Cancer Center, New York, NY, USA
[2]Body MRI, Memorial Sloan-Kettering Cancer Center, New York, NY, USA

Definition
Infections caused by pathogens (bacterial, viral, fungal, or protozoan) that usually do not cause disease in a healthy host, that is, one with a healthy immune system. A compromised immune system, however, presents an "opportunity" for the pathogen to infect.

Cross-References
▶ AIDS
▶ Chemotherapy
▶ Human Immunodeficiency Virus (HIV)
▶ Imaging in Oncology

Orchiectomy

JOHANNES CLASSEN
Department of Radiation Oncology, St. Vincentius-Kliniken Karlsruhe, Karlsruhe, Germany

Definition
Surgical removal of the testis.

Cross-References
▶ Prostate
▶ Testes

ORN

THEODORE E. YAEGER
Department Radiation Oncology, Wake Forest University School of Medicine, Winston-Salem, NC, USA

Definition
Bone necrosis resulting from exposure to high dose radiation.

Cross-References
▶ Osteoradionecrosis (also ORN or Osteonecrosis)
▶ Sarcoma
▶ Sarcomas of the Head and Neck

Oro-Hypopharynx

VOLKER BUDACH, CARMEN STROMBERGER
Department of Radiotherapy and Radiation
Oncology, Charité - University Hospital Berlin,
Berlin, Germany

Description

Nonsurgical treatment of oro-hypopharyngeal and oral cavity cancer is stage dependent. Early stage tumors (T1/2 N0/1) can be cured by either surgery or radiotherapy depending on age, performance status, comorbidities, and choice of the patient. Combined modality treatment based on surgery followed by adjuvant radiotherapy is generally required for T2/3 N0/1 tumors. For locally advanced disease (T3/4 and T4b, N2/3), R0/1 tumor resections without mutilation and substantial functional loss might only be achieved in individual cases. For locally advanced and/or unresectable tumors definitive concurrent chemoradiation (CRTX) is the treatment of choice. Alternatively, ▶ induction chemotherapy (ICT) using TPF (taxane, cis-platinum, 5-flurouracil) followed by chemo- or bio-radiation using monoclonal antibodies (e.g., cetuximab) or hyperfractionated radiation therapy alone can also be considered. Palliative chemo- or cetuximab therapy is indicated for primarily disseminated disease or pre-irradiated locoregional tumor recurrences. During the last decade, considerable advances have been made in surgery, radiation therapy, drug therapy, and molecular targets development leading to an improved therapeutic outcome.

Etiology and Epidemiology

Tumors of the head and neck region represent 6% of the worldwide cancer incidence and about a third of these tumors are diagnosed at the pharynx and oral cavity. Carcinoma of the palatine tonsil and the tonsillar pillars has an incidence of 0.5:100,000, base of tongue tumors occur in 2:100,000 with a male predominance of 3:1. The overall survival rate at 5 years for oropharyngeal tumors is about 55% and 41% at 10 years. For hypopharyngeal tumors the male predominance is 5:1 and represents approximately 7% of all cancers of the upper aerodigestive tract. All pharyngeal subsites accounted for approximately 124,000 cancer cases worldwide in 2002. At diagnosis 25% of hypopharyngeal tumors are almost incurable (low performance score, T4b, N3, M1). Second primary tumors in the lung and upper aerodigestive tract occur in 25% of patients. Ninety to ninety-five percent of the tumors are of squamous cell carcinoma (SCC) origin, less common tumors include the salivary glands respectively adenoid cystic, mucoepidermoid, and adenocarcinoma histologies.

The etiology appears to be multifactorial in origin and includes consumption of tobacco, alcohol, chewing of betal nuts, and HPV-infection (serotype 16, 18). For the development of an oral cavity tumor, poor oral hygiene seems to be an additional risk factor. A latent tumor infection by the ▶ human papilloma viruses (HPV) is associated with a better prognosis than nonviral-associated SCC. The highest prevalence of HPV infection has been observed in oropharynx tumors, especially tonsillar tumors, with 21–100%, whereas oral cavity tumors are weakly associated with HPV infection. Sexual practices such as oral sex is thought to be a major source for the transmission of a HPV infection. Oral leukoplakia can progress into an invasive tumor in 10–17% of patients. Tumors of the soft palate and anterior tonsillar pillars are more likely to be differentiated and less aggressive while tumors of the base of tongue have a high potential for lymphogenic spread. Most frequently, distant metastases occur in the lungs (>50%), bones (20%), and liver (6%).

Anatomy

The oropharynx connects the nasopharynx with the oral cavity and the hypopharynx. Oropharyngeal subsites are the soft palate, the tonsils, the tonsillar pillars, the lateral and posterior pharyngeal wall, the base of tongue, and the valleculae. The N. glossopharyngeus (IX), N. vagus (X), N. hypoglossus (XII), and the second and third branch of the N. trigeminus (V) innervate the oropharynx. The lymph node drainage from the oropharynx extends from levels IB-V including the retropharyngeal lymph nodes.

The hypopharynx is the part of the pharynx from the pharyngoepiglottic fold to the caudal border of the cricoid and the esophageal entrance. Hypopharyngeal subsites are the posterior and lateral pharyngeal wall, the pyriform sinuses, and the postcricoid area. The plexus pharyngeus (pharyngeal branch of the N. glossopharyngeus, branches of the N. vagus, and sympathetic fibers of the superior cervical ganglion) and the cranial part of N. accessorius (XI) and N. vagus (X) innervate the hypopharynx. The lymph node drainage from the hypopharynx extends from levels II–V, the retropharyngeal lymph nodes and the para-tracheal and paraesophageal lymph nodes (invasion of the lowest part of the hypopharynx and the postcricoid region).

Different anatomical sites are defined as parts of the oral cavity: the lips, the gingivo-buccal sulcus, the buccal mucosa, the gingiva with the alveolar ridge, the retromolar trigone, the floor of mouth, the hard palate, and the anterior two thirds of the tongue. Motor innervation of the tongue is provided by the N. hypoglossus (XII), the sensory innervation by a branch of the N. lingualis (V). The taste for the anterior two third of the tongue is mediated by the N. facialis (VII; chorda tympany branch) and for the posterior part of tongue by the N. glossopharyngeus (IX). The muscles of the floor of mouth are innervated by C1. The sensory innervation for the tooth, the gingiva, and oral mucosa is mediated by the second and third branch of the N. trigeminus (V). The lymph node drainage extends from level IA–VI, and for the upper lip to the periauricular and peri-parotid nodes and level IB.

Clinical Presentation

Most common oro-hypopharyngeal tumors present with a sore throat, otalgia (N. tympani IX. via Ganglion petrosi), a dysphagia, a hot potato voice (base of tongue invasion), odynophagia, hoarseness (larynx invasion), trismus (invasion of masseter muscle and pterygoideus muscle), large cervical tumor, with or without a weight loss. Additional symptoms for tumors of the oral cavity might be bleeding out of the oral cavity (ulcerated tumor growth), deviation of the tongue, and an increase of saliva.

Diagnostics

- Medical history
- Physical examination including tumor consistence and mobility, and cervical lymph nodes
- Inspection (symmetry of the head, mouth opening, dental status, movement of the tongue and tonsillar pillars, color and surface appearance of the tumor, ulceration or bulky growth of the mucosa)
- Indirect mirror examination, flexible endoscopy
- Panendoscopy with biopsy
- Contrast media-enhanced CT or MRI of the head and neck region
- Ultrasound of the abdomen
- CT or X-ray of the chest
- Optional: PET-CT scan
- Panorex if indicated
- Preventive dental care with potential tooth extraction at least 10 days prior to the start of radiotherapy
- Speech and swallowing evaluation
- HPV status

Differential Diagnosis

Ninety to ninety-five percent of the tumors are SCC, others histologic types are rare and include adenocarcinoma, mucoepidermoid, adenoid cystic, small cell carcinoma, non-Hodgkin lymphomas, melanoma, and sarcomas.

Therapy

Surgery and radiotherapy with or without chemotherapy are the main treatment options for a potential cure. Based on multiple phase-III clinical trials ▶ concurrent chemoradiation has evolved to be the most important worldwide treatment standard for locally advanced SCC (LA SCC) of the oro-hypopharynx and oral cavity (Pignon et al. 2007). Neoadjuvant chemotherapy (ICT) with a triplet (cis-platinum, 5-fluorouracil and docetaxel; TPF) has been investigated in the last years and turned out to be superior when compared to a doublet with cis-platinum and 5-fluorouracil paralleled by a loss of compliance for subsequent radiotherapy (Vermorken et al. 2007; Posner et al. 2007). Adjuvant chemoradiation is indicated for high-risk situations characterized by an extracapsular node extension (ECE) and/or microscopically involved surgical margins (Bernier et al. 2005). Chemotherapy alone is used for palliative treatment only. All treatment options have to be presented and discussed at an interdisciplinary tumor board.

Surgery

Early stage tumors of the oro-hypopharynx and oral cavity carrying a minor risk of local recurrence or lymphatic spread can be resected and cured by surgery. For tumors of the floor of mouth surgery is the preferred treatment modality over radiotherapy if the tumor reaches the mandibular bone or invades the gingiva.

T3/4 primaries of the tonsils require radical tonsillectomy often with partial mandibulectomy. For base of tongue lesions partial or total glossectomy and myocutaneous flap reconstruction is often needed. Resection margins of 2 cm should be acquired for hypopharyngeal tumors. T2 tumors of the posterior pharyngeal wall need a partial pharyngectomy. The classical surgical approach for these tumors requires partial pharyngectomy combined with total laryngectomy (T2-3) or total pharyngolaryngectomy with myocutaneous flap reconstruction (up to T4a). Resection of the tongue is stage dependent ranging from laser resections to hemi- or even total glossectomy.

Radical neck dissections remove nodal levels I–V, the sternocleidomastoid muscle, the omohyoid muscle, the internal and external jugular veins, the N. accessorius (XI), and the submandibular glands. Modified neck dissection leaves one or more of the following structures: the sternocleidomastoid muscle, the internal jugular vein, or the XI nerve. Selective neck dissection does not resect complete lymph node levels from I–V. Supraomohyoid or lateral neck dissections remove levels I–III and II–IV, respectively.

Salvage surgery supplements chemoradiation for selected cases of persistent bulky or residual lymph nodes and low-volume local or regional relapse. It should be carried out >12 weeks following chemoradiation.

Radiotherapy

Early stage tumors can be cured by radiotherapy (TD 66–70 Gy). Small T1/2 N0 tumors of the oropharynx and oral cavity can be treated with interstitial high-dose rate brachytherapy using Ir-192. Adjuvant radiotherapy alone is indicated for node levels carrying an intermediate risk of failure such as multiple or large positive lymph nodes (≥N2a) and ≥T3 at diagnosis (dose prescription: TD 50–60 Gy). Treatment planning in this case should be based on preoperative imaging, e.g., MRI, CT, or PET-CT. Adjuvant chemoradiation with cis-platinum ± 5-fluorouracil is indicated for node levels carrying a high risk of extracapsular spread (ECE) and/or microscopically involved surgical margins (R1, dose prescription: TD 64–66 Gy). The gold standard for the curative treatment of locally advanced tumors of the oro-hypopharynx and oral cavity is concurrent chemoradiation with cis-platinum or mitomycin C ± 5-fluorouracil containing chemotherapy in conventional fractions (SD: 1.8–2 Gy, TD 70–72 Gy) or accelerated hyperfractionation (dose prescription: TD 72 Gy). The floor of mouth has a lower radiation tolerance due to an increased risk of mandibular osteoradionecrosis and potential soft tissue injury. Split course radiotherapeutic schemes showed unfavorable results due to intermittent tumor cell repopulation. Modern radiotherapy is based on the acquisition of a volumetric data set derived from a CT scanning in each individual patient. These data are used to generate 3D ▶ conformal therapy or ▶ Intensity Modulated Radio-Therapy (IMRT) treatment plans. The ▶ dose calculation algorithms used for the customized planning systems are based on either the "pencil beam" or the "Monte Carlo" algorithms. For quality assurance purposes most departments use an individual case verification of the dose distributions of the treatment plans (preferred method for dynamic irradiation procedures like the "sliding window," "dynamic IMRT," or "Rapid Arc or VMAT" therapies) whereas others also use a machine-based general dose verification of the linacs each morning prior to treatment of the patients. External beam radiotherapy for head and neck tumors is delivered by linear accelerators. Precise delivery of radiotherapy in daily routine is extremely important as a prerequisite for generating adequate outcomes in terms of tumor control and can be provided by means of image guidance (IGRT) procedures. These rely nowadays besides the "portal beam" kilovoltage imaging also on megavoltage "cone beam" imaging. Moreover, for moving targets, e.g., in the lung, liver, and abdomen, different methods of a 3D focussing of the respective targets during the fractionation period are available like the "breath hold technique," "Gating," (formally: 4D treatment planning/respiratory gating) and "Tracking" supplemented by manual, semiautomatic, or automatic correction algorithms. In most of these cases for dynamic image guidance, high-density metal fiducials (generally gold markers) have to be inserted into the respective tumors for matching the planning CT images with the actual patients' position during irradiation. With IMRT a complex tumor of the oro-hypopharynx (Fig. 1) or of the oral cavity and the cervical lymph node levels can be irradiated while organs at risk like salivary glands, spinal cord, etc. can be spared and side effects such as ▶ xerostomia can be substantially reduced to improve the quality of life in those patients. In addition, IMRT offers the opportunity for the delivery of a ▶ simultaneous integrated boost (SIB). This facilitates various risk levels in the target to receive different dose levels within a single fraction. IMRT delivered via dynamic arcs (Rapid arc, VMAT) can reduce treatment time and monitor units. IGRT can be carried out on a daily basis by using integrated megavolt (MV) CT scanners from the ▶ IGRT tomotherapy or kilovolt (kV, cone beam) CT scanners from linear accelerators (Figs. 2 and 3).

Chemotherapy

Cis-platinum, ±5-fluorouracil, carbo-platinum, or mitomycin C ± 5-fluorouracil are the most common drugs used for chemoradiation. ICT uses platinum-based agents, 5-fluorouracil, and docetaxel with subsequent radiotherapy or chemoradiation.

First-line palliative chemotherapy for recurrent or metastatic squamous-cell carcinoma of the head and neck is carried out with platinum-based agents, 5-fluorouracil, and cetuximab (Vermorken et al. 2008).

Targeted Therapies

The monoclonal antibody cetuximab blocks the extracellular domain of the epidermal growth factor receptor and thus tyrosine kinase activation and tumor cell proliferation. For patients with LA head and neck tumors, concurrent

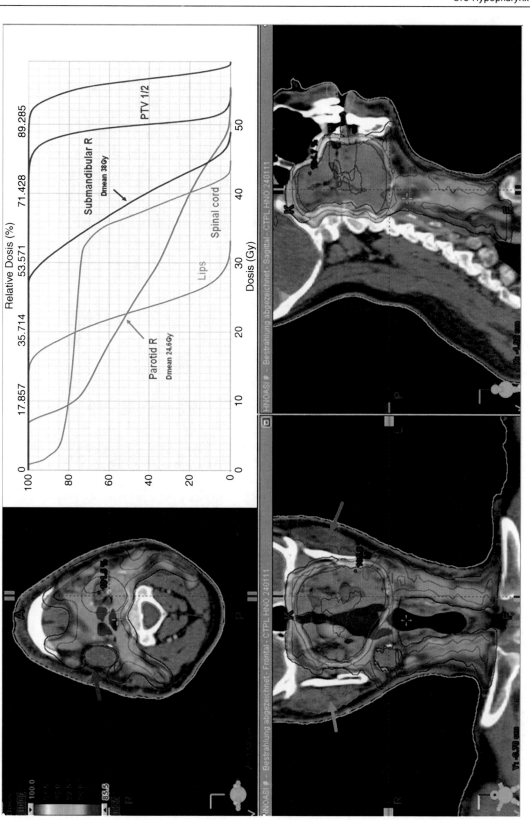

Oro-Hypopharynx. Fig. 1 Example for dose distribution and DVH for a patient with a SCC of the left tonsil; pT3, pN0 (0/18), M0, R0; postoperative radiotherapy with SIB (IMRT); dose prescription: SD 2/2.24 Gy to a TD of 50/56 Gy with sparing of the right submandibular gland and right parotid gland

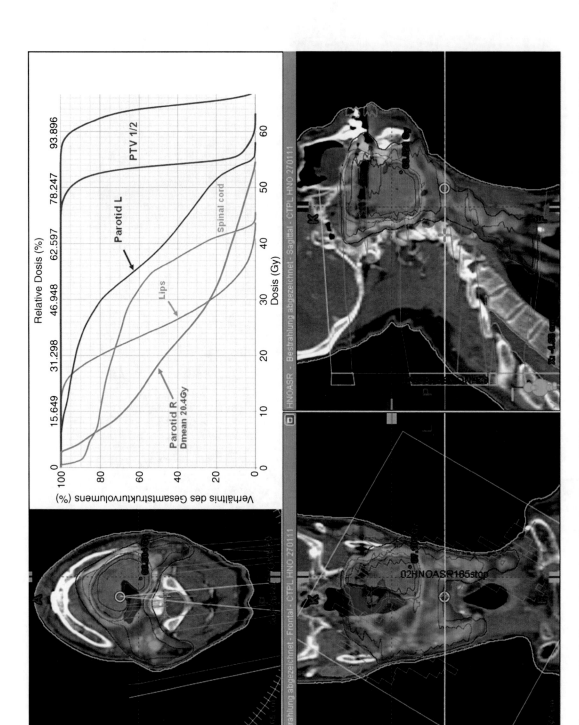

Oro-Hypopharynx. Fig. 2 Example for dose distribution and DVH for a patient with a SCC left base of tongue; pT2, pN0 (0/9), M0, R1; postoperative chemoradiation with SIB (RapidArc® technique); dose prescription: SD 2/2.13 Gy to a TD of 54/63 Gy with sparing of the right parotid gland

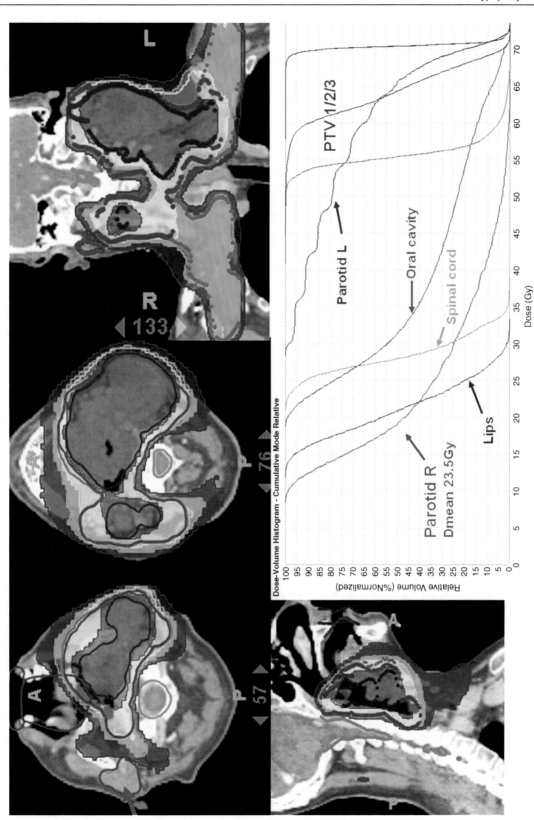

Oro-Hypopharynx. Fig. 3 Example for dose distribution and DVH for a patient with a SCC of the left tonsil; cT3, cN3, M0; definitive chemoradiation with SIB (TomoTherapy®); dose prescription: SD 1.7/1.9/2.2 Gy to a TD of 54.4/60.8/70.4 Gy with sparing of the right parotid gland

Oro-Hypopharynx. Table 1 UICC, TNM staging system (7th Edition, 2010)

Stage 0	Tis	N0	M0
Stage I	T1	N0	M0
Stage II	T2	N0	M0
Stage III	T1, T2	N1	M0
	T3	N0, N1	M0
Stage IVA	T1, T2, T3	N2	M0
	T4a	N0, N1, N2	M0
Stage IVB	T4b	any N	M0
	any T	N3	M0
Stage IVC	any T	any N	M1

Oropharynx tumor (T)

T1: Tumor $\leq$ 2 cm in greatest dimension

T2: Tumor $\geq$ 2–4 cm in greatest dimension

T3: Tumor > 4 cm in greatest dimension or extension to the lingual surface of the epiglottis

T4a: Tumor invades adjacent structures e.g. larynx, hard palate, deep muscle of tongue, lamina medialis of pterygoid plates, or bone of mandible

T4b: Tumor invades adjacent structures e.g. lateral pterygoid muscle, lamina lateralis of pterygoid plates, skull base and/or encases internal carotid artery

Hypopharynx tumor (T)

T1: Tumor limited to one subsite of the hypopharynx and < 2 cm in greatest dimension

T2: Tumor invades more than one subsite of the hypopharynx or an adjacent site, or measures > 2–4 cm in greatest diameter without fixation of hemilarynx

T3: Tumor measures > 4 cm in greatest dimension or with fixation of hemilarynx

T4a: Tumor invades thyroid/cricoid cartilage, hyoid bone, thyroid gland, esophagus, or central compartment soft tissue (including prelaryngeal strap muscles and subcutaneous fat)

T4b: Tumor invades prevertebral fascia, encases internal carotid artery, or involves mediastinal structures

Oral cavity tumor (T)

T1: Tumor $\leq$ 2 cm in greatest dimension

T2: Tumor $\geq$ 2–4 cm in greatest dimension

T3: Tumor > 4 cm in greatest dimension

T4a: Tumor invades adjacent structures e.g. cortical bone, deep muscle of tongue, maxillary sinus, or skin of face

T4b: Tumor invades masticator space, pterygoid plates, skull base, encases internal carotid artery

Regional lymph nodes (N)

N0: No regional lymph node metastasis

N1: Metastasis in a single ipsilateral lymph node, < 3 cm in greatest dimension

N2a: Metastasis in a single ipsilateral lymph node > 3–6 cm in greatest dimension

N2b: Metastasis in multiple ipsilateral lymph nodes, $\leq$ 6 cm in greatest dimension

N2c: Metastasis in bilateral or contralateral lymph nodes, $\leq$ 6 cm in greatest dimension

N3: Metastasis in a lymph node > 6 cm in greatest dimension

Distant metastasis (M)

M0: No distant metastasis

M1: Distant metastasis

bio-radiation with cetuximab significantly improves overall survival at 5 years compared with radiotherapy alone (Bonner et al. 2010).

Side Effects

Surgery

Perioperative complications include hemorrhage, bleeding, infections, prolonged wound healing, edema, and airway obstruction. Long-term postoperative complications of surgery include stenosis, fistula, and aspiration with consecutive pneumonia.

Radiotherapy

Early side effects include different degrees of hoarseness, dermatitis, mucositis, dysphagia, sticky saliva, xerostomia, taste alteration, and consecutive weight loss. Late side effects of radiotherapy (>90 days) include fibrosis of the soft tissues, xerostomia, hyperpigmentation, submental edema, upper limb plexopathy, ▶ Lhermitte's sign, ▶ trismus, long-term tube feeding, tracheostomy, stenosis of the esophageal entrance, and ▶ osteoradionecrosis.

Chemotherapy and Targeted Therapy

Complications are drug dependent. Hematologic and gastrointestinal side effects (nausea and vomiting), mucositis, and transient infertility are most common. Cis-platinum causes severe nausea and vomiting, anemia, neutropenia, and thrombocytopenia, and affects the kidney function and can potentially compromise the hearing qualities permanently. 5-flurouracil can cause neurologic impairments (hand-foot syndrome) and coronary spasms. The taxanes have been related to allergic reactions. This also applies for cetuximab leading to an anaphylactic shock exceptionally, skin rash (acne-like), and hair and nail alterations.

Prognosis

The TNM-staging system (Table 1) could clearly establish by multivariate analyses the major prognostic factors. These are the T-, N-, and M-stages, sites, grading, age, and the performance score. Postoperatively, positive resection margins (R1, R2) and ECE are the prognostic factors of highest predominance. The disease-free survival is negatively influenced by a positive nodal status. A latent HPV infection is a positive prognostic factor. No overall survival benefit has been observed for adjuvant chemotherapy, but a significant survival benefit was observed with concurrent chemoradiation in the order of 7% with 5 years follow-up from the meta-analysis of Pignon et al. (2009). However, high-dose hyperfractionated radiation therapy also confirmed an 8% survival benefit in the same patient population (Bourhis et al. 2006). Furthermore, a diminishing effect of chemotherapy was observed with increasing age.

References

Bernier J, Cooper JS, Pajak TF et al (2005) Defining risk levels in locally advanced head and neck cancers: a comparative analysis of concurrent postoperative radiation plus chemotherapy trials of the EORTC (#22931) and RTOG (# 9501). Head Neck 27:843–850

Bonner JA, Harari PM, Giralt J et al (2010) Radiotherapy plus cetuximab for locoregionally advanced head and neck cancer: 5-year survival data from a phase 3 randomised trial, and relation between cetuximab-induced rash and survival. Lancet Oncol 11:21–28

Bourhis J, Overgaard J, Audry H et al (2006) Hyperfractionated or accelerated radiotherapy in head and neck cancer: a meta-analysis. Meta-Analysis of Radiotherapy in Carcinomas of Head and neck (MARCH) Collaborative Group. Lancet 368:843–854

Pignon JP, le Maître A, Maillard E et al (2009) MACH-NC Collaborative Group. Meta-analysis of chemotherapy in head and neck cancer (MACH-NC): an update on 93 randomised trials and 17,346 patients. Radiother Oncol 92:4–14

Posner MR, Hershock DM, Blajman CR et al (2007) TAX 324 Study Group. Cisplatin and fluorouracil alone or with docetaxel in head and neck cancer. N Engl J Med 357:1705–1715

Vermorken JB, Remenar E, van Herpen C et al (2007) EORTC 24971/TAX 323 Study Group (2007) Cisplatin, fluorouracil, and docetaxel in unresectable head and neck cancer. N Engl J Med 357:1695–1706

Vermorken JB, Mesia R, Rivera F et al (2008) Platinum-based chemotherapy plus cetuximab in head and neck cancer. N Engl J Med 359:1116–1127

Orthovoltage Therapy

BRANDON J. FISHER
Department of Radiation Oncology,
College of Medicine, Drexel University,
Philadelphia, PA, USA

Definition
Orthovoltage therapy, also known as deep therapy, is a type of X-ray therapy used to treat tumors of a depth of about 2–3 cm. Typical X-ray energies are 200–300 kV_p, with a skin-to-source distance of roughly 50 cm. The treatments usually incorporate a movable diaphragm and lead plates for size adjustments.

Cross-References
▶ Skin Cancer

Osteonecrosis

THEODORE E. YAEGER
Department Radiation Oncology, Wake Forest University School of Medicine, Winston-Salem NC, USA

Definition
Bone death secondary to vascular insufficiency.

Cross-References
▶ ORN
▶ Osteoradionecrosis (also ORN or Osteonecrosis)

Osteoradionecrosis (also ORN or Osteonecrosis)

JAMES H. BRASHEARS, III
Radiation Oncologist, Venice, FL, USA

Synonyms
ORN; Osteonecrosis

Definition
Devitalized bone occurring as a late effect after radiotherapy. It frequently involves the mandible after treatment with >60 Gy and can occur subsequent to minor dental trauma. Intimal fibrosis and thrombosis are identified on microscopy affecting the inferior alveolar artery.

Cross-References
▶ Oro-Hypopharynx
▶ Supportive Care and Quality of Life

Osteosarcoma

▶ Sarcoma

Ovarian Cancer

▶ Ovary

Ovarian Malignancy

▶ Ovary

Ovary

MICHELLE KOLTON MACKAY[1],
CHRISTIN A. KNOWLTON[2]
[1]Department of Radiation Oncology, Marshfield
Clinic, Marshfield, WI, USA
[2]Department of Radiation Oncology,
Drexel University, Philadelphia, PA, USA

Synonyms

Ovarian cancer; Ovarian malignancy

Definition

Ovarian cancer encompasses a group of malignant histologic entities that arise from diverse types of tissues contained within the ovaries. This group of diseases includes epithelial ovarian cancer, germ cell neoplasms of the ovary, carcinosarcomas (malignant mixed müllerian tumors of the ovary), and ovarian stromal tumors.

Background

Ovarian cancer is the second most common gynecologic cancer diagnosis, following ▶ endometrial cancer, and is the leading cause of gynecologic cancer death (American Cancer Society 2011). It is the fifth leading cause of cancer death in women. The median age at the time of an ovarian cancer diagnosis is 63 years, and approximately 70% of patients present with advanced disease at diagnosis.

It is important to understand the anatomy of the ovary and its relationship to the gynecologic tract to appreciate ovarian cancer. The ovaries are a pair of organs located in the female pelvis that are solid and oval in shape. They are connected to the broad ligament, which is a reflection of the peritoneal lining that connects laterally to the side wall of the pelvis. Medially, the ovaries connect to the uterus by the utero-ovarian ligament. The arterial blood supplies to the ovaries are the ovarian arteries, which arise from the aorta inferior to the renal vessels. The venous drainage mirrors the drainage of the testes, with the left ovarian vein draining to the left renal vein and the right ovarian vein draining to the inferior vena cava. The first echelon of lymphatic drainage from the ovaries is by way of the infundibulopelvic and round ligament to the external iliac regional lymph nodes. Drainage proceeds into the internal iliac, obturator, common iliac, and para-aortic regions.

Ovarian cancer tends to be predominant in more affluent societies with longer life expectancies. Risk factors for ovarian cancer include nulliparity, older age at first birth, use of ovulation-inducing medications, and diet including high fat and high lactose. Decreased risk of ovarian cancer is associated with younger age at first birth, multiparity, use of oral contraceptive medication, and breast feeding.

Only approximately 5% of ovarian cancer diagnoses are thought to result from genetic predisposition, although family history also represents a risk factor. Familial syndromes include linkage with the ▶ BRCA1 and BRCA2 genotypes and with hereditary nonpolyposis colorectal cancer.

Diagnosis of ovarian cancer is difficult because of the wide range of vague symptoms at presentation, and therefore the disease tends to present in later stages. No practical, effective screening technique exists, which also makes early detection of the disease difficult. Cancer antigen 125 (▶ CA 125) and ultrasound are techniques that have been studied for screening, but without satisfactory results.

Histologic diagnosis is necessary in establishing an ovarian cancer diagnosis. The World Health Organization classifies ovarian cancers into three main categories including epithelial, sex-cord stromal tumors, and germ cell tumors. The majority of ovarian cancers (more than 85%) are epithelial in origin. Epithelial cancers include a variety of histologic subtypes such as endometrioid, serous, mucinous, clear cell, Brenner (transitional cell), squamous cell, mixed epithelial, and undifferentiated tumors. Histologic diagnosis helps determine treatment course and outcomes.

The stage of cancer is another major factor that determines treatment course and outcome. Two staging systems are used in staging, the American Joint Committee on Cancer (AJCC) staging with tumor-node-metastasis (TNM) classification and the Federation Internationale de Gynecologie (FIGO) classification. Table 1 details the staging for these systems. Ovarian cancer is a surgically/pathologically staged disease.

Ovary. Table 1 Staging for ovarian cancer according to AJCC and FIGO

Primary Tumor		
TNM	FIGO	
TX		Primary tumor cannot be assessed
T0		No evidence of primary tumor
T1	I	Tumor limited to ovaries (one or both)
Tia	IA	Tumor limited to one ovary; capsule intact, no tumor on ovarian surface. No malignant cells in ascites or peritoneal washings
T1b	IB	Tumor limited to both ovaries; capsules intact, no tumor on ovarian surface. No malignant cells in ascites or peritoneal washings
T1c	IC	Tumor limited to one or both ovaries with any of the following: capsule ruptured, tumor on ovarian surface, malignant cells in ascites or peritoneal washings
T2	II	Tumor involves one or both ovaries with pelvic extension and/or implants
T2a	IIA	Extension and/or implants on uterus and/or tube(s). No malignant cells in ascites or peritoneal washings

Ovary. Table 1 (continued)

T2b	IIB	Extension to and/or implants on other pelvic tissues. No malignant cells in ascites or peritoneal washings
T2c	IIC	Pelvic extension and/or implants (T2a or T2b) with malignant cells in ascites or peritoneal washings
T3	III	Tumor involves one or both ovaries with microscopically confirmed peritoneal metastasis outside the pelvis
T3a	IIIA	Microscopic peritoneal metastasis beyond pelvis (no macroscopic tumor)
T3b	IIIB	Macroscopic peritoneal metastasis beyond pelvis 2 cm or less in greatest dimension
T3c	IIIC	Peritoneal metastasis beyond pelvis more than 2 cm in greatest dimension and/or regional lymph node metastasis

Note: Liver capsule metastasis T3/Stage III; liver parenchymal metastasis M1/Stage IV.

Pleural effusion must have positive cytology for M1/Stage IV.

Regional Lymph Nodes		
TNM	FIGO	
NX		Regional lymph nodes cannot be assessed
N0		No regional lymph node metastasis
N1	IIIC	Regional lymph node metastasis
Distant Metastasis		
TNM	FIGO	
M0		No distant metastasis (no pathologic M0; use clinical M to complete stage group)
M1	IV	Distant metastasis (excludes peritoneal metastasis)

Used with the permission of the American Joint Committee on Cancer (AJCC), Chicago, Illinois. The original source for this material is the AJCC Cancer Staging Manual, Seventh Edition (2010) published by Springer Science and Business Media LLC, www.springer.com (American Joint Committee on Cancer 2010)

Ovary. Table 2 Stage/prognostic grouping for ovarian cancer

Group	T	N	M
I	T1	N0	M0
IA	T1a	N0	M0
IB	T1b	N0	M0
IC	T1c	N0	M0
II	T2	N0	M0
IIA	T2a	N0	M0
IIB	T2b	N0	M0
IIC	T2c	N0	M0
III	T3	N0	M0
IIIA	T3a	N0	M0
IIIB	T3b	N0	M0
IIIC	T3c	N0	M0
	Any T	N1	M0
IV	Any T	Any N	M1

Used with the permission of the American Joint Committee on Cancer (AJCC), Chicago, Illinois. The original source for this material is the AJCC Cancer Staging Manual, Seventh Edition (2010) published by Springer Science and Business Media LLC, www.springer.com (American Joint Committee on Cancer 2010)

The TNM staging furthermore categorizes patients into groups according to the TNM classification as described in Table 2.

Initial Evaluation

The first step in evaluation for ovarian cancer is to perform a thorough history and examination including evaluation for abdominal bloating, abdominal or pelvic pain, vaginal bleeding or discharge, pain with sexual intercourse, urinary symptoms including frequency, urgency, hematuria, and rectal bleeding. Obtaining history of the patient's gastrointestinal habits is also important, including factors such as difficulty with eating, bloating, and early satiety.

A physical examination should focus on examination of the abdomen, pelvis, gynecologic examination, and rectovaginal examination to assess extent of the disease clinically. Findings may include adnexal mass, ascites, and pleural effusion. Attention should be paid to signature findings in ovarian cancer including appearance of the ▶ Sister Mary Joseph nodule, which presents as a palpable nodule at the umbilicus representing an underlying abdominal malignancy. A Blumer's shelf tumor, which is palpable in the anterior rectal wall, may also represent an ovarian malignancy. Ovarian cancer can also be associated with paraneoplastic syndromes including hypercalcemia and subacute cerebellar degeneration. The Leser-Trélat sign, which is the explosive presence of multiple seborrheic keratoses, has been known to herald ovarian cancer diagnosis in rare cases. This is thought to be a paraneoplastic syndrome in which cytokines and growth factors from the neoplasm stimulate the growth of the lesions.

Differential Diagnosis

A differential diagnosis for ovarian cancer includes ovarian cyst, irritable bowel syndrome, ascites, malignancy from another origin, including ▶ colorectal or ▶ pancreatic cancer, and benign adnexal tumors.

Imaging Studies

Imaging studies for ovarian cancer include the use of transvaginal ultrasound to visualize the adnexa and assess characteristics of lesions. A computed tomography (CT) scan or magnetic resonance imaging of the pelvis is helpful in determining extent of disease preoperatively. Cystoscopy and sigmoidoscopy may assist in determining possible disease involvement of the bladder or rectum. Upper gastrointestinal (GI) evaluation with endoscopy or upper GI series will help in ruling out metastatic disease from a GI primary tumor, known as a Krukenberg tumor. Metastatic workup can be obtained with a CT scan of the chest, abdomen, and pelvis.

Laboratory Studies

Important laboratory work to obtain includes a complete blood count and metabolic panel with liver function tests. Tumor markers to obtain include CA 125, which is the most useful for following disease status and is elevated in most epithelial ovarian malignancies. Other tumor markers include CA 19-9 and carcinoembryonic antigen (CEA). α-Fetoprotein and β-human chorionic gonadotropin are helpful markers with ovarian cancers of germ cell origin.

Treatment

Tissue confirmation is necessary to establish an ovarian malignancy diagnosis, and surgical/pathologic staging is necessary to determine course of treatment. Treatment of ovarian cancer usually begins with surgical management, which acts as a diagnostic and treatment tool. A vertical midline abdominal incision is generally used in patients with a suspected ovarian malignancy. For earlier-stage disease confined to the ovary or pelvis, surgery beginning with aspiration of ascites or peritoneal lavage is performed and the specimens sent for cytologic evaluation. Careful evaluation of the peritoneal surface should be performed next and excisions or biopsies taken. If there are no areas of visible or palpable concern, random peritoneal biopsy specimens should be taken. The standard surgery for removal of the neoplasm and adjacent structures is the total hysterectomy, bilateral ▶ salpingectomy, bilateral ▶ oophorectomy, and omentectomy (National Comprehensive Cancer Network 2010). A unilateral salpingoophorectomy can be considered in selected patients with early-stage disease as a method for preserving fertility. Minimally invasive techniques can also be considered. Lymph node dissection will also be performed at the time of surgery with removal of pelvic lymph nodes in the regions of the common iliac, external iliac, and hypogastric vessels and the region of the obturator fossa. Aortic lymph nodes are dissected superiorly to the level of the inferior mesenteric artery or renal vessels.

For patients with more advanced disease, surgery begins in the same manner as with early-stage disease; however, debulking is also performed in an effort to achieve maximum cytoreduction with an attempt to leave less than 1 cm of residual disease. To achieve maximum debulking, surgery may need to include procedures such as radical pelvic dissection, bowel resection, stripping of diaphragm or peritoneal surfaces, or splenectomy.

Following surgery, patients may be eligible for either intravenous or ▶ intraperitoneal chemotherapy (Gerhig 2008). Standard recommendations include using intravenous chemotherapy with a taxane/carboplatin combination for three to six cycles in stage IC disease. Intraperitoneal chemotherapy can be offered to patients with stage II and III disease who have had optimal debulking and have less than 1 cm of residual disease. The alternative in stage II, III, and IV disease is intravenous ▶ chemotherapy with a taxane/carboplatin combination for a total of six to eight cycles. Following the six to eight cycles of chemotherapy, completion surgery should be considered to assess further potential resectability in these patients.

In patients with recurrent disease, further surgery should be considered. Chemotherapy including platinum-based doublets or single agents as well as single agents that are non-platinum based can also be considered if the disease becomes platinum resistant. Hormonal therapies including aromatase inhibitors, tamoxifen, leuprolide acetate, and megestrol acetate can be incorporated. Targeted therapy such as bevacizumab may also be used.

Radiation therapy historically had a prominent role in the definitive treatment of ovarian cancer. Previously, adjuvant ▶ whole abdominal radiation therapy (WART) following maximal surgical resection was found to be superior to older types of chemotherapy. With improvements in the delivery and toxicity profile of

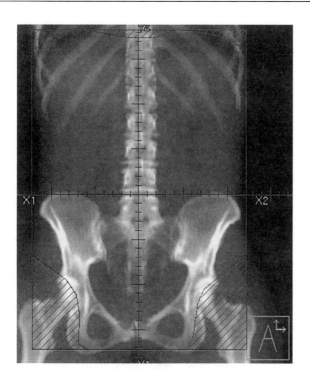

Ovary. Fig. 1 Anterior beam view of a whole abdominal radiation therapy (WART) field

chemotherapy, results with chemotherapy for consolidation were found to be equivalent to WART with less toxicity. WART is associated with a high rate of acute gastrointestinal side effects and myelosuppression. Late-term side effects include transient elevation in liver function tests, chronic diarrhea, and bowel obstruction. While WART is no longer commonly employed in the definitive treatment of ovarian cancer, there has been a recent resurgence in the technique. At some institutions, WART is used for stage III patients who demonstrate a complete clinical response following maximal surgical resection and chemotherapy. In addition, WART remains an option for patients with less than 2 cm of residual disease following maximum surgical resection who are deemed poor candidates for chemotherapy.

WART can be performed with external beam radiation therapy using opposed anterior and

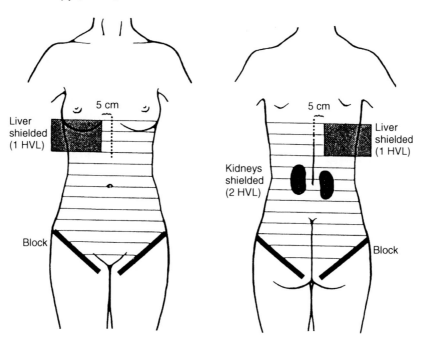

Ovary. Fig. 2 Technique used in moving strip for whole abdominal radiation therapy. Figure from Brady, LW et al: Treatment Planning in the Radiation Therapy of Cancer. Front Radiat Ther Oncol 1987, Vol. 21, pp 302–332, published by S. Karger AG, Basel. Used with permission

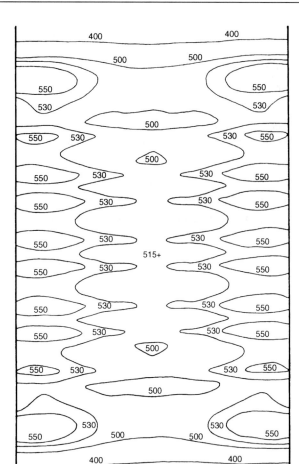

Ovary. Fig. 3 Isodose summation curves for whole abdominal radiation therapy using the moving strip technique. Figure from Brady, LW et al: Treatment Planning in the Radiation Therapy of Cancer. Front Radiat Ther Oncol 1987, Vol. 21, pp 302–332, published by S. Karger AG, Basel. Used with permission

posterior beams (Fig. 1). The borders of the field include above the domes of the diaphragm superiorly, below the obturator foramen inferiorly, and covering the peritoneal reflection laterally. The dose to the field is 30 Gy in 1.2–1.5 Gy fractions to the abdominal field with a para-aortic region boost to 45 Gy and pelvis boost to 45–55 Gy. Kidney blocks are generally placed in the field after approximately 15 Gy and a liver block is placed after 25 Gy. This blocking allows for preservation of organ function in a large treatment field. The moving strip technique can also be used in an effort to treat the above fields with less toxicity. The abdomen is divided into 2.5 cm horizontal strips. On day one, the most caudal strip is treated to 375 cGy using opposed anterior and posterior beams. Each day, the adjacent superior strip is added to the treatment field, until a maximum of four strips are included in the treatment field. Each strip is treated to 3,000 cGy in eight fractions over 10 days. Once the dose has been reached in the most inferior strip, it is dropped from the treatment field and the adjacent cephalad strip is added (Brady et al. 1987; Friedman et al. 1970). The moving strip technique has been largely replaced by the open field technique (Figs. 2 and 3). ▶ Intensity-modulated radiation therapy (IMRT) is currently being explored as a means to limit the toxicity of WART.

Radiation therapy also plays a role in localized palliative treatment of ovarian cancer including problematic deposits in the abdomen or pelvis and in distant metastatic disease involving sites such as the brain, bone, or lung. External beam radiation is delivered using a ▶ conformal therapy technique directed to the region of concern. Radiation therapy can also be considered in locally recurrent disease that is not amenable to surgery.

Cross-References

▶ Brachytherapy: High Dose Rate (HDR) Implants
▶ Cervical Cancer
▶ Endometrium
▶ Uterine Cervix
▶ Vagina

References

American Cancer Society (2011) Ovarian cancer. American Cancer Society Cancer Statistics 61(4), July/August 2011, Atlanta, GA

American Joint Committee on Cancer (2010) Ovary and primary peritoneal carcinoma. In: Edge SB, Byrd DR, Compton CC, Fritz AG, Greene FL, Trotti A (eds) AJCC cancer staging manual, 7th edn. Springer, New York

Brady LW, Markoe AM, Micaily B et al (1987) Clinical treatment planning in gynecologic cancer. Front Radiat Ther Oncol 21:302–332

Friedman AB, Benninghoff DL, Alexander LL, Aron BS (1970) Total abdominal irradiation using cobalt 60 moving strip technique. Am J Roentgenol Radium Ther Nucl Med 108:172–177

Gerhig PA, Varia M, Apisarnthanarax S (2008) Ovary. In: Halperin EC, Perez CA, Brady LW (eds) Principles and practice of radiation oncology, 5th edn. Wolters Kluwer/Lippincott Williams & Wilkins, Philadelphia

National Comprehensive Cancer Network (2010) NCCN clinical practice guidelines in oncology: ovarian cancer including fallopian tube cancer and primary peritoneal cancer, V.1.2010. Available at http://www.nccn.org/professionals/physician_gls/PDF/ovarian.pdf. Accessed on 31 January 2010

Oxidative Stress

Susan M. Varnum, Marianne B. Sowa, William F. Morgan
Biological Sciences Division, Fundamental & Computational Sciences, Directorate Pacific Northwest National Laboratory, Richland, WA, USA

Definition

Damage that can occur to cells resulting from an imbalance between the production of reactive oxygen species and a biological system's ability to readily detoxify the reactive intermediates or easily repair the resulting damage.

Cross-References

▶ Radiation-Induced Genomic Instability and Radiation Sensitivity

P

1p16q

Larry C. Daugherty[1], Brandon J. Fisher[2]
[1]Department of Radiation Oncology,
College of Medicine, Drexel University,
Glenside, PA, USA
[2]Department of Radiation Oncology,
College of Medicine, Drexel University,
Philadelphia, PA, USA

Definition

An important genetic marker in Wilm's tumor which has prognostic implications. Loss of heterozygosity of this chromosome results in increased risk of relapse and death from Wilm's tumor.

Cross-References

▶ Wilm's Tumor

Paclitaxel

Christin A. Knowlton[1], Michelle Kolton Mackay[2]
[1]Department of Radiation Oncology, Drexel University, Philadelphia, PA, USA
[2]Department of Radiation Oncology, Marshfield Clinic, Marshfield, WI, USA

Definition

Paclitaxel is a chemotherapy agent in the taxane class, derived from the yew tree. Paclitaxel binds to tubulin, inhibiting disassembly of microtubules and causing stabilization of microtubules and preventing cell division. Paclitaxel is commonly used in the treatment of ovarian cancer, often in combination with carboplatin. Side effects of paclitaxel include nausea, loss of appetite, brittle and thinned hair, discoloration of the nails, and tingling in the hands or toes.

Cross-References

▶ Lung Cancer
▶ Ovary
▶ Principles of Chemotherapy

Paget's Disease

David E. Wazer[1,3], Anthony E. Dragun[2]
[1]Radiation Oncology Department, Tufts Medical Center, Tufts University School of Medicine, Boston, MA, USA
[2]Department of Radiation Oncology, James Graham Brown Cancer Center, University of Louisville School of Medicine, Louisville, KY, USA
[3]Radiation Oncology Department, Rhode Island Hospital, Brown University School of Medicine, Providence, RI, USA

Synonyms

Paget's disease of the nipple

Definition

A clinical presentation of nipple eczema and superficial epidermal scaling which can progress to crusting, erosion, and exudates. Histologically characterized by the presence of Paget's cells,

L.W. Brady, T.E. Yaeger (eds.), *Encyclopedia of Radiation Oncology*, DOI 10.1007/978-3-540-85516-3,
© Springer-Verlag Berlin Heidelberg 2013

described as large, round-to-oval cells that contain hyperchromatic nuclei and prominent nucleoli, scattered throughout the epidermis, this process is often associated with underlying DCIS or invasive carcinoma.

Paget's disease is a rare presentation of breast cancer involving inflammation, crusting, and eczematous changes of the nipple and areola. It is associated with an underlying papable mass in 40–50% of cases, which will contain invasive cancer approximately 90% of the time. Cases which are not associated with an underlying papable mass will contain ductal carcinoma in situ in approximately 75% of the time. Histologic analysis shows Paget's cells in the epidermis. Stage-for-stage, the prognosis is similar to that of early stage breast cancer in general. Workup, diagnosis, and therapy are similar as well, with breast conserving therapy as an option. Conservative treatment involves removal of the nipple-areola complex with negative surgical margins and adjuvant whole breast radiation therapy.

Cross-References
▶ Cancer of the Breast Tis
▶ Early-Stage Breast Cancer

Paget's Disease of the Nipple

▶ Paget's Disease

Pain

James H. Brashears, III
Radiation Oncologist, Venice, FL, USA

Definition
An unpleasant sensory and emotional experience associated with actual and potential tissue damage, or described in terms of such damage or both (from the International Association for the Study of Pain).

Cross-References
▶ Pain Management

Pain Flare

James H. Brashears, III
Radiation Oncologist, Venice, FL, USA

Definition
An initial, transient worsening in pain and/or increased need for analgesics as a result of therapy. This can be seen in the palliative setting with intravenous radionuclide or large fraction external beam therapy for bone metastases. The process is usually self-limited to less than one week.

Cross-References
▶ Pain Management
▶ Palliation of Bone Metastases

Pain Management

James H. Brashears, III
Radiation Oncologist, Venice, FL, USA

Synonyms
Algiatry; Cancer quality of life; Palliation

Definition/Description
The vast majority of patients with cancer will experience some form of ▶ pain. Pain can come from a variety of contributing sources with a corresponding array of interventions to alleviate

symptoms. Biomedical and nontraditional techniques are discussed.

Background

Pain is "an unpleasant sensory and emotional experience associated with actual and potential tissue damage, or described in terms of such damage or both," according to the International Association for the Study of Pain (NCCN 2009). The vast majority of patients with cancer suffer at least some form of pain during their disease process. Most sources find that this pain is insufficiently addressed by care providers for a variety of posited reasons including: discrepancies in understanding the severity and presence of pain between the patient and physician, conservative prescription practices of pain relievers for fear of drug diversion, patient anxiety of drug addiction, difficulties in objectively measuring pain, and confusing the different etiologies of pain with resultant misstargeting of therapies. The cause of a particular patient's pain can be either simple or complex; owing to this, early consultation with ▶ pain management specialists when pain does not respond as expected to traditional therapies or there is suspicion of a multifactorial process is encouraged.

Anatomy and Taxonomy

Even at the most simplistic, the perception of pain from the body is a complicated process that usually involves several layers of neural connections in the central and peripheral nervous systems. Pain resulting from tissue damage in the body is mediated by nociceptors that transmit signals through the spinothalamic tract for higher processing via the ventral posterolateral thalamus or reticular formation. In keeping with our ontogeny, cranial nerves responsible for sensation also carry the signals for pain for a given territory via the medial lemniscus to the thalamus (the trigeminal nerve covers much of the face, though the seventh, ninth, and tenth cranial nerves also carry pain impulses from the ear and

pharynx). The degree of pain is moderated both cortically and at the level of the spinal cord by way of axons coming from the pontine periaqueductal gray matter. To complicate matters, human experience also teaches that pain can be moderated and even elicited by emotional stimuli and the ▶ psychosocial state of an individual.

Since a precise explanation for the myriad of peoples' experience of pain is wanting, categorization of pain remains imprecise, so a system based on the probable etiology that may in turn guide therapy seems reasonable. Generally, pain can be either local or generalized. Beyond this rudimentary taxonomy, somatogenic pain, as the name implies, manifests from insult to the body and can be divided into nociceptive and neuropathic pain. Nociceptive pain is detected by specialized detectors (nociceptors) in tissue that are connected to A-delta fibers or unmyelinated C-fibers. A-delta fibers are associated with sharp or stabbing pain as well as intense temperatures that can localize the site of the noxious stimuli and these are also incorporated into reflex arcs. C-fibers tend to carry the dull, nonspecific pain that can follow more acute pain. Furthermore, nociceptive pain can be superficial (usually from receptors on the outer layers of the body and carried by A-delta fibers), deep somatic (from nociceptors in tendons, ligaments, fasciae with resulting poorly localized pain), and visceral pain (from organs within the body that can be crampy and mistakenly localized, as is the case with ▶ referred pain syndromes). Neuropathic pain results from dysfunction of either peripheral or central nerves and can be tingling or numb and can be associated with specific nerve distributions (as with trigeminal neuralgia). Non-somatogenic pain is classified as psychogenic (or somatoform) and is pain caused or exacerbated by mental, emotional, or behavioral factors while pain without identifiable cause can be said to be idiopathic. Each of the pain types is usually amenable to different therapies and they may not occur in isolation in the cancer patient, so a multidimensional treatment approach is appropriate when a patient is experiencing pain from a multifactorial process (mixed pain).

Evaluation

Several scales and measurement tools have been developed to quantify pain and make recommendations regarding treatment. These should be employed supplementary to the complete history and physical examination of the patient paying particular attention to the pain's intensity, location, quality, and moderating factors. In addition, managing the patient's expectations regarding pain control and any side effects of the therapy is crucial to success.

A three-step pain ladder was created by the World Health Organization (WHO) that recommends incremental escalation of pharmaceutical therapeutic strength to achieve pain control (Deng 2008). This pain ladder is the cornerstone for most pain-control recommendations by various organizations. Adjuvant therapies including non-analgesic medications like antidepressants and steroids as well as nontraditional approaches are permitted at all levels. At the first rung, mild pain is addressed by non-opioid analgesics often in the form of nonsteroidal anti-inflammatory drugs (NSAIDs) like acetaminophen, aspirin, ibuprofen, and COX-2 (cyclooxygenase-2 isoenzyme) inhibitors. If adequate relief is not reached, pain is said to be moderate and second tier, or weak opioid medications can be added. Such agents include: codeine, tramadol, hydrocodone, and propoxyphene. Nonresponsive, severe cancer pain reaches tier three and strong opioids may be used in place of weak opioid medications. Examples of strong opioids are: morphine, oxycodone, hydromorphone, fentanyl, heroin, and buprenorphine. The WHO approach is roughly 85% effective and has been applied successfully in large medical centers (Deng 2008).

The National Comprehensive Cancer Network (NCCN) has also set forth guidelines for pain management that is both useful and available gratis online (NCCN 2009). Beginning with the screening of all cancer patients, the guidelines set out a decision-tree-based approach to managing pain, which is described by the patient on an ascending 0–10 scale using writing, verbal questioning, nonverbal signs (the faces pain rating scale), or behavior. Tools exist even for assessing pain in demented patients. In addition, the disabling impact of pain can also be measured, again using a 0–10 scale. Based on patient desires, etiology, and the acuity of symptoms, a pain management plan is formulated with the goal of achieving pain relief without unmanageable side effects. For severe chronic, opioid-requiring pain, escalating doses of short-acting opiates are initially utilized based on regularly spaced reevaluations. Similarly, use of patient-controlled analgesia can also be employed to get an idea of a patient's opioid requirements. Once adequately addressed, the patient can be transitioned to an equi-analgesic dosage of a long-acting opioid with a short-acting medication available for ▶ breakthrough pain. This rescue dose should be around 15% of the analgesic activity of the 24 h dose for oral medicine or start with the lowest dose if the transmucosal route is used (e.g., fentanyl lozenges, lollipops, or buccal tablets). In addition, recommendations for adjuvant therapies include ▶ psychosocial support and education as well as information regarding management of medication side effects.

Treatment

Nociceptive pain tends to respond to both NSAIDs and opioid medications. As per the NCCN and WHO, any nociceptive pain that is more than mild (scored greater than 3) makes the patient a candidate for treatment with opioids. Neuropathic pain from inflammation or pressure on a nerve may be addressed with NSAIDs and glucocorticoids initially; when caused by a specific identifiable lesion, localized interventions like radiotherapy or surgical extirpation may become appropriate. Antidepressants, anticonvulsants, and topical anesthetics may also be used to address neuropathic pain. Psychogenic pain may also benefit from antidepressants in addition to referral for specialized psychiatric and psychologic treatment. Patient and family education with marshaling of social resources can also meliorate a patient's psychogenic pain.

NSAIDs and opioids are powerful and oft-used tools for pain management. Aside from the selection of the specific agent and titration of the appropriate dose, the formulation and means of delivery of the medication bears consideration. NSAIDs and opioids are available for rectal, intravenous, epidural, intramuscular, topical, transdermal, and trans-oral administration. Input from a capable pharmacist can also be invaluable as many medications can be compounded on custom order. Potential side effects will also influence the choice of treatment. Nonselective cyclooxygenase inhibitor NSAIDs like aspirin, indomethacin, or ibuprofen have several potential side effects including gastric ulceration, renal toxicity, and risk of bleeding. COX-2 inhibitors like celecoxib also pose the risk of gastric ulceration in addition to the well-publicized cardiovascular risk (Deng 2008). Acetaminophen (or paracetamol) also acts through COX inhibition, but presents less risk of bleeding or renal disorders, though it has an increased risk of hepatic toxicity. The opioid class of drugs have a myriad of side effects, perhaps the most prevalent being constipation, so patients require an effective bowel regimen that allows for titration of both the dosage of the opioid and whatever medicines are being used to stay regular (laxatives, stool softeners, etc.). Other potential side effects include disturbance of the mood and sensorium, confusion, drowsiness, nausea, vomiting, dry mouth, and respiratory depression (which can all be reversed emergently by opioid antagonism with naloxone or naltrexone) (NCCN, 2009).

Beyond pure analgesics, antidepressants can be tried to lower opioid requirements with neuropathic pain or used alone for psychogenic pain. Duloxetine, venlafaxine, and bupropion are available and may have a preferable safety profile compared with the anticholinergic effects of tricyclic antidepressants. Treatment with gabapentin, pregabalin, or other anticonvulsants may also be appropriate for neuropathic pain, though they too can cause drowsiness and changes in patients' sensorium and mood. Muscle relaxants including the benzodiazepines may be beneficial if muscle spasm or anxiety is contributing to pain, but they present many of the same risks as anticonvulsants and can be habit forming. Topical medicines like capsaicin cream or lidocaine gel or patch can provide site directed treatment with little risk of systemic side effects so long as the skin barrier is intact. Short-term use of glucocorticoids like prednisone or dexamethasone may also be appropriate for acute inflammation, though chronic use may lead to immunosuppression, changes in the sensorium and mood, insomnia, osteoporosis, truncal obesity, glaucoma, and fatigue.

Non-pharmacologic approaches are also important in the pain management armamentarium and can be used to decrease medication usage, complement medical therapy, or when such medications are not effective. Radiotherapy can be applied both locally and systemically through an array of techniques including intravenous administration, brachytherapy with a high- or low-dose rate source, or teletherapy. The latter approach is most prevalent and tends to be applied locally. Typically, a target representing a pathologic process is defined by physical examination or imaging and treated with the goal of eventual alleviation or avoidance of symptoms. Careful and reproducible patient positioning is required so analgesic medications may be

P

necessary before and during treatment. Ablation of peripheral nerves, ganglia, and even segments of the spinal cord are another means of pain control. In these procedures, an attempt is made to interrupt the flow of information sent from the painful area to the higher regions of the central nervous system by the chemical, thermal, or physical destruction of the offending nerve or nervous structure. Drug delivery systems or electrical stimulation devices may also be implanted to directly affect the central nervous system in an effort to interfere with pain pathways. Less intrusive, but still efficacious, are behavioral, cognitive, and social interventions. Encouraging physical activity, perhaps with the help of physical or occupational therapy, can help relieve pain and improve quality of life as can participating in support group, learning healthy coping skills, or utilizing psychological support services. The use of heat and/or ice, massage, and proper patient positioning may also be beneficial along with spiritual counseling or nontraditional techniques.

Alternative, or nontraditional, medicine has been growing in popularity in the Western world despite concerns regarding safety and efficacy – ▶ acupuncture is a nice illustration. With more than two millennia of use in Asia, acupuncture has a long history and has been gaining increasing acceptance in western ▶ biomedicine, though its effectiveness is controversial. Some insurers cover the procedure while others do not. The National Institutes of Health (NIH), NCCN, and WHO at least tacitly acknowledge the effectiveness, and rising popularity, of acupuncture and support ongoing research while the American Medical Association (AMA) finds that evidence for acupuncture (and other alternative therapies) is wanting and encourages more rigorous testing (Zhang 2003; NCCAM 2006; AMA 1997; NCCN 2009). Though incompletely understood, neurochemical and functional imaging suggest that acupuncture interferes with the transmission of the sensation of pain to the cortex at the level of the thalamus and periaqueductal gray matter by release of endogenous opioids in addition to increasing local circulation by increasing nitric oxide concentration (Zhang 2003). There are also questions about what exactly the technique represents, since techniques involving application of electric current, laser, and massage (without any needles) may all pass under acupuncture's aegis and certification for acupuncturists varies significantly state by state. Such confusion and the inherent nature of such nontraditional techniques as standing outside of the typical Western medical curriculum put professionals of biomedicine in a difficult position. How best to advise patients in light of evidence-based practice regarding yoga, Tai Chi, music therapy, guided imagery, hypnosis, relaxation/distraction training, cognitive behavioral training, and a myriad of other remedies that may each have a role in managing a particular individual's pain presents a quandary, thus a pragmatic, patient-focused approach to such therapies is recommended.

Cross-References

▶ Clinical Research and the Practice of Evidence-Based Medicine in Radiation Oncology
▶ Economics
▶ Palliation of Bone Metastases
▶ Palliation of Visceral Recurrences and Metastases
▶ Principles of Chemotherapy
▶ Supportive Care and Quality of Life
▶ Targeted Radionuclide Therapy

References

AMA (1997) Report 12 of the Council of Scientific Affairs (A-97) – alternative medicine. American Medical Association, Chicago
Deng GA (2008) Pain management. In: Halperin PA (ed) Principles and practice of radiation oncology, 5th edn. Lipincott Williams & Wilkins, Philadelphia, pp 2005–2009
NCCN (National Comprehensive Cancer Network) (2009) NCCN Clinical Practice Guidelines in Oncology: Adult Cancer Pain v1.2009. National Comprehensive Caner Network, Fort Washington

NCCAM (2006). Acupuncture for pain. Retrieved march 13, 2010, from National Center for Complementary and Alternative Medicine. http://nccam.nih.gov/health/acupuncture/introduction.htm

Zhang X (2003) Acupuncture: review and analysis of reports on controlled clinical trials. World Health Organization, Geneva

Pain Management Specialist

JAMES H. BRASHEARS, III
Radiation Oncologist, Venice, FL, USA

Definition

A physician or other health care provider that focuses their practice on alleviating chronic or acute pain and improving or maintaining patients' quality of life. Though not a requirement, the American Board of Pain Medicine certifies physicians after at least 2 years of pain management–related experience.

Cross-References

▶ Pain Management

Palliation

JAMES H. BRASHEARS, III
Radiation Oncologist, Venice, FL, USA

Synonyms

Cancer quality of life

Definition

Derived from the Latin, palliare, a verb meaning to cloak. Palliative therapy attempts to cloak the symptoms of a disease process and promote quality of life instead of trying to achieve cure.

Cross-References

▶ Pain Management
▶ Palliation of Bone Metastases

Palliation of Bone Metastases

JAMES H. BRASHEARS, III
Radiation Oncologist, Venice, FL, USA

Synonyms

Dissemination or involvement; Management or treatment of osseous disease

Definition/Description

The majority of patients with metastatic cancer have bone involvement. There are numerous tools to manage bone metastases including interventional procedures like surgical stabilization and percutaneous vertebroplasty, radiation therapy, and systemic agents. The goals and potential morbidity of palliative treatments should be reconciled with each patient's desires and clinical circumstance.

Background

The term ▶ palliation is appropriately derived from the Latin, *palliare*, a verb meaning to cloak. The aim of palliative treatment is just that, to cloak the symptoms of a disease and promote quality of life instead of trying to achieve cure. In the case of bone metastases, the goals of radiation therapy may be to manage pain, maintain function, contribute to structural stability, or delay the development of such problems. Over 100,000 people in the United States develop bone metastases each year and some estimate that 350,000 die annually with bone metastases. Osseous involvement is the most common cause of cancer pain. Bone metastases most frequently involve the red marrow of the axial skeleton with the five lumbar spine segments having the highest proportion. For the appendicular skeleton, involvement around the hips at the femur and/or pelvic girdle occurs most often. Malignancies most associated with osseous involvement include: prostate, breast, kidney, thyroid, lung, melanoma, and multiple myeloma (Ratanatharathorn and Powers 2008). The prognosis for such patients is varied and depends on patient factors as well as histology, extent of nonosseous disease, and the extent of bone involvement. Whereas patients with lung primaries tend to succumb within several months of diagnosis with osseous metastases, patients with hormone-responsive tumors like prostate or breast cancer may survive for several years, hence there is the potential for significant palliative benefit in terms of ▶ quality-adjusted life years for those with symptoms.

Initial Evaluation and Imaging

Bone metastases commonly present with pain that can take protean forms. Discomfort may be progressive and localizable (thought to be from pressure or inflammation of the periosteum), radiating (with pressure on nearby nerves or muscle spasm), or sharp when accompanied by fracture. Pain may be worse with weight bearing or use of the muscle groups near the affected bone. Function may also be sacrificed by nerve impingement, bone fracture, or severe pain itself. In a patient suspected of harboring bone metastases, radiographic workup is often appropriate and biopsy may be required if this is the first sign of metastatic disease. Detection by plain skeletal radiographs generally requires a 50% loss in bone mineralization and lesion size of at least 1 cm to show an abnormality, though expansile lesions or fractures can sometimes be detected without the accompanying loss of radio-opacity. For solid-organ malignancies, bone radioscintigraphy with metastable technetium-99 (Tc-99m bone scan) is an effective means to screen for metastatic bone disease. This technique relies on deposition of the metastable radioisotope through increased osteoblastic (bone building) activity at the site of metastasis, so false-positive results can come from any process causing bone turnover as with

arthritis, injury repair, or Paget's disease; therefore confirmatory imaging is helpful. Bone involvement with multiple myeloma or any aggressively osteolytic cancer may not appear on bone scan; in these cases, skeletal survey is an appropriate screening test. Alternatively, using increased metabolic activity as a proxy for bone breakdown, positron emission tomography (PET) imaging with radio-labeled 18-fluorodeoxyglucose (in combination with a co-registered computed tomography, or CT scan to aid in lesion localization) can preferentially identify osteolytic metastases. CT scans are more adept at identifying cortical breakdown than plain radiographs, while magnetic resonance imaging, or MRI, is able to more accurately evaluate the central areas of red marrow versus Tc-99m radioscintigraphy, CT, or plain films (Ratanatharathorn and Powers 2008). Each of these modalities can subsequently be used to target lesions for biopsy or local therapy.

Differential Diagnosis

Bone metastases may be mistaken for areas of infection (abscess), trauma, or new primary neoplasm. If the patient is stable and the diagnosis is in question, biopsy or excision may be reasonable.

Treatment

The loss of function and pain associated with the pathologic fracture of an extremity requires careful consideration for the stability of any long bone affected by neoplasm in all but the most dire of circumstances. Prophylactic surgical stabilization is preferred over repair after a pathologic fracture and such surgery generally takes precedence over other forms of local intervention like radiation. More than 50% of pathologic fractures involve the femur and the bone cortex is responsible for bone strength; risk factors for fracture include cortical lesion greater than or equal to 2.5 cm or if the cortex is eroded more than halfway. Mirel's scoring system can be used to evaluate the structural integrity of an affected long bone in a quantitative fashion by summing point values for the following four factors (points = 1/2/3): pain (mild/moderate/severe), location (upper limb/lower limb/peritrochanteric), cortical destruction ($<\frac{1}{3}/\frac{1}{3}-\frac{2}{3}/>\frac{2}{3}$), and appearance on plain film (blastic/mixed/lytic) (Ratanatharathorn and Powers 2008). The numerical result is from 4 to 12 with surgical intervention considered for a score of 9 or more (since a score of 8 points is said to carry a 15% fracture risk versus 9 points with 33% risk). While normally not functionally debilitating, pathologic fracture of the axial skeleton, particularly the vertebrae, can cause pain and alter body stature. Open or percutaneous vertebroplasty with methylmethacrylate can be effective, though caution is appropriate to ensure that the cementing agent does not enter the spinal canal.

After an appropriate time for healing from such invasive procedures, patients may be considered for a course of local radiation therapy. In situations where surgical stabilization is not performed, radiation therapy can be used to lower the risk for subsequent pathologic fracture and decrease pain. When applied to discrete, symptomatic lesions, roughly 70% of patients receive at least partial alleviation of pain and about half of these experience complete resolution after a course of external beam treatment. The question of dose and fractionation is left to the discretion of the treating physicians and should be individualized based on considerations of life expectancy, treatment area, patient desires or expectations, and remaining quality of life. Several randomized trials worldwide have explored single and multifraction treatment paradigms that have been the subject of many consequent reviews (Hartsell 2005; Rasmusson and Vejborg 1995; Sze and Shelley 2003). Predictably, breast, lung, and prostate cancer affecting the spine, pelvis, or extremities accounted for the lion's share of treatments, so dose recommendations

may not apply to relatively radioresistant or responsive tumors. The overriding conclusions from these investigations are that similar pain relief occurs with absolute doses over 8 Gy regardless of the total dose or fractionation and the following thus provide equivalent analgesia: 8 Gy in 1 fraction, 20 Gy in 4 or 5 fractions, and 30 Gy in 10–15 fractions with the caveat that there is a 2–3 times higher rate of retreatment noted in those receiving a single fraction (Ratanatharathorn and Powers 2008). From this, some radiation oncologists hold that the increase in the need for retreatment justifies the higher cost of administering multiple fractions, particularly in patients with a longer life expectancy, while other practitioners will accept this retreatment rate and prefer single-fraction treatment to moderate the initial use of scarce resources (be it the patient's time or the direct cost of therapy). Interestingly, radiation oncologists in the United States were significantly more likely to prefer multifraction therapy versus their Canadian equivalents who generally recommended a single fraction (Fairchild and Barnes 2009).

Aside from dose and fractionation issues, the delineation of the target volume or radiation treatment portals offers the potential for significant individualization of therapy, notably when there are multiple sites of osseous disease. For example, using a half-beam block or angling beams to decrease divergence inferiorly or superiorly when treating spine metastases, may allow for further treatment to nearby areas at a later date with less concern for potential overlap from the original treatment field(s). Also helpful, accurate and readily available record keeping can precisely identify collateral areas treated in previous fields that might be less radiation-tolerant than bone which can then impact therapy recommendations. Regardless of the situation, the goals of therapy should be clearly managed and articulated to the patient and family along with realistic estimations of success whenever possible. The threshold for treatment-related morbidity should be low and prophylactic or as-needed medications should be available. The target should always be treated with a minimum of risk. Toward this end, build-up regions may be shortened and treatment breaks necessary. When multiple areas of treatment are required that may endanger hematologic reserves from the amount of bone marrow radiated or threaten too much gastrointestinal morbidity, a stepwise method to therapy is appropriate or systemic approaches can be employed. Additionally, the timing of radiotherapy is important; initiating treatment at a lower pain threshold or before narcotic analgesics are employed both increases analgesic response while protecting against structural breakdown and possible failure.

When initial radiation therapy fails, retreatment of previously radiated bones, particularly in the spine, introduces the specter of severe radiation-induced ▶ myelopathy. Thankfully, such events are rare enough that construction of precise dose–volume relationships for human subjects has been impossible. We are left with using animal models, imaging (rather than clinical findings) and amalgamating such data with case and series reports of myelopathy in the human literature. To wit, the risk of Grade 2 or higher myelopathy with treatment of the full cervical spinal cord thickness and length of less than 5 cm at 1.8–2 Gy is less than 1% at 54 Gy, less than 10% at 61 Gy, and 50% at 69 Gy with a recently reported $\alpha/\beta = 0.87$ Gy (which predicts more damage at higher dose per fraction versus the more accepted $\alpha/\beta = 2$–4 Gy (Kirkpatrick and van der Kogel 2010)). As a late reacting tissue, the spinal cord does have delayed radiation repair capacity and most would agree that allowing 6 months or longer to pass from the initial therapy is optimal before retreating an area of the cord (Nieder and Grosu 2005). Clearly then, it would not be appropriate to treat an area of the spinal cord with two courses of 30 Gy over

10 fractions, particularly if only a short time has intervened, unless life expectancy was severely abrogated. The remaining options are to alter the treatment, total dose, and/or fractionation, defer therapy, or employ stereotactic body radiotherapy (SBRT or ▶ stereotactic radiosurgery – extracranial or ▶ robotic radiosurgery). SBRT has been used effectively for various lesions in close proximity to the spinal cord with only occasional reports of myelopathy which seem related to the maximum point doses within the thecal sac (danger when exceeding 10 Gy in 1 fraction or a biologically equivalent dose of 30–35 Gy for up to 5 fractions) (Sahgal and Ma 2010). Groups have reported satisfactory results treating spinal metastases recurring in previously treated fields by single and multifraction approaches with few instances of severe myelopathy (Choi and Alder 2010). Detailed dose–volume recommendations are still being worked out as is application into the community, but SBRT seems to have potential to help with this very complicated patient subset.

Systemic therapy has the potential to reach all areas of metastases concurrently and does not have the same anatomical restrictions as external beam radiation. Depending on the type of cancer, any of a number of cytotoxic chemotherapeutic agents may be germane. Traditionally, success or response is measured by serial imaging exams, however achievement of pain relief or more general improvement in quality of life may be a more reasonable alternative measure of the attainment of palliative therapy. Hormone blockade or modulation can also be extremely effective, particularly with metastatic prostate and breast cancer. In keeping with the philosophy of early intervention, it may be better to initiate hormone therapy soon after the diagnosis of metastatic disease rather than waiting for more severe symptoms to develop. Through their protective effects on bone density, and perhaps intrinsic antitumor activity, ▶ bisphosphonates are employed in patients with osteolytic bone metastases (particularly breast cancer) to decrease skeletal complications and maintain quality of life. Adverse effects associated with bisphosphonates include renal toxicity and mandibular osteonecrosis.

Intravenously introduced ► targeted radionuclide therapy, like strontium-89 (Sr-89), samarium-153 ethylenediaminetetramethylenephosphoric acid (Sm-153), and historically phosphorus-32 (P-32), are preferentially deposited into newly forming bone. Once incorporated, beta rays (for Sr-89, Sm-153 and P-32) and/or gamma rays (Sm-153) are emitted as part of the normal decay process and elicit the palliative effect. Localized uptake on Tc-99m bone scan is a good surrogate for the likely effectiveness of Sr-89 or Sm-153 since the biochemical mode of isotope localization is shared. Likewise, the concurrent use of a bisphosphonate could limit the deposition of the isotopes and hence therapeutic benefit by decreasing pathologic bone turnover. Naturally, radiopharmaceutical research has focused on metastatic prostate carcinoma given its prevalence and predilection for multiple osteoblastic, Tc-99m bone scan avid lesions. As might be expected, the main side effect from these medicines is hematologic, though renal and hepatic dysfunction are possible as well.

Sr-89 has a half-life of 50.6 days and emits electrons only, so supplementary functional imaging (with Tc-99m bone scan) is required to show areas of probable deposition if posttreatment scanning is desired. The majority of energy from Sm-153 (physical half-life 1.9 days and effective half-life less than 8 hours with normal renal function) is transmitted by electrons while a low energy gamma ray (0.1 mm lead half value layer) is helpful for imaging after therapy, so no posttherapy Tc-99m injection is needed. Electrons from Sr-89 are more energetic (average 583 keV) than with Sm-153 (average 233 keV) with a mean range of 3 mm and 0.5 mm in soft tissue, respectively (Finlay and Mason 2005). Hematologic reserve limits treatment with both

► radiopharmaceuticals. Caution is advised for Sr-89 therapy when platelets are below 60,000/µl and white cell count below 2,400/µl; for Sm-153, the limits are 100,000/µl and 3,000/µl, respectively. Precaution with Sm-153 is also appropriate in patients with disseminated intravascular coagulation, absolute neutrophil count less than 1,500/µl, hemoglobin less than 10 g/dL, or renal insufficiency – such conditions may also give pause before therapy with Sr-89. Sr-89 is given either as a 148 MBq (4 mCi) slow IV injection over 1–2 min or calculated as 1.5–2.2 MBq/kg (40–60 µCi/kg) versus 37 MBq/kg (or 1 mCi/kg) of Sm-153 given IV over 1 min with oral or IV hydration before and after to aid in efficient renal clearance. Roughly 14 days posttherapy, weekly or biweekly complete blood counts are monitored until bone marrow recovery. Owing to the different decay kinetics, the nadir platelet levels for Sr-89 are reached between 12 and 16 weeks after treatment in contrast to the most severe thrombocytopenia or neutropenia which is regularly seen at 4–6 weeks for Sm-153 (Finlay and Mason 2005). Roughly 15% of patients will experience a ► pain flare, or transient worsening in bone pain, that should subside within one week (ad hoc analgesics can be prescribed for this). Pain relief is generally noted to begin in one to two weeks and reach a plateau in four to six weeks; as a conservative guideline, 25% of patients are expected to have no response to the drug, 50% will have a partial decrement in pain, and 25% will have complete resolution of pain with the response lasting around three to four months (Ratanatharathorn and Powers 2008). Both agents have shown similar efficacy in reducing pain associated with diffuse osseous metastases and can be used more than once and/or in concert with a course of localized external beam radiation; trials have also shown response with concurrent use of chemotherapy, usually for metastatic prostate cancer (Finlay and Mason 2005). The shorter half-life, and therefore less onerous

P

radiation safety measures, required capability of functional imaging soon after the procedure without additional radionuclide injection, less penetrating beta particle, and faster recovery of bone marrow function are advantages with Sm-153. The longer experience and pure beta particle emission are benefits of Sr-89.

Cross-References

► Economics
► Pain Management
► Palliation of Brain and Spinal Cord Metastases
► Principles of Chemotherapy
► Robotic Radiosurgery
► Stereotactic Radiosurgery: Extracranial
► Supportive Care and Quality of Life
► Targeted Radionuclide Therapy

References

Choi C, Alder J (2010) Stereotactic radiosurgery for treatment of spinal metastases recurring in close proximity to previously irradiated spinal cord. Int J Radiat Oncol Biol Phys 78:499–506

Fairchild A, Barnes E (2009) International patterns of practice in palliative radiotherapy for painful bone metastases: evidence-based practice. Int J Radiat Oncol Biol Phys 75:1501–1510

Finlay I, Mason M (2005) Radioisotopes for the palliation of metastatic bone cancer: a systemic review. Lancet Oncol 6:392–400

Kirkpatrick J, van der Kogel A (2010) Radiation dose-volume effects in the spinal cord. Int J Radiat Oncol Biol Phys 76:S42–S49

Nieder C, Grosu A (2005) Proposal of human spinal cord reirradiation dose based on collection of data from 40 patients. Int J Radiat Oncol Biol Phys 61:851–855

Rasmusson B, Vejborg I (1995) Irradiation of bone metastases in breast cancer patients: A randomized study with 1 year follow-up. Radiother Oncol 34:179–184

Ratanatharathorn V, Powers W (2008) Role of radionuclide therapy as adjuvant to external beam. In: Brady L, Perez C (eds) Principles and practice of radiation oncology, 5th edn

Sahgal A, Ma L (2010) Spinal cord tolerance for stereotactic body radiotherapy. Int J Radiat Oncol Biol Phys 77:548–553

Sze W, Shelley M (2003) Palliation of metastatic bone pain: single fraction versus multifraction radiotherapy – a systemic review of randomized trials. Clin Oncol 12:345–352

Palliation of Brain and Spinal Cord Metastases

JAMES H. BRASHEARS, III
Radiation Oncologist, Venice, FL, USA

Synonyms

Treatment or management of central nervous system involvement or dissemination

Definition/Description

Metastases to the central nervous system (CNS) are an increasingly identified cause of severe morbidity in cancer patients. Anatomically confined and serially organized, the brain and spinal cord are exquisitely sensitive to space-occupying lesions and inflammation. Involvement of the brain and spinal cord compression frequently require prompt multimodality management, with medical, surgical, and radiation interventions including whole brain radiation therapy (WBRT) and/or stereotactic radiosurgery (SRS).

Background

Of the roughly half million people who die from cancer annually, up to 30% have brain metastases and 10% have involvement of the spinal cord. Ten times more common than primary CNS neoplasm, the vast majority of brain metastases are from lung cancer, while breast cancer and melanoma account for the second and third most frequent primary sites, respectively (Kwok and Patchell 2008). Half of brain metastases are solitary and the rest multiple, the majority located supratentorially (Videtic and Gaspar 2009). Metastatic spinal cord compression is mostly related to breast, lung, or prostate carcinoma. Excepting small cell lung cancer, the median survival after radiation therapy with brain metastases or metastatic spinal cord compression is 3–6 months, though certain subsets like the chemotherapy naïve may survive longer than 1 year (Linskey and Andrews 2010). Goals of therapy are to limit or improve symptoms that are predominantly related to effects from tumor growth, inflammation, vascular compromise, or structural instability, thus contributing both to quality of life and potential longevity.

Initial Evaluation

Brain metastases can present with hemiparesis, headache, focal weakness, ataxia, seizure, aphasia, and cognitive, mental, or sensory changes. Patients with emergent spinal cord compression may have localized or diffuse back pain, weakness (even to the point of paralysis), sensory alterations, urinary/fecal incontinence, erectile dysfunction, and abnormal reflexes. Such symptoms and signs should trigger suspicion in any patient with a previous history of cancer, long-term cigarette use, genetic predilection, or significant environmental exposure. The most important prognostic variable is performance status, while age, extra-CNS disease, number of CNS metastases, and histology may also be used to estimate overall survival (NCCN 2010). Functional outcome also depends on time to development of severe symptoms, specifically, a longer period of time elapsing from first symptom (often pain) to motor deficits before therapy for metastatic spinal cord compression portends a higher likelihood of improvement and maintenance of ambulatory ability (Kwok and Patchell 2008).

Differential Diagnosis

Circulatory compromise, abscess, trauma, or primary neoplasm affecting CNS structures may yield similar symptoms and imaging findings as CNS metastases depending on location of the pathology.

Imaging Studies

With suspicion for brain metastases and if the patient meets safety criteria, magnetic resonance imaging (MRI) of the head with standard dose contrast is most appropriate (high-dose contrast is appropriate if SRS is contemplated) (ACR 2009). Probably, the most useful sequences are the contrast-enhanced T1 and fluid-attenuated inversion-recovery (FLAIR) data sets. Similarly, MRI of the spine with standard dose contrast should be performed when there is concern for metastatic spinal cord compression. ▶ Epidural spinal cord compression, as the name implies, requires compression of the contents of the dural sac by an extrinsic mass for diagnosis. Identification of any metastatic CNS lesion, particularly in the spinal cord, prompts MRI of the entire CNS axis owing to the risk of concurrent, multifocal involvement (NCCN 2010). In cases where patient or institutional factors preclude MRI, the less sensitive contrast-enhanced computed tomography (CT) scan should be carried out; in the case of metastatic spinal cord compression, consideration of CT myelography is appropriate. Similarly, follow-up after treatment is based on regular history and physicals and contrast-enhanced MRI every 3 months or as clinically indicated (NCCN 2010).

Treatment

Corticosteroids are the cornerstone of initial therapy for symptomatic CNS metastases, though it may mask an underlying lymphoproliferative disorder if there is a question as to the pathologic diagnosis. A loading dose of 10 mg intravenous dexamethasone and subsequent maintenance with 4 mg every 6 h or 6 mg every 8 h and concurrent antiulcer medication is acceptable (Kwok and Patchell 2008). The steroid can be transitioned to an equipotent oral form with an appropriate taper once symptoms are controlled. Anticonvulsant therapy is necessary for patients presenting with seizures, but should not be given in a prophylactic fashion. Institution of cytotoxic chemotherapy may also be useful for extremely chemo-sensitive malignancies like myeloma, lymphoma, or germ cell tumors when there is a paucity of symptoms and structural integrity is not an issue (NCCN 2010).

Importantly, neurosurgical intervention should be considered early since resection can yield immediate relief of pressure exerted from extrinsic or intrinsic masses, stabilize potential skeletal fragility, and promote rapid restitution of compromised neural function in addition to providing specimens for pathologic examination. Thanks, in no small part, to Patchell's yeoman service, we know that:

1. Patients with ▶ single brain metastasis benefit from surgical resection and subsequent WBRT versus WBRT alone in terms of median overall survival, local recurrence, time-to-local failure, time to neurologic death, maintenance of Karnofsky performance status (or KPS), and maintenance of functional independence – good surrogates for quality of life.
2. Postoperative WBRT after surgical extirpation of single brain metastasis increases local control at the site of resection and in other areas of the brain, but does not change the length of overall survival or functional independence.
3. Patients with paraplegia from metastatic spinal cord compression benefit from decompressive surgery (not posterior laminectomy alone) with spinal stabilization and radiation therapy versus radiation therapy alone in terms of maintenance or recovery of the ability to walk, continence, pain control, and overall survival.

Taken together, surgical resection of patients with single brain metastases followed by whole brain radiation therapy is preferable in patients with a reasonable life expectancy and good performance status. Likewise, surgical decompression and stabilization followed by local radiation is recommended for operable patients with metastatic spinal cord compression.

External beam radiation therapy remains standard for the management of metastases to the CNS. The target volume for whole brain treatment is all intracranial contents inclusive of the cribriform plate and temporal fossa. Traditionally, WBRT is accomplished by opposed lateral fields with some consideration given to avoiding divergence into the lenses of the eyes. The portals extend inferiorly to somewhere between the foramen magnum and the second cervical vertebrae and flash in the anterior, posterior, and superior dimensions. Conventional radiation fields for metastatic spinal cord compression extend superiorly and inferiorly for one vertebral body (about 2 cm) and are wide enough to cover the entire affected vertebral body or lesion with room for build up (usually at least 8 cm wide). Depending on body habitus and lesion location, opposed lateral beams are often appropriate for targets in the cervical spine, a single posterior (PA) field for the thoracic spine, and an anterior/posterior pair (AP/PA) for the lumbar spine. As always, modern treatment planning systems allow for more accurate dose-volume evaluation and can help appraise the relative benefits of each approach vis-à-vis coverage of the lesion and potential overdosage of the spinal cord or other normal structures. The standard dose and fractionation scheme is 30 Gy in 10 fractions (Kwok and Patchell 2008). More abbreviated courses for CNS radiotherapy are possible (20 Gy in 5 fractions for WBRT or 8 Gy in 1 fraction for metastatic spinal cord compression) when life expectancy of the patient obviates any risk of late radiation neural toxicity and with the caveat that there is an increased rate of retreatment with hypofractionation. So far, no concurrent radiosensitizer has been shown conclusively as an effective adjunct to radiation therapy though studies are ongoing (Kwok and Patchell 2008).

In lieu of open surgery, SRS offers a noninvasive opportunity to deposit a large biological equivalent dose of radiation to tumor with millimeter or submillimeter accuracy with a single treatment. Using a variety of different methods, SRS can address one or multiple tumors so long as each is less than 10 cc in volume (typically less than 3 cm in average diameter) with a single fraction. Recommended doses often depend on target diameter – less than 2 cm, 24 Gy; 2–3 cm, 18 Gy; 3–4 cm, 15 Gy (NCCN 2010). Maximum point dose to the optic nerves should be kept less than 8 Gy while the brainstem and visual pathways should be kept less than 12 Gy. Lesion-specific local control with SRS and whole brain local control with SRS and WBRT are comparable to surgery with and without WBRT in newly diagnosed patients with single lesions less than 2–3 cm in diameter causing minimal mass effect and KPS of at least 70 (Linskey and Andrews 2010). For this subset of patients, the use of SRS after WBRT appears to yield improved survival versus WBRT alone. In general, when SRS is used for brain metastases without WBRT, there is an increased risk of intracranial failure, though this may not change survival; therefore, careful surveillance is advised in circumstances when WBRT is neglected. About 5% of patients have symptomatic radiation-related brain necrosis that is usually addressed satisfactorily with anti-inflammatory medications like corticosteroids with surgery reserved for intractable cases (Linskey and Andrews 2010).

For recurrent or residual brain and spinal cord metastases, the decision of how to proceed depends on previous treatment, disease response to previous treatment, the amount of time intervening since therapy, the clinical situation, patient/caregiver desires, and resource availability. The decision to retreat an area of the CNS should not be taken lightly owing to the critical role these normal structures play in maintaining functionality and quality of life; however, this risk is moderated by the truncated life expectancy typical in this clinical situation. Late radiation-induced neural toxicity usually takes from 6 to 18 months to begin; tolerance doses to treatment given at 1.8–2 Gy per fraction giving 5% or less risk of severe side effects are thought to be 45 Gy for the whole brain, 60 Gy for partial brain

volumes, and 50–54 Gy for lengths of the spinal cord less than 10 cm. These estimates are affected in unknown ways based on patient factors, background therapy, and repair of radiation damage that takes 6 months or more to complete. For brain metastases, previous WBRT does not preclude a repeat of therapy albeit with an attenuated dose and fractionation (at least 20 Gy in 1.8–2 Gy fractions) (Kwok and Patchell 2008). When lesion size, location, and number are appropriate, SRS or surgery may also be used after previous WBRT, SRS, and/or surgery (NCCN 2010). Corticosteroids will often be used for symptom management. When asymptomatic, chemotherapy or other systemic agents can be attempted to control CNS metastasis. Likewise, with careful consideration, surgery with further stabilization, conventional external beam radiotherapy, and extracranial SRS may have a role in managing recurrent metastatic spinal cord compression.

Cross-References

▶ Pain Management
▶ Principles of Chemotherapy
▶ Robotic Radiosurgery
▶ Stereotactic Radiosurgery – Cranial
▶ Stereotactic Radiosurgery: Extracranial
▶ Supportive Care and Quality of Life

References

ACR (2009) ACR appropriateness criteria: pre-irradiation evaluation. American College of Radiology

Kwok Y, Patchell R (2008) Palliation of brain and spinal cord metastases. In: Perez C, Halperin E (eds) Principles and practice of radiation oncology, 5th edn. Lippincott Williams and Wilkins, Philadelphia, pp 1974–1985

Linskey M, Andrews D (2010) The role of stereotactic radiosurgery in the management of patients with newly diagnosed brain metastases: a systemic review and evidence-based clinical practice guidelines. J Neurooncol 96:45–68

NCCN (2010) Central nervous system cancers v.1.2010. National Comprehensive Cancer Network, Fort Washington

Videtic G, Gaspar L (2009) American College of Radiology appropriateness criteria on multiple brain metastases. Int J Radiat Oncol Biol Phys 75:961–965

Palliation of Metastatic Disease to the Liver

Lydia T. Komarnicky-Kocher[1], Fiori Alite[2]
[1]Department of Radiation Oncology,
College of Medicine, Drexel University,
Philadelphia, PA, USA
[2]College of Medicine, Drexel University,
Philadelphia, PA, USA

Synonyms

Colorectal metastases to liver; Hepatic metastasis

Definition/Description

The liver's rich dual blood supply predisposes it to metastases from essentially every organ, and the large flow of blood from the gastrointestinal tract via the portal circulation makes it particularly susceptible to metastatic spread from primary gastrointestinal malignancies. Liver metastases are a significant cause of morbidity and mortality in cancer patients, particularly in ▶ colorectal cancer. Symptoms can include abdominal pain, referred right shoulder pain, nausea, and vomiting. A colorectal primary most commonly manifests with liver metastases, yet breast cancer, lung cancer, melanoma, and other GI malignancies also often metastasize to the liver. The presence of liver metastases was classically considered as a very poor prognostic factor and many times treatment was not pursued. Recently, success from local and systemic therapies has lead to a paradigm shift where carefully selected patients can be cured by the treatment of hepatic metastases. Still, median survival without treatment currently ranges between 5 and 10 months. The management of liver metastases spans several modalities including surgery, chemotherapy, radiation, and several novel techniques like chemoembolization, *radioembolization*, ▶ radiofrequency ablation, cryoablation, and ethanol injection. Carefully selected patients can be surgically resected and exhibit a 5 year survival of 30–40%. Radiation therapy plays an important and growing palliative role when patients are not candidates for any form of surgical or other invasive procedure. Recent advances in stereotactic body radiosurgery (▶ SBRT) and cyberknife ▶ robotic radiosurgery offer a more targeted, noninvasive anticancer option in the management of liver metastases.

Clinical Presentation

Liver metastases are most often detected after a metastatic workup for a primary malignancy, but patients can also present with liver metastases with a primary malignancy that is detected thereafter. As many as 15% of patients with colorectal cancer can present with liver metastases, and as many as 60% develop them during the course of their disease. Presentation can include right upper quadrant abdominal pain, anorexia, weight loss, nausea, and vomiting. Extensive liver dissemination by metastases or biliary obstruction can result in jaundice, confusion, and lethargy. Laboratory studies can suggest liver metastases but are not as sensitive as the multiple modalities that have been developed to image the liver. On physical exam, hepatomegaly may be appreciated and nodularity may be palpated on the free edge of the liver.

Work Up

Detecting liver metastases early and accurately has gained clinical importance since the advent of new local management modalities. Computerized tomography, abdominal ultrasound, and magnetic resonance imaging have improved in sensitivity and specificity for detecting and quantifying liver metastases, and it is important to employ imaging appropriately in order to qualify patients for surgical resection or the various ablative therapies.

Ultrasonography is a cost-effective and efficient instrument in detecting liver metastases and is the most often used test to screen for metastases in a cancer patient. It is most useful for detecting superficial lesions, and often the sensitivity and specificity of ultrasound is operator dependant. Computerized tomography (CT) has been used for many years to visualize liver metastases and has proven to be a very sensitive instrument for detection. Noncontrast CT lacks specificity and is not as sensitive in detecting hypovascular lesions, but the addition of radiopaque intravenous contrast improves detection. Intravenous contrast is usually infused over a 2 min timeframe, with repeated imaging to capture any enhancing lesions in different phases of enhancement. The arterial phase occurs 25 s after infusion and the portal venous phase requires a 60 s delay. Most metastases can be visualized during the venous filling phase, since the normal liver parenchyma enhances, and hypovascular lesions such as colorectal metastases do not and often display contrast filling defects. Scanning a patient after a 4–6 h delay from contrast infusion (delayed contrast CT) can be useful in identifying metastatic lesions which appear hypodense, since most do not retain contrast when compared with surrounding normal liver parenchyma. Magnetic resonance imaging (MRI) can detect liver metastases with similar sensitivity and specificity to CT, and together the two modalities can detect up to 2/3 of liver metastases. T2-weighted images with gadolinium enhancement display metastatic lesions as less bright and heterogeneous than benign cysts, hemangiomas, or normal liver parenchyma.

Both CT and MR angiography can also be employed to evaluate the liver vasculature in relation to metastases.

Positron emission tomography (PET) can be employed to evaluate for extrahepatic metastasis when staging patients for surgical resection or to evaluate response after treatment.

Laboratory Studies

Although not as sensitive as imaging modalities, perturbations in laboratory analysis of liver function may suggest the presence of liver metastases or a malignancy in a patient, and can often prompt imaging which identifies the liver metastases. The basic liver function tests include alkaline phosphatase, bilirubin, ▶ albumin, prothrombin time, lactate dehydrogenase, alanine aminotransferase, and aspartate aminotransferase. Carcinoembryonic Antigen (CEA) is a very sensitive oncofetal serum marker that is often elevated in the setting of colorectal cancer with liver metastases. Although the liver can sustain a significant destruction of its parenchyma with neoplasm without detectable changes of liver function, extensive dissemination or biliary tract obstruction can result in nonspecific elevated liver enzymes, or a cholestatic pattern. Elevated liver enzymes in the setting of iron deficiency anemia in an older patient suggest the possibility of a colorectal primary with liver metastases, and workup should focus on ruling out malignancy with a colonoscopy and CEA.

Epidemiology

Liver metastases are the most common type of liver malignancy. The true prevalence is difficult to establish since most case series are derived from autopsies of patients dying at the end stage, disseminated point of their disease. Approximately 30–70% of patients dying of cancer exhibit metastases to the liver. In a prospective series by Bydder et al. (2003) in 28 patients with symptomatic liver metastases causing either pain, abdominal distention, night sweats or nausea and vomiting, 39% were due to colorectal cancer. There are approximately 50,000 cases of liver metastases from colorectal cancer every year in the United States.

Differential Diagnosis

Involvement of the liver by a metastatic neoplastic process is far more common than a primary neoplasm of the liver. In the setting of a known primary malignancy, especially colorectal, multiple lesions detected by imaging in the liver is highly suggestive of metastases. Still, when patients present with a liver lesion, it is important to consider the extensive radiographic differential which includes many benign liver lesions. Normal vascular anatomy can be confused with small metastatic lesions, and hemangiomas and cysts appear similar to highly vascular tumors (islet cell, renal, carcinoid) on MRI. On CT, fatty infiltration appears similar to metastases or hepatocellular carcinoma and abscesses can appear similar to adenomas. If the identity of the liver lesion(s) still remains nebulous after considering the clinical evidence and imaging, a liver biopsy to confirm the diagnosis can be considered.

Treatment

When considering the management of liver metastases, an important distinction must be made considering the goal of treatment. Colorectal metastases without signs of dissemination are managed by surgical resection, higher doses of radiotherapy, and other techniques like radiofrequency ablation since the goal is prolonging survival. When considering other primary neoplastic sites with liver metastasis or in more extensive metastatic disease, adjuvant radiotherapy, chemotherapy, and other techniques can be employed with the goal of palliating symptoms.

Surgery

Resection of hepatic metastasis has emerged as a growing form of management in carefully selected patients, and offers the best chance for prolonging survival. The emerging literature shows that as much as 25% of patients with colorectal metastases can be cured by surgical resection, but the data is disappointing when considering other primary sites. Resection of liver metastases from breast cancer primaries is currently controversial, with a recent case series showing that only 18 out of 108 patients were alive at 5 years after resection of breast cancer liver metastases (Pocard et al. 2000).

Preoperative evaluation of patients is crucial in identifying candidates that will benefit from resection and includes evaluating patient medical fitness for surgery, the tumor biology, as well as the anatomical position of the tumor. Resectability for colorectal metastases is defined based on the ability to obtain a wide (>1 cm) resection margin while being able to preserve two contiguous hepatic segments with adequate vascular flow and biliary drainage and/or the ability to preserve at least >20% healthy liver remnant. The presence of extrahepatic disease is no longer an absolute contraindication if margin-free resection is feasible for both the intrahepatic and extrahepatic disease. Earlier techniques focused on resection of larger liver components with lobectomies being the standard of care. Recent advances in surgical techniques, like ▶ total vascular exclusion and intraoperative ultrasound, as well as minimally invasive techniques have allowed for greater preservation of liver parenchyma and offer patients a more effective operation with less perioperative morbidity.

Outcomes after surgical resection continue to improve as techniques advance with a focus toward qualifying more patients for resection. Five-year survival has increased from 31% to 58% from the 1980s to patients treated from 1993 to 1999. The most favorable patients are those with solitary liver metastases, enjoying overall 5 year survival as high as 71%. Fong et al. (1999) have developed a clinical score, based on five preoperative risk factors that incorporate tumor biology, as a prognostic assessment tool. Node positivity, disease-free interval less than 12 months, more than one tumor, size greater than 5 cm, and CEA greater than 200 ng/mL all add points to the clinical score and higher scores correlate with decreased survival.

Chemotherapy

Chemotherapy is readily employed when there is disseminated disease outside the liver or the number of metastatic lesions is too numerous to control by local means. Delivery methods include systemic chemotherapy or via direct delivery into the hepatic artery. Since liver metastases are preferentially perfused by the hepatic artery, and normal liver parenchyma is usually supplied by the portal vein, direct delivery into the hepatic artery can be exploited to achieve higher drug levels at the tumor site and to minimize systemic toxicity.

The local response rate with intravenous chemotherapy varies depending on the primary site and the extent of disease, with ranges of response rates of 40–50% in patients with breast cancer, gastric cancer, and colon cancer. Utilizing direct hepatic artery infusion of chemotherapeutic agents results in 20–30% improvement in local control rates. Infusion is achieved via an injection pump which is attached to a surgically implanted hepatic artery catheter. The most readily utilized agent is 5-fluoro-2′-deoxyuridine (floxuridine, FUDR), which is usually delivered slowly over a period of 2 weeks.

The differential vascularity of liver malignancies has also been exploited with hepatic artery ligation and hepatic artery embolization which cuts off blood supply to the tumor. An extension to these methods is hepatic artery chemoembolization which involves the local entrapment of a chemotherapeutic drug in the embolization agent or microspheres, in an attempt to provide prolonged local exposure of the chemotherapeutic agent to the tumor. Chemoembolization with the preferential hypoxic cell killer mytomycin C has been employed to target difficult-to-treat hypoxic tumor cells. Monoclonal antitumor antibodies have also been attached to microspheres and continue to be employed in therapy.

Radiation Therapy

Historically, radiation therapy has played a minor role in the management of hepatic metastases due to the low tolerance of the liver to radiation. Yet, just as the guidelines for liver resection have broadened, the emergence of more conformal radiotherapy techniques and the various ablative procedures have allowed for a greater amount of previously unresectable patients to be considered for definitive treatment. This has moved the role of radiotherapy in the management of hepatic metastases from a palliative modality to a more definitive form of management. As with surgery, a sharp distinction must be made between colorectal metastases and those from other cancers, since the response to radiotherapy is greater with colorectal metastases, and more varied and indeterminate with other cancers. Conventional radiotherapy, stereotactic body radiotherapy, cyberknife robotic radiosurgery, as well as yttrium-90 microspheres radioembolization are methods available for definitive treatment in selected patients.

The initial experience with conventionally fractionated external beam radiation therapy to the whole liver was often successful in palliating symptoms in most patients, but the relative radiosensitivity of the normal liver parenchyma often limited the cumulative dose due to accumulated toxicity. The development of ▶ Radiation-Induced Liver Disease (RILD) is a dose-limiting complication of radiotherapy, which can progress to fulminant liver failure and death. RILD usually develops several weeks to months after radiation treatment and is a clinical syndrome comprised of pain, hepatomegaly, ascites, and elevated liver enzymes. Tissue tolerance of the liver demonstrates that 5% of patients develop RILD when 1/3rd reaches 5000 cGy, 2/3rds reach 3500 cGy and whole liver reaches 5000 cGy exposure within five years of treatment. Plus 50% of patients exposed to more than 4000 cGy to the whole liver will suffer RILD and liver failure within five years. Thus whole liver radiotherapy is generally limited to palliation.

Just as surgical techniques evolved away from anatomical resections toward metastatectomies in order to spare normal liver parenchyma, 3D conformal planning has moved radiotherapy toward delivering higher doses to precisely defined portions of the liver. In this way, the percentage of normal liver receiving radiation can be quantified, evaluated with a dose–volume histogram and limited to prevent RILD. With regard to liver tolerance, a normal tissue complication probability model has been developed to predict volumes of normal liver that must be spared to prevent development of RILD. The use of this model as well as more advanced conformal treatment planning has allowed for the delivery of much higher doses (70–90 Gy) to tumor volumes safely. With regard to colorectal metastases, conformal treatment planning has allowed for delivery of tumoricidal doses of 70 Gy and long-term follow-up has shown 1 year and 2 year overall survival of 80 and 30%, respectively. Improved local control rates have also been reported with the incorporation of hepatic artery delivery of fluorodeoxyuridine (FUdR) concurrently with radiation therapy since it exploits the circulatory dependence of liver tumors on the hepatic arterial system and FUdR acts as a radiosensitizer (Swaminath and Dawson 2011).

Palliation

External beam radiotherapy can also be employed for palliative goals. Most of the studies on palliation of liver metastases have been conducted in patients where survival is judged to be at least 3 months, and when used appropriately, relief of symptoms can be accomplished within weeks of treatment with limited toxicity. Patients that expect to enjoy the most benefit are usually ambulatory, have a bilirubin level below 1.5 mg/dl, and have significant pain secondary to liver metastases. Pain relief as a result of radiotherapy has been reported subjectively as mild-moderate for as many as 60–80% of patients meeting the above criteria. In prospective trials where 10 Gy was delivered in 2 fractions to the symptomatic portion of the liver within 6–24 h, symptoms, pain, nausea, and vomiting were reported as improved in 63%, 44%, and 100%, respectively. When asked if patients believed the treatment had been helpful to them, 75% reported in the affirmative (Bydder et al. 2003).

Cross-References

▶ Colon Cancer
▶ Esophagus Cancer
▶ External Beam Radiation Therapy
▶ Liver and Hepatobiliary Tract
▶ Lung Cancer
▶ Melanoma
▶ Palliation
▶ Pancreatic Cancer
▶ Radiation-Induced Liver Disease (also RILD)
▶ Radioactive Microsphere Embolization (of Liver Tumors)
▶ Radiofrequency Ablation
▶ Rectal Cancer

References

Altekruse SF, Kosary CL, Krapcho M et al (2010) SEER cancer statistics review, 1975–2007, National Cancer Institute. Bethesda. http://seer.cancer.gov/csr/1975_2007/, based on Nov 2009 SEER data submission, posted to the SEER web site

Brown BE, Bower MR, Martin RCG (2010) Hepatic resection for colorectal liver metastases. Surg Clin N Am 90:839–852

Bydder S, Spry NA, Christie DH et al (2003) A prospective trial of short-fractionation radiotherapy for the palliation of liver metastases. Aust Radiol 47:284–288

Charnsangavej C, Clary B, Fong Y, Grothey A, Pawlik TM, Choti MA (2006) Selection of patients for resection of hepatic colorectal metastases: expert consensus statement. Ann Surg Oncol 13(10):1261–1268

Dawson L, Lawrence T (2004) The role of radiotherapy in the treatment of liver metastases. Cancer J 10(2):139–144

Fong Y, Fortner J, Sun RL et al (1999) Clinical score for predicting recurrence after hepatic resection for metastatic colorectal cancer: analysis of 1001 consecutive cases. Ann Surg 230:309

Gaspar LE (2008) Liver metastases. In: Halperin EC, Perez CA, Brady LW (eds) Principles and practice of radiation oncology, 5th edn. Wolters Kluwer/Lippincott Williams & Wilkins, Philadelphia

Kemeny N, Kemeny M, Dawson L (2009) Liver metastases. In: Abeloff's clinical oncology, 4th edn. Churchill Livingstone/Elsevier, Philadelphia

National Comprehensive Cancer Network (2010) NCCN clinical practice guidelines in oncology: colon Cancer, V.3.2011. http://www.nccn.org/professionals/physician_gls/pdf/colon.pdf Accessed 17 Mar 2010

Pocard M, Pouillart P, Asselain B, Salmon R (2000) Hepatic resection in metastatic breast cancer: results and prognostic factors. Eur J Surg Oncol 26:155–159

Swaminath A, Dawson LA (2011) Emerging role of radiotherapy in the management of liver metastases. Cancer J 16(2):150–155

Palliation of Visceral Recurrences and Metastases

James H. Brashears, III
Radiation Oncologist, Venice, FL, USA

Synonyms

Chest, abdominal, and pelvic tumor metastases; Treatment or management of liver, splenic, lung, and pelvic metastases

Definition/Description

Visceral tumor recurrence and metastases present a myriad of problems and potential therapies based on the location, primary malignancy, clinical circumstances, and patient/caregiver desires. Computed tomography (CT) is often integral to the delineation of intra-corporeal lesions. Multidisciplinary management with surgeons, medical oncologists, radiation oncologists, and radiologists can help provide an array of palliative tools to aid the patient suffering from terminal cancer affecting the chest, abdomen, or pelvis. Before undertaking any intervention, techniques and realistic goals should be clearly articulated to all those involved while care should be taken to minimize collateral damage to normal structures and manage expected complications in a prophylactic manner.

Background

Regardless of the area of origin, almost all malignancies have the capacity for dissemination to the core of the body and owing to therapeutic and diagnostic difficulties, there is often a high rate of local recurrence in those cancers originating therein. The chest, abdomen, and pelvis house several critical organs whose continued function is vital to preserve homeostasis through their complex interactions. Tumors in these areas produce their detrimental effects, including pain, by impairing these interactions through a few relatively easily understood phenomena:

1. Obstruction, which frequently occurs in the chest and abdomen. Examples are ► Superior vena cava and airway, biliary, or intestinal obstruction.
2. Bleeding or discharge from breakdown of tissue linings or excrescence, which is often associated with locally recurrent tumor in the pelvis that may affect the vulva, vagina, cervix, anus, or rectum.
3. Tumor replacement of normal parenchyma, which causes functional difficulties as with infiltration of the liver and spleen.

With this understanding, general principles of therapy for specific areas might be reasonably applied to patients who do not meet the specific entry criteria for certain trials or guidelines. Obstruction is most expeditiously addressed by prompt reestablishment of flow (by stenting, bypass, medications, or radiation). Abolishing low-pressure bleeding or fluid loss is achieved by pressure dressings and reestablishment of a tissue lining by managing local tumor invasion. Similarly, delivery of cytotoxic therapy to tumors in ► parallel organs like the liver aims to halt or slow the loss of normally functioning subunits. Reaching any of these objectives may thus improve the quality of life in the terminally ill.

Initial Evaluation

The evaluation of visceral tumor begins with an accurate history and physical examination where suspicion will be high in those with a previous history of cancer either in the area of symptoms or with a predilection for spread to that region. Evaluation of vital signs and clues to nutritional status must not be neglected. Next, germane laboratory and imaging exams can be ordered.

For tumors involving the inside of the chest, obstructive phenomena dominate. There can be compression of blood vessels, airways from the trachea distally or of the esophagus and gastroesophageal junction. Flow can be impeded and fistulization is possible between these structures as well. Extrinsic compression of the SVC requires particular attention and is accompanied by intracaval thrombus about half the time (Gaspar 2008). Patient's with SVC syndrome show varying degrees of facial edema, arm swelling, headache, respiratory compromise, jugulovenous distention, and evidence for cephalad collateral circulation; they frequently have lung cancer, though other histologies are possible. The extent of workup will depend on the severity of the respiratory and/or circulatory compromise. When pathology is unknown and the patient is stable, biopsy should be undertaken because chemosensitive and benign tumors are known to occur (e.g., lymphoma, small cell lung cancer, or germ cell tumor and thymoma or goiter, respectively). Otherwise, treatment can be commenced on a presumptive basis. Patients suffering from airway compromise may complain of cough, hemoptysis, or shortness of breath and have stridor on auscultation. Esophageal obstruction can cause difficulty swallowing, emesis, and weight loss; fistula with the trachea can lead to severe cough and recurrent pneumonia. Upper aerodigestive obstruction can be investigated by endoscopic techniques that can provide tissue for diagnosis, fiducial information about the extent of tumor,

and potentially provide therapy through dilation, debulking, and/or stenting (Kyale and Selecky 2007).

Symptomatic abdominal tumors may be related to blockage of the biliary and intestinal tract or infiltration of the liver or spleen. Biliary obstruction may lead to pruritus, stool changes, and appetite/weight loss; seen in combination with jaundice and abnormal liver function tests, there is risk for diffuse hepatic malignancy (Gaspar 2008). Abdominal distention, pain, and absence of bowel sounds coupled with appetite/weight loss may be a clue to intestinal obstruction that can occur from obstructive tumor itself or the mass acting as a point for volvulus or adhesion formation. Depending on underlying pathology and volume of disease, splenic involvement may cause pain, lack of energy (from anemia), and easy bleeding or bruisability from thrombocytopenia.

Uncontrolled pelvic tumors are known to be painful and can cause bleeding or malodorous discharge with subsequent diminution in quality of life. For gynecologic tumors or those of the low rectum/anus, complete physical examination (including pelvic exam or anoscopy as appropriate) with careful inspection and palpation can yield important information as to the extent of disease and what kinds of therapy might be most appropriate.

Differential Diagnosis

Metastases or recurrences in the chest, abdomen, or pelvis may be mistaken for areas of infection (abscess), rheumatologic condition, trauma, foreign body, or new primary neoplasm. If the patient is stable and the diagnosis is in question, biopsy or excision is appropriate.

Imaging Studies

The need for imaging will be guided by the patient's oncologic history, location and nature of complaint, or symptoms and the acuity of the clinical circumstances. In the thorax, direct visualization is possible for the proximal airways and the distensible esophagus, otherwise contrast-enhanced computed tomography (CT) scan will show lesions that are large enough to cause obstruction. In SVC syndrome, a tissue density mass is generally identifiable in the area of the right paratracheal or precarinal lymph nodes (Laskin and Cmelak 2004). Esophageal obstruction will show as luminal narrowing on barium swallow and fistula with the trachea or bronchi may allow barium into the lungs. CT of the chest may also reveal lung or hilar masses that appear to produce atelectasis distally. In these cases, combination positron emission tomography (PET)-CT scan can provide information differentiating the malignancy from collapsed lung (which can also be used for radiation treatment planning).

Contrast-enhanced CT scan is also applicable for evaluation of intra-abdominal and pelvic neoplastic lesions. CT can reveal organomegaly, lymphadenopathy, and sometimes identify areas of possible intestinal obstruction. Specialized contrast CT sequences, CT angiography, CT portography, intraoperative ultrasound, PET scan, and contrast-enhanced magnetic resonance imaging (MRI), including magnetic resonance cholangiopancreatography (MRCP), are also able to evaluate intrahepatic pathology (Kemeny and Kemeny 2004). Assessment of the biliary tree can be undertaken by more interventional and potentially therapeutic means with endoscopic retrograde cholangiopancreatography (ERCP) or percutaneous cholangiopancreatography. Within the pelvis, CT displays the internal extent of tumors that are appreciated on physical examination which can have import for the choice of treatment (e.g., brachytherapy with a vaginal cylinder versus wide field external beam therapy depending on the depth of tumor).

Laboratory Studies

Laboratory investigations will be guided by the clinical situation. That said, a complete blood count (CBC) is needed to ascertain the hematologic status of anyone suspected of significant bleeding, hepatomegaly, or splenomegaly. A complete metabolic panel with liver function tests (CMP) is reasonable for anyone with liver metastases. When initially abnormal, both CBC and CMP can be monitored to quantify effectiveness of or adverse reactions to therapy. Serum tumor markers can help in the diagnosis of metastases if in question.

Treatment

In clinically stable patients, obstructive phenomena from a known malignancy are best relieved by timely interventional means whenever possible. Corticosteroids may be used to reduce contributing inflammation, but it is incumbent to recognize there will be a lag in response to radiotherapy and/or chemotherapy. For obstruction of the trachea or bronchi, bronchoscopy is critical for evaluation and treatment. Palliative bronchoscopic procedures designed to alleviate dyspnea or hemoptysis can be used in concert with later radiation therapy and include: balloon dilation, endotracheal intubation, debulking of intraluminal tumor, photodynamic therapy, laser, electrocautery, cryotherapy, argon coagulation, and stent placement (Kyale and Selecky 2007). In addition, bronchoscopists can deploy a catheter for afterloading with a high or low dose rate radioactive source. Similarly, esophagoscopy allows for direct visualization of the obstructed area and allows the same opportunity for therapy, though there may be a higher risk for fistula formation. In the case of tracheoesophageal fistula, an esophageal stent, and/or palliative surgery may be appropriate. When areas of obstruction are not traversable by the endoscope, palliative gastrostomy is an option. There is debate as to whether SVC compression is an emergency since treatment outcome seems not to be related to symptom duration so pathologic diagnosis can often be secured (Kvale and Selecky 2007). Medical management includes head elevation, diuretics, and corticosteroids. For chemotherapy-responsive tumors like small cell lung cancer, either chemotherapy and/or radiation therapy relieve symptoms in at least three quarters of patients while for non–small cell lung cancer and metastases from solid organ malignancies, initial external beam radiation has usually been preferred. Not surprisingly, the most rapid symptom relief is achieved with successful intravascular stent placement (Laskin and Cmelak 2004).

With its dual vascular supply, the liver is the second most common organ to be affected by metastases (after lymph nodes) and there are numerous local therapies designed to prolong the quality and/or quantity of life (Gaspar 2008). Nearly 15% of colorectal cancer patients have liver involvement at the time of diagnosis and another 60% will develop it subsequently (Kemeny and Kemeny 2004). Pathology, the nature and onset of symptoms, responsiveness to therapy, life expectancy, and resource availability impact the specific choice of therapy which includes endoscopic, percutaneous, open, and noninvasive approaches. Endoscopic or percutaneous methods with use of radiopaque contrast can identify areas of biliary obstruction ripe for palliation. With severe compression, percutaneous drainage may be necessary, but the physiological flow of bile might be reestablished with balloon dilation and stent placement in the biliary tree. Percutaneous placement of an appropriate blind-ended catheter can allow for intraluminal brachytherapy to help maintain bile duct patency either as monotherapy or as a boost treatment with external beam radiation. Locally ablative therapies like surgery, cryotherapy, ► radiofrequency ablation, ethanol injection, ► radioactive microsphere embolization, dose-escalated conformal radiation, or extracranial stereotactic radiosurgery may be attempted to prolong the normal

5–10 months median survival depending on the number, location, and size of hepatic metastases as well as the remaining normally functioning liver. Hepatic reserve is often quantified based on the serum bilirubin and the amount of normal appearing liver on imaging studies. If needed, selective pre-therapy embolization of hepatic vasculature can increase the volume of normal liver potentially changing the candidacy of patients for subsequent interventional procedures. In cases where the liver is replete with metastases and pain control is the overriding concern, palliative external beam radiation can be administered to the entire liver with proper allowance for the kidneys and lungs. The risk of ► radiation-induced liver disease is 5% with 30 Gy in 15 fractions to the entire organ so 21 Gy in 7 fractions is a reasonable whole liver prescription while the maximal point dose should be kept less than 90 Gy for conformal or stereotactic radiation therapy (Gaspar 2008). Splenomegaly from malignant infiltration can also cause pain. If related to a myeloproliferative process, 5–10 Gy given at 1 Gy per fraction three times per week with close clinical and hematologic monitoring can be attempted.

Palliative surgery is appropriate for malignant bowel obstruction in patients with a significant life expectancy. For more terminal patients or those refusing open surgery, symptoms can be medically managed with antiemetics and opioids. The subject of parenternal nutrition can be discussed. If the area of obstruction can be reached endoscopically, dilation and stent placement may provide temporary relief. For traversable tumors involving the distal colon, brachytherapy may be possible though there is the risk of fistulization.

Symptomatic recurrent or metastatic pelvic tumors often respond well to external beam radiation. If the site of venous bleeding is from the vagina or vulva, pressure dressings and initiation of radiation are warranted. Anemia can be treated by transfusion. In the radiation naïve with a short life expectancy, a single 10 Gy fraction to the whole pelvis (repeatable 1 month later) provides reduction in bleeding for the majority of patients. Regrettably, patients that live long enough often show severe late radiation toxicity with such high single doses, so many opt for lower individual doses including 3.7 Gy twice daily (with at least a 6-h interfraction interval) for two days (total 14.4 Gy) that can be repeated at 2 week intervals twice or more traditional fraction schemes with 30–37.5 Gy in 10–15 fractions (Gaspar 2008). For less acute bleeding or discharge, CT scan can help determine the depth of the cancer and whether brachytherapy or treatment with an electron cone could be appropriate. For recurrent pelvic tumors, like rectal cancer, where radiation was applied previously, retreatment can be given at 1.8–2 Gy once per day or 1.2 Gy twice daily with at least 6 h between treatments to a total of between 30 and 30.6 Gy (Gaspar 2008).

Cross-References

▶ Imaging in Oncology
▶ Nuclear Medicine
▶ Pain Management
▶ Principles of Chemotherapy
▶ Robotic Radiosurgery
▶ Stereotactic Radiosurgery: Extracranial
▶ Supportive Care and Quality of Life

References

Gaspar L (2008) Palliation of visceral recurrences and metastases. In: Halperin E, Perez C (eds) Principles and practice of radiation oncology, 5th edn. Lippincott Williams and Wilkins, Philadelphia, pp 2000–2003

Kemeny N, Kemeny MM, Lawrence TS (2004) In: Abeloff MD, Armitage JO, Niederhuber JE et al (eds) Clinical Oncology. Liver metastases. Third Edition. Philadelphia, Elsevier, pp 1141–1178

Kyale P, Selecky P (2007) Palliative care in lung cancer: ACCP evidence-based clinical practice guidelines (2nd edition). Chest 132:368S–403S

Laskin J, Cmelak A (2004) Superior vena cava syndrome. In: Armitage J, Abeloff M (eds) Clinical oncology, 3rd edn. Elsevier Churchill Livingstone, Philadelphia, pp 1047–1059

Pancoast Syndrome

FENG-MING KONG, JINGBO WANG
Department of Radiation Oncology, Veteran Administration Health Center and University Hospital, University of Michigan, Ann Arbor, MI, USA

Definition

The classic Pancoast syndrome presents symptoms and signs that include shoulder and arm pain along the distribution of the eighth cervical nerve trunk and first and second thoracic nerve trunks, Horner's syndrome, and weakness and atrophy of the muscles of the hand caused by lower brachial plexopathy. This syndrome is most commonly caused by local extension of an apical lung tumor at the superior thoracic inlet and such tumor is called superior pulmonary sulcus tumor or Pancoast's tumor.

Cross-References

▶ Lung

Pancreatic Cancer

▶ Cancer of the Pancreas

Pap Smear

▶ Papanicolaou Smear

Pap Test

▶ Papanicolaou Smear

Papanicolaou Smear

CHRISTIN A. KNOWLTON[1], MICHELLE KOLTON MACKAY[2]
[1]Department of Radiation Oncology, Drexel University, Philadelphia, PA, USA
[2]Department of Radiation Oncology, Marshfield Clinic, Marshfield, WI, USA

Synonyms
Pap smear; Pap test

Definition
The Papanicolaou test is a screening test for cervical cancer that is performed with a pelvic examination to allow for cytologic evaluation of the cells at the cervical transformation zone. This test has greatly decreased cervical cancer incidence in the United States as it also detects premalignant changes.

Cross-References
▶ Uterine Cervix

Papillary Carcinoma

▶ Bladder
▶ Thyroid Cancer

Papilloma

▶ Bladder
▶ Colon Cancer

Parallel Organ

JAMES H. BRASHEARS, III
Radiation Oncologist, Venice, FL, USA

Definition
A term from radiobiology that is based on an analogy with electrical circuits and can be contrasted with serial organs. A parallel organ, like the liver or kidney, has redundancy built in, and a certain fraction of the organ parenchyma (or functional subunits) can be sacrificed and the organ will maintain function. Classic serial organs are the spinal cord and intestinal tract where loss of function will occur if even a small length of either structure is sacrificed.

Cross-References
▶ Palliation of Visceral Recurrences and Metastases

Paranasal Sinuses

FILIP T. TROICKI
College of Medicine, Drexel University, Philadelphia, PA, USA

Definition
Paranasal sinuses are any of the paired cavities in the anterior skull and adjacent to the nasal cavity. These are lined with mucous membrane and include the maxillary, ethmoid, sphenoid, and frontal sinuses.

Cross-References
▶ Nasal Cavity and Paranasal Sinuses

Paraneoplastic Syndromes

FENG-MING KONG, JINGBO WANG
Department of Radiation Oncology, Veteran
Administration Health Center and University
Hospital University of Michigan, Ann Arbor,
MI, USA

Definition
These syndromes are collections of symptoms that result from substances (hormones or cytokines) produced by the tumor cells or by an immune response against the cancer, rather than by the direct invasion of tumor. Generally, these disorders are divided into the following categories: (1) miscellaneous (nonspecific), (2) rheumatologic, (3) renal, (4) gastrointestinal, (5) hematologic, (6) cutaneous, (7) endocrine, and (8) neuromuscular.

Cross-References
▶ Lung

Parenteral Nutrition

FILIP T. TROICKI[1], JAGANMOHAN POLI[2]
[1]College of Medicine, Drexel University,
Philadelphia, PA, USA
[2]Department of Radiation Oncology,
College of Medicine, Drexel University,
Philadelphia, PA, USA

Definition
Nutrition directly into the vein, bypassing the gastrointestinal system.

Cross-References
▶ Stomach Cancer

PARP Inhibitors (Poly(ADP-Ribose) Polymerase Inhibitors)

RENE RUBIN
Rittenhouse Hematology/Oncology,
Philadelphia, PA, USA

Definition
BRCA1/2 are genes that regulate DNA repair. The mutated genes lead to errors in DNA repair. Therefore, inhibition of PARP, which is an important protein for DNA repair, can prevent the repair of DNA in these mutated genes and therefore prevent cell repair and then ultimately cell death. PARP inhibitors (iniparib, olaparib) may be quite effective in combination with radiation therapy. There is evidence that the combination may lead to more effective DNA damage and prevention of repair, giving way to synergy. These agents are not yet commercially available; their use is therefore experimental. Up to now, promising results in BRCA1/2 breast cancer and ovarian carcinoma have been demonstrated.

Cross-References
▶ Principles of Chemotherapy

Passive Scattering

DANIEL YEUNG[1], JATINDER PALTA[2]
[1]Department of Radiation Oncology,
Univeristy of Florida Proton Therapy Institute,
Jacksonville, FL, USA
[2]Department of Radiation Oncology,
University of Florida Health Science Center,
Gainesville, FL, USA

Definition
A technique to generate a broad beam by using passive scatterers to increase the lateral spread of a narrow proton beam.

Cross-References

▶ Proton Therapy

PCa

▶ Prostate

Pediatric Ovarian Cancer

▶ Juvenile Granulosa Cell Tumors

Pencil-Beam Dose Kernel

CHARLIE MA, LU WANG
Department of Radiation Oncology, Fox Chase
Cancer Center, Philadelphia, PA, USA

Definition
The dose distribution resulting from scattered
photons and secondary electrons set in motion
by a single ray of primary photons.

Cross-References
▶ Dose Calculation Algorithms

Pencil-Beam Scanning (PBS)

DANIEL YEUNG[1], JATINDER PALTA[2]
[1]Department of Radiation Oncology,
Univeristy of Florida Proton Therapy Institute,
Jacksonville, FL, USA
[2]Department of Radiation Oncology,
University of Florida Health Science Center,
Gainesville, FL, USA

Definition
A technique that uses magnets to sweep a
narrow proton pencil-beam and allows precise
three-dimensional dose deposition. Both the
intensity and energy of the protons can be manipulated throughout the scan.

Cross-References
▶ Proton Therapy

Penile Cancer

STEPHAN MOSE
Department of Radiation Oncology,
Schwarzwald-Baar-Klinikum,
Villingen-Schwenningen, Germany

Synonyms
Carcinoma of the penis; Penile carcinoma

Definition/Description
Penile carcinoma is a rare tumor in old men.
Although the carcinogenesis is not clearly defined,
it is stated that in many cases ▶ human papilloma
virus (HPV) 16 plays an important role. The
tumor is often initially confined to the organ
itself. Therefore, organ-preserving therapies
are important in small and well-differentiated
tumors achieving local control and additionally
preserving sexual function. In those patients,
penile conserving surgery is an excellent option
that may be replaced in well-selected patients by
brachytherapy because of similar results. However, there are no prospective studies comparing
these different therapies. In larger tumors,
total penectomy is the gold standard although
a radiotherapeutic approach may be considered
as well. The main prognostic factor is the status of
lymph nodes.

Anatomy
The paired root of the penis is embedded into
the superficial perineum, covered by muscles

(m. bulbospongiosus and ischiocavernous) and thus fixed to the osseous pelvis. The pendulous body (shaft) includes the two corpora cavernosa and the corpus spongiosum encased in a dense deep fascia, which itself is surrounded by a layer of connective tissue and then covered by the skin. The corpora cavernosa contain sponge-like erectile tissue (collagen fibers, elastic tissue, and smooth muscles), which is filled with blood during penile erection. The corpus spongiosum, which is initially covered by the bulbospongiosus muscle, proximally begins under the urogenital diaphragm and distally ends as expanded cap (glans penis). It contains dense venous plexus and includes the urethra that ends within the glans (fossa navicularis and external meatus). The glans is covered by a retractable double-layered fold of skin and mucous membrane (foreskin, prepuce). Glans and body are arbitrarily separated by the coronal sulcus or the balanopreputial area.

The subfascial penile vessels arise from the internal pudendal arteries. Most of the penile veins drain to the internal pudendal vein; only small dorsal superficial veins empty into the external pudendal vessels. The lymphatic vessels of the foreskin and the skin of the body proceed into the superficial inguinal nodes whereas the glans, corpora cavernosa, and body mainly drain into the deep inguinal, obturator, and iliac nodes.

Epidemiology

Penile carcinoma accounts for 0.5% of all cancers and 0.1–1.0% of all malignancies in men. The tumor mostly occurs between 60 and 70 years of age although it is observed in younger men as well as in children. It is a relatively rare disease in Europe and the USA (age-standardized incidence: 0.3–1/ 100,000 men) whereas in some parts of South America and Africa the incidence can reach up to 4/100,000 men. In Europe, each year approximately 4,000 men are diagnosed with penile cancer.

Although the precise mechanisms of the carcinogenesis are largely unknown, there are (multifactorial) risk factors that are associated with penile cancer: history of phimosis (in 20–75%), smoking, poor penile hygiene, leukoplakia, ▶ balanitis xerotica obliterans, and lack of circumcision during childhood. It is important to note that adult circumcision has no preventive effect suggesting that a long time of exposure to smegma might be necessary for carcinogenesis although definitive evidence is still missing. An association with sexual transmitted diseases could not be verified. Premalignant lesions (i.e., bowenoid papulosis, condyloma, pseudoepitheliomatous keratotic, and micaceous balanitis) and carcinoma in situ (▶ Morbus Bowen, ▶ Erythroplasia de Queyrat) are found in 10–35%. Due to recent molecular and serologic findings, it is clearly demonstrated that in more than 50% of cases human papilloma virus 16 acts as a carcinogenic factor in penile cancer whereas the contribution of HPV 18 and HPV 6 is not finally defined. Furthermore, patients with psoriasis who were exposed to ultraviolet-A photochemotherapy (PUVA) without shielding their genitals may have a higher risk to develop penile cancer (Heideman et al. 2007).

Clinical Presentation

In most patients, the tumor is slowly progressive and in 66–75% initially confined to the organ. Because of fear, embarrassment, ignorance, and/ or disregard, diagnosis and subsequent treatment are delayed in 15–50% of patients. Neglecting the tumor leads to death within 2 years without treatment. A careful clinical examination is mandatory because the tumor may be initially diagnosed as a subtle induration, small papule or pustule, or as warty lesion combined with itching and burning. At a later point in time, the typically seen infiltrative ulcerations and larger exophytic papillary lesions cause pain (12%), bleeding (7%), and urinary symptoms (7%) (Fig. 1).

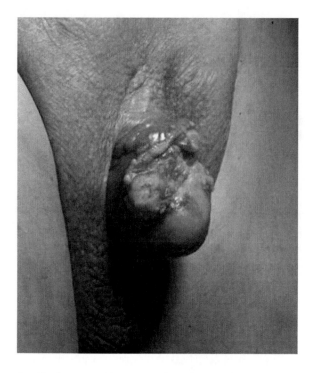

Penile Cancer. Fig. 1 Locally advanced penile carcinoma (With courtesy of A. Lampel, MD, Professor and Head of Department of Urology and Paediatric Urology, Schwarzwald-Baar-Klinikum Villingen-Schwenningen, Germany)

An untreated phimosis may mask an underlying tumor growth, which itself may lead to secondary infections and foul-smelling discharge. The tumor is located at different sites that may be combined: glans (66–83%), prepuce (21–55%), coronal sulcus (6%), and shaft (2–14%).

In 17–50% inguinal lymph nodes are palpable whereas 45–50% of nodes are enlarged because of secondary inflammatory lymphadenopathy. In approximately 50% of positive inguinal nodes, bilateral disease and/or iliac nodes are diagnosed; the incidence of positive pelvic lymph node metastases depends on the number of positive inguinal nodes (1–3 nodes: 12–22%, >3 nodes: 57–87%). Furthermore, the incidence of lymph node metastases is correlated to the grade of tumor differentiation (6–16%, 12–35%, and 60–80% in T1 G1, T1 G2, and T1 G3 tumor,

respectively) and the T-stage (16%, 30–50%, <80% in Tis/Ta, T1, and T2–4). At time of diagnosis, distant metastases (overall incidence <10%) are unusual in the absence of regional lymphatic disease whereas it is more often described in patients with positive lymph nodes (lung, liver, bone, and brain). In dependence on risk factors, occult inguinal disease is present in 16–73% of clinically node negative patients; distant metastases should be suspected in 15–20% of lymph node positive tumors.

In 90–95% of all penile carcinomas, a squamous cell carcinoma is found. Of these different subtypes are: usual, basaloid, verrucous, warty (condylomatous), papillary, sarcomatoid, adenosquamous, and mixed. Other histologies occur very seldom (angiosarcoma, leiomyosarcoma, basal cell carcinoma). Likewise, lymphomas that may be cured by radiotherapy are rare (Misra et al. 2004; Guimarães et al. 2009).

Differential Diagnosis

As some symptoms resemble those of benign diseases, a careful diagnosis and examination are to be done. Erythema, itching, and pain may be seen in infectious diseases (balanitis, candidiasis) as well as in dermatological lesions (psoriasis, contact dermatitis, lichen sclerosus et athrophicus). Scaly and crusted plaques may indicate Bowen's disease and/or Erythroplasia de Queyrat. Furthermore, benign condylomata acuminata should be considered.

Imaging Studies

In addition to careful physical examination, a biopsy is mandatory to histologically assure the diagnosis. To evaluate the invasion into the tunica or corpora cavernosa and to detect (non-)palpable inguinal lymph nodes potentially completed by a fine-needle aspiration ultrasound is a reliable method. Furthermore, it helps to assess the possibility of organ-preserving therapies. Endoscopy of the urethra will give further information regarding deep tumor infiltration. Computed tomography (CT) is

Penile Cancer. Table 1 TNM-classification and staging in penile cancer. Recent evaluations discussed a modified TNM-classification in order to better differentiate tumors in terms of survival and prognostic stratification of patients: T2 = invasion of corpus spongiosum, T3 = invasion of corpus cavernosum, T4 = invasion of adjacent structures; N1 = unilateral inguinal metastases mobile, N2 = bilateral inguinal metastases mobile, N3 = fixed inguinal metastases or metastases in pelvic lymph node(s) (Leitje et al. 2008)

TNM	
Ta	Noninvasive verrucous carcinoma
Tis	Carcinoma in situ
T1	Invasion of the subepithelial connective tissue
T2	Invasion of the corpus spongiosum or cavernosum
T3	Invasion of urethra or prostate
T4	Invasion of adjacent structures
N0	No regional lymph node metastases
N1	Metastasis in a single superficial inguinal lymph node
N2	Metastases in multiple or bilateral superficial inguinal lymph nodes
N3	Metastases in deep inguinal or pelvic lymph nodes, uni-/bilateral
M0	No distant metastases
M1	Distant metastases
Staging	
Stage 0	Ta/Tis N0 M0
Stage I	T1 N0 M0
Stage II	T1 N1 M0
	T2 N0−1 M0
Stage III	T1−2 N2 M0
	T3 N0−2 M0
Stage IV	T4 any N M0
	Any T N3 M0
	Any T any N M1

usually performed for detection of pelvic lymph nodes although its sensitivity is relatively low. Therefore, magnetic resonance imaging may provide better information; further optimization of MRI techniques is in progress (i.e., lymphotropic ultrasmall superparamagnetic particles). CT scanning of liver and upper abdominal region, chest radiography, and bone scan are performed for exact staging (Table 1) as clinically indicated. A promising diagnostic tool is scanning with ^{18}F-FDG-PET/CT to detect pelvic lymph node metastases as well as distant metastases. However, regarding improved MRI techniques and PET/CT scanning, further results with a larger number of patients are needed (Graafland et al. 2009).

Laboratory Studies

Laboratory studies that have no pathognomic value with regard to penile cancer include the blood count and the chemistry profile of liver and kidneys as well as a urine analysis. In case of pathologic results, they may give information about organ function (e.g., kidney) or may eventually indicate osseous metastases (e.g., alkaline phosphatase). Tumor markers have no diagnostic relevance.

Treatment

Because penile cancer represents a primarily locoregional problem, the major goal of treatment is the complete removal or destruction of the tumor. The traditional gold standard is the partial or total penectomy. However, the functional and psychological problems of these procedures have always supported the efforts toward organ-preserving techniques (laser surgery, micrographic surgery, glansectomy, brachytherapy, external radiation). Up to now, there are no studies comparing these therapies; retrospective data lead to the presumption that the results of organ-preserving surgery and radiotherapy are almost equivalent. The question of how to deal with inguinal and pelvic lymph nodes is still debatable.

The prognosis principally depends on the absence or existence of lymph node involvement, the size of the primary tumor, its grading, and histology (Tables 2 and 3). Furthermore, there is a strong association of positive lymph nodes and high mortality rate in sarcomatoid histology whereas less metastases and better survival were seen in verrucous, mixed, papillary, and warty cancers.

Surgery

If the tumor is small and confined to the prepuce, a wide circumcision may be indicated. In experienced hands, the same seems to hold true for tumors of the glans where glansectomy combined

Penile Cancer. Table 2 Overall and disease-free survival and dependence on T, N, Grading, and vascular invasion

	Five-year overall survival (%)	Ten-year overall survival (%)	Five-year disease-free survival (%)
N0	80–90	59	95
N 1–3	36–50	18	
N + (pelvic)	<20		
N1–2			60–75
N3			12
Ta/Tis			89
T1–2			63–75
T3–4			28–46
G1			86
G2			78
G3			65
With vascular invasion			89
Without vascular invasion			69

Penile Cancer. Table 3 Adverse prognostic factors and the corresponding incidence of histological subtypes (in %) of penile squamous cell carcinoma

	Basaloid, sarcomatoid, adenosquamous	Usual, mixed	Verrucous, warty, papillary
Adverse prognostic factors (in %):			
– T3	50–100	41–46	12–44
– N+	50–75	9–28	0–17
– G3	75–100	22–47	0–22
– Vascular invasion	33–75	23–28	0–12
– Perineural invasion	50–67	23–35	4–12
Recurrence (%)	25–67 (more often systemic recurrence)	19–28%	0–12 (more often locoregional/local recurrence)

with a reconstruction with a skin graft yields good functional and cosmetic results with recurrences in only 0–6%. Micrographic surgery can be performed in superficial lesions (diameter < 1 cm); the reported 5-year overall survival is 81% with local recurrences in 0–32% of the case. Likewise, laser surgery (CO_2 and NdYAG laser) aims to preserve the organ function and structure, which is obtained in 67–82%. In carcinomas in situ cure is obtained in 100%; in T1–2 tumors, recurrences are reported in 15–34%. However, glansectomy, micrographic surgery, which is a time-consuming procedure from the technical point of view, and laser surgery, which is probably the most preferable procedure in small, superficial, and well-differentiated tumors (pTa–T1, G1–2), have not entirely been proven; most data were reported by single institutions. It is important to discuss especially in patients who do not want to maintain the penile sexual function that a partial or complete penectomy yield lower recurrences rates.

In pT1 G3 and ≥pT2 tumors, a partial or a complete penectomy is the surgical gold standard, which is also reasonable in recurrent patients initially treated by organ-preserving procedures. A partial penectomy is done if an arbitrarily communicated 2 cm tumor-free margin can be obtained. Recently published data discussed a 10 mm and a <15 mm free margin in G1–2 tumors and G3 tumors, respectively. The local recurrence rate is 0–13%; in absence of inguinal lymph nodes, the 5-year overall survival is 80%. In 25–64%, this therapy permits normal micturition and sexual function. In larger tumors, a total penectomy combined with a perineal urethrostomy has to be performed. Irrespective of organ-preserving or radical surgery, the reported 5-year overall survival is 72–77%, 55–70%, 0–10% in T1, T2, and T3–4, respectively.

There are no evidence-based data considering prophylactic lymphonodectomy in clinically lymph node negative patients. Furthermore, because of the morbidity of lymphadenectomy, efforts were made to evaluate the usefulness of sentinel node biopsy in penile cancer. This comes along with the retrospective evidence that elective lymph node dissection yields better survival compared to surgical removal at the time of clinical occurrence (3-year overall survival 35% versus 84%). In recent years, the technique of dynamic sentinel node biopsy was improved (complication rate <5%) and better standardized leading to a reduction of false-negative results from 22% to 7% in experienced urologists. The sentinel node is found in up to 97%; occult lymph node metastases are diagnosed in up to 15% by this technique. In doing so, an elective lymph node dissection could be unnecessary simultaneously avoiding morbidity. Up to now, it may be reasonable to perform a sentinel lymph node dissection in those patients having a low grade (pTis, TaG1–2, T1G1) – otherwise surveillance is recommended in these patients – and/or intermediate risk (pT1G2) for occult inguinal lymph nodes. However, conclusive data are yet not available.

Keeping in mind the guidelines of the European Urology Association, in patients with a high risk of (i.e., proximal shaft tumors, ≥pT2, G3, vascular and lymphatic invasion) or definitive positive inguinal metastases, a modified lymphadenectomy is important considering improved survival and curability. Nevertheless, the further risk of having microscopic and/or macroscopic pelvic disease is consequently high, leading to reduced survival although pelvic lymphadenectomy may be added. A benefit of neoadjuvant/adjuvant modalities is not clearly reported (Schlenker et al. 2008; Angerer-Shpilenya & Jakse 2009; Leitje et al. 2009).

Radiotherapy

External radiotherapy and brachytherapy are discussed as alternative modalities in order to preserve organ function equivalent to surgical methods due to the exemplified fact that retrospective data comparing irradiated patients with/without salvage surgery and surgically treated patients with/without postoperative radiotherapy yield fairly similar 10-year cancer-specific survival rates (56% and 53%) with equivalent organ-preservation rates (52%). However, prospective studies are yet not available. In addition, many reports concerning radiotherapy include only a few patients, data were partially recruited from orthovolt series, and different therapies were statistically combined. This hampers the comparison with surgical data and with radiotherapeutic results obtained with modern techniques.

Today curative brachytherapy can be considered in selected, especially sexual active patients with small (<4 cm diameter, <1 cm invasion), superficial lesions of the glans or coronal sulcus without corpus cavernosum involvement. In those patients, tumor size, depth of invasion, and needle spacing due to the implant geometry are predictive regarding local control. In contrast, histopathology does not seem to play an important role. Circumcision should be performed prior to brachytherapy to reduce radiogen-induced sequelae and to allow optimal tumor assessment and determination of the target volume. This is defined as the macroscopic tumor plus 5–10 mm. According to ICRU 58, the reference dose should encompass the tumor with its microscopic extensions. Using LDR (low-dose-rate) or PDR (pulsed-dose-rate) brachytherapy with ^{192}Iriduim, a total dose of 60–70 Gy (0.4–0.5 Gy/h) should be delivered; the maximum urethral dose is 50 Gy. The experiences with interstitial HDR (high-dose-rate) brachytherapy (45–54 Gy, single dose 3 Gy) are limited in case reports. In superficial non-infiltrating tumors (<5 mm), an external mold technique is possible necessitating a reproducible fixation of the applicators. Performing interstitial brachytherapy, two templates are used that are perforated by holes (distance 5 mm) to allow the implantation of needles (recommended space: 12–18 mm, medium number of needles: 5–6). This system enables a homogenous dose distribution according to the Paris System rules.

Brachytherapy leads to a 5- and 10-year penile preservation rate of 85–88% and 67%. However, in literature sexual function is often not documented but seems to be maintained in the majority of irradiated patients. Local control is obtained in 90–100% (superficial T1 tumors), in 70–90% (T1–2), and in <20% (T3–4).

In cT1–2 N0 tumors penile recurrences, which often occur within the first 3 years comparable to surgical series, are reported in 0–20% (follow-up <10 years). Inguinal node recurrences occur in 10–20%; metastases are seldom (6–8%). Salvage surgery (i.e., partial/total penectomy ± lymph node dissection) with/without external radiotherapy is reasonable leading to an overall control in 44–86%. The 5- and 10-year overall survival is 78–90% and 59–65% in primarily node negative patients.

If external radiotherapy is to be delivered, three-dimensional planning is obligatory. Usually, specially designed accessories (e.g., wax or Perspex block, water bath) are needed to obtain a uniform dose distribution. A total dose of 50 Gy (1.8–2.0 Gy, 5×/week) is given to the tumor, which is boosted (60–70 Gy) to a reduced field. With definitive external radiotherapy preservation of the penis is possible in 50–66%. After 5 years, the local control is 44–65% and therefore worse compared to surgical organ sparing series; the 5-year overall survival ranges from 62% to 88%.

The role of radiotherapy in the management of lymph nodes remains controversial and is discussed similar to the surgical procedure. In T1 and small well-differentiated T2 tumors, close follow-up is suggested whereas, if surgery is not done, in T1 G3 and ≥T2 tumors elective radiotherapy of the inguinal lymph nodes is recommended. Preoperative irradiation (50 Gy) may allow lymph node dissection in fixed nodes and may be beneficial with regard to local control as it is reported in postoperative lymph node irradiation (50 Gy). Because of the high incidence of combined side effects and its questionable effect on survival, pre- or postoperative radiotherapy of inguinal and pelvic lymph nodes should be carefully indicated in highly selected patients with extensive disease (5-year overall survival 25–38%). Definitive curative radiotherapy of positive inguinal lymph nodes seems to be of no benefit and is only recommended in a palliative setting.

Retrospective data suggest a role of postoperative radiotherapy (external beam on primary tumor and/or inguinal lymph nodes ± brachytherapy) in R1-resected, individually selected patients (pT1–3 N0–1 G1–3) (5-year local control rate: 75%, 5-year disease-free and overall survival: 65% and 57%) (Strnad et al. 2005; de Crevoisier et al. 2009; Crook et al. 2009).

Chemotherapy

Considering chemotherapy, only very small, nonrandomized collectives were published; therefore, all data are still preliminary. Apart from palliative situations, adjuvant and neoadjuvant chemotherapy has been used limited by its toxicity (≤10% G3–4 hematological and non-hematological side effects) and the multimorbidity of the typically older patients. Adjuvant chemotherapy may be discussed if the risk of failure is thought to be extensively high although it is unknown if the survival rate will be optimized. In a neoadjuvant setting, survival may be improved if the tumor becomes operable. The traditionally given combination of cisplatin, bleomycin, and methotrexate yields response rates of up to 72% combined with severe toxicity. Paclitaxel and cisplatin containing regimens demonstrated a response in 20–60% of patients with bulky disease. There are no reliable data about the combination of radiotherapy and chemotherapy.

Sequelae of Therapy

Side effects of surgery include postoperative wound infections, seroma, and skin necrosis. In case of lymph nodes dissection, the morbidity is relatively high (<25%) additionally including lower-limb edema. A mortality rate of up to 3% is reported. Acute and late sequelae of irradiation are more often induced by brachytherapy than by external radiotherapy. Acute moist desquamation and penile swelling are reversible. Summarizing all data including old series, radionecrosis with secondary penectomy is seen in 0–23%; urethral strictures are reported in

10–45% necessitating dilation with symptomatic relief in 90% of patients. Using modern techniques, these chronic side effects can be reduced.

Cross-References
► Brachytherapy
► Carcinoma of the Male Urethra

References

Angerer-Shpilenya M, Jakse (2009) Der Stellenwert der Lymphknotenchirurgie beim Peniskarzinom. Urologe 48:54–58

de Crevoisier R, Slimane K, Sanfilippo N, Bossi A, Albano M, Dumas I, Wibault P, Fizazi K, Gerbaulet A, Haie-Meder C (2009) Long-term results of brachytherapy for carcinoma of the penis confined to the glans (N0 or NX). Int J Radiat Oncol Biol Phys 74:1150–1156

Crook J, Ma C, Grimard L (2009) Radiation therapy in the management of the primary penile tumor: an update. World J Urol 27:189–196

Graafland NM, Leitje JAP, Olmos RAV, Hoefnagel CA, Teertsrta HJ, Horenblas S (2009) Scanning with 18F-FDG-PET/CT for detection of pelvic nodal involvement in inguinal node-positive penile carcinoma. Eur Urol 56:339–345

Guimarães GC, Cunha IW, Soares FA, Lopes A, Torres J, Chaux A, Velazquez EF, Ayala G, Cubilla AL (2009) Penile squamous cell carcinoma clinicopathological features, nodal metastasis and outcome in 333 cases. J Urol 182:528–534

Heideman DAM, Waterboer T, Pawlita M, Delis-van Diemen P, Nindl I, Leitje JA, Blonfrer JMG, Horenblas S, Meijer CJLM, Snijders PJF (2007) Human papilloma virus-16 is the predominate type etiologically involved in penile squamous cell carcinoma. J Clin Oncol 24:4550–4556

Leitje JAP, Gallee M, Antonini N, Horenblas S (2008) Evaluation of the current TNM classification of penile carcinoma. J Urol 180:933–938

Leitje JAP, Hughes B, Graafland NM, Kroon BK, Olmos RAV, Nieweg OE, Corbishley C, Heenan S, Watkin N, Horenblas S (2009) Two-center evaluation of dynamic sentinel node biopsy for sqaumous cell carcinoma of the penis. J Clin Oncol 27:3325–3329

Misra S, Chaturvedi A, Misra NC (2004) Penile carcinoma: a challenge for the developing world. Lancet Oncol 5:240–247

Schlenker B, Gratzke C, Tilki D, Hungerhuber E, Schneede P, Reich O, Stief CG, Seitz M (2008) Organerhaltende Chirurgie des Peniskarzinoms. Urologe 47:803–808

Strnad V, Pötter R, Kovács G (2005) Peniskarzinom. In: Strnad V, Pötter R, Kovács G (eds) Stand und Perspektiven der klinischen Brachytherapie, 1st edn. Science UniMed Bremen, Boston/London

Penile Carcinoma

► Penile Cancer

Perigastric Lymph Nodes

FILIP T. TROICKI[1], JAGANMOHAN POLI[2]
[1]College of Medicine, Drexel University, Philadelphia, PA, USA
[2]Department of Radiation Oncology, College of Medicine, Drexel University, Philadelphia, PA, USA

Definition
Lymph nodes located within close proximity to and drain from the stomach.

Cross-References
► Esophagus Cancer
► Pancreatic Cancer
► Sister Mary Joseph Nodule
► Stomach Cancer

Perineural Invasion

FILIP T. TROICKI[1], JAGANMOHAN POLI[2]
[1]College of Medicine, Drexel University, Philadelphia, PA, USA
[2]Department of Radiation Oncology, College of Medicine, Drexel University, Philadelphia, PA, USA

Definition
Cancerous invasion into nerve cells.

Cross-References

▶ Esophageal Cancer
▶ Head and Neck Cancer
▶ Palliation of Brain and Spinal Cord
▶ Salivary Gland Cancer
▶ Sinus Cancer
▶ Stomach Cancer

Perioperative Brachytherapy

FELIPE A. CALVO
Department of Oncology, Hospital General
Universitario Gregorio Maranon, Madrid, Spain

Definition

The catheters are implanted during the surgical procedure, but the radiation dose planning and delivery is performed after the patient's recovery from anesthesia; the radiation therapy generally employs hypofractionated schemes.

Cross-References

▶ Intraoperative Irradiation

Periosteal Reaction

HEDVIG HRICAK[1], OGUZ AKIN[2], HEBERT ALBERTO VARGAS[2]
[1]Department of Radiology, Memorial Sloan-Kettering Cancer Center, New York, NY, USA
[2]Body MRI, Memorial Sloan-Kettering Cancer Center, New York, NY, USA

Definition

Production of new bone by the periosteum in response to injury or irritation.

Cross-References

▶ Imaging in Oncology

Peripheral Nerve Tumors

▶ Soft Tissue Sarcoma

Peripheral Primitive Neuroectodermal Tumor

DANIEL J. INDELICATO[1], ROBERT H. SAGERMAN[2]
[1]Department of Radiation Oncology, University of Florida Proton Therapy Institute, University of Florida College of Medicine, Jacksonville, FL, USA
[2]Department of Radiation Oncology, SUNY Upstate Medical University, Syracuse, NY, USA

Definition

A peripheral primitive neuroectodermal tumor (pPNET) is a neural crest tumor arising outside the central nervous system. Current evidence indicates that both Ewing sarcoma and PNET have a similar neural phenotype and, because they share an identical chromosome translocation, they should be viewed as the same tumor, differing only in their degree of neural differentiation. Tumors that demonstrate neural differentiation have been traditionally labeled PNETs, while those that are undifferentiated have been diagnosed as Ewing sarcoma.

Cross-References

▶ Ewing Sarcoma

Peritoneal Cavity

Filip T. Troicki[1], Jaganmohan Poli[2]
[1]College of Medicine, Drexel University,
Philadelphia, PA, USA
[2]Department of Radiation Oncology,
College of Medicine, Drexel University,
Philadelphia, PA, USA

Definition

Abdominal cavity that contains all of the abdominal contents (stomach, liver, intestines, pancreas, etc.).

Cross-References

► Colon Cancer
► Ovarian Cancer
► Stomach Cancer

Perivascular Tumors

► Soft Tissue Sarcoma

Permanent Implants

Erik van Limbergen[1], Yan Yu[2], Laura Doyle[2]
[1]Department of Radiation Oncology, University Hospital Gasthuisberg, Leuven, Belgium
[2]Department of Radiation Oncology, Thomas Jefferson University Hospital, Philadelphia, PA, USA

Definition

Usually a single procedure in which radioactive material is permanently implanted in tissue.

Activity of radioactive sources decreases exponentially over time and continuously delivers radiation.

Permanent low-energy and low-active iodine-125 or palladium-103 seeds can be implanted and are mainly used for treatment of early stage prostate cancer. The sources deliver their dose, over weeks while the sources are decaying. Because the low activity and the low-emitted energy, patients can leave the hospital shortly after implantation without causing a problem for radioprotection for their family.

Cross-References

► Clinical Aspects of Brachytherapy (BT)
► High-Dose Rate (HDR) Brachytherapy
► Low-Dose Rate (LDR) Brachytherapy

Pernicious Anemia

Filip T. Troicki[1], Jaganmohan Poli[2]
[1]College of Medicine, Drexel University,
Philadelphia, PA, USA
[2]Department of Radiation Oncology,
College of Medicine, Drexel University,
Philadelphia, PA, USA

Definition

Low red blood cell count due to inability of the body to absorb vitamin B12 from the gastrointestinal tract.

Cross-References

► Stomach Cancer

PET Scan

► Positron Emission Tomography

Pilocytic Astrocytoma

▶ Primary Intracranial Neoplasms

Pitch

Darek Michalski[1], M. Saiful Huq[2]
[1]Division of Medical Physics, Department of Radiation Oncology, University of Pittsburgh Cancer Centers, Pittsburgh, PA, USA
[2]Department of Radiation Oncology, University of Pittsburgh Medical Center Cancer Pavilion, Pittsburgh, PA, USA

Definition

For helical CT it is the ratio d/SC where d is table feed per 360° rotation of the tube/detector array and SC is the total slice collimation, which is the number of slices specific to a given scanner times a nominal slice width.

Cross-References

▶ Four-Dimensional (4D) Treatment Planning/Respiratory Gating

Pituitary

Theodore E. Yaeger, Cheri Yaeger
Department Radiation Oncology, Wake Forest University School of Medicine, Winston-Salem, NC, USA

Definition

The pituitary is a systemic, multifunctional hormone regulating gland. It is located in the sella turcica just inferior to the optic chiasm in the anterior base of brain. The optic chiasm is where the individual optic nerves from each eye cross below the hypothalamus as they trace posteriorily toward the brainstem.

Etiology

Embyrology: There are two parts to the main pituitary body. The pars tuberalis (or infundibularis), the pars intermedia, and the pars distalis are components of the adenohypophysis. The neural lobe, the median eminence, and the infundibular stem form the neurohypophysis. The median eminence is commonly described as the infundibulum or neural stalk but the hypophyseal stalk typically refers to the pars infundibularis of the posterior aspect of the gland. Normal developmental functions result in the adenohypophysis developing from a diverticulum of the buccopharyngeal region. This makes up about 80% of the total gland size (Ramzi et al. 1999). In contrast, the neurohypophysis develops from a diverticulum from the floor of the third ventricle. Realistically it functions as a storage gland for secretions produced by the hypothalamus. It is the axona of the supra-opticohyphophyseal tract that serves as the conduit for the secretions traveling to the neurohypophysis from the hypothalamus The distribution of pituitary adenomas are described in Table 1 (Burger et al. 1991).

Pituitary. Table 1 Tumor Frequency

Type	Frequency
Prolactinoma	20–30%
Null cell adenoma	20%
Gonadotroph adenoma	15%
ACTH adenoma	10–15%
Growth hormone adenoma	5%
Mixed growth/prolactin adenoma	5%
Plurihormone adenoma	1–5%
TSH adenoma	1%

Clinical Presentation

Generally, pituitary adenomas are benign tumors that come to medical attention as a result of abnormal hormone secretions, physical compression of adjacent normal anatomic structures, or displacement of the pituitary stalk resulting in Hypopituitarism.

Therapy

Primary medical interventions are designed to decrease the physical size of the pituitary typically by a trans-sphenoidal resection directly via the sphenoidal air sinus. Most patients will quickly normalize hormone levels. Radiation therapy is reserved for non-operable patients or those with risk of postsurgical residual functional disease. Radiation doses in the range for 45 Gy at 1.8 Gy per fraction over 25 fractions can achieve good local control with very low risk of complications such as optic neuropathy (Tsang et al. 1996). With radiation alone, however, normalization of hormones may take months to years to achieve; thus, medical agents such as a dopamine agonist are typical adjuvant therapies.

Prognosis

Radiation late effects are usually the potential of radiation-induced optic neuropathies, hypopituitarism, and secondary brain tumors. The incidence of optic neuropathy is consistently reported very low, ranging from 0.7% to 2.0% and is known to be dose-dependent for both total dose and dose per fraction (McCord et al. 1994). Likewise, secondary brain tumors have a very low incidence (Brada et al. 1992). It has been reported generally ranging from 1% to 3% over a 15–20-year period. More substantial is the risk of ultimately developing hypopituitarism. This has a potential risk of about 50% of patients ultimately developing at least one pituitary hormone deficiency at about 5 years from definitive radiotherapy and rarely causing an empty sella syndrome (Zierhut et al. 1995). As such, follow-up is lifelong with secondary interventions and supportive therapies as appropriate.

Cross-References

▶ Conformal Therapy: Treatment Planning, Treatment Delivery, and Clinical Results
▶ Intensity-Modulated Proton Therapy (IMPT)
▶ Palliation of Brain and Spinal Cord Metastases
▶ Primary Intracranial Neoplasms
▶ Radiotherapy of Nonmalignant diseases

References

Boyd WH (1960) Anat Rec 137:437
Brada M et al (1992) Risk of secondary brain tumor after conservation surgery and radiotherapy for pituitary adenoma. Br Med J 304:1343
Burger PC et al (1991) Pituitary neoplasia: Surgical pathology of the nervous system and its coverings, 3rd edn. Churchill Livingstone, New York
Ferner H (1960) Z Anat EntwGesch 121:407
McCord MW et al (1994) Radiotherapy for pituitary adenoma: long-term outcome and sequelae. Int J Radiat Oncol Biol Phys 30:557
Ramzi S et al (1999) Robbins pathologic basis of disease. Saunders, Philadelphia
Sutherland S (1945) J Anat Lond 79:33
Tsang RW et al (1996) Role of radiation therapy in clinical hormonally active pituitary adenomas. Radiother Oncol 41:45
Zierhut D et al (1995) External radiotherapy of pituitary adenomas. Int J Radiat Oncol Biol Phys 33:307

Planning Target Volume (PTV)

BRANDON J. FISHER[1], LARRY C. DAUGHERTY[2],
JAY E. REIFF[1]
[1]Department of Radiation Oncology, College of Medicine, Drexel University, Philadelphia, PA, USA
[2]Department of Radiation Oncology, College of Medicine, Drexel University, Glenside, PA, USA

Definition

PTV includes the gross tumor volume (GTV), the clinical target volume (CTV), and a margin to account for setup error, movement, and any possible geometric variations.

The volume that includes the CTV with any ITV (if present) as well as a setup margin to account for patient movement and daily setup uncertainties.

Cross-References
▶ Conformal
▶ Nasopharynx

Plasma Cell Myeloma

JO ANN CHALAL
Department of Radiation Oncology, Fox Chase Cancer Center, Philadelphia, PA, USA

Synonyms
Malignant myeloma; Myeloma; Plasma cell neoplasm; Plasmacytoma; Solitary plasmacytoma

Definition/Description
Multiple Myeloma is a malignant disorder of the plasma cell, which is involved in antibody production and immunologic response and is the final differentiated cell in the B-cell lineage. Plasma cells are produced in the bone marrow and can circulate through the lymphatic system. The proliferation of a clone of plasma cells results in bone destruction and bone marrow failure. End organ damage may also occur. Multiple myeloma accounts for 22% of plasma cell neoplasms, making it the most common of the plasma cell neoplasms.

Multiple myeloma is not curable. However, it is the advent of new drug therapy combinations as well as the role of stem cell transplants which have changed the landscape for those diagnosed with the disease. Now, its endpoints are commonly durable remissions and longer survivals.

Epidemiology and Etiology
Multiple Myeloma is the most common of the plasma cell neoplasms, accounting for 20,580 new cases in the United States in 2009. It accounts for 10,580 deaths. Its 5-year survival rate has increased from 25% in 1975 to 34% in 2003. More common in men (11,680 new cases versus 8,900 for women), slightly more common in African Americans with higher mortality rates, more common with advancing age with a median age of 70 at diagnosis, its incidence exceeds that of Hodgkins Lymphoma. The rate of myeloma is 25% of that of non-Hodgkins Lymphoma. The five year survival rate may be as high as 35%.

There is no known cause of myeloma. Possible predisposing factors may include radiation exposure (Hiroshima atomic bomb survivors) and environmental exposures (benzene, petroleum). Formerly herpes simplex virus 8 was thought to be a risk factor, but this has not been demonstrated to be a causal effect. Oncogenes such as c-myc as well as P-53 tumor suppressor gene changes may occur.

Differential Diagnosis
Since plasma cell ▶ dyscrasias are a spectrum of diseases, multiple myeloma (MM) needs to be distinguished from other disorders such as monoclonal gammopathy of uncertain significance (MGUS), solitary plasmacytoma, as well as Waldenstrom's Macroglobulinemia (WM). It must also be distinguished from chronic lymphocytic leukemia as these patients may also have monoclonal gammopathies.

Bone Marrow Pathology
Usually distinctive in MM and WM. Plasma cells constituting more than 20% of nucleated marrow cells (excluding erythoblasts) are characteristic but not diagnostic of MM (Figs. 1 and 2)

MGUS: normal plasma cells rarely >10% of bone marrow cells

MM: plasma cells are 20–95% of marrow cells

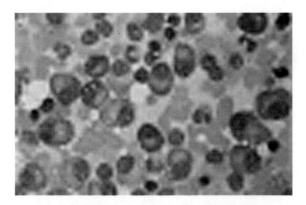

Plasma Cell Myeloma. Fig. 1 Multiple myeloma. A bone marrow aspirate shows a predominance of plasma cells. (Image reproduced with permission from Goldman: Cecil Medicine, 23rd edition, 2007)

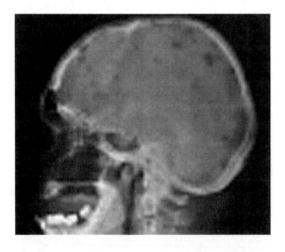

Plasma Cell Myeloma. Fig. 2 Skull radiograph showing multiple lytic lesions (Image reproduced with permission from Goldman, Cecil Medicine, 23rd edition, 2007)

WM: BM contains 10–19% plasmacytoid lymphocytes or small mature lymphocytes

Reactive plasmacytosis occurs in viral illness, including HIV, serum sickness, and plasma cell leukemia (very rare disease). Bone marrow plasmacytosis that is not due to myeloma is characterized by diffuse distribution and alignment of mature plasma cells along blood vessels or near marrow reticulum cells. It is seen in these settings: viral infections, serum sickness, collagen vascular disease, ► granulomatous disease, liver cirrhosis, and marrow hypoplasia.

Presentation

Fatigue, anemia, osteopenia, lytic bone lesions, hypercalcemia, renal insufficiency and/or failure, immunodeficiency, spinal cord compression, and pathologic fracture may or may not be present at the time of diagnosis.

Diagnostic Workup

This should include a history and physical with attention to symptoms of bone pain, fatigue, weakness, performance status, history of bone fractures, and number and frequency of infections. Laboratory work must include CBC with differential and platelets, BUN, serum creatinine, serum electrolytes, serum calcium, albumin, total protein, LDH, and beta-2 microglobulin level. The beta-2 microglobulin level reflects tumor mass and it is the standard measure of tumor burden. Serum protein electrophoresis (SPEP), serum immunofixation electrophoresis (SIFE), 24 h urine for protein, urine protein electrophoresis (UPEP), and urine immunofixation electrophoresis (UIFE) are all required for standard workup and evaluation. Most patients have serum proteins whether or not they have urinary proteins. Some 20% will have urinary proteins but fewer than 3% will have a nonsecretory myeloma where no serum or urine proteins are found.

Imaging studies are a key component to the workup as well. Skeletal surveys are standard. Findings include well-defined, rounded, punched out lesions and tend to be located in the skull, spine, and pelvis. Other bone findings include osteopenia osteoporosis, cortical erosions, and osteolysis with trabecular patterns. Since myeloma bone lesions are lytic, bone scans are not recommended since the lesions are frequently not visualized easily. MRI and CT scans are recommended to evaluate lesions involving the spine to rule out large endplate depressions, spinal cord compression, or epidural encroachment. For extraosseous presentations, MRI and/or CT may be essential to establish extent of involvement. PET scans may show asymptomatic bone involvement but are not typically routine. Baseline bone densitometry may be done if biphosphonates are going to be administered.

A bone marrow biopsy and aspirate is essential to the diagnostic workup. Cytogenetics and FISH (fluorescence in situ hybridization) may determine chromosomal abnormalities now linked to myeloma. A deletion of chromosome 13 (del(13)), p53 deletion, and a translocation between chromosomes 4 and 14 (t(4;14)) are all associated with a poor prognosis. Improved survival may be noted with a translocation between 11 and 14 (t(11;14)). Other chromosomal abnormalities include a deletion in chromosome 17 (del(17)) and a translocation between chromosomes 14 and 16 (t(14;16)). A biopsy of an ▶ extramedullary mass may be essential to the diagnosis.

Other nonstandard tests may include plasma cell labeling index to identify the fraction of proliferating myeloma cells, staining for ▶ amyloid, as well as measure of serum viscosity where appropriate.

Staging: Diagnostic Categories

Smoldering (asymptomatic disease)
Active (symptomatic) disease

The older Durie and Salmon Staging System incorporates baseline hemoglobin, serum calcium, bone involvement, renal function, and M-component. The newer International Staging System is based on serum albumin and beta-2 microglobulin making it easier to use than the older Durie and Salmon System (Tables 1–3); (Anderson 2009).

Plasma Cell Myeloma. Table 1 Durie and Salmon staging system

Stage I	All of the following: – Hemoglobin > 10 mg/dl – Serum calcium normal – Normal bones or solitary plasmacytoma only – Low M-component (IgG < 5 g/dl, IgA < 3 g/dl, urine light chains < 4 g/24 h)
Stage II	Fits neither Stage I or Stage III
Stage III	One or more of the following: – Hemoglobin > 8.5 g/dl – Serum calcium > 12 mg/dl – Advanced lytic lesions – High M-component (IgG > 7 g/dl; IgA > 3 g/dl; urine light chains > 12 g/24 h)
Subclassification: A: Normal renal function B: Abnormal renal function	Serum creatinine < 2 mg/dl Serum creatinine > 2 mg/dl

Plasma Cell Myeloma. Table 2 International Staging System (ISS)

Stage I	Serum beta-2 microbulin < 3.5 mg/l, Serum albumin > 35 g/L
Stage II	Neither I or III
Stage III	Serum beta-2 microglobulin > 5.5 mg/l

Treatment

Smoldering (Asymptomatic) Myeloma

This disease is often quiescent with an indolent course which may last many years. NCCN guidelines advise observation for this group with either Durie–Salmon classification with hemoglobin > 10 g/dl, serum calcium < 12 mg/dl, absence of bone lesions on x-ray, and low

Plasma Cell Myeloma. Table 3 Adverse prognostic factors

ECOG performance status of 3 or 4
Serum albumin < 3 g/dl
Serum creatinine > 2 mg/dl
Platelets < 150,000
Age > 70
B2-Microglobulin > 4 mg/l
Plasma cell labeling index > 1%
Serum calcium > 11 mg/dl
Hemoglobin < 10 g/dl
Bone marrow plasma cell > 50%

M-protein production or ISS Stage I with beta-2 microglobulin <3.5 mg/l and serum albumin > 3.5 g/dl without symptoms or end organ damage. These patients generally have low M-protein concentrations, and bone marrow infiltration is <10% plasma cells. These include Durie–Salmon Stage I. Periodic surveillance monitoring is advised with evaluation of CBC, LDH, calcium, creatinine, Beta-2 microglobulin, SPEP, and SIFE. Other studies such as bone marrow biopsy and imaging studies are guided by symptoms.

Disease Progression: >25% increase in plasma cells or >25% increase in M-protein in serum or urine, bone lesions increasing in size and/or number, and hypercalcemia. When Stage II or greater, treatment may be recommended.

Active (Symptomatic) Multiple Myeloma

These patients have symptoms such as bone pain, renal compromise, hypercalcemia, hyperviscosity, and hypercoagulability. Typically, anemia with hemoglobin < 10 g/dl, serum calcium > 12 mg/dl, lytic bone lesions, and renal insufficiency with creatinine > 2 mg/dl should receive treatment. In addition to receiving treatment for the underlying myeloma, many also require treatment directed at correction of these symptomatic and concurrent medical problems.

The best treatment for any patient should be enrollment in a clinical trial if one is available. Treatment should be in a clinical trial which consists of induction chemotherapy followed by high-dose chemotherapy and autologous stem cell support in select patients. Formerly, melphalan and prednisone were favored agents in early management. Then vincristine, adriamycin, and dexamethasone (VAD) were used in combination. When VAD was compared with TD, thalidomide (Thalomid) and dexamethasone, the TD regimen provided superior results with a 64% response rate. However, there is a significant risk of deep vein thrombosis (DVT) of 12% and peripheral neuropathy but little myelosuppression.

With the introduction of lenalidomide (Revlimid), when paired with dexamethasone, superior results and lower incidence of thromboembolic events have been seen. However, progenitor cell collections must be performed no later than after four cycles of therapy to prevent interference with their mobilization. In the untreated pre-transplant patient, Revlimid and dexamethasone appear to be the safest combination in patients with standard-risk disease. Low dose dexamethasone is preferred over standard dose in combination with lenalidomide.

Bortezomib (Velcade) introduction has led to even greater response rates along with complete remissions of 20–30%. For those patients with high-risk disease with a guarded prognosis, use of borezomib-containing regimens is advised.

For those nontransplant eligible patients, the regimen of choice is melphalan, prednisone, and thalidomide in standard-risk patients. For high-risk patients, the addition of bortezomib is recommended to the standard melphalan and prednisone.

Relapsed disease can be treated on a clinical trial. If this is not a possibility, then the use of any of the newer agents alone or in combinations may result in more durable responses.

▶ Autologous stem cell transplant (ASCT) has become the standard of care for eligible patients as it increases the probability of complete response, prolonged disease-free survival, and has extended overall survival. Mortality due to the procedure is now about 2% and the transplant can be performed as an outpatient.

Double transplantation or tandem transplantation is a second transplant after recovery from the first. However, the patients who benefit from the second transplant are those who only achieve a suboptimal response to the first transplant.

Radiation Treatment of Multiple Myeloma

The main use for radiation is for palliation of painful bony disease. Some 40% of patients will likely receive palliative radiation during the course of their disease. Treatment of long bones can be to the area of involvement rather than to the whole bone, as rarely are there relapses beyond the site of involvement. Doses of 10–20 Gy generally are sufficient. Spine involvement requires doses of 30 Gy in 10 fractions to provide a more durable response, relief of pain, and prevention of neurologic sequelae. More generous volumes should be considered with spine irradiation but must be balanced by a consideration of the marrow effects of the radiation. Concurrent treatment with bortezomib and radiation leads to severe enteritis and should be avoided. Prophylactic use of biphosphonates was shown to reduce the need for palliative radiation treatment in at least one study. TBI and hemi-body radiation are not standard regimens in the treatment of myeloma patients.

Solitary Plasmacytoma

These are collections of plasma cells which may be osseous or extraosseous in origin. When present in a bone without other evidence of disease, a solitary plasmacytoma is osseous. Extraosseous plasmactyomas are derived from soft tissue. A thorough systemic evaluation is mandatory in order to rule out the presence of occult disease which would indicate systemic multiple myeloma.

The presence of an osseous plasmacytoma, as opposed to an extraosseous presentation, is associated with a 76% risk of development of myeloma within 10 years. Another poor prognostic is the presence of subclinical bony disease, and rapid progression to symptomatic myeloma is predicted.

Treatment for these lesions is generally radiation with a dose of 40–45 Gy to the involved field. This is considered to be definitive treatment. The role of systemic treatment is reserved for systemic and symptomatic relapse. However, follow-up surveillance is necessary to determine if the patient remains in remission or develops stigmata of progression to full-blown multiple myeloma. High local control rates exist and overall survival is 50% at 10 years. Unfortunately, more than 60% with solitary lesions progress to myeloma, with a median of 2–3 years after treatment.

The M-protein level is very significant. If elevated prior to treatment, systemic relapse is much more likely if it remains elevated following treatment.

With extraosseous plasmacytomas, surgery may be sufficient for smaller lesions. But, larger lesions as well as incompletely excised lesions also receive radiation treatment. Progression to myeloma is much less common. Many are cured of their disease.

Extent of the radiation field has been discussed with regard to inclusion of nodal-bearing areas. However, it is not common to include nodal areas for soft tissue plasmacytomas.

Doses over 40 Gy are necessary for control with a local failure rate of 6% which increases with lower doses. For bulky tumors, doses above 45 Gy may be necessary if tumors are bulky and over 5 cm in size.

Follow-up consists of blood and urine tests every 4 weeks to assess response. Periodic radiographic studies at intervals of 4–6 months. Residual abnormalities may persist beyond treatment and are not necessarily indicative of persistent disease. An M-protein increase can precede clinical development of disease progression.

Cross-References

▶ Leukemia
▶ Non-Hodgkins Lymphoma
▶ Pain Management
▶ Palliation of Bone Metastases
▶ Supportive Care and Quality of Life

References

Anderson KC, Bensinger W, Richardson PG (2008) Impact of the 2009 NCCN guidelines on the diagnosis, staging and treatment of multiple myeloma. In: Abeloff (ed) Clinical Oncology, 4th edn. Update, 2008, 3

Anderson KC et al (2009) NCCN clinical practice guidelines in oncology: multiple myeloma. J Natl Compr Cancer Netw 7(9):908–942

Dingli D, Rajkumar SV (2009) Emerging therapies for multiple myeloma. Oncology 23(5): 407–415

Gleason C, Nooka A, Lonial S (2009) Supportive therapies in multiple myeloma. J Natl Compr Cancer Netw 7(9):971

Harousseau JL (2009a) Hematopoietic stem cell in multiple myeloma. J Natl Compr Cancer Netw 7(9):961–970

Harousseau JL (2009b) Autologous hematopoeitic stem-cell transplantation for multiple. N Engl J Med 360:2645–2654

Hodgson DC, Mikhael J, Tsang RW (2008) Plasma cell myeloma and plasmacytoma. In: Halperin EC, Perez CA, Brady LW (eds) Perez and Brady's principles and practice of radiation oncology, 5th edn. Lippincott Williams & Wilkins, Philadelphia, p 1790

Katzel JA et al (2007) Multiple Myeloma: charging toward a bright future. CA Cancer J Clin 57: 301–318

Laubach JP et al (2009) Novel therapies in the treatment of multiple myeloma. J Natl Compr Cancer Netw 7(9):947–960

Rajkumar SV, Kyle RA (2007) Plasma cell disorders. In: Goldman L, Ausiello D (eds) Cecil Medicine, 23rd edn. Saunders Elsevier, Philadelphia

Plasma Cell Neoplasm

▶ Plasma Cell Myeloma

Plasmacytoma

▶ Leukemia
▶ Leukemia in general
▶ Multiple Myeloma
▶ Plasma Cell Myeloma

Platinum Analogs

RENE RUBIN
Rittenhouse Hematology/Oncology,
Philadelphia, PA, USA

Definition

The platinum analogs (cisplatin, carboplatin) covalently bind to the DNA and work nonspecifically regarding the cell cycle. A lot of tumors are treated with these drugs (non-small cell lung cancer, small cell lung cancer, carcinoma of the head and neck, esophageal cancer, bladder cancer, ovarian cancer, germ cell carcinoma, non-Hodgkin's lymphoma). They enhance the tumor activity of etoposide and are widely used (cisplatin) as radiosensitizers. Amifostine and mesna may ameliorate the nephrotoxicity.

Side Effects

- Nephrotoxicity (cisplatin)
- Marrow suppression (carboplatin)
- Nausea and vomiting
- Neurotoxicity
- Ototoxicity
- Alopecia
- Schwarz-Bartter-Syndrome (SIADH) (cisplatin)
- Hepatoxicity and abnormalities in liver function tests

Cross-References

▶ Principles of Chemotherapy

Pleomorphic Adenoma

LINDSAY G. JENSEN, LOREN K. MELL
Center for Advanced Radiotherapy Technologies,
Department of Radiation Oncology, San Diego
Rebecca and John Moores Cancer Center,
University of California, La Jolla, CA, USA

Definition

Most common benign tumor of the salivary glands and also most common salivary gland tumor overall. Occurs more commonly in younger patients and is usually treated with superficial parotidectomy (Terhaard 2008).

Cross-References

▶ Salivary Gland Cancer
▶ Sarcomas of the Head and Neck

Pleural Mesothelioma

RAMESH RENGAN[1], CHARLES R. THOMAS, JR.[2]
[1]Department of Radiation Oncology, Hospital of
the University of Pennsylvania, Philadelphia,
PA, USA
[2]Department of Radiation Medicine, Oregon
Health Sciences University, Portland, OR, USA

Synonyms

Malignant mesothelioma

Definition/Description

Pleural mesothelioma is an aggressive cancer that originates from the serosal cells of the pleural cavity. It is linked epidemiologically to exposure to asbestos. The latency period from exposure to clinical presentation can often be decades, suggesting that other modulatory factors may contribute. Pleural mesothelioma has also been linked to radiation exposure with increased incidence in children treated with radiation for Wilm's tumor or lymphoma. Histologically, mesotheliomas are divided into an epithelial subtype (~50%), a sarcomatoid subtype (~10%), a mixed/biphasic subtype (~30%), and a desmoplastic subtype. The sarcomatoid subtype is particularly aggressive. Unfortunately, the treatment options for malignant mesothelioma, regardless of subtype, that are currently available for this disease are largely ineffective (Eng et al. 2007).

Anatomy

The thoracic pleura consists of a solitary serosal membrane that folds to cover both the lung (visceral pleura) and lines the thoracic cavity (parietal pleura). The parietal pleura contains sensory fibers and is sensitive to pain, while the visceral pleura does not contain pain receptors. The space between the parietal and the visceral pleura is known as the pleural cavity and is invisible in health as the two layers are in complete apposition. Pleural fluid, which is produced by the parietal circulation, is continuously circulated within the pleural space. Regional lymph nodes include intrathoracic, scalene, supraclavicular, internal mammary, and peridiaphragmatic.

Epidemiology

In 1960, Wagner et al. showed that South African mine workers who had been exposed to crocilodite asbestos were dying of pleural mesothelioma (Wagner et al. 1960). Unfortunately, it was not until approximately 15 years later that crocilodite mining and usage was discontinued. Based upon the predicted 30–40 year lag in presentation, it is expected that mesothelioma rates will continue to rise in the USA until approximately 2020. In the New York city area, there was considerable exposure to asbestos on September 11, 2001. It is unclear the impact that this exposure will have on mesothelioma rates. The annual incidence of mesothelioma in the

USA is approximately 2,000 new cases per year (Antman 1993). There is a strong male predominance (3:1) with the median age at presentation being ~60 years of age. Unfortunately, there are still some regions of the world that continue to use asbestos today. In addition to asbestos, radiation exposure has been shown to be causatively linked to mesothelioma with increased incidence identified in adults with previous thoracic radiation treatment or exposure to thoratrast.

Clinical Presentation

The majority of patients present with non-pleuritic chest pain and dyspnea. Most patients will present with an associated pleural effusion. Cytologic confirmation of malignancy is only achieved in approximately 60% of cases and therefore a pleural biopsy remains the gold standard for diagnosis. The duration of symptoms can range from weeks to years with a median time to diagnosis from the onset of symptoms being 3 months.

Differential Diagnosis

The differential diagnosis for pleural mesothelioma is an adenocarcinoma of the lung with pleural dissemination or solitary fibrous tumors of the pleura.

Imaging Studies

Chest X-ray is often part of the initial evaluation of symptoms. This study may reveal the presence of a pleural effusion or diffuse pleural thickening. Contrast-enhanced computed tomographic scan of the thorax is the diagnostic chest of choice. This allows for density resolution and three-dimensional visualization not possible with a chest X-ray. A CT scan may reveal plaque-like pleural thickening as well as intrapulmonary nodules (Fig. 1). Magnetic resonance imaging may be useful to identify diaphragmatic invasion. Finally, PET/CT is gaining acceptance for identification of extrathoracic disease, however, its role in identification of mediastinal nodal disease remains to be defined (Flores et al. 2003). The updated IMIG staging system for pleural mesothelioma is shown in Table 1.

Laboratory Studies

There are no laboratory aberrations that are specific to mesothelioma. The patient may have nonspecific findings such as anemia of chronic disease or vitamin B12 or B6 deficiency. Additionally, thrombocytosis is often seen in patients with mesothelioma with 15% of patients having counts above 1,000,000.

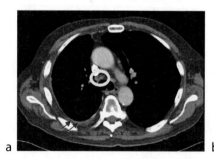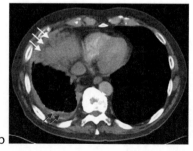

Pleural Mesothelioma. Fig. 1 CT scan of patient with right pleural mesothelioma with pleural thickening (*red arrows*) and (**a**) mediastinal adenopathy (*yellow circle*) and (**b**) right hemidiaphragmatic invasion (*white arrows*)

Pleural Mesothelioma. Table 1 International mesothelioma interest group staging system for pleural mesothelioma (AJCC Cancer Staging Manual 2010)

Tumor (T)	
Tx	Primary tumor cannot be assessed
T0	No evidence of primary tumor
T1	Tumor involves ipsilateral parietal pleura, with or without focal involvement of visceral pleura
T1a	Tumor involves ipsilateral parietal (mediastinal, diaphragmatic) pleura. No involvement of the visceral pleura
T1b	Tumor involves ipsilateral parietal (mediastinal, diaphragmatic) pleura, with focal involvement of the visceral pleura
T2	Tumor involves any of the ipsilateral pleural surfaces with at least one of the following: – Confluent visceral pleural tumor (including fissure) – Invasion of diaphragmatic muscle – Invasion of lung parenchyma
Resectable	
T3[a]	Tumor involves any of the ipsilateral pleural surfaces, with at least one of the following: – Involvement of endothoracic fascia – Invasion into mediastinal fat – Solitary focus of tumor invading the soft tissues of the chest wall – Non-transmural involvement of the pericardium
T4[b]	Tumor involves any of the ipsilateral pleural surfaces with at least one of the following: – Diffuse or multifocal invasion into soft tissues of the chest wall – Any involvement of rib – Invasion through the diaphragm to the peritoneum – Invasion of any mediastinal organ(s) – Direct extension to the contralateral pleura – Invasion into the spine – Extension to the internal surface of the pericardium – Pericardial effusion with positive cytology – Invasion of the myocardium – Invasion of the brachial plexus

Pleural Mesothelioma. Table 1 (continued)

Nodes (N)	
NX	Regional lymph nodes cannot be assessed
N0	No lymph node metastases
N1	Metastases in ipsilateral bronchopulmonary and/or hilar lymph node(s)
N2	Metastases in the subcarinal lymph node(s) and/or the ipsilateral mediastinal, peridiaphragmatic, or internal mammary node(s)
N3	Metastases in the contralateral mediastinal, internal mammary, or hilar lymph node(s) and/or the ipsilateral or contralateral supraclavicular or scalene lymph node(s)

Metastasis (M)	
Mx	Distant metastases cannot be assessed
M0	No metastases
M1	Distant metastases

Stage	Grouping		
I			
Ia	T1a	N0	M0
Ib	T1b	N0	M0
II	T2	N0	M0
III	T3	N0, N1, N2	M0
	T1, T2	N1	M0
	T1,T2	N2	M0
IV	T4	Any N	M0
	Any T	N3	M0
	Any T	Any N	M1

[a]T3 describes locally advanced, but potentially resectable tumor
[b]T4 describes locally advanced, technically unresectable tumor

Diagnostic Approach

A pleural biopsy represents the gold standard for diagnosis. A thoracentesis with cytologic examination of the pleural fluid, if positive, is diagnostic. Multiple pleural biopsies must be taken in order to avoid sampling error. Pleural biopsy may be achieved either through a thoracentesis with closed pleural biopsy, through video-assisted thoracoscopy, or an open procedure. If an open procedure is required, care must be taken to ensure that the scar can be incorporated into the major incision for the major resection, if performed.

Treatment

Surgery

There is no current established standard of care for resectable pleural mestheliona. Surgical resection, either through an extrapleural pneumonectomy (EPP) or pleurectomy decortication are the treatment approaches that are most commonly employed. The approach chosen is influenced by extent of disease and pulmonary and overall functional status of the patient and philosophy and experience of the physician. Long-term survival rates after EPP are disappointing with a median survival of 10 months. Patients usually succumb to locoregional relapse. These results have ushered in interest in multimodality approaches to the treatment of this disease.

Radiotherapy

Radiotherapy has been utilized both as a sole modality for the treatment of inoperable patients and as an adjuvant treatment after surgery. Definitive radiotherapy alone is hampered by the risk of normal tissue injury to the underlying lung. IMRT or Arc-based treatment approaches have been employed to deliver 40–55 cGy to the pleural space. Adjuvant radiotherapy may be effective; however, care must be taken to minimize the dose to the contralateral lung to limit the risk of potentially fatal radiation pneumonitis (Allen et al. 2006). IMRT has been commonly employed, however, a matched electron-photon technique may have dosimetric advantages (Hill-Kayser et al. 2009).

Chemotherapy

Single agent chemotherapy has poor activity in this disease. However, combination approaches with platinum-based regimens have shown activity. The combination of cisplatin and pemetrexed has recently been shown to be superior to cisplatin monotherapy with a 41% response rate and median survival of 12.1 months. These numbers compare favorably with other platinum-based doublets (Vogelzang et al. 2003).

Intrapleural Photodynamic Therapy

Photodynamic therapy utilizes light activation of sensitized tumor cells to achieve sterilization. The patient is infused with a photosensitizer that accumulates in malignant tissue in vivo. This sensitizer is then activated by 630 nm light in the operating room producing reactive oxygen species. This is an attractive approach in that it confers specificity of therapy thorough placement of light at the time of surgical resection, allowing for direct visualization of regions at risk for recurrence. Studies validating this approach are ongoing.

In short, the treatment of mesothelioma requires a multidisciplinary approach with an experienced team consisting of a pulmonary specialist, thoracic surgeon, thoracic radiation oncologist, and a medical oncologist.

References

AJCC Cancer Staging Manual (2010) Heidelberg, Springer

Allen AM, Czerminska M et al (2006) Fatal pneumonitis associated with intensity-modulated radiation therapy for mesothelioma. Int J Radiat Oncol Biol Phys 65(3):640–645

Antman KH (1993) Natural history and epidemiology of malignant mesothelioma. Chest 103(4 Suppl): 373S–376S

Eng TY, Stevens CW et al (2007) Uncommon thoracic malignances. In: Gunderson LL, Tepper JE (eds) Clinical radiation oncology. Churchill Livingston/Elsevier, Philadelphia, pp 973–1005

Flores RM, Akhurst T et al (2003) Positron emission tomography defines metastatic disease but not locoregional disease in patients with malignant pleural mesothelioma. J Thorac Cardiovasc Surg 126(1):11–16

Hill-Kayser CE, Avery S et al (2009) Hemithoracic radiotherapy after extrapleural pneumonectomy for malignant pleural mesothelioma: a dosimetric comparison of two well-described techniques. J Thorac Oncol 4(11):1431–1437

Vogelzang NJ, Rusthoven JJ et al (2003) Phase III study of pemetrexed in combination with cisplatin versus cisplatin alone in patients with malignant pleural mesothelioma. J Clin Oncol 21(14): 2636–2644

Wagner JC, Sleggs CA et al (1960) Diffuse pleural mesothelioma and asbestos exposure in the North Western Cape Province. Br J Ind Med 17:260–271

PNET Tumor

▶ Extraskeletal Small Cell Tumors

Pneumoperitoneum

HEDVIG HRICAK[1], OGUZ AKIN[2], HEBERT ALBERTO VARGAS[2]
[1]Department of Radiology, Memorial Sloan-Kettering Cancer Center, New York, NY, USA
[2]Body MRI, Memorial Sloan-Kettering Cancer Center, New York, NY, USA

Definition
Refers to the presence of air within the peritoneal cavity. The most common cause is a perforation of the bowel. Other causes include recent surgical procedures, infection, or trauma.

Cross-References
▶ Imaging in Oncology

Pneumothorax

HEDVIG HRICAK[1], OGUZ AKIN[2], HEBERT ALBERTO VARGAS[2]
[1]Department of Radiology, Memorial Sloan-Kettering Cancer Center, New York, NY, USA
[2]Body MRI, Memorial Sloan-Kettering Cancer Center, New York, NY, USA

Definition
Collection of air in the pleural space (between the lung and the chest wall) resulting in collapse of the lung in the affected side.

Cross-References
▶ Imaging in Oncology

Point A

CHRISTIN A. KNOWLTON[1], MICHELLE KOLTON MACKAY[2]
[1]Department of Radiation Oncology, Drexel University, Philadelphia, PA, USA
[2]Department of Radiation Oncology, Marshfield Clinic, Marshfield, WI, USA

Definition
Point A is a dose point used in brachytherapy treatment planning in the treatment of cervical cancer and medically inoperable uterine cancer. It is located 2 cm superior to the cervical os along the tandem and 2 cm lateral to the plane of the tandem. It represents the lateral cervix/medial parametrium at the approximate location where the uterine vessels cross the ureter.

P

P

Cross-References

▶ Brachytherapy: High Dose Rate (HDR) Implants
▶ Endometrium
▶ Low-Dose Rate (LDR) Brachytherapy
▶ Uterine Cervix

Point Dose Kernel

Charlie Ma, Lu Wang
Department of Radiation Oncology, Fox Chase Cancer Center, Philadelphia, PA, USA

Definition

Point dose kernel: The dose distribution in water resulting from both scattered photons and secondary electrons set in motion by primary photon interactions at one particular point.

Cross-References

▶ Dose Calculation Algorithms

Population

Edward J. Gracely
Department of Epidemiology and Biostatistics, College of Medicine, Drexel University, Philadelphia, PA, USA

Definition

The group of all individuals to which study results are intended to apply. Estimated by sample data.

Cross-References

▶ Statistics and Clinical Trials

Positron Emission Tomography

Feng-Ming Kong[1], Jingbo Wang[1], Christin A. Knowlton[2], Michelle Kolton Mackay[3]
[1]Department of Radiation Oncology, Veteran Administration Health Center and University Hospital University of Michigan, Ann Arbor, MI, USA
[2]Department of Radiation Oncology, Drexel University, Philadelphia, PA, USA
[3]Department of Radiation Oncology, Marshfield Clinic, Marshfield, WI, USA

Synonyms

PET scan

Definition

Positron emission tomography is a type of nuclear medicine imaging based on the four-dimensional (spatial and time) distribution of a given radiotracer within human body and can reveal the metabolic function such as glucose metabolism. Therefore, it is often referred to as a functional imaging modality. Positron emission tomography (PET) scan is a nuclear medicine test that creates three-dimensional images according to metabolic uptake in cells. It is very useful in cancer staging, as malignant cells are PET avid. Fluorodeoxyglucose is the radioactive tracer administered for this examination.

Cross-References

▶ Bladder
▶ Esophageal Cancer
▶ Hodgkin's Lymphoma
▶ Lung
▶ Melanoma
▶ Non-Hodgkin's Lymphoma
▶ Sarcomas of the Head and Neck
▶ Uterine Cervix

Positron Emission Tomography (PET)

HEDVIG HRICAK[1], OGUZ AKIN[2], HEBERT ALBERTO VARGAS[2]
[1]Department of Radiology, Memorial Sloan-Kettering Cancer Center, New York, NY, USA
[2]Body MRI, Memorial Sloan-Kettering Cancer Center, New York, NY, USA

Definition

Nuclear medicine imaging technique that produces a three-dimensional image or picture of functional processes in the body. The system detects pairs of photons emitted indirectly but simultaneously by a positron-emitting radionuclide (tracer), which is introduced into the body on a biologically active molecule.

Cross-References

▶ Imaging in Oncology

Post Mastectomy Reconstruction

ANTHONY E. DRAGUN
Department of Radiation Oncology, James Graham Brown Cancer Center, University of Louisville School of Medicine, Louisville, KY, USA

Synonyms

Autologous tissue reconstruction; Immediate-delayed reconstruction

Definition

Post mastectomy reconstruction is an important offering for any patient who chooses or requires mastectomy for the treatment of her primary disease. Ideal techniques of reconstruction and the integration with adjuvant treatment are subjects of debate. In general, reconstruction may be considered immediate (at the time of mastectomy) in order to avoid the risks of multiple major surgeries, or delayed after adjuvant therapy has been completed. Best outcomes are obtained in patients who are nonsmokers and who have a low volume of disease at the time of diagnosis. Immediate-delayed reconstruction consists of the insertion of a temporary tissue expander with a eventual exchange for the permanent implant. Autologous tissue reconstruction consists of the use of the trans rectus abdominal (TRAM), deep inferior epigastric pedicle (DIEP), or latisimus dorsi flap techniques.

Cross-References

▶ Stage 0 Breast Cancer

Potassium Iodide

JOHN P. CHRISTODOULEAS
The Perelman Cancer Center, Department of Radiation Oncology, University of Pennsylvania Hospital, Philadelphia, PA, USA

Definition

Potassium iodide is an FDA-approved medicine that may be used to protect the thyroid gland from I-131 contamination during power-plant accidents. Potassium iodide can saturate the thyroid and thus inhibit thyroid uptake of ingested or inhaled I-131 allowing the radioactive isotope to be excreted.

Cross-References

▶ Radiation-Induced Genomic Instability
▶ Short-Term and Long-Term Health Risk of Nuclear Power Plant Accident

Power

Edward J. Gracely
Department of Epidemiology and Biostatistics,
College of Medicine, Drexel University,
Philadelphia, PA, USA

Definition

The probability that a study will obtain evidence for a true difference or effect of a certain magnitude, if in fact such a difference or effect exists.

Cross-References

▶ Statistics and Clinical Trials

Predictive In vitro Assays in Radiation Oncology

Claudia E. Rübe
Department of Radiation Oncology, Saarland University, Homburg/Saar, Germany

Predictive Assays for Normal Tissue Reactions

The maximum dose of radiotherapy that can be given during cancer therapy is determined by the tolerance of normal tissues within the irradiation field. Patients vary considerably in their response to radiation and it is the tolerance of the more sensitive subjects that limits the dose that can be given to the population as a whole; this may limit the chance of tumor cure in some cases. Predictive assays that accurately determine normal tissue tolerance in individual patients permit modification of the treatment in radiosensitive individuals to prevent severe side effects, and to intensify radiotherapy in relatively resistant patients, thereby improving the therapeutic ratio in cancer treatment.

In the past decades, our understanding of normal tissue responses to radiation damage has advanced enormously. It is now widely recognized that the pathogenesis of ▶ radiation-induced normal tissue injury is a highly complex process, whereas tissue-specific characteristics have profound impact on normal tissues responses. Radiation induces an orchestrated response cascade at the molecular, cellular, and tissue level involving ▶ DNA damage response, cell cycle arrest, induction of apoptosis, loss of reproductive capacity, premature senescence, cytokine cascades, tissue remodeling, etc. Predictive in vitro assays try to target different variables known to determine normal tissue reactions.

Intrinsic Radiosensitivity

In the 1980s and early 1990s, the target cell hypothesis reigned supreme in radiation biology. This hypothesis stated that killing and depletion of critical target cells based on their ▶ intrinsic radiosensitivity is the main effect of ionizing radiation. The long latent time, in which damage was not overtly expressed for months after radiotherapy, was assumed to be due to the long cycle time of the target cells. The most reliable in vitro assay for monitoring intrinsic cellular radiosensitivity is the ▶ clonogenic survival assay. In this test, cells are grown in soft agar, which reduces cell movement and allows individual cells to develop into cell clones that can be identified as single colonies. Survival dose-response curves after irradiation with different doses have been thoroughly analyzed with different cell types, but were most frequently carried out using skin fibroblasts. The surviving fraction of normal cells in vitro after irradiation doses of 2 Gy (SF2) was thought to be a useful estimate of the effect of clinical dose fractions. However, clinical studies on the possible predictive value of the in vitro radiosensitivity of normal human skin fibroblasts reported varying associations with normal tissue side effects. Moreover, clonogenic survival assays are of limited value for predictive testing in the clinic setting, because these assays need culture periods of several weeks and are not feasible for cell types that display low cloning efficiency.

Biomarkers

▶ Biomarkers measured in blood and other samples have been analyzed to potentially predict how certain tissues might respond to treatment. Most biomarkers studies (▶ Molecular Markers in Clinical Radiation Oncology) so far have been based on the specific detection of proteins with defined biological functions during radiation-induced tissue reactions. It is likely however that any single marker may not suffice in capturing the complexities of normal tissue responses to radiation therapy. Most of these biomarker studies have been carried out to predict the radiation-induced reactions of the lung. The pathogenesis of radiation-induced lung injury comprises an inflammatory process involving a complex interplay of cellular interactions mediated through a variety of ▶ cytokines, chemokines, adhesion molecules, etc. Animal data have shown an early overproduction of both pro-inflammatory and pro-fibrogenic cytokines in lung tissue during thoracic irradiation and have suggested a role of the sustained production of these cytokines in the development of acute and late pulmonary toxicities. Consequently, cytokines have been used in clinical studies to evaluate their potential as biomarkers for radiation-induced injury. Some clinical reports have shown changes in the plasma concentration of TGF-β1 and IL-6 during radiotherapy and suggested that these variations could identify patients at risk of radiation pneumonitis. Other investigators, however, could not confirm that cytokine levels, neither their absolute nor any relative values, may identify patients at increased risk for normal tissue injury (Rübe et al. 2008). Accordingly, it cannot be concluded with certainty, that cytokine plasma levels can be used as biomarkers for radiation-induced lung injury.

DNA Damage Repair

Exposure of cells to ionizing radiation results in the induction of DNA damage, and processes responding to that damage that serve to maintain DNA integrity lie at the core of the cellular response to radiation (▶ Radiation-induced Genomic Instability and Radiation Sensitivity). By the mid 1970s, it was appreciated that, although single-strand breaks (SSB) arise more frequently than double-strand breaks (DSB), the latter represent the most significant lethal lesion. Central to these studies were emerging methods to monitor SSB and DSB induction and repair. An early technique was sucrose gradient sedimentation, which separated DNA fragments based on size. The analysis was carried out under alkaline or neutral conditions to detect SSB or DSB, respectively. Radiation was shown to reduce the sedimentation rate of DNA, which following incubation, returned to that observed in nonirradiated cells. The alkaline and neutral DNA elution technique and the DNA unwinding technique were additional approaches exploited to measure SSB and DSB induction and repair. However, many limitations existed with the standard protocols in that it was unable to separate large molecules of DNA effectively. Subsequently, ▶ pulsed field gel electrophoresis emerged as an even more sensitive methodology, by introducing an alternating voltage gradient leading to a better resolution of larger molecules. These methods have limitations, however. First, they necessitate the use of high radiation doses, usually >10 Gy, precluding an examination of DNA repair following therapeutically relevant doses. Second, these techniques are not readily able to detect subtle repair defects. Third, apoptosis also causes DNA breakage and the techniques do not readily facilitate a distinction between breakages arising as a consequence of radiation-induced apoptosis versus directly induced DNA breaks.

A more recent approach for quantifying the induction and repair of DNA damage encompass the neutral ▶ comet assay, a versatile technique for the detection of SSB and DSB at the single cell level. It involves the encapsulation of cells in low-melting-point agarose suspension, lysis of the cells under neutral or alkaline conditions, and electrophoresis of the suspended lysed cells. This is followed by visual analysis with staining of DNA and calculating fluorescence to determine the extent of DNA damage. However, comet analysis of in vitro irradiated cells did not correlate well with the occurrence of acute or late normal tissue reactions after therapeutic radiotherapy, suggesting that these DNA damage assays are not suitable for predicting the risk or severity of radiation-induced normal tissue responses (Fernet et al. 2008).

Over the past several years, γH2AX expression has been established as a sensitive indicator of DSB. At sites of radiation-induced DSB, histone H2AX becomes rapidly phosphorylated, extending several megabase pairs from the site of the DSB, and can be visualized by immunofluorescence as discrete nuclear foci (referred as γH2AX-foci). The number of foci visualized closely correlates with current estimates of DSB formation, and their rate of loss closely parallels the rate of DSB repair monitored by the methods described above. Thus, ▶ γH2AX foci analysis is an exquisitely sensitive technique to monitor DSB repair, amenable for use with very low doses. There are limitations to the technique, however. H2AX phosphorylation can also arise from single-stranded regions of DNA generated following replication fork stalling or during the processing of bulky lesions. It is an indirect method that monitors the consequence of the lesion rather than the lesion itself; and finally, there may be a delay between DSB repair and loss of H2AX phosphorylation or circumstances when γH2AX loss does not occur. Currently, the γH2AX assay is investigated as a predictive test for the development of normal tissue complications. Recent evidence suggests that genetically defined DSB repair

capacities determine the individual risk of developing severe treatment-related side effects. In first clinical studies, γH2AX analysis of blood lymphocytes allowed the detection of DSB repair deficiencies and thus enabled clinicians to identify patients at risk for high-grade toxicities (Rübe et al. 2010).

Genetic Variants

Over the last decade, many studies have addressed possible associations between various genetic sequence alterations (single-nucleotide polymorphisms, SNPs) and risk of normal tissue complication after radiotherapy (▶ Radiation-induced Genomic Instability and Radiation Sensitivity). Most studies were based on a candidate gene approach, which means that, the investigated sequence alterations were selected based on functional knowledge about the gene product. The published studies can be broadly divided based on the mechanisms of the genes in the pathogenesis of radiation toxicity. Most studies have addressed genes involved in DNA damage response and reactive oxygen species (ROS) scavenging, as well as radiation-induced fibrogenesis (Andreassen et al. 2009). First insights into the underlying molecular mechanisms of radiosensitivity are coming from studies that assess associations between common polymorphisms in DNA damage detection and repair genes and the development of adverse reactions to radiotherapy. The presence of such variants may alter protein function and an individual's capacity to repair damaged DNA by modifying the response of the normal tissue. However, while some of these studies found clear associations between genetic variants in selected genes and normal tissue radiosensitivity, the attempts to identify robust genetic markers for the patient population as a whole have been disappointingly unrewarding. This finding probably reflects our insufficient understanding of the biology underlying the development of radiation-induced normal tissue damage. Genome-wide association studies may help to successfully unravel the genetic background for differences in radiation sensitivity (Bentzen et al. 2008).

Differential Gene Expression

Over the past decade, there has been a rapid expansion in the use of microarray technology to identify genes involved in normal tissue responses to radiotherapy. ▶ Gene expression profiling is the measurement of the activity of thousands of genes at once, to create a global picture of cellular functions. With respect to normal tissue radiation injury, microarrays have been used to generate gene signatures to identify radio-sensitive and radioresistant populations (thereby defining predisposition markers for radiation sensitivity), as well as to identify genes and pathways involved in tissue responses to unravel molecular mechanisms leading to acute and late tissue toxicity. Rather than focusing on individual genes, researchers focus on gene sets, based on functionally defined biochemical pathways. These gene sets allow the detection of coordinated changes in the expression of groups of functionally related genes, and thus facilitates the interpretation of large-scale experiments. Many of the genes identified showing differential expression were those involved in known radiation response pathways like DNA damage response, cell cycle arrest, proliferation, reactive oxygen scavenging, and extracellular matrix remodeling. A number of studies have investigated the transcriptional response to ionizing radiation in peripheral blood lymphocytes or cell cultures obtained from patients. Some studies have demonstrated a relationship between certain gene expression profiles for lymphocytes irradiated ex vivo and the development of acute or late radiation injury suggesting that with further optimization such an experimental approach may generate profiles that could be used to predict susceptibility. Gene expression profiling may become an important diagnostic test to predict clinical response to radiotherapy (Bentzen et al. 2008). However, none of the approaches developed so far have become routine in the clinic.

Collectively, substantial research efforts into predictive radiation oncology have so far produced very little terms of clinically applicable assays. This may change with the development of novel high-throughput assays, which facilitate the simultaneous collection of many thousands of biological data items from a single biopsy or blood sample from an individual. The introduction of these assays may open intriguing possibilities for a comprehensive biology approach to radiation effects in normal tissues. Although the technological possibilities seem endless, the practical implementation of these assays in the clinic appears to be some way into the future.

Predictive Assays for Tumors

The development of a successful clinical assay to predict tumor response to radiation therapy is a major clinical goal in radiation oncology. Such an approach could result in better selection of patients for radiotherapy protocols, could improve assessment of individual response and prognosis, and could lead to the personalization of radiation dose parameters.

Traditional in vitro assays to predict tumor response to radiotherapy assessed mainly the parameters intrinsic radiosensitivity, oxygenation status, and proliferative potential (Torres-Roca et al. 2008).

Intrinsic Radiosensitivity

Tumors of different histology differ considerably in their response to radiotherapy; and beyond that, tumors of the same histological type differ in their intrinsic radiosensitivity. The clonogenic cell survival assay, determining the survival fraction at 2 Gy (SF2), has been the gold standard to measure cellular tumor response to ionizing radiation. Studies on experimental tumors in animals have shown that SF2 measured in vitro can predict response to in vivo irradiation. These studies raised the possibility that measurements of individual tumor radiosensitivity might be used to predict response to clinical radiotherapy. However, the clinical application of the clonogenic cell survival assay has been hindered by technical difficulties of plating tumor cells ex vivo, with only about 1% plating efficiency. Furthermore, the results of this assay are not available at the time of treatment decision since plating and enumerating the clonogenic assays usually take several weeks. Another growth assay that has been used to determine radiosensitivity is the MTT (3-(4,5-dimethylthiazol-2-yl)-2,5-diphenyltetrazolium) assay. The ▶ MTT assay estimates cell survival based upon the capacity of living cells to reduce a tetrazolium compound to a colored product that can be measured spectrophotometrically. These reductions take place only when reductase enzymes are active, and therefore conversion is often used as a measure of viable (living) cells. However, it is important to keep in mind that other viability tests sometimes give completely different results, as many different conditions can increase or decrease metabolic activity.

Tumor Oxygenation Status

Hypoxic areas, resulting from an imbalance between the supply and consumption of oxygen, are a characteristic property of solid tumors. Major pathogenic mechanisms for the emergence of hypoxia are structural and functional abnormalities in the tumor microvasculature, an increase in diffusion distances, and tumor- or therapy-associated anemia leading to a reduced O_2 transport capacity of the blood. There is a pronounced inter-tumor variability in the extent of hypoxia, which is independent of clinical size, stage, histopathology type, or grade. ▶ Tumor hypoxia is a therapeutic problem, as it makes solid tumors resistant to ionizing radiation. The correlation between radiosensitivity and the pressure of oxygen is generally referred as "oxygen effect." Hypoxia as a predictor of radiation response has been studied in different cancer entities, and has been shown to be an independent prognostic factor in cervix cancers, carcinomas of the head and neck, and in soft-tissue sarcomas. Hence, the tumor oxygenation status plays a central role in tumor physiology and cancer treatment and is therefore an independent prognostic factor of overall and disease-free survival. The routine evaluation of the pretherapeutic tumor oxygenation status may facilitate the establishment of individual therapeutic strategies, including the use of antiangiogenic agents to target the tumor vasculature (Hypoxic Radiosensitizers and Cytotoxins in Radiation Oncology). Many independent studies involving various techniques have measured different parameters to define the tumor oxygenation status. The ▶ Eppendorf microelectrode has been considered the "gold standard" for several decades, as it has been the only technique that could directly measure the oxygen tension in tumor tissue. Eppendorf electrodes have been applied to accessible tumors, but this invasive approach is unfeasible for the most deep-seated tumors, where potential tissue damage by the Eppendorf needle is a problem. To address these practical issues, several studies have used hypoxia markers (e.g., hypoxia-inducible factor HIF-1α) to identify hypoxic tumor regions. However, tumor oxygenation is heterogeneous and cannot be described by single parameters. It is influenced by multiple factors including microvessel density, blood flow, blood oxygen saturation, tissue pO_2, oxygen consumption rate, and hypoxic fraction. An assessment combining several different methods is desirable to define the oxygen profile of a tumor for diagnostic and prognostic purposes. However, due to the technical demands and/or their invasive nature, none of these approaches have so far led to routine clinical use.

Tumor Proliferative Potential (Tpot)

Cell kinetic measurements have been used to predict which tumors will rapidly proliferate during treatment and thus are likely to benefit from accelerated radiotherapy. Among various cell kinetic parameters the ▶ tumor potential doubling time (Tpot) has been postulated to be a predictor of the tumor's proliferative capability, thus representing a potential predictive factor of local control after irradiation. Tpot is defined as the time within which the cell population of a tumor would double if there were no cell loss. Tpot can be calculated knowing the bromodeoxyuridine labeling index (proportion of cells incorporating the DNA precursor BrdU) and the DNA synthesis time measured by flow cytometry. Multicenter analysis has shown that pretreatment Tpot measurements using flow cytometry provide only a weak predictor of outcome after radiotherapy in head and neck cancer. Pitfalls associated with cell kinetic measurements such as assay variability, intratumor and intertumor variability, interlaboratory variability, and the problem of an admixture of normal and malignant cells make Tpot not accurate and reproducible enough for a robust predictive assay.

Over the past decade, research in molecular oncology has focused on the underlying mechanisms of carcinogenesis, tumor progression, and metastasis. Knowledge gained from this research has led to the development of new classes of drugs that target specific pathways known to be involved in one or more of the processes that may be altered as part of the tumor biology. The development of disease-specific anticancer drugs is advancing the treatment of many malignancies, generally referred as "▶ molecular targeting." The idea behind molecular targeting is to design drugs that specifically attack the molecular pathways that cause malignant disease, without disrupting the normal functions in other cells and tissues. In radiotherapy, there is a great need to identify new molecular targets that will allow the specific inactivation of tumor cells. In this context, certain receptors such as ▶ epidermal growth factor receptor (EGFR) are considered of great relevance. This receptor is involved in several important endpoints such as proliferation and differentiation, angiogenesis, metastasis, and in the DNA damage response after both radio-and chemotherapy. In many tumors, this receptor is over expressed and, most importantly, upregulated after irradiation. This upregulation is suggested to stimulate the respective DNA repair pathways, leading thus to radioresistance. Therefore, inhibition of EGFR either by antibodies or by specific tyrosine-kinase inhibitors was found to inhibit DNA repair and to enhance cell killing. Hence, modulation of tumor response to radiotherapy by targeting specific growth factor signaling pathways may establish new treatment options for various tumors. Rational strategies for combining radiotherapy with molecular therapeutics depend on finding which patients will respond to which targeted therapies and on developing assays to identify patients who might benefit from combined therapy modalities. However, to date no predictive tests are routinely used in the clinical setting to predict the clinical outcome of cancer patients after targeted therapy. More work is needed to conclusively characterize the parameters determining the tumor response to combined treatment modalities, and consequently, to develop strategies for the implementation of more personalized cancer therapies.

References

Andreassen CN, Alsner J (2009) Genetic variants and normal tissue toxicity after radiotherapy: a systematic review. Radiother Oncol 92:299–309

Bentzen SM (2008) From cellular to high-throughput predictive assays in radiation oncology: challenges and opportunities. Semin Radiat Oncol 18:75–88

Fernet M, Hall J (2008) Predictive markers for normal tissue reactions: fantasy or reality? Cancer Radiothér 12:614–618

Rübe CE, Palm J, Erren M, Fleckenstein J, König J, Remberger K, Rübe C (2008) Cytokine plasma levels: reliable predictors for radiation pneumonitis? Plos one 3(8):e2898

Rübe CE, Fricke A, Schneider R, Simon K, Kühne M, Fleckenstein J, Gräber S, Graf N, Rübe C (2010) DNA repair alterations in children with pediatric malignancies: novel opportunities to identify patients at risk for high-grade toxicities. Int J Radiat Oncol Biol Phys. [Epub ahead of print]

Torres-Roca JF, Stevens CW (2008) Predicting response to clinical radiotherapy: past, present, and future directions. Cancer Control 15:151–156

Preoperative (Preplan)

YAN YU, LAURA DOYLE
Department of Radiation Oncology, Thomas Jefferson University Hospital, Philadelphia, PA, USA

Definition

Dosimetric calculation based on TRUS images from a prostate volume study prior to implant procedure, determines the location of needles and seeds necessary to provide target coverage before the day of the implant.

Cross-References

▶ Brachytherapy: Low Dose Rate (LDR) Permanent Implants (Prostate)

Primary Cancer of The Duodenum

PAUL J. SCHILLING
Community Cancer Center of North Florida, Gainesville, FL, USA

Definition

A carcinoma arising in the proximal small intestine.

Introduction

Intra-abdominal gastrointestinal cancer most commonly occurs in the duodenum with an incidence of 50% of small bowel tumors, followed by the jejunum with 23% of primary tumors, followed by the ileum with 15%. The majority of patients present with node-positive disease (Howe 1999). The overall 1-year survival rate is 60.2%; 2-year survival rate is 44.2%; 3-year survival rate is 37%; and 5-year survival rate is 30%. Mean survival was 9.7 months (Howe 1999; Lai 2007). Adenocarcinoma arising in the duodenum shares many morphologic characteristics and risk factors of colorectal carcinoma. The tumors arise from preexisting polyps. Polyposis is associated with increased risk in patients with a familial polyposis, hereditary nonpolyposis colorectal cancer syndrome, and inflammatory bowel disease (Cheung 2003).

Diagnosis and Symptoms

Patients present with gastrointestinal hemorrhage, unresolved weight loss, epigastric pain, or malabsorption syndrome. The mean duration of symptoms in patients with primary duodenal cancers is 10.4 months (Kerremans 1979). Early diagnosis is certainly the key for curative surgical treatment and possible postoperative adjuvant treatment to improve regional control. In patients with primary duodenal cancer, the resectability is approximately 66%. If a tumor is suspected, the patient should undergo an upper GI, biopsy, and colonoscopy. CT scans are usually helpful to rule out hepatic or other abdominal metastasis or peritoneal carcinomatosis. The role of positron emission tomography is likely helpful, but currently unstudied.

Histologic Subtypes of Primary Duodenal Carcinoma

The most common histologic type is adenocarcinoma; other histologic types include non-Hodgkin's lymphoma, gastrointestinal stromal tumors, and carcinoid tumors. Each will be considered separately with respect to treatment.

Adenocarcinoma Arising in the Duodenum

Ninety percent of patients with familial polyposis syndrome including Gardner syndrome develop duodenal polyps. These polyps have malignant potential, and 2–5% of all patients with familial polyposis syndrome develop adenocarcinoma of the duodenum at some time in their lifetime. Adenocarcinoma of the duodenum is the leading cause of death among patients with familial polyposis syndrome who have had a proctocolectomy (Vasen 1997).

Surgery is the mainstay of treatment, with complete surgical resection with negative margins remaining the single best curative option for patients. Surgery may include segmental duodenal resection, pancreaticoduodenectomy, or pancreas-preserving duodenal resection. Less than complete excision of the duodenum appears to reduce overall survival (Sohn 1998; Crawley 1998). Prognostic features indicating the need for adjuvant treatment include positive regional nodes, positive margins, and transmural penetration (Lai 2007). For patients who have negative nodes, median survival is 42 months; for patients with regional nodal involvement, the median survival is 16.5 months. For patients with distant lymph nodes outside the peri-duodenal region, the survival is 6 months (Lai 2007).

Postoperative adjuvant treatment of primary adenocarcinoma of the duodenum after resection appears to improve regional control and reduce local recurrence. In reviewing the literature, Howe surveyed the National Cancer Database and found that 15.6% of patients with regional nodal involvement received radiation treatment. This is a very similar percentage to those who received chemotherapy, and these patients probably received combination treatment. There

appears to be improved survival and regional control for patients receiving concurrent 5-fluorouracil plus radiation treatment. In a retrospective study by Swartz, patients who received adjuvant chemoradiation who had positive lymph nodes with tumor completely resected had improved median survival to 41 months from 21 months after surgery alone. Overall 5-year survival for both groups was similar, however. (Swartz 2007). Reports in the literature from the National Cancer Institute Data Base indicate improved survival for patients receiving 5-fluorouracil and regional radiation treatment possibly increased the adjuvant use of radiation treatment plus chemotherapy which increased from 8.1% of patients undergoing surgical resection in 1985 to 23.8% in 2005 (Bilimoria 2009).

Recommendations for treatment of primary duodenal carcinoma with positive nodes or positive margins include radiation treatment with continuous infusion of 5-fluorouracil. Radiation treatment should be given with either intensity-modulated therapy or 3-dimensional conformal therapy to a total dose of approximately 50 Gy (range 40–57) (Swartz 2007; Sohn 1998).

Carcinoid Tumor Arising in the Duodenum

Within the small intestine, the majority of carcinoid tumors are found in the ileum with second most common site being the duodenum. There is a significantly higher incidence of tumors arising in Meckel's diverticulum. The mainstay of management for patients with carcinoid tumor of the duodenum is complete resection including resection of any potentially involved lymph nodes. Carcinoid syndrome is a constellation of symptoms including flushing, diarrhea, and wheezing caused by release of serotonin, bradykinin, prostaglandin, and catecholamines. Approximately 10% of patients with small bowel carcinoids present with carcinoid syndrome. Octreotide can be helpful in treating carcinoid syndrome. It is unclear whether any adjuvant treatment after resection of duodenal carcinoid tumors improves survival in a nonmetastatic setting (Shebani 1999).

Non-Hodgkin's Lymphoma of the Duodenum

Lymphoma limited to the duodenum and its regional nodes is rare with fewer than 100 cases reported in the English literature (Najen 1984). Once diagnosed, microscopic examination should also include flow cytometry to determine the histologic subtype and biologic behavior. Diffuse large B-cell non-Hodgkin's lymphoma is the most common lymphoma occurring in the small intestine. Treatment is usually directed by stage with radiation treatment being employed curatively in stage I and stage II patients after systemic chemotherapy and to preserve the integrity of the small bowel tract.

Mucosa-associated lymphoid tissue lymphoma (MALT) also known as marginal zone B-cell lymphoma can be associated with other autoimmune diseases including Sjögren's syndrome or Hashimoto's thyroiditis. The majority of patients with MALT tumors of the duodenum present with localized stage I or stage II extranodal disease and treatment is radiation therapy, with or without chemotherapy. Survival is reported to be better with MALT tumors arising in the duodenum than in the stomach (Nakamura 2000).

Gastrointestinal Stromal Tumors of the Duodenum

Treatment for gastrointestinal stromal tumors arising in the duodenum is complete surgical resection. The tumors are soft and fleshy and sometimes prone to rupture and lead to diffuse intra-abdominal recurrence. En bloc resection should be accomplished if possible. Lymph node metastases are rare and lymph node dissection is not recommended. In patients who underwent complete surgical excision of their tumors at Memorial Sloan-Kettering, the survival rates were 88% at 1 year, 65% at 3 years, and 54% at 5 years (Miettinen 2002). Positron emission tomography may form an imaging modality which is complementary for these patients. Early studies of Imatinib (Gleevec) were performed in patients with unresected tumors and response to Imatinib was documented with positron emission tomography. Adjuvant Imatinib may be helpful in patients who have had complete resections, and should be considered.

In conclusion, primary duodenal cancers are more treatable today. Complete surgical resection is the mainstay of therapy, with the possible exception of non-Hodgkin's lymphoma. Adjuvant treatment improves outcome for adenocarcinoma, non-Hodgkin's lymphoma, and gastrointestinal stromal tumors.

Cross-References

▶ Carcinoid Tumor
▶ Colon Cancer
▶ Hodgkin's Lymphoma

References

Bilimoria KY (2009) Small bowel cancer in the United States: changes in epidemiology, treatment, and survival over the last twenty years. Ann Surg 249(1):63–71

Cheung O (2003) Primary duodenal carcinomas showing divergent growth patterns as determined by microdissection-based mutational genotype. Arch Pathol Lab Med 127:861–865

Crawley C (1998) The Royal Marsden experience of small bowel adenocarcinoma treated with protracted venous 5-fluorouracil infusion. Br J Cancer 78:508–513

Howe JR (1999) American College of Surgeons Commission on Cancer and the American Cancer Society: adenocarcinoma of the small bowel. Review of the National Cancer Data Base, 1985–1995. Cancer 86:2693–2700

Kerremans RP (1979) Primary malignant duodenal tumors. Ann Surg 3:179–191

Lai EC (2007) Primary adenocarcinoma of the duodenum: analysis of survival. World J Surg 12(5):695–699

Miettinen M (2002) Evaluation of malignancy and prognosis of gastrointestinal stromal tumors. A review. Hum Pathol 133:478–492

Najen AZ (1984) Primary non-Hodgkin's lymphoma of the duodenum. Cancer 54:895–898

Nakamura S (2000) A clinicopathologic study of primary small intestine lymphoma—prognostic significance of mucosa-associated lymphoid tissue-derived lymphoma. Cancer 88:286–293

Santoro E (1997) Primary adenocarcinoma of the duodenum: treatment and survival in 89 patients. Hepatogastroenterology 44:1157–1163

Shebani KO (1999) Prognosis and survival in patients with gastrointestinal tract carcinoid tumors. Ann Surg 229:815–823

Sohn TA (1998) Adenocarcinoma of the duodenum: factors influencing long term survival. Journal of Gastrointestinal Surgery 2(1):79–87

Swartz MJ (2007) Adjuvant concurrent chemoradiation for node-positive adenocarcinoma of the duodenum. Arch Surg 142(3):285–288

Vasen HF (1997) Decisional analysis in the management of duodenal adenomatosis in familial polyposis. Gut 40:716–718

Primary Cardiac Tumors

RAMESH RENGAN[1], CHARLES R. THOMAS, JR.[2]
[1]Department of Radiation Oncology, Hospital of the University of Pennsylvania, Philadelphia, PA, USA
[2]Department of Radiation Medicine, Oregon Health Sciences University, Portland, OR, USA

Synonyms

Atrial myxoma

Background

Primary cardiac tumors are rare, with metastases outnumbering primary tumors by a ratio of approximately 1,000:1 (Chiles et al. 2001). Atrial myxomas are the most common primary cardiac tumor accounting for 40–50% of all primary cardiac tumors. The mortality of patients with atrial myxomas does not differ significantly from that of the general population (Attar et al. 1980). This entry will focus primarily on non-myxomatous primary cardiac tumors (nMPCT). These tumors are divided into benign (70% of all primary cardiac tumors) and malignant tumors (30% of all primary cardiac tumors). Benign tumors include rhabdomyoma, fibroma, fibroelastoma, hemangioma, lipoma, teratoma, and hamartoma; malignant tumors are primarily sarcomas (including angiosarcoma, osteosarcoma, malignant fibrohistiocytoma, leiomyosarcoma, and rhabdomyosarcoma), lymphomas, and pericardial mesothelioma (Cameron et al. 2008). In autopsy series, the incidence of primary cardiac neoplasms range from 0.001% to 0.003% (Butany et al. 2005). The mainstay of therapy is complete surgical resection. The prognosis for benign nMPCTs is excellent; however, the prognosis for malignant nMPCTs is extremely poor with a median survival of 10–24 months.

Anatomy

The heart is positioned obliquely within the middle mediastinum. The heart consists of four chambers: right and left atria and ventricles. These chambers are divided into three layers: the epicardium (outer layer), the myocardium (middle layer), and the inner endocardium. The base of the heart lies posteriorly and primarily consisting of the left atrium. It is located between the T5 and T9 vertebral bodies. The anterior surface of the heart is formed primarily by the right ventricle and is bounded by the posterior surface of the sternum. The apex of the heart is formed by the left ventricle and is bounded inferiorly by the diaphragm. The heart is surrounded by the pericardium that serves to anchor the heart and prevents overfilling. Additionally, the pericardial sac minimizes friction against the surfaces of the heart.

Epidemiology

Primary cardiac neoplasms are exceedingly rare with an autopsy incidence of 0.001–0.003%.

The most common of these are benign atrial myxomas. Of nMPCTs, benign tumors predominate comprising 70% of all tumors with malignant nMPCTs the remaining 30%. The vast majority malignant nMPCTs are sarcomas.

Clinical Presentation

The clinical presentation of nMPCTs can vary based upon the size and location of the tumor. The classic clinical triad of presentation consists of signs of intracardiac obstruction, systemic embolization, and systemic or constitutional symptoms. Most patients present with dyspnea or orthopnea secondary to pulmonary venous hypertension or pulmonary edema. Tumors of the AV nodal system can present with arrhythmias, often bradycardia.

Differential Diagnosis

The primary differential diagnosis for primary cardiac neoplasms is ▶ Carney Complex. This is an autosomal dominant disorder that accounts for 7–10% of all cardiac myxomas. Carney Complex findings include cardiac myxomas, cutaneous myxomas, spotty pigmentation of the skin, endocrinopathy, and both endocrine and nonendocrine tumors.

Imaging Studies

The diagnostic test of choice is transthoracic echocardiography. These studies can provide a high level of anatomic detail as well as functional evaluation (Thomas et al. 1995). Transesophageal echocardiography, although invasive, can potentially provide greater anatomic detail. Additionally, a transvenous biopsy can be performed via transesophageal echocardiography in the case of right-sided lesions. A contrast-enhanced computed tomographic scan of the chest should be performed to assess for metastatic dissemination. Magnetic resonance imaging (MRI)

can also be used. It has the advantage of multiplanar imaging is superior to computed tomography in identifying vessel invasion. Additionally, MRI can be used with greater latitude in the setting of renal insufficiency or allergy to iodinated contrast dye.

Laboratory Studies

An erythrocyte sedimentation rate should be ordered as it may be elevated in the setting of nMPCT. This is a nonspecific finding.

Treatment

The mainstay of therapy for benign nMPCTs is complete surgical resection. Palliative debulking may relieve symptoms in some patients. There is no established role for chemotherapy or radiation in the treatment of benign tumors. Malignant tumors, which are predominantly sarcomas, are usually treated with a multimodal approach. Systemic chemotherapy, usually anthracycline based, is employed for cytoreduction prior to surgical resection and the treatment of disseminated disease. In rare situations of localized, unresectable disease cardiac transplantation has been used. The clinical benefit of this approach is unclear. The prognosis for malignant tumors is almost uniformly poor.

Cross-References

▶ Mediastinal Germ Cell Tumor
▶ Soft Tissue Sarcoma
▶ Thymic Neoplasms

References

Attar S, Lee YC et al (1980) Cardiac myxoma. Ann Thorac Surg 29(5):397–405

Butany J, Nair V et al (2005) Cardiac tumours: diagnosis and management. Lancet Oncol 6(4):219–228

Cameron RB, Loehrer PJ et al (2008) Neoplasms of the mediastinum, Chap. 38. In: DeVita VT Jr, Lawrence TS, Rosenberg SA, Principles and practice of oncology. Lippincott-Raven, Philadelphia, pp 973–988

Chiles C, Woodard PK et al (2001) Metastatic involvement of the heart and pericardium: CT and MR imaging. Radiographics 21(2):439–449

Thomas CR, De Vries B et al (1995) Cardiac Neoplasms. In: Wood DE, Thomas CR (eds) Medical radiology – diagnostic imaging and radiation oncology volume: mediastinal tumors: update 1995. Springer, Heidelberg

Primary Intracranial Neoplasms

TONY S. QUANG

Department of Radiation Oncology, VA Puget Sound Health Care System University of Washington Medical Center, Seattle, WA, USA

Synonyms

Anaplastic astrocytoma; Astrocytoma with anaplastic foci (AAF); Glioblastoma multiforme; Oligoastrocytoma; Oligodendroglioma; Pilocytic astrocytoma

Definition

Primary brainy tumors are a heterogeneous group of diseases arising from different cells of origin and exhibiting characteristic age distributions. They represent less than 1% of all cancers in Western countries. Primary brain tumors include low-grade astrocytomas (pilocytic astrocytomas, oligodendrogliomas, and oligoastrocytomas), malignant high-grade gliomas (astrocytoma with anaplastic foci and glioblastoma multiforme), ependymomas, meningiomas, and central nervous system (CNS) lymphomas. They present asymptomatically until growth to a certain size to impinge on and infiltrate into the brain parenchyma, which disrupts function at that particular location. Pathogenesis is largely unknown but is associated with the activation of cellular oncogenes and the loss of tumor suppressor genes. Multimodality therapy includes maximal safe resection followed by observation or radiation and/or chemotherapy. Novel therapies including biological agents, radiolabeled monoclonal antibodies, and radiosurgical technology show promise in therapeutic efficacy and warrant further investigation. Because the natural history, prognosis, and patterns of failures of various primary intracranial neoplasms are a diverse heterogeneous group, only low- and high-grade gliomas are the focus of discussion here since they represent the majority of primary intracranial neoplasms. The role of interdisciplinary management of more rare primary brain tumors and pediatric primary brain tumors is not discussed here.

Anatomy

The brain is the center of the central nervous system (CNS). It is situated in the cranium. The brain measures on average 16 cm anterior-posteriorly, 14 cm transversely, and 12 cm superior-inferiorly. It weighs about 1,500 g.

The CNS is composed of 60% white matter and 40% gray matter. It is enveloped by the meninges, including the dura mater, the pia mater, and the arachnoid mater. Between the pia mater and the arachnoid mater is the subarachnoid space, which is filled with cerebrospinal fluid (CSF). The falx cerebri is the dural fold that separates the brain into two hemispheres of the cerebrum. The tentorum cerebelli separates the cerebrum from the cerebellum and brain stem.

The cerebral cortex with left and right hemispheres is responsible for cognitive and behavioral functions. Each hemisphere is divided into four lobes, the frontal lobe, parietal lobe, temporal lobe, and occipital lobe. Underneath the cerebrum lies the brain stem, pons, medulla, and cerebellum, which are relay centers of motor and sensory signals from the brain to the rest of the body. These structures also play an important role in the regulation of the CNS system, cardiac and respiratory function, maintenance of consciousness, and the sleep cycle.

The brain receives its arterial supply from the internal carotids (anterior circulation) and the vertebral vessels, which join to form the basilar artery (posterior circulation). One anterior communicating and two posterior communicating arteries produce communication between the anterior and posterior circulations and form the circle of Willis. The anterior cerebral artery, middle cerebral artery, and posterior cerebral artery supply the mesial interhemispheric surface, lateral surface, and the parietal and occipital lobes of the brain, respectively.

The ventricular system is filled with CSF, which bathes and cushions the brain and spinal cord within their bony confines. CSF is made by modified ependymal cells of the choroid plexus found in all components of the ventricular system, except for the cerebral aqueduct and the occipital and frontal horns of the lateral ventricles. CSF flows from the lateral ventricles via the foramina of Monro into the third ventricles, and then the fourth ventricle via the aqueduct of Sylvius. CSF flows out of the fourth ventricle through the midline foramen of Magendie and lateral foramina of Luschka to the subarachnoid space that widens into several cisterns. CSF then flows around the superior sagittal sinus to be reabsorbed by the arachnoid granulations into the venous system.

Background

In 2011, an estimated 22,340 new cases of primary brain and other nervous system neoplasms will be diagnosed in the USA. These tumors will be responsible for approximately 13,110 deaths (American Cancer Society 2011). Because of the heterogeneity in these brain neoplasms, the natural history, patterns of failure, and prognosis should be considered for each patient. The involvement of an interdisciplinary team, which includes the radiation oncologists, neurosurgeons, medical oncologists, neurologists, neuroradiologists, and pathologists, is the key to successful and optimal management of these patients.

The majority of CNS tumors in adults arises supratentorially in the brain parenchyma. The most common glioma histology is the astrocytoma, which can be classified as low grade or high grade. Low-grade gliomas are a heterogeneous group of uncommon malignancies. Of these malignancies, 70% are diffuse astrocytomas of the fibrillary, protoplasmic, and gemistocytic types. They include the World Health Organization (WHO) grade I pilocytic astrocytoma and WHO grade II includes low-grade astroctyoma, oligodendroglioma, oligoastrocytoma, pleomorphic xanthoastrocytoma, subependymal giant cell astrocytoma, and subependymoma. The mean age at presentation for these tumors is about 40 years. The most powerful prognostic factor is age with younger age associated with higher survival rate. Although low-grade astrocytomas are commonly thought to be benign, 25–40% of these tumors can behave aggressively when they transform into malignant astrocytomas during a period of 5–10 years. Other low-grade CNS tumors are managed similarly to low-grade gliomas.

In contrast, high-grade gliomas include WHO grade III astrocytoma with anaplastic foci (AAF) and grade IV glioblastoma multiforme (GBM). Collectively, they are the most common primary tumors in adults and account for 2.3% of all cancer-related deaths. GBM accounts for more than 50% of all gliomas and 85% of all high-grade gliomas. Peak incidence occurs in 50–70-year-old patients for GBM, whereas less-malignant forms occur at least a decade earlier. They usually present as unifocal lesions, but less than 1% are multifocal. The median survival for GBM and AAF is 10–15 months versus 30–50 months despite maximal surgical resection, postoperative radiation, and chemotherapy. While CNS lymphoma, pinealblastoma, anaplastic ependymoma, and medulloblastoma are not classified as a glioma, they are aggressive (if not more so) than high-grade gliomas.

The development of brain gliomas is sporadic without any genetic predisposition. However, certain occupational and environmental exposures have been implicated. A possible viral cause includes the SV40 or cytomegalovirus. Petrochemical such as polyvinyl chloride appears to be linked. Prior exposure to ionizing radiation including long-term survivors among children given prophylatic cranial irradiation for acute lymphocytic leukemia shows increase over the expected incidence. The connection between cellular phone use and brain gliomas is controversial, but probably nonexistent.

Development of brain gliomas has been described as a part of hereditary cancer syndromes including neurofibromatosis type 1 and 2, von Hippel–Lindau disease, ► tuberous sclerosis, retinoblastoma, ► Turcot syndrome, and ► Li–Fraumeni syndrome. Other risk factors include male gender, age >50 years, ethnicity (Caucasians, Asians, and Latinos), and having a low-grade astrocytoma with its potential for transformation into a high-grade glioma.

Although the exact pathogenesis of carcinogenic events leading to brain glioma development is unknown, it is generally accepted that the accumulation of genetic alterations that lead to the acquisition of a malignant phenotype through activation of cellular oncogenes and loss of cellular tumor suppressor genes is the etiology. Whether the process is malignant transformation from a low-grade glioma to an astrocytoma with anaplastic or de novo GBM, the genes TP53, Rb, PTEN, CDK4, EGFR, EFGRvIII, VEGF, and other protein kinases are implicated.

Clinical Presentation

The presenting symptoms of a brain glioma can be classified as generalized or focal. Common generalized symptoms of the disease include seizure, nausea, vomiting, and headache. It is suggested that headache is more prevalent in patients with faster growing, high-grade gliomas, and seizures are more common in patients with lower grade gliomas, but it can be variable. Because brain parenchyma is anesthetic, headaches associated with gliomas may be due to increased intracranial pressure secondary to ventricular obstruction or to local compressive pressure on intracranial structures. Headaches associated with increased intracranial pressure occur in the morning after the patient has been recumbent from the night (effects of gravity on CSF) and subside as the day progresses. Associated with increased intracranial pressures may be findings of focal neurologic deficits, sensory and motor impairment, cognitive and behavioral changes, and papilledema. Cushing's triad classically consists of increased intracranial pressure with attendant hypertension, bradycardia, and respiratory irregularity. Long-standing increased intracranial pressure may lead to optic atrophy and subsequent blindness because of compression of the optic nerves.

Seizures are common in patients with brain gliomas, and can in fact, be a symptom that heralds the presence of the glioma, which may lead to early diagnosis. They most likely originate from the brain adjacent to the glioma nidus. Seizures may be partial (simple, complex, or secondarily generalized) or generalized (tonic–clonic or absence).

Other impairments include progressive memory, personality, endocrine disorders, fatigue, or focal neurological deficits, which for instance, implicate temporal and frontal lobe involvement. The specific kind of symptoms produced depends highly on the location of the tumor, and is usually clinically apparent when the brain lesion grows into a large mass. CSF dissemination of glioma cells should be suspected in patients who exhibit symptoms that cannot be explained by the location of the brain glioma.

Differential Diagnosis

The initial work-up of a patient with brain tumors includes a complete history and general physical examination with particular attention to the neurologic examination. A complete neurologic exam includes assessment of mental condition, coordination, sensation, reflexes, motor, and cranial nerves. Ophthalmoscopy is important to check for papilledema as a sign of increased intracranial pressure and attendant optic nerve atrophy. Patients in whom signs, symptoms, or imaging suggest systemic spread of disease outside the CNS, pathological confirmation via biopsy is recommended.

When patients present with new or persistent neurologic findings, the use of imaging such as CT or MR is indicated, to determine the nature of space-occupying lesions. The etiology could be neoplastic (primary vs. metastatic), infectious (abscess, cerebritis, or meningitis), vascular (ischemia, infarct, or hemorrhage), or treatment-related necrosis (chemotherapy and/or radiation therapy). When a neoplasm is suspected, the following aside from gliomas should be included in the differential diagnosis: germ cell tumors, pineal tumors, meningiomas, pituitary tumors, schwannomas, choroid plexus tumors, gangliogliomas, neurocytomas, mesenchymal tumors, hemangioblastomas, plasmacytomas, lymphomas, craniopharyngiomas, and embryonal tumors.

Imaging Studies

The imaging modality of choice for primary brain tumors is MRI and is considered the gold standard. It can demonstrate neuroanatomy and local pathologic processes such as edema due to the extravasation of cellular fluid in the interstitial space. MRI also allows better delineation of a brain glioma with respect to normal neuroanatomy because it offers views from three planes (transverse, sagittal, and coronal). Higher-grade tumors usually enhance. The most useful imaging studies are the MR T1-weighted with and without gadolinium along with T2-weighted and FLAIR sequences. T1-weighted with and without gadolinium sequence allows for exquisite delineation of anatomy and area of contrast enhancement. Gadolinium leaks into the brain parenchyma when the blood-brain barrier breaks down due to glioma growth and infiltration. T2-weighted and FLAIR sequences are more sensitive for detecting edema. When there is a suspicion of neuroaxis spread, MRI of the complete cervical, thoracic, and lumbar spine should be performed. However, the limitations to MRI are that it is sensitive to movement, metallic objects causing artifacts, and patients with implantable devices and claustrophobia.

Enhanced CT of the brain and spine is useful in instances where patients cannot undergo an MRI due to implantable devices such as a pacemaker or paramagnetic surgical clips or unwilling because of claustrophobia. Studies with intravenous contrast are most helpful in this instance. An important limitation is the lack of resolution compared to MRI, especially in the posterior fossa.

Positron emission tomography (PET) can give information on metabolic and BBB function but of limited value except in the setting where it is necessary to distinguish tumor from necrosis. Tumor would usually be PET avid whereas necrosis would be to the contrary. However, the accuracy of interpretations and the availability of isotopes are potential limitations.

MR spectroscopy also assesses metabolites with tumors and normal tissue, while MR perfusion measures cerebral blood volumes in tumors. They are useful in differentiating between tumor recurrence and necrosis. Their limitations rest on tumors near vessels, air spaces, bone and small volume lesions.

Laboratory Studies

Pathological confirmation is required to diagnose most primary brain tumors. Tissue can be obtained via a stereotactic biopsy or a craniotomy. High-grade gliomas under histologic examination would reveal cellular atypia, increased mitoses, and endothelial proliferation. Pseudopa-lisading necrosis is pathognomonic for GBM. If brain metastases are suspected with a high index of suspicion in the setting of active systemic disease or if radiographic findings are suggestive of a brainstem glioma, optic nerve meningioma, or CNS lymphoma suspected in an HIV+patient, then biopsy would not be necessary. If neuraxis spread is suspected, then a lumbar puncture to obtain CSF cytology is recommended.

Treatment

General

Several fundamental principles govern the management of patients with primary brain tumors. Regardless of tumor histology, surgical resection of the lesions generally provides the best outcome and accurate confirmation of the pathological diagnosis. The decision to recommend surgery for a patient depends on the following factors: Performance status of the patient, proximity to eloquent (functionally critical areas) of the brain, ability to relieve mass effect due to tumor impingement, resectability of the lesion, de novo vs. recurrent tumor, and suspected pathology (benign vs. malignant). The administration of adjuvant therapy including chemotherapy and radiation therapy depends on postoperative pathological status, disease type, and patient tolerability.

Medical

The medical management of patients with primary brain tumors includes control of cerebral edema, increased intracranial pressure, and neurologic symptoms. The common symptoms of seizures, headaches, and nausea and vomiting are usually first to be addressed. Glucocorticoids are used before surgery and during radiotherapy to control symptoms due to cerebral edema. Dexamethasone 4 mg PO QID is commonly prescribed initially after a 10 mg loading dose. Because of the numerous side effects attendant with prolonged steroid use, it should be tapered slowly over several weeks when neurologic symptoms abate. Anticonvulsants such as carbamapezine, phenobarbital, and valproate are commonly prescribed for patients presenting with seizures. Liver function enzymes should be monitored as many first-generation anticonvulsants induce hepatic cytochrome P450 isoenzymes, which may affect metabolism of certain chemotherapeutic agents. Prophylatic anticonvulsant remains controversial and should not be routinely administered. Nonsteroid anti-inflammatory agents, opioids, and antiemetics should be given for headaches and nausea. Endocrinopathies are common among patients, and the hypothalamic–pituitary–adrenal axis should be addressed with the appropriate repletion. Fatigue and depression are not uncommon and can be severe, persistent, and emotionally overwhelming. Therefore, the referral of the patient to a psychologist would be appropriate to address this symptom with coping skills, which may include psychotropics and moderate exercise.

Surgery

Surgical options include stereotactic biopsy, open biopsy, or debulking procedure, and maximally safe resection. Review of pathological specimens by an experienced neuropathologist is highly preferable. A postoperative MRI scan with and without gadolinium should be obtained 24–72 h after surgery to document the extent of surgical resection lest edema may confound the picture of residual disease. If an MRI scan cannot be obtained in this time window, an MRI done at 2 weeks postoperatively is also acceptable. The extent of resection should be judged on the postoperative MRI and used as a baseline to assess therapeutic efficacy and disease progression.

Surgery plays a significant role in the interdisciplinary management of primary brain tumors, except for CNS lymphomas. Maximal tumor resection with minimal surgical morbidity for accurate diagnosis is the goal. Stereotactic biopsy is helpful for diagnosis. With a stereotactic head frame, a CT or an MRI is performed and the images are loaded into an image-guidance system. An entry point is determined on the scalp and a burr hole is made. The biopsy needle is then placed through the burr hole to the appropriate depth using the image-guidance system. Samples of tissues are then obtained and sent to the neuropathologist for histological confirmation. If a diversion procedure is necessary to relieve increased intracranial pressure or hydrocephalus, endoscopy can be used to this end.

If a patient requires surgical debulking to relieve mass effect-related symptoms, CT- and MR-guidance systems offer neurosurgeons intraoperative navigation in order to precisely locate anatomical structures and to map out the safest approach. If possible, a complete surgical resection is done as it offers the best chance for cure and is associated with a survival advantage.

Chemotherapy

Many chemotherapy agents have been ineffective in the management of primary brain tumors except for CNS lymphomas and high-grade gliomas. It was thought that the reason was due to their inability to cross the BBB. But even when agents are delivered in adequate doses to the brain parenchyma, the gliomas or meningiomas appear to be resistant to them. Alkylating agents, such as nitrosoureas, BCNU (carmustine), and CCNU (lomustine) given either locally via wafers at the surgical bed or intravenously appear to confer a modest survival advantage while almost all other chemotherapy agents offer negligible efficacy.

However, for GBM, a recent randomized trial demonstrated that temozolomide confers a survival benefit if used concurrently ($75\,mg/m^2$ daily $\times$ 7 days per week for 6 weeks) with radiation therapy and in the adjuvant setting ($150–200\ mg/m^2$ daily $\times$ 5 days every 28 days for six cycles) for patients diagnosed with GBM (Stupp et al. 2009). Temozolomide is a methylating agent whose cytotoxic product is O^6-methylguanine-DNA adducts and works by causing futile mismatch repair and resultant apoptotic GBM cell death. Temozolomide's unique mechanism of action is particularly effective in patients with GBM containing a methylated O^6-methylguanine-DNA-methyltransferase (MGMT) promoter. MGMT reverses alkylation at the O^6 position of guanine, preventing cell death in tumors. High MGMT levels cause resistance to alkylating agents, whereas low MGMT levels cause tumors to be susceptible to alkylating drugs. Therefore, patients in whom MGMT promoters were highly methylated and were treated with temozolomide were observed to have a higher median survival compared to patients in whom MGMT promoters were unmethylated (Heigi et al. 2005). Because of temozolomide's efficacy in the treatment of GBM, its efficacy has been extrapolated for use in treating patients diagnosed with astrocytomas with anaplastic foci.

Investigational Agents

As the search for more effective treatment ensues, new agents are being evaluated for use in patients with newly diagnosed high-grade gliomas. Targeted therapies designed to target-specific biological mechanisms of high-grade glioma cell growth, proliferation, and angiogenesis show potential. These novel agents include vascular endothelial growth factor receptor (VEGF-R), mammalian target of rapamycin (mTOR), integrin inhibitor (cilengitide), farnesyltransferase, and histone deacetylase (HDAC).

Furthermore, efforts are made to evaluate the efficiency of monoclonal antibodies in immunologic mediated processes. Epidermal growth factor receptor variant III (EGFRvIII) appears to enhance immune response in newly diagnosed GBM. Radiolabeled ^{125}I-EGFR MAb 425 has been shown to increase median survival in patients diagnosed with AAF and GBM (Quang & Brady 2004). These new therapies should be considered in selected patients.

Radiotherapy

The role of radiotherapy in the treatment of low-grade gliomas and meningiomas is appropriate for a select group of patients, especially those with residual disease after maximally safe resection. The role of radiotherapy is well-established in high-grade gliomas and CNS lymphomas. The evolution of conventional extern beam radiation therapy delivered to the whole brain to highly conformal intensity-modulated radiation therapy (IMRT) to the partial brain has allowed a definitive dose to be delivered to the tumor while minimizing critical structure toxicities. Late injury with the end point being glial cell necrosis for 5% and 50% risk level at 5 years ($TD_{5/5}$ or $TD_{50/5}$) is 60 Gy and 70 Gy, respectively for whole brain fractionated radiotherapy given at 2 Gy per fraction. With partial brain, it is conceivable highly by 10 Gy. However, early trials by the Brain Tumor Study Group failed to show a survival difference in escalating dose beyond 60 Gy. Various fractionation schemes have been explored. Intracavitary placement of iodine-125 radiocolloids has been used. Stereotactic radiosurgery using a Gamma Knife or Cyber Knife and fractionated stereotactic radiotherapy (FSRT) have been tried (Souhami et al. 2004). However, none of these approaches have increased median survivals. Perhaps heavy-charged particles and proton therapy may yield better results in the near future.

For low-grade gliomas, no consensus exists regarding the proper timing of posteroperative radiation in low-grade gliomas or meningiomas (The NCCN Clinical Practice Guidelines in Oncology Central Nervous System Cancers 2009). If residual disease is present and the decision is to offer radiotherapy therapy, 50–54 Gy to the PTV (planned target volume) is usually delivered 4–6 weeks postoperatively. From randomized controlled studies, RT prolongs progression free survival. A three-dimensional conformal (3D conformal) or intensive modulated radiation therapy (IMRT) should be used. In the era of IMRT and image-guided radiation therapy (IGRT), the PTV is a construct and volume, which consists of a margin for random and systematic error and the clinical target volume (CTV). CTV in turn consists of a margin for microscopic disease based on the pattern of spread and the gross tumor volume (GTV). With that in mind, the GTV should be contoured as the enhancement volume on T1-weighted MR imaging with gadolium (or FLAIR for oligodendrogliomas). CTV is obtained by expanding the GTV plus 1–2 cm. A tighter margin of 0.5–1 cm can be used for meningiomas. PTV is generated by adding 0.5 cm. Critical structure tolerances ($TD_{5/5}$) such as lens, optic nerve, retina, optic chiasm, brain stem, pituitary, and temporal lobe should be observed and the doses that they receive usually depend on the proximity to the PTV and the beam arrangements used.

For high-grade gliomas, the current recommended regimen for a patient who has been recommended to undergo definitive postoperative radiation therapy 4–8 weeks after a maximally safe resection is 60 Gy to the PTV (planned target volume) with concurrent and adjuvant temozolomide. A 3-dimensional conformal (3D conformal) or intensive modulated radiation therapy (IMRT) should be used with a shrinking field technique or a concomitant boost, respectively. While there are variations in how the PTV is defined, a surgical-pathological imaging series has established that 97% of GBM recurrence is within 3 cm of the edge of the tumor by CT or MRI with gadolinium (Wallner et al. 1989). In the era of IMRT and image-guided radiation therapy (IGRT), the PTV is a construct and volume, which consists of a margin for random and systematic error and the clinical target volume (CTV). CTV in turn consists of a margin for microscopic disease based on the pattern of spread and the gross tumor volume (GTV). With that in mind, the GTV should be contoured as the enhancement volume on T1-weighted MR imaging with gadolium. CTV should be contoured as the enhancement volume that includes the gross tumor and surrounding edema on T2-weighted imaging with gadolinium plus 1.5 cm margin to take into account microscopic glioma cells in proximity to the edema. PTV can then be expanded by another 0.5 cm. This initial PTV should be treated to 46 Gy with multiple beam arrangements (at minimum 3, but preferably 3–7 for better conformality). After 46 Gy, the remaining boost volume should be given the remaining 14 Gy to a cumulative total dose of 60 Gy. Dosimetrically, the 95% isodose line (IDL) should cover the initial PTV and the boost volume for the respective plans. Dose inhomogeneity of 5–7% should be the goal, but the acceptability beyond that is up to the discretion of the treating physician. Because local recurrence is high in high-grade gliomas, the recommendation for follow-up is to see the radiation oncologist every 3–4 months for the first 2 years, and every 4–6 months until year 5, and annually thereafter with serial MR brain done at each visit. Since this close follow-up with imaging has not been shown to increase patient survival, the need for this approach is being heavily debated upon in the neuro-oncology community. Furthermore, many MR brains done in follow-up show changes in the brain that are difficult to distinguish between radiation changes versus brain necrosis versus glioma recurrence. A PET scan is typically used to help better define MR findings. The argument for close follow-up, however, may be justified as it allows the radiation oncologist to detect recurrence early and to be able to intervene early whether it is to institute therapeutic and/or supportive measures for the patient. Since there are long-term survivals, albeit few, further therapies including re-resection, investigational chemotherapy or biologic agents, stereotactic radiosurgery, and radiolabeled monoclonal antibodies may have an impact on certain patients.

For patients with other malignant primary brain tumors such as patients who are considered for palliative radiation therapy usually because of poor Karnofsky Performance Status (KPS), many fractionation schemes and total dose could be used. These palliative regimens have been shown to marginally increase median survivals. The PTV is usually the enhancing volume (tumor and edema) plus 2 cm. Various regimens include 30 Gy in ten fractions, 20 Gy in five fractions, 40 Gy in 15 fractions, but any single fraction 8 Gy or more should be avoided as it may cause cerebral edema. Supportive and symptoms management should be included alongside palliative radiation treatment.

High-grade gliomas are almost uniformly fatal. This disease should be treated with available full therapy, including maximally safe resection followed by radiation therapy with concurrent and adjuvant chemotherapy. In selected patients, additional therapy should be offered to maximize survival.

Cross-References

▶ Palliation of Brain and Spinal Cord Metastases
▶ Soft Tissue Sarcoma

References

American Cancer Society (2011) Cancer facts and figures. American Cancer Society 61(4):212, July/August 2011, Atlanta, GA

Heigi ME et al (2005) MGMT gene silencing and benefit from temozomide in glioblastoma. N Eng J Med 352:997–1003

Quang TS, Brady LW (2004) Radioimmunotherapy as a Novel Treatment Regimen: 125I-labeled monoclonal antibody 425 in the Treatment of High-Grade Gliomas. Int J Radiat Oncol Biol Phys 58(3):972–975

Siker ML et al (2008) Primary Intracranial Neoplasms. In: Halperin EC, Perez CA, Brady LW (eds) Principles and practice of radiation oncology, 5th edn. Wolters Kluwer/Lippincott Wiliams and Wilkens, Philadelphia

Souhami L et al (2004) Randomized comparison of stereotactic radiosurgery followed by conventional radiotherapy with carmustine to conventional radiotherapy with carmustine for patients with glioblastoma multiforme: report of the Radiation Therapy Oncology Group 93-05 Protocol. Int J Radiat Oncol Biol Phys 60:853–860

Stupp R et al (2009) Effects of radiotherapy plus concomitant and adjuvant temozolomide versus radiotherapy alone on survival in a glioblastoma in a randomized phase III study: 5-year analysis of the EORTC-NCIC trial. Lancet Oncol 10:459–466

The NCCN Clinical Practice Guidelines in Oncology Central Nervous System Cancers (Version V.3.2009). (© 2009 National Comprehensive Cancer Network, Inc. Available at: NCCN.org. Accessed January 25, 2009). To view the most recent and complete version of the NCCN Guidelines, go online to NCCN.org

Wallner KE et al (1989) Patterns of failure following treatment for glioblastoma multiforme and anaplastic astrocytoma. Int J Radiat Oncol Biol Phys 16:1405–1409

Principles of Chemotherapy

Rene Rubin[1], Theodore E. Yaeger[2], Stephan Mose[3], Cheri Yaeger[2]

[1]Rittenhouse Hematology/Oncology, Philadelphia, PA, USA

[2]Department Radiation Oncology, Wake Forest University School of Medicine, Winston-Salem, NC, USA

[3]Department of Radiation Oncology, Schwarzwald-Baar-Klinikum, Villingen-Schwenningen, Germany

Introduction

The definition of chemotherapy is quite different from the colloquial use of the term.

In the simple definition it is the treatment of diseases with chemicals. The true first chemotherapeutic agent was asphenamine discovered in 1909 – an arsenic derivative used to treat syphilis. In modern times, the term has become synonymous with cancer treatment. Most modern chemotherapy agents act by killing rapidly diving cells. Cancer cells divide more rapidly than normal cells so they are more susceptible to these drugs.

Historical Overview

The first anticancer agent was aminotepin given by Dr. Sidney Farber to children with leukemia. It was an antifolate folic acid that made the bone marrow proliferate when given to people with folic acid deficiency. When folic acid was given to children with leukemia, it accelerated the growth of the leukemia. Therefore, it made sense to try an antifolate. This primitive drug produced some short-lived remissions. Nondividing cancer cells are not killed by these drugs.

It should also be mentioned that the first chemotherapeutic agent was derived out of chemical warfare. Mustard gas, which was used to cause blistering in the soldiers, was also found to lower their lymphocytes. By 1942, the first human clinical trials were performed on patients with blood malignancies. However, thousands of compounds had to be proven to develop one useful chemotherapeutic agent. It takes an average of 10–15 years to bring a drug to the market, and their steadfastness should be noted.

Use of Chemotherapy Today

Modern chemotherapy consists of many types of medications that kill eukaryotic dividing cancer cells. They have a toxic specificity that is limited to killing only actively dividing cells. The mechanism of action can inhibit the synthesis of DNA (antimetabolites), prevent microtubulin formation (vinca alkaloids), or prevent microtubule separation (taxanes). Some chemotherapeutic agents are actually in the class of herbal remedies. For instance, the vinca alkaloids are derived from the vinca rosacea plant and taxol and taxotere from the bark and pine needles, respectively, of the pacific yew tree. Then there are hormonal treatments and antihormonal treatments; these work by blocking cell function. Newer biologic agents and treatments include monoclonal antibodies, kinase inhibitors, immune modulation, anti-angiogenesis medication, and VEGF inhibition.

Treatment of solid cancers with chemotherapy needs to be segregated into adjuvant treatment for curative intent and palliative treatment to palliate the symptoms of metastatic cancer. When discussing chemotherapy with the aim for cure, the treatment usually consists of several chemotherapeutic agents given simultaneously. The rationale for this is to attack the cancer cell from multiple points along its cell cycle growth pathways. The intent is to prevent the cells from genetic repairing between treatments and to prevent resistance development. When treating metastatic carcinoma, the goal is palliation of symptoms with both quantity and quality of life. In the palliative setting, single agent treatment is most commonly given until there is evidence of disease progression. Subsequently, other agents with different mechanisms of action are tried hoping for secondary or more responses, typically with shorter duration of positive effect over time.

Side Effects of Chemotherapy

Normally dividing cells are also killed by these medications and are the mainstay of chemotherapy-associated side effects. Hair, bone marrow, and the digestive tract also have cells that divide rapidly. Hence, side effects such as baldness, neutropenia, infection, diarrhea, and mucositis are frequent in patients active on chemotherapy. For the sometimes devastating side effects there are a myriad of supportive medications and interventions that ameliorate the toxic effects. If not for these supportive medications, the ability to give effective chemotherapy in dosages to effect a cure, or even adequate palliation, could cause injury or death. Support can include antibiotics to prevent infections, antiemetics to prevent nausea and vomiting

that is centrally mediated from the chemotherapy trigger zone in the brain, chemoprotective agents (amifostine, mesna, dexrazoxane) to capitalize on the ability that some normal cells can repair themselves, and bone marrow rescuing agents (neupogen, erythropoietin, etc.) as these hormones and cytokines can stimulate the bone marrow to get stem cells into active cell division.

Effect of Chemotherapy on the Cell Cycle

Drugs are either cell cycle dependent or cell cycle independent. They may be specific for a certain phase or all dependent on the proliferation index. Nondividing cells are rarely damaged by chemotherapy.

The choices of chemotherapy drugs are in part based on the knowledge of the specific cancer and its cellular function. The other components consist of understanding the toxicity of the drugs. For example, one can deliver different chemicals if they affect the normal host cells differently. Likewise, two myelosuppressive agents may be too toxic, but a myelosuppressive agent and a neurotoxin may be tolerated well together.

More recently, the emphasis has been on the cell cycle (see Table 1) and the cell function, and its metabolic pathways. It has been learned in the last 60 years that it takes multiple steps to develop a cancer cell and for most cancers approximately 10–50 mutations have taken place before there is uncontrolled proliferation (e.g., cancer). It has

Principles of Chemotherapy. Table 1 Cell cycle

G0 (gap phase)	Nondividing, resting cell, reserve pool
G1 gap phase	Replication of chromosomes – DNA replication and synthesis
G2	Pre-mitosis
M mitosis	Cell division

most of the normal cell characteristics but is mutated sufficiently enough to develop uncontrolled growth and the independent ability to form its own blood vessels and sustained divisions.

Classes of Chemotherapeutic Drugs

Table 2 is not meant to be an exhaustive review of chemotherapy but rather an introduction to the subject. It will give the reader an insight into the use of the drugs.

Principles of Chemotherapy. Table 2 Classes of chemotherapeutic drugs

▶ ALK inhibitors
▶ Alkylating agents
▶ Antimetabolites/antifolates
▶ Antiangiogenesis inhibitors
▶ Antifolates
▶ Anti-EGFR
▶ Biological response modifiers
▶ BRAF inhibitors
▶ Epothilones
▶ Hedgehog pathway inhibition
▶ HER 2 inhibitors
▶ Histone deacetylase inhibitors
▶ Hormonal agents
▶ Monoclonal antibodies
▶ mTOR inhibitors
▶ PARP inhibitors
▶ Platinum analogues
▶ Signal transduction inhibitors
▶ Taxanes
▶ Topoisomerase inhibitors
▶ Vinca alkaloids
▶ Various drugs

Cross-References

▶ Bladder
▶ Colon Cancer
▶ Hodgkin's Lymphoma
▶ Leukemia
▶ Lung Cancer
▶ Non-Hodgkins Lymphoma
▶ Rectal Cancer
▶ Sarcoma
▶ Sarcomas of the Head and Neck
▶ Stage 0 Breast Cancer
▶ Testes

References

Chang AE, Ganz PA, Hayes DF, Kinsella TJ et al (2006) Oncology an evidence-based approach. Springer, New York

DeVita VT Jr, Hellman S, Rosenberg SA (eds) (1997) CANCER principles and practice of oncology, 5th edn. Philadelphia, Lippincott-Raven

Lenhard RE Jr, Osteen RT, Gansler T (eds) (2001) Clinical oncology. American Cancer Society, Atlanta

Page R, Takimoto C (2003) Principles of chemotherapy, Chapter 3. In: Padzur R, Coia LR et al (eds) Cancer management: a multidisciplinary approach, 7th edn. The Oncology Group, New York

P

Principles of Surgical Oncology

Ari D. Brooks
College of Medicine, Drexel University, Philadelphia, PA, USA

Definition

Surgical oncology is defined as the practice of surgery with specialty focus on malignancy in one or more organ systems.

Introduction

There is currently no board exam or training requirement, over and above a general surgery residency, for the title of surgical oncologist. The main specialty society for Surgical Oncology in the United States is called the Society for Surgical Oncology (www.surgonc.org), and membership is open to all general, urologic, ENT, thoracic, neurosurgeons, and GYN surgeons who provide specialty care in cancer. Members of the Society for Surgical Oncology may have reciprocal membership in the American Society of Clinical Oncology (www.asco.org) and/or the American Society for Radiation Oncology (www.ASTRO. org). In addition, surgical oncologists with special focus in breast cancer may belong to the Society of Breast Surgeons, and other breast specialty societies. There are specialty societies for colorectal (American Society for Colorectal Surgery, ASCRS), hepatobiliary (American Hepato-Pancreatico-Biliary Association), endocrine (American Association of Endocrine Surgeons), urology (American Urological Association), and GYN (Society of Gynecologic Oncologists) as well.

These specialty societies serve to promote education and awareness among the membership regarding the latest trends and developments in surgical management, diagnosis, and multimodality treatment. Most organizations have their own publications (Ann Surg Onc, Breast J, etc.) (Annals of Surgical Oncology: Copyright by Society of Surgical Oncology; The Breast Journal: Shala Masood). They also serve to regulate the fellowship training programs that have emerged across the country.

Most of these societies have representation at the American College of Surgeons and on the American Board of Surgery to help guide policy and regulation of the specialty.

Implementation of Practice

With regard to practice, the main difference between general surgery and surgical oncology is the focus on multimodality management. Collaborative efforts in oncologic surgery have led to the development of the National Surgical Adjuvant Bowel and Breast Project (NSABP) (National Surgical Adjuvant Bowel and Breast Project: East Common Professional Building) and its groundbreaking studies in adjuvant, neoadjuvant, and prevention therapy for breast and colorectal cancers. The American College of Surgeons Commission on Cancer (COC) (American College of Surgeons Commission on Cancer: 633 N. Saint Clair St.), which certifies the majority of hospital based cancer programs is run by surgical oncologists, and is designed to emphasize teamwork and quality measures in these programs. All general surgeons are trained in the surgical management of common tumors; however, the specialty fellowships just increase the volume of cases seen and introduce the concepts of collaborative multidisciplinary management and clinical research. Many training programs also emphasize training in leadership and education, ensuring a key leadership role for surgical oncologists at most medical centers and on the national medical scene.

Specialty Training

The fellowship training programs in general surgical oncology are available upon completion of a general surgery residency. All involve clinical rotations in head and neck, thoracic, GI, hepatobiliary, colorectal, melanoma, sarcoma, breast, endocrine, and GYN oncology. Rotations in pathology, medical oncology, and radiation oncology are also required. Many programs offer elective rotations as well. Some exposure to clinical research is essential, and all programs have basic research experiences available. These general surgical oncology fellowships are 2–3 years in length.

The specialty fellowships are usually 1 year in length at the completion of a general surgery residency and provide immersion in the field of choice along with exposure to pathology, medical oncology, radiation oncology, and clinical research opportunities. Although all cardiothoracic surgeons get experience in lung cancer and mediastinal tumors during their fellowship, the specialized thoracic surgical oncology fellowship is a 2-year fellowship with 6 months of cardiac surgery and the remainder in thoracic. Lastly, gynecologic (GYN) oncology training is a 3-year program at the completion of GYN residency with significant time spent in medical oncology (or the chemotherapy side of GYN oncology) and time spent in surgery, pathology, and radiation oncology.

Another key characteristic of surgical oncology is the emphasis on outcomes. The National Cancer Data Base (The National Cancer Data Base: The American College of Surgeons) was created by surgical oncologists at the American College of Surgeons to track management trends and outcomes across the country. Participation in this database is a mandatory requirement for COC accreditation, and this effort has helped boost the state cancer registries over the past few decades. Surgical oncologists are at the center of the current debate about the relationship between case volume and quality of outcomes. This emphasis on benchmarking outcome quality has helped increase adoption of multimodality care in common cancers, and will probably be responsible for regionalizing the management of rarer or more difficult cases to high volume centers.

Surgical oncology has been a driving force in pushing the limits of multidisciplinary clinical care, quality measurement, research, education, and leadership for decades. The next decade will see challenges in the rise of subspecialty training programs that reduce exposure to less common or more complex cases during general surgical residency, the push for a board certification in surgical oncology that may cause problems for unity among general surgeons, and encroachment by other specialties such as interventional radiology, dermatology, and transplantation.

Surgical Oncology Procedures

The oncologic approach to surgical management of disease has led to the evolution of procedures and protocols to maximize cure. Several examples are described in this section.

1. Breast Cancer: The original management of breast cancer in the twentieth century included a mastectomy including all the skin of the breast down to and including the entire pectoralis major muscle and the lymph nodes of the axilla. Reconstruction with a skin graft was standard. In the 1970s, the NSABP (1) performed several groundbreaking trials, first randomizing radical versus modified radical mastectomy for the management of breast cancer. In this trial, the modified radical mastectomy was found to be equivalent for survival and became the standard treatment, where the pectoralis muscle is preserved and most of the skin of the breast is conserved for primary closure. A second trial showed that for tumors smaller than 5 cm, partial mastectomy (lumpectomy) was equivalent to modified radical mastectomy for survival. Adding adjuvant radiation to lumpectomy was shown to reduce the recurrence rate to an acceptable level in a subsequent NSABP trial. More recently, sentinel node dissection was added to the management of early breast cancers, and now a majority of women with breast cancer are managed without axillary dissection. Also, plastic and reconstructive surgeons have joined in the evolution of breast cancer management and there are a multitude of flaps, implants, and staged techniques for breast reconstruction that are available for our patients with breast cancer. In the last decade, working closely with oncologic surgeons, radiation oncologists have begun to offer partial breast irradiation using brachytherapy catheters, external beam, or intraoperative

radiation, reducing posttreatment morbidity and shortening treatment times for good risk patients.

2. Colorectal Cancer: The recognition that an anatomic approach to colon resection improves local recurrence rates led to a major advance in surgical management in the 1980s. The surgical management dictates a removal of the entire right/transverse, left/transverse, left/sigmoid, or total mesorectal excision for tumors in those regions. These anatomic resections are facilitated by taking the entire blood supply and mesentery at their origin. There are two byproducts of performing resections this way, one is that there is less handling of the colon/tumor itself, and the second is a larger yield of lymph nodes for pathologic examination. Clearly, in the area of rectal cancer, a wide radial margin, including all the fat and vessels supplying the rectum and heading distally to include the length of the mesorectum in the specimen, has been shown to reduce local recurrence and increase lymph node yield. NSABP and other cooperative studies performed in the 1980s and 1990s also demonstrated a significant downstaging and reduction in local recurrence when neoadjuvant radiation is added to rectal resection, although a survival advantage has not been demonstrated (2).

3. Gastric Cancer: Malignancies of the stomach were traditionally managed by total or distal gastrectomy without lymph node dissection. In the 1970s and later, many prospective studies of surgical management indicated that proximal gastrectomy, distal gastrectomy, and total gastrectomy can be selectively used to manage gastric cancer with lower local recurrence rates. A prospective trial comparing aggressive lymphadenectomy to standard resection for gastric cancer showed no survival advantage but did show that the lymph node information obtained from aggressive lymphadenectomy is a key to accurate staging in this disease (3). Now, with encouraging results from the adjuvant and neoadjuvant trials of chemotherapy combinations in gastric cancer, this staging information is more relevant and may lead to better outcomes.

4. Esophageal Cancer: There are many approaches to esophageal resection, to date; aggressive surgical resection with en bloc lymphadenectomy has not demonstrated significant improvement in survival or local recurrence. No matter which surgical approach is used, a multimodality treatment course is usually applied, either with or without neoadjuvant chemotherapy or chemo-radiotherapy.

5. Liver Tumors: Advances in knowledge of the anatomy of the liver combined with improved technologies have led to significant improvements in survival post liver resection (4). Also, high volume liver surgeons have moved to a multimodal approach to liver surgery in metastatic disease, often using combinations of chemotherapy, resection, and ablation for these patients. Several prospective series have demonstrated a survival advantage to chemotherapy plus resection in stage IV patients over chemotherapy or surgery alone. New techniques for ablation using cryosurgery, radiofrequency, and microwave have opened therapeutic options for those who are unable to benefit from a liver resection. Interventional transcatheter techniques include embolization and chemo-embolization of liver tumors. The availability of yttrium-90 spheres has also improved control of intrahepatic disease and reduced recurrence of hepatocellular cancers after resection. Lastly, the addition of transplantation as a viable treatment for hepatocellular cancers has opened new options for management of these difficult tumors.

6. Skin Cancer and Sarcoma: A majority of melanomas and sarcomas are managed by oncologic surgeons. Randomized trials completed in the 1980s determined the ideal margins for melanoma surgery (5), and demonstrated that

limb-preserving radical resection plus radiation is equivalent to amputation for survival for soft tissue sarcomas of the extremity (6). Sentinel node became standard for melanomas in the 1990s and continues to be essential in separating the high-risk patients from the low-risk patients to this day.

7. Multimodalities: As adjuvant chemotherapy continues to evolve into patient-specific molecular-based regimens (e.g., Herceptin, Gleevec, Nexavar, and Sutent) (Herceptin (Trastuzumab – Genentech, USA), Gleevec (Imatinib mesylate – Novartis Pharmaceutical Corporation), Nexavar (Sorafenib – Bayer HealthCare Pharmaceuticals) and Sutent (Sunitinib Malate – Pfizer Oncology Inc)), and radiation options evolve for directed therapy (brachytherapy or transcatheter options), the surgeon must be a well-informed member of the multidisciplinary team to ensure that their patients get access to the most advanced and least morbid therapeutic regimens. This has been a traditional advantage of surgical oncology training, and a well-trained team remains the mainstay of multimodality cancer treatment nationwide.

Cross-References

▶ Pain Management
▶ Skin Cancer
▶ Stage 0 Breast Cancer

References

American College of Surgeons Commission on Cancer: 633 N. Saint Clair St., Chicago, IL 60611

Annals of Surgical Oncology: Copyright by Society of Surgical Oncology, Springer (pub.)

Chapter 1, The history of breast therapy: 20th century. In: Bland KI, Copeland EM, editors. The breast. 4th ed. Philadelphia: Saunders; 2009

Chapter 61, Adenocarcinoma of the stomach, duodenum and small intestine: gastric adenocarcinoma, treatment. In: Yeo CJ, editor. Shackelford's surgery of the alimentary tract. 6th ed. Philadelphia: Saunders; 2007. p. 908–911.

Chapter 73, Melanoma. In: Abeloff MD, editor. Abeloff's clinical oncology. 4th ed. Philadelphia: Churchill Livingstone; 2008. p. 1238.

Chapter 73a, Surgical treatment of metastatic metastases from colorectal cancer. In: Blumgart LH, editor. Surgery of the liver, biliary tract and pancreas. 4th ed. Philadelphia: Saunders; p. 1187–1191

Chapter 82, Rectal cancer: preoperative therapy: results of clinical trials. In: Abeloff MD, editor. Abeloff's clinical oncology. 4th ed. Philadelphia: Churchill Livingstone; 2008. p. 1544–1549.

Chapter 97, Sarcomas of soft tissue. In: Abeloff MD, editor. Abeloff's clinical oncology. 4th ed. Philadelphia: Churchill Livingstone;2008. p. 2009.

Herceptin (Trastuzumab – Genentech, USA), Gleevec (Imatinib mesylate – Novartis Pharmaceutical Corporation), Nexavar (Sorafenib – Bayer HealthCare Pharmaceuticals) and Sutent (Sunitinib Malate - Pfizer Oncology Inc)

National Surgical Adjuvant Bowel and Breast Project: East Common Professional Building, Four Allegheny Center, Pittsburg, PA 15212

The Breast Journal: Shala Masood (ed.), Wiley-Blackwell (pub.)

The National Cancer Data Base: The American College of Surgeons, 633 N. Saint Clair St., Chicago, IL 60611

Prostate

T. Wiegel[1], D. Bottke[1], A. Al Ghazal[2], M. Schrader[2]
[1]Klinik für Radioonkologie und Strahlentherapie, Universitätsklinikum Ulm, Ulm, Germany
[2]Urologische Universitätsklinik, Ulm, Germany

Synonyms

Adenocarcinoma of the prostate; PCa; Prostate cancer; Prostatic adenocarcinoma; Prostatic carcinoma; RFA

Definition

The prostate is a compound tubuloalveolar exocrine gland of male reproduction. It is located in the pelvis posterior to the bladder and anterior to the rectum.

Introduction

Prostate cancer (PCa) is considered as the most common solid neoplasm of the male population. It is currently the second most common cause of cancer death in men. PCa affects elderly men more often than young men. The risk factors of developing a clinical relevant PCa are not well known. Anyway a few have been identified. Three well-established risk factors for PCa are: increasing age, ethnical origin, and heredity.

Treatment of PCa has become increasingly complex due to the various therapeutic options available, which have similar oncological efficacy but significantly different, treatment-related side effects. Therapeutic management options vary from deferred conservative management strategies of "watchful waiting" and "active surveillance" in case of small, localized, well-differentiated PCa up to definitive radiation therapy or radical prostatectomy in case of localized prostate cancer. In case of advanced/metastatic disease hormonal therapy in terms of androgen-suppressing strategies has become the mainstay of palliative management. In case of "hormone-refractory" prostate cancer therapeutic management becomes even more complex and often requires switching to an alternative anti-androgen therapy or addition of a non-hormonal therapy with cytotoxic agents.

Anatomy

The prostate in shape and size resembles a chestnut and weighs about 20 g. It is a fibromuscular gland that is placed in the pelvic cavity behind the symphysis pubis, posterior to the deep perineal fascia and upon the rectum separated from it by the Denonvillier's fascia. Posterior and superiorly the seminal vesicles and the vasa deferentia are placed. The prostate surrounds the neck of the bladder and commencement of the urethra. On its ventral site it is fixed to the posterior part of the symphysis pubis by the puboprostatic ligaments. It is also held in its position by the posterior layer of the deep perineal fascia and by the anterior portion of the Levator ani muscle. In its posterior site the prostate is perforated by the common seminal ducts (ejaculatory ducts) that pass forward obliquely and open into the prostatic portion of the urethra. The prostate consists of three lobes: two lateral and a middle lobe.

The muscular tissue of the prostate is arranged in the form of circular bands around the urethra that derive from the smooth muscle fibers of the detrusor muscle of the urinary bladder wall. These circular bands form the sphincter internus vesicae.

The arteries supplying the prostate are derived from the inferior vesical, internal pudendal, and medial rectal arteries. Its veins communicate with the dorsal vein of the penis and form a plexus (Santorini) around the sides and the base of the gland that terminates in the internal iliac vein.

The nerves are derived from the pelvic and vesical plexus of sympathetic and parasympathetic nerves. The neurovascular bundle lies on either side of the prostate on the rectum. It is derived from the pelvic plexus and is important for erectile function. The lymph drainage of the prostate is to the sacral, vesical, obturator, and internal and external iliac lymph nodes.

Epidemiology

Prostate cancer is considered as the most common solid neoplasm of the male population with an incidence rate in Europe of 214 cases per 1,000 men. Furthermore, PCa is currently the second most common cause of cancer death in men. International studies show that at age between 60 and 70 years prevalences differ from about 124/100.000 (African-American men in the USA) to 14/100.000 (Greek men). Prostate cancer affects elderly men more often than young men. The risk of being diagnosed with prostate cancer increases with age, from 1 in 2,500 at age 45, to

1 in 9 at age 75. For men in the general population, the overall risk of being diagnosed with prostate cancer is 1 in 6. The risk of dying is 1 in 35.

It is therefore a bigger health concern in developed countries with their greater proportion of elderly men. Thus, about 15% of male cancers are PCa in developed countries compared to 4% of male cancers in undeveloped countries.

A so-called *stage-shift* to lower, localized stages of prostate cancer can be observed.

This effect is apparently is attributed to the measurement of the prostate-specific antigen (PSA).

Approximately 40% of the male population in the western industrialized countries carry the risk to develop prostate cancer in course of a lifetime. Only about 10% show clinically manifest disease, and 3% decease. Prostate cancer is also found during autopsies performed following other causes of death. The rate of latent or autopsy cancer is much greater than that of clinical cancer. In fact, it may be as high as 80% by age 80 years.

The risk factors of developing a clinical relevant PCa are not well known. Anyway a few have been identified. Three well-established risk factors for PCa are: increasing age, ethnical origin, and heredity.

Exogenous factors seem to affect the risk of progression from so-called latent PCa to clinical PCa. Factors such as food consumption, pattern of sexual behavior, alcohol consumption, exposure to ultraviolet radiation, and occupational exposure have all been discussed as being of etiological importance, but no real evidence-data so long exists.

Clinical Presentation

Due to the common peripheral localization of prostate cancer in the prostate gland itself it may not cause signs or symptoms in its early stages. About 40–50% of the patients are asymptomatic. More often advanced stages may cause signs and symptoms mostly related to urination, i.e., decreased urinary stream or urinary retention. Nonspecific symptoms that may accompany urinary symptoms include: pelvic pain, back or hip pain in case of bone metastases, or weight loss as an unspecific sign of disease. Also erectile dysfunction, anemia, lymphatic edema of the lower limbs, or hydronephrosis in advanced stage may occur.

The primary extension assessment of prostate cancer is usually made by digital rectal examination, prostate-specific antigen (PSA) measurement, and bone scan, supplemented with computed tomography (CT) or magnetic resonance imaging (MRI) and chest X-ray in specific situations. UICC-classification should be consulted (Table 1).

Histologic Findings

A biopsy confirms the diagnosis of prostatic cancer. The most common used system of classifying the histologic characteristics of prostate cancer is the *Gleason score*, which is determined using the glandular architecture within the tumor.

The predominant pattern and the second most common pattern are given grades from 1 to 5. The addition of these two grades is referred to as the *Gleason score*. Scoring based on the two most common patterns is an attempt to factor in the considerable heterogeneity within cases of prostate cancer. In addition, this scoring method was found to be superior for predicting disease outcomes compared with using the individual grades alone (Table 2).

Differential Diagnosis

Other diseases which are more common may cause symptoms related to urination are, for example, benign prostatic hypertrophy, prostatic cysts, or acute or chronic prostatitis. They are possible alternative diagnoses to consider during the diagnostic process for prostate cancer. A biopsy of the prostate with positive histologic findings confirms the diagnosis of prostatic cancer.

Prostate. Table 1 TNM classification of prostate cancer (UICC, 7th edition)

TNM	
Tx	Primary tumor cannot be assessed
T0	No evidence of primary tumor
T1	Clinically inapparent tumor (not palpable or visible by imaging)
T1a	Incidental tumor, histological finding in less than 5% of resected tissue
T1b	Incidental tumor, histological finding in more than 5% of resected tissue
T1c	Tumor identified by needle biopsy because of elevated PSA
T2	Tumor confined to the prostate
T2a	Tumor involved half a lobe or less of prostate
T2b	Tumor involved more than half a lobe but not both lobes
T2c	Tumor involved both lobes
T3	Tumor extends through prostatic capsule
T3a	Extracapsular extension (unilateral or bilateral) including microscopic bladder neck involvement
T3b	Tumor invades seminal vesicle
T4	Tumor involves structures other than seminal vesicle
T4a	Tumor Invades bladder neck, external sphincter, or rectum Invades
T4b	Muscles and/or pelvic wall
Nx	Lymphnodes cannot be assessed
N0	No regional node metastases
N1	Regional lymph node metastases
Mx	Distant metastases cannot be assessed
M0	No distant metastases
M1	Distant metastases
M1a	Non regional lymph nodes
M1b	Bone metastases
M1c	Other sites

Prostate. Table 2 Gleason score for histological grading (*SIU* 2005)

Gleason score	
2–4	Is considered as low-grade carcinoma or well differentiated
5–7	Is considered moderate grade or moderate differentiated
8–10	Is considered high-grade or poorly differentiated

Imaging Studies

The main diagnostic tools to obtain evidence of PCa include digital rectal examination (DRE), serum concentration of PSA, and transrectal ultrasonography (TRUS). A prostate biopsy confirms the definite diagnosis depending on the presence of adenocarcinoma in prostate biopsy cores or operative specimens. Transrectal ultrasonography can show the classic picture of a hypoechoic area in the peripheral zone of the prostate but will not always be seen. So TRUS does not detect areas of PCa with adequate reliability. It also is no more accurate in showing organ-confined disease as DRE. It is therefore not useful to replace systematic biopsies with targeted biopsies of suspect areas. However, additional biopsies of suspect areas may be useful.

Local staging (T-staging) of PCa is based on findings from DRE and possibly MRI. Conventional endorectal MRI is helpful for localizing cancer within the prostate and seminal vesicles and to determine infiltration, i.e., into the urinary bladder or neurovascular bundles (sensitivity about 40–70% and specificity about 60–95%). Dynamic contrast-enhanced MRI and MR spectroscopic imaging are also complementary in local staging, but so long their use in most cases is currently limited to a research setting. MR spectroscopic imaging (MRSI) allows for the assessment of tumor metabolism by displaying the relative concentrations of citrate, choline, creatinine, and polyamines. Differences in the concentrations of these metabolites between normal and malignant prostate tissues allow potentially tumor localization within the prostate (specificity 75–90% and sensitivity 63–91%). Difficulties in interpreting signal changes related to post-biopsy hemorrhage and inflammatory changes of the prostate, and the unquantifiable but significant inter- and intra-observer variability seen between both non-dedicated and dedicated radiologists may lead to under- or overestimation of tumor presence and the local extent.

The overall accuracy of ^{11}C-choline positron emission tomography (PET) in defining local tumor stage has been reported to be around 70%. PET tends to under stage PCa. On the other hand it can be useful for diagnostic of local or distant failure in case of post-therapeutic PSA-elevation in terms of tumor recurrence. Recurrent disease can be localized reliably in patients with PSA levels of >2 μg/L.

CT scanning or MRI are not recommended to be used to determine if lymph nodes are reactive or contain malignant deposits. Actually the gold standard for N-staging is operative lymphadenectomy.

Skeletal metastasis (M-staging) is best assessed by bone scan. This may not be indicated in asymptomatic patients if the serum PSA level is less than 20 ng/mL and in the presence of well or moderately differentiated tumors.

Besides bone, PCa may metastasise to any organ, but most commonly it affects distant lymph nodes, lung, liver, brain, and skin. Clinical examination, chest X-ray, ultrasound, CT, and MRI scans are appropriate methods of investigation, but only if symptoms suggest the possibility of metastases.

Laboratory Studies

Prostate-specific antigen (PSA) is a kallikrein-like serine protease produced almost exclusively by the epithelial cells of the prostate. It is organ-specific but not cancer-specific. Serum levels may be elevated in the presence of benign prostatic hypertrophy (BPH), prostatitis, and other nonmalignant conditions. Several modifications of serum PSA value have been described, which may improve the specificity of PSA in the early detection of PCa. They include: PSA density, PSA density of the transition zone, age-specific reference ranges, and PSA molecular forms.

A prostate-specific noncoding mRNA marker, PCA3, is measured in urine sediment after prostatic massage. The main advantages of PCA3 over PSA are its higher sensitivity and specificity and that is not influenced by prostate volume or prostatitis. Although PCA3 may have potential value for identifying prostate cancer in men with initially negative biopsies in spite of an elevated PSA, the determination of PCA3 remains still experimental.

Elevated alkaline phosphatase levels and a positive bone scan point to bone metastasis.

Treatment

Treatment of PCa has become increasingly complex due to the various therapeutic options available. Treatment decisions for each clinical stage and risk group of PCa should be based on the actual guidelines. A multidisciplinary approach in patients with high-risk PCa from the beginning is recommended in case if adjuvant treatment will be necessary for locally advanced disease. Different types of treatment options according to the clinical stage and condition of the patient are used.

Deferred Treatment

The incidence of small, localized, well-differentiated PCa is increasing, mainly as a result of prostate-specific antigen (PSA) screening and prostate biopsy. Data shows that patients with localized PCa would not, in fact, benefit from a definitive treatment. For reducing the risk of overtreatment in this subgroup of patients, two conservative management strategies of deferred treatment like "watchful waiting" and "active surveillance" have been proposed.

Watchful waiting is closely monitoring a patient's condition without giving any treatment until symptoms appear or change. This is usually used in older men with other medical problems and a limited life expectancy and for older patients with less aggressive cancers or early-stage disease. The rationale behind this strategy is the observation that PCa often progresses slowly. Studies with a follow-up of up to 25 years show an overall survival and disease-specific survival at 10 years ranging from 82% to 87%. Beyond 15 years survival-rates between 58% and 80% and after 20-years disease-specific survival-rates of 32–57% have been reported.

Active surveillance (or expectant management) includes an active decision not to treat the patient immediately and to follow him with close surveillance with the aim of reducing the ratio of overtreatment in patients with clinically confined low-risk PCa (cT1c/T2a, Gleason score 6 and PSA levels ≤10), without giving up radical treatment and the intention to treat at predefined thresholds that classify progression (i.e., short PSA doubling time and deteriorating histopathologic factors on repeat biopsy). In these cases, the treatment options are intended to be curative. Only non-mature randomized clinical trials with a follow-up <10 years are currently available to stratify survivals-rates under active-surveillance strategy.

At a median follow-up of 8 years, overall survival-rates up to 85% were reported, while disease-specific survival and metastasis-free survival were 99%. A multicentre clinical trial active surveillance versus immediate treatment was opened in the USA in 2006. Results are expected in 2025.

Surgery

In patients with low risk (cT1c/T2a, Gleason score 6 and PSA levels ≤10) and intermediate risk (T2b or Gleason score ≥7 and PSA ≥10 and ≤20) localized PCa and a life expectancy >10 years surgical treatment of prostate cancer consists of radical prostatectomy (RP).

Optional selected patients with low-volume high-risk localized PCa (cT3a or Gleason score ≥8 or PSA ≥20) and highly selected patients with very high-risk localized PCa (cT3b-T4N0 or any TN1) in the context of multimodality treatment can be treated by radical prostectomy.

It involves the removal of the entire prostate gland between the urethra and the bladder, and resection of both seminal vesicles along with sufficient surrounding tissue to obtain a negative margin. Nerve-sparing RP can be performed safely in most patients but may have a higher chance of local disease recurrence and therefore should be selected carefully. Clear contraindications are those patients in whom there is a high risk of extracapsular disease, such as any cT3 PCa, cT2c, anyGleason score >7 on biopsy, or more than one biopsy >6 at the ipsilateral side. Often, radical prostatectomy is accompanied by a bilateral pelvic lymph node dissection. No age threshold for RP is given and a patient should not be denied this procedure on the grounds of age alone.

Radical retropubic prostactectomy (RRP) and perineal prostatectomy are performed through open incisions, while more recently minimally invasive laparoscopic (LRP) and robot-assisted radical prostatectomy (RALP) have been developed.

After performing radical prostatectomy in organ-confined disease the 10 year cancer-specific survival is up to 94–98%. Ten-year PSA-free survival is 60–75%.

Experimental Local Treatment of Prostate Cancer

Focal therapy of prostate cancer cannot be recommended as a therapeutic alternative outside clinical trials.

Cryosurgery

Cryosurgery is a treatment that uses an instrument to freeze and destroy prostate cancer cells. This type of treatment is also called cryotherapy. Freezing of the prostate is ensured by placement of 12–15 17 G-cryoneedles under transrectal ultrasound (TRUS) guidance, placement of thermosensors at the level of the external sphincter and the bladder neck, and insertion of a urethral warmer. Two freeze-thaw cycles are used under TRUS guidance, resulting in temperature of $-40°C$ in the mid-gland and at the neurovascular bundle.

Impotence and leakage of urine from the bladder or stool from the rectum may occur in men treated with cryosurgery.

High-Intensity Focused Ultrasound (HIFU)

High-intensity focused ultrasound consists of focused ultrasound waves emitted from a transducer, which cause tissue damage by mechanical and thermal effects as well as by cavitation. The goal of HIFU is to heat malignant tissues above $65°C$ so that they are destroyed by coagulative necrosis. The available evidence on efficacy and safety of *HIFU* in prostate cancer is of very low quality.

Hormone Therapy

After definite surgical therapy or radiotherapy there still remains a significant risk of cancer recurrence. Between 27% and 53% of all patients undergoing radiation therapy or RP will develop local or distant recurrences within 10 years of initial therapy, and 16–35% of patients will receive second-line treatment within 5 years of initial therapy.

In case of advanced/metastatic disease hormonal therapy in terms of androgen-suppressing strategies has become the mainstay of palliative management. The indication of hormone therapy is to palliate symptoms and to reduce the risk for potentially severe complications in advanced or metastatic disease (spinal cord compression, pathological fractures, ureteral obstruction, extraskeletal metastasis).

Prostate cells are physiologically dependent on androgens to stimulate growth, function, and proliferation. Testosterone, although not tumorigenic, is essential for the growth and perpetuation of prostate tumor cells. The testes are the source of most of the androgens, with only 5–10% (androstenedione, dihydroepiandrosterone, and dihydroepiandrosterone sulfate) being derived from adrenal biosynthesis.

Hormone therapy is a cancer treatment that removes hormones or blocks their action and stops cancer cells from growing.

Drugs, surgery, or other hormones are used to reduce the production of male hormones or block them from working.

Hormone therapy used in the treatment of prostate cancer may include the following:

Orchiectomy is a surgical procedure to remove one or both testicles, the main source of male hormones, to decrease hormone production.
Luteinizing hormone-releasing hormone agonists (LHRH-agonists) can prevent the testicles from producing testosterone. Examples are leuprolide, goserelin, and buserelin.
Antiandrogens can block the action of androgens. Two examples are flutamide and nilutamide.
Drugs that can prevent the adrenal glands from making androgens include ketoconazole and aminoglutethimide.

Chemotherapy

In case of "hormone-refractory" and metastatic prostate cancer palliative therapeutical management becomes even more complex and often requires switching to an alternative anti-androgen therapy, combined androgene blockade (CAB) or addition of a non-hormonal therapy with cytotoxic agents, i.e., mitoxantrone or docetaxel.

Application of bisphosphonates like zoledronic acid or Denosumab, a fully human monoclonal antibody, which targets RANKL *(receptor activator of nuclear factor-kappa-B-ligand*, a protein that acts as the primary signal to promote bone removal; in many bone loss conditions, RANKL overwhelms the body's natural defense against bone destruction), can be proposed to patients with bone metastases to prevent skeletal complications. Pain due to osseous metastases is one of the most debilitating complications. Bisphosphonates seem to be highly effective with a response rate of 70–80% to pain reduction. Palliative external beam radiation of bone metastases can be added to reduce symptoms and prevent pathological fractures.

Radiotherapy

Localized Prostate Cancer T1–2cN0M0

For patients with a low-risk prostate cancer (<T2b, Gleason Score <7, PSA <10 ng/mL) prospective randomized clinical trials have shown that biochemical disease-free survival (bNED) and prostate cancer-specific mortality is significantly improved with a radiation dose ≥72 Gy. However, the best dose is not known until yet. In randomized trials doses between 74 and 79 Gy have been used. An additional hormonal treatment is not recommended.

For patients with intermediate risk (T2b or PSA 10–20 ng/mL or Gleason Score 7) the same advantage has been demonstrated. For this group, too, a total dose >74 Gy for the prostate is recommended. On the other hand, in the intermediate risk group it has also been shown, that an additional neoadjuvant and/or adjuvant hormonal treatment using LHRH-analogons over a period of 6 months improves biochemical progression-free survival and metastates-free survival compared with radiation alone. It is an alternative treatment compared with dose escalation alone.

In the high-risk group (T2c or Gleason Score >7 or PSA >20 ng/mL) the combination of a short-term hormonal androgen deprivation therapy in combination with external beam radiation has been shown superior survival outcome compared with radiation therapy (70 Gy) alone. Therefore, in patients with localized prostate cancer in the high-risk group at least a short-term hormonal treatment in addition to radiotherapy is recommended. On the other hand, the data from the EORTC-22961 randomized phase-III trial comparing 36 months of hormonal treatment plus radiotherapy with 6 months of hormonal treatment plus radiotherapy showed that increased hormonal treatment improved overall survival.

The role of prophylactic irradiation of pelvic lymphnodes in localized PCA is not clearly defined until yet. It seems possible to treat patients of the intermediate und high-risk group with a total dose of 50.4 Gy (single dose 1.8 Gy) to the pelvic lymphatics but clear data are lacking.

Locally Advanced PCA: T3–4N0M0

For locally advanced PCA the standard remains the combination of long-term hormonal treatment with LHRH-analogons (at least 2 years, better 3 years) in combination with percutaneous irradiation to the prostate and the seminal vesicles to a dose of at least 72 Gy. This combination significantly increases overall survival compared with irradiation alone. Prophylactic treatment of pelvic lymph nodes remains a possible way of treatment; however, it is no standard procedure due to lacking data of randomized clinical trials. Neoadjuvant hormonal treatment as used in the RTOG studies 86–10 and 92–02 is often used in the high-risk group to reduce the size of the gland and to reduce the number of clonogenic tumor cells at the start of irradiation and is then combined with an adjuvant hormonal treatment as stated before.

Patients with cN1 or pN1 with pelvic lymph node involvement lower than the iliac regional nodes seem to stand to profit from external beam radiation therapy (EBRT) plus immediate long-term hormonal manipulation for at least 3 years. This should be concluded from the RTOG 85–31 randomized phase-III trial. However, this finding was not the primary endpoint of this study. A summary of definitive radiation therapy shows Table 3 as defined by the Guidelines of the European Association of Urology (EAU).

Comparing radical prostatectomy with either external beam radiation therapy (EBRT) or brachytherapy (permanent seed implantation) for localized prostate cancer, EBRT offers the same long-term survival results as surgery. For example, 5-year biochemical progression-free survival for the low-risk group is about 90–95%, for the intermediate risk group about 80–85%, and for the high-risk group about 60–70%. Ten-year cancer-specific survival for localized PCA is about 85–90% and for locally advanced PCA between 60% and 75%. The data suggest that EBRT provides a quality of life at least as good as that provided for surgery. Prospectively collected data of quality of life demonstrated after a time period of about 1 year comparable long-time quality of life outcomes for all three treatments. An additional option as stated before is an active-surveillance policy in selected patients.

Radiotherapy After Prostatectomy

Following radical prostatectomy depending on tumor stage up to 50–70% of patients develop a PSA increase or a persisting PSA following RP as a sign of tumor progression. Due to these findings, immediate adjuvant radiotherapy after RP in selected patients at high risk of tumor progression or salvage RT (SRT) for patients with increasing PSA after RP offers a second chance of cure.

Immediate postoperative external beam irradiation after RP for patients with pathological tumor stage of pT3N0M0 seems to improve overall survival, biochemical and clinical disease-free

Prostate. Table 3 Guidelines of the EAU

	LE
– In localized prostate cancer T1c-T2bNoMo, 3D-CRT with or without IMRT is recommended even for young patients who refuse surgical intervention. There is fairly strong evidence that low-, intermediate-, and high-risk patients benefit from dose escalation.	1a
For patients in the high-risk group, short-term ADT prior to and during radiotherapy results in increased overall survival, but three years of adjuvant ADT are better according to the results of EORTC 22961.	2a
– Transperineal interstitial brachytherapy with permanent implants is an option for patients with cT1-T2a, Gleason Score < 7 (or 3 + 4), PSA $\leq$ 10 ng/mL, prostate volume $\leq$ 50 mL, without a previous TURP and with a good IPSS.	2b
– Immediate postoperative external beam irradiation after RP for patients with pathological tumor stage T3N0M0 improves overall survival, biochemical and clinical disease-free survival with the highest impact in cases of positive margins (R1).	1d
An alternative option is to give radiation at the time of biochemical failure, but before PSA rises above 0.5 ng/mL.	3
– In locally advanced prostate cancer T3–4 N0 M0, overall survival is improved by concomitant and adjuvant hormonal therapy for a total duration of 3 years, with external beam irradiation for patients with a WHO 0–2 performance status.	1a
For a subset of patients with T2c-T3N0-x and a Gleason Score of 2–6, short-term ADT before and during radiotherapy may favorably influence overall survival.	1b
– In very high-risk prostate cancer, c-pN1M0 with no severe comorbidity, pelvic external irradiation and immediate long-term adjuvant hormonal treatment improve overall survival, disease-specific failure, metastatic failure and biochemical control.	2b

LE Level of evidence

survival with the highest impact in cases of positive surgical margins (R1). For these patients with positive surgical margins the results of 3 randomized prospective phase-III trials have shown an increase of about 30% of bNED after 5 years. For patients with pT3-tumors and other risk factors as invasion of the seminal vesicles and/or a Gleason Score ≥7 this advantage seems to be about 10% after 5 years. In the German ARO-trial it has been shown in a randomized setting that this fact even appears for patients with R1-resection whose PSA after RP achieved the undetectable range (<0.1 ng/mL). Subgroup analyses of the EORTC-trial of adjuvant radiotherapy suggest the same effect of about 30% better bNED after 5 years also for pT2R1-patients. In this case, an immediate irradiation 6–12 weeks following RP is directed to the prostatic bed with a single dose of 2 Gy and a total dose of 60–64 Gy.

In contrast to immediate radiotherapy after RP an alternative setting is clinical and biological monitoring followed by salvage radiotherapy when the PSA increases out of the undetectable range or persists after RP. Tumor progression is still defined in most guidelines as a PSA increase over 0.2 ng/mL. However, radiotherapy is also possible, when the PSA increases out of the undetectable range (>0.05 ng/mL). In this case, the risk of residual nonmalignant prostate tissue remains higher than in the situation of an increase above 0.2 ng/mL.

Over the last years, it has been shown that an early start of irradiation remains the best way of achieving an undetectable PSA after SRT again. Achieving an undetectable PSA after SRT gives a second chance of cure of about 80% of bNED 5 years following SRT and is the most independent factor of tumor control. When starting with a PSA <0.5 ng/mL, about 50–60% of the patients achieve an undetectable PSA again. The results are dependent from other risk factors as Gleason Score >7 and/or infiltration of seminal vesicles

at time of RP, giving a lower chance of about 30–40% in these patients. Standard of cure in these patients is to treat the prostatic fossa with a total dose of at least 66 Gy and a single dose of 1.8–2 Gy. The role of irradiation of the pelvic lymphatics remains controversial as prospective phase-III data are lacking but seems reasonable in selected high-risk patients (for example patients with a higher PSA, Gleason Score 8–10). The role of neoadjuvant or adjuvant hormonal treatment is not proven until yet. Therefore, radiotherapy alone remains standard.

Prospective data comparing adjuvant radiotherapy with salvage radiotherapy are not available. Two randomized clinical phase-III trials are on the way but the results should be awaited in about 5–10 years. Therefore, the best treatment remains to be established in an individual setting between the patient, the urologist, and the radiation oncologist.

Interstitial Brachytherapy

Transperineal Interstitial Brachytherapy with Permanent Seeds

Transperineal interstitial brachytherapy with permanent seeds (iodine-125 in granular form is the radioelement of reference while palladium-103 may be used for less differentiated tumors with a high doubling time) implanted transperineal into the prostate is an option for patients with cT1-T2a, Gleason score <7 (or 3 + 4), PSA <10 ng/mL, prostate volume <50 mL, without a previous TURP and with a good IPSS. Patients with low-risk PCa are the most suitable candidates for low-dose rate (LDR) brachytherapy. The dose delivered to the planning target volume is 160 Gy for iodine-125, and 120 Gy for palladium-103.

In cases of intermediate- or high-risk localized PCa, brachytherapy in combination with supplemental external irradiation or neoadjuvant hormonal treatment may be considered.

High-dose rate brachytherapy (HDR) may be considered as treatment in patients with locally advanced tumors and cN0-stage. In most cases, two single fractions of about 8–9 Gy to the prostate using ultrasound-guided transperineal implantation followed by a homogenious treatment of the prostate with EBRT up to a total dose of about 50 Gy is used. One prospective phase-III trial suggested at least comparable results of this treatment compared with EBRT alone. The role of adjuvant hormonal treatment in these patients remains uncertain.

Technical Aspects

Three-dimensional conformal radiotherapy (3D-RT) is the gold standard and intensity-modulated radiotherapy (step-and-shoot-technique and sliding-window-technique) are gaining ground in standard procedure therapies in most cases (Fig. 1: typical IMRT treatment plan). Dose escalation is mostly used in combination with intensity-modulated radiotherapy also including the delivery of IGRT (image guided RT) with cone beam CT, fiducial markers, or stereotactic ultrasound. Some data suggest an increase of radiation-induced secondary tumors following IMRT. However, this point remains controversial and needs further investigation. In the treatment of prostate cancer using dose escalation schemes, the use of dose constraints remain necessary. Typical dose constraints for the rectum are, for example, not more than 20% of the rectum achieves more than 70 Gy, not more than 40% of the rectum more than 60 Gy, and not more than 20% of the bladder more than 70 Gy. Using these dose constraints, the risk of severe late side effects grade III or IV seems to be below 5%.

Proton Beam or Carbon Ion-Beam Therapy

In theory, proton beams are an attractive alternative to photon beam radiotherapy for PCA because they deposit almost all the radiation dose at the end of the particles path in tissue (the Bragg peek), in contrast to photons which deposit radiation belong the path. Additionally, there is a very sharp fall-off for proton beams beyond the tumor depth, meaning that critical normal tissues beyond these depths could be effectively spared. However, this theoretical advantage focusing on the lower rate of acute and late side effects has not been proven in randomized clinical phase-III trials until yet. Until yet, published data do not show any advantage in tumor control or biochemical progression-free survival following proton treatment compared with high end photon treatment. Theoretically, proton therapy might be associated with a lower risk of secondary cancers compared with IMRT because of the lower integral dose of radiation, but there are no data in patients treated for PCA to support this.

For the moment, proton beam therapy remains a treatment option in definitive irradiation of prostate cancer but has not proven advantage until yet.

Side Effects and Quality of Life

The potential risk of late genito-urinary or gastrointestinal toxicity as well as the impact of irradiation on erectile function depends on the dose

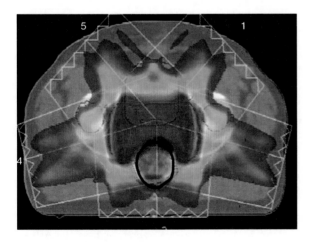

Prostate. Fig. 1 Typical IMRT treatment plan using five fields

and treatment technique. With modern treatment techniques like IMRT and IGRT using cone beam CT, goldmarkers, or BAT-ultrasound the risk of severe late side effects for rectum and bladder using total doses up to 78 Gy seems to be beyond 5%. An important fact is the use of dose constraints for rectum and bladder. Radiotherapy effects erectile function to a lesser degree than surgery according to retrospective surveys of patients. Up to 50% of patients depending on the stage of erectile function before start of treatment maintain their erectile function following RT.

Recent studies have demonstrated a significantly increased risk of developing secondary malignancies of the rectum and bladder following EBRT and also brachytherapy. However, this risk seems to be low and smaller than 0.5% of radiation-induced malignant tumors for 10-year survivors.

Cross-References

▶ Bladder Cancer
▶ Brachytherapy
▶ Image-Guided Radiotherapy (IGRT)
▶ IMRT
▶ Rectal Cancer

References

Bott SR, Birtle AJ, Taylor CJ, Kirby RS (2003) Prostate cancer management: (1) an update on localised disease. Postgrad Med J 79(936):575–580

Bottke D, de Reijke TM, Bartkowiak D, Wiegel T (2009) Salvage radiotherapy in patients with persisting/rising PSA after radical prostatectomy for prostate cancer. Eur J Cancer 45(Suppl 1):148–157

Boyle P, Ferlay J (2005) Cancer incidence and mortality in Europe 2004. Ann Oncol 16(3):481–488

Chun FK, Graefen M, Zacharias M et al (2006) Anatomic radical retropubic prostatectomy-long-term recurrence-free survival rates for localized prostate cancer. World J Urol 24:273–280

Fuchsjager M, Shukla-Dave A, Akin O, Barentsz HH (2008) Prostate cancer imaging. Acta Radiol 49:107–20

Heidenreich A, Bellmunt J, Bolla M, Joniau S, Mason M, Matveev V, Mottet N, Schmid HP, van der Kwast T, Wiegel T, Zattoni F (2010) EAU-guidelines on prostate cancer. Update Apr 2010

Heidenreich A, Bellmunt J, Bolla M, Joniau S, Mason M, Matveev V, Mottet N, Schmid HP, van der Kwast T, Wiegel T, Zattoni F (2010b) EAU guidelines on prostate cancer. Part 1: screening, diagnosis, and treatment of clinically localised disease. Eur Urol 59(1):61–71. [Epub ahead of print]

Hessels D, van Gils MP, van Hooij O, Jannink SA, Witjes JA, Verhaegh GW, Schalken JA (2010) Predictive value of PCA3 in urinary sediments in determining clinico-pathological characteristics of prostate cancer. Prostate 70(1):10–16

Huang J, Kestin LL, Ye H, Wallace M, Martinez AA, Vicini FA (2011) Analysis of second malignancies after modern radiotherapy versus prostatectomy for localized prostate cancer. Radiother Oncol 98(1):81–86

Jemal A, Siegel R, Ward E, Hao Y, Xu J, Murray T, Thun MJ (2008) Cancer statistics, 2008. CA Cancer J Clin 58(2):71–96

Michalski JM, Lawton C, El Naqa I, Ritter M, O'Meara E, Seider MJ, Lee WR, Rosenthal SA, Pisansky T, Catton C, Valicenti RK, Zietman AL, Bosch WR, Sandler H, Buyyounouski MK, Ménard C (2009) Development of RTOG consensus guidelines for the definition of the clinical target volume for postoperative conformal radiation therapy for prostate cancer. Int J Radiat Oncol Biol Phys 2010(76):14–22

Stephenson AJ, Scardino PT, Kattan MW et al (2007) Predicting the outcome of salvage radiation therapy for recurrent prostate cancer after radical prostatectomy. J Clin Oncol 25:2035–2041

Wenz F, Martin T, Böhmer D, Martens S, Sedlmayer F, Wirth M, Miller K, Heidenreich A, Schrader M, Hinkelbein W, Wiegel T (2010) The German S3 guideline prostate cancer: aspects for the radiation oncologist. Strahlenther Onkol 186:531–534

Widmark A, Klepp O, Solberg A, Damber JE, Angelsen A, Fransson P, Lund JA, Tasdemir I, Hoyer M, Wiklund F, Fosså SD, Scandinavian Prostate Cancer Group Study 7, Swedish Association for Urological Oncology 3 (2009) Endocrine treatment, with or without radiotherapy, in locally advanced prostate cancer (SPCG-7/SFUO-3): an open randomised phase III trial. Lancet 373(9660):301–308

Wiegel T, Bottke D, Steiner U, Siegmann A, Golz R, Störkel S, Willich N, Semjonow A, Souchon R, Stöckle M, Rübe C, Weissbach L, Althaus P, Rebmann U, Kälble T, Feldmann HJ, Wirth M, Hinke A, Hinkelbein W, Miller K (2009) Phase III postoperative adjuvant radiotherapy after radical prostatectomy compared with radical prostatectomy alone in pT3 prostate cancer with postoperative undetectable prostate-specific antigen: ARO 96–02/AUO AP 09/95. J Clin Oncol 27(18):2924–2930

Prostate Seed Implants (PSI)

▶ Brachytherapy: Low Dose Rate (LDR) Permanent Implants (Prostate)

Prostatic Adenocarcinoma

▶ Prostate

Prostatic Carcinoma

▶ Prostate

Proton Therapy

Daniel Yeung[1], Jatinder Palta[2]
[1]Department of Radiation Oncology, University of Florida Proton Therapy Institute, Jacksonville, FL, USA
[2]Department of Radiation Oncology, University of Florida Health Science Center, Gainesville, FL, USA

Definition
Proton therapy is a form of radiation treatment that uses high-energy proton beams to irradiate cancers and other diseased tissues.

Background
The principal feature and physical advantage of proton therapy is the finite range of protons in the patient. Protons deliver a reduced dose proximal to the target volume and essentially no dose beyond the end of their range (Fig. 1). In 1946, Robert Wilson of Harvard University (Cambridge, MA, USA) was the first to realize these advantages when he proposed the use of accelerated protons for cancer treatment.

The first proton therapy treatment, which was conducted in 1954 at UC Berkeley (Berkeley, CA, USA), resulted in good clinical response for advanced breast cancer. Using a 185 MeV synchrocyclotron targeted at a variety of disease sites, Uppsala University (Uppsala, Sweden) followed suit in 1957. In 1961, using 160 MeV protons, the Harvard Cyclotron Laboratory (HCL) and Massachusetts General Hospital (Boston, MA, USA) started a highly successful clinical program that lasted 4 decades and clearly established the efficacy of proton therapy.

These early experiences (1954–1990) with proton therapy were primarily in the realm of high-energy physics research laboratories. However, since 1990, a number of hospital-based proton therapy facilities were built (http://ptcog.web.psi.ch/ptcentres.html) and several others are under construction (http://ptcog.web.psi.ch/newptcentres.html). Thus, protons have entered the cancer treatment armamentarium.

Basic Characteristics
As protons pass through tissues and undergo atomic and nuclear interactions, they lose energy and slow down. Consequently, they have increased interactions with electrons, which results in a higher rate of energy loss. Therefore, the linear energy transfer (LET) increases (albeit slowly) with the depth of penetration. The LET rises sharply as particles are near the end of their range, resulting in maximum energy transfer and dose deposition. This phenomenon is reflected in the proton depth-dose curve, which exhibits a relatively low-dose plateau at the entrance, a sharp rise forming the Bragg peak, and a rapid distal falloff (Fig. 1). For protons in the clinical energy range (60–250 MeV), the latter translates to a negligible exit dose beyond the range.

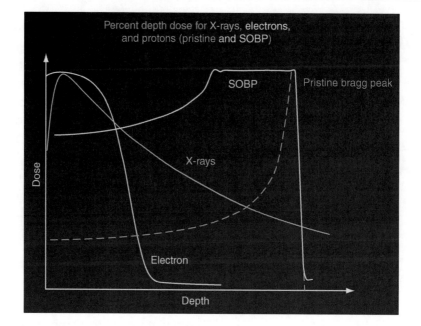

Proton Therapy. Fig. 1 Comparison of the percent depth-dose characteristics for high-energy X-rays, electron and proton beams. For the latter, the depth doses for both the pristine and spread-out Bragg peaks (*SOBPs*) are shown. Note the sharp distal falloff for the proton beam beyond its range. The width of the SOBP was chosen to cover the longitudinal dimension of the target volume along the beam direction

Protons also suffer deflections from multiple Coulomb scattering (MCS) with atomic nuclei, which results in angular and radial spread and ▶ range straggling.

The spread of the Bragg peak of a monoenergetic proton beam is too narrow to cover a typical lesion. To form a uniform dose region covering the depth dimension of the tumor, a ▶ spread-out Bragg peak (SOBP) is generated by stacking multiple Bragg peaks of different energies and intensities (Fig. 2). For lateral coverage, the dose distribution is broadened using either a ▶ passive scattering or a scanning beam technique.

The relative biological effectiveness (RBE) for proton beams is defined as the ratio of the photon dose from 250 kV_p X-rays to the proton dose required to produce the same biological effect. Based on published data and clinical

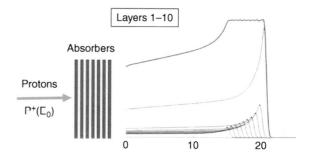

Proton Therapy. Fig. 2 A spread-out Bragg peak (SOBP) to extend the uniform dose region in depth can be formed by energy stacking. Ten layers are shown in this illustration (Courtesy of R. Slopsema, UFPTI, USA)

observations, a mean RBE value of 1.1 is adopted as the current standard (ICRU 2007). However, near the peak and toward the end of the range, the LET rises sharply and the RBE can reach a value as high as 1.5. These higher RBE values extend the biological effective range of the beam by 1–2 mm, which can be clinically significant.

Proton Therapy System (PTS)

The three major equipment components of a proton therapy system are the accelerator, the beam transport system (BTS), and the treatment delivery system. Clinical proton energies typically range from 60 to 250 MeV to support treatments of various disease sites. The most common accelerators for clinical proton facilities are cyclotrons and synchrotrons. Cyclotrons accelerate protons in a circular path and offer protons with fixed energy, a continuous current, and inherently higher beam output. Synchrotrons are the most flexible machines in terms of energy variation, which can be accomplished pulse by pulse, but beam intensities are limited.

Protons extracted from the accelerators are transported through a beam line for treatment delivery. For a fixed energy cyclotron, a variable energy degrader reduces the proton energy to match the required clinical range. Figure 3 illustrates a typical beam transport system (BTS) with a gantry room. A series of bending and focusing magnets are used to transport the beam. At strategic points along the BTS, the beam current, its horizontal and vertical position, and its profile are monitored. Automatic steering and tuning are used to maintain high-precision beam characteristics. An energized switching magnet diverts the beam into the treatment room where the transport is continued through a gantry (TR1) or a fixed beam to reach the beam-delivery nozzle, which

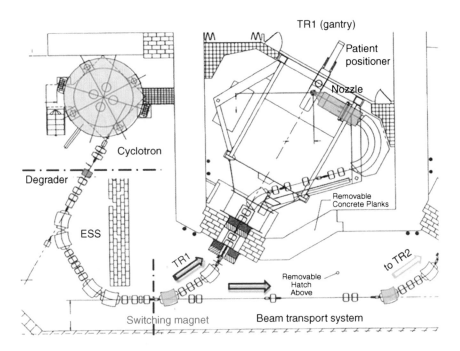

Proton Therapy. Fig. 3 An example of the beam transport system (BTS). Accelerated protons extracted from the cyclotron pass through the degrader and energy selection system (*ESS*) are transported along the beam line. Switching magnets are used to direct the beam to the treatment rooms (Courtesy of IBA, Belgium)

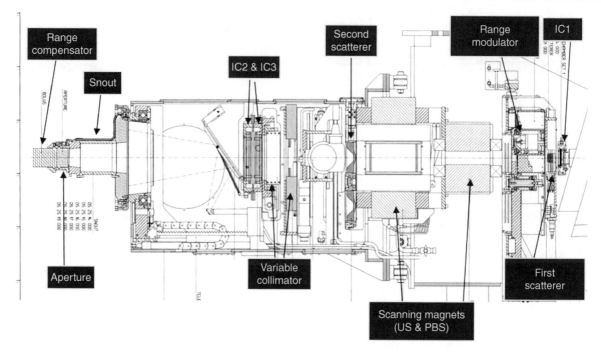

Proton Therapy. Fig. 4 The IBA Universal Nozzle supports passive scatterings (SIS, DS) and uniform (US) and pencil-beam scanning (PBS). A snout designed for different field sizes can be attached to end of the nozzle to house the aperture and compensator (Courtesy of IBA, Belgium)

houses elements to shape and deliver the proton beam (Fig. 4).

For passive scattering, a single (SIS) or double scattering (DS) system is used to generate a uniform beam profile in the transverse direction. The longitudinal (in depth) beam spread or SOBP is achieved through a rotating range modulator (Fig. 5) or a stationary ridge filter. For active scanning or ► pencil-beam scanning (PBS), the nozzle houses the scanning magnets to allow the beam to be swept in the lateral directions. The energy layers of the SOBP are generated sequentially by changing the beam energy upstream. Both raster and spot scanning can be used, and dose optimization can be achieved with intensity modulation. ► Uniform scanning (US) sweeps a larger beam spot across in a fixed pattern to generate a broad lateral profile

and offers a deeper range and a larger field size than DS. Scanning can be achieved with a dedicated nozzle design optimized for PBS or a "universal" nozzle (Fig. 4) that can support both scanning and passive scattering. To ensure high precision in treatment delivery, image guidance and a robotic couch capable of six degrees of freedom (three translations plus pitch, roll, and rotation) are often used for precise patient positioning and setup correction.

Current Knowledge

Proton Equipment and Delivery

Passive Scattering: Passive scattering (Fig. 6) is a standard technique for proton beam delivery that is reliable due to its simplicity. For single scattering, a series of lead foils (or similar

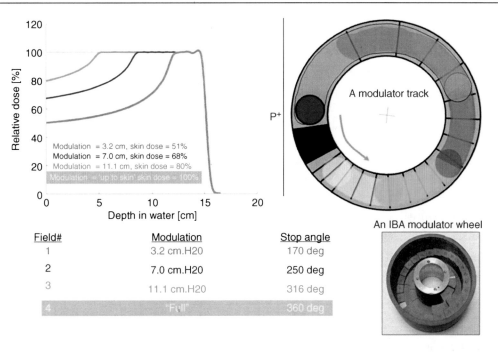

Proton Therapy. Fig. 5 Generation of a SOBP using a rotating modulator wheel. The width of the SOBP is controlled by the number of the steps included in the track when the beam is on. Note that the skin dose increases with the SOBP width. The insert is an IBA modulator wheel designed with three tracks (Courtesy of R. Slopsema, UFPTI, USA)

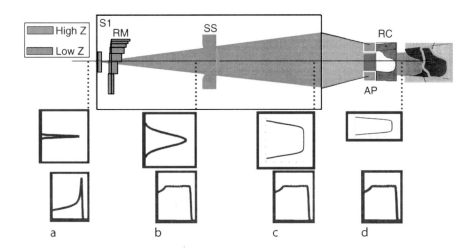

Proton Therapy. Fig. 6 A schematic diagram showing the double scattering (DS) technique to generate a broad beam. Legend: *S1* – first scatterer, *SS* – second scatterer, *RM* – range modulator, *AP* – aperture, *RC* – range compensator. The shape of the lateral (*blue*) and longitudinal (*red*) profiles of the beam at positions a, b, c, and d in relation to the nozzle elements are also plotted (Courtesy of IBA, Belgium)

high-Z materials) are used to transform the pencil beam to a Gaussian-shaped profile. For double scattering, a much thicker second scatterer is added to yield a broad uniform beam. The design and selection of these scatterers are optimized and beam-energy specific. Longitudinal spread is achieved with either a ridge filter or a rotating modulator. Uniformity of $\pm 2\%$ is achievable in lateral and longitudinal beam profiles – a result comparable to that achieved with photons. Brass (or cerrobend) apertures and range compensators (typically lucite or wax) are used for the field shaping and distal conformance of the SOBP. The "continuous" temporal delivery of the SOBP makes passive scattering less sensitive to organ motion; however, field size and useful range are limited.

Uniform Scanning (US): US, which is used in several proton centers, uses scanning magnets to spread a beam laterally. US offers several advantages: a larger range (~ 32 g/cm^2 versus ~ 28 g/cm^2), a large field size (30×40 cm versus 25 cm diameter), and a slightly smaller penumbra. By indexing to a modulator track in static mode, the SOBP is delivered layer by layer. Because of the segmented delivery of the SOBP temporally, US is sensitive to patient or organ motions that result in tissue-depth changes. Each energy layer is delivered by scanning a fairly large beam spot in a fixed pattern with two scanning magnets housed inside the nozzle (Fig. 4). The beam spot and scanning amplitude are optimized for the required field size to achieve dose uniformity and the smallest lateral penumbra. With deeper ranges and large field sizes, US can be used to treat prostate cancers for obese patients and sarcomas with extensive size. It also allows fewer spine fields for craniospinal irradiation (CSI).

Pencil-Beam Scanning (PBS): In PBS, a narrow proton pencil beam is scanned under magnetic control to deliver a true three-dimensional (proximal, lateral, and distal) conformal dose distribution. The composite dose is the result of the superposition of many small pencil beams. High conformality (close to physical limits) is due to the finite penetration of the Bragg peak, the limited scatter, and the fact that the modulation width of the SOBP for each pencil is independently matched to the dimension of the target along the beam axis. The typical pencil beam has a spot size of 6–7 mm full width at half maximum (FWHM), resulting in a relatively sharp lateral penumbra. To minimize the multiple Coulomb scattering (MCS) in the air, the beam transport vacuum system is extended as close as possible to the patient. PBS also exhibits a sharper distal falloff. The beam current required is low (< 0.5 nA), which reduces the neutron dose from activation and the risk of radiation-induced secondary malignancies. For statistical accuracy, a delivery of 10,000 beam spots to a one liter volume (or its equivalent) in a few minutes is necessary. Delivery of PBS can be continuous, using raster scans or static, using discrete beam spots (Pedroni 2008). Spacing between energy layers depends on the spot size and the number of layers intended; 5 mm spacing is typical. Energy selected for each layer is set upstream at the degrader for precision. Fast energy switching (~ 200 ms) would be desirable and multiple repaintings are used to improve accuracy in delivery.

▶ Intensity-modulated proton therapy (IMPT) can be achieved by intensity-modulated scanning. Active beam-current modulation on the timescale of 100 μs with an intensity control precision of 2–5% is desirable. Because beam scanning is sensitive to organ motion during delivery, only well-immobilized tumors located in the head and neck, spinal cord, and lower pelvis are treated with PBS. Finally, PBS eliminates the need for field-specific apertures and range compensators. For a range of 10 cm or larger, edge enhancement with scanning by optimizing the individual spot weights can achieve a sharper lateral penumbra

(~1.4 times steeper) than resulted with the use of collimation by aperture (Pedroni 2008).

Treatment Planning

The clinical implementation of treatment planning for proton therapy presents unique opportunities and challenges. Its finite range and sharp distal falloff allow for sparing of critical structures and flexibilities in beam arrangements. However, because of the inherent uncertainties in range, the proton dose is highly dependent on the accuracy of stopping powers determination, tissue heterogeneities, patient alignment and motion, and other uncertainties (Palta and Yeung 2011). Several key concepts and various treatment planning issues are discussed below.

- *Clinical range and modulation:* For each treatment field, these two key clinical parameters define the beam energy and SOBP required for adequate penetration and longitudinal coverage. Margins are often added to account for uncertainties in the calculation and delivery.
- *Range compensator:* To achieve distal dose conformance to the target, a compensator can be designed for range compensation. The range pullbacks are converted to physical thicknesses based on the stopping power of the compensator material used. Compensators are milled out of lucite or other low-Z materials to minimize degradation in the penumbra.
- *Dosimetric considerations:* To avoid dose spilling to proximal tissues in passive scattering and US where the modulation width is constant across the beam, one should select a beam angle in which the modulation variations are small.
- *Air gap:* Since the penumbra due to scatter from the compensator will be magnified with skin gap, the air gap to the patient should be minimized.

- *Compensator design:* A sharp gradient in the compensator profile will induce fluence perturbations. Although hot and cold spots of 10–20% in dose can result near the slope, a tapered drill bit (~3 degree tapering) can be used to reduce these effects.
- *Beam incidence:* One should avoid beam angles that will result in a sharp gradient, such as those tangential to a bony ridge, large air cavities, or a significant amount of metal implants. Often, a change of even a few degrees can alleviate such problems.
- *Smoothing:* This process is used to smooth out the compensator thickness profile in the field-margin area. It helps to remove sharp gradients (near vertical walls) and allow for adequate penetration, even in the case of misalignment or patient motion.
- *Smearing:* Setup errors or motion can cause misalignment of the compensator with the expected patient anatomy during delivery. This can cause underdosing of the target or overdosing of organs-at-risk (OARs) if the intended depths (ranges) shift significantly. In smearing, the thickness of each grid point is replaced with the thinnest value found within a specified region. This modification ensures adequate range coverage at the expense of lesser distal conformance.
- *Match and patch fields:* These techniques are often used to avoid OARs that are adjacent to the target volume which might otherwise be difficult to spare. The target volume is partitioned into segments (sub-targets) and each is treated with individual sub-beams that combine to cover the entire target. Using sub-beams from different directions makes it possible to avoid the OARs. In the simplest approach, which involves a pair of beams, one beam partially treats the target, while the residual volume is either treated with a match (Fig. 7) or a patch beam

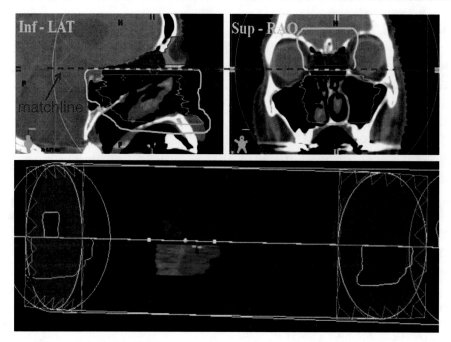

Proton Therapy. Fig. 7 Illustration of the match field technique. The superior aspect of the target (shown in *red*) is treated with a right anterior oblique (RAO) field to allow sparing of the orbits and optic nerves. The residual inferior target (*green*) is covered with a lateral field designed to abut the RAO field at the match line. With a much smaller divergence (SAD > 200 cm) and a finite range, protons offer a clear advantage over photons: a wider choice in beam angulations, especially in noncoplanar configurations

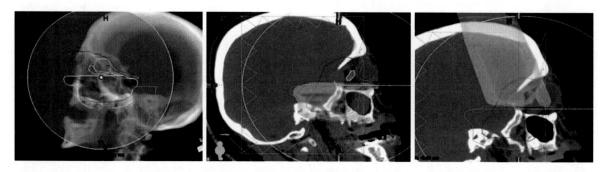

Proton Therapy. Fig. 8 Illustration of the patch-field technique. The inferior aspect of the target (*red contour*) is treated with a left posterior oblique (LPO) field, namely, the through beam (*left*); dose in color wash (*middle*). The residual target (*superior aspect*) is patched with a superior posterior oblique (SPO) field; dose in color wash (*right*)

(Fig. 8). More complex cases involve combinations of match and patch trios or multiple pairs. Match fields are commonly used in conventional therapy, but with their much smaller divergence (SAD >200 cm) and finite range, protons offer a clear advantage: a wider choice in beam angulations, especially in noncoplanar configurations. In the patch-field technique, the 50% lateral penumbra of the first field (the through beam) is matched by the distal falloff of the patch beam. This is achieved with a range pullback such that the distal 50% coincides with the match line. Patch field should avoid passing through sharp gradient of heterogeneities since fluence perturbations (Goitein 2008) will cause the dose distribution to be wavy and highly irregular and result in significant hot and cold areas in the composite dose.

- *Distal blocking:* This technique can be used to limit the dose to OARs that are distal to the target. It allows selective pullback of the range near distal OARs (Fig. 9). Instead of reducing the range of the beam as a whole, distal blocking does not compromise target coverage in areas where pullback is unnecessary. The user can select which OAR and margins to use. However, one may need to create pseudo-structures to "trick" the planning system and achieve the desired dose distribution (Fig. 10).

- *Intensity-modulated proton therapy:* Because of the finite range of protons, IMPT enjoys an additional degree of freedom (depth) for dose optimization as compared to that of IMRT. With the ability to manipulate the energy and fluence for the field(s), one can achieve a true 3D dose optimization. There are two modes of planning optimizations: (a) single-field uniform dose and (b) simultaneous optimization of multiple fields to achieve the desired composite dose distribution. With the added complexities and inherent uncertainties, the "plan robustness" (Pedroni 2008; Lomax 2008) should be carefully considered in IMPT planning and treatments.

Clinical Treatments

The ability of proton therapy to spare critical structures in close proximity to the target and substantially reduce the dose to normal tissues holds the key to improve outcomes and lower acute and long-term toxicities. Selected clinical cases are discussed below to highlight the current practice of proton therapy.

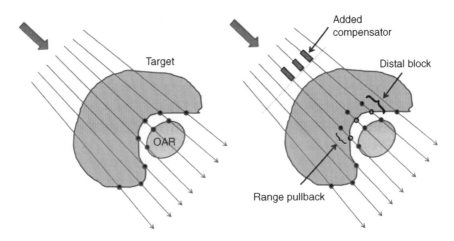

Proton Therapy. Fig. 9 An illustration of the distal blocking technique. The range pullbacks specified to spare the critical structure(s) distal to the target are achieved by adding the required thicknesses in the compensator design

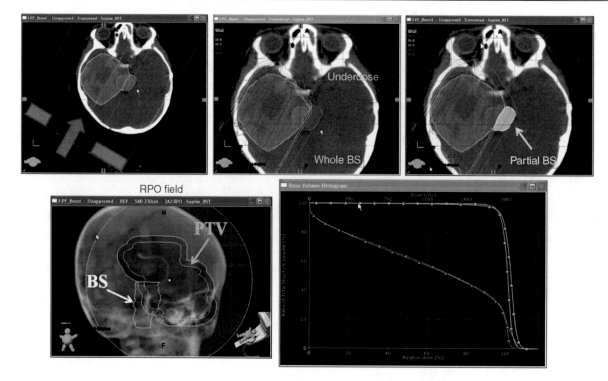

Proton Therapy. Fig. 10 An illustration of using a pseudo structure for distal blocking. Since the brainstem (BS) overlaps with the target volume, distal blocking to lower the dose to BS can lead to underdosing of the target. By using a partial BS that excludes the target for distal blocking, same sparing effect to BS can be achieved without compromising target dose as shown in the dose volume histogram (DVH) plots

Adult Cancers

Base of skull, paraspinal tumors: Chordomas and chondrosarcomas of the base of skull and spine are rare, locally aggressive tumors. Total gross resections with negative margins are infrequently performed because of their invasive nature and the tendency of these tumors to wrap around the brain stem, optic chiasm, optic nerves, or spinal cord. Based on clinical evidence, proton therapy represents the most promising adjunctive treatment owing to its ability to deliver very high doses (~72 ▶ Cobalt Gray Equivalent (CGE) averaged) while limiting morbidity.

Paranasal sinus (PNS): Tumors in this anatomical area are late in developing metastatic disease. Increased local control, therefore, may translate to increased survival. Figure 11 presents a case of esthesioneuroblastoma treated with protons (Rx: 50.4 CGE with a boost to 74.4 CGE). Despite the high-target dose, the brain stem, chiasm, and optic nerves are all within dose constraints. The lower neck was treated with photons to 50 Gy.

Prostate cancers: Proton therapy has the potential to reduce dose to the bladder, rectal walls, and bowels. Reductions in grades 2 and 3 gastrointestinal (GI) and gastrourinary (GU)

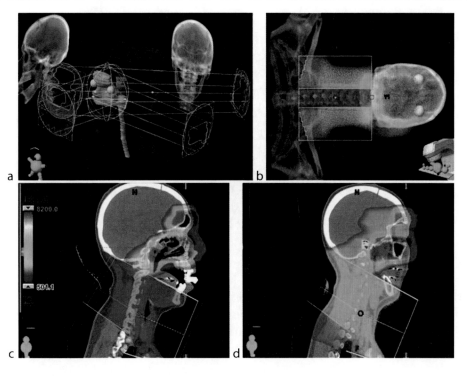

Proton Therapy. Fig. 11 Esthesioneuroblastoma. Rx: Protons – 74.4 CGE; Photons (lower neck) – 50 Gy. (**a**) Proton field arrangement for the initial target volume (PTV5040): superior anterior oblique (SAO), left posterior oblique (LPO), and anterior posterior (AP) (superior)+left lateral (LLAT) (inferior) match pair. (**b**) BEV of the inferior anterior oblique (IAO) photon field with composite dose (proton+photon) in color wash. (**c** & **d**) Sagittal views with composite dose; (**c**) near mid-plane; (**d**) off-axis. Use of protons and match fields allow sparing of the brain stem and visual structures. The lower neck photon fields are also matched to the 50% isodose level from the proton plans

P

toxicities have been reported in early outcome studies. Treatments using lateral or oblique beams with either one field (alternating between left and right) or two fields a day are most common (Fig. 12). Consistent patient setup (e.g., skin folds, hip positions, bladder filling, and rectal and bowel contents) is crucial. Any significant deviations in proton ranges can have detrimental effect on the dose delivered. For high-risk patients, protons are combined with IMRT treatments of the pelvic nodes (Fig. 13). Dosage and fractionation schemes are similar to those of conventional therapy.

Pediatric Cancers

In the proton treatments of medulloblastoma (the most common malignant brain tumor in children) using craniospinal irradiation (CSI), the absence of exit dose to the heart, mediastinum, bowel, bladder, and other tissues significantly reduces the risks of potential complications. For central nervous system (CNS) tumors, clinical observations and dose-effects models indicate that dose reduction to normal brain tissues with proton treatments improves posttreatment IQ and reading scores. Other benefits include lowering the severity of

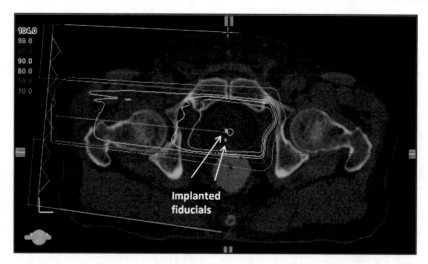

Proton Therapy. Fig. 12 Single-field proton plan for prostate treatment. Common beam angles used are laterals or obliques. A right anterior oblique (*RAO*) field is shown with relative dose in percentage. Anterior obliques are preferred to posterior angles since significant changes in skin folds in the posterior aspect of the body during setup (> 1 cm change in range) can occur. For one field a day treatments, fields are alternating between coming from the left and the right. Implanted fiducials inside the prostate are often used for image guidance

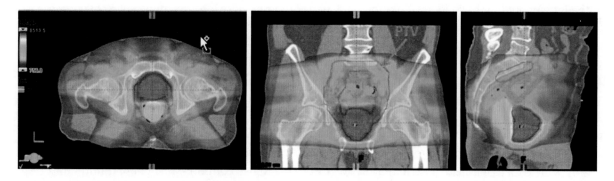

Proton Therapy. Fig. 13 Composite dose plan for a high-risk prostate patient. Protons are used to treat the prostate and seminal vesicles. Intensity-modulated proton therapy (IMRT) is used to treat the pelvic nodal area. The case shown has an IMRT dose of 45 Gy and a proton dose of 25.2 CGE, yielding a total of 79.2 CGE

growth hormone deficiency and the incidence of hearing loss.

Craniopharyngiomas: Although these are benign tumors, their close proximity to the pituitary gland and the hypothalamus may cause blindness, permanent hormonal insufficiency, or even death. Conservative surgery combined with radiation therapy is effective for long-term

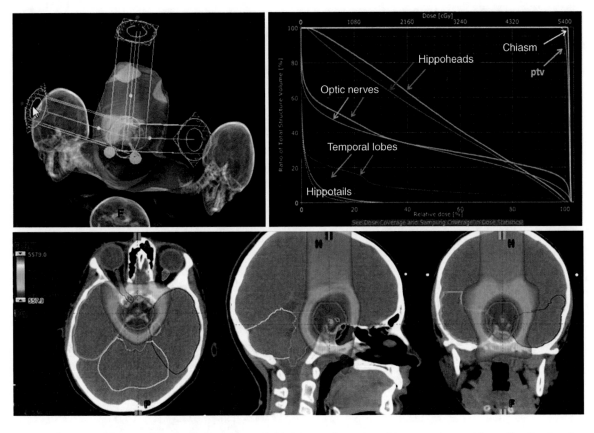

Proton Therapy. Fig. 14 Craniopharyngioma. A highly conformal and homogeneous dose distribution is achieved with a three-field (right superior oblique (*RSO*), left superior oblique (*LSO*), and superior posterior oblique (*SPO*)) proton plan (Rx: 54 CGE), sparing most of the normal brain and critical structures. The noncoplanar field arrangements minimize dose to the temporal lobes and hippocampuses

P

disease control. Protons, with their clear dosimetric advantage (Fig. 14), can minimize long-term side effects of radiotherapy.

Paraspinal Ewing's sarcoma: This rare disease is often adjacent to organs with low-dose tolerance, such as the lung or kidney. Figure 15 presents a case of two patients with near identical gross tumor volumes and anatomical locations; one was treated with IMRT, while the other was treated with protons. The proton plan delivered significantly lower doses to the kidneys as compared to IMRT. Both patients were disease free at 2 years post-RT follow-up; however, the patient treated with IMRT developed a failure in the right kidney (Fig. 16).

Other disease sites: Lung, lymphoma, and abdominal cancers have been investigated for their response to proton therapy. Each site presents its own challenges, but they share the problem of organ motion. Before any potential clinical benefits for these disease sites can be realized, better treatment techniques are necessary.

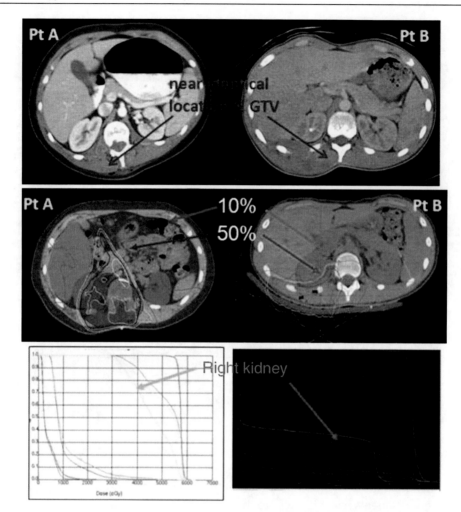

Proton Therapy. Fig. 15 Paraspinal Ewing sarcoma: two patients presented with lesions with near identical location and gross tumor volume (GTV) (*top*). Pt A was treated with IMRT (55.2 Gy at 1.2 Gy/fx) and Pt B was treated with proton (55.8 CGE, 1.8 CGE/fx). Protons offered significant dose reduction to kidney over IMRT (*bottom*). Both patients were disease free in 24 months post-RT follow-up but IMRT patient developed kidney failure (see Fig. 16) (Courtesy of S Keole, formally at UFPTI, USA)

Summary

Compared to photon therapy, proton therapy delivers less dose to adjacent normal tissues; therefore, proton therapy holds the promise of less toxicity and potentially higher cure rates than those achievable with X-ray therapy. Nonetheless, proton therapy, with its huge potential, is still in its infancy. The state of the art still requires the fabrication of patient-specific compensators and apertures. Even though these beams spare a significant amount of normal tissue, they do not provide conformal radiation dose to the tumor. Through the development of IMPT, we should be able to deliver highly conformal radiation to the tumor while sparing the healthy normal tissue. IMPT will likely rival any advanced technology used in conventional radiation therapy treatments.

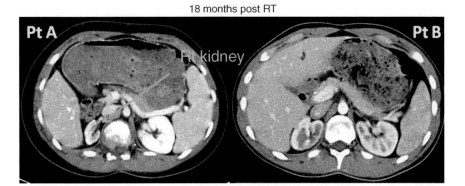

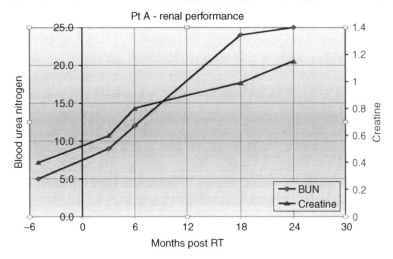

Proton Therapy. Fig. 16 Post-RT follow-up. Both the post-RT follow-up CT and renal performance indicated failure of right kidney for the patient treated with IMRT (Pt A). Patient treated with proton maintained normal kidney function

Proton therapy is less tolerant to uncertainties in both treatment planning and delivery than photon therapy. These uncertainties arise from several sources: dose-calculation approximations, biological considerations, setup and anatomical variations, and internal movements of low- and high-density organs into the beam path. Organ motion also has a major impact on the proton range, which is managed by adding a distal safety margin. These margins reduce the benefit of proton therapy in treatment sites where the physical properties of protons could make a significant difference, such as the lung. Therefore, in order for proton therapy to be beneficial, one must understand: (a) the potential sources of dosimetric uncertainties; (b) the impact of these uncertainties in the accuracy and conformity of dose delivered to patients; and (c) potential strategies that translate the physical advantage of proton therapy into a maximized dosimetric benefit in the patient.

Cross-References

▶ Conformal Therapy: Treatment Planning, Treatment Delivery, and Clinical Results
▶ Four-Dimensional (4D) Treatment Planning/Respiratory Gating
▶ Image-Guided Radiotherapy (IGRT)
▶ Intensity Modulated Radiation Therapy (IMRT)
▶ Radiation Oncology Physics

Acknowledgments

The authors would like to thank their colleagues at UF and UFPTI for their comments and suggestions.

References

Goitein M (2008) Radiation oncology: a physicist's-eye view. Springer, New York

International Commission on Radiation Units and Measurements (2007) ICRU report 78: prescribing, recording and reporting proton-beam therapy. International Commission on Radiation Units and Measurements, Inc., Bethesda

Lomax AJ (2008) Intensity-modulated proton therapy. In: DeLaney TF, Kooy HM (eds) Proton and charged particle radiotherapy. Wolters Kluwer, Lippincott Wiliams & Wilkens, Philadelphia

Palta J, Yeung D (2011) Precision and uncertainties in proton therapy for non-moving targets. In: Paganetti (ed) Proton Therapy Physics (in press)

Pedroni E (2008) Pencil beam scanning. In: DeLaney TF, Kooy HM (eds) Proton and charged particle radiotherapy. Wolters Kluwer, Lippincott Wiliams & Wilkens, Philadelphia

Proto-oncogene

Bradley J. Huth
Department of Radiation Oncology,
Philadelphia, PA, USA

Synonyms

Oncogene

Definition

Genes involved in cellular and genetic replication which when upregulated increase cellular proliferation. Proto-oncogenes become oncogenes after mutation. Mutation can take many forms such as increased transcription and translation and single-peptide errors which alter or block a regulatory binding site on the protein. Examples of oncogenes include epidermal growth factors and receptors, tyrosine kinases, and regulatory GTPases such as ras.

Cross-References

▶ Colon Cancer

Psychosocial State

James H. Brashears, III
Radiation Oncologist, Venice, FL, USA

Definition

The psychological well-being, development, and internal challenges of an individual as they interact within their social context or environment. The term was first used by Erik Erikson to define stages of development, but also relates to the dynamic interplay between a person and others like families, friends, and care providers.

Cross-References

▶ Pain Management

Psychosocial Support

James H. Brashears, III
Radiation Oncologist, Venice, FL, USA

Definition

An approach designed to help patients by fostering resilience and participating as much as possible in their normal lives. Hence it addresses the problems of the patient, their family, friends, and care givers. Examples of psychosocial support include mental health or spiritual counseling, group therapy, and helping provide a safe and nurturing environment at home.

Cross-References

▶ Complimentary Medicine
▶ Pain Management

Pulmonary Embolism

HEDVIG HRICAK[1], OGUZ AKIN[2],
HEBERT ALBERTO VARGAS[2]
[1]Department of Radiology, Memorial Sloan-
Kettering Cancer Center, New York, NY, USA
[2]Body MRI, Memorial Sloan-Kettering Cancer
Center, New York, NY, USA

Definition
Obstruction of the arterial supply to the lung by a substance that has migrated from elsewhere in the body through the bloodstream (embolism). Usually this is due to embolism of a thrombus from the deep veins in the legs. A small proportion is due to the embolization of air, fat, or amniotic fluid. The risk of PE is increased in various situations, such as cancer and prolonged bed rest.

Cross-References
▶ Imaging in Oncology

Pulmonary Toxicity

ANTHONY E. DRAGUN
Department of Radiation Oncology, James
Graham Brown Cancer Center, University of
Louisville School of Medicine, Louisville,
KY, USA

Synonyms
Radiation pneumonitis

Definition
Symptomatic radiation pneumonitis (dry cough, dyspnia on exertion, and shortness of breath) is a clinical syndrome that is rarely associated with breast cancer treatment. The overall risk is less than 1% in patients treated with modern radiotherapy techniques. Radiation pneumonitis is generally considered a diagnosis of exclusion, and clinicians are obliged to rule out infectious causes or causes related to metastatic tumor spread. The risk is generally increased with regional lymph node irradiation (especially inclusion of the internal mammary chain) and concurrent chemotherapy (especially those that include a taxane). Treatment typically consists of oral steroid therapy and oxygen delivered in the outpatient setting. The need for hospitalization in the otherwise healthy breast cancer patient is extraordinarily rare.

Cross-References
▶ Stage 0 Breast Cancer

Pulsed Field Gel Electrophoresis

CLAUDIA E. RÜBE
Department of Radiation Oncology, Saarland
University, Homburg/Saar, Germany

Definition
Gel electrophoresis technique with an alternating voltage gradient which allows to separate very large DNA molecules.

Cross-References
▶ Predictive In vitro Assays in Radiation Oncology

Pulsed-Dose Rate (PDR) Brachytherapy

ERIK VAN LIMBERGEN
Department of Radiation Oncology, University
Hospital Gasthuisberg, Leuven, Belgium

Definition

The dose is delivered by a stepping source afterloader (link) usually loaded with 37 GBq Iridium 192 at >12 Gy h^{-1} (>10 Gy/min) in hyperfractionated hourly- or two-hourly pulses with incomplete repair in between fractions in order to mimic the radiobiological effects of low-dose rate irradiation (link) while having the advantages of dwell time optimization of a stepping source afterloader.

Cross-References

► Clinical Aspects of Brachytherapy (BT)
► High-Dose Rate (HDR) Brachytherapy
► Low-Dose Rate (LDR) Brachytherapy

Pure Red Cell Aplasia

RAMESH RENGAN[1], CHARLES R. THOMAS, JR.[2]
[1]Department of Radiation Oncology, Hospital of
the University of Pennsylvania, Philadelphia,
PA, USA
[2]Department of Radiation Medicine, Oregon
Health Sciences University, Portland, OR, USA

Definition

Is an autoimmune disorder characterized by loss of erythrogenic precursors in the bone marrow. Thrombocytopenia and leukopenia may be present in a minority of patients. Thymectomy produces remission in approximately one-third of patients.

Cross-References

► Thymic Neoplasms

PUVA

CURT HEESE
Department of Radiation Oncology, Eastern
Regional Cancer Treatment Centers of America,
Philadelphia, PA, USA

Definition

PUVA is a ► Psoralen + UVA treatment for ► Eczema, ► Psoriasis and Vitiligo, and ► Mycosis Fungoides. The Psoralen is applied or taken orally to sensitize the skin, then the skin is exposed to UVA.

Cross-References

► Cutaneous T-Cell Lymphoma

p-value

EDWARD J. GRACELY
Department of Epidemiology and Biostatistics,
College of Medicine, Drexel University,
Philadelphia, PA, USA

Definition

A probability statistic used to determine whether a result could easily be due to chance.

Cross-References

► Statistics and Clinical Trials

Pylorus of Stomach

FILIP T. TROICKI[1], JAGANMOHAN POLI[2]
[1]College of Medicine, Drexel University, Philadelphia, PA, USA
[2]Department of Radiation Oncology, College of Medicine, Drexel University, Philadelphia, PA, USA

Definition

Most distant section of the stomach through which food contents exit to the small intestine, specifically to the duodenum.

Cross-References

▶ Stomach Cancer

P

Q

QOL

► Supportive Care and Quality of Life

Quality Assurance (QA)

THEODORE E. YAEGER
Department Radiation Oncology, Wake Forest
University School of Medicine, Winston-Salem,
NC, USA

Definition

In radiotherapy, QA is the process of evaluating
all components for the delivery of radiation so
that it conforms with the intent of the treatment
prescription.

Cross-References

► Brachytherapy
► Dose Calculation Algorithms
► Linear Accelerators
► Quality Control

Quality Control (QC)

THEODORE E. YAEGER
Department Radiation Oncology, Wake Forest
University School of Medicine, Winston-Salem,
NC, USA

Definition

In radiotherapy, QC is the evaluation of all
linear accelerator components to ensure the
proper computer functions, radiation outputs
and mechanical positioning that will safely and
properly deliver the radiation prescription.

Cross-References

► Brachytherapy
► Linear Accelerators
► Quality Assurance

Quality-Adjusted Life Year (Also QALY)

JAMES H. BRASHEARS, III
Radiation Oncologist, Venice, FL, USA

Definition

The quality of life year metric is based on the
number of years of life that would be added to a
living person if a proposed intervention was successfully performed. It is designed to evaluate the
effectiveness of any treatment as well as any side
effects; when considered with the monetary cost
of the intervention, cost effectiveness can theoretically be calculated.

Cross-References

► Palliation of Bone Metastases
► Statistics and Clinical Trails

L.W. Brady, T.E. Yaeger (eds.), *Encyclopedia of Radiation Oncology*, DOI 10.1007/978-3-540-85516-3,
© Springer-Verlag Berlin Heidelberg 2013

R

Radial Dose Function

NING J. YUE
The Department of Radiation Oncology, The
Cancer Institute of New Jersey, UMDNJ-Robert
Wood Johnson Medical School, New Brunswick,
NJ, USA

Definition

A quantity describing the relative dose change due
to photon attenuation and scatter in the medium
along the source central transverse axis.

Cross-References

▶ Brachytherapy: Low Dose Rate (LDR) Temporary Implants

Radiation Dermatitis

▶ Acute Radiation Toxicity

Radiation Detectors

KENT LAMBERT
Radiation Oncology, College of Medicine, Drexel
University, Philadelphia, PA, USA

Introduction

Because ionizing radiation cannot be sensed by
humans (except at very, very high doses) it is
necessary to use other means to perceive its presence. If you think about it, radiation detectors
existed before the discovery of radiation. It was,
after all, necessary for Wilhelm Roentgen to
observe the rays created from the Crookes tube
in his physics laboratory. A detector is a device
that converts an event that cannot be observed to
one which can. A variety of radiation detection
mechanisms exist; virtually all rely on sensing
either chemical or electrical changes caused by
ionization events within the detection system.

Gas-Filled Detectors

Ionization Chambers

Gas-filled radiation detectors use the electron-ion
pairs produced by ionizing radiation to create an
electric current which is then measured. Figure 1
is a simple schematic diagram of a gas-filled radiation detector, in which a gas-filled cylinder has
a central electrode connected to the positive contact of a direct current (DC) voltage supply and
the cylinder itself is connected to the negative
contact. (Note that actual detectors can take
a variety of shapes.) A resistor completes the
circuit and an amplifier and voltage measuring
circuitry provides the output.

With the proper voltage, the liberated electrons will move to the central electrode and the
positive ions will move toward the outer wall of
the detector, creating an electric current which will
produce a voltage across the resistor. If the applied
voltage is too low (below 200 V), the electrons
and positive ions can recombine so that no current
is produced. If the applied voltage is too high,
electrical arcing will occur. Somewhere between

L.W. Brady, T.E. Yaeger (eds.), *Encyclopedia of Radiation Oncology*, DOI 10.1007/978-3-540-85516-3,
© Springer-Verlag Berlin Heidelberg 2013

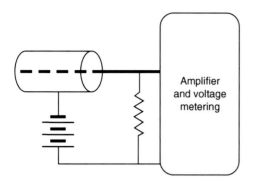

Radiation Detectors. Fig. 1 Gas-filled radiation detector schematic

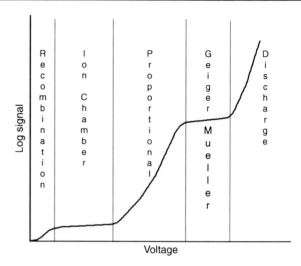

Radiation Detectors. Fig. 2 Ion pairs produced as a function of applied voltage

these two extremes are voltages that can be used. Figure 2 shows the signal response (i.e., number of ion pairs) as a function of voltage.

At lower applied voltages, on the order of 300 V, recombination does not occur to any significant degree and a current is created. The more radiation there is, the more ion pairs are created, and the more current is produced. Radiation detectors which operate in this fashion are called ionization chambers. The current created is directly related to the charge produced by the ionization of the detector gas, which, in the case of ionization chambers, is air. For ionization chambers that are open to the atmosphere which are used for calibration purposes, corrections for the ambient temperature and air pressure must be made as this affects the mass of air that is in the active volume of the ionization chamber. The quantity exposure is defined as the absolute value of the total charge of the ions of one sign produced in air when all the electrons liberated by photons in air are completely stopped in air. The unit of exposure is the Roentgen (1 Roentgen = 2.58×10^{-4} C kg^{-1}). This means that an ionization chamber directly measures exposure.

The energy response of ionization chambers is relatively flat over a large energy range. It is limited at the lower end (below 100 keV) by absorption of photons in the detector walls and at the upper end by the lack of electronic equilibrium (i.e., the range of secondary electrons exceeds the size of the detector).

As previously mentioned, ionization chambers come in many shapes and sizes and are designed for various purposes. Described below are just a few types of ionization chambers currently in use.

Free-air ionization chamber – an open air ionization chamber designed as a primary standard. As such, it is used at national standard laboratories for calibration of secondary instruments. These chambers are large and are impractical for use in radiation oncology clinics.

Thimble chamber – this ionization chamber is shaped like a sewing thimble (hence its name) with a chamber wall that is often made of air equivalent material to simulate a free-air ionization chamber; however chamber walls may also be composed of tissue equivalent plastic, acrylic, or graphite. The inside of the chamber wall is coated with an electrically conducting material. Common thimble chambers include condenser chambers and Farmer chambers.

Condenser chamber – this chamber is a thimble chamber connected to an electrical condenser, or capacitor, which stores charge. An electrometer is used to both charge the condenser and to measure the charge on it. Approximately 400 V are applied to the condenser. Then, as ionizations occur in the chamber, the electron is attracted to the positive electrode and the positive ion is attracted to the negative electrode, resulting in a reduction of the charge on the condenser. The reduction in charge is measured by the electrometer.

Farmer chamber – this is a thimble chamber with specific dimensions, originally designed by Farmer and later modified by Aird and Farmer. The design of the chamber provided for a 0.6 cm^3 collecting volume with a flat energy response over the range of energies of interest in radiation therapy. This chamber is commonly used to calibrate linear accelerators used for patient treatment.

Parallel-plate chamber – also known as a plane-parallel chamber, this is a pancake-shaped ionization chamber with a thin foil for the chamber wall (called a window) through which the radiation enters the chamber. The positively charged collection electrode is typically just a few millimeters below the window. Parallel-plate chambers are used in regions where the volume of a Farmer chamber is too large, such as in regions of rapidly changing dose with depth as in the buildup region of therapeutic beams or in electron beams.

Well chamber – this is a chamber typically used to calibrate or assay sources used for brachytherapy applications (either high-dose rate or low-dose rate sources) or nuclear medicine. As the name implies, this ionization chamber is shaped like a well into which the radioactive source is placed.

Survey meters – this type of ionization chamber is used to detect the presence of radiation and provide a measure of the exposure rate. These meters are typically handheld devices with collection volumes on the order of 500 cm^3. Such a large volume makes this meter a very sensitive survey instrument. The response of a typical survey meter as a function of incoming photon energy is shown in Fig. 3.

Proportional Counters

Proportional counters operate at a higher applied voltage than ionization chambers. With this increased voltage, the electrons gain sufficient energy as they are accelerated to the positive electrode (anode) that they create new ion pairs as they collide with gas molecules in their path. This is known as gas multiplication. These ion pairs will also contribute to the pulse of electric current. The amplitude of the pulse is proportional to the energy of the initiating event. Detectors operated in this fashion are called proportional counters. It is critical that the gas used in the detector has a low electron capture affinity. Noble gases are often used; however, they need a polyatomic gas to act as a stabilizer. A common mixture is 90% argon and 10% methane, known as P-10 gas. Proportional counters can be used for charged particle spectroscopy, although they are limited by their resolution. Proportional counters are used as survey meters and as analytical instruments for measuring low activity samples of alpha and/or beta emitters. Proportional counters are not commonly used in radiation oncology.

Geiger-Mueller (GM) Detectors

At applied voltages on the order of 900 V, an ionization event in the detector triggers an avalanche of electrons and the complete discharge of the detector. The pulses are counted and the electronics give output in units of counts or counts per unit time. The amplitude of the pulse is independent of the energy or number of initiating events. The large pulse size allows for simple circuitry, resulting in a relatively inexpensive radiation detection meter. Instruments which operate this way are called Geiger-Mueller or G-M detectors. The primary gas in G-M detectors is a noble gas, usually helium or argon. But

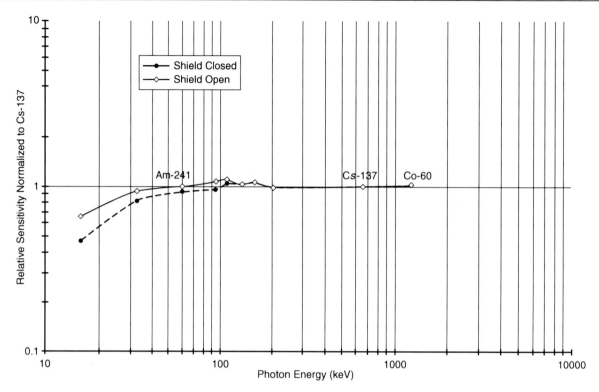

Radiation Detectors. Fig. 3 Energy response curve for a common ion chamber survey meter (Energy response curves used with permission of Ludlum Measurements, Inc.)

a quench gas is needed to allow the detector to recharge after the discharge pulse. An organic molecule (e.g., ethyl alcohol) or halogen gas (e.g., chlorine or bromine) may be used as a quench gas. Geiger-Mueller detectors are used for detection of radiation, often as survey meters. Because the pulse amplitude is independent of energy deposited in the detector, information about the type of radiation and its energy is lost. These instruments cannot, therefore, measure exposure unless calibrated to the specific energy of the radiation being measured. Typical independent radiation detectors used to signal whether radiation is present in a linear accelerator or high-dose rate remote afterloader vault utilize Geiger-Mueller detectors. It should be noted, however, that G-M and other pulse counting detectors should not be used to measure radiation levels from pulsed radiation sources such as clinical linear accelerators because they count the pulse rate of the source rather than provide a measure of the amount of radiation. As G-M detectors are commonly used to detect radiation they may be used to detect radioactive contamination, dropped brachytherapy sources, etc. The response of a typical Geiger-Mueller detector as a function of incoming photon energy is shown in Fig. 4.

Scintillation Detectors

Certain materials produce light, that is, scintillate, when an ionizing event occurs. Roentgen's "detector" was a scintillator. The resultant light can be converted to an electrical signal (with, e.g., a photomultiplier tube), which is then used as a part of a radiation detection system. Sodium iodide activated (doped) with thallium, NaI(Tl), cesium iodide activated with sodium, CsI(Na), calcium tungstate, $CaWO_4$, and zinc sulfide

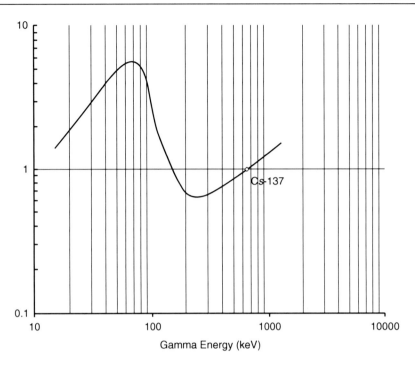

Radiation Detectors. Fig. 4 Energy response curve for a common G-M detector (Energy response curves used with permission of Ludlum Measurements, Inc.)

doped with silver, ZnS(Ag) are examples of these materials. Of course, each has its own interaction and light output characteristics. Scintillation detectors are used for a variety of medical, industrial, and general applications. For example, in simple film radiology, the radiographic film is sandwiched between two flat scintillating screens. The light output from the screen exposes the film in addition to the direct exposure of the film to x rays. As a result, much less radiation is needed to obtain a good quality image and the dose to the patient can be significantly reduced. (Film radiography is rapidly being replaced with digital imaging.) Nuclear medicine cameras are NaI(Tl) scintillation crystals connected to photomultiplier tubes and then to signal processing computers to reconstruct 2D and 3D images. Image receptors used in fluoroscopy are scintillation detectors. The input phosphor, typically a CsI(Na) crystal, creates light which is converted to an electrical signal by a

photodiode. The electrical signal is amplified while maintaining the geometry of the image and is made to strike an output phosphor creating a much brighter image, hence the name image intensifier. The output image is typically routed through a video camera to a television monitor.

Because these scintillators have a greater mass density than gas-filled detectors, and because generally they consist of materials with higher atomic numbers, interactions between x and gamma rays and the detection medium are much more likely to occur. The scintillating material is often encased to protect it from damage. With these detectors, charged particles and very low energy photons can be attenuated in the encasement. This means that these detectors are more efficient for x and gamma radiation than the gas-filled detectors, but may not be well suited for detecting alpha and beta radiation. (This is not to say that alpha scintillation detectors and beta scintillation detectors do not exist, but that they are specialized detectors.)

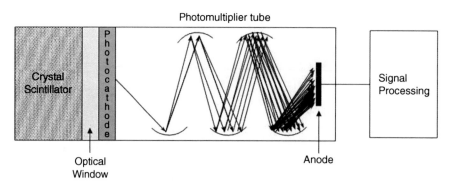

Photomultiplier tube

Crystal Scintillator | Photocathode | Anode | Signal Processing

Optical Window

Radiation Detectors. Fig. 5 Schematic of crystal scintillator with photomultiplier tube

The light emitted from a scintillator as a result of absorption of energy from ionizing particles is converted to an electrical signal in a photomultiplier tube (PMT). A PMT consists of a photosensitive cathode and a sequence of dynodes. The cathode emits electrons when light from the scintillator impinges on it. The number of electrons emitted is proportional to the amount of light incident upon it. The electrons are accelerated within the PMT and strike the first dynode which is a biased with approximately +100 V. For each electron that strikes the dynode, several additional electrons are emitted. The electrons from the first dynode are accelerated to collide with successive dynodes, each with a charge of +100 V more than the previous one. Thus, a PMT consisting of 10 dynodes has a total charge of +1,000 V across it and have multiplication factors on the order of 10^6. At the distal end of the PMT, the electrons are collected at the anode where they produce a signal for subsequent processing and analysis. A schematic diagram of a photomultiplier tube is shown in Fig. 5.

The amount of light produced by the scintillator is proportional to the energy deposited in it. This energy information is retained by the photomultiplier tube so the amplitude of the pulse is directly related to the energy deposited in the detector. It is, therefore, possible to use these detectors for x and gamma ray spectroscopy.

Two of the three types of digital radiography systems use a scintillator. In the first type, light is produced and channeled into an amorphous silicon photodiode layer where it is converted to an electrical signal which is then converted to a digital signal by a thin-film transistor array. A second type used an older technology, a charge-coupled device (CCD) to convert scintillations to a digital signal. The third type converts the radiation to an electrical signal directly with an amorphous selenium photoconductor.

Some scintillators can be dissolved in a suitable solvent. The liquid scintillation fluid is mixed with a sample to be measured in a transparent or translucent vial which is then placed in front of a photomultiplier tube. Because the sample is mixed with the detector, complications can arise, for example, colored samples can reduce the amount of light, certain chemicals can inhibit the transfer of energy from solvent to fluor (quench), some chemicals can create light (chemiluminescence), ultraviolet light can stimulate the solvent (photoluminescence), etc. These detectors, however, have great utility as there is no barrier between the detector and the sample being measured. Radiation with low penetrating abilities can be easily detected using a liquid scintillation counter.

Chemical Detectors

Chemical detectors work by measuring the chemical changes that result from irradiation of the chemical. The most common chemical detector is the Fricke dosimeter which measures the conversion of ferrous ions (Fe^{+2}) to ferric ions (Fe^{+3}) by ionizing radiation. The increase in concentration of the ferric ions generates a blue color that can be quantified with a spectrophotometer. Because the solution is mostly water, the attenuation of radiation resembles that of tissue. Due to the inherent insensitivity of the detector (one must be able to detect a change on the order of 1 part per billion) this detector is useful only for high dose (it is linear up to about 400 Gy) and high-dose rate applications.

Film

Radiographic and other radiation detection films are also chemical radiation detectors. The basic structure of the film is outlined in Fig. 6.

The film base provides the structural strength for the film. However, the base must be flexible to allow for processing, essentially transparent to light, free of artifacts, and dimensionally stable over time. A thin layer of adhesive binds the emulsion layer to the base. Covering the emulsion is a protective coating or supercoat to prevent mechanical damage to the emulsion.

The two principal components of a photographic emulsion are gelatin and silver halide. Most (but not all) x-ray film has emulsion on both sides of the film. The gelatin serves as a suspension medium for the grains of silver halide crystals. Silver halide (a mix of silver bromide and silver iodide) is the light sensitive material in the emulsion. The crystals are activated with the inclusion of silver sulfide on the surface of the crystal. The silver sulfide is referred to as the sensitivity speck. The sensitivity speck traps electrons to begin formation of the latent image where the silver ions are reduced to become metallic silver atoms. The number of crystals, crystal size, and thickness of the emulsion layers all play a part in the sensitivity (speed) and resolution of the film. The film goes through chemical

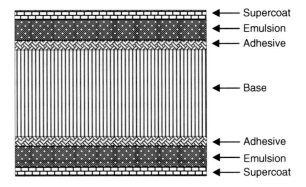

Radiation Detectors. Fig. 6 Structure of double emulsion radiographic film

processing to change the latent image to an actual image on the film. In addition to imaging, radiographic film is used in personal radiation dosimetry.

Radiochromic Film

Radiochromic film works differently than radiographic film. There is no latent image requiring processing to create an actual image. Instead, a thin layer of microcrystals (a radiation-sensitive monomer) are dispersed on a flexible film base. Irradiation results in polymerization of the microcrystals which changes the optical density of the film proportionately with the radiation dose. Typical radiochromic film is not sensitive to light and humidity but it is affected by temperature. A disadvantage of radiochromic film with respect to traditional film is that it is rather insensitive. Radiochromic film requires much higher doses in order to get a reasonable image.

Thermoluminescent Dosimeters (TLDs) and Optically Stimulated Luminescent (OSL) Dosimeters

In the scintillation detectors section discussed previously, the scintillating crystal, when stimulated by ionizing radiation, gives off light photons promptly. Many materials can trap a portion of the radiation energy until stimulated with heat at which point the crystal gives up this trapped energy in the form of light. Only a handful of these materials can do so in a reliably quantifiable way as to make them useful as radiation dosimeters. This phenomenon is called thermoluminescence. Basically, irradiation of a thermoluminescent material results in storage of energy in a metastable state. This happens when an orbital electron absorbs enough energy to be raised to a higher energy state and then get "trapped" in the crystal lattice. The traps are created by impurities in the crystal structure. These impurities may occur naturally or may be intentionally included during crystal production. When the crystal is heated, the crystal vibrates, releasing the trapped electron. The electron returns to its equilibrium (i.e., ground) state with the release of stored energy in the form of light. A glow curve is created by plotting the light output with temperature (or time) as the temperature is increased. The TLD crystal is heated under a photomultiplier tube where the emitted light is converted into an electrical signal as previously discussed.

TLD characteristics of importance are:

- Dose response – the relationship between absorbed dose and light output, ideally a linear response over a large absorbed dose range.
- Energy response – the dependence of output based on the photon energy for a given absorbed dose. Ideally, the TLD would be independent over the range of photon and electron energies of interest in radiation oncology.
- Sensitivity – output per unit absorbed dose. Higher sensitivities allow for lower detection limits, while lower sensitivities allow for high-dose applications.
- Fade – the reduction of output with time between irradiation and processing.

As stated previously, there are many thermoluminescent materials. Lithium fluoride (LiF) crystals, however, are the most popular for medical and health physics applications. Useful characteristics of LiF include an effective atomic number of 8.2 (soft tissue has an effective atomic number of 7.4), it is useful for measuring doses from hundreds of microgray up to thousands of Gray, will fade by less than 5% over a 3-month period, and is available in as a powder or a crystal for patient in vivo dosimetry.

Certain crystals can release stored energy with stimulation by light rather than heat, specifically Al_2O_3:C. These are known as optically stimulated luminescent (OSL) dosimeters. These crystals re used for health and medical physics applications as well.

Semiconductor Detectors

Diodes

When an ionization or excitation event occurs in most liquids or solids, the resulting freed electron cannot travel any significant distance; therefore, cannot be collected to produce a signal. The exception is semiconductors. Semiconductor detectors are made from silicon or germanium crystals.

In semiconductors, almost all of the orbital electrons are in the valence band within the crystal lattice. A few electrons will randomly gain sufficient thermal energy to jump from the valence band into the higher energy conduction band. For each electron in the conduction band, there is an electron vacancy in the valence band. This electron vacancy is called a hole. Obviously, in a solid the positively charged atom is not free to move as it is in a gas-filled detector. In this case, the hole is filled by an electron from a nearby atom, resulting in an electron vacancy in that nearby atom. Consequently, the hole moves. Applying a voltage causes electrons in the conduction band to travel to the positive electrode and the holes to travel toward the negative electrode.

Ionizing radiation produces free electrons and electrons at higher energy states. (Remember ionizing radiation loses energy through ionization and excitation.) Electron holes are also created as described above. The number of electron–hole pairs created is proportional to the energy transmitted by the radiation to the semiconductor. Applying a voltage and collecting the charge results in an electrical pulse (or current) that can be measured. In many ways, a semiconductor detector is similar to an ionization chamber. In a semiconductor detector electron–hole pairs are collected; in an ionization chamber ion pairs are collected.

It turns out that the magnitude of the electric pulse created in a semiconductor detector is about ten times larger than the pulse created in a typical ion chamber. This is because it takes approximately 3 eV to produce an electron–hole pair, whereas it takes almost 34 eV to create an ion pair in a gas. This means that the signal-to-noise ratio is much better. It also means that the statistical fluctuations in the number electron–hole pairs per pulse is smaller, resulting in much better energy resolution. Furthermore, because the density of silicon (the most commonly used diode) is on the order of 1,000 times that of air, diodes can be made much smaller than ion chambers to maintain an equivalent sensitivity.

Semiconductor detectors, being a solid, offer the advantage of higher radiation absorption. All the energy from alpha particles is deposited in a fraction of a millimeter. Of more practical value is that the range of even very energetic electrons or beta particles is just few millimeters in silicon as opposed to meters in air. This also improves the energy resolution.

Since the amount of energy required to create an electron–hole pair is known, measuring the number of electron–hole pairs provides energy information about the incident radiation. Basically, the pulse amplitude provides radiation energy information and pulse frequency provides radiation intensity information. Consequently, these types of semiconductor detectors lend themselves very nicely to spectrometry applications.

Another type of semiconductor radiation detector involves observing the change in conductivity in a semiconductor due to the creation of additional electron–hole pairs by radiation. These devices are classified as photoconductors.

MOSFET Detectors

MOSFET (metal oxide semiconductor field effect transistor) detectors fall into the photoconductor category. Ionizing radiation produces changes to the semiconductor such that a shift in the threshold voltage is measured. This shift is proportional to the radiation dose. Their small size, relatively low cost, ability to be read immediately, reusability, and ability to respond to high-dose rates make MOSFET detectors useful for confirming treatment doses in radiation therapy.

Germanium Detectors

Current manufacturing methods permit highly purified germanium (HPGe) crystals to be produced. Before this, the impurities in the germanium crystals trapped the electrons and holes, effectively prohibiting their use as spectroscopy detectors. Doping the germanium crystal with lithium (GeLi, pronounced, "jelly") permitted the electrons and holes to reach to the electrodes and create a signal.

Germanium detectors have a much lower detection efficiency than NaI(Tl) detectors because the effective atomic number of the detector is lower. Another disadvantage of germanium detectors is that they must be operated at very low (liquid nitrogen, 77° K) temperatures. At higher temperatures, electrons can reach the conduction band creating electrical noise that masks the signal. HPGe detectors must operate at these temperatures, but GeLi detectors have to be kept at this temperature to prevent the lithium from

R

drifting out of the crystal. Current refrigeration techniques now provide an acceptable alternative to using liquid nitrogen.

Polymer Gels

Polymer gels are gelatin-based materials which are radiologically tissue equivalent. They can fill spherical containers and may be used to verify the full 3D dose distribution in a phantom. The radiation causes polymer chains to form in the gel. This is useful for validating complex and/or high-dose treatment plans used in radiosurgery, stereotactic body radiation therapy, IMRT, etc. The results may be obtained via an MRI scan of the gel after irradiation.

Cross-References

▶ Brachytherapy: High Dose Rate (HDR) Implants
▶ Brachytherapy: Low Dose Rate (LDR) Temporary Implants
▶ Electronic Portal Imaging Devices (EPID)
▶ History of Radiation Oncology
▶ Linear Accelerators (LINAC)
▶ Radiation Therapy Shielding

References

Cember H (1996) Introduction to health physics, 3rd edn. McGraw-Hill, New York
Cember H (ed) (2001) Radiation instruments: Health Physics Society 2001 summer school. Medical Physics, Madison, Wisconsin
Chabot G Jr, CHP, Ph.D. Health Physics Society Ask the Experts Question 534 Alpha, beta, and gamma detectors http://hps.org/publicinformation/ate/q534.html
Encyclopædia Britannica (2011) Radiation measurement. Encyclopædia Britannica. Encyclopædia Britannica Online. Web, 29 Sept 2011 http://www.britannica.com/EBchecked/topic/1357248/radiation-measurement
Higginbotham J (1996) Applications of new technology: external dosimetry: Health Physics Society 1996 summer school. Medical Physics, Madison, Wisconsin
Knoll GF (1979) Radiation detection and measurement. Wiley, New York
Recommendations of AAPM Radiation Therapy Committee Task Group 55, Azam Niroomand-Rad, Chair American
Association of Physicists in Medicine 1998. Radiochromic Film Dosimetry. © 1998 American Association of Physicists in Medicine. [S0094-2405(98)00211-9]
Spieler H (1998) Introduction to radiation detectors and electronics. Lecture Notes – Physics 198, Spring Semester 1998, UC Berkeley
Thiel CW An introduction to semiconductor radiation detectors (1999) Montana State University, Bozeman Montana http://www.physics.montana.edu/students/thiel/docs/Detector.pdf

Radiation Induced Gene Expression

▶ Jun Gene Expression

Radiation Oncology Physics

JAY E. REIFF
Department of Radiation Oncology, College of Medicine, Drexel University, Philadelphia, PA, USA

Synonyms

Radiation therapy physics; Therapy physics; Therapeutic radiological physics

Introduction

Radiation oncology physics is the branch of ▶ medical physics which relates to the radiological procedures that are prescribed by a qualified practitioner for therapeutic purposes. In particular, this field of physics pertains to the safe and effective delivery of therapeutic applications of x-rays, gamma rays, charged and uncharged particle beams, as well as radiations emanating from sealed radionuclide sources.

Medical physicists are predominantly involved in the areas of clinical service, research and development, and/or teaching. The ▶ American Association of Physicists in

Medicine (AAPM) is a scientific, educational, and professional organization made up of over 7,000 medical physicists. This organization helps guide and promote the practice of medical physics. Among the goals of the AAPM are to "promote the highest quality medical physics services for patients, encourage research and development to advance the discipline, disseminate scientific and technical information in the discipline, foster the education and professional development of medical physicists, and support the medical physics education of physicians and other medical professionals." (AAPM goals website) Although each of these areas will be described in more detail, a brief description of these fields is included here.

Clinical service responsibilities include, but are not limited to, consultation with physicians on appropriateness of treatments, accurate measurement and calibration of radiation outputs from external radiation beams as well as brachytherapy sources, and equipment performance evaluation.

The role radiation therapy physicists play in research and development is seemingly boundless. From designing new and improved treatment machines for the delivery of external beam as well as brachytherapy treatments, to developing new techniques and equipment for the precise measurement of radiation, to the refinement of computer programs for improved dose calculation algorithms, to designing and improving new instrumentation and technology, medical physicists alongside engineers from various disciplines have significantly improved and will continue to improve the way radiation treatments are administered and monitored.

Medical physicists often hold academic appointments at colleges, universities, or medical schools. As such, they are often involved in teaching in undergraduate and graduate physics and medical physics programs. They also teach radiation oncology residents, medical physics residents, medical students, radiation therapy students, and future dosimetrists.

Clinical Service

Medical physicists have the overall responsibility for all the technical aspects of patient treatment in radiation oncology. For example, before a linear accelerator is ever used for patient treatment, it is the responsibility of the physicist to ensure the treatment delivery system is working properly and is characterized appropriately. This is done through the procedure known as ► acceptance testing and commissioning. The AAPM has published a report which can help guide a medical physicist through this procedure (Das et al. 2008). Of course acceptance testing is not limited to linear accelerators. Whenever any new piece of equipment is obtained, it is the responsibility of the physicist to ensure that it is working properly prior to it being implemented in the clinic.

After verifying that a piece of equipment is working properly, it often needs to undergo some type of calibration. For some equipment, such as in vivo diodes or detector arrays, a calibration procedure is supplied by the manufacturer. For ionization chambers and electrometers that are to be used to calibrate linear accelerators and high dose rate brachytherapy afterloader sources, certain calibration factors are determined by an ► accredited dosimetry calibration laboratory (ADCL). Based on these factors as well as characteristics of the treatment machine to be calibrated, specific protocols are used to calibrate the radiation beams to be used in the clinic (Almond et al. 1999).

Once equipment has been implemented in the clinic, it is the responsibility of the physicist to ensure it keeps working properly with the maximum accuracy and precision possible. To this end, the AAPM publishes and updates reports on the quality assurance of many types of equipment used in a radiation oncology clinic. Included in these reports is the quality assurance of linear accelerators, brachytherapy systems, and equipment involved in various procedures, as well

R

as quality assurance of a radiation oncology department as a whole. Two incredibly useful examples of these are those reports from Task Groups 40 (Kutcher et al. 1994) and 142 (Klein et al. 2009). The reader is highly encouraged to view a complete list of the AAPM reports by going to their website (AAPM reports website). These reports are all written by medical physicists for medical physicists.

When a department wishes to start a new program, such as intensity-modulated radiation therapy (IMRT), image-guided radiation therapy (IGRT), total body irradiation (TBI), or total skin electron treatment (TSET) to name a few, it is up to the physicist to lay the technical ground work upon which these programs will be based. Getting new programs off the ground can sometimes take many weeks of measurements by a qualified physicist. Once all the measurements have been completed, it is up to the physicist to establish the technical and quality assurance procedures by which these programs will be implemented clinically. Once again, AAPM reports provide an invaluable source of information as to how to go about establishing such programs.

While keeping all the equipment in a radiation oncology clinic operating at peak performance is certainly an important responsibility of the therapy physicist, it is by no means the only one. Fostering a collegial and professional relationship with the radiation oncologists whereby each party respects the role of the other is crucial in order to provide the best possible treatment of the patient. Whether discussing the modality or energy of the treatment beam to be used, or which beam orientation will best accomplish the goals of treatment, whether or not to use bolus (which type or how much to use), or deciding upon which immobilization technique will be most beneficial for the patient, medical physicists can offer a unique perspective on how best to attain the aims of therapy.

Additional responsibilities of the therapy physicist include, but are not limited to, checking the treatment plan for accuracy, verifying the monitor units for external beam plans, verifying the time of treatment for brachytherapy plans, performing regular periodic chart checks, acting as or working with the institution's radiation safety officer (RSO) as necessary, and offering any advice or insight as requested by the treating physician.

Research and Development

Physicists have always played a vital role in the realm of medical research. Since Roentgen's discovery of x-rays in 1895 and Becquerel's discovery of natural radioactivity in 1896, physicists have been major players in the discoveries and applications of radiation to medicine. In an article which appeared on the occasion of the 25th anniversary of the AAPM, Dr. John Laughlin chronicles the achievements of medical physicists and the subsequent advancements in the field of radiation oncology (Laughlin 1983).

A physicist in 1983 could not have imagined the technological advances that would invade and improve the field of radiation oncology over the next three decades. Advances in computed tomography (CT) imaging technology followed by three-dimensional treatment planning, the use of inhomogeneity corrections, and improved dose calculation algorithms increased patient response rates. Image fusion between different modalities such as magnetic resonance imaging (MRI) and positron emission tomography (PET) with CT has made delineating the tumor volume much more exact. Computer-controlled linear accelerators fit with multileaf collimators (MLCs) were the first steps in developing advanced treatment techniques that would ultimately result in IMRT. Advances in imaging such as the development of electronic portal imaging devices (EPIDs) and amorphous silicon technology have resulted in the development and wide spread use of IGRT. The implementation of this technology involves the use of faster and more powerful computers and more elegant computer codes. The development and proper use of all these advanced technologies demand that medical physicists be at the forefront.

Education

Many medical physicists are involved in some type of formal education. Those who work in teaching hospitals often hold a faculty appointment and have the responsibility of formally teaching the physics of radiation oncology to resident physicians entering the field. This is often accomplished by leading structured physics classes. To this end, in 2004, the ▶ American Society for Radiation Oncology developed a core curriculum for the physics education of radiation oncology residents (Klein et al. 2004). Some institutions augment the classroom lectures by placing the resident physicians on a physics rotation at some point in their training.

In addition to training physicians in radiation oncology physics, therapy physicists participate in a variety of academic degree and training programs available to aspiring medical physicists. Such programs include graduate education programs, residency education programs, and professional degree programs. Guidelines for these programs have been laid out in several AAPM reports (Paliwal et al. 2009; Lane et al. 2006; Maughan et al. 2011). These programs, which are generally accredited by ▶ the Commission on Accreditation of Medical Physics Education Programs, Inc. (CAMPEP), offer a structured clinical medical physics education.

Cross-References

▶ Brachytherapy
▶ Dose Calculation Algorithms
▶ Electronic Portal Imaging Devices (EPID)
▶ High-Dose Rate (HDR) Brachytherapy
▶ Image-Guided Radiotherapy (IGRT)
▶ Imaging in Oncology
▶ Intensity Modulated Radiation Therapy (IMRT)
▶ Linear Accelerators (LINAC)
▶ Radiation Detectors
▶ Three-Dimensional Conformal Radiation Therapy
▶ Total Body Irradiation (TBI)
▶ Total Skin Electron Therapy (TSET)

References

AAPM goals website. http://aapm.org/org/objectives.asp. Accessed 14 May 2011

AAPM reports website. http://aapm.org/pubs/reports/. Accessed 14 May 2011

Almond PR, Biggs PJ, Coursey BM et al (1999) AAPM's TG-51 protocol for clinical reference dosimetry of high-energy photon and electron beams. Med Phys 26(9): 1847–1870. http://aapm.org/pubs/reports/RPT_67.pdf. Accessed 14 May 2011

Das I, Cheng C-W, Watts RJ et al (2008) Accelerator beam data commissioning equipment and procedures: report of the TG-106 of the therapy physics committee of the AAPM. Med Phys 35(9):4186–4215. http://aapm.org/pubs/reports/RPT_106.pdf. Accessed 14 May 2011

Klein EE, Balter JM, Chaney EL et al (2004) ASTRO's core physics curriculum for radiation oncology residents. Int J Radiat Oncol Biol Phys 60:697–705

Klein EE, Hanley J, Bayouth J et al (2009) Task group 142 report: quality assurance of medical accelerators. Med Phys 36(9):4197–4212. http://aapm.org/pubs/reports/RPT_142.pdf. Accessed 14 May 2011

Kutcher GJ, Coia L, Gillin M et al (1994) Comprehensive QA for radiation oncology: report of AAPM radiation therapy committee task group 40. Med Phys 21(4): 581–618. http://aapm.org/pubs/reports/RPT_46.pdf. Accessed 14 May 2011

Lane RG, Stevens DM, Gibbons JP et al (2006) Essentials and guidelines for hospital-based medical physics residency training programs. AAPM Report No. 90, American Association of Physicists in Medicine, College Park, Maryland. http://aapm.org/pubs/reports/RPT_90.pdf. Accessed 14 May 2011

Laughlin JS (1983) History of medical physics. Phys Today 36(7):26–33

Maughan RL, Burmeister JW, Gerbi BJ et al (2011) The essential medical physics didactic elements for physicists entering the profession through an alternative pathway: a recommendation from the AAPM working group on the revision of reports 44 & 79, AAPM report no. 197S, American Association of Physicists in

Medicine, College Park, Maryland. http://aapm.org/pubs/reports/RPT_197S.pdf. Accessed 14 May 2011

Paliwal BR, DeLuca PM Jr, Grein EE et al (2009) Academic program recommendations for graduate degrees in medical physics. AAPM report no. 197, American Association of Physicists in Medicine, College Park, Maryland. http://aapm.org/pubs/reports/RPT_197.pdf. Accessed 14 May 2011

Radiation Pneumonitis

▶ Pulmonary Toxicity

Radiation Recall Reaction

ANTHONY E. DRAGUN
Department of Radiation Oncology, James Graham Brown Cancer Center, University of Louisville School of Medicine, Louisville, KY, USA

Synonyms
Recall phenomenon

Definition
This refers to the reappearance of skin inflammation in a previously irradiated field, brought on by the subsequent administration of chemotherapy or other pharmacologic agent. Etiology is thought to be due to a hypersensitivity reaction and is mediated by the inflammatory cascade. Recall reactions were originally described in the 1950s in association with the antineoplastic and antifungal agent, actinomycin D. Today, it is most often associated with post-radiation therapy delivery of adriamycin in the treatment of advanced breast cancer, where the risk is as high as 15–20%. This phenomenon is generally prevented by the sequencing of adjuvant radiation therapy after adjuvant systemic chemotherapy. Treatment consists of corticoid steroid therapy and withdrawal of the offending drug.

Cross-References
▶ Stage 0 Breast Cancer

Radiation Safety

NING J. YUE
The Department of Radiation Oncology, The Cancer Institute of New Jersey, UMDNJ-Robert Wood Johnson Medical School, New Brunswick, NJ, USA

Definition
Procedures, documentations, and regulations that ensure safe use of radioactive materials for the protections of professional personnel, patients, general public, and environment.

Radiation Therapy Oncology Group (RTOG)

JAY E. REIFF
Department of Radiation Oncology, College of Medicine, Drexel University, Philadelphia, PA, USA

The Radiation Therapy Oncology Group is a national clinical cooperative group which consists of clinical and laboratory investigators from over 360 institutions across the United States and Canada. Its mission is fourfold:

A) To improve the survival outcome and quality of life of adults with cancer through the conduct of high-quality clinical trials

B) To evaluate new forms of radiotherapy delivery, including stereotactic radiotherapy, brachytherapy, three dimensional conformal radiotherapy, and intensity modulated radiotherapy in the context of clinical research

C) To test new systemic therapies in conjunction with radiotherapy, including chemotherapeutic drugs, hormonal strategies, biologic agents, and new classes of cytostatic, cytotoxic, and targeted therapies

D) To employ translational research strategies to identify patient subgroups at risk for failure with existing treatments and identify new approaches for these patients.

Cross-References

▶ American Society for Radiation Oncology (ASTRO)
▶ History of Radiation Oncology
▶ Radiation Oncology Physics
▶ Stereotactic Radiosurgery :Extracranial

Radiation Therapy Physics

▶ Radiation Oncology Physics

Radiation Therapy Shielding

Jean St. Germain
Department of Medical Physics, Memorial Sloan-Kettering Cancer Center, New York, NY, USA

This section is intended to explain the general principles used in designing treatment facilities and provide information regarding the decisions to be made by the radiation oncologist and on-site physicist which will affect the overall facility design. The design of structural shielding for treatment facilities may appear to be a daunting task, not to be undertaken by someone who has not attempted such a design previously. This section is not intended to be used by the professional medical physicist, the qualified expert who is designing a treatment facility. It is intended to remove some of the confusion regarding how shielding designs are decided. This section is not a substitute for the information and calculations found in the reports of the National Council on Radiation Protection and Measurements which detail the calculations to be used and the design criteria [NCRP 147 (2004), 151 (2005) and 155 (2006)]. Shielding design will require a qualified expert who should not only participate in the design process, but who will be available as questions arise during construction. The term "qualified expert" in this entry is defined as a medical physicist or health physicist who is competent to design radiation shielding in radiotherapy facilities, and who is certified by the American Board of Radiology (ABR), American Board of Medical Physics (ABMP), American Board of Health Physics (ABHP), or Canadian College of Physicists in Medicine (CCPM). Such an expert may exist at the facility, be hired as a consultant to the facility, or be hired by the architectural firm to oversee the design. A number of states specify in their regulations the qualifications of such experts and may require that these experts be registered or licensed. The qualified expert should be consulted during the early planning stages since the shielding requirements may affect the choice of location and type of building construction.

The accelerator manufacturer will supply a design or installation package to the facility or to the owner which contains specifications for the placement of the accelerator and room layout. These packages may include typical shielding designs and show minimum room dimensions required to place the machine in a treatment room. Such shielding designs typically carry a disclaimer that the design for a facility must be evaluated individually by a qualified expert and

R

that the design supplied by the manufacturer is only a template to be considered for further evaluation.

Dose Limits for Controlled and Uncontrolled Areas

A controlled area is a limited-access area in which the occupational exposure of personnel to radiation-producing equipment or radioactive materials is under the supervision of an individual in charge of radiation protection (NCRP 151 2005). For radiation oncology facilities, such areas typically include the treatment room, control console, and adjacent treatment rooms. An uncontrolled area would include any other area in the environs. Examples include lobbies, offices, waiting areas, examining rooms, rest rooms, and outside areas.

Employees in controlled areas are trained in radiation protection techniques. NCRP 151 recommends an annual dose limit of 50 mSv/year for individuals in such areas with the cumulative dose not to exceed the product of 10 mSv times the worker's age in years. That notwithstanding, NCRP recommends that for design of new facilities, the total dose in a year should be a fraction of 10 mSv. Therefore, NCRP 151 recommends a shielding design goal of 5 mSv/year. For uncontrolled areas, the design goal recommended is 1 mSv/year. The numbers recommended in the recent NCRP reports are more conservative than those that appeared previously in NCRP Reports 49 and 51 and reflect the dose limit recommendations published in NCRP Report number 116. After publication of this report and the revision of Part 20 by the US Nuclear Regulatory Commission [USNRC], it might be expected that there would be a requirement for the shielding of installations constructed using NCRP Reports number 49 and 51 to be upgraded. However, there was no such recommendation because it was recognized that virtually all of these designs had been done conservatively. As older facilities are renovated or as

new facilities are designed, the most recent revisions should be applied.

It is certainly possible that recommended occupational and general public dose limits will continue to decrease, both as a result of new evaluations of exposed populations and as the profession shows that lower limits can be achieved without detriment. A word of caution is necessary. Since it is always more expensive to renovate a facility, a realistic estimate of future patient load is necessary. Although the initial load for a treatment unit may be lighter than the final operating load as the facility ramps up its treatment schedule, the final anticipated treatment load must be used to calculate the shielding. One cannot change barriers with any degree of ease, and the space to "correct" any problems may shrink the size of the room and possibly compromise the couch extension or the viability of radiation treatments which depend on large room dimensions such as ▶ total body irradiation and ▶ total skin electron therapy. Thus, an element of balanced conservatism is appropriate when evaluating and/or designing shielding for radiation treatment facilities.

Primary and Secondary Barriers

Radiation within the treatment room arises from the machine itself, from leakage radiation transmitted through the head of the treatment unit and from radiation scattered from objects in the path of the primary beam. The primary beam, alternately called the useful beam, is emitted directly from the accelerator and is "aimed" at the patient, that is, at the treatment field. Barriers that intercept the primary beam are called primary barriers. Typically, the accelerator will rotate in a 360° circle with the isocenter as the central point of the circle. Portions of the floor, ceiling, and sidewalls will generally receive the primary beam and are primary barriers. Radiation is also emitted through the treatment head of the unit, the so-called leakage radiation, and these emissions are limited by regulation and recommendation. Typically, the value of the leakage radiation emission is designed to meet the standards of the International Electrotechnical Commission (IEC) and the NCRP, namely, to be less than 0.1% of the primary beam dose rate at 1 m. The remaining radiations found in the treatment room arise from radiation scattered from the patient and other objects in the path of the primary beam. Barriers which receive only the leakage radiation from the treatment head and/or scattered radiation from the patient are called secondary barriers.

In order to reduce primary beam shielding requirements, some installations have made use of "beam stops," devices which intercept the primary beam of radiation; therefore, other barriers may be shielded as secondary barriers. The beam stop is part of the treatment gantry and will rotate with the treatment head. In some machines, the beam stop may be retractable, that is, the operator can select the angles at which the beam stop is present. Consideration of the use of a beam stop must reflect any constraints on the treatments to be given as well as the overall facility design.

Workload and Its Modifiers

One of the significant factors used in calculating shielding is the evaluation of the workload, W, anticipated in the facility. The workload is defined as the time integral of the absorbed dose rate [cGy/min or rad/min] determined at the depth of maximum absorbed dose, 1 m from the "source" (NCRP 151). Typically, the workload is specified over a period of 1 week. The values for W are usually taken as the absorbed dose from photons delivered to the isocenter in 1 week. The value chosen must necessarily be a function of the amount of time that the beam is "on," that is, in a treatment mode. For machines capable of operating at more than one photon energy, for example, 6 MV, 10 MV, 15 MV, and 18 MV, the shielding calculation for the higher energy mode

will usually determine the required shielding. However, in some cases, it may be desirable to calculate the shielding separately for each treatment modality. The original workloads specified in NCRP Reports 49 and 51 were revised upward in Reports 147 and 151 to reflect the introduction of ▶ Intensity Modulated Radiation Therapy [IMRT] and ▶ Image Guided Radiation Therapy [IGRT] techniques. These techniques generally require larger workloads and consequently, higher values for leakage radiation values to be used in secondary barrier calculations (Mechalakos and St Germain 2002; Mechalakos et al. 2004).

Use Factor, U, and Occupancy Factor, T

The definitions of the use factor, "U," and the occupancy factor, "T," are given in the NCRP reports (NCRP 151 2005). Both of these factors are intended to modify the workload so that the person performing the calculations can more realistically estimate the actual radiation doses likely to be delivered in the areas to be shielded. The use factor, U, requires that one knows the fraction of the "beam-on" time, that is, the workload, that the beam is pointed toward the area to be shielded. Use factors only apply to the primary beam. Typical values for "U" and "T" can be found in NCRP Report number 151. Unpublished data from Kleck et al. may also be available. It is usual for the physicist to assume that the beam points at the lateral walls about 25% of the total beam-on time; however, if total body irradiation is the most common treatment in the room being designed, this number needs to be evaluated and probably increased for a particular wall. It is, therefore, essential that the overall treatment pattern be known and if not, that more conservative assumptions be used.

The occupancy factor, T, refers to the fraction of time that the space being shielded is occupied. This is the typical reason that treatment vaults are placed in the lowest floor of buildings, namely, there is no occupancy below and in most cases, no shielding may be required, only structural material. It may also be possible to place the vault so that one or more of the walls abut earth, reducing the number of shielded barriers to be constructed. The occupancy factor for controlled areas must always be one. In considering occupancy around the vault, the designer may wish to consider future use of the space above and around the vault. For example, if a garden or public space is placed above the ceiling, is it likely or possible that another building or space may be built using the shielding walls as foundation for that building? Is it possible to make the area above the vault, that is, the area above the ceiling, an exclusion area, thus reducing the value of the occupancy factor? How likely is it that this condition will remain indefinitely? Occupancy above the shielded vault, if it is located on the lowest level of the facility, may have a public access area directly above such as a lobby, cafeteria, or other uncontrolled area. It may be possible in the case where access to an area is strictly controlled to designate the area as a controlled space. Examples might include the roof of a single-story structure or a mechanical room. How such access is controlled and the practicality of such a designation should be discussed with the qualified expert and the facility radiation safety officer.

Distance (d)

Rooms should be designed to take the maximum advantage of the inverse square reduction in radiation intensity. The manufacturer's packages will recommend minimum distances required for placement of the machine, access to the machine controls inside the treatment room, and requirements for couch movement. In addition, the package will specify the minimum distances required to get the machine into the room including the minimum dimensions and weight of the machine as it is delivered. Typical clear dimensions would include a doorframe height of 7 ft.

and a clear width of 4 ft. Because of the weight of the accelerator and its associated shielding, it is usually necessary to provide rigging to place the accelerator. Advice from a structural engineer may be necessary to plan the delivery route as it may traverse locations where the floor loading may need to be enhanced.

Reduction of radiation intensity by increasing distance is always more effective than additional shielding. Architects often use English units so conversion to metric units will be necessary to use the shielding paradigms in the NCRP reports. Treatment accessories such as molds, blocks, and electron applicators will be stored in the treatment room as well as alignment devices, cameras, and other items. These items will add to the overall interior space needed.

Shielding Calculations

The variables discussed above will be used in equations to calculate shielding. The following equation is used in the NCRP reports to calculate shielding for primary barriers:

$$B = Pd^2/WUT$$

where "B" is transmission through the barrier, given the values of the factors used in the equation. P is the desired permissible dose level at a distance, d, in meters from the source or isocenter to the point to be shielded. W is the workload at the isocenter in cGy per week, and U and T are the use factor and occupancy factors chosen as described above. Once the transmission factor is calculated, the amount of shielding necessary can be evaluated. For example, for a value of B equal to 10^{-6}, 6 tenth value layers will be necessary. Using the values in Table 2, for 15 MV photons, a shield of 6×44 cm of concrete, 264 cm or slightly more than 8.5 ft of concrete would be required. Table 1 is intended to give some idea of typical shielding barriers that may be encountered. The values shown are in concrete only and a shield of concrete combined

Radiation Therapy Shielding. Table 1 Sample values for accelerator shielding

Energy (MV)	Primary barrier (ft of concrete)	Secondary barrier (ft of concrete)
6	6	3–4
15	7–9	4–5

Values shown are for concrete with a density of 2.35 g/cm³ or 147 lb/ft³. These values should not be quoted or used for specific installations. Considerations for each installation need to be calculated separately and reviewed by a qualified expert

Radiation Therapy Shielding. Table 2 Tenth value layers [TVLs] in concrete, lead, and steel at various energies

Energy (MV)	Tenth value layer (TVL) in cm		
	Concrete	Steel	Lead
^{192}Ir (0.2–0.9)	17.6	–	1.1
6	30	9.9	5.7
10	41	11	5.7
15	44	11	5.7
18	45	11	5.7

Concrete density is 2.35 g cm⁻³. Steel density is 7.87 g cm⁻³. Lead density is 11.35 g cm⁻³
Table adapted from Table B.2 in NCRP Report No. 151 and Table D.1 in NCRP Report No. 155

with steel or lead will take less space. Values are shown in English units since architects still use these units.

Mazes and Doors

Many radiation installations, particularly those with photon energies above 6 MV, use a maze design The maze design will reduce the thickness of the shielded door required and will serve to reduce the neutron dose when neutrons are present. A typical door will contain a steel case, from 0.25 to 0.5 in thickness into which shielding plates or blocks will be loaded. For installations where neutrons are present, both lead and borated polyethylene sheets will be loaded into the door.

Depending on the weight of the door, a mechanized operator may be required. It should always be possible to open a door mechanically. Different door manufacturers use various methods to accomplish this. There have been circumstances where a patient is trapped in a treatment room due to a power failure or other event. The therapist or nursing staff should be able to enter the room and escort the patient from the treatment room using mechanical assists. The possibility of such an event should be included in the emergency training of the treating staff.

Mazes take space and where the room size cannot accommodate a maze, a directly shielded door may be necessary. These doors are placed in secondary barriers and receive both leakage radiation and scattered radiation. These doors may move on a system of rollers which move the door into a pocket when it is not needed. These pockets also take space so some facilities prefer a hinged door. The hinges on these doors need to be carefully placed to balance the weight of the door and there are specialized manufacturers who deal with these placements. The experience of the supplier should be a major consideration since if the weight of a shielded door caused the hinges to pull away from the doorframe, a patient could be trapped for some time until the weight of the door could be shifted to allow entrance by rescuers. Maze and door designs are discussed by McGinley (2002) in his text.

Penetrations of the Shielding

It will be necessary to penetrate the shielding at certain locations to bring in services such as plumbing, ventilation, and power supplies. The installation package from the manufacturer will detail the number and size of penetrations necessary for the operation of the accelerator. In addition to these, there will be physics ports, plumbing lines, and conduits for other systems.

The largest penetration will usually be for ventilation ductwork. If possible, these penetrations should be placed as close to the ceiling as possible and in the secondary barriers. If they need to be placed at a lower elevation, they should be angled such that there is no direct path of radiation through the opening. It is usually necessary that shielding of the ducts be provided for both neutrons and photons. The geometry of how the ducts are placed will determine the dimensions of the required shielding. A discussion of barrier penetrations and the associated geometry can be found in NCRP 151 and in the book by McGinley. Shielding designs for penetrations should be reviewed by a qualified expert.

Barrier Materials

Typical shielding materials for the construction of shielding barriers include concrete, steel, lead, and borated polyethylene. The amount of material needed to reduce the radiation intensity by a factor of ten is called the tenth value layer [TVL]. The thickness of material needed is a function of the beam energy. Table 2, adapted from NCRP Reports 151 and 155, shows the tenth value layers in concrete, steel, and lead for typical beam energies used with medical linear accelerators. Concrete is the least expensive material used; however, it takes up space. To reduce the space constraints, the density of the concrete can be increased by the addition of high atomic number materials to the concrete. Materials used may include barium and more typically, iron ore. It is difficult to achieve a uniform distribution of the added materials since their heavier weight means that they would sink in a concrete mix. These materials are, therefore, commonly supplied as shielding blocks, the so-called high-density concrete. Whether such blocks offer advantages in a shielding design needs to be determined by a qualified expert. In the event that there is insufficient space for the amount of concrete shielding specified, it may be necessary to substitute lead or steel for some thickness of concrete. This type of problem is most often encountered in shielding of the ceiling where available space may be limited.

As the photon energy increases above 6 MV, neutrons will be produced by gamma, neutron [γ, n] reactions in the high atomic number materials of the accelerator head with the largest contribution coming from the target and flattening filter. Unlike photons, neutrons do not travel in straight lines, but more properly resemble a gas as they move from the point of origin to the shielding barrier. The high water content of concrete means that hydrogen atoms are available to interact with neutrons, and a sufficient thickness of concrete could be an adequate neutron shield. As neutrons encounter other atoms, particularly atoms of hydrogen, their energy may be reduced by scattering. If the neutron energy is sufficiently reduced, the neutron can be captured by boron atoms dispersed in a plastic matrix. Boron has a very high capture cross section [approximately 2,500 barns] for thermal neutrons, and the daughter product is an alpha particle which has a very limited range and does not generally escape from the matrix.

$$\left[_5B^{10} + {}_0n^1 = {}_2\alpha^4 + {}_3Li^7 \right]$$

Polyethylene sheets used for neutron shielding are loaded with boron compounds. A 5% boron loading is the most common shielding material, although larger boron loadings are available.

Width and Length of the Primary Barrier

The maximum field size of most accelerators is 40 cm by 40 cm at the isocenter. Projecting this beam size onto the primary barrier will give some idea of the width of the beam at the barrier. An additional 1 ft of width for primary beam barrier is added to remove any radiation from small angle scatter and to prevent the possibility of radiation leaking through the secondary barrier as it abuts the primary barrier. For some applications, this width may need to be increased and reviewed by the qualified expert. Rotating the collimator by 45° from the zero position as might be done for total body irradiations will predict the maximum height of the primary beam at the barrier. Many physicists prefer to carry the height of the primary beam at the wall from the floor to the under slab to ensure that there is no leakage through the abutment of the wall and the ceiling.

Special Considerations

In addition to shielding evaluations, the following considerations should also be part of the overall design. Door switches should be placed on both the inside and outside of the door to the treatment room. It is recommended that the interior switches be "open" only, so that there is no possibility of someone being caught by the vault door as it is closing. Safety edges should be placed for the full height and full width of the door. Significant injuries have occurred when a body part, typically a limb, has been caught in a door as it is being closed or opened. Safety edges ensure that the door will stop when the switch is engaged. Emergency off-switches should be placed in easily visible and accessible locations to avoid injury to the patient and the therapists.

High Dose Rate (HDR) Remote Afterloader Facilities

The installation of a High Dose Rate [HDR] remote afterloader in a facility will depend on the expected patient load as well as the type of practice expected. Most modern HDR units use ^{192}Ir sources, and the half-value layer and tenth value layer for ^{192}Ir sources are given in Table 2. A discussion of the calculations and planning for the shielding of HDR rooms can be found in Appendix D of NCRP Report number 155. The situation most often encountered is the placement of the HDR unit within a treatment room (e.g., a linear accelerator room). The number of treatment hours available for HDR treatments will be limited by the patient schedule for all treatment modalities. When an HDR unit is placed within an accelerator room, the shielding for the high-energy photons will be sufficient to shield the HDR unit. Some facilities have placed HDR units within rooms previously designed for ^{60}Co teletherapy, particularly when these facilities could not be renovated to accept linacs. The shielding in these facilities should be adequate for the HDR units. Some larger academic centers have created stand-alone HDR facilities where the shielding is designed by a qualified expert to suit the needs for HDR treatment only.

Proton Accelerators

It is to be expected that technology will continue to advance. The ^{60}Co units of the 1960s were replaced by linear accelerators, and the design of these machines continues to be a subject for research. The use of accelerators for ▶ proton therapy appears to be the most recent subject discussed as a technological advance. Proton accelerators, cyclotrons, have been available since the 1960s, but until recently, they were used primarily for the production of short-lived radiopharmaceuticals. Radiation treatment with protons was restricted to one or two centers. The interest in the use of protons for treatment has been a "hot topic" in more recent times, and proton accelerators using high-energy proton beams (150–250 MeV) have been and are being installed in selected locations across the country. These machines vary in size, but all require significant shielding. The number of treatment rooms may vary from one to five or more. The treatment gantry may rotate around the patient in a manner similar to that of conventional treatment units or the protons may be steered to a fixed nozzle which is aimed at a specific location.

R

The fixed nozzle is most often used with treatments of the head and neck. Shielding of the largest proton machines may require yards (not feet) of concrete. The calculation of proton shielding is usually performed using Monte Carlo computer techniques and is a very specialized field (Agosteo et al. 2011).

Post-Installation Evaluations

The final assessment of the adequacy of the design and construction of protective shielding can only be based on a post-construction radiation survey performed by a qualified expert. In order to avoid any problems which may be uncovered during such a survey, it is advisable for the qualified expert to review the installation during its construction, and particularly before any finishes are applied. The report of the survey should remain with the installation and the construction company. Such a report is also usually required by the regulatory agencies.

References

Agosteo S, Magistris M, Silari M (2011) Shielding of proton accelerators. Radiat Prot Dosim 145:414–424

Kleck JH, Elsalim M (1994) Clinical workload and use factors for medical linear accelerators (abstract). Med Phys 21:952–953

McGinley PH (2002) Shielding techniques for radiation oncology facilities, Expanded 2nd edn. Medical Physics, Madison

Mechalakos JG, St Germain J (2002) Estimation of shielding factors for linear accelerators. Oper Radiat Saf 83(11): S65–S67

Mechalakos JG, St Germain J, Burman C (2004) Results of a one year survey of output for linear accelerators using IMRT and non-IMRT techniques. J Appl Clin Med Phys 5(1):64–72

National Council on Radiation Protection and Measurements (1976) Structural shielding design and evaluation for medical use of x-rays and gamma rays up to 10 MeV. NCRP Report No.49. National Council on Radiation Protection and Measurements, Bethesda

National Council on Radiation Protection and Measurements (1977) Radiation protection design guidelines for 0.1–100 MeV particle accelerator facilities. NCRP Report No. 51. National Council on Radiation Protection and Measurements, Bethesda

National Council on Radiation Protection and Measurements (1993) Limitation of exposure to ionizing radiation. NCRP Report No. 116. National Council on Radiation Protection and Measurements, Bethesda

National Council on Radiation Protection and Measurements (2004) Structural shielding design for medical x-ray imaging facilities. NCRP Report No. 147. National Council on Radiation Protection and Measurements, Bethesda

National Council on Radiation Protection and Measurements (2005) Structural shielding design and evaluation for megavoltage x- and gamma ray- radiotherapy facilities. NCRP Report No. 151. National Council on Radiation Protection and Measurements, Bethesda

National Council on Radiation Protection and Measurements (2006) Management of radionuclide therapy patients. NCRP Report No. 155. National Council on Radiation Protection and Measurements, Bethesda

Radiation-Induced Genomic Instability

SUSAN M. VARNUM, MARIANNE B. SOWA, WILLIAM F. MORGAN

Biological Sciences Division, Fundamental & Computational Sciences, Directorate Pacific Northwest National Laboratory, Richland, WA, USA

Definition

Radiation-induced genomic instability can occur following cellular irradiation and is characterized by an increased rate of acquisition of genomic rearrangements in the progeny of irradiated cells. These genomic alterations may include cytogenetic abnormalities, mutations, gene amplifications, transformation, and cell death in the progeny of the irradiated cells' multiple generations following the initial exposure.

Cross-References

Radiation-Induced Genomic Instability and Radiation Sensitivity

Susan M. Varnum[1], Marianne B. Sowa[1]
Grace J. Kim[2], William F. Morgan[1]
[1]Biological Sciences Division, Fundamental & Computational Sciences, Directorate Pacific Northwest National Laboratory, Richland, WA, USA
[2]Department of Radiation Oncology, University of Maryland, Baltimore, MD, USA

Definitions

Bystander effects describe the ability of an irradiated cell to send a signal capable of eliciting a response in a nonirradiated cell. This signal may be communicated via cell-to-cell gap junction communication and/or from secreted or shed factors from irradiated cells.

Radiation-induced genomic instability can occur following cellular irradiation and is characterized by an increased rate of acquisition of genomic rearrangements in the progeny of irradiated cells. These genomic alterations may include cytogenetic abnormalities, mutations, gene amplifications, transformation, and cell death in the progeny of the irradiated cells multiple generations following the initial exposure.

Nontargeted effects of ionizing radiation is an all embracing concept that describes responses in nonirradiated cells (hence the term nontargeted) after receiving signals from an irradiated cell (i.e., a targeted cell). These nontargeted effects include, but are not limited to, bystander effects and radiation-induced genomic instability.

Bystander Effects, Radiation Sensitivity, and the Radiation Oncology Patient

Bystander effects are those effects occurring in nonirradiated cells that received a signal from an irradiated cell that can cause the nonirradiated cell to exhibit many of those phenotypes associated with an irradiated cell. Such effects can manifest as induced DNA damage, chromosomal changes, mutation, transformation, and even cell killing. The concept of radiation-induced bystander effects is summarized in Fig. 1. Bystander effects have been demonstrated in vitro (Morgan 2003a) and in vivo (Morgan 2003b), but as with the majority of biological systems and processes, they do not occur universally in all biological systems. The bulk of evidence suggests that bystander effects are detrimental to the bystander cell, e.g., a mutation or chromosomal change. Because bystander effects have been the subject of recent reviews (Hei et al. 2008; Morgan and Sowa 2009), the details are not considered further here.

By definition, bystander effects suggest that the risk to the tissue, organ, and organism is greater than the volume actually irradiated. So how does this impact the radiation oncology patient? To the best of the abilities of the radiation oncologist(s), the medical physicist, and the nursing staff, the tumor is identified, localized, and a conformal therapy strategy devised. The tumor gets the highest radiation dose possible within acceptable limits to the surrounding normal tissue. While modern conformal radiotherapy technologies achieve this goal with impressive results, these new radiation modalities often expose more normal tissue than conventional radiation therapy. For example, intensity modulated radiation therapy (IMRT) is a treatment modality that uses a larger number of radiation beams than conventional therapy to allow for greater conformality of the dose to the target. In the case of IMRT for prostate cancer, the total dose

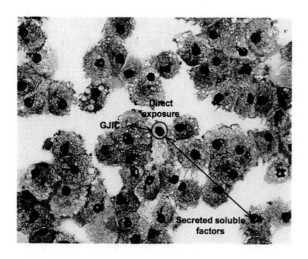

Radiation-Induced Genomic Instability and Radiation Sensitivity. Fig. 1 The radiation-induced bystander effect. The central circle illustrates the field of direct radiation exposure. A larger volume may be affected by signal secreted via soluble/shed factors and/or gap junction intercellular communication (GJIC)

to the target, the prostate, could be more than 75 Gy – a high dose. Through IMRT, the dose fall off from the prostate is rapid and the rectum and bladder can be spared from excessive doses of radiation thereby reducing toxic side effects such as diarrhea or dysuria. High-dose conformality and thus tumor control however comes at the cost of increased exposure of normal tissue to lower doses of radiation. The volume of tissue encompassed by the "5% isodose line" is usually considered to receive a "low dose." This dose level is frequently considered trivial by radiation oncologists and often does not even appear on the patient dosimetric records. Nevertheless this dose may be between 4 and 10 Gy.

The dose received outside the target volume for 3D conformal radiotherapy and IMRT is not likely to be significant but the whole body is nevertheless irradiated. For IMRT, other normal tissue exposure to low-dose radiation derives from increased scatter from the larger number of beams used as well as radiation leakage from the multileaf collimators. Other sources of radiation scatter include the devices used in delivering 3D conventional radiotherapy including physical wedges, blocks, block holders etc. Head leakage is probably the main contributor to the whole body exposure in most situations using IMRT. If it is assumed that this is 0.1% of the total dose delivered, the maximum allowable leakage from a typical linear accelerator, then the whole body would receive a dose of 0.76 Gy (total dose = 76 Gy × 0.1% head leakage = 0.076 Gy or 7.6 cGy). In radiation therapy, but not in the real world, this would be considered to be a "very low dose." Potential biological effects at these low doses remain a subject of considerable controversy (Fig. 2).

Please note: it is not the intent here to confuse a definition of "low dose" for the radiation oncologist with a "low dose" for regulators, the public and occupational exposures. A "low dose" for this latter community is <100 mGy as defined by the US Department of Energies "Low Dose Radiation Research Program" [http://lowdose.energy.gov/].

If, according to the definition presented here, bystander effects occur in nonirradiated cells, tissues, organs etc., then there cannot be bystander effects in the clinical situation because the whole body is irradiated. Instead, any potential out-of-field effects should be considered a "very low dose" effect. There is a long literature on out-of-field effects and their potential role in induced second cancers observed in radiotherapy patients, particularly children. However, it is beyond the scope of this document to address the debate on the role of radiation in second cancers.

There is an interesting and provocative literature on radiation-induced "abscopal effects." An abscopal effect can be described as "a significant tissue response to radiation in tissues definitively separate from the radiation-exposed area." An

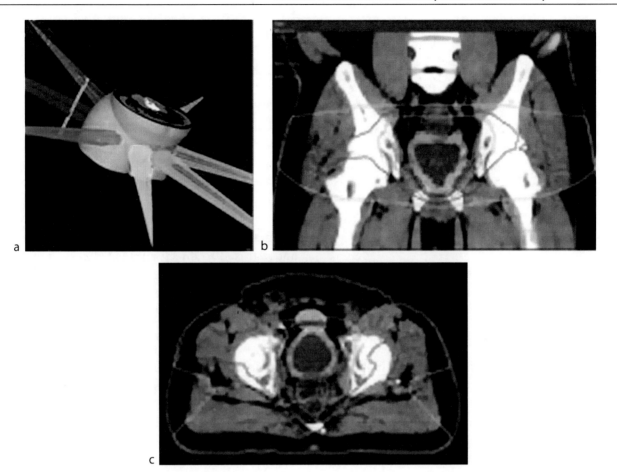

Radiation-Induced Genomic Instability and Radiation Sensitivity. Fig. 2 (**a**) The 3D figure represents a gross view of seven IMRT beams, all low dose and centered on the prostate, which leads to a high dose at the tumor and low doses to the rest of the body. (**b**) and (**c**) Prostate IMRT plan. Axial and coronal views the prostate (*red*) and seminal vesicles (*green/tan*) and the appropriate margin (*teal*) is covered by 75.6 Gy (*red line*) and other isodose curves representing varying doses show the dose fall off from the prostate. Most of the bladder (*yellow*) and rectum (*brown*) are spared excess high doses of radiation

example of an experimental abscopal effect is provided by Camphausen et al. (2003). In an effort to understand the mechanism of the abscopal effect, Camphausen and colleagues irradiated nontumor-bearing legs of C57BL/6 (wild-type p53) and p53 null B6.129 S2-Trp53(tm1Tyj) mice to determine whether an abscopal effect could be observed against Lewis lung carcinoma (LLC) and T241 (fibrosarcoma) implanted at a distant site, i.e., into the midline dorsum of the mouse gut. In mice with wild-type p53, both LLC and T241 tumors grew at a significantly slower rate when the leg of the animal was exposed to five 10 Gy radiation fractions compared with sham-irradiated animals. When the radiation dose to the leg was reduced to 12 fractions of 2 Gy, the inhibition of LLC tumor growth was decreased indicating a radiation-dose

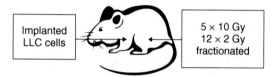

Radiation-Induced Genomic Instability and Radiation Sensitivity. Fig. 3 Tumor cells are implanted into the midline dorsum of the mouse gut and the irradiated leg. Tumor cell growth is measured and is significantly delayed in the irradiated animals compared with the control

dependency for the abscopal effect. This experimental protocol is summarized diagrammatically in Fig. 3. In contrast, when the legs of p53 null animals or wild-type p53 mice treated with pifithrin-alpha, a p53 blocker were irradiated (5 × 10 Gy fractions), tumor growth was not delayed. These data implicated p53 as a mediator of the radiation-induced abscopal effect and suggest that pathways downstream of p53 are important in eliciting this response. Further evidence for the abscopal effect in animal models and human patients is summarized in Morgan (2003b).

While an out-of-field effect, such as suppression of carcinoma cell growth, might be considered beneficial to the animal, out-of-field very low radiation-dose effects have also been shown to lead to oncogenic effects in the cerebellum of cancer-prone Patched heterozygous mice after hind body irradiation (Mancuso et al. 2008). It should be stressed that in a review of the clinical literature on "out-of-field" (bystander effects and/or abscopal) effects, Goldberg and Lehnert (2002) concluded that there is no strong evidence for such effects in the clinical literature. This is not to say they do not exist. But until careful prospective trials are undertaken that involve dose information, detailed field dosimetries and

patient risk factors, no definitive conclusion on such effects in the clinic are possible (Goldberg and Lehnert 2002).

Radiation-Induced Genomic Instability and the Radiation Oncology Patient

A central paradigm of radiation science has been that the initial genetic changes caused by radiation occur as a consequence of direct DNA damage in irradiated cells. However, many observations indicate that genetic alterations are not restricted to directly irradiated cells. Radiation-induced genomic instability can occur in the progeny of the irradiated cell multiple generations after exposure to the initial insult. Genetic alterations observed as a consequence of radiation-induced genomic instability include chromosomal aberrations, aneuploidy, micronuclei, gene mutations and amplifications, and cell death.

Like bystander effects, radiation-induced genomic instability has been the topic of a number of reviews (Morgan 2003a, b), so is not considered in detail here except to speculate upon its implications for the radiation oncology patient. In the preceding paragraphs, we have argued that the radiotherapy patient is subject to whole body radiation exposures, high doses, low doses, and very low doses that vary with tumor location. Thus all cells in the body are at risk to carry the legacy of radiation exposure and have the potential to exhibit radiation-induced instability. Thus there exists the potential for radiation-induced second cancers in surviving patients treated with radiotherapy.

The vast majority of tumors show genomic instability as a consequence of their transformed state. Since radiation can induce a similar phenotype, it has been argued that radiation-induced genomic instability is a significant contributor to radiation-induced carcinogenesis (Huang et al. 2003).

Traditional views of radiation carcinogenesis implicate a mutation in a critical gene as the first step in the process of transforming a normal cell to a neoplastic clone exhibiting tumorigenic potential. However, for a cell to become carcinogenic, typically, 4–6 mutations in genes critical for cancer development occur in the cell (Hanahan and Weinberg 2000). The radiation-induced mutation rate is so low as to make it highly unlikely that the carcinogenic process will reach completion within a human life span. While ionizing radiations have been commonly studied as human carcinogens, the causal mechanisms at the molecular and cellular levels are not fully understood. It is attractive to speculate that radiation induces genomic instability in a population of cells, and that is the source of the multiple mutational events that appear to be required for carcinogenesis (Huang et al. 2003). But it is unlikely that a single mutation, such as in a DNA repair gene, would account for this phenomena as the frequency of ionizing radiation-induced genomic instability (ranging from 35% to 40%) is orders of magnitude greater than that of conventional gene mutation frequencies. While it is reasonable to expect genes from the radiation response pathways to be involved in radiation-induced genomic instability, there must be additional underlying mechanisms. These are discussed in the following section.

Nontargeted Effects and the Radiation Oncology Patient

Bystander effects and radiation-induced genomic instability can both be considered nontargeted effects of exposure(s) to ionizing radiation. That is, they occur in either nonirradiated cells (bystander effects) or the nonirradiated progeny of an irradiated cell (induced instability). So

what are the implications of nontargeted effects for the patient? In the true sense of the definition of nontargeted effects, there is probably little impact, either detrimental or beneficial.

Potential Mechanisms Contributing to Nontargeted Effects

Epigenetic Mechanisms

There is evidence from animal models that nontargeted effects can involve epigenetic mechanisms, such as changes of the methylation of cytosine residues located within CpG dinucleotides (reviewed in Kovalchuk and Baulch 2008). Ionizing radiation can affect DNA methylation patterns in a dose- and tissue-dependent manner, possibly through radiation-induced alterations in the expression of DNA methyltransferases. Studies have demonstrated a widespread dysregulation of CpG methylation persisting in human keratinocytes under conditions where the cells exhibit a genomic instability phenotype. In vivo mouse studies found that chronic low-dose radiation exposure resulted in global methylation changes that were sex- and tissue-specific. Thus epigenetic modifications either directly or indirectly induced by irradiation may contribute to the reported nontargeted effects associated with exposures to ionizing radiation.

Alterations in Reactive Oxygen/ Nitrogen Species and Subsequent Cellular Responses

Exposure of cells to ionizing radiation results in the formation of free radicals due to the radiolysis of water. These reactive species persist for milliseconds and can result in oxidative damage to biomolecules such as DNA, proteins, and lipids. Conventional wisdom suggests that because of their short half-lives and the efficient cellular

R

DNA repair mechanisms, these directly induced free radicals do not contribute significantly to the delayed effects of radiation exposure. Nevertheless, there is increasing evidence for a role for delayed reactive oxygen/nitrogen species appearing and persisting after radiation exposure (reviewed in Morgan 2003a; Kim et al. 2006). These appear to play a role in radiation-induced nontargeted effects associated with radiation exposures. In addition, the generation of reactive oxygen species following irradiation has been documented in various cell-types exhibiting radiation-induced genomic instability (reviewed in Morgan 2003a) suggesting that reactive oxygen species may play a role in genomic instability. Furthermore, studies have demonstrated that irradiated cells treated with free radical scavengers or under hypoxic conditions results in a reduced incidence of radiation-induced genomic instability.

Such studies suggest a mode of action for such reactive molecules (Hei et al. 2008). New data implicate dysfunctional mitochondria driving the persistent contribution of these reactive molecules to ultimately contribute to the observed nontargeted effects of exposure to ionizing radiation (Kim et al. 2006). The mitochondria are a likely source of radiation-induced reactive oxygen species, as they are responsible for the generation of most of the total cellular reactive oxygen species. Damaged mitochondria can generate even higher levels of free radicals when the electron transport chain is impaired. If radiation-induced damage resulted in mutations to the genes encoding the electron transport chain, or the genes required for the proper assembly of the electron transport chain, the resulting condition of a permanently increased state of metabolic stress could become a heritable trait. The resulting pro-oxidant intracellular environment could then perpetuate the process of mutagenesis, leading to genomic instability.

Inflammatory Type Responses

Inflammatory type responses are well documented following radiation exposure (reviewed in Lorimore and Wright 2003). It has been suggested that inflammatory processes either leading to, or as a consequence of, oxidative stress might be a mechanism common to both bystander responses and induced genomic instability. Hematopoietic tissue exposed to ionizing radiation resulted in increased macrophage activation, a hallmark of the inflammatory response. They also demonstrated that increased macrophage activation is the indirect consequence of the recognition and clearance of radiation-induced apoptotic cells. More recent studies (Lorimore et al. 2008) compared the radiation response in two mouse strains, CBA/Ca mice and C57BL/6 mice that are, respectively, susceptible or resistant to the development of radiation-induced acute myeloid leukemia. They found that macrophages from the bone marrow of irradiated CBA/Ca, but not C57BL/6 mice, were able to induce chromosomal instability as a consequence of pro-inflammatory cytokine signaling.

Interestingly, in the context of this discussion are the reports of persistent long-term increase in inflammatory responses in Japanese A-bomb survivors >50 years after their radiation exposure. A recent review summarizes the long-lasting alterations in immunological functions associated with A-bomb irradiation, and discusses the likelihood that damaging effects of radiation on the immune system may be involved in disease development in the A-bomb survivors (Kusunoki and Hayashi 2008).

Reactive Chemokines and Cytokines

A role for chemokines and cytokines in nontargeted effects of ionizing radiation was recently reviewed by Laiakis et al. (2006), so are not discussed in detail here. A number of reactive chemokines and cytokines have been implicated in inducing and/or perpetuating nontargeted effects including interleukin 8, transforming growth factor beta-1, tumor necrosis factor alpha, and nuclear factor kappa-B.

Relationship to Radiosensitivity

The potential for radiotherapy to increase therapy-related carcinogenesis has been documented in a number of studies (Allan and Travis 2005). While it would be expected that radiosensitivity in the human population would follow a binomial distribution, carriers of certain genetic alterations appear particularly sensitive. These include increased risk for breast cancer in BRCA1/2 carriers and young women treated for Hodgkins disease and neurofibromatosis patients treated for optic glioma and retinoblastoma. In addition, individuals with polymorphisms in various DNA damage and response genes, the ataxia telangiectasia mutated gene, apoptosis and proliferation related genes, and estrogen biosynthesis and metabolism-related genes all appear to demonstrate increased risk of radiation sensitivity. For further discussion see (Hall et al. 2005). Whether or not these radiosensitivities are modulated by nontargeted effects remains to be seen, but detailed prospective trials will be required to address this question.

Conclusions

The obvious relationships between reactive oxygen and nitrogen species, mitochondrial dysfunction, inflammatory type responses and reactive chemokines and cytokines suggest that a general stress response induced by ionizing radiation most likely leads to the nontargeted effects described after radiation exposure.

It is unlikely that true bystander effects do not occur in the radiation therapy clinic. But there is no question that effects outside the target volume do occur. These "out-of-field effects" are considered very low-dose effects in the context of therapy.

So what are the implications of nontargeted effects on radiation sensitivity? The primary goal of therapy is to eradicate the tumor. Given the genetic diversity of the human population, lifestyle, and environment factors, it is likely that some combination of these will influence patient outcome. Nontargeted effects may contribute to a greater or lesser extent. But consider the potential situation involving a partial body exposure due to a radiation accident or radiological terrorism. Nontargeted effects suggest that the tissue at risk for demonstrating possible detrimental effects of radiation exposure might be greater than the volume actually irradiated.

Cross-References

▶ Brachytherapy: High Dose Rate (HDR) Implants
▶ Brachytherapy: Low Dose Rate (LDR) Temporary Implants
▶ Breast Cancer: Locally Advanced and Recurrent Disease, Postmastectomy Radiation and Systemic Therapies
▶ Conformal Therapy: Treatment Planning, Treatment Delivery, and Clinical Results
▶ Intensity Modulated Radiation Therapy (IMRT)
▶ Prostate
▶ Radiation Oncology Physics
▶ Stereotactic Radiosurgery – Cranial
▶ Stereotactic Radiosurgery: Extracranial
▶ Total Body Irradiation (TBI)

References

Allan JM, Travis LB (2005) Mechanisms of therapy-related carcinogenesis. Nat Rev Cancer 5(12):943–955
Camphausen K, Moses MA, Menard C, Sproull M, Beecken WD, Folkman J, O'Reilly MS (2003) Radiation abscopal antitumor effect is mediated through p53. Cancer Res 63(8):1990–1993
Goldberg Z, Lehnert BE (2002) Radiation-induced effects in unirradiated cells: a review and implications in cancer. Int J Oncol 21(2):337–349

Hall EJ, Brenner DJ, Worgul B, Smilenov L (2005) Genetic susceptibility to radiation. Adv Space Res 35(2): 249–253

Hanahan D, Weinberg RA (2000) The hallmarks of cancer. Cell 100(1):57–70

Hei TK, Zhou H, Ivanov VN, Hong M, Lieberman HB, Brenner DJ, Amundson SA, Geard CR (2008) Mechanism of radiation-induced bystander effects: a unifying model. J Pharm Pharmacol 60(8):943–950

Huang L, Snyder AR, Morgan WF (2003) Radiation-induced genomic instability and its implications for radiation carcinogenesis. Oncogene 22(37):5848–5854

Kim GJ, Chandrasekaran K, Morgan WF (2006) Mitochondrial dysfunction, persistently elevated levels of reactive oxygen species and radiation-induced genomic instability: a review. Mutagenesis 21(6):361–367

Kovalchuk O, Baulch JE (2008) Epigenetic changes and nontargeted radiation effects – is there a link? Environ Mol Mutagen 49(1):16–25

Kusunoki Y, Hayashi T (2008) Long-lasting alterations of the immune system by ionizing radiation exposure: implications for disease development among atomic bomb survivors. Int J Radiat Biol 84(1):1–14

Laiakis EC, Baulch JE, Morgan WF (2006) Cytokine and chemokine responses after exposure to ionizing radiation. Implications for the astronauts. Adv Space Res 39(6):1019–1025

Lorimore SA, Chrystal JA, Robinson JI, Coates PJ, Wright EG (2008) Chromosomal instability in unirradiated hematopoietic cells induced by macrophages exposed in vivo to ionizing radiation. Cancer Res 68(19):8122–8126

Lorimore SA, Wright EG (2003) Radiation-induced genomic instability and bystander effects: related inflammatory-type responses to radiation-induced stress and injury? A review. Int J Radiat Biol 79(1):15–25

Mancuso M, Pasquali E, Leonardi S, Tanori M, Rebessi S, Di Majo V, Pazzaglia S, Toni MP, Pimpinella M, Covelli V, Saran A (2008) Oncogenic bystander radiation effects in Patched heterozygous mouse cerebellum. Proc Natl Acad Sci USA 105(34): 12445–12450

Morgan WF (2003a) Non-targeted and delayed effects of exposure to ionizing radiation: I. Radiation-induced genomic instability and bystander effects in vitro. Radiat Res 159(5):567–580

Morgan WF (2003b) Non-targeted and delayed effects of exposure to ionizing radiation: II. Radiation-induced genomic instability and bystander effects in vivo, clastogenic factors and transgenerational effects. Radiat Res 159(5):581–596

Morgan WF, Sowa MB (2009) Non-targeted effects of ionizing radiation: implications for risk assessment and the radiation dose response profile. Health Phys 97(5): 426–432

Radiation-Induced Liver Disease (also RILD)

JAMES H. BRASHEARS, III[1], LYDIA T. KOMARNICKY-KOCHER[2]

[1]Radiation Oncologist, Venice, FL, USA
[2]Department of Radiation Oncology, College of Medicine, Drexel University, Philadelphia, PA, USA

Synonyms

RILD

Definition

Occurs after the tolerance dose of radiation for the liver has been reached (>35 Gy whole organ equivalent). Symptoms begin as right upper quadrant pain, and anicteric ascites evolve in roughly 3 months with eventual liver failure. Microscopic evaluation shows central venoocclusive disease.

Cross-References

▶ Metastatic Disease to the Liver
▶ Palliation of Visceral Recurrences and Metastases

Radiation-Induced Normal Tissue Injury

CLAUDIA RÜBE
Department of Radiation Oncology, Saarland University, Homburg/Saar, Germany

Definition

Radiation induces a complex tissue-specific response cascade at the molecular, cellular, and tissue level involving DNA damage response, cell cycle arrest, induction of apoptosis, loss of reproductive capacity, premature senescence, cytokine cascades, tissue remodelling, etc. Predictive in vitro assays try to target different variables known to determine normal tissue reactions.

Cross-References

▶ Predictive In vitro Assays in Radiation Oncology

Radiation-Induced Sarcoma

ANTHONY E. DRAGUN
Department of Radiation Oncology, James Graham Brown Cancer Center, University of Louisville School of Medicine, Louisville, KY, USA

Definition

Despite an increased use of breast-conserving therapy (with post operative radiation therapy) and post mastectomy radiation therapy over the last few decades, radiation-induced tumors remain extraordinarily rare. Radiation-induced sarcomas are most often malignant fibrous histiocytoma (MFH), angiosarcoma, or fibrosarcoma. The risk of a radiation-induced solid tumor is estimated to be approximately 1% over the course of 20 years and the average latency period is approximately 10 years. Standard treatment involves surgical resection with adjuvant local and systemic therapies depending on histologic grade and margin status. Overall, prognosis is poor with 5-year survival rate of approximately 30%.

Cross-References

▶ Stage 0 Breast Cancer

Radical Hysterectomy

CHRISTIN A. KNOWLTON[1], MICHELLE KOLTON MACKAY[2]
[1]Department of Radiation Oncology, Drexel University, Philadelphia, PA, USA
[2]Department of Radiation Oncology, Marshfield Clinic, Marshfield, WI, USA

Synonyms

Class III hysterectomy

Definition

A radical hysterectomy is the surgical removal of the uterus, cervix, upper quarter to third of the vagina, and parametrial tissues to the pelvic sidewall. Care is taken to mobilize the ureters, rectum, and bladder from the parametrial tissues. Pelvic lymphadenectomy and para-aortic lymph node sampling are often included with this procedure.

Cross-References

▶ Endometrium
▶ Uterine Cervix

Radical Trachelectomy

CHRISTIN A. KNOWLTON[1], MICHELLE KOLTON MACKAY[2]
[1]Department of Radiation Oncology, Drexel University, Philadelphia, PA, USA
[2]Department of Radiation Oncology, Marshfield Clinic, Marshfield, WI, USA

Definition

A radical trachelectomy is the surgical removal of the cervix and surrounding parametrial tissues.

The uterus is left intact. This procedure is an option for surgical treatment of early-stage cervical cancers in patients who are considering preserving fertility.

Cross-References
► Uterine Cervix

Radioactive Microsphere Embolization (of Liver Tumors)

James H. Brashears, III
Radiation Oncologist, Venice, FL, USA

Definition
An invasive procedure typically involving interventional radiology, radiation oncology, and/or nuclear medicine, wherein a catheter is introduced under angiographic guidance into the arterial supply of tumor by way of the hepatic artery, and beta emitting Yttrium-90 (Y-90) is introduced. The Y-90 is attached to either glass or resin microspheres, and secondary bremsstrahlung photons can be detected after therapy by gamma cameras to help evaluate the technical success of the procedure.

Cross-References
► Palliation of Visceral Recurrences and Metastases

Radioactive Plaque Therapy

► Eye Plaque Physics

Radioactivity

Hedvig Hricak[1], Oguz Akin[2], Hebert Alberto Vargas[2]
[1]Department of Radiology, Memorial Sloan-Kettering Cancer Center, New York, NY, USA
[2]Body MRI, Memorial Sloan-Kettering Cancer Center, New York, NY, USA

Definition
Radioactivity is the spontaneous disintegration of atomic nuclei. The nucleus emits α particles, β particles, or electromagnetic rays during this process.

Cross-References
► Brachytherapy: High Dose Rate (HDR) Implants
► Brachytherapy: Low Dose Rate (LDR) Permanent Implants (Prostate)
► Brachytherapy: Low Dose Rate (LDR) Temporary Implants
► Eye Plaque Physics
► Imaging in Oncology

Radiodensity

Darek Michalski[1], M. Saiful Huq[2]
[1]Division of Medical Physics, Department of Radiation Oncology, University of Pittsburgh Cancer Institute, Pittsburgh, PA, USA
[2]Department of Radiation Oncology, University of Pittsburgh Medical Center Cancer Pavilion, Pittsburgh, PA, USA

Definition
The relative transparency to the passing of X-rays.

Cross-References
► Four-Dimensional (4D) Treatment Planning/Respiratory Gating

Radiofrequency Ablation (also RFA)

JAMES H. BRASHEARS, III
Radiation Oncologist, Venice, FL, USA

Synonyms
RFA

Definition
A percutaneous or open procedure where tumor or other pathologic tissue is selectively targeted and then thermally eradicated with high-frequency alternating current electricity. The minimally invasive probes can be unipolar or bipolar and may inject saline to increase the volume of the thermal lesion.

Cross-References
▶ Palliation of Visceral Recurrences and Metastases

Radioimmunotherapy (RIT)

▶ Targeted Radioimmunotherapy

Radionecrosis

BRANDON J. FISHER
Department of Radiation Oncology, College of Medicine, Drexel University, Philadelphia, PA, USA

Definition
Radionecrosis is any necrosis caused by radiation. Each tissue has a biological tolerance for radiation prior to the initiation of necrosis. Radionecrosis is typically thought to be a late reaction to radiation.

Cross-References
▶ Skin Cancer

Radiopharmaceuticals

JAMES H. BRASHEARS, III
Radiation Oncologist, Venice, FL, USA

Definition
Unencapsulated radioactive agents used in imaging and treating diseases. Examples include technetium-99m, samarium-153, strontium-89, and iodine-131.

Cross-References
▶ Palliation of Bone Metastases

Radiosensitizer

FILIP T. TROICKI[1], JAGANMOHAN POLI[2]
[1]College of Medicine, Drexel University, Philadelphia, PA, USA
[2]Department of Radiation Oncology, College of Medicine, Drexel University, Philadelphia, PA, USA

Definition
A substance capable of increasing the radiosensitivity of a cell or tissue, making radiation therapy more effective.

Cross-References
▶ Stomach Cancer

Radiosurgery

MARY ELLEN MASTERSON-MCGARY
CyberKnife Center of Tampa Bay, Tampa, FL, USA

Definition

A procedure by which a localized volume of tissue is destroyed by ionizing radiation rather than by surgical excision using extremely focused fields and high fractional doses.

Cross-References

▶ Robotic Radiosurgery

▶ Stereotactic Radiosurgery – Cranial

▶ Stereotactic Radiosurgery: Extracranial

Radiotherapy of Nonmalignant Diseases

LUTHER W. BRADY, MICHAEL L. WONG
Department of Radiation Oncology, College of Medicine, Drexel University, Philadelphia, PA, USA

Synonyms

Benign tumors; Nonmalignant disease

Definition

Nonmalignant diseases are benign diseases that involve inflammatory, degenerative, hyperproliferative, or functional processes.

Background

The role of radiation is usually thought of for the treatment of malignant diseases but it also has an important role in the treatment of benign diseases. Radiotherapy has been utilized in the treatment of a variety of benign diseases ranging from pterygium of the eye to the prevention of vascular restenosis. Of the almost 100 benign diseases that have been documented, several are treated with greater frequency, such as: heterotopic ossification, keloids, gynecomastia, macular degeneration and meningiomas.

Keloids are fibrous tissue formed in response to infections, burns, traumatic or surgical wounds. They are a result of overgrowth of granulation tissue at the site of the injury that is eventually replaced by collagen forming a scar that extends beyond the boundaries of the original wound. Keloids can be pruritic, painful, restrict skin movement and for many patients cosmetically unacceptable. Keloid formation most frequently occurs in African-Americans.

Heterotopic ossification (HO) is a dystrophic calcification after injury to soft tissue. The etiology is either traumatic, neurogenic, or genetic. Heterotopic ossification occurs most commonly at joints, especially at the hip after an ORIF or total hip arthroplasty, but can occur in soft tissue sites as well. It has been shown to occur as frequently as 30% of patients who have undergone hip arthroplasty. The greatest risk factor for this aberrant formation is a previous history of HO that translates to a 60–90% risk. Other risk factors are hypertrophic osteoarthritis, ankylosing spondylitis, and diffuse idiopathic skeletal hyperostosis.

Gynecomastia is a frequent side effect of androgen deprivation therapy for prostate cancer that is often cosmetically unacceptable for men but can also have associated breast tenderness. In fact, the EPC Program has shown that of the men who developed gynecomastia, 74% of the men had breast pain.

Meningiomas comprise approximately 20% of all primary brain tumors and are the most common benign brain tumors. As the name implies, the tumor originates from the meninges, specifically the arachnoid cap cells. Although 90% of these tumors are benign, a small percentage are malignant. The WHO classification of meningiomas is graded I, II, and III for benign, atypical, and anaplastic, respectively. The disease occurs twice as often in women than men and the typical age range is between 40 and 70 years. Known risk factors are previous radiation to the head and neurofibromatosis.

Initial Evaluation

A thorough history and physical examination is essential for any disease whether benign or malignant.

For patients with heterotrophic ossification, a decreased range of motion can be seen on examination that can be severe enough to cause complete ankylosis.

Symptoms of meningioma are related to the mass effect on the brain tissue possibly manifesting as headaches, vomiting, papillary edema, etc., depending on the size and location of the tumor.

Imaging Studies

If not treated prophylactically, heterotrophic ossification is often found incidentally on plain radiographs. The Brooker Classification is used to stratify heterotrophic ossification on radiographic imaging from stages I to IV denoting changes that are clinically silent to clinically significant, respectively.

Meningiomas are distinguished from other intracranial neoplasms by CT and MRI. CT imaging shows meningiomas as well-defined extra-axial lesions that are sometimes calcified. An MRI is preferred for meningiomas because it shows the dural origin of the lesion. The lesions appear hyperintense if IV contrast is used with both CT and MRI.

Treatment

Radiation oncologists have a diversity of opinion in regards to the technique for treating nonmalignant diseases with radiation. Although there are differences in fractionation, dosing, and radiation modality used, the thought process between clinicians is similar. The aim is to select a radiation technique to deliver a therapeutic dose to the intended area while maximally sparing adjacent normal tissues.

Treatments for keloids include intra-lesion corticosteroids, silicone gel sheeting, cryosurgery, and pulsed dye laser treatments. However, the preferred treatment for keloids involves excision followed by modalities such as radiotherapy aimed at reducing the possibility of recurrence by inhibiting fibroblast proliferation. Radiotherapy is typically employed in cases of repeated recurrences after excision, marginal resection, large lesion, or unfavorable location. Radiation is typically delivered within 24 h of surgery using kilovoltage x-rays or low-energy electrons to a total dose of 10–15 Gy in 2–5 fractions. Excellent cosmetic outcomes with low rates of recurrence have been documented following radiation treatment. Radiotherapy alone has also been use for inoperable keloids and is much less effective than if given in combination with surgery, but some response has been shown as long as it is initiated soon after the initial trauma.

Heterotrophic ossification is usually treated prophylactically after traumatic injury or surgery with nonsteroidal anti-inflammatory drugs and/or radiotherapy. Radiation is typically delivered in 1 fraction of 7–8 Gy to the area of concern within 48–72 h postoperatively. In the case of radiotherapy to the hip for young men, testicular shielding is important in reducing the possibility of azospermia.

Prophylactic radiotherapy can also be effective for gynecomastia. Radiotherapy is less effective once androgen deprivation therapy has been started. Different fractionation schedules exist that involve delivering 10–15 Gy in 1–3 fractions. Radiotherapy modalities can involve orthovoltage, 6–12 MeV electrons, ^{60}Co, or 4-MV photon beam. Prophylactic Tamoxifen of 20 mg daily has also shown efficacy. Surgery is available for cases refractory to more conservative management.

The management of meningioma depends on the size of tumor.

Nevertheless, for any of these diseases, an honest discussion of the risks and benefits of

R

radiotherapy is imperative. The potential side effects of treatment must be well delineated as these are benign diseases in which treatment is not always necessary.

Cross-References
▶ Eye and Orbit
▶ Palliation of Brain and Spinal Cord Metastases
▶ Primary Intracranial Neoplasms
▶ Prostate
▶ Skin Cancer
▶ Spinal Canal Tumor

References
Brady LW et al (2008) In: Lu JJ, Brady LW (eds) Radiation oncology, an evidence-based approach. Springer, Berlin
Chao KS et al (2011) Radiation oncology management decisions, 3rd edn. Lippincott Williams & Wilkins, Philadelphia
Levitt SH et al (2012) In: Brady LW, Heilman HP, Molls M, Nieder C (eds) Technical basis of radiation therapy, 5th edn. Springer
Order SE, Donaldson SS (1998) In: Brady LW, Heilman HP (eds) Radiation therapy of benign diseases. Springer, Berlin
Perez CA, Brady LW (2004) In: Halperin EC, Perez CA, Brady LW (eds) Principles and practice of radiation oncology, 5th edn. Lippincott Williams & Wilkins, Philadelphia
Seegenschmiedt MH, Katalinic A, Makoski H et al (2000) Radiation therapy for benign diseases: patterns of care study in Germany. Int J Radiat Oncol Biol Phys 47(1):195–202

Randomization=Random Assignment

Edward J. Gracely
Department of Epidemiology and Biostatistics, College of Medicine, Drexel University, Philadelphia, PA, USA

Definition
Process of assigning subjects to different treatment or prevention groups by chance (randomly).

Cross-References
▶ Statistics and Clinical Trials

Randomized Clinical Trial

Edward J. Gracely
Department of Epidemiology and Biostatistics, College of Medicine, Drexel University, Philadelphia, PA, USA

Definition
Clinical trial in human subjects in which random assignment to groups is utilized.

Cross-References
▶ Statistics and Clinical Trials

Range Straggling

Daniel Yeung[1], Jatinder Palta[2]
[1]Department of Radiation Oncology, Univeristy of Florida Proton Therapy Institute, Jacksonville, FL, USA
[2]Department of Radiation Oncology, University of Florida Health Science Center, Gainesville, FL, USA

Definition
The variations in the expected depth traversed in a medium by protons of a given energy due to the statistical fluctuations in energy loss and trajectories as well as the small inherent energy spread in the beam.

Cross-References
▶ Proton Therapy

Reactor Accidents

▶ Short-Term and Long-Term Health Risk of Nuclear Power Plant Accident

Reactor Explosions

JOHN P. CHRISTODOULEAS
The Perelman Cancer Center, Department of Radiation Oncology, University of Pennsylvania Hospital, Philadelphia, PA, USA

Definition
Reactor explosions can occur when there is a buildup of excessive hydrogen in the setting of high temperatures and pressures within a reactor core. Importantly, explosions that are seen in reactor accidents are fundamentally different from those seen with nuclear weapons. Explosions that result from the detonation of nuclear weapons involve highly enriched uranium or plutonium isotopes in concentrations and forms that are not present in power plants.

Cross-References
▶ Short-Term and Long-Term Health Risk of Nuclear Power Plant Accident

Real-Time Planning

YAN YU, LAURA DOYLE
Department of Radiation Oncology, Thomas Jefferson University Hospital, Philadelphia, PA, USA

Definition
Dynamic dosimetric calculations performed on live TRUS images to determine needle and seed placement. Advantages include constant feedback from live images and dosimetry updates throughout the implant procedure.

Cross-References
▶ Brachytherapy: Low Dose Rate (LDR) Permanent Implants (Prostate)

Recall Phenomenon

▶ Radiation Recall Reaction

Record-and-Verification (R&V)

TIMOTHY HOLMES
Department of Radiation Oncology, Sinai Hospital, Baltimore, MD, USA

Definition
Modern radiotherapy systems include an R&V system that monitors the execution of the treatment under computer control and interrupts the treatment if any deviation in machine parameters is detected. The R&V system records the treatment parameters in a database for later review by the medical physicist as part of a quality assurance program.

Cross-References
▶ Image-Guided Radiation Therapy (IGRT): TomoTherapy
▶ Radiation Oncology Physics

R

Rectal Cancer

Claus Rödel
Department of Radiotherapy and Oncology,
Johann Wolfgang Goethe-University Frankfurt,
Frankfurt, Germany

Description

The treatment of rectal cancer is as variable as its clinical presentations. It can occur as an early tumor suitable for local excision, a locally advanced tumor that requires major surgery plus (neo)adjuvant therapy, one invading adjacent organs with no evidence of distant metastases, and lastly, presenting with distant metastases. New data have been collected, and progress has been made both in surgery as well as in radio- and chemotherapy. Better knowledge of radial spread within the so-called mesorectum has led to the use of total mesorectal excision (TME). With this type of surgery, local control rates have been markedly increased. Technical advances in radiotherapy, and improvements in the sequencing of radiotherapy, chemotherapy, and surgery have further allowed to increase the therapeutic ratio. Newer generation chemotherapy and targeted agents are incorporated into the multimodality treatment. In addition, advances both in pathology and imaging have further contributed to the multidisciplinary management.

Anatomy

The rectum is approximately 16 cm in length. Because of differences in treatment and prognosis, the rectum is subdivided into three parts, according to the distance of the lower margin of the tumor from the anal verge (assessed by rigid rectoscopy): upper third 12–16 cm, middle third 6– $\leq$12 cm, and lower third <6 cm. The anterior peritoneal reflexion represents the point at which the rectum exits the peritoneal cavity and becomes retroperitoneal (approximately 8–12 cm from the anal verge, extremely variable between females and males). Below this level, there is a mesorectal, or circumferential, resection margin all around the rectum. A layer of visceral fascia (fascia propria) encloses both rectum and mesorectum and thus forms a separate compartment within the pelvis. The major portion of the lymphatic drainage of the rectum passes along the superior hemorrhoidal arterial trunk toward the inferior mesenteric artery. Only a few lymphatics follow the inferior mesenteric vein. The pararectal nodes above the level of the middle rectal valve drain exclusively along the superior hemorrhoidal lymphatic chain. Below this level (approximately 7–8 cm above the anal verge), some lymphatics pass to the lateral rectal pedicle. These lymphatics are associated with nodes along the middle hemorrhoidal artery, obturator fossa, and hypogastric and common iliac arteries. Extensive lymphatics are also present in women contiguous with the rectovaginal septum, and in men along Denonvilliers' fascia. The venous drainage of the upper rectum is to the inferior mesenteric vein via the superior hemorrhoidal and then to the portal system, whereas the lower rectum can, in addition, drain to the internal iliac veins and inferior vena cava.

Epidemiology and Etiology

Colorectal cancer is the third most frequently diagnosed cancer in men and women in Europe and the USA, with an estimated 40,840 new cases diagnosed in the USA in 2009. High incidence rates are found in North America, Western Europe, and Australia ($\approx$40–45 cases/100,000 population), and intermediate rates in Eastern Europe ($\approx$ 26/100,000), with the lowest rates found in Africa ($\approx$3–8/100,000). Approximately two thirds of cases occur in the colon and one third in the rectum. Within the United States, little difference in incidence exists among whites,

African Americans, and Asian Americans. The occurrence of sporadic colorectal cancer increases continuously above the age of 45–50 years for both genders and peaks in the seventh decade. Subgroups of patients, including those with inherited syndromes, such as ▶ familial adenomatous polyposis (FAP) or ▶ hereditary nonpolyposis colorectal cancer (HNPCC), can experience colorectal cancer at a much earlier age. The etiology appears to be multifactorial in origin and includes both environmental factors and a genetic component. Approximately 75–85% of colorectal cancers are sporadic, 15–20% develop in those with either a positive family history or a personal history of colorectal cancer or polyps. The remaining cases occur in people with certain genetic predispositions, such as HNPCC (4–7%), FAP (1%), or in people with inflammatory bowel disease, particularly chronic ulcerative colitis (1%).

Clinical Presentation

Rectal cancer is usually symptomatic prior to diagnosis. Common symptoms include gross red blood (mixed or covering stool, or by itself, sometimes accompanied by the passage of mucus), a change in bowel habits such as unexplained constipation, diarrhea, or reduction in stool caliber. Hemorrhoidal bleeding should always be a diagnosis of exclusion. Obstructing rectal cancers frequently present with diarrhea rather than constipation. In cases of locally advanced rectal cancer with circumferential growth and extensive transmural penetration, urgency, inadequate emptying, and tenesmus are seen. Urinary symptoms, buttock or perineal pain from posterior extension are grave signs.

Differential Diagnosis

The vast majority (over 90%) of rectal cancers are adenocarcinoma. Mucinous and signet ring carcinoma are both variants of adenocarcinoma and account for some 10% of all rectal cancer. This subdivision appears to confer no independent prognostic value. Other histologic types are rare and include carcinoid tumors, leiomyosarcomas, lymphoma, and squamous cell cancers.

Diagnostic Evaluation and Imaging

The standard workup for rectal cancer is seen in Table 1. The pretreatment evaluation should include a careful history and physical examination. Through digital rectal examination (DRE, the average finger can reach approximately 8 cm above the anal verge), tumors can be assessed for size, ulceration, and fixation to surrounding structures. DRE also permits a cursory evaluation of the patient's sphincter function, which is critical when determining whether a patient is a candidate for a sphincter-sparing procedure. Rigid proctosigmoidoscopy allows direct visualization of the lesion and provides an estimation of the size of the lesion and degree of obstruction. This procedure is used to obtain biopsies and gives an accurate measurement of the distance of the lesion from the anal verge and the dentate line. A complete evaluation of the large bowel, preferably by colonoscopy, should also be done to rule out synchronous intraluminal neoplasms.

The primary imaging modalities to assess the extent of the primary tumor are endorectal ultrasound (ERUS), multidetector 4–16 slice CT, and phased-array MRI. ERUS is the most accurate tool in predicting T stage of rectal cancers, especially T1 vs T2. ERUS cannot be reliably used in patients with high or stenosing tumors. Because of limited acoustic penetration by ERUS, invasion of bulky tumors into the perirectal fat and adjacent organs and pelvic sidewalls is better evaluated by multislice-CT scan and phased-array MRI. The involvement of the anal sphincter and levator ani muscles cannot be truly seen on CT scans, whereas high-resolution MRI techniques using phased-array coils have led to better spatial resolution and particularly have been shown to

Rectal Cancer. **Table 1** Workup for rectal cancer

History	Including family history of colorectal cancer or polyps
Physical Exam	Including assessment of size, minimum diameter of the lumen, mobility, distance from the anal verge and cursory evaluation of sphincter function
Rigid Rectoscopy	Including assessment of mobility, minimum diameter of the lumen, and distance from the anal verge. Allows diagnostic biopsy of the primary tumor (preferably performed after or 1 week before rectal ultrasound to avoid false-positive classification of lymph nodes in the mesorectal compartment)
Colonscopy	To detect possible synchronous neoplasm; barium is only allowed if there is no stenotic tumor! In cases of stenotic tumor, enema with water soluble contrast is favored
Endorectal ultrasound	Considering a local excision or preoperative therapy; allows determination of the infiltration depth into the rectal wall and LN status, offers the surgeon, who should perform the endorectal ultrasound, the possibility to clarify the surgical strategy (low anterior resection with sphincter preservation or coloanal anastomosis, abdominoperineal resection)
Pelvic CT or MRI	To assess the extent of the primary tumor and lymph node involvement
Abdominal/ Lung-CT	To detect possible metastatic disease

Rectal Cancer. **Table 1** (continued)

CEA	To obtain baseline CEA level (a prognostic factor and important for follow-up)
Complete blood count	Anemia secondary to bleeding
Blood chemistry profile	Liver and renal function

identify the anal sphincter, puborectalis, and particularly the mesorectal fascia. This latter is an important feature to predict negative circumferential margins, and makes phase array MRI superior to CT especially for lower third rectal tumors. The identification of positive lymph nodes is more difficult. Involvement is mainly assessed by size criteria (>8 mm), although enlarged lymph nodes are not pathognomonic of tumor involvement, and morphological features such as the presence of mixed signal intensity and irregularity of the borders of the lymph nodes may be more reliable. The overall accuracy in detecting positive lymph nodes with the above techniques is approximately 60–75%.

Screening for distant metastatic disease is accomplished routinely by abdominal contrast-enhanced CT or MRI and thoracic CT. Bone scan and brain imaging are required for clinical symptoms only. The major advantage of a positron emission tomography (PET) scan is to differentiate between recurrent tumor and scar tissue by measuring tissue metabolism of an injected glucose-based substance. Scar tissue is inactive, whereas tumor generally is hypermetabolic. This test generally is not used in a routine preoperative metastatic workup. Routine laboratory studies should include a complete blood cell count, blood chemistry profile (including liver and renal function studies), and the carcinoembryonic antigen value. The most recent TNM staging system is given in Table 2.

Rectal Cancer. Table 2 AJCC TNM staging system (7th edn, 2010)

Primary tumor (T)	
Tx	Primary tumor cannot be assessed
T0	No evidence of primary tumor
Tis	Carcinoma in situ: intraepithelial or invasion of the lamina propria
T1	Tumor invades submucosa
T2	Tumor invades muscularis propria
T3	Tumor invades through the muscularis propria into the pericolorectal tissues
T4a	Tumor penetrates to the surface of the visceral peritoneum
T4b	Tumor directly invades or is adherent to other organs or structures
Regional lymph nodes (N)	
Nx	Regional lymph nodes cannot be assessed
N0	No regional lymph node metastasis
N1a	Metastasis in one regional lymph node
N1b	Metastasis in 2–3 regional lymph nodes
N1c	Tumor deposit(s) in the subserosa, mesentery, or nonperitonealized pericolic or perirectal tissues without regional nodal metastasis
N2a	Metastasis in 4–6 regional lymph nodes
N2b	Metastasis in seven or more regional lymph nodes
Distant Metastasis (M)	
M0	No distant metastasis
M1a	Metastasis confined to one organ or site
M1b	Metastases in more than one organ/site or the peritoneum

Treatment

Surgery

"Low-risk" pT1 (<3 cm, <30% circumference of bowel, well or moderately differentiated, no lymphovascular or perineural invasion) cancers can be cured by local removal of the full thickness of the rectal wall, accomplished either by transanal endoscopic microsurgery (TEM) for lesions localized 5–16 cm above the anal verge or with transanal excision alone (0–5 cm above anal verge). In other T1 and ≥T2 rectal cancers, the standard transabdominal resection (anterior or low anterior resection and abdominoperineal resection) including total mesorectal excision (TME) is the adequate treatment. The TME procedure is recommended for patients with rectal cancer localized in the middle and lower third of the rectum. It is known that metastatic involvement of lymph nodes and other tumor deposits can be found in the mesorectal compartment up to 4 cm distally from the lower pole of the rectal cancer. Therefore, complete removal of the mesorectum is always indicated for these tumor locations, and should be further extended in cases of sphincter infiltration as wide abdomino-perineal excision. In rectal cancer of the upper third of the rectum, a partial mesorectal excision (PME) extending 5 cm below the lower tumor margin (as measured intraoperatively) while sparing the distal part of the mesorectum is feasible. It is important to avoid coning with the remaining mesorectal tissue, because this could contain cancer clusters or satellites. In both, TME and PME, circumferential excision needs to be performed in an anatomically defined plane (including the mesorectal fascia), and with a sharp dissection. T4 cancers are defined as lesions extending beyond the rectal wall with infiltration to surrounding organs or structures, and/or perforation of the visceral peritoneum. In these cases, the evaluation of resectability depends on the extent of the operation the surgeon is able to perform as well as the degree of morbidity the patient is willing to accept. From both the surgical as well as the oncological point of view, histologically confirmed R0 resection represents the most important parameter to achieve the best long-term outcome.

Radiotherapy and Concurrent Chemotherapy

Historically, the combination of postoperative radiotherapy (RT) and 5-FU-based chemotherapy has been shown in several randomized trials to reduce local recurrence rates and to improve overall survival compared with (conventional, i.e., non-TME) surgery alone in locally advanced rectal cancer (defined as pT3-4 and/or pN+). The standard design of postoperative chemoradiotherapy (CRT) is to deliver six cycles of 5-FU chemotherapy with concurrent RT (45–50 Gy; 1.8–2.0 Gy, 5×/week, +/−boost) during cycles 1 and 2 or 3 and 4. During RT, continuous infusion 5-FU regimens are recommended. The main advantage with the postoperative approach is the better selection of the patients based on pathologic staging (i.e., exclusion of patients with early pT1-2 pN0 disease). The primary disadvantages include an increased toxicity related to the anastomosis and the amount of small bowel in the radiation field, a potentially more radio-resistant hypoxic postsurgical bed and, if the patient has undergone an abdominoperineal excision, the radiation field has to be extended to include the perineal scar.

The optimum sequence of RT/CRT and surgery has been addressed in several randomized trials, and preoperative RT/CRT has been shown to be superior to postoperative treatment for a variety of endpoints, including local control, acute and chronic toxicity, and, according to some, sphincter preservation in low-lying tumors. Given these advantages, preoperative RT/CRT is now the preferred treatment for patients with locally advanced rectal cancer (cT3-4 and/or cN+). There are two approaches to preoperative therapy. The first, used most commonly in Northern Europe and Scandinavia, is the short-course RT (25 Gy in five fractions) with immediate surgery. In contrast, most other investigators recommend standard course (45–50.4 Gy in 25–28 fractions) combined with concurrent 5-FU chemotherapy. Surgery is performed 4–6 weeks after completion of CRT.

With optimized local treatment, achieved through preoperative RT/CRT and TME surgery, local recurrence rates are less than 10%. The development of distant metastasis is now the predominant mode of failure in rectal cancer. Integrating more effective systemic therapy into combined modality programs is the challenge. Newer generation chemotherapeutics, such as oral fluoropyrimidines, oxaliplatin, irinotecan as well as molecularly targeted agents (cetuximab, bevacizumab), have been incorporated into phase I–III studies for preoperative CRT protocols. Long-term results are awaited.

Adjuvant Chemotherapy

Generally, there are no sufficient data on postoperative 5-FU chemotherapy after preoperative treatment with RT or CRT. Whether positive results from adjuvant colon cancer chemotherapy can be extrapolated to adjuvant rectal cancer is unknown. Most investigators feel it is reasonable and use the same adjuvant chemotherapy for adjuvant colon and rectal cancers. FOLFOX has replaced bolus 5 FU/leucovorin as a standard postoperative chemotherapy treatment. For patients who receive preoperative CRT and are selected to receive postoperative adjuvant chemotherapy, 4 month (eight cycles) of mFOLFOX6 is recommended in the USA. A recent European consensus conference failed to reach a definitive recommendation regarding the use of postoperative chemotherapy after preoperative CRT/RT and surgical resection.

Many controversies remain and a bundle of further questions need to be addressed in upcoming trials. These include the role of short-course RT versus CRT, the omission of preoperative RT/CRT for selected patients or applying neoadjuvant chemotherapy alone without RT, less radical surgery or even a wait-and-see strategy for responding patients. Moreover, clinical factors beyond the TNM stage, e.g., the circumferential resection margin, as assessed on MRI, and molecular markers that may help to stratify patients for the respective alternatives, remain active and promising areas of clinical investigation.

Cross-References
▶ Anal Carcinoma
▶ Colon Cancer

References
Minsky BD, Rödel C, Valentini V (2010) Combined modality therapy for rectal cancer. Cancer J 16:253–261
Peeters KC, Marijnen CA, Nagtegaal ID et al (2007) The TME trial after a median follow-up of 6 years: increased local control but no survival benefit in irradiated patients with resectable rectal carcinoma. Ann Surg 246: 693–701
Rodel C, Sauer R (2007) Integration of novel agents into combined-modality treatment for rectal cancer patients. Strahlenther Onkol 183:227–235
Sauer R, Becker H, Hohenberger W et al (2004) Preoperative versus postoperative chemoradiotherapy for rectal cancer. N Engl J Med 351:1731–1740
Schmiegel W, Pox C, Reinacher-Schick A et al (2010) S3 guidelines for colorectal carcinoma: results of an evidence-based consensus conference on February 6/7, 2004 and June 8/9, 2007 (for the topics IV, VI and VII). Z Gastroenterol 48:65–136
Valentini V, Aristei C, Glimelius B et al (2009) Multidisciplinary rectal cancer management: 2nd European Rectal Cancer Consensus Conference (EURECA-CC2). Radiother Oncol 92:148–163

Referred Pain (or Reflective Pain)

James H. Brashears, III
Radiation Oncologist, Venice, FL, USA

Synonyms
Reflective pain

Definition
The perception of pain at some distance away from the origin of injury. A classic example is left shoulder pain with a myocardial infarction.

Cross-References
▶ Pain Management

Reflective Pain

▶ Referred Pain (or Reflective Pain)

Re-irradiation

Carsten Nieder[1], Johannes A. Langendijk[2]
[1]Radiation Oncology Unit, Nordlandssykehuset HF, Bodoe, Norway
[2]Department of Radiation Oncology, University of Groningen, University Medical Center Groningen, Groningen, The Netherlands

Definition
Re-irradiation is defined as repeat administration of radiotherapy to a previously exposed region of the body, e.g., for locoregional tumor recurrence or second primary cancers arising months or years after an initial course of radiotherapy that has not exceeded tolerance of critical tissues or organs.

Purpose
Depending on disease extent and other patient- and tumor-related prognostic factors, in some instances curative re-irradiation might be pursued. In the majority of scenarios, the aim of re-irradiation is palliation of symptoms and prolongation of survival.

Principle

A clear treatment aim has to be defined upfront, e.g., palliation of pain from previously irradiated bone metastases or local control of chest wall relapse from breast cancer. Multidisciplinary expert teams should assess whether or not other, more effective or less toxic, treatment approaches exist, and if participation in a prospective clinical trial is feasible. In some cases, re-irradiation might be part of a multimodal approach, e.g., neoadjuvant treatment for rectal cancer or adjuvant therapy for head and neck tumors. A thorough review of the previous course of radiotherapy is mandatory (dose, fractionation, isoeffect calculations as shown in Table 1, target volumes, fields, dose-volume histograms, interval to re-irradiation, acute and long-term toxicity of the previous course, residual organ function). If feasible, co-registration of the initial treatment with actual planning scans may provide valuable information. Figure 1 summarizes the biological heterogeneity of tumors treated with repeat radiotherapy. Experimental data suggest long-term recovery of occult radiation injury in some organs such as spinal cord (Nieder and Langendijk 2011). However, toxicity progresses rather than recovers with time in the kidneys, bladder, and heart. Therefore, re-irradiation of these organs might cause considerable late side effects. Acute reactions in skin and mucosa are often indistinguishable from those of first-line radiotherapy. However, late fibrosis, mucosal necrosis, fistulas, and osteoradionecrosis have been described in a large number of clinical studies. One has to consider combinations of re-irradiation with chemotherapy and/or ▶ hyperthermia, which have the potential to broaden the therapeutic window. New investigational agents should preferably be evaluated within well-defined study protocols. Hyperfractionated re-irradiation might theoretically improve the ▶ therapeutic ratio. Prospective trials comparing different fractionation regimens are not available.

Given the need to provide very conformal treatment, which limits the volumes of normal tissues receiving high cumulative radiation doses as much as possible, optimal techniques of imaging for target volume definition, intra-fractional motion control, and immobilization to allow for tight margins should be used. Image guidance (IGRT), intensity modulation (IMRT), stereotactic techniques, and brachytherapy are among the technologies that might improve normal tissue sparing. Typically, elective nodal irradiation is avoided as this would result in larger irradiated volumes with a higher risk of severe complications. Some types of palliative re-irradiation do not require advanced planning and delivery techniques, e.g., in patients with bone metastases where moderate cumulative doses are used. Monitoring and documentation of toxicity is of great importance since limited data on re-irradiation in humans are available in the literature. Given the potential for serious late toxicity, the benefits and risks of re-irradiation must be considered carefully.

Indication

Primary Brain Tumors

Re-irradiation of brain tumors is attracting more interest as our understanding of the tolerance of the brain to radiation evolves, and developments in radiation technology and imaging make highly accurate targeting of biologically relevant tumor volumes possible. Relevant prognostic factors include performance status, initial histology, age, time interval, and tumor location (frontal tumors more favorable). Various brachytherapy techniques, 3-D conformal RT, stereotactic RT, and IMRT have been used by different groups. No head to head comparison or prospective phase III trials are available. Thus, there is no standard protocol. When aiming to keep the total dose of both treatment courses <100 Gy to limit the risk of necrosis, external beam doses of 30–36 Gy are often administered. Even fraction sizes of 3–5 Gy

Re-irradiation. Table 1 Isoeffect calculations: The biologically effective dose (BED) of different fractionation regimens is shown (formula $n \times d \times (1+ d \div$ alpha/beta ratio) where n is the number of fractions and d the dose per fraction as described in Nieder and Langendijk 2011)[a]

	Tumor cells and acute responding normal tissues (alpha/beta ratio 10 Gy)	Spinal cord (alpha/beta ratio 2 Gy)	Other late responding normal tissue (alpha/beta ratio 3 Gy)	Other late responding normal tissue (alpha/beta ratio 4 Gy)
First course, 60 Gy in 30 fractions of 2 Gy, once daily	72 Gy$_{10}$	Exceeds commonly accepted constraints	100 Gy$_3$	90 Gy$_4$
Same fractionation, but normal tissue sparing[b]		79 Gy$_2$[b] Equivalent to 40 Gy in 2-Gy fractions	67.5 Gy$_3$[b] Equivalent to 40 Gy in 2-Gy fractions	62 Gy$_4$[b] Equivalent to 42 Gy in 2-Gy fractions

[a]It is assumed that acute responding tissues react to re-irradiation in the same manner as to first-line radiotherapy. Regarding late responding tissues, it has been demonstrated that the fractionation sensitivity of the rat cervical spinal cord during re-irradiation was not significantly different from the fractionation sensitivity of not previously irradiated control rats, with an alpha/beta ratio of 2.3 Gy in control rats and 1.9 Gy during re-irradiation of the spinal cord. The alpha/beta ratio of tumors might vary. A second primary squamous cell carcinoma in the aerodigestive tract might have the same alpha/beta ratio as a squamous cell carcinoma treated several years earlier in the same patient. However, that might not necessarily be true for a locally recurrent squamous cell carcinoma arising from malignant cells that survived a radical course of radiotherapy and where the surviving clonogens might be biologically different from the ones that could be eradicated.

[b]The maximum normal tissue dose in this example is 30 fractions of 1.5 Gy, i.e., 75% of the prescription dose of 2 Gy.

appear to be well tolerated in limited-volume recurrences as long as the total dose is limited to 30–35 Gy.

Head and Neck Cancer

Re-irradiation for locoregional failure or second primary tumors is an area where more evidence than in other anatomical regions has been collected (McDonald et al. 2011). However, salvage surgery remains the standard of care. Curatively intended (chemo-) radiation should be considered in well-selected cases and can be administered safely with a reasonable chance of long-term survival (approximately 15–20%) but at the cost of increased acute and late toxicity. New induction chemotherapy regimens and the addition of ► cetuximab to radiation are of interest as these approaches might improve locoregional control

without increasing morbidity. Relevant prognostic factors include comorbidity, organ dysfunction prior to re-irradiation, isolated neck recurrence, tumor bulk, and time interval. It has also been suggested that prior chemoradiotherapy adversely impacts outcome, possibly because tumor cells surviving such aggressive treatment are relatively resistant to re-irradiation even if combined with chemotherapy again. Recent studies have used conventional, hyper- or hypofractionated (stereotactic or robotic image-guided) regimens, often with concomitant chemotherapy. Re-irradiation with 30 Gy in fractions of 5–6 Gy to small target volumes or conventionally fractionated regimens (cumulative doses of 110–130 Gy) might be considered. However, severe morbidity remains of major concern both after postoperative or primary re-irradiation (Janot et al. 2008).

R

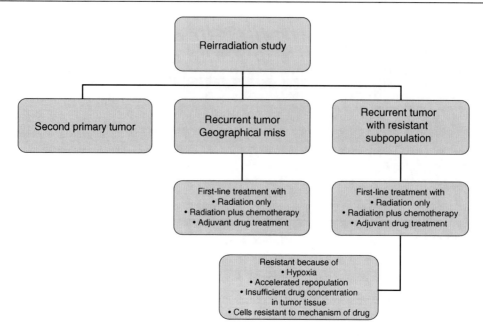

Re-irradiation. Fig. 1 In clinical re-irradiation studies, the situation is complicated by very complex and heterogeneous tumor biology and changes in physiological and microenvironmental parameters resulting from the first course of radiotherapy, e.g., fibrosis and impaired tissue perfusion. It has been suggested that human tumor cells derived from radiotherapy failures (head and neck carcinomas) are relatively radioresistant. Importantly, some radiosensitive tumors from previously irradiated patients were also found in previous studies

Lung Cancer

Re-irradiation has typically been considered for symptom palliation, especially in patients with non-small cell histology. Doses of 30 Gy or less were often prescribed, e.g., in 2.5–3.0 Gy-fractions. With stereotactic and IMRT techniques, more aggressive approaches might be feasible in selected cases (Fig. 2). Endobronchial recurrences should be considered for brachytherapy. The risk of fatal bleeding is estimated to be 0–7%. Performance status and time interval are prognostic factors for survival after re-irradiation.

Breast Cancer

Chest wall recurrence generally portends a worse prognosis than in-breast local recurrences. A subset of patients may be long-term survivors in the absence of metastasis. Experiences with chest wall re-irradiation show high response rates with acceptable late toxicity, but follow-up is limited. Local control is in the range of 43–85%. In selected cases, salvage breast conserving surgery with breast re-irradiation (various techniques of partial breast radiotherapy) appears feasible. A prospective phase II trial is being performed by the Radiation Therapy Oncology Group (RTOG). Toxicity increases with re-irradiation doses above 46 Gy and cumulative doses above 100 Gy, but is also volume-dependent. Additional hyperthermia might increase the likelihood of local response. Response rate also varies with recurrent tumor size.

Prostate Cancer

Salvage radiotherapy for locally recurrent prostate cancer after primary radiation is generally performed by brachytherapy, e.g., with

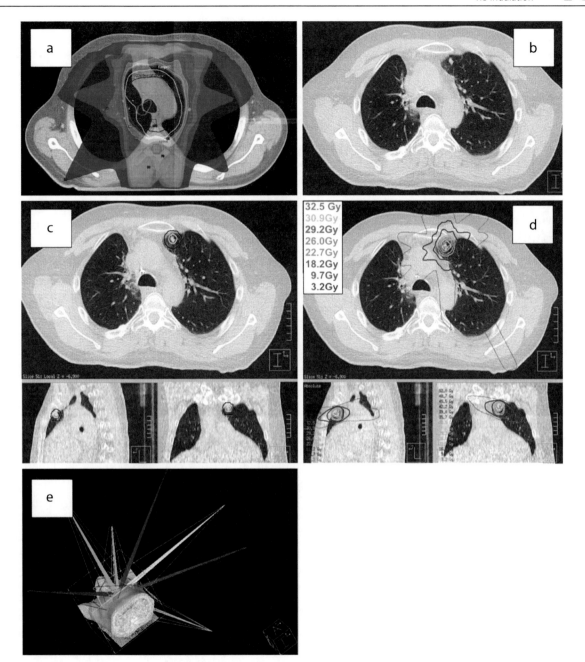

Re-irradiation. Fig. 2 Case example of retreatment for a solitary lung metastasis with stereotactic body radiotherapy (SBRT). Medical history: 2007 – Primary NSCLC (adenocarcinoma) right lower lobe, three cycles of neo-adjuvant chemotherapy, surgery with lobectomy and mediastinal lymph node dissection, tumor stage: ypT2 ypN2 M0, postoperative adjuvant chemotherapy, postoperative radiotherapy to the mediastinum (55.8 Gy). 2008 – Solitary brain metastasis treated with radiosurgery. 2009 – Solitary lung metastasis treated with radiosurgery of 26 Gy. (**a**) Adjuvant radiotherapy after surgical treatment of N2 disease. (**b**) Solitary lung metastasis (**c**) Target volume for SBRT GTV (*yellow*) and PTV (*red*). (**d**) Dose distribution of SBRT with delivery of a single fraction of 26 Gy to the 80% isodose. (**e**) Beam arrangement for SBRT

permanent seeds. Only a limited amount of small studies has been performed, all retrospective. In these studies, the rate of severe toxicity (especially genitourinary side effects) was high and outcome was poorer than expected (5-year biochemical no evidence of disease 20–65%). Furthermore, it is unclear whether salvage treatment will improve disease-specific or overall survival. A prospective phase II trial is being performed by the RTOG. Selecting patients with organ-confined disease is not trivial. Salvage currently can be considered in patients with a pathology proven local recurrence after an interval of at least 2–3 years after primary treatment, together with a limited and nonaggressive tumor presentation at the time of salvage. Equal doses to primary treatment to the entire prostate are often recommended. Current developments in PET and MRI imaging give the possibility to localize the macroscopic recurrent tumor in the prostate. This enables future focal salvage techniques which can be expected to reduce severe toxicity rates.

Rectal Cancer

Re-irradiation combined with chemotherapy for patients developing recurrent rectal cancer after radiation or chemoradiation is feasible and provides high chances for cure and palliation of symptoms, such as pain or bleeding. Classification of recurrence is based on localization and regions of tumor fixation, e.g., to the pelvic side wall, or organ invasion. Nearly one half of patients who also undergo resection of recurrent disease achieve long-term pelvic control and 5-year survival might reach up to 65%. Even in unresected patients, long-term control can be achieved in about 20% of cases with one out of five patients surviving after 5 years (median survival 14–16 months). Prognosis depends on performance status, initial disease extent, resectability, and time interval. Acute and late toxicity are not prohibitive if proper attention is paid to both radiation technique and surgical technique. The major side effects include small bowel obstruction, fistula, and postoperative complications. Use of small radiation fields, exclusion of bowel and bladder, and use of radiation doses up to 40 Gy are recommended. Data from a non-randomized study suggest that hyperfractionation (1.2 Gy BID) might reduce toxicity risk.

Gynecological Tumors

Patients who present with an isolated recurrence after having undergone definitive radiation treatment pose a therapeutic dilemma, balancing risks of re-treatment with a desire to optimize local control. A patient's suitability for a radical approach to re-treatment is determined by multiple factors: their clinical performance status and symptomatology, previous radiotherapy and radiation-related toxicities, and disease extent. An aggressive approach is worth pursuing in carefully selected patients, where not only palliation of local symptoms is possible but long-term local control can be a realistic aim. Prognostic factors include time interval, resectability, and performance status. Interstitial brachytherapy, intraoperative RT, robotic image-guided external beam RT, IMRT, and other techniques have been used. However, numbers of patients were small and re-irradiation doses and fractionation varied considerably. Table 2 shows fractionation schedules used by different groups. Decision making is highly complex and requires multidisciplinary tumor boards. An algorithm, which is also relevant to other re-irradiation scenarios in different primary disease sites, is presented in Fig. 3.

Bone Metastases

There are three clinical situations where retreatment for pain caused by bone metastases may be considered:

1. Patients who experience no pain relief or even pain progression after initial radiotherapy

Re-irradiation. Table 2 Suggested re-irradiation fractionation schedules for gynecological tumors

Location of recurrence	Radical dose/fractionation schedules (highly conformal techniques)	Palliative – High dose palliative dose/ fractionation schedules
Pelvic side-wall recurrence	EBRT	EBRT
	50 Gy/25 fx	40 Gy/20 fx
	45 Gy/25 fx	25–30 Gy/10–15 fx
	40 Gy/20 fx	
Vaginal-vault recurrence	EBRT + brachytherapy	EBRT
	50 Gy/25 fx	40 Gy/20 fx
	40 Gy/20 fx	30 Gy/20 fx
	+brachy to total dose 65–75 Gy	Brachytherapy alone
		20–25 Gy HDR/3 fx
	EBRT alone	
	45 Gy/25 fx	
	40 Gy/20 fx	
	Brachytherapy alone	
	35–50 Gy LDR over 4–6 days	
	20–25 Gy HDR/4–5 fx BID/2–2.5 days	

2. Patients who have a partial response with initial radiotherapy and hope to achieve further pain reduction with more radiotherapy
3. Patients with a partial or complete response with initial radiotherapy but subsequent recurrence of pain during follow-up

Because the response to initial treatment takes about 3–4 weeks to occur, it is recommended to consider re-irradiation after a minimum interval of 4 weeks. It appears from a variety of data sets, largely retrospective in nature, that 40–70% of patients experience pain relief. Both single fraction and multiple fraction regimens might be effective. Even second re-irradiation might palliate pain in patients who responded previously. Spinal retreatment might be effective in patients with metastatic spinal cord compression. Published tolerance limits should be observed (Nieder et al. 2006). IMRT or stereotactic RT might allow for lower doses to critical structures in cases were high cumulative doses must be avoided.

Brain Metastases

Re-irradiation with radioactive implants, stereotactic radiosurgery (SRS), fractionated stereotactic RT, and whole-brain radiotherapy (WBRT) might be considered, depending on the key questions shown in Table 3. Salvage WBRT after previous SRS is a common treatment option with survival results indistinguishable from those of first-line WBRT, i.e., usually 3–6 months of median survival. A repeat course of WBRT is used only if salvage SRS or other focal treatment is not feasible. Response rates of 27–42% have been reported in retrospective studies. Often 25 Gy in 10 fractions of 2.5 Gy or lower equivalent doses were used. The RTOG performed a prospective phase I dose escalation trial of SRS

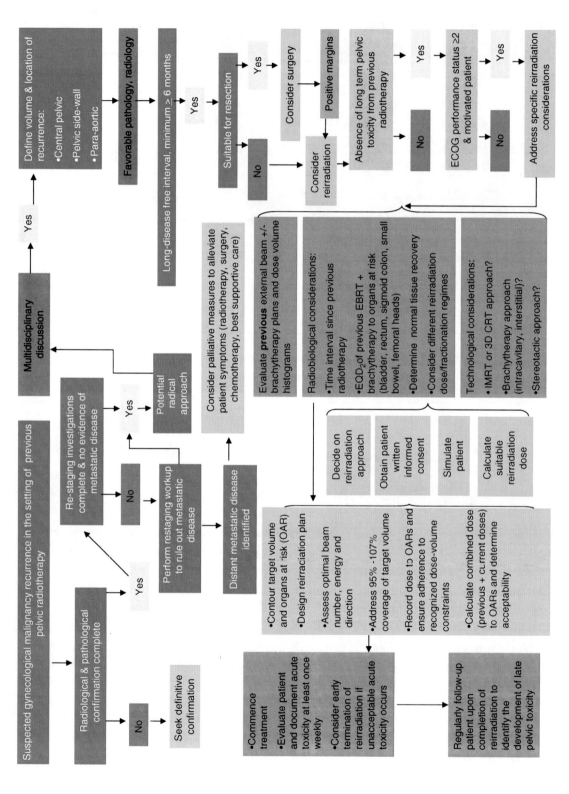

Re-irradiation. Fig. 3 Re-irradiation algorithm

Re-irradiation. Table 3 Key questions when selecting between the different treatment options for recurrent brain metastases

• Is the patient's performance status after initiation of steroid treatment at a level that justifies initiation of radiation therapy?
• Do laboratory tests point to advanced extracranial disease status and poor tolerability/ efficacy of the planned therapy?
• Are extracranial disease sites absent or controlled and if so, does one expect continued extracranial disease control?
• Will systemic treatment be offered or are there no more options left?
• Will brain control impact on the survival of the patient or is treatment focused on palliation of symptoms?
• Will surgical intervention lead to rapid symptom improvement or effective local control, if co-morbidity and other factors allow for consideration of invasive measures? Could the same goals be achieved without surgery?
• Might the cumulative radiation dose to critical normal tissue structures result in serious toxicity in patients with expect prolonged survival?
• What would be the functional consequence of treatment-induced injury?
• How did the lesion(s) respond to initial radiotherapy and how long is the interval?

in recurrent, previously irradiated ▶ primary intracranial neoplasms and brain metastases (RTOG 90–05). Eligible patients had received first-line radiotherapy at least 3 months prior to study entry (Shaw et al. 2000). Their Karnofsky performance status was ≥60 and life expectancy ≥3 months. Dose was determined by the maximum diameter of the tumor. Initial doses were 18 Gy for lesions ≤20 mm, 15 Gy for lesions measuring 21–30 mm, and 12 Gy for lesions measuring 31–40 mm. Dose was prescribed to the 50–90% isodose line, which was to encompass the entire enhancing target volume. The trial

eventually defined the maximum acutely tolerable SRS dose in this setting, except for lesions ≤20 mm where the dose was not escalated beyond 24 Gy because of investigators' reluctance. While small lesions ≤20 mm can be treated with up to 24 Gy to the margin of the lesion, those that measure between 21 and 30 mm might receive 18 Gy, and those that measure between 31 and 40 mm, 15 Gy. Combined radionecrosis data on patients with brain metastases and primary brain tumors were published. The actuarial incidence was 8% and 11% at 12 and 24 months, respectively.

Other Indications

Regarding lymph node metastases from different primary tumors, skin cancer, eye tumors, lymphoma, sarcoma, and other entities, very limited evidence from small studies exists. Basically these data suggest that carefully selected patients might benefit from re-irradiation after favorable disease-free intervals. However, serious late toxicity might occur after high cumulative doses.

Cross-References
▶ Accelerated Partial Breast Irradiation
▶ Boost to Breast
▶ Brachytherapy
▶ Brachytherapy: High Dose Rate (HDR) Implants
▶ Brachytherapy: Low Dose Rate (LDR) Permanent Implants (Prostate)
▶ Breast Cancer Risk Models
▶ Breast Cancer: Locally Advanced and Recurrent Disease, Postmastectomy Radiation and Systemic Therapies
▶ Breast Conservation Therapy
▶ Breast Lymphoma
▶ Breast Tumor Markers
▶ Cancer of the Breast Tis
▶ Conformal Therapy: Treatment Planning, Treatment Delivery, and Clinical Results
▶ Diffuse Large B Cell Lymphoma of the Breast

R

► Early-Stage Breast Cancer
► Hyperthermia
► Image-Guided Radiation Therapy (IGRT): kV Imaging
► Image-Guided Radiation Therapy (IGRT): MV Imaging
► Imaging in Oncology
► Intensity Modulated Radiation Therapy (IMRT)
► International Breast Cancer Intervention Survey (IBIS) Models
► Intraoperative Irradiation
► Intraoperative Radiation Therapy (IORT)
► Noninvasive Breast Cancer
► Palliation of Bone Metastases
► Palliation of Brain and Spinal Cord Metastases
► Primary Intracranial Neoplasms
► Rectal Cancer
► Robotic Radiosurgery
► Salvage Treatment
► Stage 0 Breast Cancer
► Stereotactic Radiosurgery – Cranial
► Stereotactic Radiosurgery Extracranial
► Whole Breast Radiation

References

Janot F, de Raucourt D, Benhamou E et al (2008) Randomized trial of postoperative reirradiation combined with chemotherapy after salvage surgery compared with salvage surgery alone in head and neck carcinoma. J Clin Oncol 26:5518–5523

McDonald MW, Lawson J, Garg MK et al (2011) ACR appropriateness criteria® retreatment of recurrent head and neck cancer after prior definitive radiation Expert Panel on Radiation Oncology-Head and Neck Cancer. Int J Radiat Oncol Biol Phys 80(5):1292–1298

Nieder C, Grosu AL, Andratschke NH, Molls M (2006) Update of human spinal cord reirradiation tolerance based on additional data from 38 patients. Int J Radiat Oncol Biol Phys 66:1446–1449

Nieder C, Langendijk JA (2011) Re-irradiation: new frontiers. Springer, Berlin/Heidelberg

Shaw E, Scott C, Souhami L et al (2000) Single dose radiosurgical treatment of recurrent previously irradiated primary brain tumors and brain metastases: final report of RTOG protocol 90–05. Int J Radiat Oncol Biol Phys 47:291–298

Relative Biological Effectiveness (RBE)

George E. Laramore[1], Jay J. Liao[1], Jason K. Rockhill[1], Lydia T. Komarnicky-Kocher[2]
[1]Department of Radiation Oncology, University of Washington Medical Center, Seattle, WA, USA
[2]Department of Radiation Oncology, College of Medicine, Drexel University, Philadelphia, PA, USA

Definition

The ratio of physical doses between two different types of radiation required to produce the same biological endpoint. Typically, the comparison is made to 250 kV_p x-rays. The specific RBE depends upon the specific tissue and endpoint chosen. Although clinical usage tends to describe RBEs as single numbers, they are actually better represented by families of curves. RBE is LET dependent, rising to a maximum at approximately 100 keV/μm as this is the diameter of a DNA double helix.

Cross-References

► Melanoma
► Neutron Radiotherapy

Remote Control Afterloaders

Erik Van Limbergen
Department of Radiation Oncology, University Hospital Gasthuisberg, Leuven, Belgium

Definition

A remote afterloading machine transfers the source(s) from the shielded source container to the patient and vice versa. Transport is secured by a pneumatic or mechanical system. The most modern machines are stepping source afterloaders. The miniaturized but highly active source (usually Ir-192) is driven by a flexible cable into the different channels, toward preprogrammed dwell positions. Optimal dwell positions as well as dwelling times can be planned by a 3D planning system in order to optimize dose distribution to cover the PTV and spare the OAR.

These machines ensure accurate source positioning, a time control structure, and automatic source retraction. This provides complete radioprotection for the personnel and any visitor.

Cross-References
▶ Clinical Aspects of Brachytherapy (BT)
▶ High-Dose Rate (HDR) Brachytherapy
▶ Low-Dose Rate (LDR) Brachytherapy

Renal Cell Carcinoma

▶ Kidney

Renal Pelvis and Ureter

STEPHAN MOSE
Department of Radiation Oncology,
Schwarzwald-Baar-Klinikum,
Villingen-Schwenningen, Germany

Synonyms
Carcinoma of the upper urinary tract; Upper tract urothelial carcinoma; Upper urinary tract carcinoma; Ureter cancer; Urothelial carcinoma; Urothelial carcinoma of upper urinary tract

Definition/Description
Urothelial tumors of the upper urinary tract are rare. Men are more often affected than women. Considering etiological factors there is a strong association to those factors inducing bladder cancer and to bladder cancer itself. Forty-five to sixty percent of tumors have a risk of <10% to be diagnosed with positive lymph nodes; therefore, an early diagnosis accompanied with a low grading, the absence of negative prognostic factors (i.e., lymphangiosis, tumor necrosis) leads to an improved outcome. The gold standard is radical nephroureterectomy. However, laparoscopic nephroureterectomy as well as endoscopic organ sparing approaches are gaining increased acceptance in well-selected patients although randomized data are not available. (Neo) adjuvant therapies (chemotherapy, radiotherapy) are seldom used because – due to the paucity of data – the beneficial effect although theoretically present in advanced tumor stages, is still missing.

Anatomy
The renal pelvis is the funnel-shaped central part of the paired kidney, which both is retroperitoneally and paravertebrally located within perinephric fat at the level between the 11th rib and the transverse process of the third lumbar vertebral body. It is the proximal part of the urine transporting system that collects the urine produced by the renal papillae. The urine is then propelled through the renal hilum into the ureter. The ureter is a muscular tube (25–30 cm, 3–4 mm in diameter) paralleling on both sides the lateral border and front of the psoas muscle and crossing the pelvic brim near the bifurcation of the iliac arteries until they curve anteriormedially toward the bladder fundus. The course through the bladder wall is approximately 2 cm long where the ureter is closed by nonvoluntary bladder muscles (ureterovesical valves) preventing the backflow of urine.

The mucous surface of the renal pelvis and the ureter is covered with transitional epithelium, with underlying loose connective tissue and a spiraliform layer of smooth muscles which are – with regard to the ureter – divided into an inner loose longitudinal spiral and outer more circular layer. The ureter is surrounded by fibrous connective tissue.

The renal pelvis and the ureter are supplied by the renal arteries, the arteries of the testicular duct and the ovarian arteries, respectively, and drains to the correspondent veins. The lymphatic vessels empty to the paraaortic nodes and – due to the abdominal course of the ureter – to the common iliac, internal and external iliac nodes.

Epidemiology

Carcinoma of the renal pelvis and ureter accounts for 3–6% of all urothelial malignancies and for 10% of all renal carcinomas. Men are more often affected than women (1.5–2:1); however, women are more likely to be diagnosed with advanced disease, larger tumor size, and higher tumor grade. The average age at diagnosis is 60–70 years although in adults tumors are found in every life decade.

The etiologic factors resemble those of bladder cancer due to the similar embryological origin: nicotine abuse that is presumably responsible for 50–65% of tumors in men and for 20–30% in women. Also, phenacetin abuse, and aminophenol exposure have been implicated. Furthermore, there is a strong association with the ▶ Balkan Endemic Nephropathy. Nearly 2–4% of patients with bladder cancer develop a carcinoma of the upper urothelial tract. In contrast, in 15–50% of patients with urothelial cancer develop a metachronous bladder carcinoma which is interpreted as a result of multifocality, an unstable urothelium field effect, and/or an intraluminal tumor seeding. This observation is mainly documented within the first 2 years after diagnosis, although a lifelong risk is supposed (Zigeuner & Pummer 2008; Margulis et al. 2009).

Clinical Presentation

The most frequently seen symptom is macrohematuria (60–90%). In 10–20% of patients, pain in the laterocaudal region due to tumor mass and/or hydronephrosis is documented; 5–10% of patients suffer from bladder irritation. However, some carcinomas are asymptomatic (10–15%) or only lead to weight loss and weakness (2–7%).

Most tumors are located in the renal pelvis (48–64%) (Fig. 1) and 21–40% in the ureter (Fig. 2), where in approximately 20% a multifocality is diagnosed; 2–8% of all tumors are bilateral. In 94–99% of all tumors, a transitional cell carcinoma is found; of these, 64–72% and 28–35% are papillary and sessile in architecture, respectively. Adeno cell carcinoma (1%), squamous cell carcinoma (7–8%), and

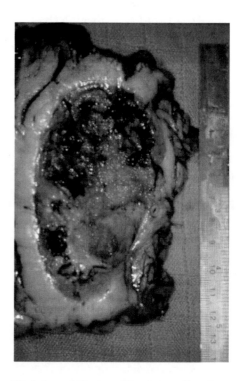

Renal Pelvis and Ureter. Fig. 1 Locally advanced carcinoma of the renal pelvis (With courtesy of A. Lampel M.D., Professor and Head of Department of Urology and Paediatric Urology, Schwarzwald-Baar-Klinikum Villingen-Schwenningen, Germany)

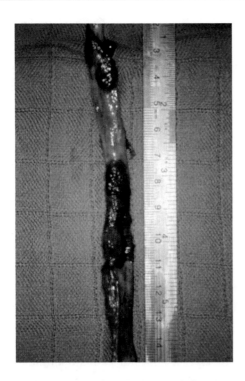

Renal Pelvis and Ureter. Fig. 2 Multifocal carcinoma of the ureter (With courtesy of A. Lampel M.D., Professor and Head of Department of Urology and Paediatric Urology, Schwarzwald-Baar-Klinikum Villingen-Schwenningen, Germany)

Renal Pelvis and Ureter. Table 1 TNM-classification and staging of upper urothelial tract carcinoma

TNM	
Ta	Papillary noninvasive carcinoma
Tis	Carcinoma in situ
T1	Invasion of the subepithelial connective tissue
T2	Invasion of the muscularis
T3	*For renal pelvis only*: Invasion beyond the muscularis into peripelvic fat or the renal parenchyma
	For ureter only: Invasion beyond the muscularis into periureteric fat
T4	Invasion of adjacent organs or through the kidney into perinephric fat
N0	No regional lymph node metastases
N1	Metastasis in a single lymph node, ≤2 cm in greatest dimension
N2	Metastases in a single lymph node, >2 but ≤5 cm in greatest dimension, or multiple lymph nodes, ≤5 cm in greatest dimension
N3	Metastasis in a lymph node, >5 cm in greatest dimension
M0	No distant metastases
M1	Distant metastases
Staging	
Stage 0a	Ta N0 M0
Stage 0is	Tis N0 M0
Stage I	T1 N0 M0
Stage II	T2 N0 M0
Stage III	T3 N0 M0
Stage IV	T4 N0 M0 Any T N1–3 M0 Any T any N M1

sarcoma (<1%) rarely occur. In approximately one-third of tumors, a tumor necrosis (21–39%), a lymphangiosis (25–39%), or a concomitant carcinoma in situ (28–36%) is diagnosed. Sixty-four to eighty-two percent of tumors are high-grade carcinomas, whereas 18–36% are classified as low-grade tumors.

At initial diagnosis (Table 1), most tumors are staged ≥pT2 (pTa 15–19%, pTis 1–2%, pT1 18–22%, pt2 16–21%, pT3 32–34%, pT4 5–11%). Lymph-node-negative and -positive tumors occur in 33–52% and 10–20% of patients, respectively; due to the inconsistently performed lymphadenectomy in 28–56% of tumors the nodal status is not known. The incidence of positive lymph nodes as well as of metastases depends on tumor stage (Table 2); pTa and pTis have

Renal Pelvis and Ureter. Table 2 Incidence of nodal and distant metastases and dependence on tumor stage

	pTa/-pT2	pT3	pT4
pN1	2.4–9.6%	17–32%	46–84%
cM1	2.4–4.9%	15%	35%

a negligible risk to be diagnosed with lymph node metastases. Positive lymph nodes are more often associated with advanced tumor stage, high-grade tumors, lymphangiosis, tumor necrosis, and concomitant carcinoma in situ. Furthermore, tumors with sessile architecture are frequently found in lymph-node-positive carcinomas (Lughezzani et al. 2009; Margulis et al. 2009).

Differential Diagnosis

Other diseases which may induce hematuria are to be taken under consideration. These may be nephrolithiasis, renal cancer, papilloma, infectious diseases of the renal pelvis, the ureter, the bladder, as well as the urethra. Furthermore, renal cysts and/or stenosis within the course of the upper urinary tract may cause hydronephrosis and pain.

Imaging Studies

Besides the clinical investigation, the initial diagnostic algorithm contains cystoscopy, ultrasound, and intravenous urography. This may be completed by a retrograde pyeloureterography. However, ultrasound is of limited value due to anatomical reasons. Urography enables visualization of tumor lesions but is not argumentative. Having a higher sensitivity nowadays computed tomography and magnet resonance imaging mainly add to the locoregional tumor staging and to the diagnosis of metastases (liver, bone, lung, brain). Recent data demonstrate that the multidetector computerized tomography urography is more accurate than excretory urography in adults with hematuria due to better sensitivity and higher specificity, although small

or noninfiltrating tumors < 1 cm are still difficult to find. Conclusive data considering the role of magnet resonance urography are not yet available. Therefore, diagnostic ureterorenoscopy combined with biopsy verifies the suspected diagnosis and may enable the physician to further select tumors probably suitable for organ sparing surgery.

The most important problem in imaging studies is the limitation of the correct nodal staging particularly when nodes are not enlarged. Newer scanning techniques and magnetic resonance contrast agents may help address some of these limitations (Vikram et al. 2009).

Laboratory Studies

Blood count, urine analysis, and chemistry profile of kidney and liver are routinely taken although there is no pathognomic value. In contrast, urine cytology serves as the gold standard although this technique highly depends on the experience of the investigator; sensitivity in low-grade tumors is 20–60%, whereas it is >90% in high-grade tumors. Recent results with respect to urine tumor markers are still experimental.

Treatment

In upper urinary tract carcinoma, surgical treatment is the therapy of choice although prospective randomized trials are not available regarding the surgical approach (open radical vs. laparoscopic nephrouretherectomy vs. organ sparing endoscopic procedures). The reported incidence of neoadjuvant (chemotherapy 3%) or adjuvant therapies (chemotherapy 13%, radiotherapy 2%) is low because there is no beneficial evidence. Small nonrandomized series regarding immunotherapy recommend its use only in carcinoma in situ. Gene and molecular-targeted therapy is expected but conclusive data are not available. In analogy to bladder carcinoma, chemotherapy is indicated in a palliative setting as well as radiotherapy in localized painful recurrent tumors and distant metastases.

The incidence of local (4–28%), nodal (15–18%), and distant (31–54%) failures depends on some tumor and patient-specific characteristics. In high-grade tumors, a local failure occurs more often than in low-grade carcinomas (76% vs. 40%). Tumor necrosis, sessile architecture, lymphangiosis, higher age at diagnosis, and microscopic residual disease (R1 resection) are associated with increased recurrences and decreased survival. There is no influence on recurrence and/or survival regarding the localization of the primary tumor and gender.

Surgery

Open radical nephrouretherectomy with resection of distal ureter with a bladder-cuff is the gold standard in upper urinary tract carcinoma although it may result in an overtreatment in patients with small and low-grade tumors. The complete removal of the ureter is derived from high recurrence rates in the remaining distal ureter and the high incidence of multifocality if the ureter is left; in contrast, this radical procedure is efficient in achieving negative margins and to decrease the risk of seeding. In the last years, laparoscopic nephroureterectomy has gained popularity as well as hand-assisted laparoscopic nephroureterectomy. Endourologic nephron-sparing techniques were initially developed to treat patients with renal insufficiency, significant comorbidities, and/or solitary kidneys. Encouraged by the success of ureterscopic treatments with holmium or neodymium yttrium-aluminum-garnet lasers (Nd:YAG; Ho:YAG) in selected patients with well differentiated and small tumors, the available data are yielding promising results in patients with normal contralateral kidney function.

After performing a radical nephrouretherectomy, the 5-year cancer-specific survival is 62–78%. In tumors < pT1 it is 94–100%. Mortality is reported to be < 4%. After surgery,

Renal Pelvis and Ureter. Table 3 Survival data in dependence of tumor stage, nodal status, grading, lymphangiosis (L1), and histological characteristics

	5-year cancer-specific survival (%)	10-year cancer-specific survival (%)	10-year recurrence free survival (%)
Overall	62–78	67	65
pT1 N0	94		
pT2 N0	86		
pT3 N0	65		
pT4 N0	55		
Any TN1–3	35		
pT1–2 N1–3	69		
pT3–4 N1–3	29		
pT0 Ta Tis	94–100	89	90
pT1	92–94	85	81
pT2	72–82	71	70
pT3	40–56	45	41
pT4	0–16	6	5
Low grade		85	85
High grade		56	52
Nx/N0		71	96
N+		32	25
L1 absent		75	72
L1 present		43	39
Papillary histology		77	75
Sessile histology		36	35

survival is strongly associated with tumor stage, nodal status, grading, and the absence or presence of negative histological factors (Table 3). These data apply for other (endoscopic) therapies as a benchmark and must be compared with in the absence of randomized trials.

After ureterscopic treatment, favorable results are obtained with disease-specific survival rates ranging from 81% to 100% and therefore reflect the proper selection of patients. However, high ipsilateral local recurrence rates (25–93%) are observed in these patients demonstrating the risk of understaging (i.e., inadequate tumor sampling from the tumor base) necessitating the life-long responsibility of close endoscopic follow-up. In 2% of all patients ureteral perforations and in 5–14% ureteral strictures are reported. Furthermore, there is a theoretical risk of tumor seeding via ureteroscopic therapy.

Considering the other surgical approach, data demonstrate that the laparoscopic procedure with open distal ureterectomy is a safe and acceptable alternative to the gold standard open surgery. Cancer control rates seem to be similar with superior convalescence. However, laparoscopic surgery is not yet standard and should be selectively performed. Likewise, endourologic therapies are highly selective (low-grade, non-muscle invasive) and limited to solitary tumors <1.5 cm in diameter. High-grade tumors are not advised to be treated with organ sparing surgery, because this is less likely to be curative.

In 26–48% of patients, a lymph node dissection is performed although there are no valid data concerning the indication and extent of dissection. These patients are mainly those in whom a muscle invasive tumor is diagnosed. Typically, in case of renal pelvis and proximal ureter tumors, paraaortic, paracaval, and interaortocaval lymph nodes from the renal hilum to the inferior mesenteric artery were removed. In case of mid- and lower-uretral tumors, the nodes from the renal hilum to the bifurcation of the common iliac artery and ipsilateral pelvic nodes were removed. If the nodes are positive, the dissection enables a prognostic statement; however, the dissection itself has no relevance with regard to survival because of the high risk of distant metastases in node-positive patients. On the other hand, there are recent data suggesting an improved cancer-specific survival after lymph node dissection and removal of at least eight lymph nodes; it is hypothesized that in node-negative patients, the survival benefit may be related to the removal of otherwise undetected lymph node micrometastases. However, randomized trials are yet not available (Bader et al. 2009; Cai et al. 2009; Lughezzani et al. 2009; Margulis et al. 2009; Roscigno et al. 2009).

Radiotherapy

Conclusive data regarding the efficacy of irradiation cannot be drawn due to the paucity of studies analyzing adjuvant radiotherapy and the small number of treated patients, although theoretically there is an indication for local adjuvant therapy considering the incidence of local recurrences in high-risk tumors (pT3–4 and/or N+ and/or R1 resection). Retrospective data both support and reject the influence of radiotherapy on local control. An overview showed that local recurrences and 5-year overall survival is 9–38% and 21–49% in adjuvant irradiated patients, respectively, whereas the corresponding data were 45–65% and 17–33% in nonirradiated patients suggesting a debatable role. This role may be optimized if adjuvant radiotherapy is simultaneously given with chemotherapy. In a retrospective study including only locally advanced tumors, the 5-year overall and disease-specific survival was 67% and 76% in the adjuvant treated group compared to 72% and 41% in the observation group with surgery only.

However, the indication of radiotherapy has to be scrutinized because of the accompanying inefficiency of chemotherapy prohibiting occult metastases, the high incidence of subsequent metastases in node-positive patients, and the prognostic significance of high-grade tumors in contrast to the low incidence of local recurrences in node-negative patients (Latchamsetty & Porter 2006; Margulis et al. 2009).

If radiotherapy will be used, three-dimensional conformal treatment planning is mandatory. Theoretically, intensity-modulated radiotherapy can offer a more conformal dose delivery. The planning target volume should encompass the renal fossa, the course of the ureter to the bladder wall at the ipsilateral trigone. The paracaval, paraaortic, and ipsilateral iliacal lymph nodes should be covered. The total dose is 45–50 Gy (1.8–2.0 Gy, 5x/week); if tumor is microscopically left and ideally marked with clips, this region may be additionally treated with 5–10 Gy. Side effects of treatment mainly include diarrhea, cystitis, and nausea.

Chemotherapy

Neoadjuvant or adjuvant chemotherapy is infrequently used. The reported response rates vary between 30% and 70%; median survival in treated patients who suffered mainly from high-risk tumors (pT3–4 N0–3 G3) was 14–24 months. The traditionally given combination including methotrexate, vinblastine, doxorubicine, and cisplatin yielded the best results in advanced and/or metastasized tumors although the toxicity profile of combined cisplatin and gemcitamine demonstrates an improved tolerability. However, chemotherapy confers minimal impact on overall or cancer-specific survival.

Cross-References

► Bladder
► Kidney

References

Bader JM, Sroka R, Gratzke C, Seitz M, Weidlich P, Staehler M, Becker A, Stief CG, Reich O (2009) Laser therapy for upper urinary tract transitional cell carcinoma: indications and management. Eur Urol 56:65–71

Cai G, Liu X, Wu B (2009) Treatment of upper urinary tract urothelial carcinoma. Surg Oncol (Epub ahead)

Latchamsetty KC, Porter CR (2006) Treatment of upper tract urothelial carcinoma: a review of surgical and adjuvant therapy. Rev Urol 8:61–70

Lughezzani G, Jeldres C, Isbarn HM, Sun M, Shariat SF, Alasker A, Pharand D, Widmer H, Arjan EP, Graefen M, Montorsi F, Perrotte P, Karakiewicz P (2009) Nephroureterectomy and segmental ureterectomy in the treatment of invasive upper tract urothelial carcinoma: a population-based study of 2299 patients. Eur J Cancer 45:3291–3297

Margulis V, Shariat SF, Matin SF, Kamat AM, Zigeuner R, Kikuchi E, Lotan Y, Weizer A, Raman JD, Wood CG, Upper Tract Urothelial Carcinoma Collaboration (2009) Outcomes of radical nephroureterectomy: a series from the Upper Tract Urothelial Carcinoma Collaboration. Cancer 115:1224–1233

Roscigno M, Shariat SF, Margulis V, Karakiewicz P, Remzi M, Kikuchi E, Zigeuner R, Weizer A, Sagalowsky A, Bensalah K, Raman YD, Bolenz C, Kassou W, Koppie TM, Wood CG, Wheat J, Langner C, Ng CK, Capitanio U, Bertini R, Fernandes MI, Mikami S, Isida M, Stroebel P, Montorsi F (2009) The extent of lymphadenectomy seems to be associated with better survival in patients with non metastatic upper-tract urothelial carcinoma: how many lymph nodes should be removed? Eur Urol 56:512–519

Vikram R, Sandler CM, Ng CS (2009) Imaging and staging of transitional cell carcinoma: part 1/part 2, lower/upper urinary tract. AJR Am J Roentgenol 192:1481–1487, and 1488–1493

Zigeuner R, Pummer K (2008) Urothelial carcinoma of the upper urinary tract: surgical approach and prognostic factors. Eur Urol 53:720–731

Retinoblastoma

R

JOHN P. LAMOND
Department of Radiation Oncology, Temple University Crozer-Chester Medical Center, Upland, PA, USA

Definition

Rare malignant retinal tumor seen in young children commonly associated with a genetic mutation.

Cross-References

► Eye and Orbit
► Eye Plaque Physics
► Soft Tissue Sarcoma

Retropharyngeal Nodes

Brandon J. Fisher[1], Larry C. Daugherty[2]
[1]Department of Radiation Oncology, College of Medicine, Drexel University, Philadelphia, PA, USA
[2]Department of Radiation Oncology, College of Medicine, Drexel University, Glenside, PA, USA

Definition

These nodes lie medial to the internal carotid arteries and extend from the base of the skull to the bottom of the hyoid bone. Their anterior anatomic boundary is the fascia of the pharyngeal mucosa and their posterior boundary is the prevertebral muscles.

Cross-References

▶ Nasopharynx

RFA

▶ Prostate
▶ Radiofrequency Ablation (RFA)

Rhabdomyosarcoma

Robert H. Sagerman
Department of Radiation Oncology, SUNY Upstate Medical University, Syracuse, NY, USA

Definition

Rhabdomyosarcoma is a tumor of unusual characteristics, highly malignant, involving soft tissues and arises from unsegmented, undifferentiated mesoderm. It can also arise from myotome-derived skeletal muscle.

Introduction

These sarcoma tumors may occur in any part of the body, but are most frequently seen in the orbit, head and neck, parameningeal tissues, genitourinary tract, extremities, trunk, and retroperitoneum. Most patients are children, less than 10 years old, with smaller numbers in adolescents, and much less common in adults. Caucasians are involved more frequently than African Americans and males more than females.

Presentations

The clinical presentation is highly dependent upon the primary site of tumor involvement. In the eye, it commonly presents with proptosis and ophthalmoplegia. Other sites of presentation give rise to symptoms relating to that site. Table 1 illustrates the recommended workup for tumors at various primary sites (Breneman and Donaldson 2007).

The patterns of spread relate to the primary site at presentation. Metastatic lesions are rare for orbital primaries but metastases occur in about 15% of head and neck tumors, 25% of paratesticular tumors, and 20% of extremity and truncal tumors. Spread may occur by direct extension into surrounding tissues and organs and to regional lymph nodes. Hematogenous dissemination most commonly involves the lung and bones. The most important prognostic factors are related to primary site, tumor size, histological type, presence or absence of metastatic disease, and age (Breneman et al. 2003; Joshi et al. 2004). The intergroup Rhabdomyosarcoma pretreatment staging system is shown in Table 2 (Mauer 1980).

From a histologic point of view, classical pathology consisted of four histologic subtypes, embryonal, botryoid subtype of embryonal, alveolar, and pleomorphic. More recent data suggests that there is another subtype with a solid alveolar pattern. The wide variation of opinion among pathologists contributed to the development of a new international classification for rhabdomyosarcoma,

Rhabdomyosarcoma. Table 1 Recommended workup for tumors at various sites

All patients	Optional
All sites	
History	
Physical examination by several observers	Examination under anesthesia for infants and youngsters
Laboratory studies	
Complete blood cell count	
Liver function tests	
Renal function tests	
Urinalysis	
Imaging studies	Plain films of bones, abnormal on scan
Chest X-ray	Abdomen/pelvis CT, MRI, or ultrasound
Thoracic CT scan	
Bone scan	
MRI or CT of primary tumor	
Bone marrow biopsy and aspirate	
Head and neck	
MRI or CT of primary tumor (with contrast)	Plain films of area
	Dental films
	Paranasal sinus and skull films
Lumbar puncture with cytologic examination of fluid in parameningeal	MRI of spine if cerebrospinal fluid is positive or patient is symptomatic
Genitourinary	
CT or MRI of abdomen/pelvis (with contrast)	Ultrasound of pelvis
Pelvic examination under anesthesia	Cystoscopy
Extremity and truncal lesions	

Rhabdomyosarcoma. Table 1 (continued)

All patients	Optional
MRI or CT of primary lesion (with contrast)	Plain films of primary site
	Ultrasound
	Barium gastrointestinal contrast studies

Rhabdomyosarcoma. Table 2 IRS clinical grouping classification

Group I	Localized disease, completely resected
A	Confined to organ or muscle of origin
B	Infiltration outside organ or muscle of origin; regional nodes not involved
Group II	Compromised or regional resection
A	Grossly resected tumor with microscopic residual disease
B	Regional disease with involved nodes, grossly resected, in which nodes may be involved, or extension of tumor into adjacent organ may exist
C	Regional disease with involved nodes, grossly resected, but with evidence of microscopic residual disease
Group III	Incomplete resection or biopsy with gross residual disease
Group IV	Distant metastases at diagnosis

based upon review of IRS-II data illustrated in Table 3 (Asmar et al. 1994; Qualman et al. 1998).

Therapy

The diversity of sites of origin, histological types, modes of spread from direct invasion to lymphatic and hemotogenous dissemination, and therapeutic interventions including surgery, radiation therapy, and chemotherapy, employed individually and in varying combinations, was, and still is, best reserved for a multifaceted group able to insure a thorough diagnostic evaluation and therapeutic intervention. This has led to the

Rhabdomyosarcoma. Table 3 International Classification of Rhabdomyosarcoma

I.	Superior prognosis
	(a) Botryoid rhabdomyosarcoma
	(b) Spindle cell rhabdomyosarcoma
II.	Intermediate prognosis
	(a) Alveolar rhabdomyosarcoma
III.	Poor prognosis
	(a) Alveolar rhabdomyosarcoma
	(b) Undifferentiated sarcoma
	(c) Anaplastic rhabdomyosarcoma
IV.	Subtypes whose prognosis is not presently evaluable
	(a) Rhabdomyosarcoma with rhabdoid features

remarkable increase in patient outcomes affecting survival, preservation of tissue, and minimization of deleterious treatment after effects.

Orbit

The value of the multidisciplinary approach is illustrated by the evolution of therapy for orbital rhabdomyosarcoma from surgery (exenteration), to irradiation after biopsy only, to biopsy followed by irradiation, and chemotherapy with long-term survival increasing from 10–20% to 70–90% and with preservation of the globe with useful vision (Sagerman 1993). This occurred because of the rapid, visible enlargement of the primary lesion in young children often noticed by parents, leading to ophthalmologic consultation, the low incidence of lymphatic spread, and in more recent years, the evolution of imaging and irradiation technologies and techniques, as well as of chemotherapeutic agents and their value when employed independently and in multimodal therapy, so that current results are better than 90% (Crist et al. 1990, 1995). Chemotherapy alone has been employed in selected, early stage patients but with a higher incidence of local relapse and a diminished

survival, as well as greater loss of functional vision after retreatment (Oberlin et al. 2001).

Head and Neck – Parameningeal Sites

Non-orbital rhabdomyosarcomas of the head and neck are grouped into various parameningeal sites including nasopharynx, nasal cavity, paranasal sinuses, middle ear, pterygopalatine fossa, and infratemporal fossa, which illustrate the many differences in the natural history, as well as treatment possibilities and prognosis for the various sites. These tumors may involve the base of the skull resulting in cranial nerve palsies and direct extension into the central nervous system. Complete tumor resection is often difficult and cosmesis impaired so that surgery is often limited and radiation therapy programs recommend that adequate local tumor control can be achieved with precisely defined radiotherapy fields without the necessity of irradiating the whole brain, so long as one includes the original tumor volume as demonstrated on imaging studies (Benk et al. 1996; Crist et al. 1995). Whole brain irradiation may not be required for local extension so long as one encompasses the original tumor volume (Raney et al. 2002). Those patients with known meningeal involvement require craniospinal irradiation.

Head and Neck – Nonparameningeal Sites

Tumors of the nonparameningeal sites may be more amenable to complete gross total excision than parameningeal tumors. They tend to have a better outcome and may involve the scalp, parotid gland, oral cavity, larynx, oropharynx, and cheek. Lymph node involvement occurs in about 15% of the patients. Radiation therapy is based upon the characteristics at the time of initial presentation and the adequacy of the surgical resection. Therefore, it is necessary to design the treatment program in such a way as to include adequate margins around the initial presentation, as well as the findings demonstrated at the time of surgery, and chemotherapy may be recommended.

Pelvis

Pelvic tumors are divided into anatomic subgroups including the bladder, prostate, paratesticular areas, gynecologic areas, and other pelvic sites. In large measure, surgical resection with postoperative radiation therapy and chemotherapy would be the recommended program of management.

Extremity

Extremity tumors are often of the alveolar or undifferentiated subtypes, tending to be large and deeply invasive at the time of diagnosis, and are associated with a high probability of lymphatic and hematogenous dissemination. Adequate surgical resection is mandatory, with postoperative radiation therapy and chemotherapy, to maximize the potential for long-term control.

Treatment Sequelae

Treatment sequelae are related to the primary site of presentation as well as the utilized combination of surgery, radiation therapy, and chemotherapy. Therefore, exquisite attention should be directed toward developing a treatment program which mitigates the after-effects of treatment from each of the therapeutic modalities and recognizes late effects in growing children such as epiphyseal bone centers, primary site organ function, and overall growth potential (Heyn et al. 1992; Michalski et al. 2004; Sung et al. 2004).

Cross-References

▶ Eye and Orbit
▶ Nasopharynx
▶ Soft-Tissue Sarcoma

References

Asmar L, Gehan EM, Newton WA et al (1994) Agreement among and within groups of pathologists in the classification of rhabdomyosarcoma and related childhood sarcomas: report of an international study of four pathology classifications. Cancer 74:2579–2588

Benk V, Rodary C, Donaldson SS et al (1996) Parameningeal rhabdomyosarcoma: results of an international workshop. Int J Radiat Oncol Biol Phys 36:533–540

Breneman JC, Donaldson SS (2007) Rhabdomyosarcoma. In: Perez CA, Brady LW, Halperin EC (eds) Principles and practice of radiation oncology, 5th edn. Lippincott Williams & Wilkins, Philadelphia, pp 1872–1885

Breneman JC, Lyden E, Pappo AS et al (2003) Prognostic factors and outcome in children with metastatic rhabdomyosarcoma: a report from the intergroup rhabdomyosarcoma study IV. J Clin Oncol 21:78–84

Crist WM, Garnsey L, Beltangady MS et al (1990) Prognosis in children with rhabdomyosarcoma: a report of the intergroup rhabdomyosarcoma studies I and II. J Clin Oncol 8:443–452

Crist W, Gehan EA, Ragab AH et al (1995) The third intergroup rhabdomyosarcoma study. J Clin Oncol 13:610–630

Heyn R, Raney RB, Hays DM et al (1992) Late effects of therapy in patients with paratesticular rhabdomyosarcoma. J Clin Oncol 10:614–623

Joshi D, Anderson J, Paidas C et al (2004) Age is an independent prognostic factor in rhabdomyosarcoma: a report from the soft tissue sarcoma committee of the children's oncology group. Pediatr Blood Cancer 42:64–73

Mauer HM (1980) The intergroup rhabdomyosarcoma study: objectives and clinical staging classification. J Pediatr Surg 15:371–372

Michalski JM, Meza J, Breneman JC et al (2004) Influence of radiation therapy parameters on outcome in children treated with radiation therapy for localized parameningeal rhabdomyosarcoma in intergroup rhabdomyosarcoma study group trials II through IV. Int J Radiat Oncol Biol Phys 59:1027–1038

Oberlin O, Rey A, Anderson J et al (2001) Treatment of orbital rhabdomyosarcoma: survival and late effects of treatment. Results of an international workshop. J Clin Oncol 19:197–204

Qualman SJ, Coffin CM, Newton WA et al (1998) Intergroup rhabdomyosarcoma study: update for pathologist. Pediatr Dev Pathol 1:550–561

Raney RB, Meza J, Anderson JR et al (2002) Treatment of children and adolescents with localized parameningeal sarcoma: experience of the intergroup rhabdomyosarcoma study group protocols IRS-II through –IV, 1978–1997. Med Pediatr Oncol 38:22–32

Sagerman RH (1993) Orbital rhabdomyosarcoma: a paradigm for irradiation. Radiology 187:605–607

Sung L, Anderson JR, Donaldson SS et al (2004) Late effects occurring five years or more after successful therapy for childhood rhabdomyosarcoma: a report from the soft tissue sarcoma committee of the children's oncology group. Eur J Cancer 40:1878–1885

R

Richter Transformation

CASPIAN OLIAI
Department of Radiation Oncology, College of
Medicine, Drexel University, Philadelphia, PA,
USA

Definition

The development of high-grade NHL in a patient
with CLL or small lymphocytic lymphoma. It
usually manifests as diffuse B-cell NHL. Symptoms include fever, loss of weight and muscle
mass, and LAD. An increased serum LDH occurs
in the majority of patients. Survival is poor, usually between 5 and 8 months. Five percent to ten
percent of CLL patients will experience this
transformation.

Cross-References

▶ Leukemia in General
▶ Non-Hodgkins Lymphoma

RILD

▶ Radiation-Induced Liver Disease (also RILD)

Robotic Radiosurgery

MARY ELLEN MASTERSON-McGARY
CyberKnife Center of Tampa Bay, Tampa, FL, USA

As of 2011, there is only one commercially available robotic radiosurgery (cf. ▶ Stereotactic
Radiosurgery – Cranial and Stereotactic Radiosurgery -Extracranial) device, the CyberKnife®
System (Accuray Incorporated, Sunnyvale, CA).
Therefore, this article is primarily concerned with
describing the design, functionality, and clinical

accuracy of the current version (version 9.0) of
CyberKnife (CK).

Historically, CK was designed to be
a frameless, whole-body alternative to other
forms of cranial radiosurgery, which have been
in use since the late 1960s (Lasak and Gorecki
2009). The earlier technologies are based on
either the use of gamma radiation produced by
radioactive Cobalt 60 in the case of Gamma
Knife® (Elekta AB, Stockholm, Sweden) or X-rays
by conventional linear accelerators (cf. ▶ Linear
Accelerators). These technologies use small-
diameter, cylindrical collimators to produce
beamlets of radiation. They rely on a
frame screwed into the cranium to establish
a stereotactic coordinate system. This coordinate
system allows users to accurately register the location of a malignant or benign tumor in the brain
to the geometry of the treatment machine. The
introduction of the stereotactic frame significantly improved the accuracy of the treatment
delivery over the conventional radiotherapy
methods available at the time. The improved
spatial accuracy provided by stereotaxy allowed
practitioners to deliver higher single doses of
radiation to the tumor, with significantly lower
doses to the adjacent normal tissues than had
been previously possible.

The robotic radiosurgery system consists of
a megavoltage linear accelerator (linac) (cf.
▶ Linear Accelerators) attached to a robot that
delivers very precise, noncoplanar, non-
isocentric beams of X-rays to a specified target
volume. The incorporation of a precise image
guidance system allows for submillimeter target
accuracy without the use of head frames or other
immobilization devices. Furthermore, robotic
radiosurgery is not confined to intracranial
applications, but is widely used for the treatment
of extracranial targets, for example, lung, prostate, spine, pancreas, liver, and head and neck
(cf. ▶ Stereotactic Radiosurgery – Extracranial).
It can be effectively applied to treatment of tissue

targets anywhere in the body, as long as the target can be accurately visualized and contoured on a volumetric imaging study, for example, CT, MRI, PET/CT, or 3D angiography (cf. ▶ Imaging in Oncology). Finally, because there is no frame, robotic radiosurgery readily allows for multifraction (multistage) treatments to be delivered. For most anatomic sites, practitioners believe that multi-fraction treatments are advantageous from a radiobiological perspective (Tubiana 1988).

Treatment Overview

Once a patient is deemed to be a candidate for robotic radiosurgery, image data sets are acquired for treatment planning. As with most radiotherapy planning, the primary dataset must be a CT dataset due to the correspondence between the CT numbers for a volume of interest (VOI) and its electron density. If CT does not provide sufficient information for the practitioner to contour the target volume(s) and adjacent organs at risk (OARs) confidently, then other imaging modalities, for example, MRI, PET/CT, and 3D angiography, are obtained (cf. ▶ Imaging in Oncology). The data sets are imported into the treatment planning system, and automatically fused (cf. ▶ Conformal Therapy: Treatment Planning, Treatment Delivery and Clinical Results). The CT coordinate system is registered to the robot coordinate system in one of the several manners specific to the treatment site (tracking methods for different disease sites will be discussed in detail later in this article). With the aid of the fused data sets, the practitioner contours the volume to be targeted, as well as the surrounding normal structures to which radiation dose should be limited. The treatment planner specifies mathematical constraints on dose to the VOIs in order to calculate an optimized array of beam angles and weights to achieve the desired dose distribution. A typical treatment plan on the robotic radiosurgery unit requires 100–300 noncoplanar, non-isocentric beams to deliver a dose distribution that conforms highly to the 3D shape of the target(s), while keeping the dose to the OARs below toxic dose levels. Isocentric planning is also available with the system, and is useful for spherical target volumes. Because robotic radiosurgery does not require a frame, imaging and planning can be performed on the days prior to the treatment. Stereotactic radiosurgery systems that rely on rigidly attached frames require that frame placement, imaging, planning, and treatment be done on the same day.

When the patients arrive for their first treatment fraction, they lie on the treatment couch. An initial pair of stereotactic images is acquired using the X-ray tubes on the ceiling and image detectors flush with the floor. The couch is moved in six directions (three translations and three rotations) to place the patient in approximately the same position as he was during the CT study. The final corrections for translations and angles are accomplished by the image guidance system (cf. ▶ Image Guided Radiation Therapy (IGRT) – kV Imaging) feeding back angular and translational corrections to the robot, which adjusts the aim of the MV X-ray beam to correct for these variations. Treatment is initiated and the robot moves the linac around the patient under computer control, stopping to deliver a precise dose from those optimized trajectory angles determined in the treatment plan. Throughout treatment, the image guidance system continues to acquire images and feedback corrections to the robot. The couch remains stationary during treatment. In this way, each beam intersects the target at the precise point specified by the treatment plan, even if the target is moving. Treatment can be interrupted by the operator at any time, and resumed when ready. Treatment times on the CK have been reduced significantly over the years through the introduction of technical refinements. With the current system, treatment times, including setup and imaging, generally range from 20 to 45 min per session.

R

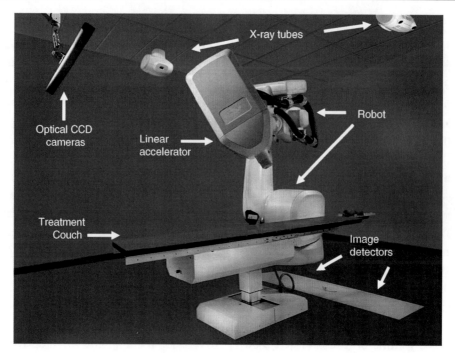

Robotic Radiosurgery. Fig. 1 Typical robotic radiosurgery (Accuray CyberKnife) room showing the elements of the treatment delivery system (linear accelerator and robot) and of the image guidance system (ceiling-mounted x-ray tubes, in-floor image detectors, and CCD camera array in ceiling-mounted boom)

Hardware System Overview

Linear Accelerator

A typical treatment room is depicted in Fig. 1. The linear accelerator (cf. ▶ Linear Accelerators) is a compact, 6-MV, standing-wave, side-coupled accelerating waveguide that does not have a flattening filter or any bending magnets. Microwave power is supplied by an X-band cavity magnetron. As with conventional medical linacs, dose is quantified through the use of two independent downstream monitor ionization chambers, sealed to the atmosphere. The current version produces 1,000 monitor units per minute, which corresponds to 1,000 cGy per minute at 80 cm from the source. Beam size is set by a secondary collimation system. The user can opt to use one or more fixed collimators or a motor-controlled variable collimator (called the Iris® collimator). The fixed collimators are divergent and made of

tungsten. They range in diameter from 5 to 60 mm, measured at 80 cm from the source. The Iris collimator consists of two divergent hexagonal tungsten collimator banks. One bank sits on top of the other and is rotated 15° relative to the lower bank, creating an effective beam aperture that is 12-sided. This dodecagon approximates a circle, mimicking the fixed circular collimators in shape and size. A single motor controls the aperture of both banks, making the system mechanically simpler than a conventional multileaf collimator with dozens of individual motors. The reproducibility of the Iris aperture size is 0.2 mm (Echner et al. 2009).

Robot

The linac is attached to a KR240-2 robot (Kuka Roboter GmbH, Augsburg, Germany). The manufacturer's specification for position repeatability is 0.12 mm. The robot has six joints which provide a great deal of geometric flexibility. In principle, the robot could position and angle the linac virtually anywhere in a wide workspace around the patient. In reality, however, a finite number of nodes (positions in the room at which the robot is allowed to place the linac target) is established for each installation in order to make the mathematical optimization problem manageable. Although finite, a large number of beam positions and angles is available during the treatment planning process. For a typical installation, approximately 5,000 beam orientations are available. For patient (and machine) safety, the robot is pre-programmed to walk specific "paths" from node to node. Different path sets are provided with the machine that are designed to provide a large number of noncoplanar beam angles for both extra- and intracranial targets. Robot path selection is done by the practitioner during treatment planning.

Imaging System Hardware

The imaging system consists of two kilovoltage (kV) X-ray tubes (cf. ▶ Image Guided Radiation Therapy (IGRT) – kV Imaging) rigidly attached to the vault ceiling and two image detectors embedded in the floor. A third element of the imaging system is a set of three optical charge-coupled device (CCD) cameras attached to a boom at the end of the couch. These cameras are used when treating lesions that move with respiration and will be discussed later in the article. The X-ray tubes are aligned such that the central axis of each X-ray field is at 45° to the vertical, and their center lines intersect at 90° to each other at the "reference point" of the room geometry. To obtain true stereoscopic images, the tubes are controlled to fire simultaneously. The robot is calibrated to the room reference point for each installation. The kV X-ray field size at the plane of the reference point is 15 × 15 cm. The image detectors consist of cesium iodide scintillators deposited on amorphous silicon photo-diodes. They generate images with 1,024 × 1,024, 16-bit resolution. The fixed geometry of the imaging system allows for stereoscopic reconstruction of the patient geometry relative to the room geometry and the robot coordinate system. During treatment, imaging frequency can be set by the operator or modulated by a computer which adapts the imaging frequency based on the magnitude of the detected motion of the target.

Other Hardware

Much of the robotic radiosurgery system hardware is housed in a room close to, but separated from, the treatment vault. This includes all of the electronics associated with the linac and the robot, as well as the central database computer, image guidance computer, motion tracking computer, robot computer, associated communication links, X-ray tube generators, a chiller/gas controller, and a power conditioner. Treatment planning computers are located separately and networked to the central database computer. The operator's station contains a simple control module, as well as two computer monitors, which allow for visual monitoring of all aspects of the treatment as it progresses. One monitor displays and plots the translational and angular motion corrections against time, as well as live images with their associated digitally reconstructed radiographs (DRRs). A second monitor displays plots and data related to the motion tracking accuracy and modeling for targets that move with respiration. Finally, the control console has equipment which provides real-time visual monitoring and audio communication with the patient.

Treatment Delivery Methodologies

As shown in Table 1, there are five different tracking methods available on the robotic radiosurgery system that enable the system to detect and correct for motion throughout treatment. Each method is

Robotic Radiosurgery. Table 1 Tracking methodologies for robotic radiosurgery

Method	Clinical sites	Requirements
Fiducial tracking	Soft tissues, e.g., prostate, bladder, head and neck, extremities	Implanted fiducial markers
Skull tracking	Brain and other tissues that move rigidly with cranium	No frame, no fiducial markers
Spine tracking	Cervical, thoracic and lumbar spine, and tissues that move rigidly with spine	No frame, no fiducial markers
Respiratory motion tracking with fiducial markers (Synchrony)	Selected lung lesions, liver, kidney (organs that move with respiration)	Implanted fiducial markers
Respiratory motion tracking without fiducial markers (X-Sight Lung)	Selected lung lesions visible on real-time images	No frame, no fiducial markers

premised on knowing how the position and orientation of the target at any point in time compares with the target position and orientation on the treatment planning CT study. For this purpose, DRRs are generated by the treatment planning system, which uses the volumetric CT data to generate planar radiographs of patient anatomy taken under the geometric conditions of the treatment room kV X-ray imaging system. In this way, the target in the CT reference frame can be registered to the room coordinate system. Since the image guidance system is calibrated to the room coordinate system, information from the live in-room images obtained before and during treatment can be compared with the DRRs. Using the

methods described below, the differences in the location and orientation of the target in real time and the location and orientation of the target in the CT dataset can be precisely determined. These translational and angular differences are fed back to the robot, which then corrects the aim of the MV X-ray beam, so that it hits the target precisely according to the treatment plan.

For all of the tracking methods, initial setup of the patient is managed by a radiation therapist, using the image guidance system from the control console. The therapist obtains an initial pair of images, these images are compared with the DRRs, and angular and translational differences are calculated (see Fig. 2). Then the therapist activates the couch to move to make the necessary corrections, and another pair of live images is obtained. Once the patient is approximately aligned such that corrections are within the robot's ability to correct for them, the treatment is initiated. The couch remains stationary, and all motion correction is accomplished by the robot during the treatment. Typically, images are acquired every 15–30 s, with the robot responding to any target motion changes in approximately 1 s. If a motion occurs that exceeds the robot's ability to safely make the correction, then the operator may need to realign the patient using remotely controlled couch motion. In practice, this intervention is rarely needed unless the patient coughs or sneezes, or makes a large shift in position.

Fiducial Tracking

Fiducial tracking is used when there is insufficient contrast in the live image for the target to be reliably tracked without intervention, for example, when treating the prostate gland (cf. ▶ Prostate). It requires the implantation of radio-opaque fiducial markers in, or close to, the target volume. Commonly, gold seeds are used (approximately 1 mm in diameter and 5 mm long), although other markers have been used too. A minimum

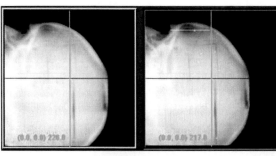
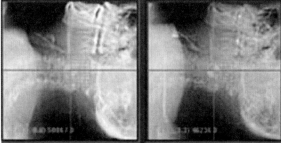

6D Skull Tracking

Xsight® Spine Tracking System

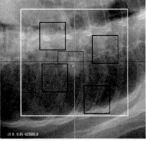
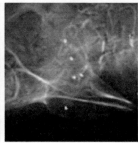
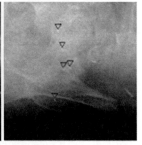

Xsight® Lung Tracking System

Fiducial Marker Tracking

Robotic Radiosurgery. Fig. 2 Examples of digitally reconstructed radiographs (*left*) compared with live X-ray images (*right*) using different CyberKnife tracking methods

of three markers is required to detect rotations as well as translations. Markers are usually implanted percutaneously under image guidance; for lung tumors (cf. ▶ Lung), bronchoscopic placement is also used. Generally, practitioners allow 1 week between implantation of the fiducials and the acquisition of the planning CT to assure marker stabilization in tissue. During treatment, the system uses the 6D coordinates of the markers as a surrogate for the location of the target. Registration is accomplished based on extraction of the fiducial locations in the live X-ray images with the corresponding DRR positions. Rigid body geometry is used to determine the positional and angular differences between the location of the markers in the DRRs and the live images to achieve submillimeter targeting accuracy.

Skull Tracking

Skull tracking is used for the treatment of intracranial targets (cf. ▶ Stereotactic Radiosurgery – Cranial), as well as head and neck targets

(cf. ▶ Eye and Orbit, ▶ Nasal Cavity and Paranasal Sinuses, ▶ Nasopharynx, ▶ Oro-Hypopharynx), which can be considered to have a fixed position relative to the skull. Like fiducial tracking, it assumes rigid body geometry. In this method, the live X-ray images are registered to the DRRs using the high-contrast information from the bones and sinuses. One can infer two translational and two rotational offsets from each X-ray image pair. Then a 3D back-projection of the 2D results provides three translational corrections, as well as pitch and yaw. To obtain the roll correction, hundreds of DRRs with different degrees of roll are calculated prior to treatment. These are compared with the live images to obtain an estimate of roll. This information is folded back into the back-projection calculation, and the process is iterated until an accurate 6D transformation is determined. Skull tracking has been demonstrated to reliably achieve its submillimeter specification (Antypas and Pantelis 2008; Fu and Kuduvalli 2008).

Spine Tracking

Spine tracking with the Xsight® Spine Tracking System is used to track targets in or near skeletal structures without the need to implant fiducial markers (cf. ▶ Spinal Canal Tumor). Rigid body geometry cannot be assumed to apply to the spine because the vertebrae can move independent of one another. However, submillimeter targeting accuracy is especially needed in paraspinal targets because of the proximity of the spinal cord. Therefore, a method has been developed which noninvasively registers nonrigid bony anatomy landmarks in the live image to the same landmarks in the DRRs. In this application, both the DRRs and the live images are electronically enhanced through the use of edge and contrast enhancement filters. Registration uses a region of interest (ROI) that covers about three vertebrae. A 9 × 9 rectilinear grid is overlaid onto the registration ROI. The places where grid lines cross are called "nodes." The scheme looks at the image intensity distribution in the vicinity of each node in the DRR images and searches for a similar local intensity distribution in the live image. A set of 2D displacement vectors is determined for each image, which provides a nonrigid transformation from the live image to the DRR image. The 3D translations and rotations are computed from the two 2D displacement fields. The roll angle needs to be approximated and iterated, as it was for skull tracking, based on a pre-computed library of DRRs with different degrees of roll (Muacevic et al. 2006).

Respiratory Motion Tracking

The tracking of targets that move with respiration, for example, lesions in lungs (cf. ▶ Lung), liver (cf. ▶ Liver and Hepatobiliary Tract), pancreas, or kidney (cf. ▶ Kidney), is accomplished without the need for the patient to hold their breath or for the treatment beam to be "gated" on and off. The treatment beam is moved dynamically, following tumor motion in real time.

Both forms of respiratory tracking described below require optical markers, that is, light-emitting diodes (LEDs), to be placed on the patient's chest during treatment. To facilitate the placement of these external markers, the patient wears a spandex vest that has Velcro strips for easy placement of the LEDs. The real-time motion of the light from the LEDs is observed by three CCD cameras mounted in a boom above the edge of the treatment couch (See Fig. 1). By taking a series of kV images at different points in the respiratory cycle at the start of treatment, the location of the lesion (derived from the stereotactic kV images) can be correlated to the location of the LEDs. The correlation model fits the tumor location to the simultaneous location of the LED markers. Separate functions are automatically fitted to inhalation and exhalation phases to account for motion hysteresis or phase shifts between internal and external motions. During treatment, the robot aims the linac beam at the target based on the position of the LEDs, with the location of the target being inferred from the correlation model. The correlation model is checked for accuracy and recalculated after each new image acquisition using the 15 most recently acquired live images (using a first-in, first-out approach). In this way, if there is a systematic change in the patient's breathing pattern during a treatment session, the correlation model will adapt to the change.

Respiratory Motion Tracking with Fiducial Markers (Synchrony®)

Synchrony® (Accuray) motion tracking is used when treating a lesion that moves with respiration that is either not in the lung (e.g., in the liver, pancreas, kidney) or is in the lung but not of sufficient size and/or density to be reliably identified by the image guidance system without the use of fiducial markers. For these cases, radio-opaque markers are implanted percutaneously or transbronchially into and/or near the target.

Just as in fiducial tracking, the image guidance system identifies the locations of the fiducials in each of the live orthogonal images, compares them with the marker locations in the DRRs, and determines the location of the target in the live images. These data are correlated with the LED positions to create the correlation model. The accuracy of this tracking method is <1.5 mm (Hoogeman et al. 2009).

Respiratory Motion Tracking Without Fiducial Markers (Xsight® Lung)

Xsight® Lung Tracking (XLT) (Accuray) is used when a lung lesion can be reliably identified in each of the live images. The ability to identify the lesion in the images depends on whether there is sufficient contrast between the lesion and the tissue surrounding it. The contrast, in turn, depends primarily on the size and location of the tumor in the lung. Lesions that are >15 mm and surrounded by normal lung tissue are the most likely candidates for this form of tracking. The image intensity pattern of the tumor in two DRRs is matched to the most similar region in the corresponding live images in order to determine the location of the tumor in real time. By correlating the tumor location with the LED locations as described above, direct tracking of the moving target is accomplished.

In practice, XLT tracking begins by globally aligning the patient using spine tracking (described above). This assures that the patient's global alignment on the treatment couch matches the alignment during the treatment planning CT study. Once this alignment is achieved, the couch automatically moves to place the centroid of the lung lesion (based on its location relative to the spine on the planning CT) at the room reference point. The system acquires a series of images at different points in the respiratory cycle. Automatic timing of the X-ray acquisitions ensures a uniform sampling over the entire respiratory cycle. The control console displays the location of the lesion in the live images, as well as in the DRRs, as it has been identified by the system. The practitioner reviews the images, and if it is ascertained that the images of the tumor are accurately identified, then the correlation model between the tumor and LED marker locations is developed as described above.

Lung-Optimized Treatment (LOT)

While Xsight Lung tracking requires the visibility of the tumor in both orthogonal live images, a recently developed refinement allows for fiducial-free tracking of lung tumors that are visible in only one of the live images, or even in neither of them. The one-view approach extracts tumor motion information that is available from the single-view image, combines it with information from previously acquired full-inhalation and full-exhalation CT scans, and advises the user on how much to expand margins to account for the missing location information. Because LOT has not yet been released for clinical use, further description will be left for a future article.

Treatment Planning

As with other contemporary treatment planning systems, the robotic radiosurgery treatment planning process consists of six steps: image acquisition, image fusion, delineation of VOIs, specification of dosimetric goals, mathematical optimization to achieve those goals, and plan evaluation.

(a) Image acquisition

A thin-slice volumetric CT scan is required for all cases. Up to three additional imaging data sets can be imported in order to assist the practitioner with contouring and plan evaluation. These data sets may be from any DICOM compliant modality, for example, MRI, PET, PET/CT, 3D angiography, or a different CT scan (e.g., with contrast). Naturally, high-resolution and high-quality images are needed to achieve submillimeter delivery accuracy.

(b) Image Fusion

Image fusion is accomplished by any of the three methods: automatic maximization of mutual information, semiautomatic point-to-point landmark registration, or manual registration.

(c) Target Delineation

Contouring of target volume(s) and OARs can be performed on any of the fused data sets and in any of the three principle planes (axial, sagittal, or coronal). An automatic segmentation option for pelvic anatomy has been made available recently, and a similar upgrade for the cranial anatomy has been announced to be released soon. Automatic segmentation is based on a shape model-based segmentation algorithm.

(d) Specification of Dosimetric Goals

As with most inverse planning systems, the planner must specify dosimetric goals that are either required to be achieved or are desirable to achieve. Depending upon which dose algorithm is used, dosimetric goals for target volumes can be specified as a combination of maximum dose, minimum dose, mean dose, and dose–volume limits. For OARs, the planner can specify maximum dose, mean dose, and dose–volume constraints. In addition, the planner specifies the maximum total number of monitor units that may be used for the plan, the maximum number of monitor units per beam, and the maximum number of monitor units per node. The number of monitor units (per plan, per beam, per node) is set by the planner for each case. It is used to reduce the probability of high dose "fingers" corresponding to too many monitor units per beam or per node from occurring in the plan. Treatment time per fraction depends in part on the total number of monitor units the planner allows.

(e) Mathematical Optimization

A variety of optimization algorithms are available for selection including Simplex, Sequential, and Monte Carlo Optimization (cf. ▶ Dose Calculation Algorithms). These have been described in detail elsewhere (Dieterich and Gibbs 2011; Heilbrun 2005). The most commonly used optimization algorithm is Sequential Optimization. There are two dose calculation algorithms available to the planner: ray-tracing and Monte Carlo. Ray tracing (also known as effective path length) includes a crude (1D) heterogeneity correction and obliquity correction for each beam. The Monte Carlo algorithm, as implemented on the CK system, is very time-efficient (typically achieving 2% uncertainty in 5 min). It has been described in detail by Deng et al. (2003). Dose optimization can be done using either ray tracing or Monte Carlo dose algorithm.

Once an acceptable dose distribution has been obtained, the system provides tools that allow for reduction of treatment time without compromising plan quality. These are called "Beam Reduction" and "Time Reduction."

(f) Evaluation

Common tools for plan evaluation are available, including visual evaluation of normalized or absolute dose distributions throughout any of the 3D datasets, dose–volume histograms (DVHs), tabular dose values, treatment time, conformality indices, and homogeneity index (cf. ▶ Radiation Oncology Physics). As of this writing, the practitioner has the ability to directly compare two treatment plans side by side, with all of their associated DVHs and dose indices.

Summary

Robotic radiosurgery enables radiation dose delivery with high geometric accuracy for both intracranial and extracranial lesions without the use of rigid immobilization. Precise spatial accuracy is made possible through the implementation of sophisticated image guidance techniques that detect and quantify any motion of the targeted tissue. This information is fed to a robot which changes the aim of the therapeutic linac beams to correct for target motion throughout the treatment session. A typical treatment session consists of 100–300 independent non-isocentric, noncoplanar beams, which produce dose distributions that conform tightly to the shape of the target tissue, while sharp gradients outside the target volume keep the dose to the surrounding normal tissues low.

Cross-References

► Conformal Therapy: Treatment Planning, Treatment Delivery, and Clinical Results
► Dose Calculation Algorithms
► Eye and Orbit
► Image-Guided Radiation Therapy (IGRT): kV Imaging
► Imaging in Oncology
► Kidney
► Linear Accelerators (LINAC)
► Liver and Hepatobiliary Tract
► Lung
► Nasal cavity and Paranasal sinuses
► Nasopharynx
► Oro-Hypopharynx
► Prostate
► Radiation Oncology Physics
► Spinal Canal Tumor
► Stereotactic Radiosurgery – Cranial
► Stereotactic Radiosurgery: Extracranial

References

Antypas C, Pantelis E (2008) Performance evaluation of a CyberKnife G4 image-guided robotic stereotactic radiosurgery system. Phys Med Biol 53:4697–4718

Deng J, Ma CM, Hai J et al (2003) Commissioning 6 MV photon beams of a stereotactic radiosurgery system for Monte Carlo treatment planning. Med Phys 30:3124–3134

Dieterich S, Gibbs IC (2011) The CyberKnife in clinical use: current roles, future expectations. Front Radiat Ther Oncol 43:181–194

Echner GG, Kilby W, Lee M et al (2009) The design, physical properties and clinical utility of an iris collimator for robotic radiosurgery. Phys Med Biol 54:5359–5380

Fu D, Kuduvalli G (2008) A fast, accurate, and automatic 2D-3D image registration for image-guided cranial radiosurgery. Med Phys 35:2180–2194

Heilbrun MP (2005) CyberKnife radiosurgery – a practical guide. CyberKnife Society Press, Sunnyvale

Hoogeman M, Prevost JB, Nuyttens J et al (2009) Clinical accuracy of the respiratory tumor tracking system of the CyberKnife: assessment by analysis of log files. Int J Radiat Oncol Biol Phys 74:297–303

Lasak JM, Gorecki JP (2009) The history of stereotactic radiosurgery and radiotherapy. Otolaryngol Clin North Am 42:593–599

Muacevic A, Staehler M, Drexler C et al (2006) Technical description, phantom accuracy, and clinical feasibility for fiducial-free frameless real-time image-guided spinal radiosurgery. J Neurosurg Spine 5:303–312

Tubiana M (1988) Repopulation in human tumors. A biological background for fractionation in radiotherapy. Acta Oncol 27:83–88

Round Blue-Cell Tumors

Brandon J. Fisher[1], Larry C. Daugherty[2]
[1]Department of Radiation Oncology, College of Medicine, Drexel University, Philadelphia, PA, USA
[2]Department of Radiation Oncology, College of Medicine, Drexel University, Glenside, PA, USA

Definition

Round blue-cell tumors are tumors, including acute leukemia, Ewing's sarcoma, small cell mesothelioma, neuroblastoma, primitive neuroectodermal tumors, Wilms' tumor, desmoplastic small round blue cell tumors, and rhabdomyosarcoma, which share the histological appearance of small, round, blue malignant cells.

Cross-References

► Neuroblastoma

S

Salivary Gland Cancer

Lindsay G. Jensen, Loren K. Mell
Center for Advanced Radiotherapy Technologies,
Department of Radiation Oncology, San Diego
Rebecca and John Moores Cancer Center,
University of California, La Jolla, CA, USA

Definition/Description

Salivary gland cancer is a rare malignancy that can occur in the major or minor salivary glands. Most salivary gland cancers occur in the parotid gland and present as a painless mass. Salivary cancers are a histologically diverse group of tumors with varying prognosis and treatment according to grade, histology, tumor extent, and stage. Treatment is primarily surgical, with postoperative radiotherapy reserved for patients with poor prognostic factors. Radiotherapy alone may be used for the treatment of inoperable tumors. Chemotherapy is not currently used in the initial management of stage I–III salivary gland cancer, but is commonly used to treat recurrent and metastatic salivary gland tumors.

Anatomy

The salivary glands consist of three paired major salivary glands: the parotid, submandibular, and sublingual glands as well as minor salivary glands.

The parotid glands are the largest salivary glands. They are situated posterior and superficial to the ramus of the mandible and masseter muscle, anterior to the sternocleidomastoid muscle and the mastoid process, inferior to the zygomatic arch, superior to the angle of the mandible, and deep to the platysma muscle. The facial and auriculotemporal nerves, the external carotid artery, and the retromandibular vein pass through the parotid gland (Carlson and Ord 2009).

The blood supply to the parotid glands is from small branches of the external carotid artery. Venous drainage is to the retromandibular veins. Primary lymphatic drainage occurs within intraparotid nodes and to the superior cervical (level II–III) nodes. Parasympathetic fibers from the glossopharyngeal nerve synapse in the otic ganglion and travel with the auriculotemporal nerve to innervate the parotids. Sympathetic fibers to the parotids arise in the superior cervical sympathetic ganglion and also travel with the auriculotemporal nerve.

The submandibular glands consist of two smaller continuous lobes: a superficial lobe in the submandibular triangle of the neck, and a deep lobe in the floor of the mouth. The blood supply to the submandibular glands is from the facial and lingual arteries. Lymphatic drainage is to the submandibular (level IB) nodes and deep cervical nodes (level II). Parasympathetic fibers to the submandibular gland travel with the chorda tympani branch of cranial nerve VII nerve and synapse in the submandibular ganglion.

The sublingual glands are located in the floor of the mouth, between the mylohyoid muscle and the mucous membrane. Minor salivary glands are distributed throughout the aerodigestive tract, including the oral cavity, pharynx, and paranasal sinuses (Carlson and Ord 2009).

L.W. Brady, T.E. Yaeger (eds.), *Encyclopedia of Radiation Oncology*, DOI 10.1007/978-3-540-85516-3,
© Springer-Verlag Berlin Heidelberg 2013

Epidemiology

Salivary gland cancer is uncommon, making up <5% of head and neck cancers (Garden 2010; Terhaard 2008). Annual incidence worldwide is between 0.4 and 2.6/100,000 (Terhaard 2008). The majority of salivary gland tumors arise within the parotid gland and are benign. Although women are more likely than men to have benign salivary gland tumors, the incidence of malignant tumors in men and women is equal. The incidence of salivary gland tumors increases with age. Mean age of diagnosis for malignant tumors is 54 (Terhaard 2008).

Environmental risk factors include radiation. Alcohol use may or may not be a risk factor for salivary gland cancer (Garden 2010; Terhaard 2008), but does not appear to be as significant as for other head and neck cancers (Laurie 2010). Tobacco is not known to be a risk factor for salivary gland cancers but is a risk factor for some benign tumors of the salivary gland, particularly ▶ Warthin's tumor (Laurie 2010). Genetic influence on salivary gland cancer is not well understood, but salivary gland cancer is more common in Inuit populations, which may be related to ▶ Epstein-Barr virus (Carlson and Ord 2009) or a diet low in vitamins A and C (Terhaard 2008). Certain occupations including hairdressing (Swanson and Burns 1997), employment in the rubber industry, and exposure to nickel (Horn-Ross et al. 1997) appear to be associated with increased risk of salivary gland cancer.

Pathology

Cytopathology of salivary gland tumors is complex, with >40 types by WHO classification (Terhaard 2008). Tumors of the sublingual and minor salivary glands are much more likely to be malignant (>50%) than submandibular (~50%) or parotid tumors (<25%) (Terhaard 2008; Carlson and Ord 2009). Pleomorphic adenomas make up 50% of all salivary gland tumors and are the most common benign tumors in the major and minor glands.

Tumors of many histologies can arise in salivary glands, including carcinomas, lymphomas, sarcomas, and metastases. Major histologies include ▶ mucoepidermoid carcinoma, ▶ adenoid cystic carcinoma, acinic cell carcinoma, adenocarcinoma, carcinoma ex pleomorphic adenoma, and squamous cell carcinoma. Mucoepidermoid carcinoma is the most common type of malignant salivary gland cancer in the parotid gland, but adenoid cystic carcinoma is the most common type for the submandibular and minor salivary glands (Terhaard 2008; Garden 2010). Squamous cell carcinomas in the salivary glands are most often metastases from a skin or head/neck primary. True primary squamous carcinomas of the salivary glands are rare (Carlson and Ord 2009).

Clinical Presentation

Major salivary gland tumors most commonly present as an enlarging mass. Up to 25% of malignant parotid gland tumors present as facial palsy as a result of facial nerve invasion (Terhaard 2008). The clinical presentation of minor salivary gland cancers depends on location, but the majority of minor salivary gland tumors are intraoral and present as a painless mass (Terhaard 2008). Pain is less commonly a presenting symptom of salivary gland cancer and may indicate a poorer prognosis (Garden 2010). Metastases are rare at presentation but are most common to lung, bone, and liver (Terhaard 2008).

Differential Diagnosis

Differential diagnosis for salivary gland mass includes sebaceous or dermoid cysts, obstructive disease such as salivary gland calculi, salivary cysts, cysts of the first branchial cleft, salivary gland stones, sarcoid, ▶ Sjögren's syndrome, secondary tumor metastases (e.g., squamous cell skin cancer, kidney, breast, and lung), lymphoepithelial cysts (particularly in an immunocompromised host), chronic sclerosing sialadenitis (Küttner's tumor), and regional lymphadenopathy from infectious, inflammatory, or malignant diseases (Laurie 2010).

Diagnostic Evaluation

Evaluation of a suspected salivary gland tumor should begin with a careful history and physical examination. The physical should include palpation of the mass, palpation of cervical lymph nodes, evaluation of cranial nerves, and screening for signs of metastasis.

Ultrasound can be used for initial evaluation of salivary gland tumors and also for guiding fine needle aspiration (FNA) for tissue diagnosis. Computed tomography (CT) and/or magnetic resonance imaging (MRI) are recommended for evaluating the extent of the tumor into surrounding structures. MRI has superior soft tissue definition relative to CT and is especially helpful for delineating tumor extent, margins, and soft tissue infiltration. CT may be superior for evaluating bone invasion. FDG-PET is not usually included in the workup of salivary gland cancers, but may be helpful in staging primary disease and detecting recurrence (Laurie 2010).

FNA is commonly used in diagnosing parotid and submandibular tumors. Sensitivity and specificity for malignancy by FNA are 80–90% and >90%, respectively (Terhaard 2008). Excisional biopsy is usually necessary to diagnose minor salivary gland tumors because they are frequently polymorphic (Terhaard 2008). Generally, no serum markers or other specific lab workup are recommended for salivary gland cancer.

Staging

Major salivary gland cancers are staged using the American Joint Committee on Cancer (AJCC) staging system, tumor, node, metastasis (TNM) staging system. T stage is dependent on the size and extent of the tumor. T1 tumors are ≤2 cm, T2 tumors are 2–4 cm, T3 tumors extend outside the gland, and T4 tumors invade skin, mandible, facial nerve, ear canal, base of skull, or pterygoid plates. N stage follows the standard system of most head and neck cancers according to size (≤3 cm, 3–6 cm, or >6 cm), multiplicity (0, 1, or >1), and presence of contralateral nodal involvement, which is rare. M1 indicates distant metastasis. Minor salivary gland cancers are staged according to their site of origin (Edge et al. 2009).

Treatment and Prognosis

At diagnosis, 35.9% of patients have stage I disease, 15.5% stage II, 4.6% stage III, 25.4% stage IV, and 18.5% unstaged (Piccirillo et al. 2007). Five-year survival rates for patients with stage I, II, III, and IV salivary gland cancer are approximately 96%, 77%, 73%, and 37%, respectively (Piccirillo et al. 2007). Distant metastasis at diagnosis is uncommon (Terhaard 2008). Poor prognostic factors include T3-4 disease, intermediate to high-grade histology, extraglandular extension, perineural or soft tissue invasion, lymph node involvement, and positive surgical margins.

Surgery: Surgery is the preferred mode of treatment for major and minor salivary gland tumors, with adjuvant postoperative radiotherapy reserved for patients at high risk of recurrence. For parotid tumors, surgical treatment usually consists of superficial or total parotidectomy. Techniques to monitor and preserve the facial nerve can usually be employed, unless the facial nerve is directly involved by tumor. For submandibular and minor salivary gland tumors, wide local excision of the tumor and gland is used. Depending on prognostic factors (in particular, high tumor grade), surgery may include selective or modified radical neck dissection to assess for presence of occult positive nodes. Local recurrence rates with surgery alone vary and depend on stage and other prognostic factors, but can be up to 40% for parotid, 60% for submandibular, and 65% for minor salivary gland tumors. Local recurrence after resection of benign pleomorphic adenoma occurs in <5% of cases (Terhaard 2008).

Chemotherapy: Chemotherapy has not been shown to be efficacious in the treatment of salivary gland cancer and should be reserved for recurrence, disease-related symptoms, and rapidly progressive disease (Lalami et al. 2006). Cisplatin is the most studied chemotherapeutic agent for salivary gland cancer, but combination chemotherapy (cisplatin, 5-fluorouracil, doxorubicin, cyclophosphamide) and docetaxel have also been administered in small series. Combination chemotherapy has had better response rates (50%) than cisplatin alone (20%). Presence of HER-2/Neu, VEGF, and EGFR receptors in salivary gland cancer presents the possibility for molecular targeted agents, some of which have been evaluated in small phase II studies. Further trials are needed to establish the role of molecular targeted agents in the treatment of salivary gland cancer (Lalami et al. 2006).

Radiotherapy: Postoperative radiotherapy should be considered for salivary gland tumors with intermediate or high grade, positive nodes, positive surgical margins, perineural invasion, extracapsular nodal extension, or for recurrent tumors. Adjuvant radiation has been shown in several retrospective studies to substantially increase local control for higher stages of disease (Terhaard 2008). One retrospective study of 498 patients treated with surgery with or without adjuvant radiotherapy found significantly improved local control at 10 years with adjuvant radiotherapy in patients with T3 or T4 disease (84% vs 18%), close resection margins (95% vs 55%), incomplete resection (82% vs 44%), bone invasion (86% vs 54%), and perineural invasion (88% vs 60%). No significant difference in 10-year local control was found for patients with T1 and T2 disease or complete resection (Terhaard

et al. 2005). No randomized trials have been conducted to determine the effect of postoperative radiation therapy specifically for salivary gland cancers. Low-grade tumors may be observed postoperatively, even when adverse features such as positive margins are present, due to their relatively indolent clinical course. Pleomorphic adenomas can also be treated with radiotherapy in the rare case that they recur after superficial parotidectomy. A series of 72 patients treated with 50–60 Gy for recurrent pleomorphic adenoma reported local control in 88% with median follow-up of 14 years (Barton et al. 1992).

Classical radiotherapy techniques may consist of either a wedged pair or opposed lateral fields – with or without a matched anterior low-neck field. Generally, contralateral neck irradiation is not necessary, as the risk of occult contralateral nodal metastasis and contralateral neck recurrence are rare. In some cases, a limited superficial target volume may be optimally treated with an en face electron beam. In the past 10–15 years, conformal radiotherapy techniques have gained greater usage, particularly intensity modulated radiation therapy (IMRT). In many cases, IMRT is superior to alternative techniques in sparing adjacent organs such as the mandible, cochlea, spinal cord, brain, and oropharynx (Terhaard et al. 2008).

Standard-risk target volumes for postoperative patients generally include the operative bed (including surgical scars and clips) and ipsilateral primary draining neck nodes (unless addressed surgically). Radiotherapy is usually delivered in standard fractionated doses of 2 Gy per day to 60 Gy over 6 weeks. For positive margins or gross residual disease, higher doses of 66 Gy (33 fractions) or 70 Gy (35 fractions), respectively, are recommended.

Radiation therapy alone is recommended for unresectable and/or unfavorably located tumors, such as massive major salivary gland tumors, or minor salivary gland tumors involving the naso-pharynx, base of skull, tongue base, hypopharynx, etc. For unresectable tumors, neutrons may provide superior locoregional control compared to photons due to their higher radiobiologic efficacy (Garden 2010); however, few centers offer this form of treatment.

Complications: ▶ Xerostomia is a common complication of surgery and radiation therapy for salivary tumors. Usually, the severity is modest since the contralateral major salivary glands can typically be spared from radiation. Tooth decay can result from poor salivary function, particularly in patients treated with radiation. The likelihood of facial nerve paralysis after surgery depends on facial nerve involvement and surgical approach (Carlson and Ord 2009). Gustatory sweating (▶ Frey's Syndrome), or sweating from a small area anterior to the ear with exposure to food or thoughts of food may occur in some patients after surgery as a result of parasympathetic nerves to the parotid gland innervating sweat gland of the overlying skin (Carlson and Ord 2009). ▶ Trismus can result from radiation to the muscles of mastication and temporomandibular joint (Terhaard 2008). Osteoradio-necrosis of the mandible is an uncommon but potentially severe late complication.

Cross-References

▶ Intensity Modulated Radiation Therapy (IMRT)
▶ Neutron Radiotherapy
▶ Principles of Chemotherapy
▶ Sarcomas of the Head and Neck

References

Barton J, Slevin NJ, Gleave EN (1992) Radiotherapy for pleomorphic adenoma of the parotid gland. Int J Radiat Oncol Biol Phys 22:925–928

Carlson ER, Ord RA (2009) Textbook and color atlas of salivary gland pathology: diagnosis and management. Wiley, Ames

Edge SB, Byrd DR, Compton CC et al (eds) (2009) AJCC cancer staging manual, 7th edn. Springer, New York

Garden A (2010) The salivary glands. In: Cox JD, Ang KK (eds) Radiation oncology, 9th edn. Mosby/Elsevier, Philadelphia

Horn-Ross PL, Ljung BM, Morrow M (1997) Environmental factors and the risk of salivary gland cancer. Epidemiology 8:414–419

Lalami Y, Vereecken P, Dequanter D et al (2006) Salivary gland carcinomas, paranasal sinus cancers and melanoma of the head and neck: an update about rare but challenging tumors. Curr Opin Oncol 18:258–265

Laurie SA (2010) In: Basow DS (ed) Salivary gland tumors: epidemiology, pathogenesis, evaluation, and staging. UpToDate, Waltham

Piccirillo JF, Costas I, Reichman ME (2007) Cancers of the head and neck. In: Ries LAG, Young JL, Keel GE et al. (eds) SEER survival monograph: cancer survival among adults: U.S. SEER program, 1988–2001, patient and tumor characteristics. National Cancer Institute, SEER Program, NIH, Bethesda

Swanson GM, Burns PB (1997) Cancers of the salivary gland: workplace risks among women and men. Ann Epidemiol 7:369–374

Terhaard CH (2008) Salivary Glands. In: Halperin EC, Perez CA, Brady LW (eds) Principles and practice of radiation oncology, 5th edn. Kluwer/Lippincott Williams & Wilkens, Philadelphia

Terhaard CH, Lubsen H, Rasch CR, Dutch head and neck oncology cooperative group et al (2005) The role of radiotherapy in the treatment of malignant salivary gland tumors. Int J Radiat Oncol Biol Phys 61:103–111

Salpingectomy

Christin A. Knowlton[1], Michelle Kolton Mackay[2]
[1]Department of Radiation Oncology, Drexel University, Philadelphia, PA, USA
[2]Department of Radiation Oncology, Marshfield Clinic, Marshfield, WI, USA

Definition

Salpingectomy is the surgical removal of the fallopian tubes. It is often performed in conjunction with an oophorectomy, together called a salpingoophorectomy, because of the organs' shared blood supply. The procedure can be done unilaterally or bilaterally. The most frequent surgical treatment for ovarian cancer is the total abdominal hysterectomy and bilateral salpingoophorectomy.

Cross-References
▶ Fallopian Tube
▶ Ovary

Salvage Treatment

FILIP T. TROICKI[1], JAGANMOHAN POLI[2]
[1]College of Medicine, Drexel University, Philadelphia, PA, USA
[2]Department of Radiation Oncology, College of Medicine, Drexel University, Philadelphia, PA, USA

Definition
Any additional treatment for cancer patients who failed a "standard" therapy.

Cross-References
▶ Early Stage Breast Cancer
▶ Gynecological Tumors
▶ Melanoma
▶ Primary Intracranial Neoplasms
▶ Sarcomas of the Head and Neck
▶ Stage 0 Breast Cancer

Sample

EDWARD J. GRACELY
Department of Epidemiology and Biostatistics, College of Medicine, Drexel University, Philadelphia, PA, USA

Definition
The data "in hand." Contrast to the population.

Cross-References
▶ Statistics and Clinical Trials

Sarcoma

CHRISTIN A. KNOWLTON[1], MICHELLE KOLTON MACKAY[2]
[1]Department of Radiation Oncology, Drexel University, Philadelphia, PA, USA
[2]Department of Radiation Oncology, Marshfield Clinic, Marshfield, WI, USA

Synonyms
Osteosarcoma; Soft tissue sarcoma

Definition
A sarcoma is a tumor that arises from connective tissue, including cartilage (chondrosarcoma), bone (osteosarcoma), fibrous tissue, and adipose/fat (liposarcoma). Tumors arising from muscle (rhabdosarcoma), nerves, and blood vessels also fall into this category. There are more than 50 different types of sarcomas, which may be benign or malignant. For low-grade sarcomas, surgery is the mainstay of treatment. Pre- or postoperative radiation therapy may play a role depending upon the grade of the tumor and the ability to obtain clear surgical margins. Chemotherapy may be offered, especially for high-grade sarcomas that have spread.

Cross-References
▶ Ewing's Sarcoma
▶ Kaposi's Sarcoma
▶ Leiomyosarcoma
▶ Rhabdomyosarcoma
▶ Sarcomas of the Head and Neck
▶ Soft Tissue Sarcoma

Sarcomas of the Head and Neck

CARLOS A. PEREZ, WADE L. THORSTAD
Department of Radiation Oncology, Siteman
Cancer Center, Washington University Medical
Center, St. Louis, MO, USA

Definition

A rare tumor of complex histologies occurring in the face, scalp, orbit, or paranasal sinuses within the head and neck region.

Sarcomas account for less than 1% of malignant neoplasms in the head and neck. The most frequent histological type is malignant fibrohistocytoma (29%), while the least common is liposarcoma (1%). Distribution of these sarcomas was 33% in the scalp or face, 26% in the orbit or paranasal sinuses, 14% arising from upper aerodigestive tract including larynx, and 27% in the neck. Synovial sarcomas are rare soft tissue in the head and neck region; they account for 3–5% of the soft tissue sarcomas. Radiation-induced sarcoma of the head and neck is a rare long-term complication of treatment. The rarity of this tumor is reflected in the very few series reported in the English language medical literature. When they do occur, most appear at least 10 years following radiation therapy. Possibility of a postirradiation sarcoma should be considered, whenever a suspicious lesion is seen, regardless of the amount of time that has passed since radiation therapy was administered. The original pathology should be reexamined to ensure that the original tumor was diagnosed correctly. Electron microscopy can be useful in differentiating sarcomatous-appearing epithelial lesions from true soft tissue sarcomas.

The incidence of radiation-induced sarcomas of the head and neck is likely to increase due to progressive aging of the population combined with improved survival in head and neck cancer patients. The period of latency between initial radiation therapy and diagnosis ranges from 9 to 45 years with a median of 17 years.

Clinical Presentation and Diagnostic Workup

Clinical presentation varies with the primary site of disease.

Tumors arising from the aerodigestive tract usually present with nasal bleeding, a palpable mass in the neck, or difficulty in swallowing or breathing. Of tumors arising from the base of skull or the nerve sheath, cranial nerve deficit is the most common presentation. Diagnostic workup follows that of soft tissue sarcomas of other sites in the body. MRI, especially with gadolinium contrast, may be used as a supplement or alternative to CT scanning. A CT scan of the chest is also mandatory for staging workup.

The American Joint Committee on Cancer (AJCC) staging system for soft tissue sarcomas is based on histologic grade, the tumor size and depth, and the presence of distant or nodal metastases. The staging system is the same as for sarcomas of other sites, although specific staging for head and neck sarcomas is not standardized (Colville et al. 2005).

Bentz et al. (2004) reviewed 111 head and neck sarcoma patients; median duration of follow-up was 51 months; the actuarial 5-year relapse-free, disease-specific, and overall survivals were 55%, 52%, and 44%, respectively.

In 109 soft tissue sarcomas of all sites, a French study demonstrated that quality of the surgery was one of the most important variables for predicting local recurrences. Tumor size, surgical margins, presence of tumor necrosis, and adequacy of the excision correlated with metastasis-free survival. In 57 patients with soft tissue sarcomas of the head and neck treated at

Massachusetts General Hospital, angiosarcoma had a considerably poorer prognosis than other histologies.

General Management

Surgery is the preferred initial treatment modality for sarcomas. Unfortunately, it is often difficult to achieve complete resection of the tumor, and a high recurrence rate has been observed with surgery alone. Extracapsular enucleation of the tumor results in 90% local recurrence because of the presence of microscopic pseudopodia, which tend to grow through the pseudocapsule into the surrounding tissue and the presence of skipped lesions some distance from the main tumor mass. Pathologic analysis of the surgical bed often discloses microscopic extension of tumor. The criteria for surgical resection are impractical for head and neck sarcomas because of anatomic limitations (Colville et al. 2005); wide local excision is rarely possible because the tumors extend beyond the confines of origin and in the proximity of vital neurovascular structures. Some retrospective studies have suggested improved local tumor control when combined surgery and external irradiation are used.

Radiation therapy, by external beam or brachytherapy, plays an important adjunctive role in the management, especially for tumors where en bloc resection with negative margin is not possible. Chemotherapy regimens for soft tissue neoplasms are primarily designed to improve local tumor control.

Radiation Therapy

A systematic review of radiation therapy trials was performed by The Swedish Council of Technology Assessment in Health Care (SBU) based on data from 39 scientific articles involving 4,579 patients (Strander et al. 2003). The results were compared with those of a similar overview from 1996 which included 3,344 patients. There was evidence that adjuvant radiation therapy improves local tumor control in combination with conservative surgery with negative, marginal, or minimal microscopic positive surgical margins. There is still insufficient data to establish that preoperative radiotherapy is favorable compared to postoperative radiotherapy in patients presenting primarily with large tumors. Preoperative irradiation results in more wound complications and delayed healing. There is no randomized study comparing external beam radiotherapy and brachytherapy. The data suggest that external beam radiotherapy and low-dose rate brachytherapy result in comparable local control for high-grade tumors. Some patients with low-grade soft tissue sarcomas benefit from external beam radiotherapy in terms of local tumor control. Brachytherapy with low- dose rate for low-grade tumors seems to be of no benefit, but data is sparse.

The general principles for radiation therapy of head and neck sarcomas are similar to those of soft tissue sarcomas. Complete coverage of the surgical bed and scar with adequate margins (3–5 cm) is required (Pellitteri et al. 2003). However, because of the proximity of critical and radiosensitive organs (eyes, spinal cord, brain stem), selecting optimal portal margins without seriously compromising the functioning of these organs is an art. Techniques similar to those used in epithelial tumors of the head and neck can be applied to sarcomas. In general, 55–60 Gy is needed for postoperative adjuvant irradiation, and an additional 10- to 15-Gy boost is recommended if the surgical margins are close (≤ 3 mm) or involved by tumor. Some institutions prefer preoperative irradiation of 45–50 Gy. Special attention should be directed to limiting the dose to critical structures.

Results of Therapy

In a retrospective report of 73 patients with sarcomas of the head and neck treated at Princess Margaret Hospital, the 5-year cause-specific survival was 62%, with a local recurrence rate of

41%, and a distant metastasis rate of 31%. Extension to adjacent structures, high-grade tumor, and tumor greater than 10 cm were associated with poor survival. Gross residual tumor after surgery was also associated with a high local recurrence rate (75%) despite the addition of radiation therapy. Patients with clear surgical margins or only microscopic involvement fared much more favorably and had a similar local tumor control rate (74% and 70%, respectively) with adjuvant irradiation. Colville et al. (2005) reported on 41 male and 19 female patients treated with head and neck soft tissue sarcomas, overall 5-year survival was 60%. With mean follow-up of almost 4 years, the 5-year local tumor control was 56% in the surgical and 40% in the nonsurgical group (more advanced and aggressive tumors). The 5-year survival was 70% and 40%, respectively.

Penel et al. (2004) in 28 adult head and neck soft tissue sarcomas recorded a 2-year overall survival of 56%. Barker et al. (2003) published a review of 44 patients diagnosed with nonmetastatic soft tissue sarcoma in a head and neck. The most common tumor histologies included malignant fibrous histiocytoma (15 patients), angiosarcoma (9 patients), fibrosarcoma (6 patients), and leiomyosarcoma (6 patients). The actuarial 5-year local tumor control was 55% and was highly correlated with the extent of surgical excision: 25% for subtotal resection/debulking, 65% for wide local excision, and 100% for radical resection. Local tumor control at 5 years was 60% for patients treated with both surgery and radiotherapy, 54% surgery alone, and 43% for radiation alone.

Rapidis et al. (2005) reported on 25 patients with head and neck sarcomas following up ranged from 8 to 144 months. Twenty-three patients were treated with surgery as the primary modality and 14 with surgery alone. Clear margins were obtained in all of them and local control was achieved in 12/13. The 5-year survival for the entire group was 40%. Farhood and coworkers (1990) in a review of

Sarcomas of the Head and Neck. Table 1 Treatment results of adult soft tissue sarcomas of the head and neck

Investigator	Number of patients	Modalities	5-year actuarial rates	
			Local control	Survival
Weber et al.	188	S, R, C	–	Overall: 49.4% <5 cm
			–	Overall: 30.4% ≥5 cm
Greager et al.	48	S, R, C	–	Disease free: 54%
Farhood et al.	176	S, R, C	–	Overall: 55%
McKenna et al.	16	S, R, C	75%	Disease free: 63%
Eeles et a1.	103[a]	S, R, C	47%	Overall: 50%
LeVay et al.	52	S, R, C	59%	Cause specific: 63%
Tran et al.	164	S, R, C	41%	Overall: 66%
Willers et al.	57	S, R, C	60%	Overall: 66%
Chao et al. (unpublished data)	33	S, R, C	49%	Disease free: 40%
Colville et al.	60	S, R, C	50%	60%

S surgery, *R* radiation therapy, *C* chemotherapy
[a]Series based on adults and children, excluding angiosarcomas

176 adult head and neck sarcomas, found that only 20% of the patients with high-grade tumors were alive 10 years after treatment,as opposed to 88% of patients with low-grade tumors. Greager and coworkers (1985) noted mean survival of 93 months in patients with low-grade tumors smaller than 5 cm versus 15 months for those with high-grade lesions larger than 5 cm. Weber and coworkers (1986) described a 45% 10-year survival rate for patients with tumors smaller than 5 cm versus 10% for those with tumors 5 cm or larger. Reported results of treatment of soft tissue sarcomas are summarized in Table 1.

Cross-References

▶ Esophageal Cancer
▶ Kaposi's Sarcoma
▶ Larynx
▶ Radiation-Induced Sarcoma
▶ Soft Tissue Sarcoma

References

Barker JL Jr, Paulino AC, Feeney S (2003) Locoregional treatment for adult soft tissue sarcomas of the head and neck: an institutional review. Cancer J 9:49–57

Bentz BG, Singh B, Woodruff J et al (2004) Head and neck soft tissue sarcomas: a multivariate analysis of outcomes. Ann Surg Oncol 11:619–28

Colville R, Charlton F, Kelly G et al (2005) Multidisciplinary management of head and neck sarcomas. Head Neck 27:814–824

Farhood A, Hajdu S, Shiu M et al (1990) Soft tissue sarcomas of the head and neck in adults. Am J Surg 160:365–369

Greager J, Patel M, Briele H et al (1985) Soft tissue sarcomas of the adult head and neck. Cancer 56:820–824

Pellitteri PK, Ferlito A, Bradley PJ et al (2003) Management of sarcomas of the head and neck in adults. Oral Oncol 39:2–12

Penel N, Van Haverbeke C, Lartigau E et al (2004) Head and neck soft tissue sarcomas of adult: prognostic value of surgery in multimodal therapeutic approach. Oral Oncol 40:890–7

Rapidis AD, Gakiopoulou H, Stevrianos SD et al (2005) Sarcomas of the head and neck. Results from the treatment of 25 patients. Eur J Surg Oncol 31:177–182

Strander H, Turesson I, Cavallin-Stahl E (2003) A systematic overview of radiation therapy effects in soft tissue sarcomas. Acta Oncol 42:516–31

Weber R, Benjamin R, Peters L et al (1986) Soft tissue sarcomas of the head and neck in adolescents and adults. Am J Surg 152:386–92

SBLA Syndrome

STEPHAN MOSE
Department of Radiation Oncology, Schwarzwald-Baar-Klinikum, Villingen-Schwenningen, Germany

Definition

This syndrome includes a variety of tumors: sarcoma, breast, lung, ACC, and other tumors.

Cross-References

▶ Carcinoma of the Adrenal Gland
▶ Soft Tissue Sarcoma

SBRT

▶ Stereotactic Body Radiation Therapy
▶ Stereotactic Radiosurgery: Extracranial

Schistosoma haematobium

CHRISTIAN WEISS, CLAUS ROEDEL
Department of Radiotherapy and Radiation Oncology, University Hospital Frankfurt/Main, Frankfurt, Germany

Definition

Schistosomiasis (also known as bilharzia, bilharziosis, or snail fever) is a parasitic disease caused by several species of fluke of the genus *Schistosoma*. The urinary form of schistosomiasis is associated with increased risks for squamous cell cancer of the bladder in adults.

Cross-References
▶ Bladder

Scrotal Shielding

JOHANNES CLASSEN
Department of Radiation Oncology,
St. Vincentius-Kliniken Karlsruhe,
Karlsruhe, Germany

Definition
Lead shielding to reduce scattered radiation to the testes.

Cross-References
▶ Testes

Secondary Tumor Induction

JOHANNES CLASSEN
Department of Radiation Oncology, St.
Vincentius-Kliniken Karlsruhe, Karlsruhe,
Germany

Definition
Malignant tumor resulting from cancer treatment usually as a long-term sequalae from chemotherapy or radiotherapy.

Cross-References
▶ Bone Marrow Toxicity in Cancer Treatment
▶ Intensity Modulated Radiation Therapy (IMRT)

▶ Malignant Neoplasm Associated with Acquired Immunodeficiency Syndrome
▶ Neutron Radiotherapy
▶ Proton Therapy
▶ Radiation-Induced Genomic Instability and Radiation Sensitivity
▶ Testes
▶ Total Body Irradiation (TBI)

Segment Weighting

▶ Forward-Planning

Senile Keratosis

▶ Actinic Keratosis

Sentinel Lymph Node

LYDIA T. KOMARNICKY-KOCHER
Department of Radiation Oncology, College of Medicine, Drexel University, Philadelphia, PA, USA

Definition
Sentinel lymph node is the theoretical first lymph node reached by metastasizing cancer cells from a primary tumor. Detected by sentinel lymph node biopsy which entails injecting a radioactive tracer and dye near the tumor and detecting the first draining lymph node(s) which are then pathologically sampled.

Cross-References
▶ Stage 0 Breast Cancer
▶ Melanoma

Serial Organ

JAMES H. BRASHEARS, III
Radiation Oncologist, Venice, FL, USA

Definition

A term from radiobiology that is based on an analogy with electrical circuits and can be contrasted with parallel organs. A serial organ, like the spinal cord, will lose function if a small length of the structure is sacrificed versus parallel organs that have redundancy built in and a certain fraction of the organ parenchyma (or functional subunits) can be sacrificed and the organ will maintain function.

Cross-References

▶ Palliation of Brain and Spinal Cord Metastases

Sezary Cells

CURT HEESE
Department of Radiation Oncology, Eastern Regional Cancer Treatment Centers of America, Philadelphia, PA, USA

Definition

Atypical T-cells in the peripheral blood that are the hallmark distinguishing finding of Sezary's syndrome in mycosis fungoides patients.

Cross-References

▶ Cutaneous T-Cell Lymphoma

Shimada Pathologic Classification System

BRANDON J. FISHER[1], LARRY C. DAUGHERTY[2]
[1]Department of Radiation Oncology, College of Medicine, Drexel University, Philadelphia, PA, USA
[2]Department of Radiation Oncology, College of Medicine, Drexel University, Glenside, PA, USA

Definition

A pathologic system which categorizes patients into favorable or unfavorable prognostic groups based upon age, amount of Schwann cell stroma, mitotic-karyorrhectic index, and histologic pattern.

Cross-References

▶ Neuroblastoma

Short-Term and Long-Term Health Risk of Nuclear Power Plant Accident

JOHN P. CHRISTODOULEAS[1], ROBERT D. FORREST[3], CHRISTOPHER G. AINSLEY[2], ZELIG TOCHNER[2], STEPHEN M. HAHN[2], ELI GLATSTEIN[2]
[1]The Perelman Cancer Center, Department of Radiation Oncology, University of Pennsylvania Hospital, Philadelphia, PA, USA
[2]Department of Radiation Oncology, University of Pennsylvania Hospital, Philadelphia, PA, USA
[3]Radiation Safety, University of Pennsylvania, USA

Synonyms

Nuclear energy accidents; Reactor accidents

Definition

The fuel of a nuclear power plant is an isotope of either uranium or plutonium. A nuclear power plant produces energy by splitting its fuel in a process termed fission. The energy released by the fission reaction is used to heat water and turn steam-driven turbine generators. In addition to the release of energy, the split fuel creates radioactive products. In the event of a nuclear power plant accident, the primary concern is that the radioactive fuel and its fission products will escape into the environment.

The International Atomic Energy Agency (IAEA) developed the International Nuclear and Radiological Event Scale to characterize the severity of nuclear reactor malfunctioning. The scale classifies these events according to seven levels ranging from an anomaly "Level 1" to a major accident "Level 7." Since the first commercial nuclear reactors began producing electricity in the mid 1950s, there have only been two events classified as Level 7, the accidents at Chernobyl, Ukraine in 1986 (IAEA 2006) and Fukushima, Japan in 2011.

Etiology

There are different system malfunctions that can result in the escape of radioactive materials from a power plant. The most important mechanism is failure of the core cooling system. When the cooling system fails, the nuclear reactor core and even the fuel itself can melt partially or completely. Elevated temperatures and pressures can cause chemical reactions which generate hydrogen gas. This can lead to explosions and the dispersal of radioactive materials. Most US nuclear plants safe-guard against cooling system failures by enclosing the reactor cores within a steel-walled vessel which in turn is enclosed within a sealed steel-reinforced concrete ▶ containment structure designed to contain the radioactive elements indefinitely (Fig. 1).

There are three different mechanisms by which a human being can be exposed to radiation as a result of reactor accidents: (1) total or partial body exposures due to close proximity to a radiation source, (2) external contamination and (3) internal contamination. In the event of

such an accident, a given individual is susceptible to any or all of these threats. Total or partial body exposure occurs when an external source irradiates the body superficially to the skin and/or deeply into internal organs. How deeply the radiation penetrates in a given exposure depends on the type and energy of the radiation involved. For instance, beta radiation can be a significant source of dose to skin because it travels only a short distance in tissue, depending on its energy. However, high-energy gamma radiation can penetrate deeply and affect internal organs. In past reactor accidents, only plant workers on-site at the time of the event and emergency personnel subsequently involved have received substantial total or partial body exposures. Individuals who have experienced a total or partial body exposure but no contamination are not radioactive and therefore cannot expose the emergency or healthcare workers caring for them. External contamination occurs when the radioactive material from the reactor attaches to clothing or skin of human beings, and in this manner, exposes skin and/or internal organs. Emergency authorities may advise that people living near a power plant accident to avoid being outdoors for a period of time to minimize external contamination. The most important mechanism by which large populations around a reactor accident can be exposed is internal contamination. This occurs when radioactive materials are inhaled or ingested or enter the body through open wounds. After the accident at Chernobyl, approximately five million people in the region may have received excess radiation exposure primarily through internal contamination.

Reactor accidents can release an assortment of radioactive isotopes into the environment. Most of these are unlikely to cause significant internal or external contamination because their half-lives are very short (e.g., 67 h for molybdenum-99) or very long (e.g., 24,400 years for plutonium-239) or they are released in a gaseous

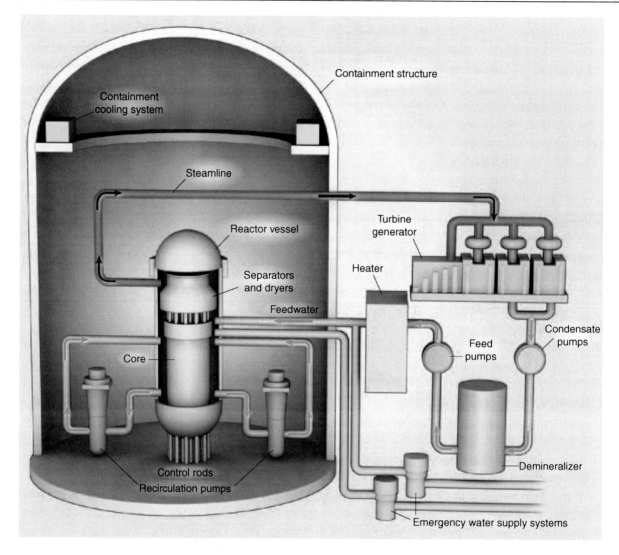

Short-Term and Long-Term Health Risk of Nuclear Power Plant Accident. Fig. 1 The figure illustrates the typical structures within a boiling water reactor, a common modern nuclear reactor design. In these reactors, the heat from nuclear fission is used to boil water and create steam which turns turbines generators and produces electricity. The temperature of the fuel and the fission products in the reactor core is carefully controlled by a water cooling system. If the water cooling system fails, the core and the fuel itself can melt partially or completely (Reproduced from Christodouleas et al. 2011 with permission)

state (e.g., xenon-133) or in very low quantities (e.g., plutonium-238). In contrast, iodine-131 (I-131) can be an important source of radiation exposure due to its intermediate half-life (8 days), its high concentrations in reactor discharges and its tendency to contaminate food and water and then concentrate in a single organ (the thyroid) when inhaled or ingested. Cesium-137 is also an important isotope dispersed by reactor accidents. Cs-137, with a half-life of 30 years, can result in prolonged low dose exposures from external sources (e.g., contaminated soil) or from ingestion of contaminated food and water. In addition, like I-131, Cs-137 can travel great distances when dispersed in the plume of a reactor explosion and contaminate large swaths of an entire country or continent. After Chernobyl, excess deposits of Cs-137 were detected as far as 3,000 km (1,800 miles) away.

Clinical Presentation

The potential health effects of radiation exposure depend on several factors, including the type of exposure, the type of tissue exposed, the type of radiation, how deeply the radiation penetrates, the total absorbed dose and the duration over which the dose is absorbed (dose rate). Importantly, the type of radiation and the dose rates involved in a power plant accident would typically be different than those seen in the detonation of nuclear weapons, so the biological consequences of these events will likely differ substantially.

Acute Radiation Sickness (ARS)

► Acute radiation sickness (ARS) can occur when most or all of a person's body is exposed to a single dose of greater than 1 Gy. National and international registries have documented over 800 cases of ARS over the past 60 years, though most of these were due to medical and not power plant accidents. Of the ARS diagnoses related to reactors, all have been diagnosed in plant workers or emergency personnel and not in the surrounding general population. Even after Chernobyl, where there were 134 confirmed cases of ARS, all occurred in individuals working at the plant or responding to the accident (IAEA 2006).

While high total or near-total body doses can affect every organ system, most of the documented morbidity and mortality is due to the acute effects on the bone marrow, gastrointestinal system and skin. Hematologic and gastrointestinal complications are common because bone marrow and intestinal epithelium are especially radiosensitive as a result of their high intrinsic replication rate. For example, after the Chernobyl accident, all 134 patients with ARS had bone marrow depression and 15 developed severe gastrointestinal complications. Cutaneous toxicity is also common because external low energy gamma and beta radiation are chiefly absorbed in the skin. Indeed, because of this effect, the absorbed dose in skin may be many times higher than the absorbed dose in bone marrow. Of the 134 patients with ARS after Chernobyl, 19 had widespread radiation dermatitis. Acute neurovascular compromise has rarely been seen, but can occur with extremely high (>20 Gy) total body doses. Even at Chernobyl, the highest absorbed dose to a worker was 16 Gy.

ARS occurs in three phases: prodrome, latency and illness. The severity of symptoms, time to onset and duration of these phases is dependent on the total body dose (Table 1). For example, mild ARS may be seen with total body doses of 1–2 Gy and is characterized by vomiting in the prodrome phase, a long latency phase of 21–35 days as the bone marrow slowly depletes and a mild illness phase from which no one would be expected to die even without medical intervention. In contrast, very severe ARS occurs with total body doses of 6–8 Gy and results in immediate and severe vomiting, diarrhea, headache, fever and altered consciousness. The latency phase is less than 7 days and the illness phase is characterized by multi-organ system dysfunction and a high estimated mortality (>50%) without medical intervention. The signs and symptoms of skin injury depend on the volume of skin exposed and the dose. With relatively low skin doses (3–15 Gy), redness and epilation may occur. With high skin doses (>15 Gy), skin may blister and ulcerate.

S

Short-Term and Long-Term Health Risk of Nuclear Power Plant Accident. Table 1 Signs and symptoms by phase of acute radiation syndrome[a]

	Prodrome	Latency	Illness
Mild (1–2 Gy)	Vomiting	21–35 days	Fatigue, weakness
	Onset 2 h		Mortality[b] 0%
Moderate (2–4 Gy)	Vomiting, mild headache	18–35 days	Fever, infections, bleeding, weakness, epilation
	Onset 1–2 h		Mortality[b] 0–50%
Severe (4–6 Gy)	Vomiting, mild diarrhea, moderate headache, fever	8–18 days	High fever, infections, bleeding, epilation
	Onset < 1 h		Mortality[b] 20–70%
Very Severe (6–8 Gy)	Vomiting, heavy diarrhea, severe headache, high fever, altered consciousness	≤7 days	High fever, diarrhea, vomiting, dizziness and disorientation, hypotension
	Onset <30 min		Mortality[b] 50–100%
Lethal (>8 Gy)	Vomiting, heavy diarrhea, severe headache, high fever, unconsciousness	No latency	High fever, diarrhea, unconsciousness
	Onset <10 min		Mortality[b] 100%

[a]Table adapted from IAEA (1998) and Christodouleas et al. (2011)
[b]Mortality estimates are for patients who do not receive medical intervention

Long-Term Cancer Risks

In addition to ARS in workers, an important concern with reactor accidents is the potential for elevated long-term cancer risks in large populations surrounding the compromised plant. In the Chernobyl region, for example, over five million people may have been exposed to excess radiation primarily as a result of I-131 or Cs-137 contamination (IAEA 2006). However, unlike ARS which has been reasonably well described, the subsequent cancer risk in a population exposed to nuclear reactor fallout is less well understood. Long-term cancer risk as a result of accidents is difficult to study because even in the worst events, the exposures that occur are low and heterogeneous. In addition, the secondary cancer, if it happens, may take decades to develop and the resulting increased incidence may be small relative to a population's baseline cancer rate. Perhaps for these reasons, epidemiologic studies of reactor accidents to date have provided strong evidence for an increased risk of only one type of cancer: secondary thyroid malignancies in children who ingest excess I-131. Studies evaluating leukemia and nonthyroid solid cancer have not found consistently elevated risks though small increases may become more apparent with improved cancer registries and/or longer follow up. In contrast, studies of the atomic bomb survivors showed clearly elevated rates of leukemia and solid cancers even at relatively low total body doses. However, there are important differences between the type of radiation and dose rate of exposure experienced by atomic bomb survivors and those experienced by populations around a reactor accident which may result in different long-term cancer risks.

Thyroid Cancer in Children

High quality studies of children who ingested excess I-131 after Chernobyl suggest that the risk of thyroid cancer increased by a factor of 2–5 per Gy of thyroid dose (Cardis et al. 2006). While the absolute number of excess pediatric thyroid cancers in the regions surrounding Chernobyl was not high, it *could* be detected because the baseline thyroid cancer incidence in children was low (<1 case per 100,000 children). Factors that have been shown to increase the carcinogenic effect of I-131 include younger age and iodine deficiency at the time of exposure. Children in regions around Chernobyl with endemic iodine deficiency were more likely to develop thyroid cancer per Gy of thyroid dose compared to those in regions with normal iodine intake. In addition, children who were provided stable iodine following the Chernobyl accident were at one-third risk of developing thyroid cancer compared to those who did not receive it. In contrast, studies of the effect of thyroid exposure in utero and in adulthood have so far been inconclusive.

Therapy

Public Health Response

A nuclear reactor accident and the potential spread of radioactive contaminants over a large area is an event that develops over days and weeks and its potential effects can last months and even years. Because reactor accidents are very rare events, few individuals have direct experience managing the overall public health response. Organizations that could be involved due to proximity to a power plant or role in the health system must therefore put detailed algorithmic response plans in place and practice them regularly. The risks to the population outside the immediate reactor area should be constantly monitored. Clear communication to the surrounding community about exposure levels and corresponding risk is of paramount importance and needs to be sensitive to widespread public apprehension and misunderstanding of ARS and long-term cancer risk. Evacuating populations from areas around a reactor accident and clear instructions to those that do not need to be evacuated will minimize risks of exposure and significantly reduce the level of anxiety and fear.

Public health response plans should identify primary hospitals in the vicinity of nuclear reactors where individuals with immediate life-threatening conventional trauma can be evacuated to and treated emergently. Secondary hospitals at greater distances from a reactor should also be identified should the primary hospitals be deemed unsafe due to contamination. These hospitals, in collaboration with public health agencies, should also have organized disaster plans. Hospitals should stockpile equipment and medication that may be required and staff should be trained regularly. The number of casualties will be a major factor in determining the response of the medical system. If only a few individuals are affected, no significant change of the system will be needed. However, if a large number (dozens or more) of casualties is suspected, significant adaptation of the medical system may be required. The U.S. Department of Health and Human Services and other organizations have produced publicly available documents summarizing steps necessary to prepare for radiation accidents (USDHHS 2011).

Initial Medical Evaluation and Treatment

In nuclear power plant accidents to date, individuals who were exposed to significant doses of radiation and were at risk of developing ARS were either workers at the reactors or emergency personnel called to the site. These people may also suffer from conventional trauma or burns and may need an immediate evacuation to a surrounding hospital for treatment. In these hospitals, a distinct decontamination area needs to be established where the initial evaluation of patients will occur. The first step in the treatment of any patient accidentally exposed to radiation is to manage immediate life-threatening injuries. The next step is to clear the patient of any on-going external or internal contamination. Detailed decontamination protocols have been developed by the International Atomic Energy Agency (IAEA). Once life threatening injuries and decontamination issues have been addressed, the presence and severity of ARS should be determined.

Acute Radiation Sickness

ARS treatment is guided by the total dose, estimated using initial clinical symptoms, lymphocyte depletion kinetics and cytogenetic analyses, when available. Patients with estimated whole body doses of ≤ 2 Gy may only require symptomatic support for nausea and vomiting. In patients with whole body doses >2 Gy, the care team may need to manage the consequences of bone marrow depletion, and gastrointestinal and cutaneous injuries. Strategies to address bone marrow suppression and consequent infections include antibiotics, antivirals and antifungals, use of hematopoietic growth factors and possibly bone marrow transplantation. High quality studies comparing different approaches to managing bone marrow depletion in this setting have not been done because of the rarity of these events. In particular, the use of bone marrow transplantation is controversial as outcomes after radiation accidents have been poor. After Chernobyl, 13 patients with ARS received bone marrow transplants and only two survived long-term. Two of the 11 patients who died appeared to have died mainly due to complications from transplantation. Gastrointestinal radiation sequelae are managed supportively and possibly with the use of prophylactic probiotics. Cutaneous radiation injuries may evolve over the course of weeks. Treatment of such lesions must balance the need to minimize acute and chronic inflammation with topical glucocorticoids with the goal avoiding secondary infections. The IAEA has developed detailed ARS treatment algorithms that are publicly available (IAEA 1998).

Thyroid Cancer Prevention

In accidents where I-131 is dispersed into the environment, individuals in affected areas should attempt to minimize or eliminate intake of locally-grown produce and groundwater. However, 2–3 months after an event, local resources will no long contain significant amounts of I-131 since its half-life is only 8 days. Public health officials may advise area residents to take ▶ potassium iodide (KI) to block uptake of the I-131 in the thyroid. Prophylactic KI is most effective when taken before or within a few hours of I-131 exposure. Consuming KI a day after the exposure probably has limited benefits unless additional or continuing exposures are expected. However, KI can have toxicity so should not be consumed by the general public without instruction from public health officials. The U.S. FDA has produced guidelines for KI dose as a function of age and expected radiation exposure. After Chernobyl, over ten million children and adolescents in Poland were given a single dose of prophylactic KI with few reported adverse outcomes.

Cross-References

▶ Bone Marrow Toxicity in Cancer Treament
▶ Leukemia in General
▶ Nuclear Medicine

▶ Sarcomas of the Head and Neck
▶ Thyroid Cancer

References

Cardis E, Howe G, Ron E et al (2006) Cancer consequences of the Chernobyl accident: 20 years on. J Radiol Prot 26(2): 127–40

Christodouleas JP, Forrest RD, Ainsley CG et al (2011) Short-term and long-term health risks of nuclear-power-plant accidents. N Engl J Med 364(24):2334–2341

IAEA (1998) Diagnosis and treatment of radiation injuries, vol 2, Safety series. International Atomic Energy Agency, Vienna. http://www-pub.iaea.org/MTCD/publications/PDF/P040_scr.pdf

IAEA (2006) Chernobyl's legacy: health, environmental and socio-economic impacts. International Atomic Energy Agency, Vienna (IAEA Publication No. IAEA/PI/A.87 Rev.2/06-0918)

USDHHS (2011) Radiation emergency medical management. http://www.remm.nlm.gov/remm_Preplanning.htm

Sigmoidoscopy

BRADLEY J. HUTH
Department of Radiation Oncology,
Philadelphia, PA, USA

Synonyms

Flexible sigmoidoscopy

Definition

Sigmoidoscopy is an endoscopic procedure similar to colonoscopy but using a shorter, narrower instrument. The procedure can be done in the office of an experienced practitioner without anesthesia and with minimal bowel preparation. This procedure can be substituted for colonoscopy in certain patients but should be combined with occult fecal blood testing.

Cross-References

▶ Colon Cancer
▶ Rectal Cancer

Signal Transduction Inhibitors

RENE RUBIN
Rittenhouse Hematology/Oncology,
Philadelphia, PA, USA

Definition

Imatinib, desatinib, and neratinib belong to the group of signal transduction inhibitors. They inhibit the BCR-ABL tyrosine kinase and induce apoptosis in BCR-ABL-positive cells. Furthermore, they inhibit tyrosine kinases for PDGFR, c-kit, and stem cell factor. The drugs are used in chronic myeloic leukemia, in Ph-positive acute lymphocytic leukemia, in gastrointestinal stroma tumors (GIST), and in hypereosinophilic syndrome.

Side Effects

- Nausea
- Edema/fluid retention
- Myalgia
- Diarrhea
- Transaminitis
- Skin toxicity – rashes

Cross-References

▶ Principles of Chemotherapy

Signal-to-Noise Ratio (SNR)

JOHN W. WONG
Department of Radiation Oncology and
Molecular Radiation Sciences, Johns Hopkins
University, Baltimore, MD, USA

Definition

The ratio of height of the useful signal to that of all other detected events which to do not contribute to the useful signal.

Cross-References

▶ Electronic Portal Imaging Devices (EPID)

Simple Mastectomy

DAVID E. WAZER
Radiation Oncology Department, Tufts Medical
Center, Tufts University School of Medicine,
Boston, MA, USA
Radiation Oncology Department, Rhode Island
Hospital, Brown University School of Medicine,
Providence, RI, USA

Definition

Simple mastectomy is the process of removal of the entire breast tissue, from the clavicle to the rectus abdominus muscle, between the sternal edge of the latissimus dorsi muscle, with the removal of the fascia of the pectoralis major muscle.

Cross-References

▶ Cancer of the Breast Tis

Simultaneous Integrated Boost (SIB)

VOLKER BUDACH
Department of Radiotherapy and Radiation
Oncology, Charité - University Hospital Berlin,
Berlin, Germany

Definition

An IMRT technique that allows the planning and irradiation of different targets at different dose levels in a single treatment session, instead of using sequential treatment plans.

Cross-References

▶ Larynx
▶ Oro-Hypopharynx

Single Brain Metastasis

JAMES H. BRASHEARS, III
Radiation Oncologist, Venice, FL, USA

Definition

One brain lesion regardless of the extent of extra-cranial disease.

Cross-References

▶ Palliation of Brain and Spinal Cord Metastases

Single Photon Emission Computed Tomography (SPECT)

HEDVIG HRICAK[1], OGUZ AKIN[2], HEBERT ALBERTO
VARGAS[2]
[1]Department of Radiology, Memorial Sloan-
Kettering Cancer Center, New York, NY, USA
[2]Body MRI, Memorial Sloan-Kettering Cancer
Center, New York, NY, USA

Definition

A nuclear medicine imaging technique performed by using a gamma camera to acquire multiple 2-D images from multiple angles. A computer is then used to apply a tomographic reconstruction algorithm to the multiple projections, yielding a 3-D dataset. This dataset may then be manipulated to show thin slices along any chosen axis of the body.

Cross-References

▶ Imaging in Oncology

Single-Nucleotide Polymorphisms (SNP)

CLAUDIA E. RÜBE
Department of Radiation Oncology,
Saarland University, Homburg/Saar, Germany

Definition

DNA sequence variation occurring when a single nucleotide in the genome differs between members of a species or paired chromosomes in an individual.

Cross-References

► Predictive In vitro Assays in Radiation Oncology

Sinonasal Cancer

► Nasal Cavity and Paranasal Sinuses

Sister Mary Joseph Nodule

FILIP T. TROICKI[1], JAGANMOHAN POLI[2], CHRISTIN A. KNOWLTON[3], MICHELLE KOLTON MACKAY[4], BRADLEY J. HUTH[5]
[1]College of Medicine, Drexel University, Philadelphia, PA, USA
[2]Department of Radiation Oncology, College of Medicine, Drexel University, Philadelphia, PA, USA
[3]Department of Radiation Oncology, Drexel University, Philadelphia, PA, USA
[4]Department of Radiation Oncology, Marshfield Clinic, Marshfield, WI, USA
[5]Department of Radiation Oncology, Philadelphia, PA, USA

Definition

Mass around the region of the umbilicus, often associated with advanced gastric cancer and abdominal malignancy. The expression refers to a surgical assistant of Dr. William Mayo who described the correlation of peri-umbilical adenopathy in the preoperative setting with advanced malignant disease within the abdomen and pelvis at the time of surgery.

Cross-References

► Cancer of the Pancreas
► Colon Cancer
► Ovary
► Stomach Cancer

Sjögren's Syndrome

LINDSAY G. JENSEN, LOREN K. MELL
Center for Advanced Radiotherapy Technologies,
Department of Radiation Oncology, San Diego
Rebecca and John Moores Cancer Center,
University of California, La Jolla, CA, USA

Definition

Autoimmune disorder characterized by dry eyes and xerostomia.

Cross-References

► Salivary Gland Cancer

Skeletal Muscle Tumors

► Soft Tissue Sarcoma

Skin Cancer

BRANDON J. FISHER[1], LARRY C. DAUGHERTY[2]

[1]Department of Radiation Oncology, College of Medicine, Drexel University, Philadelphia, PA, USA

[2]Department of Radiation Oncology, College of Medicine, Drexel University, Glenside, PA, USA

Synonyms

Carcinomas: basal cell carcinoma; Epidermoid intradermal carcinoma; Nonmelanoma skin cancer; Squamous cell carcinoma

Definition/Description

Nonmelanoma skin cancer (NMSC) includes roughly 80 different types of skin malignancies. This section focuses on the two most common types, squamous cell carcinoma (SCC) and basal cell carcinoma (BCC).

Anatomy

The skin is composed of three layers, the outermost being the epidermis, followed by the dermis, and then by the hypodermis or adnexal structures. The epidermis is mainly avascular, consisting of stratified squamous cells that vary in thickness depending on the location on the body. As cells migrate from the basal layer to the epidermis, the cells lose their nuclei and their ability to replicate and eventually are shed from the body. The dermis, on the other hand, consists of a papillary layer that is just inferior to the epidermis basement membrane and the deeper reticular layer. Last of all, the hypodermis contains connective tissue, fat, lymphatic vessels, nerves, and vessels that give structural integrity to the skin.

Background

Skin cancer is the most common cancer in the USA, with more than one million cases occurring annually. It is thought that the overall incidence has been rising steadily over the last 50 years at a rate of 3–8% per year. SCCs comprise 20–35% of NMSCs and BCCs, about 65–80%. Melanoma comprises a small percentage of skin cancer cases, approximately 3% of all skin cancers; however, melanoma does account for the majority of skin cancer deaths. Many other tumors of the skin are much less common, including ▶ Merkel cell carcinoma (MCC), all with varying degrees of prognosis.

The most common predisposing factor is exposure to ultraviolet solar radiation, especially ultraviolet B. Cutaneous skin cancers can develop on any part of the skin; however, they are most commonly seen on the areas exposed to the sun. Painful, blistering burns before the age of 20 are related to later development of premalignant lesions as well as of NMSCs and melanomas. The typical latency period is 20–40 years and tends to be cumulative over time. Risk factors that increase one's sensitivity to solar damage include fair skin, blue eyes, and multiple genetic predispositions, such as xeroderma pigmentosum, ▶ basal cell nevus syndrome, epidermodysplasia verruciformis, albinism, and phenylketonuria. Geographic latitude and ozone depletion also play a role in the incidence of skin cancer.

Other risk factors include exposure to carcinogens such as arsenic, soot, tar, and polycyclic aromatic hydrocarbons from coal. Chronic irritation, radiation, trauma, and immunodeficiencies have also been linked to the development of skin cancer.

Squamous Cell Carcinoma

Squamous cell carcinoma arises from the keratinizing cells of the epidermis and represents 20–35% of all NMSCs. It can begin as an in situ SCC prior to invasion, which is known as Bowen's disease. It typically presents as a velvety red, keratotic nodule. Progression to invasive SCC from in situ occurs in 5–20% of cases.

Invasive SCC is characterized by expansion beyond the dermal-epidermal junction. Typical lesions are round to irregular, plaque-like, or nodular and often have a wart-like appearance or a projection from the skin as a cutaneous horn, known as ▶ actinic keratosis. Surrounding erythema may be present, and bleeding can result from minimal trauma. SCCs tend to be superficial, although they can invade the subcutaneous tissue to involve nerves, lymphatics, and bone. Perineural invasion can be seen in 2–15% of cases. Tumors arising from actinic keratoses are slow-growing and rarely metastasize. If lymphatics are involved, the process tends to occur in an orderly manner, in a single regional node that eventually metastasizes to multiple nodes. It is rare to have a metastasis bypass the primary nodal echelon. Lymphatic and even distant metastases can be seen in approximately 2–10% of all cases; however, the mortality rate is low. The most common sites of metastases are the lung, liver, and bones. Recurrence risk factors for SCC include tumor size, location, positive post-surgical margin, immunosuppression, site of prior radiation, moderate-to-poorly differentiated adenoid (acantholytic), adenosquamous (with mucin production), or desmoplastic histological appearance, and perineural or vascular invasion. High-grade features, which play an important role in staging, are depth of invasion greater than 2 mm, ▶ Clark level greater than or equal to IV, perineural invasion, ear or non-hair-bearing lip as the primary site, or poorly differentiated or undifferentiated cells.

Basal Cell Carcinoma

Basal cell carcinomas arise from nonkeratinizing cells from the basal layer of the epidermis. BCCs represent about 65–80% of all NMSCs and are the most common histological patterns seen. A BCC has no unique precursor lesion. It has a typical appearance, described as a "rodent ulcer," which is a smooth nodule with a central depression secondary to necrosis, surrounded by raised pearly or translucent borders. Telangiectasias may also be seen around the lesion, and it may bleed with minimal trauma. The most common location of the tumor is in the head and neck region, especially on the cheeks. BCCs rarely spread to lymphatic regions and metastasize less than 0.1% of the time. Perineural invasion is also uncommon in BCCs, seen in only 1% of cases. Several subtypes of BCCs exist: nodular, superficial, pigmented, micronodular, and morpheaform (infiltrating, sclerosing, or desmoplastic). The most aggressive subtype is the sclerosing morphea, known for deep, diffused dermal invasion, with poorly defined margins. Risk factors for BCC recurrence after treatment include location, size, positive surgical margin, prior radiated area, aggressive histological involvement (morpheaform, sclerosing, infiltrative, micronodular), multifocality, and perineural involvement. High-grade features are the same as in SCC.

Initial Evaluation

Diagnosis and evaluation of skin cancer should begin with a thorough history and physical examination. Special attention should be paid to specific disease-related signs and symptoms. The most common presentation for skin cancer is abnormal skin changes or a nonhealing skin wound. A biopsy or excisional biopsy should be performed for all suspicious lesions. Results from the history and physical examination, in conjunction with pathological findings, are necessary to stage patients. Definitive diagnosis can only be made from biopsy results. It is also important to note several high-risk features: depth of invasion greater than 2 mm, Clark level greater than or equal to IV, perineural invasion, ear or non-hair-bearing lip as the primary site, or poorly differentiated or undifferentiated cells. Staging follows the guidelines of the American Joint Committee on Cancer (Table 1).

Skin Cancer. Table 1 American joint committee on cancer staging system for nonmelanoma skin cancer, 7th edition (Edge et al. 2010, with permission)

Primary tumor (T)	
TX	Primary tumor cannot be assessed
T0	No evidence of primary tumor
Tis	Carcinoma in situ
T1	Tumor $\leq$ 2 cm in greatest dimension with less than two high-risk features
T2	Tumor $>$ 2 cm in greatest dimension or tumor any size with two or more high-risk features
T3	Tumor invades maxilla, mandible, orbit, or temporal bone
T4	Tumor invades skeleton (axial or appendicular) or perineural invasion of the skull base
Regional lymph nodes (N)	
NX	Regional lymph nodes cannot be assessed
N0	No regional lymph node metastasis
N1	Metastasis in a single ipsilateral lymph node, 3 cm or less in greatest dimension
N2	Metastasis in a single ipsilateral lymph node, more than 3 cm but not more than 6 cm in greatest dimension; or in multiple ipsilateral lymph nodes, none more than 6 cm in greatest dimension; or in bilateral or contralateral lymph nodes, none more than 6 cm in greatest dimension
N2a	Metastasis in a single ipsilateral lymph node, more than 3 cm but not more than 6 cm in greatest dimension
N2b	Metastasis in multiple ipsilateral lymph nodes, none more than 6 cm in greatest dimension
N2c	Metastasis in bilateral or contralateral lymph nodes, none more than 6 cm in greatest dimension
N3	Metastasis in a lymph node, more than 6 cm in greatest dimension
Distant metastasis (M)	
MX	Presence of distant metastasis cannot be assessed
M0	No distant metastasis
M1	Distant metastasis

Stage grouping			
Stage 0	Tis	N0	M0
Stage I	T1	N0	M0
Stage II	T2	N0	M0
Stage III	T3	N0	M0
	T1-3	N1	M0
Stage IV	T1-3	N2	M0
	Any T	N3	M0
	T4	Any N	M0
	Any T	Any N	M1

Differential Diagnosis

Age spots or seborrheic keratoses; basal cell nevus syndrome; hemangiomas or lymphangiomas; lipomas; nevi or birthmarks; keratoacanthoma; localized scleroderma; molluscum contagiosum; psoriasis; sebaceous hyperplasia; skin tags; warts; xeroderma pigmentosa; varicose veins; furuncles; tuberculomas; gummas and granulomas from coccidioidomycosis, sporotrichosis, and other fungi; melanoma; sarcoma; metastatic nodules; Kaposi sarcoma; neurofibromatosis; dermoid cyst; leiomyoma; and mycosis fungoides. Leukemic infiltration and Hodgkin disease may cause skin nodules or plaques as well.

Imaging Studies

The routine use of imaging studies in the work-up of NMSC is not indicated; however, computed tomography (CT) and/or magnetic resonance imaging (MRI) should be considered if PNI or LN involvement is suspected or if the lesion is near the orbits. CT may also be useful in ruling out suspected bone involvement. CT and MRI are helpful in assessing deep tissue penetration. Eyelid tumors may appear superficial but may actually penetrate deeply into the globe. CT is essential for accurate determination of tumor extent.

Laboratory Studies

No routine laboratory tests are needed. However, results from routine laboratory tests such as complete blood count, electrolyte assay, liver function tests, and alkaline phosphatase assay may be useful.

Treatment

Multiple treatment options are available for the treatment of BCC or SCC lesions. Surgical treatments or radiation therapy offers equivalent cure rates of 90–95%. For the most acceptable cosmetic outcome, treatment approaches must be individualized based on specific risk factors and patient characteristics, such as age and size and location of the lesion.

Surgery

Surgery is typically the standard of care. Multiple surgical approaches are available. Cryosurgery can treat small, well-defined tumors less than 1.5 cm but is contraindicated in deeply infiltrating lesions. Cryosurgery is better suited for actinic keratoses or Bowen's disease and is rarely used for BCC or SCC. Curettage and electrodissection are also useful for small, well-defined tumors. ▶ Mohs micrographic surgery allows for maximal skin sparing through a process of fixation and mapping of the surgical margins with multiple frozen sections to obtain microscopically clear margins. This technique is preferred for deeply invasive tumors, diffuse laterally spreading tumors, perineural invasion or any tumor on the face, and recurrent tumors. With advances in surgical techniques, more and more patients are eligible for surgery. Surgical excision offers the advantage of pathological margin assessment and potential concurrent management of lymph nodes. Surgery is preferred for scalp tumors and for lesions less than 3 cm that can be removed with little cosmetic or functional impairment. Indications for surgery as the sole modality of treatment are primary or recurrent lesions on the central face, eyelids, tip of nose, and lips; lesions greater than 5 mm and lesions greater than 2 cm on the ears, forehead, and scalp; and regional lymph node involvement. These lesions pose the potential for poor functional and cosmetic outcomes after surgery.

Radiation Therapy

Radiation therapy is an important management option. In select cases, it can be the definitive treatment; however, it is most often used postoperatively. When cosmesis is not a factor, radiation is typically preferred for elderly, debilitated, or

Skin Cancer. Table 2 Comparison of different time-dose fractionation schedules for management of nonmelanoma skin cancer (Brady 2008)

Tumor characteristics	Dose fractionation
<1 cm; debilitated patient	20–24 Gy in 1 fraction
<2 cm	45 Gy in 5–9 fractions
2–4 cm or cosmetic concerns	52 Gy in 13 fractions
>4 cm	60 Gy in 20 fractions
	64 Gy in 25 fractions
≤1 cm; elderly patient	40 Gy in 8 fractions
>1–2 cm in elderly or ≤2 cm in young patient	50 Gy in 15–20 fractions
Large fields needing good cosmesis	60 Gy in 30 fractions
Large, infiltrating	64–66 Gy in 32–33 fractions
Large, untreated + bone/cartilage invasion or large, recurrent	65 Gy in 35 fractions
Large, untreated + minimal or suspected bone/cartilage invasion	60 Gy in 34 fractions
Moderate-to-large inner canthus, eyelid, nasal, pinna (20–30 cm^2)	55 Gy in 30 fractions
Small, thin (<1.5 cm) eye, nose, ear (10 cm^2)	50 Gy in 20 fractions
Moderate or postoperative cut-through on free skin	45 Gy in 15 fractions
Small (1 cm) on free skin	40 Gy in 10 fractions
	30 Gy in 5 fractions
Cosmesis not important	40 Gy in 10 fractions
	30 Gy in 5 fractions
	20 Gy in 1 fractions

medically inoperable patients because anesthesia is not necessary. Indications for postoperative radiation include positive margins, perineural invasion (including large named nerves), bone or cartilage invasion, and SCC of the parotid. Skin cancers with perineural invasion are particularly difficult to control, and salvage after surgical recurrence is unlikely. Radiation therapy may be contraindicated in young patients because of potential carcinogenesis and tendency toward cosmetic deterioration over time. Radiation is discouraged for tumors involving the thumb web space, interdigital space, or proximal digits

because such tumors are often aggressive and prone to recurrence, lymph node metastases, and ▶ radionecrosis.

Radiation Therapy Techniques

Many specialized radiation therapy techniques are used to treat skin cancer, depending on the size, depth, and anatomic location of the lesion. Radiation volumes vary depending on the size of the tumor, histopathological test results, and the extent of the disease. Radiation fields should typically encompass the gross lesion with a 1–2 cm margin and regional nodes as indicated. Margins may vary depending on tumor size and type of radiation used. Photon margins of 1 cm and electron margins of 1–1.5 cm are used for tumors up to 2 cm; photon margins of 1.5–2 cm and electron margins of 2–2.5 cm, for tumors greater than 2–7 cm. Although lymph node metastases are rare for BCCs, they are seen in 5–10% of cutaneous SCCs. Elective nodal irradiation is typically not indicated except for large infiltrative cancer, node positivity, or recurrences in the regional nodes.

Megavoltage electrons and photons generated by linear accelerators are generally used in the treatment of NMSC; however, superficial or orthovoltage x-ray therapy has been successful in the past. Typical linear accelerator electron energies used for treating NMSCs are 6–20 MeV. Electrons offer the advantage of rapid falloff of depth dose to enable sparing of underlying normal tissues. A bolus may be used to effectively draw the beam's isodose lines upward toward the skin surface, and bolus thickness must be considered in the selection of beam energy.

The region treated should be immobilized to achieve stability and maximize setup reproducibility. Shielding of surrounding normal tissues and critical structures is particularly important in the treatment of skin cancers involving head and neck regions.

Secondary beam collimation with a lead cutout placed directly on the skin surface generally is preferred. Special shielding devices are required when treating lesions involving the eye, nose, mouth, and ear. The dose threshold for cataract formation is 5–10 Gy, and a tungsten eye shield should be used.

Time-Dose Fractionation

Similar total doses and fractionation regimens are used for BCCs and SCCs of similar size and depth, although some authors advocate higher doses for SCC than for BCC. Higher doses per fraction cause greater late effects and worse cosmesis, so concern about cosmesis and late tissue damage must be weighed against considerations of patient age and comorbidity. The following treatment schemes have been proposed with varying doses (Table 2).

Cross-References

▶ Kaposi's Sarcoma
▶ Melanoma
▶ Merkel Cell Carcinoma (MCC)

References

Baert AL (2008) Encyclopedia of diagnostic imaging, vol 2. Springer, Berlin/Heidelberg

Brady LW, Lu JJ (eds) (2008) Radiation oncology, an evidence-based approach. Springer, Berlin

Brady LW, Perez CA, Halperin EC (eds) (2008) Principles and practice of radiation oncology, 5th edn. Lippincott Williams and Wilkins, Philadelphia

Edge SB et al (eds) (2010) Cancer staging handbook, 7th edn. Springer, New York

Hansen EK, Roach M III (eds) (2007) Handbook of evidence-based radiation oncology. Springer, New York

Skin-Sparing Mastectomy

ANTHONY E. DRAGUN
Department of Radiation Oncology, James Graham Brown Cancer Center, University of Louisville School of Medicine, Louisville, KY, USA

Definition

This is a technique of mastectomy that involves removal of the breast parenchyma with the maintenance as much skin as possible to be used as an envelope for breast reconstruction. This technique usually involves removal of the nipple areola complex (although nipple sparing techniques are currently under investigation) as well as any incisions left by previous excisional biopsies. This is a technique that is gaining in popularity especially when integrated with a tissue expander-based implant reconstruction.

Cross-References

▶ Locally Advanced Breast Cancer
▶ Stage 0 Breast Cancer

Slipped Capital Femoral Epiphysis

DANIEL J. INDELICATO[1], ROBERT H. SAGERMAN[2]
[1]Department of Radiation Oncology, University of Florida Proton Therapy Institute, University of Florida College of Medicine, Jacksonville, FL, USA
[2]Department of Radiation Oncology, SUNY Upstate Medical University, Syracuse, NY, USA

Definition

Slipped capital femoral epiphysis is a posterior and inferior slippage of the proximal femoral epiphysis on the metaphysis, occurring through the physeal plate. It is classified according to stability: A stable slipped capital femoral epiphysis is one in which ambulation is possible, with or without crutches, and an unstable slipped capital femoral epiphysis is one in which ambulation is not possible.

Cross-References

▶ Ewing Sarcoma

Small Cell Lung Cancer

▶ Extraskeletal Small Cell Tumors

Small Lymphocytic Lymphoma

CASPIAN OLIAI
Department of Radiation Oncology, College of Medicine, Drexel University, Philadelphia, PA, USA

Definition

An indolent form of non-Hodgkin lymphoma in which blasts accumulate in the lymph nodes causing LAD. It is regarded as CLL if malignant cells are found in the bone marrow or peripheral blood.

Cross-References

▶ Leukemia in General
▶ Non-Hodgkins Lymphoma

Soft Tissue Lymphoma

▶ Extraskeletal Small Cell Tumors

Soft Tissue Sarcoma

JOHN P. LAMOND
Department of Radiation Oncology, Temple University, Crozer-Chester Medical Center, Upland, PA, USA

Synonyms

Adipose tissue tumors; Extraskeletal small cell tumors; Fibrohistiocytic tumors; Peripheral nerve tumors; Perivascular tumors; Skeletal muscle tumors

Definition/Description

Soft tissue sarcomas are rare tumors that arise from the soft tissues of the body which derive from mesenchymal tissue. Tissues include muscle, connective tissue, fat, vascular structures, and peripheral nerves. Tumors arise from the thigh, buttock, and groin regions in almost half of cases. Less common areas include the torso, retroperitoneum, upper extremities, and head and neck. Tumor histologic grade and to lesser extent tumor size predict overall prognosis but not cellular type. It is unusual for a low-grade sarcoma to metastasize but not uncommon for a high-grade lesion to metastasize preferentially to the lungs. On occasion, tumor diagnosis is related to a genetic syndrome or environmental exposure, but in most occasions the etiology is unknown. Treatment commonly involves multiple modalities including surgery, radiation, and chemotherapy. If the soft tissue sarcoma involves a limb, limb sparing treatment is preferred. Radiation and chemotherapy may be performed prior to surgery in order to facilitate resection. In most cases, such treatment is performed after definitive surgery. Cure rates for soft tissue sarcomas of the extremity and trunk are greater than other sites, since they are generally discovered earlier and have a higher chance of complete resection.

Anatomy

The majority of the body is made up of soft tissues. They are derived from the mesenchymal tissues, with the exception being peripheral nerves, which are from ectodermal tissue. Tumor histology often depends on the predominant soft tissue within the region. For instance, liposarcoma and malignant fibrous histiocytoma (MFH) are the most common diagnoses in extremities, since fat and muscle is abundant. Liposarcomas and leiomyosarcomas are seen in the retroperitoneum. GI stromal tumors are unique to the bowel. Leiomyosarcomas can arise from the uterus, bladder, and bowel. Small cell sarcomas and primitive ectodermal tumors (PNETs) are most common in children.

Epidemiology

Despite the abundance of soft tissues throughout the body, soft tissue sarcomas comprise less than 1% of all new cancers. Most have no clear-cut etiology. Quite infrequently is a sarcoma diagnosis associated with a hereditary syndrome (▶ Li-Fraumeni Syndrome, Neurofibromastosis type 1, hereditary ▶ retinoblastoma) or environmental exposure such as previous radiation, chemotherapy, virus (HIV), chronic irritation or lymphedema.

Clinical Presentation

Patients commonly complain of a painless enlarging mass, particularly if it is located along the extremities, buttocks, head and neck, or chest wall. Pain, gastrointestinal or genitourinary symptoms may be present from tumors within the abdomen or pelvis.

Differential Diagnosis

Differential diagnosis of soft tissue sarcoma is notoriously difficult. Given the relative rarity of the diagnosis versus benign soft tissue masses, it is not surprising that many of these tumors are followed for months or longer by the patient and/or physician before a definitive diagnosis. Benign conditions such as a lipoma, fibroma, trauma, and myositis ossificans are in the differential along with metastases from lung, melanoma, kidney, breast, and other cancers. A complete history and physical examination is important. An enlarging mass should raise one's level of suspicion of possible malignancy.

Imaging Studies and Biopsy

Workup may include plain films and CT scans, but for most locations, MRI is the preferred imaging modality. If imaging studies suggest that soft tissue sarcoma is in the differential, it is important that the patient is seen by a multi-disciplinary

S

team of experienced specialists. Core needle biopsy or limited incisional biopsy are good initial biopsy choices. More extensive initial biopsies or initial attempts at complete resection (typically for a presumed benign tumor) may complicate definitive treatment. An inappropriate biopsy of an extremity may mean the difference between limb conservation and amputation. CT scans including the chest complete routine staging.

Staging

The staging of soft tissue sarcomas is unique. Tumor grade is so important prognostically that it is included in the TNM staging.

Primary tumor (T)	
T1	Tumor 5 cm or less (T1a superficial; T1b deep)
T2	Tumor greater than 5 cm (T2a superficial; T2b deep)
Regional lymph nodes (N)	
N0	No regional lymph node metastasis
N1	Regional lymph node metastasis
Histologic grade	
Grades 1–3	

Primary tumor (T)	
TX	Primary tumor cannot be assessed
T0	No evidence of primary tumor
T1	Tumor 5 cm or less in greatest dimension*
T1a	Superficial tumor
T1b	Deep tumor
T2	Tumor more than 5 cm in greatest dimension*
T2a	Superficial tumor
T2b	Deep tumor
Regional lymph nodes (N)	
NX	Regional lymph nodes cannot be assessed
N0	No regional lymph node metastasis
N1●	Regional lymph node metastasis

Distant metastasis (M)	
M0	No distant metastasis
M1	Distant metastasis
Histologic grade (G)	
GX	Grade cannot be assessed
G1	Grade 1
G2	Grade 2
G3	Grade 3

Anatomic stage/prognostic groups				
Stage IA	T1a	N0	M0	G1, GX
	T1b	N0	M0	G1, GX
Stage IB	T2a	N0	M0	G1, GX
	T2b	N0	M0	G1, GX
Stage IIA	T1a	N0	M0	G2, G3
	T1b	N0	M0	G2, G3
Stage IIB	T2a	N0	M0	G2
	T2b	N0	M0	G2
Stage III	T2a, T2b	N0	M0	G3
	Any T	N1	M0	Any G
Stage IV	Any T	Any N	M1	Any G

Treatment

Soft tissue sarcomas infiltrate into nearby normal tissues along fascial planes. High-grade tumors have a greater infiltrative capacity, with higher risk of local recurrence even after negative margins. Spread to lymph nodes is infrequent except for histologies such as rhabdomyosarcoma, synovial, epithelial, clear cell, and vascular sarcomas. Metastatic potential depends upon size and even more so on grade. Most metastases are within the lung.

Surgery

Primary surgical resection offers the patient the best chance for cure. Preoperative planning in essential, including appropriate pre-biopsy radiographic studies and biopsy techniques that help offer the best chance at complete surgical removal. Some patients benefit from preoperative chemotherapy and/or radiation therapy to help facilitate surgery or perhaps allow for limb preservation.

Radiation

Radiation treatment helps to reduce the risk of local recurrence particularly for high-grade tumors. Preoperative treatment reduces the treated volume and potentially decreases the late side effects, at the expense of higher acute wound complications. More commonly radiation is given postoperatively, either with external radiation or brachytherapy. Radiation therapy has been used as primary treatment for unresectable cases with less favorable results compared to surgery.

Chemotherapy

The role of adjuvant chemotherapy (doxorubicin and ifosfamide-based regimens) for soft tissue sarcoma is controversial. It can be useful in children with rhabdomyosarcomas or extraskeletal Ewing sarcoma. Chemotherapy is more commonly used on a palliative basis in the setting of metastatic disease.

Cross-References
▶ Clinical Aspects of Brachytherapy (BT)
▶ Endometrium
▶ Ewing Sarcoma
▶ Low-Dose Rate (LDR) Brachytherapy
▶ Neutron Radiotherapy
▶ Principles of Surgical Oncology
▶ Rhabdomyosarcoma
▶ Sarcoma

References

Edge SB, Byrd DR, Compton CC et al (eds) (2010) AJCC (American Joint Committee on Cancer) cancer staging manual, 7th edn. Springer, New York, p 291

Kepka L, Suit HD, Goldberg SI et al (2005) Results of radiation therapy performed after unplanned surgery (without reexcision) for soft tissue sarcomas. J Surg Oncol 92:39

Klepka L, Delaney TF, Suit HD, Goldberg SI (2005) Results of radiation therapy for unresected soft tissue sarcomas. Int J Radiat Oncol Biol Phys 63:852

Panicek DM, Gatsonis C, Rosenthal DI et al (1997) CT and MRI imaging in the local staging of primary malignant musculoskeletal neoplasms: report of the radiology diagnostic oncology group. Radiology 202:237

Pisters PW, Leung DH, Woodruff J et al (1996) Analysis of prognostic factors in 1,041 patients with localized soft tissue sarcomas of the extremities. J Clin Oncol 14:1679

Pollack R, Brennan M, Lawrence W Jr (1997) Society of surgical oncology practice guidelines. Oncol (Huntingt) 11:1327

Suit HD, Rosenberg AE, Harmon DC et al (1995) Soft tissue sarcomas. In: Price P, Sikora K (eds) Treatment of cancer, 3rd edn. Chapman and Hall Medical, London, p 805

Solar Keratosis

▶ Actinic Keratosis

Solitary Brain Metastasis

James H. Brashears, III
Radiation Oncologist, Venice, FL, USA

Definition
One brain lesion as the only site of metastatic disease.

Cross-References
▶ Palliation of Brain and Spinal Cord Metastases

Solitary Plasmacytoma

▶ Plasma Cell Myeloma

Somnolence Syndrome

James H. Brashears, III
Radiation Oncologist, Venice, FL, USA

Definition
An early-delayed side effect often seen in children after whole brain radiation therapy for leukemia, with symptoms ranging from drowsiness to exhaustion. Symptoms begin 1 month after radiotherapy and spontaneously improve in 1–3 weeks.

Cross-References
▶ Supportive Care and Quality of Life

SPECT/PET Studies

Patrizia Guerrieri, Paolo Montemaggi
Department of Radiation Oncology, Regional Cancer Center "M. Ascoli", University of Palermo Medical School, Palermo, Italy

Definition
Nuclear medicine studies carried out using biomolecules linked with a radioisotope which allow tracking the incorporation of the molecule in the cells by scanning the recipient through specifically arranged detectors. Positron Emission Tomography (PET) has a useful but still nonstandardized role in the delineation of tumor biological target and in the follow-up of various neoplastic diseases. The most widely used molecule in PET studies is radioactive fluorodeoxyglucose, an analog of glucose that is labeled with fluorine-18. This tracer is a glucose analog that is taken up by glucose-using cells and phosphorylated by hexokinase (whose mitochondrial form is greatly elevated in rapidly growing malignant tumors).

Cross-References
▶ Imaging in Oncology
▶ Vulvar Carcinoma

Sphenoid Sinus

Filip T. Troicki
College of Medicine, Drexel University, Philadelphia, PA, USA

Definition
Sphenoid sinus is a mucous membrane–lined cavity located deeper in the skull behind the bridge of the nose.

Cross-References
▶ Nasal Cavity and Paranasal Sinuses

Sphere Packing

Brian F. Hasson
Department of Radiation Oncology, Abington Memorial Hospital, Abington, PA, USA
Department of Radiation Oncology, College of Medicine, Drexel University, Philadelphia, PA, USA

Definition
A set of mathematical problems that are used to compute arrangements of nonoverlapping identical spheres which fill a space. Sphere packing analysis is used in stereotactic radiosurgery treatment planning to provide possible solutions for achieving the most conformal dose coverage of a target.

Cross-References

▶ Stereotactic Radiosurgery – Cranial

Spinal Canal Tumor

TONY S. QUANG[1], LINNA LI[2]
[1]Department of Radiation Oncology, VA Puget Sound Health Care System University of Washington Medical Center, Seattle, WA, USA
[2]Radiation Oncology, Fox Chase Cancer Center, Philadelphia, PA, USA

Synonyms

Anaplastic astrocytoma; Anaplastic ependymoma; Astrocytomas; Ependymomas; Fibrillary astrocytoma; Glioblastoma multiforme; Hemangioblastomas; Meningioma; Myxopapillary ependymomas; Nerve sheath tumor; Oligodendrogliomas

Definition

Tumors of the spinal cord and cauda equina are a heterogeneous group of tumors classified by their location relative to the protective layers of the spinal cord see (Fig. 1). Lesions are intramedullary, intradural-extramedullary, or extradural-extramedullary. Intramedullary tumors include gliomas such as astrocytomas, ependymomas, and oligodendrogliomas. Extramedullary tumors arise from the intrinsic substance of the spinal canal: the connective tissues, blood vessels, or coverings adjacent to the cord or cauda equina. Intradural-extramedullary tumors include ependymoma, nerve sheath tumors, meningioma, and vascular tumors. Extradural lesions may be primary tumors, but are most often metastatic. Primary extradural tumors may arise from the vertebral bodies and surrounding tissues including benign or malignant bone tumors, epidural hemangiomas, lipomas, extradural meningiomas, nerve sheath tumors, and lymphomas. Radiation therapy is an important modality in the management of both primary and metastatic spinal canal tumors; this discussion is limited to primary tumors of the spinal cord.

Anatomy

The spinal cord is a cylindrical bundle of nerve tissue and support cells that functions to transmit neural signals between the brain and the rest of the body. It originates from the brain at the foramen magnum and terminates at the conus medullaris. At the level of each vertebra, paired ventral and dorsal nerve roots exit the lateral aspect of the cord. These coalesce to form the functional segments of the spinal cord: 31 pairs of spinal nerves (8 cervical, 12 thoracic, 5 lumbar, 5 sacral, and 1 coccygeal). The spinal cord is covered by the meninges and cushioned by cerebrospinal fluid (CSF). The protective innermost meningeal layer is the pia mater, which condenses into ligaments that suspends the cord to the dura mater, a tough, fibrous barrier between the bony spinal canal and the spinal cord. Between the dura mater and the pia mater is the arachnoid mater encloses the subarachnoid space, which is filled with CSF.

Background

Primary spinal canal tumors comprise 4–6% of all primary CNS tumors. True primary spinal cord neoplasms are relatively rare and typically intradural in location. In adults, nearly two-thirds of these are extramedullary: typically nerve sheath tumors, meningiomas, or ependymomas. The remaining intradural tumors are intramedullary; the most common histology is astrocytoma or ependymoma, followed by hemangioblastomas and other tumor types. The most common spinal canal neoplasms include extramedullary nerve sheath tumors and meningiomas, followed by intramedullary ependymomas and astrocytomas.

S

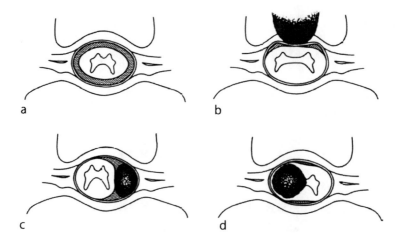

Spinal Canal Tumor. Fig. 1 Neoplasms affecting the spinal cord. (**a**) Normal transverse spine. The spinal cord is enveloped by the pia, arachnoid, and dura mater, which are housed in the spinal canal and surrounded by ligaments supporting the vertebral bony structures. The subarachnoid space contains cerebrospinal fluid. (**b**) Transverse spine with extradural mass. An extradural mass (e.g., metastasis) from the vertebral body is compressing the dural sac and the spinal cord from the anterior direction. The subarachnoid space becomes obliterated at that level, causing a myelographic block. (**c**) Transverse spine with an intradural-extramedullary mass. The mass, typically a meningioma or nerve sheath tumor, is compressing the spinal cord and roots in the dural sac, causing a myelographic block with a laterally displaced cord and, at times, producing a capping contour of contrast border. (**d**) Transverse spine with intramedullary mass. An intramedullary mass (astrocytoma or ependymoma) is infiltrating and expanding the spinal cord within the dural sac, causing a myelographic block (From Devinsky and Feldman 1988. NB: permission pending this was 34.1 in Perez Brady)

Primary spinal canal tumors are relatively more frequent in children, typically presenting at age less than 10. Intraspinal tumors in children are somewhat equally distributed between intramedullary, intradural-extramedullary, or extradural tumors.

Although most primary tumors of the spinal canal are histologically benign, they can compress or invade the spinal cord, interfering with neurologic function and causing significant disability. Mortality often results from complications of paraplegia or quadriplegia such as infection or respiratory impairment. Metastatic spread from spinal canal tumors is extremely rare. Because the CNS has no lymphatics, spread to lymph nodes does not occur. Prognostic factors include tumor type and grade, tumor extent and location,

patient age, presenting neurologic function, and tumor resectability.

Clinical Presentation

In nearly three-quarters of patients, pain is the presenting symptom, often localized to the region of involvement. Pain is often described as gnawing and unrelenting and may exist for a long time prior to the manifestation of localizing neurologic signs. Radicular pain, arising from pressure on nerve roots, is characterized by the distribution of the involved root. Recumbency may lead to venous congestion and exacerbate symptoms at night. Less commonly, pain is characterized as a burning sensation in one or more extremities, with numbness a more advanced sign that indicates compromise of spinal nerve or nerve tract conduction. CNS involvement may also manifest as weakness, sensory changes, and sphincter dysfunction. In general, symptoms have a more protracted duration in low-grade tumors than in high-grade tumors. Dysfunction in bladder or bowel is relatively uncommon except for tumors that involve the conus medullaris and filum terminale. In young children, a history of failure to achieve milestones, such as ambulation and control of bladder and bowel, or of regression of already acquired skills, may signal spinal cord or CNS pathology.

Differential Diagnosis

Diagnostic workup for primary tumors of the spinal cord requires a meticulous patient history and physical examination, and a complete neurologic examination focusing on testing motor and sensory functions and reflexes (Devinsky and Feldman 1988; Epstein et al. 1992). The differential diagnosis of a patient with a spinal cord tumor may include syringomyelia, multiple sclerosis, amyotrophic lateral sclerosis, diabetic neuropathy, viral myelitis, or paraneoplastic syndromes.

Although the level of cord compression is a few segments higher than the superior level of sensory loss, because of pathway crossing characteristics, a cutaneous sensory level may be definable. Below a specific dermatomal level, the loss of pain, heat, and cold sensation indicates compromise of the spinothalamic pathway in the lateral columns. Impaired posture, gait, and coordination and loss of vibration sense indicate that the posterior spinocerebellar pathways or posterior columns have been compromised.

Clinical findings at and below the lesion are consistent with lower and upper motor neuron involvement, respectively, and neurologic dysfunction may be asymmetric. At the lesion, flaccid weakness and loss of tendon reflexes may occur, and in acute disease stages these same signs are noticed below the lesion. In subacute and chronic stages, spastic plegia and hyperactive tendon reflexes as well as an upward Babinski's toe sign develop. A classic Brown-Séquard syndrome may exist with ipsilateral loss of motor function and fine touch sensation, and below the level of the lesion, pain and temperature sensation may be contralaterally impaired. Signs and symptoms that characterize neoplasms of the conus medullaris and filum terminale include early impairment of bladder function, saddle anesthesia, and late developing pain.

Imaging Studies

Diagnostic imaging studies should include plain radiography and magnetic resonance imaging (MRI) of the entire spine and of the brain, and intraoperative ultrasound. Myelography with computed tomography (CT) is optional.

The imaging study of choice is MRI. Almost all primary spinal cord tumors of the spine enhance with gadolinium (Greenwood 1982). Sagittal and axial images provide a three-dimensional appreciation of the patient's anatomy and help guide therapy. Some cystic tumors, vascular lesions, or lipomas can be diagnosed based on their characteristic signals on T1- and T2-weighted images without contrast injection. Administration of intravenous gadolinium improves MRI sensitivity by enhancing the solid component of intramedullary tumors and differentiating them from surrounding edema or syrinx cavities. Gadolinium also enhances sagittal T1-weighted images to localize intramedullary mass neoplasms (along with adjacent cysts), intradural-extramedullary lesions, and leptomeningeal metastases. To exclude the possibility of neuraxis seeding or the presence of an intracranial primary tumor, brain MRI should be conducted in patients with ependymoma or anaplastic ependymoma.

In approximately 50% of patients with primary spinal canal neoplasms, plain radiographs of the spine will display abnormalities. Lesions include erosion of vertebral pedicles, enlargement of the anteroposterior diameter of the bony canal, or scalloping of the posterior wall of the vertebral bodies. Plain radiographs are more likely to reveal changes in children than in adults. Calcification may be seen in extramedullary tumors, especially meningiomas, and less frequently in nerve sheath tumors. Spinal canal tumors also may be associated with scoliosis or kyphoscoliosis, especially in children.

Myelography is used in cases where MRI is contraindicated. In these patients, CT combined with myelography provides better spatial resolution. CT is most helpful in evaluating the spine for extradural pathology. Contrast-enhanced CT scans are used to detect bone tumors or paraspinal soft tissue masses that secondarily involve the spinal cord. Nerve sheath tumors can enlarge the intervertebral foramina or spinal canal and cause smooth erosion of bone, and meningiomas occasionally become calcified. Thus, both of these neoplasms are partially outlined by CSF and produce extramedullary deformity by displacing the spinal cord.

Laboratory Studies

MRI should be obtained prior to a lumbar puncture to avoid exacerbating the patient's symptoms or spinal cord shifting and incarceration. Cytological examination of the cerebrospinal fluid should be done in patients with ependymoma, anaplastic ependymoma, or high-grade glioma. Cerebrospinal fluid chemistry testing is optional. Suspected primary cord tumors should be confirmed pathologically. Diagnosis of a metastatic extradural or epidural tumor may be established via percutaneous needle biopsy under fluoroscopic or CT guidance. In patients presenting with spinal cord compression without a prior diagnosis of cancer, a surgical decompression by laminectomy or anterior corpectomy may

confirm the diagnosis and provide immediate relief of the presenting neurologic deficit. Rarely, emergency radiation therapy may be indicated to relieve spinal cord compression in the absence of a confirmed cancer diagnosis.

Treatment

General

Typically, surgery with preservation of neurologic function is the preferred treatment approach. Approximately two-thirds of all spinal canal ependymomas occur in the lumbosacral region, and 40% arise from within the filum terminale. In children, a great number of tumors are low-grade, fibrillary, or juvenile pilocytic astrocytomas, which are noninfiltrative, whereby more radical resections are possible. Complete resection of infiltrative fibrillary or anaplastic astrocytomas and glioblastoma multiforme carries a significant risk for neurologic disability; thus, a subtotal resection or biopsy may be the only safe surgical option.

Most intradural-extramedullary ependymomas in the lumbosacral spine are of the myxopapillary type which often can be completely excised. When these tumors tightly envelop the nerve roots of the cauda equina, piecemeal removal is necessitated. Because late recurrences can occur even after complete gross excision, long-term follow-up of these patients is required.

Benign vascular neoplasms, including arteriovenous malformations, hemangiomas, and hemangioblastomas, can also arise from within the spinal cord. They are well circumscribed and amenable to surgery. Most intradural-extramedullary neoplasms are meningiomas, nerve sheath tumors, or myxopapillary ependymomas, which are usually amenable to complete surgical excision. Nerve sheath tumors are typically benign, well-encapsulated, and amenable to total surgical excision. The rare malignant nerve sheath tumors are treated similarly to soft tissue sarcomas.

Finally, unusual intradural-extramedullary tumors that are categorized as miscellaneous tumors include lipomas, dermoids, and epidermoid tumors. Incomplete excision can lead to recurrence. The slow-growing dermoids are very rare. Epidermoid tumors can be seen anywhere along the spinal canal and are usually benign. Lipomas account for approximately 1% of spinal canal primary neoplasms. Small tumors are often amenable to complete removal with excellent neurologic results.

Medical

The medical management of patients with primary spinal canal tumors includes control of cerebral edema, increased intracranial pressure, and neurologic symptoms. The common symptoms of seizures, headaches, and nausea and vomiting are usually first to be addressed. Glucocorticoids are used before surgery and during radiotherapy to control symptoms due to cerebral edema. Dexamethasone 4 mg PO QID is commonly prescribed initially after a 10 mg loading dose. Because of the numerous side effects attendant with prolonged steroid use, it should be tapered slowly over several weeks when neurologic symptoms abate.

Surgery

For all tumors, the treatment of choice is total or near-total surgical excision with preservation of neurologic function. Surgical interventions for spinal canal tumors have been benefited with the introduction of the operating microscope, Cavitron ultrasonic surgical aspirator (CUSA), intraoperative ultrasonography, laser coagulation, and evoked potential monitoring, thus making complete resections more feasible with less complications. For intradural-extramedullary tumors in adults, most benign nerve sheath tumors and meningiomas can be completely resected using a posterior approach with a standard posterior laminectomy. Nerve sheath tumors are far less likely to recur than spinal meningiomas. Although piecemeal resection of ependymomas of the filum terminale can be performed with little neurologic disability, the risk of recurrence is significant, and adjuvant radiation therapy is warranted. In young children, posterior laminotomy is the treatment of choice.

For intramedullary tumors, the vast majority of which are astrocytomas and ependymomas, complete excision is the treatment of choice if it can be achieved without compromising neurologic function. Surgical advancements have assisted this goal, including microsurgical techniques, the use of intraoperative ultrasonography, and the use of CUSA and the carbon dioxide laser.

Complete excision of spinal cord tumors obviates the use of postoperative therapy. In cases of recurrence, tumor regrowth is often slow and second resection may be possible. For an intramedullary tumor, if complete surgical excision is not feasible without sacrificing neurologic function, subtotal excision may be sufficient. The benefits of postoperative radiation therapy should be weighed against the risk of late sequelae. Because many of these tumors are slow growing, radiation therapy can sometimes be delayed. Deferring the use of adjuvant radiation therapy is particularly important in children because of the effects on vertebral body growth. In children, an osteoplastic laminotomy may reduce the risk of spinal deformity, and reconstructive procedures, such as Harrington rod or Cotrel–Dubousset system placement, may prevent significant damage.

Chemotherapy

The absolute benefits of chemotherapy for ependymoma or low-grade astrocytomas have not yet been established, although some have advocated the use of chemotherapy in children. Ongoing clinical trials are investigating the use of temozolomide and lomustine in patients with high-grade spinal cord gliomas and astrocytomas.

Spinal Canal Tumor. Table 1 Radiotherapy management of spinal cord tumors

Type	Clinical target volume (CTV)	Radiation treatment
Low-grade glioma or ependymoma – total resection	–	Observation
Low-grade glioma – incomplete resection	Preoperative tumor volume + residual tumor + 1 cm	50.4 Gy
Ependymoma – incomplete resection	Preoperative tumor volume + residual tumor + 1 cm	50.4 Gy
High-grade glioma	Preoperative tumor volume + residual tumor + 1.5–2 cm	50.4 Gy
Malignant ependymoma, multifocal ependymoma, disseminated high-grade glioma	Entire spinal axis	Cranial spinal radiation to 45 Gy, with 5.4–9 Gy boost to tumor + 2 cm
Meningioma – incomplete resection	Preoperative tumor volume + residual tumor + 1 cm	Observation versus 50.4 Gy

Radiotherapy

The role of radiotherapy in the treatment of spinal canal tumors is appropriate for a select group of patients. Considerations for the use of radiation therapy include the type of tumor, tumor grade, age of the patient, extent of prior surgical excision, goal of local control and prolonged survival, and the risk for radiation-related injury see (Table 1). For patients with intramedullary low-grade astrocytomas and ependymomas who have undergone complete resection, the prognosis is excellent with no additional therapy (Larson 1996; Linstadt et al. 1989). At the time of progression or recurrence, a second surgery and/or radiation therapy may be indicated. In patients with incomplete or piecemeal resection, the addition of radiation therapy improves the local recurrence rate to that equal to rates of gross total resection. Regardless of the extent of resection, postoperative radiation is indicated for all patients with high-grade glioma or anaplastic ependymomas where local recurrences are more common and aggressive. Intradural-extramedullary tumors rarely recur after total excision and have an excellent prognosis. Data do not exist to support the routine use of radiation therapy in the management of patients with nerve sheath tumors, vascular malformations, lipomas, hemangiomas, teratomas, and dermoids. Because subtotally resected meningiomas may recur late after surgery, postoperative radiation therapy may be beneficial.

Radiation therapy in young children who are diagnosed before their pubertal growth spurt are at particular risk for developing radiation-induced deformity, and thus therapeutic options must be carefully considered in this population (Merchant et al. 1999; Merchant et al. 2000). The pediatric guideline for the treatment of a spinal cord astrocytoma and ependymomas is total resection with second surgery if postoperative MRI shows residual tumor. Radiation therapy is withheld if gross total resection achieved in low-grade astrocytomas and myxopapillary ependymomas (Michalski 2008). Due to frequent recurrence of non-myxopapillary ependymomas in children, postoperative radiation after total resection is indicated (Nadkarni and Rekate 1999; Schultheiss et al. 1984).

Sequelae of radiation therapy are contingent upon spinal cord tolerance (Schultheiss et al. 1984; Wara et al. 1975). A reversible myelopathy may manifest within 2–6 months post therapy as ▶ L'Hermitte's sign: shock-like sensations radiating to the hands and feet when the neck is flexed. This syndrome usually lasts a few weeks, is not associated with chronic progressive myelitis, and resolves without therapy. Chronic progressive myelopathy is rare, but can occur months to years after radiation therapy. The occurrence of chronic progressive myelopathy depends on total dose, fraction size, volume, and region irradiated. The risk of causing myelopathy post therapy must be weighed against the risk of progressive tumor resulting in severe neurologic dysfunction.

The use of intensity-modulated radiotherapy technique (IMRT) is typically preferred over conformal techniques to reduce the risk of acute and long-term toxicities to normal structures such as gastrointestinal tract, lungs, kidney, and liver. Additional radiation techniques such as stereotactic radiotherapy with Cyberknife or linear accelerator may further decrease dose to normal organs and decrease toxicity. Cyberknife has additional advantages of real-time tumor detection and tracking to increase treatment accuracy.

Outcome after postoperative radiation is generally excellent, with long-term survival rates of 70–100% in patients with low-grade astrocytoma and ependymoma. Recurrences are local, occurring in up to 30% of ependymomas and 50% of low-grade astrocytomas. Late local recurrence can be seen more than 5 years after initial treatment in ependymomas and 2–3 years in low-grade astrocytomas. In high-grade astrocytomas, long-term results are dismal with extreme rapid local recurrence, CSF dissemination, and short survival times of less than 1–2 years.

Cross-References

▶ Image-Guided Radiation Therapy (IGRT): kV Imaging
▶ Image-Guided Radiation Therapy (IGRT): MV Imaging
▶ Image-Guided Radiation Therapy (IGRT): TomoTherapy
▶ Image-Guided Radiotherapy (IGRT)
▶ Intensity Modulated Radiation Therapy (IMRT)
▶ Robotic Radiotherapy
▶ Spinal Canal Tumor
▶ Stereotactic Radiosurgery: Extracranial

References

Devinsky O, Feldman E (1988) Examination of the cranial and peripheral nerves. Churchill Livingstone, Philadelphia

Epstein FJ, Farmer JP, Freed D (1992) Adult intramedullary astrocytomas of the spinal cord. J Neurosurg 77:355–359

Greenwood J (1982) Spinal cord tumors. In: Youman JR (ed) Neurological surgery. W.B. Saunders, Philadelphia

Larson DA (1996) Radiation therapy of tumors of the spine. In: Youman JR (ed) Neurological surgery. W.B. Saunders, Philadelphia

Linstadt DE, Wara WM, Leibel SA et al (1989) Postoperative radiotherapy of primary spinal cord tumors. Int J Radiat Oncol Biol Phys 16:1397–1403

Merchant TE, Nguyen D, Thompson SJ et al (1999) High-grade pediatric spinal cord tumors. Pediatr Neurosurg 39:1–5

Merchant TE, Kiehna EN, Thompson SJ et al (2000) Pediatric low-grade and ependymal spinal cord tumors. Pediatr Neurosurg 32:30–36

Michalski JM (2008) Spinal canal. In: Halperin EC, Perez CA, Brady LW (eds) Perez and Brady's principles and practice of radiation oncology, 5th edn. Lippincott Williams & Wilkins, New York

Nadkarni TD, Rekate HL (1999) Pediatric intramedullary spinal cord tumors. Childs Nerv Syst 15:17–28

Schultheiss TE, Higgins EM, El-Mahdi AM (1984) The latent period in clinical radiation myelopathy. Int J Radiat Oncol Biol Phys 10:1109–1115

Wara WM, Phillips TL, Sheline GE et al (1975) Radiation tolerance of the spinal cord. Cancer 35:1558–1562

Spread-Out Bragg Peak (SOBP)

Daniel Yeung[1], Jatinder Palta[2]
[1]Department of Radiation Oncology, Univeristy of Florida Proton Therapy Institute, Jacksonville, FL, USA
[2]Department of Radiation Oncology, University of Florida Health Science Center, Gainesville, FL, USA

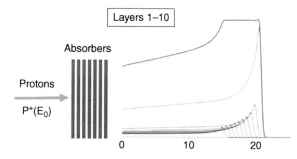

Spread-Out Bragg Peak (SOBP). Fig. 1 A spread-out Bragg peak (SOBP) to extend the uniform dose region in depth can be formed by energy stacking. Ten layers are shown in this illustration (Courtesy of R. Slopsema, UFPTI, USA)

Definition

The extended uniform dose region in depth formed by the optimal stacking of multiple depth dose curves of pristine peaks of different energies.

Cross-References

▶ Proton Therapy

Squamous Cell Carcinoma

FILIP T. TROICKI[1], JAGANMOHAN POLI[2]
[1]College of Medicine, Drexel University, Philadelphia, PA, USA
[2]Department of Radiation Oncology, College of Medicine, Drexel University, Philadelphia, PA, USA

Definition

A cancer that arises from squamous cells that have been damaged and/or mutated.

Cross-References

▶ Esophageal Cancer
▶ Lung Cancer
▶ Nasal Cavity and Paranasal Sinuses
▶ Sarcomas of the Head and Neck
▶ Skin Cancer

Stage 0 Breast Cancer

▶ Cancer of the Breast Tis

Statistically Significant

EDWARD J. GRACELY
Department of Epidemiology and Biostatistics, College of Medicine, Drexel University, Philadelphia, PA, USA

Definition

A result with *p*-value small enough that chance is considered an unlikely explanation.

Cross-References

▶ Statistics and Clinical Trials

Statistics and Clinical Trials

EDWARD J. GRACELY
Department of Epidemiology and Biostatistics, College of Medicine, Drexel University, Philadelphia, PA, USA

Introduction

This contribution is an overview of some concepts and issues in statistics and research design especially relevant to research in radiation oncology. It differs from other Encyclopedia entries in that there is, of course, no "disease" entity to define and no specific technique to elucidate. Rather, a variety of topics in the area will be presented.

Hypothesis Testing

Concepts: Null and Alternative Hypotheses, p-Values, Alpha and Beta, Type I and Type II Errors, Statistical Significance

Most clinical research compares a ▶ sample of patients given a treatment to a similar group receiving a different (or no) treatment. In the best designs, treatment assignment is randomized, although other designs are also used.

Any of these designs has the potential for producing invalid results due to flaws in the research itself ("biases") or due to unintended differences between naturally occurring populations ("confounding"). These concerns will be discussed in more detail in the research design section below.

For the topic of hypothesis testing, the main concern is that the results may be misleading because of *chance*. The observed data is from a sample, which is subject to random variation. For example, just by chance, the patients more likely to recover (or to die) could be assigned to one treatment group. The response rates in the treatment or control group (or both!) may differ in nontrivial ways from what the true, long-run response rate would be of patients in that same condition. So, the sample results do not tell the whole story. In the jargon of statistics, the true, "long-run" response pattern in each group, and the comparison, is referred to as the "▶ population" pattern, in contrast to the mere "sample" results that the researcher has in hand.

For example, researchers were studying patients with mobile rectal cancer undergoing total mesorectal excision, some of whom received preoperative radiotherapy while others did not (Peeters et al. 2007). These authors found a 5-year local recurrence rate of 5.6% in the radiotherapy group versus 10.9% in the group without it. How would we determine if this rate difference could easily be chance?

A statistical analysis of this study would begin by stating a null and alternative hypothesis. Both refer to the population state of affairs. The ▶ null hypothesis says that in the population (which, you recall, means "in the long run" or "in truth"), there is *no difference* between the radiation and non-radiation treatments on 5-year local recurrence rates. The *alternative hypothesis* says that there is a difference.

The next step is to assess the compatibility of the observed results with that null hypothesis. Using one of a variety of statistical techniques (beyond the scope of this chapter) one calculates a "▶ p-value" for the observed difference. The p-value is defined as the probability of seeing a difference as large as that observed (or larger) if there was, in truth, no real difference (equivalent to saying, "If the null hypothesis was true"). A small p-value says, in effect, "Your results would be difficult to obtain by chance alone, hence chance is not a good explanation for them." While large p-values do not demonstrate that chance is the cause, they also do not enable the researcher to argue against it.

The cutoff for a strong argument against chance (referred to as a *statistically significant result*) is set by the researcher in advance of data analysis. It is referred to as alpha (α), and is usually 0.05 in the absence of a good reason to do otherwise. Thus, normally, $p \leq 0.05$ is required to declare a result difficult to explain by chance, and thus ▶ statistically significant.

In the example above, the authors reported $p < 0.001$, which means that given their sample size, a difference as great as that observed would occur by chance alone less than once in a thousand similar studies. Thus chance is NOT a good explanation, and the result is statistically significant.

Since chance can never be completely eliminated, there is always a possibility that a researcher will obtain a statistically significant result even though there is no true difference in the population. Such a false significance is referred to as a ► type I error. The opposite error is also possible – a real effect is missed (also by chance). The latter is a ► type II error. These terms are often used in critiques of studies. For example, someone who finds no benefit to an intervention, but has a small sample size, may be challenged by a reviewer as high risk for type II error.

The probability of a type I error is alpha, as defined above. The probability of a type II error is symbolized beta (β) and is inversely related to the ► power of a study (more on that below).

Methods for Showing the Absence of a Difference or Association (Rather than for Demonstrating One)

Sometimes a researcher wants to show that there is no difference between a new treatment and an established standard. In other cases, it may be of interest to show that two treatments do not differ by what would be regarded as a clinically important amount.

There are a number of approaches that are sometimes used.

Two simple ones are commonly employed. Perhaps the least efficient is to demonstrate that one has a large sample size (and thus low probability of type II error, and a high power) and therefore should be able to find any important differences. If, in fact, no difference is found, this creates an argument that no such difference exists. While often used, at least in ad hoc analyses, this is a very indirect approach which does not give a well-defined idea how large a difference might be consistent with the obtained results.

A second simple approach, much better than the first, is to provide an indication of the largest and smallest differences that would be consistent with the observed data, based on a 95% ► confidence interval (see below). This approach allows the researcher to say something like, "Given our

data, the largest benefit for the old treatment over the new would be an absolute 5% decrease in recurrence rates." Then the reader can judge whether that is convincing evidence of lack of meaningful difference.

But if showing the absence of a difference is truly critical to the study, there are more specific methods designed to achieve that purpose. Terms like "equivalency trials" and "non-inferiority trials" are used. It is beyond the scope of this chapter to describe them in detail, but the basic idea would be something like this. Say the current standard of care requires 12 radiation treatments for a certain cancer, and a researcher is confident that 9 would work equally well at local control. Assume that the benefits of a shorter course would be sufficient to justify its use as long as it causes less than an absolute 5% increase in local recurrences. The statistical model would consist in taking as the null hypothesis *not* the absence of a difference (the usual case), but rather the existence of a 5% difference in favor of the longer course of therapy. You then design the study with enough subjects that you will be able to reject this null hypothesis in favor of less than that as the true difference. A small p-value indicates that your result is so far less than 5% in favor of the standard therapy that chance cannot explain it.

The Problem of Multiple Comparisons

A single test of a hypothesis for which there is no true difference may still result in a statistically significant result, a type I error, as described above. This is considered one of the unavoidable risks of science with variable data.

Unfortunately, some research practices can drastically multiply this risk. Too often researchers do one or more of the following:

- Test numerous, catch-all, comparisons as part of the same study ("Let's see if any of these variables is correlated with success...")

- Perform multiple subgroup analyses in the study ("Maybe the treatment will work in the elderly female subgroup with gingivitis...")
- Develop outcome measures as they go along, combining several outcomes into a "composite" that may capitalize on chance ("Treatment failure was defined as less than 5 months until recurrence, or the presence of kidney failure, or a blood pressure at any time over 130/90...")
- Report only the comparisons that were significant or nearly so, and don't "bother" to mention the things they tried but which did not produce any interesting findings

Needless to say, all of this is problematic. Here are some guidelines:

- Identify key and primary hypotheses, with pre-specified outcome variables, in advance of data analysis (or collection).
- Perform only subgroup analyses that are clearly relevant and were planned in advance.
- Avoid "data fishing" such as looking for subgroups or combinations of variables in which significance may be found.
- Report all analyses done, significant or not.
- If multiple analyses need to be reported, take that fact into account in reporting the results.

The last bullet needs a bit of elaboration. There are many ways to take multiple analyses into account. The simplest is the so-called Bonferroni correction (or one of its many variants, some of which are popular in some circles today). Basically you drastically drop the alpha level at which significance will be declared as a direct function of the number of analyses. So, for 10 comparisons, each must be significant at $p \leq 0.005$, instead of 0.05.

Some researchers will prefer to identify a single, primary hypothesis in advance, and test that at 0.05, then use a much stricter alpha for the rest. In other cases, the researcher will test all

hypotheses at 0.05 but make clear in advance that only a pattern of significance will be interpreted, not isolated results.

In general, in combination with the other bullet points above, almost any halfway reasonable method of avoiding type I error is probably acceptable. But researchers must take the issue seriously, or the literature will be cluttered with a large number of barely significant results, many of which would never have seen print but for a bit of data fishing, and whose results will not be replicable. What did you say? The literature sometimes looks like that now? Exactly!

Confidence Intervals

As noted above, the results obtained in a sample are always subject to random variation from other samples and the underlying population. Confidence intervals provide a means of indicating the extent to which such variation may reasonably have shifted the observed statistic away from the population statistic.

For example, Bartelink et al. (2001) looked at the impact of additional radiotherapy on prevention of local recurrences. They report, "The 5-year actuarial rates of local recurrence were 7.3% (95% confidence interval, 6.8–7.6%) and 4.3% (95% confidence interval, 3.8–4.7%), respectively (P < 0.001)." The two percentages refer to the standard and additional radiation groups, respectively. The quote could be interpreted as follows: In the standard therapy sample, using methods that account for losses to follow-up (actuarial) the best estimate of the 5-year local recurrence rate is 7.3%. This is just a sample rate, and is subject to chance variation. We can be 95% sure that the population rate of local recurrence is between 6.8 and 7.6%.

Of course, a confidence interval only considers chance deviations from the population value. If the sample was biased in some way, for example, by unintentionally oversampling patients with more severe disease, a 95% confidence interval cannot correct for that!

The most common uses for 95% confidence intervals are around statistics of comparative risk. There are a number of these, all of which are a ratio of some kind of rate or probability in the numerator representing one group or condition to the same statistic in the denominator representing another. In particular:

- *Relative risk*: ratio of the respective incidence rates for the outcome of interest
- *Odds ratio*: ratio of the odds of the outcome of interest between two conditions
- *Hazard ratio*: a more complex statistic that assesses the incidence in the two groups but also takes into account the pattern over time

Readers may have noted in the above example that the two 95% confidence intervals are not even overlapping. That's pretty good evidence that the percentages are different in the population. But a more direct method of assessing possible differences is to calculate one of the ratio statistics and put a confidence interval around it. Thus, Bartelink et al. reported, "a hazard ratio for local recurrence of 0.59 (99% confidence interval, 0.43–0.81) associated with an additional dose." This is pretty close to the ratio of the 5 year hazard rates above (4.3/7.3) although it is not calculated in exactly that manner. The 95% confidence interval shows that *at worst* the increased dose would still have a local recurrence of 0.81 times as great as the lesser dose (a 19% decrease), but the increase due to increased dose could be much greater!

It is common to interpret 95% confidence intervals for such ratio statistics by checking whether 1.0 is in the interval. Since a ratio of two identical values would be 1, failure to include 1 in the interval suggests a difference beyond chance, and implies a statistically significant result. Readers should also examine the width of the interval and the closeness of it to 1. Thus, a report that says the following is pretty convincing: "The relative risk of local recurrence in the condition with more radiation compared to standard was 0.4, 95% confidence interval 0.3–0.5." By contrast, "The relative risk of more radiation was 0.4, 95% confidence interval 0.05–0.95" is consistent with such a wide range as to be barely interpretable, although technically it is statistically significant.

The comparison to 1 only applies to ratio type comparative statistics, of course. If a researcher compares two percentages by calculating a risk *difference*, then the absence of an effect would be seen by a difference of 0, not of 1. Otherwise, these principles work in a similar manner.

Power and Sample Size

As noted above, chance is the ever-present lurker in all statistical analyses. One possible effect of chance is to produce false positive results, in which there is an apparent difference or effect in the study although there is no true difference in the population. We dealt with this above by setting an alpha level for an "acceptable" probability of a false positive (a type I error).

The other possibility is that chance could lead a researcher to miss a real and relevant result, a "false negative" (type II) error. The main bulwark against this risk is ensuring that the study has an adequate sample size. Our quantification of this risk is based on calculating beta (β), as defined above, or its inverse, the power of the study.

Power is defined as the probability the study will attain statistically significant results *if* a specific magnitude of effect or difference exists in the population. It is dependent on the sample size (of course!), the exact differences of interest, and sometimes other factors (most notably the variability of any numeric data being analyzed).

An example: A researcher approaches a statistician with a study design to compare two methods of administering radiotherapy in patients who have a specific type of leukemia.

The outcome variable is the rate of remission. After a bit of discussion, the two might agree that a plausible and clinically important effect would be a 60% remission rate in one method versus 75% in the other.

The statistician would then pull up a spreadsheet or calculator, and determine an appropriate sample size for that kind of effect. In this example, he or she would recommend about 304 subjects in total, 152 per group. The interpretation would be, "If there truly is a 60% rate of remission in one of the methods, and 75% in the other, and if you have about 152 subjects per group, it is about 80% probable that you will find a statistically significant result in the study. If you want to be 90% sure that the study would find significance for the difference postulated, you would need approximately 406 in total."

The 80% and 90% in the above example are the power of the study for the two sample sizes. Power and/or the necessary sample size to attain significance can be calculated in a straightforward fashion in order to compare of means or percentages, or to assess the significance of a correlation coefficient or relative risk, etc.

After a study is completed, it is sometimes necessary to recalculate the power available, especially if the study was not significant. As noted above, the power can be helpful, albeit roughly, in interpreting a negative result. Why might it be necessary to redo the power calculation? Among the likely reasons: The expected sample size was not attained (or, you got lucky and exceeded it!), the variability of a numeric outcome was quite different from what was expected, etc.

One mistake to avoid is to determine the sample size which is needed in order to call the observed difference significant. The observed difference is subject to random error and has no theoretical meaning. It is much better to assess the power needed for a clinically important difference (the definition of which has probably not changed from before the study was run).

A few other observations on sample size determination:

- Consider the likely attrition (loss of subjects after enrollment) in the sample size estimation process. If you enroll 50 subjects but ten drop out early before providing any data, you effectively have 40 subjects.
- Consider ▶ intention to treat in the calculation (see below under research design for the definition): If some subjects have to be counted in a treatment group for a treatment they did not receive, this will inevitably reduce the power.
- Researchers routinely overestimate the number of subjects they can recruit, or the number that will be available in the charts. Don't be overly optimistic in your planning!

Some Common Statistical Tests and Their Uses

This section will be a *very* brief overview of some commonly encountered statistical tests. There are many of them, and even a professional statistician sometimes encounters a test he or she has never heard of. Nowadays, you can find a review of almost anything with a web search! A good overview of basic statistical methods is Dawson and Trapp (2004).

S

Comparing Averages on a Numeric Variable Between Two or More Groups or Conditions

- Just two groups or conditions, comparison variable is normally distributed or adequately close to normally distributed (bell curve…): The analysis will probably be some kind of *t-test*.
- Two groups or conditions, for which the data is *not* very normally distributed (or other assumptions of a *t*-test are not met): Probably a test based on ranking the data, one class of the so-called "*nonparametric tests*," all of

which are designed for situations when the data is non-normal or has other features that render more standard approaches unsuitable. If there were two groups, the comparison would typically use a *Mann-Whitney U* (also known as a *Wilcoxon Rank Sum test*). If subjects were observed twice, such as before and after an intervention, or in two different conditions in the same subjects, the test would probably be a *Wilcoxon Signed Ranks test.*

- If there are more than two groups or two conditions, or if the design is more complex, but still basically comparing averages, the analysis will be an *analysis of variance* or a more modern and sophisticated version like a *mixed models analysis* (especially good with several observations per subject, some of them missing, etc.).

Predicting a Variable or Looking for Associations Involving Numeric Variables

- To quantify the association between two numeric variables you can use a *Pearson correlation* for normally distributed data or a *Spearman Rank Correlation* for other data.
- To predict one variable from another, *simple linear regression* (one predictor) can be used. If you have more than one predictor, *multiple linear regression* would serve.

Comparing Groups or Conditions on a Non-numeric Outcome

- Commonly *Chi-square*, sometimes with a correction for "continuity" when sample sizes are small, although some statisticians prefer to use the *Fisher Exact test* when they don't trust ordinary Chi-square

If you need to control for possible confounding by third variables, you will probably need to do some kind of multivariate analysis. The four most common for this are:

- *Multiple linear regression*: Like simple linear regression but with more than 1 predictor. Used when the outcome or predicted variable is numeric.
- *Logistic regression:* Used when the outcome or predicted variable is yes/no.
- *Cox model (proportional hazards)*: Used when the outcome or predicted variable is time to an event (like death) especially when not all subjects will experience the event during the study time frame.
- *Analysis of covariance*: A version of analysis of variance for comparing means between groups or conditions but while simultaneously holding constant other variables than might confound the associations seen.

It is beyond the scope of this chapter to explain in detail how these methods work or are interpreted.

Clinical Trial Design

The design of clinical trials could (and has) fill (ed) entire books, so it is not possible to do it full justice in a single chapter. Here are a few basic aspects of the topic. A good standard reference to the mechanics of a clinical trial is Pocock (2002).

Official Phases of Clinical Therapeutic Research

There are four "phases" of clinical research studies, referred to as phases I to IV. You can find the basic NIH definitions on their glossary page: http://clinicaltrials.gov/ct2/info/glossary

Since these are formal, legal definitions, here is a quote from that web page (bullets added for clarity): "A clinical trial is a research study to answer specific questions about vaccines or new therapies or new ways of using known treatments. Clinical trials (also called medical research and research studies) are used to determine whether new drugs or treatments are both safe and effective. Carefully conducted clinical trials are the fastest and safest way to find treatments that work in people. Trials are in four phases:

- Phase I tests a new drug or treatment in a small group;
- Phase II expands the study to a larger group of people;
- Phase III expands the study to an even larger group of people; and
- Phase IV takes place after the drug or treatment has been licensed and marketed."

Although Phase I trials are often done in healthy volunteers, they can also be done in patients with cancer, generally looking for very preliminary information, such as whether or not there is an immune response or certain biochemical effects.

Both randomized and nonrandomized cancer studies can be classified as phase II. Sometimes they are uncontrolled (thus comparing to historically expected outcomes), which is obviously not a very convincing design unless the effect is dramatic. The randomized phase II trials are typically small, and do not provide good enough evidence to lead to approval.

Phase III trials are often the ones that lead to actual FDA approval (if the drug works!).

Basic Terms and Concepts in Clinical Trials: Randomization, Types of Randomization, Blinding, Placebos, etc.

Some basic terms:

Randomization (also called random assignment): Placing subjects into treatment groups by a random process. A dice toss could be used for small studies, but there are formal random number generators and random numbers tables that are more appropriate for larger studies. A randomized study with clinical outcomes is known

as a *Randomized Clinical Trial*, the gold standard for most clinical prevention and treatment research.

Note that the process can be complex – for example, randomization may be done separately within key subgroups, set up to ensure equal distribution of, say, older and younger patients into treatment and control groups. It is also sometimes necessary to prepare the entire randomization plan in advance, and file it in such a way that the subject's assignment is not visible to the person assessing him or her for eligibility.

Do not confuse randomization with random *sampling*, which is a method of selecting subjects, not a way to assign them.

▶ Blinding (also called masking): Blinding is the process of concealing group assignment (or other information) from subjects or researchers to reduce potential bias.

Single blinding means that the subject does not know his or her treatment assignment (although the researcher may).
Double blinding means that neither subject nor researcher knows the treatment assignment.

In some cases, other kinds of blinding can be used. For example, the radiologist reading an x-ray can be blinded as to the treatment assignment of the subjects in the study, even if the subjects and researchers both know.

Blinding is most helpful when there are subjective components to the evaluation, but it can be helpful even in cases where the outcome is objective. For one thing, few outcomes are totally objective. Thus, recurrence may be detected sooner by someone looking harder for it! And subjective factors may affect the patient's response to treatment even if the evaluation was not affected by it (say, more attention from a physician leads to longer survivals).

Placebo: A placebo is an ineffective treatment that the subject believes to be effective (or possibly effective). In most cases placebos are indistinguishable from the active treatment, although a distinct but believable alternative can sometimes be used. Even surgery can have an indistinguishable placebo – sham surgery. But this is rather rare.

The placebo effect is the apparent benefit to therapy that results from belief in it. If one group is subject to the placebo effect (say, the active treatment group) whereas the other was not (say, a no-treatment, no-placebo, control), it becomes impossible to say whether the observed differences are due to real treatment effects or placebo effects. Obviously this is more an issue if the outcome is subjective (pain, disability) than objective (recurrence, death).

Issues in Evaluating a Clinical Trial: Biases of Many Sorts

This is a topic for a book, not a book chapter, but a few key issues in evaluating a clinical trial are easily described. The focus in this chapter is on a randomized comparison of two groups, perhaps the most common and basic clinical trial design. The one most fundamental principle of research design is that a good study *rules out* (or at least provides a good argument against) *alternative* explanations for the results. The assertion that the treatments are different, say, should be the only conclusion truly consistent with the data.

A good first place to start with *any* study is to determine whether the results would be relevant to you, by changing (or perhaps, confirming) your practice. For example, if you don't see the kind of patients studied or would not use the treatment modalities investigated, this study is not relevant to your practice. Also, are the differences reported big enough as to encourage you to switch to the new treatment if you thought the study was well designed? If not, why do you care about the results?

The second question to ask yourself about a comparative study is whether there are any

factors other than the intended intervention that differ between the groups and could explain the results. The alternative explanations principle comes in directly.

One set of possible differences involves subject and/or researcher awareness of treatment assignment, and possible biases resulting from that. Placebo effects can result from subject expectations of benefit (avoided by a proper placebo control group, as noted above). Researchers can respond to or evaluate patients in different groups differently. Blinding, especially double blinding, helps avoid these problems.

But the groups can become different in other ways as well. Perhaps the randomization did not create truly comparable groups – always check the table showing the characteristics of the two groups to assess that. Sometimes subjects drop out of the study in different patterns in the two groups, which can make them non-comparable. For example, suppose that the most severely ill subjects withdraw from the placebo group (because they get no benefit) whereas less ill subjects drop out of the treatment group (because the benefit doesn't outweigh the side effects). At the end, the researcher has two non-comparable groups.

Attrition bias results when those who remain in the study over time differ in relevant ways from those who drop out or otherwise leave the study before reaching an appropriate end point. It can affect the combined study group as a whole (making the results doubtfully generalizable and thus threatening *external validity*) or one group more (or differently) than another, rendering the basic conclusions dubious (a loss of *internal validity*). Any study with a substantial number of subjects lost to follow-up or not continuing until the end (or until a study outcome occurs) should be viewed critically.

Of course, the biggest source of non-comparability of groups is found in studies that are not randomized. While a bit out of the main focus of this chapter, note that in nonrandomized studies the single biggest problem is *confounding*, that is, the possibility of naturally occurring or self-selected differences between treatment groups. For example, a common simple study design is a chart-review in which patients given one treatment are to be compared to patients given a different one. The key question in such cases becomes, "Is the choice of treatment at the whim of the doctor, say, *or* are there good reasons for patients to get one rather than the other treatment?" In either case, it is important to look closely for unintended differences, but especially the latter case. If one treatment is routinely given to patients who are more ill, have more comorbidities, etc., than the other treatment, it may not be possible to meaningfully compare the two due to these confounding variables that may affect the outcome. There are a variety of methods to deal with or reduce confounding in a non-randomized study, such as the multivariate analyses described above. None of these methods are as good as randomization!

A third key type of question concerns *the outcome variables selected for study*. They should be defined in advance, with primary outcomes selected in advance, independently of any observed patterns. All variables should be *reliable* (that is, repeatable and consistent between evaluators or equivalent time points) and *valid* (that is, measuring what they are intended to measure).

In addition, a study that can show an effect on outcomes a patient would directly care about (patient-centered outcomes, like pain, death, disability) is more meaningful than one that only shows an effect on "signs" or other disease-centered outcomes that doctors consider relevant (biopsy changes, immune response, microscopic metastases, etc.).

And, of course, side effects need to be monitored as well.

Closely related to the outcome variables is the *length of follow-up*. Even a very good outcome measure is not useful if the study doesn't follow patients long enough for effects on it to be observed. Alternatively, a treatment may seem to work for a short time period, but produce no meaningful benefit if patients are observed long enough.

Several potential issues relate to the *assignment variable* (treatment versus control). Look closely at the doses or amounts used – are they standard and appropriate? Some studies try to standardize dosing between treatments in a way that renders the use of one or the other meaningless. And it is possible to make a competing treatment look bad by using a dosage that is too high or too low!

Consider compliance with treatment as well. Radiotherapy is generally given under observation, so researchers in this field are better able to confirm compliance than those using drug regimens, but patients may skip treatments, fail to take important ancillary medications, and so on. Noncompliance with a treatment can make a different treatment look better. Noncompliance with both treatments can obliterate genuine differences!

Intention to treat is the term of art for an approach to dealing with certain common and frustrating research situations. In essence it means that when patients do not get the treatment to which they were assigned, their data is analyzed as though they did. The idea is to maintain the randomization to avoid biases.

For example, imagine a study in which patients are assigned to radiotherapy or surgery. Unfortunately, five of the patients in the radiotherapy group deteriorate and surgery is considered clinically necessary for them. What do you do with those five? Exclude them entirely? That would make the radiotherapy group less ill (since similar patients in the surgery group would not be excluded). Count them in surgery? That's even worse – now you have moved the five most ill patients from radiotherapy to surgery, biasing both groups! So, "intention to treat" says to grit your teeth and treat them as though they got

S

radiotherapy. That was your "intention." It makes the comparison conservative. If you find differences, in spite of intention to treat, your case is strong. If not, then you have to argue whether some alternative analysis is justifiable. Try really hard to make sure that all enrolled patients will be suitable for either treatment!

Nowadays it is becoming clear that you need to consider the sponsor of the study and the funding sources of the authors. We are all human – even a basically honest and ethical researcher may be uncomfortable publishing results that directly contradict the interests of his or her major funding source. The absence of overt pressure isn't definitive. A researcher may be concerned about getting future grants from a particular source after publishing critical studies even if not a word is ever said about it.

It is, unfortunately, very difficult to fully assess the impact of this factor. When a study author has potential conflicts of interest, you should look especially closely at ways in which data can be massaged without seeming dishonest. Data fishing as defined above is a possibility: does the study seem to spend too much time on post hoc subgroups or secondary outcomes? Selective reporting of results is possible – are the authors vague about key hypotheses? Do they seem to be reporting "interesting" findings rather than a comprehensive and well-planned analysis? Consider the doses used – could they have been selected in a way such as to favor one treatment over the other.

Of course, every now and then a story appears of a researcher caught fabricating data or lying about the conduct of the study – not much you can do about that!

What about studies trying to *prove the absence of an effect*, or the similarity of a new treatment to an established method? Here the sample size and the precision of the estimates of effect are critical. See the section above specifically devoted to this topic.

Cross-References

▶ Clinical Research and the Practice of Evidence-Based Medicine in Radiation Oncology

References

Bartelink H, Horiot J-C, Poortmans P et al (2001) Recurrence rates after treatment of breast cancer with standard radiotherapy with or without additional radiation. N Engl J Med 345(19):1378–1387

Dawson B, Trapp RG (2004) Basic and clinical biostatistics. Lange/McGraw Hill, New York

Peeters K, Marijnen C, Nagtegaal I et al (2007) The TME trial after a median follow-up of 6 years: increased local control but no survival benefit in irradiated patients with resectable rectal carcinoma. Ann Surg 246(5):693–701

Pocock SJ (2002 – original printing in 1983) Clinical trials: a practical approach. Wiley, Chichester

Stepping Source Afterloader (SSA)

ERIK VAN LIMBERGEN
Department of Radiation Oncology, University Hospital Gasthuisberg, Leuven, Belgium

Definition

A modern type of remote control afterloader which uses one source with a high specific activity of usually 10 Curie iridium-192 for HDR brachytherapy and of 0.5–1 Curie for PDR afterloaders. The source movement is controlled by a stepping motor. Depending on the type, steps of 1–5 mm in 3–40 channels are available. The machine is connected by transfer tubes to the source carriers in the patient. The dwell positions and dwell times are programmed by the brachytherapy planning system. Major advantages of SSAs are full radioprotection for personnel and visitors, as well as the possibility to perform optimization of dose distribution by putting different dwell times to different dwell positions.

Iridium-192 sources have a half-life of 72.4 days. Sources have to be replaced every 3 to 4 months.

Cobalt-60 sources have a half-life of 5.25 years and can be used during a longer time which is advantageous for countries where delivery of radioactive sources poses economical or political difficulties.

Cross-References

▶ Clinical Aspects of Brachytherapy (BT)
▶ High-Dose Rate (HDR) Brachytherapy
▶ Low-Dose Rate (LDR) Brachytherapy

Stereotactic

MARY ELLEN MASTERSON-MCGARY
CyberKnife Center of Tampa Bay, Tampa, FL, USA

Definition
Stereotactic: Relating to highly precise spatial localization (of a volume of tissue).

Cross-References
▶ Robotic Radiosurgery

Stereotactic Body Radiation Therapy

FENG-MING KONG, JINGBO WANG
Department of Radiation Oncology, Veteran Administration Health Center and University Hospital, University of Michigan, Ann Arbor, MI, USA

Synonyms
SBRT

Definition
Stereotactic body radiation therapy is a type of external beam radiation therapy that delivers very high dose of radiation to the tumor target, while sparing healthy tissue by using high conformal technique, special positioning/immobilization, and image guidance during treatment delivery. This procedure can be completed in 1–5 days rather than several weeks and is most commonly used for small tumors.

Cross-References
▶ Liver and Hepatobiliary Tract
▶ Lung
▶ Robotic Radiosurgery
▶ Stereotactic Radiosurgery: Extracranial

Stereotactic Radiosurgery – Cranial

BRIAN F. HASSON
Department of Radiation Oncology, Abington Memorial Hospital, Abington, PA, USA
Department of Radiation Oncology, College of Medicine, Drexel University, Philadelphia, PA, USA

Historical Introduction
Radiation oncology has undergone a continuous technological evolution since its inception in 1896. Parallel to advancements in radiation oncology were advancements in neurosurgery and medical imaging (see Table 1). In 1949, Leksell proposed the use of radiation in conjunction with a stereotactic reference system to accurately target and treat arteriovenous malformations (AVMs). In 1951, Leksell brought the three disciplines in concert to tackle the complexities of treating functional disorders.

Stereotactic Radiosurgery – Cranial. Table 1 The history of devices and events that have shaped the field of stereotactic radiosurgery

Year	Device/Event
1895	Roentgen discovered the x-ray
1896	First medical treatment using Roentgen rays
1906	First neurosurgery treatments of pituitary cancers
1951	Leksell defines *stereotactic radiosurgery*: treats SRS with rotating orthovoltage unit
1961	First protons are used for treating cranial tumors
1968	First Gamma Knife unit becomes operational
1974	First computed tomography scanner installed
1977	First body MRI images acquired
1982	Linear accelerators adapted for stereotactic radiosurgery
1984	Installation of commercial Gamma Knife – second generation
1986	Linear accelerator used for SRS using a standard invasive ring
1993	Relocatable fixation devices like the GTC become commercially available
1994	mMLCs – miniMultileaf collimators
1994	First Cyberknife unit is installed (frameless stereotactic radiosurgery begins)
1997	Rotating Gamma Knife unit is developed
2002	First commercially available Tomotherapy unit is installed

He began treatments in 1951 using a 300 kVp x-ray beam and a cylindrical coordinate stereotactic frame (Leksell 1951). Leksell later commented that there was a "need for higher energy for better penetration" (Leksell 1956).

The work of Leksell spurred a new technique in radiation oncology called "Stereotactic Radiosurgery" (SRS). Leksell defined Stereotactic Radiosurgery as "The non-invasive destruction of intracranial lesions that may be inaccessible or unsuitable for open surgery" (Leksell 1968). Stereotactic Radiosurgery and Stereotactic Radiotherapy (SRS/T) couples a 3-D coordinate reference frame with the delivery of highly focused radiation beams to a well-defined target within and with respect to the coordinate system. The most recent definition is: "(SRS) typically is performed in a single session, using a rigidly attached stereotactic guiding device, other immobilization technology and/or a stereotactic image-guidance system, but can be performed in a limited number of sessions, up to a maximum of five" (Barnett et al. 2007). Since its infancy, this technique has relied on a precise understanding of the location of the target to be treated. This reliance has placed a continual desire to acquire the best imaging studies to define the target to be treated. The advent and subsequent technological improvements in CT, MRI, and PET imaging provided further methods and tools to define the target with increasing precision.

In 1968, Leksell et al. designed and built the first cobalt-60 (^{60}Co) treatment machine for use in SRS. The machine provided a new generation of radiation-producing devices that could offer a higher energy and more penetrating beam than other available systems at the time. Parallel to the ^{60}Co unit was the design of the first linear accelerators by Varian (Podgorsak and Metcalfe 1999). These early machines allowed stereotactic radiosurgery (SRS) to begin to expand its use into more deeply seated and more complex targets. As the technology advanced and became more widely available, and the accuracy of treatment delivery and patient positioning became more precise, SRS began to expand to many centers around the world.

SRS/T Treatment Units

Gamma Knife

The initial ▶ Gamma Knife, designed by Leksell, was the earliest prototype cranial SRS system. The first Gamma Knife system was designed with 179 cobalt sources housed in a gantry. Each source had an activity of 30 mCi. The sources were positioned in a spherical geometry in the gantry housing. This distribution of sources provided the ability to accurately target sites within the cranium. Unfortunately, the system did not offer the flexibility that is required to treat the more complex, and less spherically shaped targets that are often encountered in cranial SRS.

The second-generation Gamma Knife (Elekta, Inc., Stockholm, Sweden) provided several significant advantages. The number of cobalt sources was increased to 201. The increased number of sources provided additional directions from which the radiation could be delivered. Another significant advantage was the addition of multiple collimators for dose delivery. Collimators of sizes 4, 8, 14, and 18 mm were designed for the system. The additional collimators provided the versatility to use multiple-beam diameters in order to more precisely shape the radiation dose distribution to the target (see Fig. 1).

In the late 1990s, the prototype of a rotating Gamma Knife unit was developed (Goetsch and Murphy 1999). The system incorporates 30 cobalt sources that rotate in the head of the machine about an isocentric point. In conjunction with rotating sources, the system has been automated to allow robotic collimator changes and robotically controlled patient shifts for those lesions whose treatment require more than one isocenter.

Linear Accelerator

Parallel to the commercialization of the second-generation Gamma Knife units, Betti et al. (1983) began investigating the possibility of using a standard ▶ linear accelerator (Linac) to treat in a stereotactic mode (Betti and Derechinsky 1983). Although the early systems used different setups, they all treated patients using non-coplanar isocentric arcs. Rectangular collimation techniques were used by the earliest systems but most went to circular tertiary collimators to better focus the beam (see Fig. 2).

Circular collimators inherently possess some limitations. For targets that are irregularly shaped, or larger than 4 cm in the greatest dimension, multiple isocenters and/or cones are required in order to provide the therapeutic dose to the entire target. The use of multiple isocenters introduces large volumes of high-dose regions. To minimize the high-dose regions and to treat larger targets, mini-multileaf collimators (mMLCs) were developed in the later part of the 1990s. All of the mMLCs were of the tertiary design in the 1990s. The AAPM published Task Group Report 42 in 1998 (Schell et al. 1995). This report recommends the use of mMLCs with a maximum leaf width of 4 mm at isocenter (see Fig. 3).

In 1994, Accuray, Inc. (Sunnyvale, CA) developed a robotically driven linac for SRS known as the Cyberknife (http://www.Accuray.com). The system is composed of a small accelerator mounted on a robotic arm. The robot can position the linac using 6 degrees of freedom within the treatment vault. The system delivers approximately 300 different shots of radiation called nodes (see Fig. 4).

In 2002, Tomotherapy, Inc. (Madison, WI) developed a linac that was mounted on the rotational ring of a CT scanner (http://www. Tomotherapy.com). The system is designed to treat patients by rotating the linac on the CT-ring while the table advances into the scanner. The system uses a binary-multileaf collimator for dose delivery. In 2008, Tomotherapy Inc. partnered with Integra-Radionics Inc. (Boston, MA) to adapt the Hi-Art Tomotherapy unit for SRS (See Fig. 5).

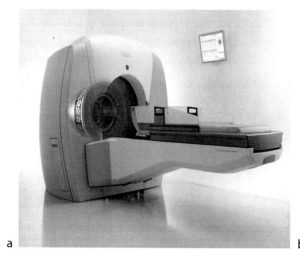
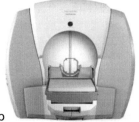

a b

Stereotactic Radiosurgery – Cranial. Fig. 1 (**a**) Gamma Knife unit and couch support exposing the central body of the system. (**b**) Gamma Knife unit showing the shielding doors closed and a Leksell ring mounted on the support assembly of the couch (Figures courtesy of Elekta Inc.)

Particles

As early as 1961, protons were used for treating cranial lesions (Noel et al. 2008). Other particles, including helium, muons, and carbon ions, began to emerge as particles that could be effective for SRS. The particles are accelerated in a cyclotron or synchrotron to energies in the 100–300 MeV range. The main advantages of particles are their characteristic ▶ Bragg Peak at the end of their range, a ▶ relative biological effective dose (RBE) > 1, and the reduction of entrance dose compared to photons. The availability of systems that can provide particles for SRS is very limited – only six centers in the United States are presently operating. There are at least four additional centers under construction (see Table 2).

Patient Immobilization

Two of the major components that facilitate a desired outcome in SRS are accurate targeting and precise dose delivery. There are three methods currently used to insure accurate targeting: invasive fixation, repeatable fixation, and frameless targeting. Each category has

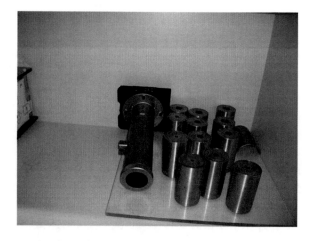

Stereotactic Radiosurgery – Cranial. Fig. 2 Picture of the linac attachment cone and multiple collimators used for cone-based stereotactic radiosurgery

multiple types of devices that have been developed and used widely in SRS/T procedures. The choice of which device to use is dependent on the SRS/T system being used, the type and location of disease, the preferred dose delivery regiment, and the specific needs of the patient.

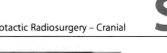

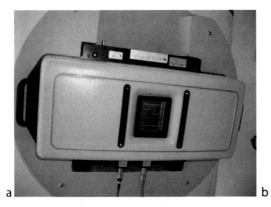
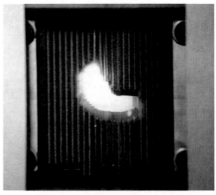

Stereotactic Radiosurgery – Cranial. Fig. 3 (**a**) Picture of an mMLC mounted on the head of a gantry. (**b**) The mMLC has 64 pairs of 4 mm leafs

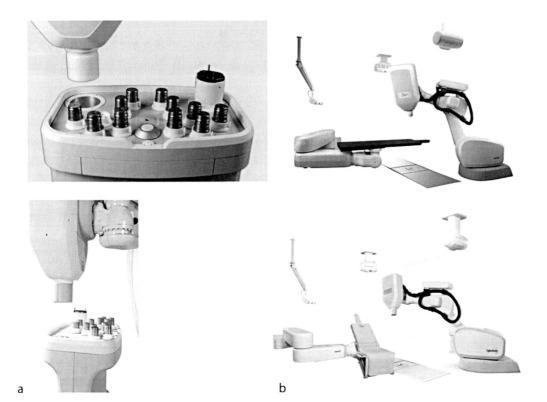

Stereotactic Radiosurgery – Cranial. Fig. 4 The Cyberknife units – (**a**) The G4 system showing the two digital cameras in the ceiling and two flat panel detectors on the floor are used for guidance during frameless stereotactic radiosurgery. The inset in the image depicts the different cone sizes that are available and loaded into the linac for treatments. (**b**) The Cyberknife VSI system (Figure courtesy of Accuray Inc.)

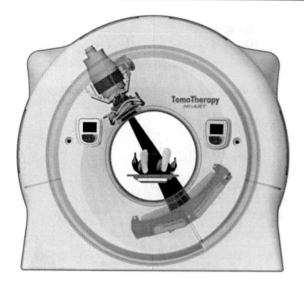

Stereotactic Radiosurgery – Cranial. Fig. 5
Diagram of the Tomotherapy Hi-Art system showing the accelerator position in reference to the patient on the treatment couch (Courtesy of Tomotherapy Inc.)

Invasive Fixation

The two most commonly used fixation devices for SRS are the Brown–Roberts–Wells (BRW) frame and Leksell frame. Both frames consist of a ring, four posts, and four screws. The four posts are connected to pins on the ring, which are driven into the outer table of the patient skull. The exact position of the pins is determined by the physical anatomy of the patient and the position of the target. The placement of the ring is critical; the ring immobilizes the cranium thereby fixing the target, and provides the basis for the coordinate system in the patient for most targeting systems. The positional accuracy of the invasive rings has an uncertainty of less than 1 mm (Marciunas et al. 1994). The system is placed once, the treatment is delivered, and the ring is removed from the patient.

Repeatable Fixation

There were two driving forces behind the design and implementation of repeatable fixation rings.

Stereotactic Radiosurgery – Cranial. Table 2 Proton facilities operating as of February, 2010

Accelerator location	Year treatments started	Accelerator type
Loma Linda University, Loma Linda, California	1990	Synchrotron
Massachusetts General Hospital Boston, Massachusetts	1961*	Cyclotron
University of Florida Gainesville, Florida	2008	Cyclotron
Indiana University, Bloomington, Indiana	1993	Cyclotron
ProCure Proton Center, Oklahoma City, Oklahoma	2009	Cyclotron
University of Pennsylvania Philadelphia, Pennsylvania	2010	Cyclotron
M.D. Anderson Cancer Center, Houston Texas	2007	Cyclotron
Outside the United States (20 facilities – approx. 40,000 treatments to date)	1961	Cyclotron/Synchrotron
The standard operating energy for stereotactic radiosurgery protons is 200–250 MeV		
New accelerating systems: lasers, dielectric wall, superconducting cyclotron		

*New system 2001

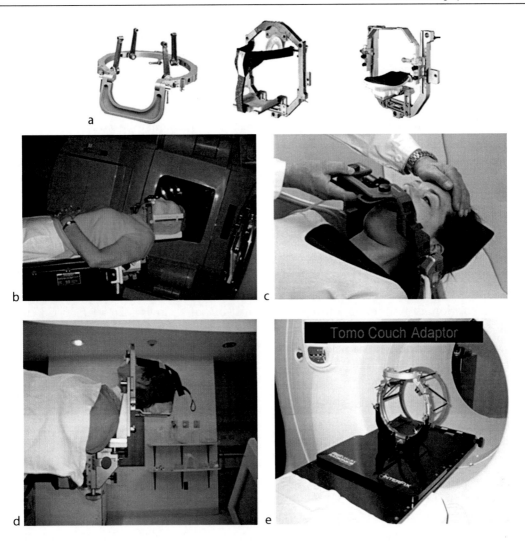

Stereotactic Radiosurgery – Cranial. Fig. 6 (**a**) BRW, GTC, and pediatric rings used for stereotactic radiosurgery procedures. (**b**) A thermoplastic mask immobilization device combined with a mouthpiece and tracking markers. (**c**) The newest relocatable immobilization device designed by Elekta is composed of a mouthpiece and back pad for fixation. (Figure courtesy of Elekta Inc.). (**d**) Patient positioned in the GTC-relocatable head ring. The ring is docked to the table support. (**e**) The Interfix adapter from Integra-Radionics mounted to a Tomotherapy Hi-Art accelerator (Figure courtesy of Tomotherapy Inc.)

S

The first was to develop a less-invasive system that could provide a comparable level of precision as the invasive systems. The second was to provide a ring that would allow for fractionated treatments while maintaining the same level of accuracy as the invasive frames. These systems provided a conduit to SRT.

Three common repeatable fixation devices are the Gill–Thomas–Cosman (GTC) device, thermoplastic masks, and the bite block mouthpiece on a rigid frame (see Fig. 6). The GTC device is composed of a molded mouthpiece, a backplate with the impression of the occipital region of the skull, and Velcro straps that place pressure on the mouthpiece pulling the ring into a fixed position. There are a number of different thermoplastic masks systems available for SRS/T. In order to achieve the greatest repositioning accuracy, most masks used for SRS/T have additional positioning/reinforcing components. A number of the systems use a bite block to facilitate the accurate positioning of the patient.

Frameless Targeting

The significant advances in image registration and technology over the past 10 years have provided the ability to position patients with submillimeter reproducibility (Murphy and Cox 1996). The patient position is monitored during the treatment to detect motion or any changes in patient position. Monitoring for frameless radiotherapy uses radiographic images, external sensors, and/or fiducial markers to determine the patient position at the time of treatment (see Fig. 7). The information is then electronically compared to the treatment planning information determined from the digitally reconstructed radiographs (DRRs) or coordinates from the treatment planning system (TPS). Any positional differences between the treatment plan and the actual patient setup are compensated for by the moving the patient couch. This ensures that the target is positioned at the exact location required for treatment. The Cyberknife unit uses multiple DRRs during the treatment to confirm the patient position. As the treatment is delivered, any change in patient position is accounted for by adjusting the attack angle of the linac (Metcalfe et al. 1997).

Patient Alignment

The initial alignment of the patient in the treatment room is critical. For ring based systems and frameless systems the patient is positioned on the table such that the target is located at the prescribed treatment location. For most targets, the position is such that the center of the target is located at the isocenter of the treatment machine. To accomplish this, the coordinates of the isocenter with respect to the localization devices are used in conjunction with lasers, DRRs, and sensors which may be attached to the fixation ring, mouthpiece, or skull. When multiple isocenters are needed, the respective coordinates for each patient position are set and verified.

Physics

Gamma Knife

^{60}Co is produced in the process of bombarding ^{59}Co with neutrons in a nuclear reactor. The half-life of ^{60}Co is 5.26 years. ^{60}Co undergoes a beta minus decay to an excited state of ^{60}Ni. The decay of ^{60}Ni is a two-step process in which two gamma rays of energy 1.17 and 1.33 MeV are emitted. In water, the dose falls off from 100% at 0.5 cm to 80% at approximately 5 cm depth.

Each source in a Gamma Knife unit is 1 mm in diameter and 2 cm in length. Each source is delivered with an initial activity of approximately 30 Ci. The total activity in the machine is approximately 6,000 Ci. The initial dose rate is approximately 300 cGy/min at the isocenter, which decreases to approximately 150 cGy/min after 5 years. The sources are exchanged every 5 years in order to maintain a significant dose rate which serves to limit the treatment time. In the standard Gamma Knife unit, the sources are housed in the central body of the machine. They are mounted in five circular arrays around the source sphere in the central body. The sources are separated along each array by 6 degree. The source to isocenter distance is 40 cm.

Linear Accelerator

The majority of SRS/T cases are treated using a 6-MV photon beam. The x-rays are produced with an approximate frequency of 3,000 MHz.

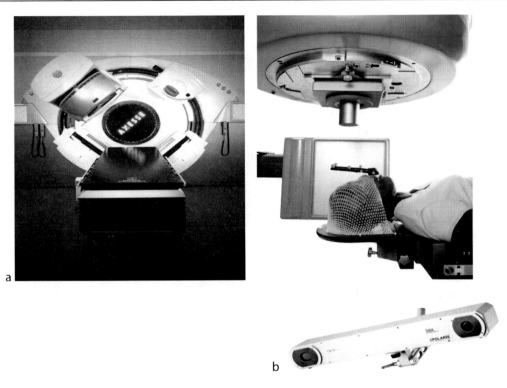

Stereotactic Radiosurgery – Cranial. Fig. 7 (**a**) Elekta Axesse has 2.5 mm MLC leafs and onboard imaging capabilities for treating stereotactic radiosurgery cases. The system is capable of delivering frameless cranial stereotactic radiosurgery (Figure courtesy of Elekta Inc.). (**b**) Optical tracking system used for frameless stereotactic radiosurgery by Varian. Via the reflectors mounted on the thermoplastic mask, the patient positions are constantly monitored by the IGRT optical camera shown below the image (Courtesy of Varian Inc.)

For a standard external beam radiation with a 10×10-cm field size, the d_{max} depth is 1.5 cm and the d_{80} is approximately 7.5 cm in water. The dose rate for modern linear accelerators is between 200 and 600 MU/min. The output as a function of rotational angle is between 0.5 and 10 MU/degree. The source to isocenter distance is 100 cm.

To use a standard linac for SRS/T procedures, there are modifications and attachments that are added to the machine. The standard collimating system for linacs is not adequate for SRS/T treatments. Tertiary collimating systems (either cones or mini-multileaf collimators) are attached to the gantry head. Tertiary collimating systems provide distinct advantages including a reduced penumbra.

The most widely used linac system for SRS/T procedures employs divergent circular cones. The cone housing is an open cylinder with a mounting plate that connects to the gantry head. The diverging cones, whose diameters range from 5 to 50 mm, are positioned in the cylinder for treatment.

Mini-Multileaf Collimators (mMLCs)

Three common commercially available mMLCs that are designed for use in SRS/T treatments are the Novalis stereotactic platform from Brainlab, Inc. (Feldkirchin, Germany) with leaf widths ranging from 1 to 3 mm, the Nomostat serial Tomotherapy unit from Best Nomos (Pittsburgh, PA) with a leaf

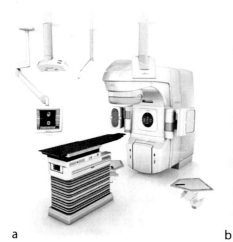

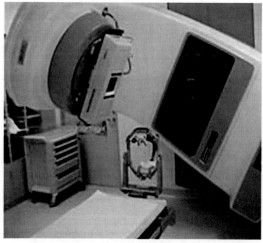

a   b

Stereotactic Radiosurgery – Cranial. Fig. 8 (**a**) The Novalis treatment machine from BrainLab has 2 mm leafs, onboard imaging capabilities and the Exact Track radiographic monitoring system for frameless radiosurgery (Figure courtesy of Brainlab Inc.). (**b**) Mini-MLC with a GTC ring connected to the couch mounts of a Varian linac (Figure courtesy of Integra-Radionics Inc.)

width of 4 mm, and the X-Knife mMLC from Integra-Radionics Inc. with a leaf width of 4 mm. The leaf widths are the size projected at the isocenter of the accelerator (SAD = 100 cm). The mMLC collimator may be permanently mounted or screwed onto the gantry head before each treatment (see Fig. 8).

Cyberknife

The small accelerator of the Cyberknife system operates at approximately 9,000 MHz. The accelerator produces a 6-MV photon beam that exits the accelerator with a dose rate of 400–600 MU/min with an SAD of 80 cm. The next-generation Cyberknife will have an increased dose rate of 1,000 MU/min. Unlike traditional linear accelerators, the isocenter is not a fixed reference point for the system. The Cyberknife has two methods of collimating the beam: (1) circular cones that range in diameter from 5 mm to 60 mm, and (2) a multileaf collimator that connects to the Cyberknife. The linac is mounted on a robotic arm (the GMF industrial robotic manipulator). The positioning accuracy of the robot is 0.5 mm

in all dimensions. The robot can deliver shots of radiation from approximately 1,200 different attack angles, or nodes.

Dosimetry

Photons

The majority of targets treated with linear accelerator systems are 2 cm or less in greatest dimension. The dosimetry of small fields (field sizes smaller than 3 × 3 cm) requires special consideration and special tools for measuring the radiation dose and distribution (Khan 2003). As the field size decreases below 2 cm, charged particle equilibrium (CPE) within the field does not exist. The result of this non-CPE causes the entire depth dose curve to shift toward the surface (see Fig. 9).

Another change in the dosimetry of small fields (i.e., field sizes where CPE does not exist) is the reduction in the width of the isodose lines. The loss of CPE causes the dose profiles to become more conical shaped, and the area under the curve that receives the full dose is significantly reduced (see Fig. 10).

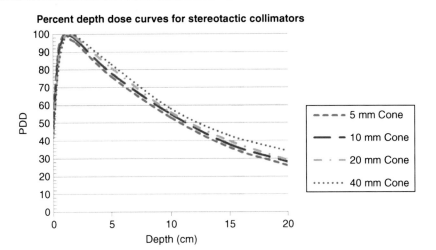

Stereotactic Radiosurgery – Cranial. Fig. 9 Percent depth dose curves for 5, 10, 20, and 40 mm stereotactic radiosurgery cones. As the cone sizes reduce, the depth of maximum dose shifts toward the surface, and the dose at depth decreases

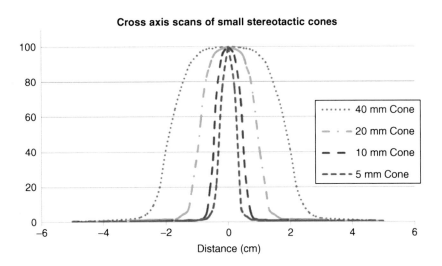

Stereotactic Radiosurgery – Cranial. Fig. 10 Cross axis scans of the dose profiles for 5, 10, 20, and 40 mm stereotactic radiosurgery cones. As the diameter of the cone decreases, the dose profiles become more cone shaped and the area under the curve for the 100% dose is reduced

Ascertaining the relevant dosimetric quantities of small fields is complicated due to the lack of CPE and the rapid dose fall off in the penumbral region. Many detectors such as diamond detectors, small field diodes, gafchromic film, aluminum oxide radiation detectors (Alora's), TLDs, ion chambers, and gel dosimeters are used to measure the output and dose distributions of small radiation fields (see Table 3). One of the main limitations for each detector is the size.

Stereotactic Radiosurgery – Cranial. Table 3 Properties of small chambers that are used for measuring the dosimetric characteristics of small (<2 cm) stereotactic fields

Detector	Dose/energy range	Volume (mm³)	Linearity (%)
Diode (Scanditronix)	1–20 MeV	0.10	2
Diamond detector	1–20 MeV	0.0125	2
TLDs	1 cGy–50 Gy	0.10	3
Pinpoint chamber (PTW, Germany)	1–50 MeV	0.015	2
Edge detector (Sun nuclear)	1–20 MeV	0.0019	3
Gafchromic film	1–100 Gy	0.01*	3
Bang gel (MGS Systems Inc.)	1–50 Gy	1.0*	3

*scanner resolution

Small field dosimetry requires chambers that are small and create a minimal perturbation of the radiation field.

The present dosimetric measurement uncertainty is >5% with small detectors (Mack et al. 2002; Das et al. 2008). In an effort to reduce this large uncertainty, there has been a concerted effort in determining the dosimetric quantities of small fields utilizing Monte Carlo models. The Monte Carlo simulations have the capability of accounting for dosimeter dimensions, non-CPE regions, source size, and the energy spectrum of the beam. However, Das et al. state that "at this time Monte Carlo cannot be assumed to invariably provide a Gold Standard without appropriate experimental validation" (Das et al. 2008). Future developments using Monte Carlo codes will provide correction factors for the specific detectors and the measurement conditions thereby reducing the measurement uncertainties.

Particles

The first particles used for SRS were helium ions used in Berkeley, CA in 1957 (Podgorsak and Podgorsak 1999). Other particles including pions, neutrons, and protons were used for treatments as early as 1961. However, as time progressed the most common particle that was used for SRS was protons. Protons are positively charged particles that originate in the nucleus of atoms. A proton is approximately 1,000 more massive than an electron. Protons with energies from 40 MeV up to 300 MeV (250 MeV being the most common) are suitable for SRS. The lowest energy protons are used for ocular diseases, while the higher energy protons are used for intracranial lesions.

Protons have specific dosimetric properties that provide distinct advantages over photons. The entrance dose for a 250-MeV proton beam is approximately 30% of the maximum dose, while 6 MV photon beams have an entrance dose of approximately 40% relative to their d_{max}. Unlike photons, the depth dose curve for protons does not decrease with depth. The depth dose is nearly constant until it reaches the depth at which the proton energy has dropped to approximately 0.15 MeV. At this depth, a large energy deposition occurs in the medium. This region on depth dose curve is defined as the Bragg Peak (see Fig. 11). The Bragg Peak occurs at

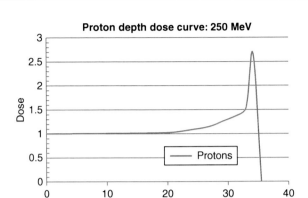

Stereotactic Radiosurgery – Cranial. Fig. 11
Relative depth dose curve of a 250 MeV proton beam in water. The curve is normalized at the surface. The sharp increase in dose at approximately 34 cm is the Bragg Peak for this beam

increasing depths as the energy of initial proton beam increases. To generate a useful proton beam, a spread-out Bragg Peak (SOBP) must be generated. The SOBP, generated by a ridge filter, creates a polyenergetic proton beam (Wilson 2004). Such a beam results in an increased entrance dose with respect to a monoenergetic beam (see Fig. 12).

Planning Tools

SRS/T procedures are intended to deliver high doses of radiation to targets that may be in very close proximity to critical structures in the cranium. There are a number of treatment planning tools that are used to analyze different plans and aid in choosing the appropriate plan for a given patient treatment. Among these tools are ▶ dose volume histograms (DVHs), tissue volume ratio (TVR), digitally reconstructed radiographs (DRRs), ▶ normal tissue complication probability (NTCP), ▶ tumor control probability (TCP), and dose tolerance tables. DVHs are graphs depicting the dose that is received by a given volume of the target or critical structure. The TVR is used to compare different plans and

determine which plan provides the best tumor coverage while limiting the dose to normal tissues. The DVHs of the critical structures and the target, and the TVR values for the prescription dose as well as doses above a certain threshold are compared for different plans to aid in deciding which plan that will provide the best clinical treatment (Bova et al. 2007).

SRS/T Delivery Paradigms

For all of the aforementioned treatment techniques and modalities, the initial step is to determine the location of the target(s) which must be treated. The immobilization device (if used) is made and placed on the patient. The ring is then connected to a support assembly on the table. A skull mapping device is placed on the ring. Measurements of the distance from the device to the skull are recorded. The mapping device is removed and a fiducial indicator is connected to the ring for scanning. The fiducial rods are used to define the 3-D space defined by the ring. The stereotactic CT scan is then performed. Stereotactic CT scans, and in most cases, MRI/MRA scans are done for each patient. The scans use slice thicknesses on the order of 1–2 mm. The CT and MRI image sets are fused within the treatment planning system (TPS). Critical structures that include but are not limited to the brain stem, optic chiasm, and optic nerves are identified and appropriately contoured. The target(s) must also be identified and contoured by either a radiation oncologist or a neurosurgeon. For most SRS/T cases, the target is not expanded into a PTV. Once all the structures identified and approved, the planning process for the delivery of the dose begins.

Gamma Knife

A critical step for Gamma Knife procedures is the placement of the fixation ring. The ring is positioned such that the intended target is centered in the ring. This is critical due to positional

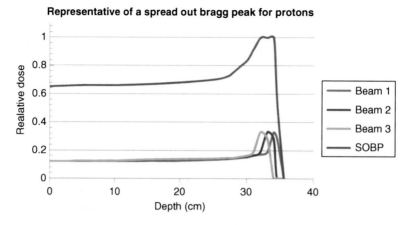

Representative of a spread out bragg peak for protons

Stereotactic Radiosurgery – Cranial. Fig. 12 A representative curve of three different energy proton beams summed to create a spread-out Bragg Peak for protons (SOBP). The entrance dose for the SOBP is higher than the entrance dose of the individual proton beams

limitations and possible collisions between the ring and the collimator (Niranjan et al. 2008). The angle, height, and anterior–posterior position of the ring must therefore be optimized.

The planning process is based on ▶ sphere packing within the target (Hartman 2008). After the size of the target is determined, the collimator size must be chosen. If the target is spherical and small such that one of the four collimator sizes covers the lesion, then a single shot may be used for the treatment. If the lesion is large or irregular then multiple shots are needed in order to provide adequate dose coverage of the target. The planner has to identify what collimator sizes, and which ports in the helmet are to be used in order to get sufficient coverage of the target while limiting the dose to the critical structures. Each of the shots with a given collimator size creates a dose sphere in the target. By summing up all of the spheres that are directed at the target, the dose distribution is calculated.

If the initial dose distribution is not adequate, there are several methods which may be used to modify the plan. Multiple small collimators may be used in place of one larger collimator. This may shape the dose distribution to better

conform to the target. Another method is to change which of the 201 ports are used for the delivery and which are plugged. A third method is to adjust the relative weighting of each of the shots. A standard plan will provide 100% dose coverage of the target and be normalized at approximately the 50% isodose level.

Once a plan is determined to be the most suitable for the given treatment, the plan is sent to the Gamma Knife treatment console. The patient is brought into the treatment room and positioned on the treatment couch. The ring is connected to the support assembly and the proper collimator helmet is connected. When the treatment is initiated, the shielding doors of the machine open and the couch slides into the treatment region of the machine. The helmet docks with the central body of the unit and irradiation begins.

After the planned treatment time for a given shot is completed, the table retracts and the shielding doors close. If multiple shots are to be delivered, the system or therapist adjusts the coordinates to position the patient so that the next isocenter may be treated. If a different collimator helmet is to be used, it is connected and the treatment is reinitiated. Once all of the shots are delivered, the patient is disconnected from the support assembly and the ring is removed.

The newest Gamma Knife unit (Perfexion from Elekta, Inc.) allows for robotic controls of the patient position and changing the collimator helmets as necessary. This automated system has significantly reduced the treatment time and improved the dose conformality within the target by eliminating the manual positioning of the patient.

Linear Accelerator Based

A common paradigm for linac SRS/T planning is to start the process with the simplest planning method and work toward a more complex method as needed. The first iteration in planning is to place an isocenter at the center of a given target. The cone size to be used is determined by the size of the target. If the target is larger than the largest cone, the largest cone is still used for planning in order to get the initial attack angles for conformal beams. Then a standard isocentric beam setup is applied. One typical method consists of using a planar arc ($>260°$), a pair of parasagittal arcs ($<120°$ each), and a sagittal arc ($<120°$) centered on the target. The next step in the process is to determine if the arcs are passing through critical structures or traversing through a large path length of normal brain tissue (>10 cm). The arcs and the attack angles are then adjusted to minimize the dose to the critical structures and to maximize the dose to the target. From this initial starting point, the main emphasis is on the dose coverage of the target, dose to the critical structures, degrees of arc for the plan (best range is $400°–700°$), hot spot location (within the target), DVHs, and the TVR. These parameters may be modified by varying the coordinates of the isocenter, adjusting the beam weights, and adding arcs from different attack angles.

For targets that are too large or irregularly shaped, the spherical dose distribution produced from a single isocenter may not be appropriate for treatment. These targets may require multiple isocenters and multiple cone sizes to produce an acceptable dose distribution. The choice of cone sizes and isocenter positioning affects the location of the hot spots, target coverage, and the TVR. A standard linac plan will provide 100% dose coverage to the target and be normalized at approximately the 80% isodose line.

Institutions that have the capability of using mMLCs start the planning process from the results of a cone-based plan. Many planning systems allow the planner to directly convert the arc plan into a conformal plan (also known as a static arc plan (SA)). By defining the angular separation of each shot to be delivered by a conformal field, each planned arc is subdivided into static conformal fields typically separated by $10°$ to $40°$. The larger the target, the larger the angular separation required to reduce the overlap exposure of normal tissue. A typical number of conformal arcs for treatment is 4–7, corresponding to 15–30 static mMLC fields.

Yet another technique that can be used to try and achieve the most appropriate dose distribution for treatment is stereotactic IMRT. Each field from the conformal plan can be modulated to determine if the desired dose distribution can be attained. However, for IMRT plans, the number of segments compared to a conformal treatment is reduced in part due to the increased number of monitor units and the overall time of delivery.

Once the desired plan is chosen and exported to the treatment console, the quality assurance procedures are initiated on the treatment machine (ACR–ASTRO 2006). For patients whose treatment calls for a relocatable ring, the ring is attached to the patient and then connected to the support assembly on the couch. The skull-mapping device is reattached to the ring and the distance measurements are verified. The acceptable reproducibility for these measurements is <1 mm based on the measurements

S

taken at the time of CT. If the criteria are not met, the mapping device is removed and the patient ring is repositioned. After all the quality assurance criteria are met, the mapping device is removed and a laser positioning device is attached. The couch is moved such that the target is positioned at the exact location in space that has been planned. Using micro adjusters, the target position is fine-tuned. The laser positioning device is then removed from the ring.

Cyberknife

The initial planning step for a Cyberknife treatment is assessing the type of fixation (ring based or frameless) that will be used for the treatment. If a frameless technique is to be used, the patient has a stereotactic CT and the images are sent to the planning computer. If a ring is to be used, then the ring is placed on the patient and the CT performed. The critical structures and target are identified and contoured by the radiation oncologist or neurosurgeon. The planning is done exclusively by inverse planning. The prescription dose and the dose constraints of the critical structures are entered into the treatment planning system (TPS). Once entered, the TPS determines the optimal beam angles and relative weight for each treatment beam.

The TPS uses up to 1,200 different possible nodes and a selection of cone sizes ranging from 5 mm to 60 mm to determine the optimal dose delivery scheme. A typical plan will use between 100 and 300 nodes to treat a given target. In general, the number of nodes increases as the irregularity and size of the target increases.

Once the desired plan is chosen and exported to the treatment console, the quality assurance procedures are initiated on the treatment machine. When all of the quality assurance procedures are complete, the patient is brought into the room. For patients who have relocatable rings, the ring is attached to the patient and connected to the support assembly on the couch. If the frameless technique is to be used, the patient is positioned on the table such that the target is located at the planned position in space. Images are acquired with the radiographic cameras and transferred to the treatment console. The digital x-rays are overlaid with the stored DRRs from the TPS. The position of the patient on the treatment couch is determined in reference to the expected position determined from the TPS DRRs. If the patient is not in the same position, the five-axis couch is adjusted to position the patient in the same position as the TPS DRRs. Once aligned, the treatment is initiated.

During treatment, the patient position is monitored and verified via digital images before the dose from each node is delivered. The images are constantly fed back to the treatment console for comparison with what was planned. If the position deviates from what was planned by 10 mm or less, the system will adjust the attack angle of the robot to account for the deviation. If deviations are greater than 10 mm, the treatment is paused and the patient couch is readjusted. After the treatment has been delivered, the patient is removed from the couch and the ring, if used, is removed.

Quality Assurance

Each SRS/T system has specific quality assurance and quality control procedures that provide confidence in the ability to deliver the prescribed dose to the correct site. Each system requires the accuracy and reproducibility of the targeting system to be within 1 mm. The total accuracy for a SRS/T system is expected to be less than 2 mm. The treatment planning systems used for SRS/T have QA procedures that quantify the image registration software, dose calculation algorithms, and machine settings for monitor units or time sets. The ▶ American Association of Physicists in Medicine (AAPM) has published extensively on the procedures and need for QA in radiation oncology. The AAPM published Task Group

Report 42 in 1995 (Schell et al. 1995). The report provides extensive information for commissioning, daily, monthly, and annual tests that are to be done for a SRS/T system. Other TG reports, TG-40 published in 1994, TG-142 published in 2009, TG-53 published in 1998, TG-108 published in 2008, TG-51 published in 1995, and TG-106 published in 2008, provide a strong base for QA procedures that can be incorporated into an SRS/T program to insure safety and reliability of treatments (American Association of Physicists in Medicine 2010).

Gamma Knife

The required QA procedures for Gamma Knife units are described in the Code of Federal Regulations Part 35. The docking mechanism, robotic positioner, and the collimator changer in the newest system are checked on a daily basis. Due to the decay of the ^{60}Co sources in the unit, the dose rate of the system must be verified each day prior to treatment. The dose rate is determined with a 16-cm diameter tissue equivalent sphere centered in the source body. Two other QA procedures that are specific to Gamma Knife units are shutter error and biannual wipe tests of the collimator helmets.

Linear Accelerator

There are multiple references that outline and explain QA procedures for each type of linac-based SRS/T systems. The unique tests that are necessary for isocentric SRS/T delivery are radiation-isocenter congruency, laser positioning, collimator holders, and the braking systems functionality. In many institutions, the radiation–isocenter congruency is confirmed using the target ball test developed by the joint centers in Boston (Lutz et al. 1988). The agreement for this test should be less than 1 mm. The laser alignment is critical as the 3 room lasers are used to transfer the isocentric coordinates of the room to the isocenter point within the patient

cranium. The tolerance for the laser alignment is less than 1 mm.

Cyberknife

The QA procedures that are associated with the Cyberknife unit are given by Mould et al. (2005) in Robotic Radiosurgery (Francescan et al. 2005). The main difference in the standard QA procedures for Cyberknife versus the standard linac are associated with the image acquisition and positioning software, and with the position accuracy and adjustment of the robot. Tests to confirm the robotic operations include the "BB" test, Mastering test, and the movement of the robot as determined from the console. The imaging alignment test is done on a daily basis to insure the imaging system is communicating appropriately with the treatment console and robot. Other individualized tests are performed to gain confidence that the delivery of the treatment can be accomplished with the robot without collisions or limitations based on the room and equipment in the room, and monitor chamber calibrations.

Cross-References

▶ Image-Guided Radiation Therapy (IGRT): TomoTherapy
▶ IMRT
▶ Linear Accelerators (LINAC)
▶ Pituitary
▶ Primary Intracranial Neoplasms
▶ Proton Therapy
▶ Radiation Detectors
▶ Radiation Oncology Physics
▶ Robotic Radiosurgery
▶ Stereotactic Radiosurgery: Extracranial

References

ACR–ASTRO (2006) Practice guideline for the performance of stereotactic radiosurgery, pp 1–6
American Association of Physicists in Medicine (2010). http://www.aapm.org/pubs/reports/
Barnett G, Linskey M et al (2007) Stereotactic-radiosurgery an organized neurosurgery sanctioned definition. J Neurosurg 106:1–5

Betti O, Derechinsky V (1983) Multiple beam stereotaxic irradiation. Neurochirurgie 29:295–298

Bova F, Meeks S et al (2007) Linac radiosurgery: system requirements, procedures, and testing. In: Kahn F (ed) Treatment planning in radiation oncology, 2nd edn. Lippincott Williams & Wilkins, Philadelphia

Das I et al (2008) Small fields: nonequilibrium radiation dosimetry. Med Phys 35:206–215

Francescan P, Coras et al (2005) Cyberknife dosimetric beam characteristics: comparison between experimental results and Monte Carlo simulation. In: Mould R (ed) Robotic radiosurgery. Cyberknife Society, Sunnyvale

Goetsch S, Murphy B (1999) Physics of rotating gamma systems for stereotactic radiosurgery. Int J Radiat Oncol Biol Phys 43:689–696

Hartman S (2008) Sorting by transpositions and reversals. In: Ming Y (ed) Encyclopedia of algorithms. Springer, New York

http://www.Accuray.com

http://www.Tomotherapy.com

Khan F (2003) The physics of radiation therapy, 3rd edn. Lippincott Williams & Wilkins, Philadelphia

Leksell L (1951) The stereotaxic method and radiosurgery of the brain. Acta Chir Scand 102:316–319

Leksell L (1956) Detection of intracranial complications following head injury. Acta Chir Scand 110:301–315

Leksell L (1968) Cerebral radiosurgery. Acta Chir Scand 134:585–595

Lutz W, Winston K et al (1988) A system of stereotactic radiosurgery with a linear accelerator. Int J Radiat Oncol Biol Phys 14:373

Mack A, Scheib S et al (2002) Precision dosimetry of narrow photon beams used in radiosurgery-determination of gamma knife output factors. Med Phys 29:2080–2089

Marciunas J, Galloway R et al (1994) The application accuracy of stereotactic frames. Neurosurgery 35:682–694

Metcalfe P et al (1997) The physics of radiotherapy x-rays and electrons. Medical Physics, Madison

Murphy M, Cox R (1996) The accuracy of dose localization for an image guided frameless radiosurgry system. Med Phys 23:2043–2049

Niranjan A, Sirin S et al (2008) Gamma knife radiosurgery. In: Chin L (ed) Principles and practices of stereotactic radiosurgery. Springer, New York

Noel G, Fitzek M et al (2008) Proton beam radiosurgery: physical bases and clinical experience. In: Chin L (ed) Principles and practices of stereotactic radiosurgery. Springer, New York

Podgorsak E, Metcalfe P (1999) Medical accelerators. In: Van Dyk J (ed) The modern technology of radiation oncology. Medical Physics, Madison

Podgorsak E, Podgorsak M (1999) Stereotactic irradiation. In: Van Dyk J (ed) The modern technology of radiation oncology. Medical Physics, Madison

Schell M, Bova F et al (1995) American Association of Physicists in Medicine (AAPM): Radiation Therapy Committee Task Group 42: stereotactic radiosurgery. American Institute of Physics Inc, College Park

Wilson R (2004) A brief history of the Harvard cyclotron. Harvard University, Department of Physics, Cambridge, MA

Stereotactic Radiosurgery: Extracranial

JAY E. REIFF
Department of Radiation Oncology, College of Medicine, Drexel University, Philadelphia, PA, USA

Synonyms

SBRT; Stereotactic body radiation therapy

Definition

Highly focused, high-dose, short-course radiation therapy to tumor sites outside of the cranium utilizing precision localization and anatomy fixation techniques.

Introduction

Extracranial stereotactic radiation therapy, also known as stereotactic body radiation therapy (SBRT), is a technique in which large doses of radiation (5–30 Gy) are delivered in only a few fractions (typically 1–5) with a very high degree of precision to a well-defined extracranial lesion. Because such high fractional doses are used, it is crucial that steep dose gradients from the target are created in order to protect the adjacent healthy tissue. Additionally, measures must be taken to not only immobilize the patient but also minimize movement of the target during the planning process and the treatment delivery.

The SBRT technique is used for lesions in multiple anatomical sites including the lung, liver, prostate, kidney, spine, and paraspinal regions (Cho et al. 2012; Martin and Gaya 2010). Doses to these regions may be delivered by conventional accelerators with or without the use of respiratory gating, or by newer technologies such as TomoTherapy or the CyberKnife (robotic radiosurgery). As the specifics of these tumors and the details of these treatment modalities are discussed elsewhere in this Encyclopedia, this entry will discuss the overall technical considerations common to all SBRT delivery systems. For a complete review, refer to Kavanagh et al. (2007), Benedict et al. (2010), and Martin and Gaya (2010) with the embedded references which give the history of SBRT.

Positioning and Immobilization

Positioning the patient in a comfortable and reproducible manner is crucial when treating a patient using SBRT. Equipment commonly used to create a customized body mold for external immobilization includes aquaplast molds, thermoplastic masks, vacuum pillows, as well as other types of immobilization cushions. These devices maintain the patient in a fairly comfortable position for the typically lengthy duration of treatment.

In the conventional three-dimensional conformal treatment planning (3DCRT) as well as with intensity-modulated radiation therapy (IMRT) treatment planning, internal tumor motion is taken into account in constructing the ▶ planning target volume (PTV). This results in treatment portals which encompass the full extent of motion which is expected during treatment. Such field sizes, however, can be unacceptably large when using the doses common to SBRT.

The most common causes of internal tumor motion are respiration, cardiac function, and digestive activity. Respiratory motion, which obviously affects the position of lung lesions, also affects the position of most abdominal tumors as well. A variety of methods have been developed to treat tumors whose position is affected by respiration. These include respiratory gating, tumor tracking, organ motion dampening, and patient-directed methods. These methods and others are described in detail in Report Number 91 from the American Association of Physicists in Medicine (Keall et al. 2006).

Patient Imaging

SBRT is an image-based treatment. As such this technique differs from conventional treatments right from the very beginning, i.e., from the time of the initial simulation/treatment planning CT scan. As noted above, the immobilization devices used are not only custom formed, but they must extend over a larger part of the body than they would if a standard treatment was being delivered. The use of additional localization markers and position monitoring devices such as implanted radiographic markers, electromagnetic transponders, and/or surface imaging techniques may be used. Imaging modalities such as MRI and PET may be obtained and fused with the planning CT.

Regardless of which body site is being treated and what type of immobilization is being used, high 3D spatial accuracy and tissue contrast definition are very important to the imaging process. The management of patient care and treatment delivery is predicated on the ability to define the localizing target and normal tissue boundaries as accurately as possible (Potters et al. 2004). If the goal of the therapy is to treat an organ that is affected by respiratory motion, then a 4D CT may be used (see "▶ Four-Dimensional (4D) Treatment Planning/Respiratory Gating" in this Encyclopedia; Keall et al. 2006; Chen et al. 2007).

It is strongly recommended that scans should extend at least 5–10 cm beyond the anticipated treatment borders for coplanar beam arrangements and up to 15 cm for noncoplanar arrangements. The slice thickness should not be greater than 3 mm. All structures (target as well as organs at risk) must be included in the imaging studies so that they may be evaluated using the resulting dose-volume histograms (DVHs) calculated by the treatment planning system (Benedict et al. 2010).

Treatment Planning

The treatment planning goal of SBRT is to deliver a very high dose which conforms tightly to the tumor volume and drops off rapidly and evenly in all directions. There are, however, some cases where an isotropic gradient is not desirable. For example, for paraspinal tumors or lung lesions close to the spinal cord, it is desirable to maintain a steeper gradient between the tumor and the spinal cord than elsewhere. Regions of high dose within the tumor volume (hot spots) are generally considered acceptable. In fact, doses for SBRT are often prescribed to isodose levels which are considered rather low (e.g., the 80% isodose surface) with respect to conventional radiation therapy. Beam directions are generally chosen such that the volume of tissue in the beam intersection region is minimized by limiting it to the target region. To accomplish this, a field arrangement using multiple non-opposed, noncoplanar beams is often used. The field size and shape from each beam coincide with the PTV as seen from the beam's eye view (BEV). By prescribing the dose to a lower isodose line, with enough fields aimed at the PTV, it is possible to cover 95% of the PTV with the prescription dose while maintaining the steep dose gradient outside this volume.

Another factor in determining the number of beams to use is the resulting entrance dose. Given the high doses prescribed to the target volume, using more beams will reduce the ▶ d_{max} dose for each entrance site. It is desirable to choose the number of beams and their relative weighting such that the d_{max} dose associated with any one particular beam is less than 30% of the cumulative dose (Benedict et al. 2010). This will prevent severe acute skin reactions and reduce late skin toxicity while maintaining the requisite steep dose gradient.

The calculation grid resolution used by the treatment planning system to generate the isodose distributions can have a profound effect on the accuracy of the dose calculation (Benedict et al. 2010). Studies have been performed where the grid resolution was varied from 1.5 up to 4 mm. Because of the extremely high dose gradients associated with SBRT, it is recommended that a grid resolution of 2 mm or less be used. Resolutions greater than 3 mm are discouraged.

Staff Responsibilities, Patient Safety, and Quality Assurance

Because of the significantly higher dose per fraction and the smaller size of the target, the margin of error associated with SBRT is significantly smaller than that for conventional radiation therapy. In fact, a small error in target localization for any given fraction risks undertreatment of portions of the tumor by 20% or more, and inadvertent overdosage of adjacent normal tissues could escalate the risk of serious injury to a much greater degree than an equivalent treatment error in a course of radiotherapy where a substantially lower dose per fraction is used (Solberg et al. 2012).

All the intricacies and fine details of an SBRT regimen necessitate full cooperation by every member of the radiation team. This includes, but is not limited to, the radiation oncologist, medical physicist, dosimetrist, radiation therapist, and diagnostic imaging physician. Each of these team members must be properly trained in their assigned roles as evidenced by certification by the appropriate medical board. Additionally, training in the various technologies used is essential.

The radiation oncologist is responsible for the overall treatment including the assessment of the patient and the determination of the appropriateness of the treatment modality. It is up to the radiation oncologist to approve the final position and immobilization of the patient including any techniques which allow for the reduction of inherent internal organ motion. The radiation oncologist also is responsible for selecting the appropriate imaging modalities to be used so that the gross tumor volume (GTV) may be demonstrated and contoured and the planning target volume (PTV) may be determined. These images will also be used to help the radiation oncologist delineate the nearby critical structures and healthy tissues.

The medical physicist is responsible for all the technical aspects of the treatment from imaging through treatment planning and dose delivery. This includes the acceptance testing and commissioning of the SBRT system, supervising the treatment planning process, and checking all the parameters of the resulting treatment plan. Designing and implementing a quality assurance program which ensures the proper functioning of the accelerator, the treatment planning system, and the entire treatment delivery process is one of the primary responsibilities of the medical physicist. Much of this is outlined in the report of the AAPM Task Group 101 (Benedict et al. 2010 and its embedded references).

The dosimetrist is responsible for devising the optimum treatment plan. This is accomplished with close consultation with the radiation oncologist and medical physicist. It is imperative that the goal of the therapy is communicated clearly to the dosimetrist by the radiation oncologist. This not only includes the prescription dose to the target but also the dose constraints to the nearby critical structures.

It is up to the team of radiation therapists to prepare the treatment room for the SBRT treatment. They will position and immobilize the patient and set up any organ-motion-restricting devices. Once the patient is ready for treatment, they will call in the radiation oncologist, medical physicist, and dosimetrist for a final review of the setup as well as approval of all the clinical and technical aspects. Once everything has been checked and double checked, it is the radiation therapists who will ultimately turn on the radiation beam to treat the patient.

Cross-References

▶ Conformal Therapy: Treatment Planning, Treatment Delivery, and Clinical Results
▶ Four-Dimensional (4D) Treatment Planning/Respiratory Gating
▶ Image-Guided Radiation Therapy (IGRT): TomoTherapy
▶ Intensity Modulated Radiation Therapy (IMRT)
▶ Kidney
▶ Liver and Hepatobiliary Tract
▶ Lung
▶ Palliation of Brain and Spinal Cord Metastases
▶ Palliation of Metastatic Disease to the Liver
▶ Prostate
▶ Radiation Oncology Physics
▶ Robotic Radiosurgery

References

Benedict SH, Yenice KM, Followill D et al (2010) Stereotactic body radiation therapy: the report of AAPM Task Group 101. Med Phys 37(8):4078

Chen GTY, Kung JH, Rietzel E (2007) Four-dimensional imaging and treatment planning of moving targets. In: Meyer JL et al (eds) IMRT, IGRT, SBRT – advances in the treatment planning and delivery of radiotherapy, Frontiers of radiation therapy and oncology. Karger, Basel

Cho LC, Fonteyne V, DeNeve W, Lo SS, Timmerman RD (2012) Stereotactic body radiotherapy. In: Levitt SH et al (eds) Technical basis of radiation therapy. Medical radiology, radiation oncology. Springer, Berlin/Heidelberg. doi:10.1007/174_2011_263

Kavanagh BD, Kelly K, Kain M (2007) The promise of stereotactic body radiation therapy in a new era of oncology. In: Meyer JL et al (eds) IMRT, IGRT, SBRT – advances in the treatment planning and delivery of radiotherapy, Frontiers of radiation therapy and oncology. Karger, Basel

Keall PJ, Mageras GS, Balter JM et al (2006) The management of respiratory motion in radiation oncology: report of AAPM Task Group 76, AAPM Report No. 91. American Association of Physicists in Medicine, College Park. http://aapm.org/pubs/reports/RPT_91.pdf

Martin A, Gaya A (2010) Stereotactic body radiotherapy: a review. Clin Oncol 22:157

Potters L, Steinberg M, Rose C et al (2004) American Society for Therapeutic Radiology and Oncology and American College of Radiology practice guideline for the performance of stereotactic body radiation therapy. Int J Radiat Oncol Biol Phys 60:1026

Solberg TD, Balter JM, Benedict SH, Fraass BA et al (2012) Quality and safety considerations in stereotactic radiosurgery and stereotactic body radiation therapy: executive summary. Pract Radiat Oncol 2:2

Stomach Cancer

FILIP T. TROICKI[1], JAGANMOHAN POLI[2]
[1]College of Medicine, Drexel University, Philadelphia, PA, USA
[2]Department of Radiation Oncology, College of Medicine, Drexel University, Philadelphia, PA, USA

Synonyms

Gastric cancer; Gastric tumor

Definition

Gastric cancer includes tumors that develop in tissues lining the stomach which begin at the ▶ gastroesophageal (GE) junction and end at the pylorus.

Background

Prior to World War II, gastric cancer was the leading cause of cancer death in the USA and worldwide. Risk factors of developing gastric cancer include dietary (high salt intake and smoked meats and fish), environmental (▶ *Helicobacter pylori* infection), smoking, previous gastric surgery, diagnosis of ▶ pernicious anemia, as well as hereditary factors (E-cadherin). The incidence of gastric cancer in the USA and Western countries has been decreasing since the 1930s. In 2009 in the USA alone, there have been an estimated 21,130 new cases and 10,620 deaths from gastric cancer, making it the 14th most common cancer in the USA. In part, the decrease in the incidence of gastric cancer can be attributed to technological advances. Refrigeration has decreased the use of salt and smoke in preservation of food products, and as a result fewer carcinogens are ingested in our diets. In addition, the increased use of antibiotics, combined with improved sanitation techniques contributed to the decrease of *H. pylori* infections. Although new cases are on the decline globally, it is still the fourth most common cancer worldwide. In fact, gastric tumors are most common type of cancer in Japanese men, and the incidence of proximal and GE junction tumors has also been on the rise in men living in Western countries.

Adenocarcinomas make up approximately 85–90% of gastric cancers and arise from premalignant ▶ villous adenomas in the ▶ gastric mucosa. Eighty percent of these adenomatous polyps originate in the pylorus or body of the stomach, and only 15% occur in the cardia. Second most common gastric malignancy is a lymphoma (mucosa-associated lymphoid tissue – MALT), occurring in up to 15% of gastric tumors. Other rare tumors found in the stomach may include ▶ leiomyosarcomas (2%), ▶ carcinoid tumors (1%), ▶ adenoacanthomas (1%), and ▶ squamous cell carcinomas (1%). Multifocal disease occurs in approximately 10% of cases on diagnosis.

As with most cancers, the most important prognostic factor for gastric cancer is the extent of the tumor. The stomach lies within the ▶ peritoneal cavity and gastric cancer can therefore spread by direct extension to the ▶ omentum, pancreas, diaphragm, transverse colon, or ▶ duodenum. In addition, lymphatic cancer spread is common due to the extensive lymphatic network within the submucosal and subserosal layers of the gastric wall. Generally, lymphatic drainage from the stomach follows gastric vascular supply of the greater and lesser curvature and most frequently terminates at the ▶ celiac axis. Nodal involvement is an important prognostic marker with local lymph node involvement having a smaller effect on prognosis than locoregional or distant lymph node positivity. Hematologic spread via the portal system is also common and up to 30% of patients have liver involvement at presentation. Unfortunately, patients who have hematogenous or transperitoneal spread at time of diagnosis have a very poor prognosis.

Initial Evaluation

Finding gastric cancer early is challenging since many early stage patients are asymptomatic, and even advanced stage patients may present with vague symptoms that may not result in a proper and timely workup. In fact, only approximately one-quarter of patients diagnosed with gastric cancer are found to have local disease and 75% being diagnosed with regional or metastatic disease. Patients with gastric cancer may present with a variety of nonspecific symptoms, such as early satiety, decreased appetite and weight loss, weakness, abdominal pain, nausea and vomiting, and black stools. Nearly 40% of patients experience the above-mentioned symptoms for less than 3 months and it is quite rare for the symptoms to extend beyond 1 year. A physical exam may reveal abdominal tenderness but only in advanced disease is an abdominal mass palpable. In advanced stages of the disease, a left supraclavicular node (▶ Virchow's node), a large anterior axillary node (▶ Irish node), or periumbilical metastatic lesion (▶ Sister Mary Joseph nodule) can also be appreciated in some advanced cancer patients.

Differential Diagnosis

Signs and symptoms of gastric cancer are nonspecific and can mimic a number of abdominal disorders. A long list of differential diagnosis includes bacterial or viral ▶ gastroenteritis, acute or chronic ▶ gastritis, gastric ulcers, esophagitis, esophageal stricture, esophageal cancer, malignant neoplasm of the small intestine, as well as non-Hodgkin's lymphoma.

Imaging Studies

In addition to a thorough history and physical exam as outlined above, a proper radiographic evaluation is imperative in any patient suspected of a gastric tumor. An abdominal CT scan with IV contrast is especially useful in determining the extent of the disease and is necessary in proper staging. In addition, a CT scan of the abdomen can dictate patient management by providing information regarding the resectability of the tumor. Metastasis to the liver can be picked up on the abdominal CT and metastasis to the lungs can often be seen on a plain chest X-ray. A helical chest CT may be necessary to identify small lung lesions or small lymph nodes in the mediastinum. A double-contrast upper GI series can also be beneficial when looking for small lesions within the gastric mucosa. In addition, ▶ esophagogastroduodenoscopy should be performed and a biopsy should be taken from any area of suspicion. Direct visualization of the gastric mucosa with an ▶ endoscopy, combined with cytology, and biopsy has a sensitivity of over 90% in patients with exophytic cancerous lesions. Unfortunately, small, infiltrative, cardia lesions are much more difficult to diagnose with endoscopy alone and ▶ endoscopic ultrasonography (EUS) looking at depth of tumor invasion may need to be used. EUS is especially useful in staging patients pre-surgically and is gaining popularity in its use.

Laboratory Studies

A complete blood count (CBC) and an electrolyte panel should be obtained on all patients with suspected gastric tumors. A CBC may reveal low hemoglobin resulting from pernicious anemia associated with gastric cancer in up to 30% of patients. An *H. pylori* test should also be ordered on any patient who presents with symptoms of a gastric ulcer such as abdominal pain, bloating, indigestion, and nausea. Although it is not standard practice, a carcinoembryonic antigen (CEA) and/or cancer antigen 19–9 (CA 19–9) can also be useful since these markers can be elevated in up to 50% and 20% of gastric cancer cases, respectively.

Staging

Primary Tumor (T)

TX Primary tumor cannot be assessed

T0 No evidence of primary tumor

Tis Carcinoma in situ: intraepithelial tumor without invasion of the lamina propria

T1 Tumor invades lamina propria, muscularis mucosae, or submucosa

T1a Tumor invades lamina propria or muscularis mucosae

T1b Tumor invades submucosa

T2 Tumor invades muscularis propria

T3 Tumor penetrates subserosal connective tissue without invasion of visceral peritoneum or adjacent structures

T4 Tumor invades serosa (visceral peritoneum) or adjacent structures

T4a Tumor invades serosa (visceral peritoneum)

T4b Tumor invades adjacent structures

Regional Lymph Nodes (N)

NX Regional lymph node(s) cannot be assessed

N0 No regional lymph node metastasis

N1 Metastasis in 1–2 regional lymph nodes

N2 Metastasis in 3–6 regional lymph nodes

N3 Metastasis in 7 or more regional lymph nodes

Distant Metastasis (M)

M0 No distant metastasis

M1 Distant metastasis

Treatment

Surgical Management

In early stage disease, surgical management is the primary treatment modality. At the time of initial presentation, curative or palliative surgical resection is possible for only 50% of gastric cancer patients, and only half of these patients will be eligible for potentially curative resection. Complete resection of the stomach with margins ≥4 cm is considered standard of care at the time of this publication. Despite the wide surgical margins required for a complete resection, negative margins are obtainable in only about 50% of patients. Due to the high morbidity of these operations, many surgeons prefer to perform a ▶ subtotal gastrectomy for distal gastric cancers and reserve total gastrectomies for large and proximal tumors. Unresectable carcinomas include those with peritoneal involvement, distant metastasis, or locally advanced disease (i.e., invasion of major blood vessels). Lymph node dissection is currently a topic of controversy, yet more extensive dissection appears to be associated with better survival. The NCCN recommendation, therefore, is for removal of at least 15 lymph nodes from the perigastric (D1), and celiac axis (D2) regions. Given that survival appears to depend on depth of tumor invasion, as well as regional lymph node involvement, it makes sense that surgical excision is a critical component in the management of gastric cancer. On the other hand, because of high rates of relapse (as high as 70% loco-regionally and 25% distally in some studies) and a poor survival with surgery alone (10–50% at 5 years even for early stage gastric cancer), adjuvant treatments with have been introduced to decrease local and systemic relapse and have proven to be vital in prolonging life in gastric cancer patients.

Radiation Therapy

Radiation is an important part of treatment for some gastric cancers, and has been used in preoperative, postoperative, and palliative settings. Preoperative radiation has been especially successful in improving survival and locoregional control over surgery alone. As described above, proper staging of gastric cancer relies heavily on accurate and detailed imaging and is especially crucial in the setting of preoperative radiotherapy. The use of EUS, upper endoscopy, and CT of abdomen with oral and/or IV contrast should be used to delineate the primary tumor and identify the pertinent lymph nodes for radiation. The patient should be simulated and treated in a supine position with the aid of immobilization devices in order to ensure daily reproducibility. The recommended radiation dose is 45–50.4 Gy delivered as 1.8 Gy per fraction. Due to the proximity of vital organs to the stomach, treatment planning should limit the radiation dose to liver, kidneys, spinal cord, heart, and lungs. Due to the acute radiation toxicity to the stomach of nausea and vomiting, supportive care must be given to patients under treatment. Special attention must be given to nutrition of these patients and enteral and/or ▶ parenteral nutrition should be considered to allow for adequate calorie intake.

Chemotherapy

There are several options for chemotherapy in the treatment of gastric cancer and appears to be advantageous for patients with locally unresectable or metastatic gastric tumors. Many different combinations of chemotherapy agents have been studied and utilized in the pre-, peri-, and postoperative setting. Currently, the best chemotherapy combination is still being investigated, but perioperative epirubicin, cisplatin, and 5-FU (ECF) has been recommended by the NCCN in medically fit patients who have a resectable gastric ▶ adenocarcinoma. In patients with metastatic or locally advanced cancer, docetaxel, cisplatin, and 5-FU (DCF) or ECF have been used successfully and are currently considered standard of care.

Combined Modality Treatments

Patients with Stage IA and node-negative gastric cancer can be observed if negative surgical margins were obtained. For patients stages IB (node positive) through stage IIIB, that is, those with cancer extending through the gastric wall and/or with positive lymph nodes, postoperative chemoradiation is the treatment of choice. Regardless of surgical margins, radiation of 45–50.4 Gy to the postsurgical tumor bed, combined with 5-FU with or without leucovorin is considered standard of care for these advanced stage patients. In a select potentially resectable patient population, preoperative chemoradiation utilizing docetaxel or paclitaxel plus a fluoropyrimidine is a reasonable option.

Palliative Care

Palliative treatment is utilized for recurrent or metastatic gastric cancer. Patient performance status is the key determining factor in deciding whether to offer best supportive care alone or combined with radiation and/or chemotherapy. Radiation is often utilized to relieve symptoms associated with obstruction, bleeding, or pain. Systemic treatments with chemotherapy agents such as ECF and DCF have been recommended by the NCCN and are now considered standard of care in the palliative setting.

Cross-References

▶ Cancer of the Pancreas
▶ Esophageal Cancer
▶ Intensity Modulated Radiation Therapy (IMRT)
▶ Non-Hodgkins Lymphoma

▶ Principles of Chemotherapy
▶ Principles of Surgical Oncology

References

Ajani J et al (2010) Gastric cancer: clinical practice guidelines in oncology. J Natl Compr Cancer Netw (NCCN) 8(4):378–409

Perez, Brady (2008) Stomach, Chapter 55. Principles and Practice of Radiation Oncology, 5th edn. Lippincott (pub)

Tepper (ed) (2002) Gastric cancer. Semin Radiat Oncol 12(2): 109–195

Stress Fracture

HEDVIG HRICAK[1], OGUZ AKIN[2], HEBERT ALBERTO VARGAS[2]
[1]Department of Radiology, Memorial Sloan-Kettering Cancer Center, New York, NY, USA
[2]Body MRI, Memorial Sloan-Kettering Cancer Center, New York, NY, USA

Definition

Overuse injuries of bone which result from repetitive loading that, over time, exceeds the bone's intrinsic ability to repair itself.

Cross-References

▶ Imaging in Oncology

Subject Contrast

JOHN W. WONG
Department of Radiation Oncology and Molecular Radiation Sciences, Johns Hopkins University, Baltimore, MD, USA

Definition

The difference in x-ray intensity transmitted through one part of the subject as compared to that transmitted through another part.

Cross-References

▶ Electronic Portal Imaging Devices (EPID)

Subtotal Gastrectomy

FILIP T. TROICKI[1], JAGANMOHAN POLI[2]
[1]College of Medicine, Drexel University, Philadelphia, PA, USA
[2]Department of Radiation Oncology, College of Medicine, Drexel University, Philadelphia, PA, USA

Definition

Surgical removal of cancer from stomach with a wide margin that includes some normal stomach tissue.

Cross-References

▶ Stomach Cancer

Superficial Therapy

BRANDON J. FISHER
Department of Radiation Oncology, College of Medicine, Drexel University, Philadelphia, PA, USA

Definition

Superficial therapy is a type of x-ray tomotherapy used to treat superficial tumors of about 5-mm depth. X-ray energies are typically 50–150 kV_p, with a skin-to-source distance of 15–20 cm. The treatments usually incorporate applicators or cones attached to the diaphragm of the treatment machine.

Cross-References

▶ Brachytherapy
▶ Skin Cancer

Superior Vena Cava Syndrome

Caspian Oliai[1], Feng-Ming Kong[2], Jingbo Wang[2]
[1]Department of Radiation Oncology, College of Medicine, Drexel University, Philadelphia, PA, USA
[2]Department of Radiation Oncology, Veteran Administration Health Center and University Hospital University of Michigan, Ann Arbor, MI, USA

Synonyms
SVCS

Definition
Compression of the superior vena cava by a mass lesion causing facial/neck/upper extremity swelling, shortness of breath, neck vein distention, coughing, and visualization of collateral veins on the chest. Common causes include lung cancers, lymphomas, thymoma, germ cell tumors, granulomatous diseases, and intravascular devices.

Cross-References
▶ Hodgkin's Lymphoma
▶ Leukemia in General
▶ Lung Cancer
▶ Non-Hodgkins Lymphoma

Supportive Care

James H. Brashears, III
Radiation Oncologist, Venice, FL, USA

Definition
The prevention and management of the adverse effects of disease and treatment whose success is not measured purely by survival. Widely conceived, this includes alleviation of symptoms from cancer and oncologic therapy, communication with patients about the disease process, easing of emotional or spiritual burdens, and helping with psychological or social difficulties.

Cross-References
▶ Supportive Care and Quality of Life

Supportive Care and Quality of Life

James H. Brashears, III
Radiation Oncologist, Venice, FL, USA

Synonyms
Cancer quality of life; QOL

Definition/Description
▶ Supportive care during curative radiotherapy is designed to increase compliance with the prescribed treatment and thereby increase the quantity and/or quality of life. After curative therapy, the goal of supportive care is to increase the quality of life and may be aimed at relieving adverse manifestations of the disease process or side effects from previous treatment. When radiation is used for palliative purposes, the radiation treatment itself might be said to be supportive. In keeping with the adage that "an ounce of prevention is worth a pound of cure," many of the negative effects on quality of life from radiotherapy can be foreseen and addressed before severe complications arise. For those complications that have no effective therapy, being forewarned about their possibility can help patients understand the body's reaction and take a more active role in care decisions and follow up.

Background

Constitutional and specific organ-system complications occur in response to treatment and to the malignancy. Multidisciplinary management before, during and subsequent to these events can lessen the impact on the patient's quality of life as can clear communication. Certainly, the quality of life for any person will depend on the individual's understanding of what it means to be "healthy" or "well" and so can be quite unique and complicated, thus any meaningful intervention aimed at fostering well-being must evaluate the potential positive and negative effects in light of the particular patient's desires. In other words, the thoughtful medical professional must negotiate care in the context of the patient's experience. Still, pragmatism dictates that some broad assumptions be made, namely, that ameliorating constitutional symptoms like fatigue, depression, and poor nutrition will contribute to quality of life. Similarly, the goal of alleviating specific organ-system complaints including xerostomia, mucositis, nausea, vomiting, diarrhea, dermatitis, and genitourinary dysfunction will support patient health (NCCN 2010a).

Evaluation of global or overall functional status may be quantified by Karnofsky performance status (KPS) or Eastern Cooperative Oncology Group (ECOG) scales (NCCN 2010b). A patient's KPS is assigned based on a 0–100 scale divided into multiples of ten with escalating numbers reflecting an increased ability to carry out activities of daily living with progressively less impairment by disease. The ECOG scale ranges from whole numbers from 0 to 5 with lower numbers representing less disability or less time spent confined to the bed or chair. For pediatric patients, the Lansky scale may be appropriate and bears much in common with KPS.

When describing organ-system side effects, grading schemes similar to the ECOG scale are used. In radiation oncology, the most prevalent is that of the Radiation Therapy Oncology Group, or RTOG, which uses whole numbers between 0 and 5 to describe escalating severity of symptoms and findings on imaging or labs (e.g., RTOG grade 0: no side effect; grade 1: mild dysfunction; grade 2: moderate dysfunction; grade 3: severe dysfunction; grade 4: life threatening dysfunction; grade 5: lethal).

Intervention

Radiation therapy prescription requires a balance between the goals of tumor control (or palliative effect) and the probability of normal tissue toxicity; toward this end, clear ideas of achievable, effective target doses and tolerance doses for normal tissues should be respected. It is here that radiation oncologists can exert the greatest influence on patient well-being, for good or ill. Obedience to sound radiation principles including reproducibility, immobilization, continuing provider education, accurate treatment planning, and rigorous quality assurance for machines and sources is incumbent. The literature is replete with data attempting to guide radiation application and cautionary instances of unintended consequences. Medications can also help reduce the risk of sustaining such injury.

While ► cancer-related fatigue is a well-recognized constitutional symptom of radiation, depression, and poor self-care (like failure to maintain proper nutrition) are not. Cancer-related fatigue or tiredness should be screened for and is under-reported, under-diagnosed, and under-treated (NCCN 2010a). The etiology of radiation-related fatigue has not been clearly defined and no dose-volume recommendations can be made, rather providers should be vigilant for patient factors that may contribute to fatigue and reduced quality of life. Underlying psychiatric issues may be addressed by medications, patient education, or psychosocial resources (e.g., support groups, exercise programs, nutritional or individual counseling). Pain can contribute to fatigue and can be dealt with by similar means in addition to more invasive approaches. Radiation at curative doses to the swallowing structures and/or upper esophagus is known to cause mucosal erosion resulting in impaired nutrition or insufficient caloric intake. In these cases, a gastrostomy tube can be inserted prior to therapy to provide an avenue for supplemental feedings when the enteral route becomes too painful thereby decreasing the probability of unwanted breaks in treatment and avoiding the excess risk of mortality associated with more than 20% weight loss (Cassileth 2008).

The risk of organ-system side effects can be reduced by attention to dose-volume constraints of uninvolved nearby tissues, medications, diet, and hygiene. Keeping the mean dose to the parotid glands $\leq$26 Gy in standard head and neck curative treatments (with the use of intensity modulated radiation therapy or IMRT) and the intravenous or subcutaneous injection of amifostine within the 30 minutes preceding radiation have been shown to reduce the risk and severity of xerostomia (Cassileth 2008). For head and neck treatments, surgical submandibular gland transfer to a location outside of the radiation fields may be also attempted. Dental evaluation and removal of imperiled teeth before starting radiation and the use of fluoride trays and good oral hygiene reduce the risk of postradiation dental carries and ▶ osteoradionecrosis (Dzuik 2005). Limiting the dose to the mandible can also truncate the risk of osteoradionecrosis. Oral mucositis can be limited by maintenance of good oral hygiene, the use of benzydamine and attention to the dose to the oral cavity and tongue on the treatment planning system. For patients with metallic dental hardware, dental trays can shield surrounding tissues from buildup and be indexed to the immobilization system to aid set-up reproducibility. Gastrointestinal (GI) mucositis, known as esophagitis, enteritis, colitis, and proctitis depending on the location of treatment, produces pain and diarrhea. Twice daily oral sulfasalazine may reduce GI mucositis, but more

effective is limiting the dose and volume of the normal enteral structures exposed to radiation by the use of image guidance, IMRT or other conformal therapy techniques and externally introduced appliances (as with rectal balloons for prostate cancer). Moreover, limiting the dose and volume of irradiated stomach and bowel can also reduce nausea, vomiting, and diarrhea. As with high and moderate emetic risk chemotherapy, patients can benefit from prophylactic anti-emetics when radiation is given to the total body or upper abdomen; serotonin (5-HT3) antagonists (dolasetron, granisetron, ondansetron, palonosetron) and/or dexamethasone are recommended (Cassileth 2008). Acute and chronic dermatitis can similarly be reduced by being mindful of the doses being administered superficially for deeper targets. When treating breast cancer, IMRT and the purposeful sparing of skin can reduce acute dermatitis. Patients should not wear aluminum-based antiperspirants in or near treatment fields (nondrying deodorants are acceptable). Moisturizers containing alcohol should likewise be avoided. The selection of appropriate photon beam energies and arrangements in addition to recognition of exit dose and bolus effects can limit radiation-related dermatitis and alopecia particularly when large fractions are given as with stereotactic body radiation therapy (SBRT or extracranial stereotactic radiosurgery). Reduction of acute and chronic urinary morbidity by decreasing the dose to the bladder wall is possible. For those considering reproduction, the radiosensitivity of germ cells calls for referral for fertility counseling and possible egg or sperm banking if the gonads will receive significant dose. Long-term androgen deprivation or anti-androgen therapy, particularly with biclautamide, can cause gynecomastia and breast pain, which can often be reduced or prevented with prophylactic hormone therapy with tamoxifen or radiation to the peri-areolar region (e.g., 10 Gy in 1 fraction or 15 Gy in 3 fractions).

Initial Evaluation

Treatment visits during radiation therapy are designed to follow the progress of patients and monitor them for side effects as well as answer any questions. The same is true for ad hoc and scheduled follow up visits. Cancer-related fatigue is experienced in more than 70% of patients undergoing multimodal treatment or with metastases (NCCN 2010a). Radiation-related fatigue should begin to remit within the first one to two months following treatment, though this will be complicated by disease, patient factors, or the use of other oncologic interventions like chemotherapy and hormone therapy. Fatigue may last longer after large areas of the brain have been treated as with ▶ somnolence syndrome. Monitoring the patient's weight and lab work can show if there are other readily correctable contributors to fatigue like inadequate nutrition or anemia. Sleep disturbance can contribute to fatigue. Careful history and physical examination, possibly with the use of standardized questionnaires, can help identify the progressive impact of therapy or disease on quality of life. Oral mucosits (and thrush), dermatitis, and treatment effects in the anogenital region are directly observable by the provider. Questionnaires filled out longitudinally may also help draw attention to symptoms that may be overlooked during the typical office visit and aid in discussing the effectiveness of previous supportive interventions. Such questionnaires are available to evaluate constitutional symptoms as well as xerostomia, nausea, vomiting, diarrhea, and genitourinary dysfunction.

Differential Diagnosis

There is an interrelationship between the constitutional and organ-system symptom. Adequately addressing one problem may lessen the burden associated with others. For example, if pain with swallowing is dealt with during radiotherapy for a thoracic malignancy, a person can have improvement in nutrition, fatigue, depression, anxiety, and nausea. The patient's prior medical and psychiatric history can give clues to factors exacerbating symptoms. Many cancer patients will also have a weakened immune system, so infection should be considered for constitutional, mucosal, GI, and genitourinary complaints.

Imaging and Laboratory Studies

Acute and unexpected symptoms during and after therapy should usually be aggressively worked up to determine if there has been changes in disease status or functionality of the organ system that is unrelated to their malignancy. Cancer and oncologic treatments may put new stresses on already frail individuals that can unmask cardiovascular, rheumatologic, psychiatric, and infectious conditions among others. Patients with new chest pain, shortness of breath, neurologic decrements, fever, or other potentially life-endangering warning signs warrant evaluation as anyone else unless there is already an understanding between the patient and providers limiting such interventions. Diagnosis with a malignancy puts a patient at risk for development of new sites of disease involvement, so there should be a low threshold for restaging. Magnetic resonance imaging (MRI) may be needed for alterations in mental status, while diagnosing new onset of severe abdominal pain with nausea, vomiting, and a paucity of bowel sounds could benefit from computed tomography (CT) of the abdomen. Suspicion for infection should be high in most cancer patients under treatment. Complete blood count (CBC) with differential can help quantify immune suppression or identify the risk of sepsis (when blood cultures should also be taken). For urinary complaints, a urinalysis with culture can confirm if a urinary tract infection exists. CBC can also reveal anemia and provide clues as to its etiology. In those with poor nutritional intake or dehydration, a complete metabolic panel may elucidate any electrolyte disturbances and guide fluid replacement while serially checking prealbumin or ▶ albumin provide clues to the efficacy of prior dietary supports.

Treatment

Management of cancer-related fatigue concentrates on addressable causes and symptom control. Patients should be educated about fatigue and provided strategies to cope including energy conservation, distraction, and encouragement of activity (NCCN 2010a). Mood disorders should receive medication, counseling, and follow-up with psychiatric professionals. Participation in support groups and exercise programs is encouraged. Sleep disturbance may be addressed through fostering better sleep hygiene, cognitive behavioral therapy, limiting napping, and medications (NCCN 2010a). Anemia can be treated with transfusions or short-term use of ▶ erythropoiesis-stimulating agents (ESAs) if related to chemotherapy being used for non-curative intent (owing to possible enhancement of tumor growth by ESAs) (NCCN 2010c). Providers should be alert for infection and treat accordingly. Dietary intake often changes for cancer patients and nutritional counseling should be considered to help manage any deficiencies in caloric, electrolyte, or fluid intake. Maintenance of a stable nitrogen balance is also critical for those with cancer (daily intake of 1.5–2.0 g of protein per kilogram per day) (Cassileth 2008). To facilitate this in patients suffering from effects of tumor growth or treatment toxicity, the consistency of foods can be altered (e.g., switching to an all liquid diet) or nasogastric, nasojejunal, gastrostomy, gastrojejunostomy, jejunostomy tubes may be placed. When unsuccessful, parenternal nutrition is a short-term fallback. If the desire to eat is lost, dronabinol, corticosteroids, and megesterol can be used to stimulate appetite.

Radiation-induced xerostomia usually begins around the third week of radiation and worsens over the course of therapy; it can become permanent and once present, therapy is composed of dietary changes, saliva stimulation, oral hygiene, and salivary replacement. Intake of cool, soft and moist foods should be favored over the hot, hard and spicy. Chilled, carbonated beverages are well tolerated (Dzuik 2005). Artificial saliva and regular use of mouthwash with baking soda, saline, and glycerol can diminish symptoms. Chewing gum or sucking on lozenges or sugar-free candy can increase residual salivary flow. The systemic saliva stimulant (sialogue) pilocarpine works through cholinergic effects, hence it may not be appropriate for those with cardiovascular disease or those taking anticholinergic medicines. Pilocarpine may take 2–3 months for maximal results at 5–10 mg, given three to four times per day (Dzuik 2005). Potential healing of the salivary glands and return to function may take years to manifest. Fluoride toothpaste and the use of fluoride trays can help maintain the health of remaining teeth as will regular follow-up with dentistry. Thrush or other oral infections should be treated and the dose of medicines with anticholinergic properties limited as far as possible.

Oral mucositis during therapy can also be managed by artificial saliva, mouthwash, dietary changes, and treatment of any local infections. Proprietary and custom prescribed topical barrier medicines and local anesthetics can reduce discomfort. Gelclair and Radiacare are popular commercial products as are physician-specified mixes of viscous lidocaine, milk of magnesia, diphenhydramine, mycostatin, chlorhexadine, tetracycline, or hydrocortisone, which are designed to be swished around the mouth and spit or swallowed as appropriate. Systemically active analgesics including opioids (frequently given in liquid formulations) are often required toward the end of therapy with a bowel regimen to avoid constipation. Acid reflux can contribute to mucositis as well, so proton pump inhibitors or type-2 histamine blockers (H-2 antagonists) may be appropriate. Certainly, patients should abstain from tobacco and alcohol.

Mucositis involving the esophagus can be managed similarly with barrier, anesthetic, analgesic, and antacid medications.

Mucositis in the remainder of the alimentary tract may manifest as nausea, vomiting, diarrhea, or proctitis. There are many therapeutic targets for anti-emetics and sometimes a combination of these works best for a particular patient. For anticipatory nausea (before the actual radiation treatment), lorazepam or another anxiolytic may be used. For intermittent postradiation nausea, prochlorperazine or promethazine can be tried and come in rectal formulations as well. Chronic nausea can be addressed with centrally acting serotonin (5-HT3) antagonists that are available in oral, IV, or transdermal forms. Corticosteroids can also relieve nausea, though long-term use carries a host of adverse effects (Dzuik 2005). Dietary change including small, frequent protein-heavy meals with fluids in between and avoidance of caffeine, alcohol, dairy products, and fat can help mild to moderate diarrhea (Cassileth 2008). Escalating doses of loperamide can be used for more severe cases and diphenoxylate/atropine may help when symptoms continue to be refractory. Acute proctitis can be addressed by topical anesthetics and hydrocortisone formulations; if complaints are chronic, endoscopic management with dilute formalin or argon coagulation may be required.

Erythema or dry desquamation can be managed with nondrying moisturizers including many commercial products containing aloe vera. Topical hydrocortisone can decrease pruritus of the skin. Hydrogel dressings and 1% silver sulfadiazine may be employed for moist desquamation. With severe dermatitis, standard wound care protocols are appropriate and may force altering the planned radiation course. Late radiation damage to subcutaneous tissue around joints can be reduced by regular stretching exercises. Vitamin E and pentoxifylline can promote healing of fibrosis and is usually well tolerated (Cassileth 2008). Lymphedema, particularly after breast cancer treatment, can be treated by complex physical decongestive therapy, which will have elements of massage, exercise, skin care, and pressure wraps.

Urinary symptoms from radiation-related cystitis usually start around the fourth week of standard fractionated treatment and can mimic those from urinary tract infection or even diabetes, so the latter causes should be ruled out (with a simple urinalysis). Frequency and/or dysuria with a good urine stream and no hesitancy can be treated with analgesics like phenazopyridine. Urgency or pain at the beginning or end of micturation, but with maintenance of a good stream argues for bladder spasm that is well treated with antispasmodics (tolterodine, oxybutynin, or flavoxate) (Dzuik 2005).

Radiation to the pelvic area and hormonal alterations may interfere with the sexual well-being of patients, decreasing libido and altering the physiological interplay necessary for coitus. Radiation to the female pelvis often brings about menopause if the ovaries are treated. The vagina and labia can also become irritated during therapy with loss of elasticity and sensation in the months and years following. Fibrosis and shortening of the vagina can be mitigated by the use of vaginal dilators and sexual function enhanced with the use of lubricants. By reducing the amount or effect of testosterone, hormone therapy for prostate cancer reduces libido and makes male sexual function difficult. Hot flashes can be treated with paroxetine, venlafaxine, depot medroxyprogesterone, or megesterol (Dzuik 2005). Radiation therapy to the prostate causes long-term vascular changes to the erectile tissues of the penis that can also lead to erectile dysfunction even when desire is present. Medications like the phosphodiesterase inhibitors (i.e., sildenafil, tadalafil, and vardenafil) and intracavernosal injection of prostaglandins are used to treat erectile dysfunction as are mechanical means including the vacuum pump and surgical implantation of prostheses in the corpora cavernosa.

Cross-References

▶ Conformal Therapy: Treatment Planning, Treatment Delivery, and Clinical Results
▶ Image-Guided Radiation Therapy (IGRT): kV Imaging
▶ Intensity Modulated Radiation Therapy (IMRT)
▶ Pain Management
▶ Principles of Chemotherapy
▶ Radiation Oncology Physics
▶ Stereotactic Radiosurgery: Extracranial

References

Cassileth D (2008) Supportive care and quality of life. In: Halperin P (ed) Principles and practice of radiation oncology, 5th edn. Lippincott Williams and Wilkins, Philadelphia, pp 2011–2018
Dziuk T (2005) Commonly prescribed medications in radiation oncology, 8th edn. South Austin Cancer Center, Austin
NCCN (2010a) NCCN clinical practice guidelines in oncology: cancer-related fatigue v.1.2010. National Comprehensive Cancer Network, Fort Washington
NCCN (2010b) NCCN clinical practice guidelines in oncology: palliative care v.1.2010. National Comprehensive Cancer Network, Fort Washington
NCCN (2010c) NCCN clinical practice guidelines in oncology: cancer and chemotheraphy-induced anemia v.2.2010. National Comprehensive Cancer Network, Fort Washington

Surface Microscopy

Lydia T. Komarnicky-Kocher
Department of Radiation Oncology, College of Medicine, Drexel University, Philadelphia, PA, USA

Definition

Surface microscopy is a method of examining the skin by utilizing a dermatoscope consisting of a magnifier (typically ×10), a non-polarized light source, and a transparent plate and a liquid medium between the instrument and the skin. This allows for inspection of skin lesions unobstructed by skin surface reflections and can be used to evaluate several features of lesions that place them at a higher risk for malignancy. Pseudopods, radial streaming, blue/gray veil, and peripheral black dots have been identified as factors suggestive of melanoma.

Cross-References

▶ Melanoma

SVCS

▶ Superior Vena Cava Syndrome

Systemic Radiation Therapy

▶ Radioimmunotherapy (RIT)

Systemic Targeted Radionuclide Therapy (STaRT)

▶ Targeted Radioimmunotherapy

T

TAH-BSO

▶ Gynecological Tumors
▶ Total Abdominal Hysterectomy

Targeted Radioimmunotherapy

TOD W. SPEER
Department of Human Oncology, University of Wisconsin School of Medicine and Public Health, UW Hospital and Clinics, Madison, WI, USA

Synonyms

Radioimmunotherapy (RIT); Systemic radiation therapy; Systemic targeted radionuclide therapy (STaRT); Unsealed source brachytherapy

Definition

Targeted radioimmunotherapy (TRIT) is a form of anticancer therapy that uses a targeting construct (antibody, antibody fragment, affibody, aptamer, peptide, nanotechnology), attached to a radionuclide (covalent bond or chelate molecule), to deliver a systemic cytotoxic dose of radiation to malignant tissue, thus representing a form of unsealed source of systemic brachytherapy. Depending upon the type of targeting construct, the immune system may have a synergistic role in inducing cell death. Intact antibodies will typically recruit elements of the immune system for cytotoxic activity (due to the Fc region of the antibody), in addition to the cell kill induced by the radionuclide. Smaller constructs, other than intact antibodies, must rely largely upon the cytotoxic power of various radionuclides to induce cell kill. The radiation delivered to the target site from TRIT is released in an exponentially decreasing low dose and low dose-rate manor. This is due to the physical half-life of the radionuclide combined with the biological half-life of the targeting construct (in combination, the effective half-life).

Background

Dr. Paul Ehrlich initially proposed the basic concept of TRIT in 1898. Although the so-called "magic bullets" of the Ehrlich era were chemical substances that were proposed to have special affinities for pathogenic organisms, his idea has been extrapolated to the concept of therapeutic compounds that specifically target pathological processes, hence potentially sparing normal tissue. This is the concept of targeted therapy. In 1908, Dr. Ehrlich received the Nobel Prize for his endeavors. As testimony to the complexities of developing these efforts into a workable form of targeted anticancer therapy, it took nearly 50 years before the first successful reports of TRIT began to show promise, as documented in published series, treating Wagner osteogenic sarcoma and melanoma patients with polyclonal antibodies, covalently bonded to I-131. Initially, antibodies were difficult to produce and isolate. As a result, the next several decades witnessed the utilization of relatively nonspecific targeting agents such as amino acids, cholesterol

L.W. Brady, T.E. Yaeger (eds.), *Encyclopedia of Radiation Oncology*, DOI 10.1007/978-3-540-85516-3,
© Springer-Verlag Berlin Heidelberg 2013

compounds, and hormones. Regardless, the cytotoxic potential of radionuclides was quite evident. In 1975, the hybridoma technique for producing monoclonal antibodies was published. Physicians and researchers had the long-awaited means to consistently produce a carrier molecule, for selected radionuclides that could accurately target tumor antigens.

The modern concept for targeting agents does not limit the use of carrier molecules to mere antibodies. Successful targeting of tumor cells, with high affinity, can also be accomplished with antibody fragments, peptides, affinity ligands and nanoparticles. As the research and clinical arena ever so modestly disengage from intact antibodies as the carrier molecule for the radionuclide, the impact of the immune system has been somewhat abrogated. Typically, the in vivo antibody-receptor complex would potentially initiate the immune effector response. However, with the aforementioned "new class" of delivery agents, this is no longer the case. Hence, the "immunotherapy contribution" of "radioimmunotherapy" is increasingly less important (the exception being intact monoclonal antibodies used as targeting agents against hematologic malignancies). Perhaps a more appropriate term for this technology would simply be "targeted radionuclide therapy." Although the goal is to deliver this form of therapy systemically, it may also be administered via intratumor or a number of intracompartmental routes. What has not changed is the availability of some of the most cytotoxic agents known. These are the radionuclides that produce beta, Auger, and alpha radiation and they are highly toxic to cells in very small amounts. For example, alpha particles have a very high ▶ linear energy of transfer (LET) with a path length measured in only several cell diameters. Only a few alpha particles need to traverse a cancer cell nucleus in order to cause a lethal event. Considering that the basic premise of successful targeted therapy is to bring the most

cytotoxic agents in close proximity to the targeted cell and spare normal tissues, it appears that there is a phenomenal potential for radionuclides as targeted anticancer agents.

To date, reasonable gains have been achieved using targeted radionuclide therapy for hematologic malignancies. Still, its acceptance into the oncology community has been somewhat tenuous. At the time of this writing, there are eight FDA-approved anticancer monoclonal antibodies. Only two of these approved drugs are radioconjugates (Zevalin; ibritumomab tiuxetan, Bexxar; tositumomab). These agents were approved by the US Food and Drug Administration (FDA) to treat non-Hodgkin lymphoma (NHL) in 1992 and 1993, respectively. There have been no further radionuclide-conjugated targeting constructs approved for therapy in the United States since this time period, although the indication for Zevalin has recently been expanded for adjuvant therapy. Progress with solid tumor-targeted radionuclide therapy has been even less sanguine. China, however, has approved Licartin (^{131}I metuximab) for Hepatoma and TNT (tumor necrosis treatment; ^{131}I-chTNT) for bronchogenic carcinoma. Still, formidable barriers remain concerning target selection, tumor penetration, dosimetry, type of radionuclide, lack of inherent radiosensitivity of tumor, heterogenic expression of tumor-associated antigens, immunogenicity of the targeting vector, aberrant tumor vascularity, elevated interstitial tumor pressure, tumor necrosis, hypoxia, an abnormal extracellular matrix, and normal tissue toxicity (acute and late radiation toxicity) of the therapeutic radioconjugate. Regardless, there is a fever-pitch burgeoning of biotechnology that will soon erupt into a plethora of exciting advancements that will move targeted radionuclide therapy to the forefront of cancer therapy, not only for metastatic disease, but more importantly into the adjuvant setting. There is a not too distant horizon when personalized cancer therapy will be standard of care. To this end, targeted radionuclide therapy will be an indispensible weapon in the armament of anticancer therapy.

Purpose

The purpose of TRIT is to safely deliver a dose or multiple doses (fractions) of a radiolabeled targeting construct. The targeting construct will exhibit a certain affinity for a tumor-associated antigen located in the malignant tissue and deliver low dose, low dose-rate radiotherapy to radiographically visible tumors and to micrometastatic disease.

Technology

Immunology and Targeting Constructs

The word "immunity" is derived from Latin, *immunitas*, meaning the protection from legal persecution, given to Roman senators while serving in office. In a medical sense, immunity signifies protection from disease or infectious agents (Abbas et al. 2007). The immune system is composed of the cells and molecules responsible for the immune response. The immune response can be divided into an early (1–12 h) reaction, termed innate immunity and a late (1–7+ days) reaction, termed adaptive immunity. The innate immune system comprises biochemical and cellular mechanisms that exist prior to the introduction of an infectious agent and results in a rapid response. The components of the innate immune system consist of epithelial barriers, phagocytic cells (neutrophils, macrophages), natural killer cells, the compliment system, and cytokines. The adaptive immune system develops over time, becoming more effective with subsequent exposures of antigen. It exhibits the ability to "remember" and to respond more quickly with continued exposures to the same antigen. The components of the adaptive immune system consist of lymphocytes and secreted antibodies. The adaptive immune system can be divided into humoral immunity and cell-mediated immunity. Concerning humoral immunity, B lymphocytes secrete antibodies for protection. Concerning cell-mediated immunity, helper T lymphocytes either activate macrophages or cytotoxic T lymphocytes, which then directly destroy pathologic (infectious or malignant) cells.

It is well known that the host's immune system is important for preventing the growth and development of cancer (Campoli and Ferrone 2011). Currently, there exists a large body of literature that supports the concept that the host immune system interacts with tumorigenesis and tumor progression (Fig. 1). It has been shown in animal models and in the clinic that cancer immune surveillance is exceedingly important. For example, mice with an impaired innate or adaptive immune system will be more susceptible for developing chemically induced or spontaneous cancers. Additionally, the malignant transformation of cells in animals and humans, due to the accumulation of somatic mutations and/or due to the deregulation of oncogenes or tumor suppressor genes results in the expression of tumor antigens (TA). These TAs are often recognized by the immune system as documented by TA-specific T-cell precursors and natural killer cells, found in the peripheral blood of cancer patients, capable of killing tumor cells. Further evidence of cancer immune surveillance exists in patients with genetic or drug-induced immunosuppression. Transplant patients exhibit a predisposition for certain malignancies (squamous cell carcinoma, basal cell carcinoma, Kaposi sarcoma, melanoma, and lymphoma). Patients with Chediak–Higashi and Wiskott–Aldrich syndrome demonstrate an increased rate of lymphoproliferative malignancies. Discontinuing immunosuppressive drugs in solid organ allograph patients with occult malignant melanoma has resulted in tumor regression.

In spite of the evidence of cancer genesis and progression in immune-compromised hosts, the

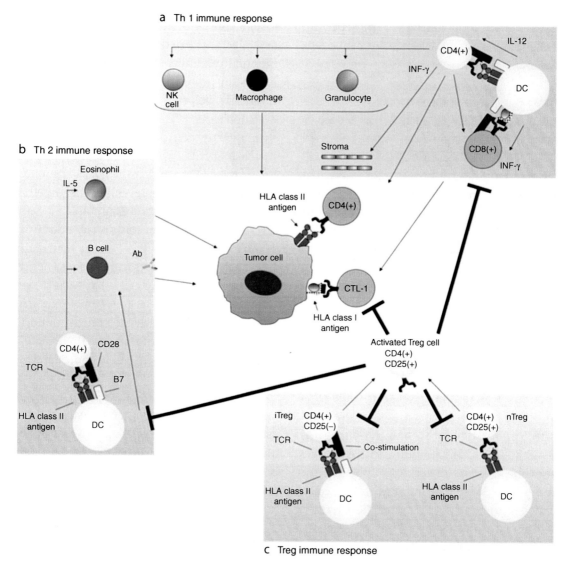

Targeted Radioimmunotherapy. Fig. 1 Generation of TA-specific T-cell-based immune responses. The immune system is believed to control tumor growth through several mechanisms. (**a**) It is thought that the most effective way of mounting a TA-specific immune response is through the combined action of CD8(+) and IFN-γ-secreting CD4(+) T helper cells (Th1). (**b**) Tumor cells can also be targeted by IL-5-secreting CD4(+) T helper cells (Th2). Antigen-presenting cells activate IL-5 Th2 cells, which induce the accumulation of eosinophils and/or provide help for the generation of a TA-specific B-cell immune response. (**c**) Treg cell-mediated suppression of TA-specific CTL responses can be accomplished through the two major types of Treg cells. nTregs do not require simultaneous TCR and co-stimulatory signals to undergo activation and clonal expansion, while iTreg require simultaneous TCR and co-stimulatory signals to be activated and expanded. iTregs primarily suppress by synthesizing suppressive cytokines while nTregs, also elaborate immunosuppressive cytokines as well as through a yet undefined contact-independent mechanism. (Abbreviations: *IFN* interferon, *IL* interleukin, *TCR* T-cell receptor, *Treg* T regulatory cells, *nTreg* naturally occurring Treg, *iTreg* induced Treg, *HLA* human leukocyte antigens, *NK* natural killer, *CTL* cytotoxic T lymphocytes)

majority of cancers develop in seemingly immune-competent individuals. The last decade of research has revealed that cancer cells have developed means to avoid immune detection and surveillance, either through the selection of nonimmunogenic tumor cells and/or the active suppression of the immune response. It has therefore been rightfully suggested that "tumor immune escape" be added to Hanahan and Weinberg's six hallmarks of cancer (self-sufficiency in growth signals, insensitivity to antigrowth signals, tissue invasion and metastasis, limitless replicative potential, sustained angiogenesis, and evasion of apoptosis).

The targets for TRIT typically consist of tumor-associated antigens (TAAs). The reason for this is because the cytotoxic radionuclide must be delivered preferentially to malignant tissue and should avoid normal tissue. To date, greater than 2000 TAAs have been identified (http://www2.licr.org/CancerImmunomeDB). One of the main methodologies used to identify TAAs is termed SEREX (serologic analysis of recombinant cDNA libraries). SEREX involves a bacteriophage recombinant cDNA expression library, prepared from various malignancies (isolated tumors or malignant cell lines) or testis tissue (Jeoung 2011; Chap. 11). This cDNA expression library is transduced in *Escherichia coli* to produce a recombinant protein library. These various proteins (clones) are then tested against the serum from autologous cancer patients. Clones that react to IgG antibodies are identified and are then further characterized as TAAs (Fig. 2). Many of these SEREX-identified TAAs have been elucidated by other processes and laboratories. This has led to the concept of a finite number of TAAs that are produced in cancer patients and are potentially identified by the immune system. These finite TAAs are collectively referred to as the "▶ cancer immunome." SEREX-defined antigens, representing broad categories, may be organized as follows: mutational antigens,

amplified or overexpressed antigens, differentiation antigens, and cancer/testis antigens. Within these categories, only a limited number of TAAs have been used as targets for TRIT (Table 1).

The ideal target for TRIT targeting constructs would be one that is overexpressed on cancer cells, is uniformly expressed, is not found to any significant level in normal tissue, is not shed into the circulation, and exhibits an important role in tumor growth and progression (Wong et al. 2011). TAAs, as the name implies, are antigens "associated" with tumors, but also are present, to some degree, in normal tissue. True tumor-specific antigens have not yet been identified and utilized. Overexpression is necessary as typical targeting constructs require antigen densities of approximately 10^5 receptors on each cell for adequate targeting. A homogeneous antigen expression is desired so that a uniform ▶ activity distribution of the radionuclide will result. Nonuniform activity distributions (heterogeneity of antigen in target tissue being one potential cause) will significantly lower the effectiveness of TRIT by subsequently resulting in nonuniform or heterogeneous dose distributions (O'Donoghue 2000). This is particularly important for radionuclides with short path lengths of the emitted particles (i.e., Auger and α particle emitters). Radionuclides with longer path lengths, such as high-energy β emitters, can partly overcome the problem of nonuniform dose distributions through the ▶ crossfire effect. If the target antigen is significantly shed into the circulation, the targeting construct may bind and "complex" with the antigen. This will result in a more rapid clearance of the TRIT agent and a much less effective treatment. If the TAA has an important signaling role, then subsequent binding of the targeting construct will most likely add to the cytoxicity of the radionuclide due to the blockade or promotion of intracellular signaling, potentially resulting in disruption of growth pathways important for tumor growth. Some TAAs

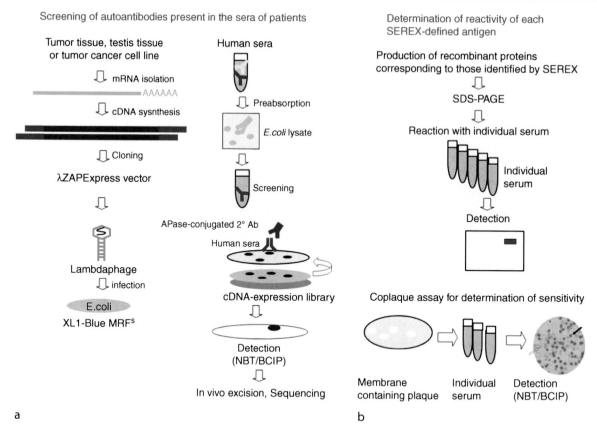

Screening of autoantibodies present in the sera of patients

Determination of reactivity of each SEREX-defined antigen

a

b

Targeted Radioimmunotherapy. Fig. 2 Identification of SEREX-defined antigens. (**a**) *Construction of cDNA expression library.* cDNA expression libraries are made from tumor tissues, tumor cell lines, or testis tissues. For this, 5 μg of poly (A)+RNA was converted into cDNA by reverse transcriptase. Thus, obtained cDNA library is cloned into λ ZAP expression vector. Each library usually consists of 2×10^6 primary recombinants, on average. A total of 5×10^5 of these recombinants are used for immunoscreening. Each of these recombinant cDNA libraries is transformed into E. coli to yield a recombinant cDNA expression library. cDNA expression libraries are screened with pooled sera of patients with cancer. Immune reactive clones are selected by reacting nitrocellulose membrane containing recombinant clones with pooled sera of patients with cancer followed by incubation with alkaline phosphatase-conjugated secondary antibody. Selected clones are subjected to in vivo excision and sequencing to determine identity of each immune reactive clone. (**b**) Sensitivity and specificity of each clone is determined by incubating each clone with individual serum of cancer patients or healthy controls

(receptors) will internalize when bound by the targeting construct. In truth, most receptors internalize, but at different rates. A rapid internalization process (internalizing receptor) will have an impact upon the type of radionuclide that is selected and potentially upon the delivery strategy of the TRIT agent.

A multitude of agents have been used as carriers (targeting constructs) for the targeted delivery of radiation to cancer. These consist of

Targeted Radioimmunotherapy. Table 1 Select monoclonal antibodies evaluated for RIT

Malignancy	Antigen	Antibody
Colorectal cancer	CEA TAG-72 A33 EpCAM DNA histone H1	cT84.66, hMN-14, A5B7 B72.3, CC49 anti-A33 NR-LU-10, NR-LU-13 chTNT-1/B
Breast cancer	MUC1 L6 TAG-72 CEA	huBrE-3, m170 chL6 CC49 cT84.66
Ovarian cancer	MUC1 Folate receptor TAG-72	HMFG1 cMov18 B72.3, CC49
Prostate cancer	PSMA TAG-72	huJ591 CC49
Lung cancer	DNA histone H1 TAG72	chTNT-1/B CC49
Head and neck cancer	CD44v6	U36, BIWA4
Gliomas	EGFR Tenascin	425 816 C, BC4
Melanoma	p97	96.5
Renal cancer	G250 Glycoprotein	cG250
Medullary thyroid	CEA	cT84.66, hMN-14, NP-4
Neuroblastoma	Ganglioside GD2 NCAM	3F8 UJ13A, ERIC-1

antibodies, antibody fragments, peptides, affibodies, aptamers, and nanostructures (i.e., liposomes, nanoparticles, microparticles, nanoshells, and minicells). By an exceedingly large margin, intact monoclonal antibodies (mAbs) have dominated the field of TRIT as targeting constructs (Fig. 3a–d) (Burvenich and Scott 2011) and will be the focus of this section. In humans, there are five classes or ▶ isotypes of antibodies (IgA, IgD, IgE, IgG, and IgM). IgG is the most commonly used mAb for TRIT because it is the most prevalent antibody in serum and has the longest serum half-life, typically measured in weeks (approximately 23 days). IgG is further divided into four subtypes, IgG1–4. IgG antibodies are large glycoprotein macromolecules, with an atomic mass of approximately 150,000 Dalton or 150 kDa. The "y-shaped structure" (Fig. 3a) consists of two Fab fragments (fragment antigen binding; ∼50,000 Da each) and an Fc fragment (crystallizable fragment; ∼50,000 Da).

The "end" or "tip" of each Fab fragment is variable in amino acid sequence, from one mAb

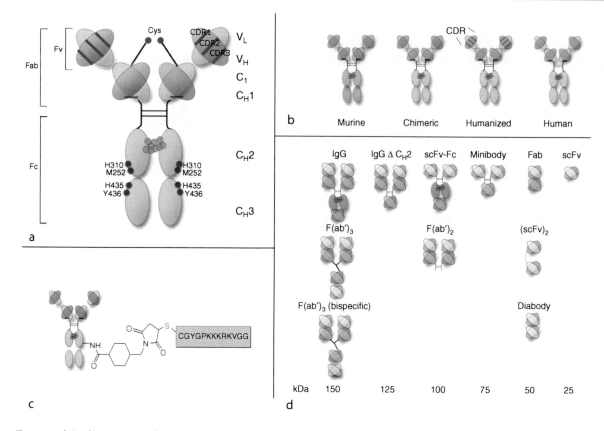

Targeted Radioimmunotherapy. Fig. 3 Antibody engineering: different strategies to improve the therapeutic index in radioimmunotherapy: (**a**) Typical structure of a humanized IgG antibody. The following engineering strategies are presented: *Black dots*, mutations in amino acids involved in FcRn binding which influence the pharmacokinetics of the IgG; *CDR1-3*, murine CDRs grafted into a human IgG backbone to humanize the antibody; *Cys*, engineered cysteine residues for site-specific conjugation (**b**) humanization strategies; *dark grey dots*, indicating the murine portion of the IgG and *light grey dots*, indicating the human portion of the IgG (**c**) introducing a nuclear localizing signal (**d**) mono-specific and bispecific fragments used in radioimmunotherapeutic strategies (Abbreviations: *CDR* complementarity-determining regions, *CH* constant domain heavy chain, *CL* constant domain light chain, *Fc* crystallizable fragment, *Fv* variable fragment)

to another. Accordingly, each "tip" is called the antigen binding site (ABS) and is responsible for antigen recognition. Each ABS forms a noncovalent bond (electrostatic forces, van der Waals forces, hydrophobic interactions, and hydrogen bonds) with the target or antigen. A specific region of an antigen, which binds to the ABS, is referred to as an ▶ epitope. It has been

proposed that a million or more different antibodies exist in various individuals. Theoretically, more than 10^9 different antibodies can be produced. The outer core of the mAb consists of two identical light chains (outer portion of the Fab fragment) designated with an "L." The inner core, consisting of the Fc region and the inner Fab region is designated as heavy or "H." Both the

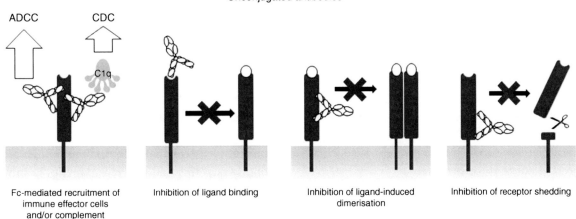

Targeted Radioimmunotherapy. Fig. 4 Potential mechanisms for antibody-mediated biological effects. The various potential mechanisms by which unconjugated antibodies, specific for cell surface receptors, may affect cell signaling

light and heavy chains contain homologous, 110 amino acid sequences that fold upon one another and are connected by a disulfide bridge, resulting in "globular" motif or loop, called an Ig domain. There are three constant heavy domains (C_H1–3) and only one constant light (C_L), one variable heavy (V_H), and one variable light (V_L) domain. The ABS consists of a V_L and a V_H region. Within each variable domain, there are three hypervariable regions (about 10 amino acid residues per hypervariable region) that form a three-dimensional surface that is "complementary" to the shape of the antigen surface; they are called complementarity-determining regions (CDRs). A total of six CDRs come together to form the ABS. There are two ABS for each IgG mAb; hence each IgG mAb is considered bivalent.

Affinity refers to the strength of the bond between the ABS and the antigen. The strength of this bond is represented by the dissociation constant (K_d). Avidity refers to the overall strength of the ABS–antigen interaction, depending upon both the affinity and the valency of the interaction. It should be noted that a high affinity interaction can improve specific delivery

of the TRIT agent and reduce overall dosing requirements. Increasing the affinity indefinitely, however, may decrease tumor penetration. It has been demonstrated that an affinity of 10^{-7} to 10^{-8} M is needed for tumor retention, but affinities in the range of $\geq 10^{-10}$ to 10^{-11} M will result in retention in normal tissue and asymmetric binding in tumor tissue, termed the "▶ binding site barrier" (DiCara and Nissim 2011). The binding site barrier may be at least partially overcome by increasing the antibody mass, the overall delivered quantity of antibody.

Unconjugated antibodies, those not attached to a radionuclide or cytotoxic agent, will also mediate biologic activities. These activities (Fig. 4) may be mediated by the Fc region of the mAb or may be Fc-independent. Fc-mediated interactions are termed effector functions and consist of ▶ antibody-dependent cell-mediated cytotoxicity (ADCC) and complement-dependent cytotoxicity (CDC) (DiCara and Nissim 2011; Abbas et al. 2007). Concerning ADCC, interaction of the Fc region of the antibody with Fc receptors (located on immune effector cells) results in the subsequent phagocytosis or lysis of the antibody-bound cancer cell. CDC is initiated by the interaction of soluble blood proteins and the Fc region. Epitope-dependent (Fc-independent) functions of the mAb may result in the inhibition of ligand binding, inhibition of ligand-induced dimerization, and inhibition of receptor shedding. These epitope-dependent functions are characteristic of modern day biologics that target growth factor receptors, such as ▶ cetuximab and trastuzumab.

The original technology that was used to produce mAbs was first published by Kohler and Milstein in 1975 (Kohler and Milstein 1975) and was called the ▶ hybridoma technique. The technique has propagated the use of murine mAbs for research and for therapy in the clinic. In fact, the two FDA TRIT agents used to treat NHL (ibritumomab tiuxetan and tositumomab) are murine mAbs. Although these agents are delivered as single instillations in patients with decreased immune recognition capabilities, there is a concern that human antiglobulin antibodies (HAGA) will develop. If this phenomenon occurs in response to murine antibodies, then the resulting HAGA will be called human antimouse antibodies (HAMA). The formation of HAMA will expedite blood clearance of the antibody and decrease targeting capabilities as well as potentially cause various adverse symptoms. Two main strategies, through the use of genetic engineering, have emerged (Burvenich and Scott 2011) that reduce the immunogenicity of mAbs: (1) the production of antibody chimeras derived from both murine and human DNA and (2) the production of humanized or fully human antibodies (Fig. 3b). Chimeric antibodies retain murine V_H and V_L domains, while humanized antibodies retain murine CDRs. Fully human antibodies retain no murine components. While the development of HAGA may not be important after a single dose of mAb in lymphoma patients, its development has a greater negative impact for patients with solid tumors (Table 2) when treated with TRIT. As can be seen in Table 2,

as the targeting construct moves from a murine to humanized forms, the immunogenicity is lessened. This concept is important in order to employ multiple doses or fractions of TRIT. Figure 3c illustrates the concept of adding a nuclear localizing signal in order to bring the mAb from the cell surface or cytoplasm into the cell nucleus.

Another factor that is critical and influences antibody targeting and pharmacokinetics is antibody molecular size (Fig. 3d). As previously stated, TRIT has been less successful for treating solid tumors than hematologic malignancies. This is largely due to the lack of radiosensitivity of epithelial tumors (compared to hematologic malignancies) and the poor penetration of mAbs into large tumors. The decreased penetration of 150 kDa antibodies into large tumors is a direct result of elevated tumor interstitial fluid pressure, an aberrant tumor vasculature and an abnormal tumor extracellular matrix. Additionally, 150 kDa antibodies need longer periods of time to accrete into tumors and have long serum half-lives. When radiolabeled, a long serum half-life of the targeting construct will increase exposure of the bone marrow to radiation which causes hematologic toxicity (bone marrow toxicity in cancer treatment) and limits the amount of antibody and radionuclide that can be given. In order to overcome some of these issues, methods have been used to generate antibody fragments of varying size and valency. These smaller fragments exhibit superior tumor penetration and clear more rapidly from the circulation. However, if clearance from the circulation is too rapid, this can further limit tumor penetration. Table 3 summarizes these basic concepts for targeting constructs of various molecular weights.

Although mAbs and their fragments represent the most commonly used targeting constructs for the delivery of a radionuclide to malignant tissue, other agents are either in use or are being investigated, consisting of

Targeted Radioimmunotherapy. Table 2 Antibody immunogenicity following a single administration (Select solid tumor RIT trials)

Study (First author and date)	Antibody	Type	No. of patients	Percent anti-antibody response
Breitz (1992)	[186]Re-NR-LU-10	Murine	15	100
Meredith (1994)	^{131}I-CC49	Murine	15	100
Welt et al. (1994)	^{131}I-mAb A33	Murine	23	100
Mulligan (1995)	^{177}Lu-CC49	Murine	9	100
Yu (1996)	^{131}I-COL-1	Murine	18	83 prevented add'n RIT in 2
Behr (1997)	^{131}I-NP-4	Murine	32	94
Juweid (1997)	^{131}I-MN-14	Murine	14	100
Meredith (1992)	^{131}I-cB72.3	Chimeric	12	58
Weiden (1993)	[186]Re-NR-LU-13	Chimeric	8	75
Meredith (1995)	[125]I-17-1A	Chimeric	15	13
Wong (2000)	^{90}Y-cT84.66	Chimeric	21	52 prevented add'n RIT in 8
Kramer (1998)	^{111}In-huBrE3	Humanized	7	14
Hajjar (2002)	^{131}I-hMN-14	Humanized	15	47
Goldsmith (2002)	^{90}Y-huJ591	Humanized	19	0
Borjesson et al. (2003)	[186]Re-BIWA 4	Humanized	20	10

Targeted Radioimmunotherapy. Table 3 Targeting and pharmacokinetics of intact IgG and various antibody fragments

	IgG	F(ab')2	CH2- deletion	Minibody	Fab	Diabody	scFv
MW	150	100	120	80	50	40–50	20–25
Serum t1/2	2–3 days[a]	1 day	Hours	Hours	Hours	Hours	Hour
Metabolism	Liver	Liver	Liver	Liver	Kidney	Kidney	Kidney
Tumor uptake	****	***	*** to **	*** to **	**	**	*
Time to accretion	Days	Day	Hours	Hours	Hours	Hours	Hour

[a]Serum half-life for fully human IgG is approximately 23 days: murine IgG serum half-life is 2–3 days
MW molecular weight (kDa), $t_{1/2}$ (half-life), tumor uptake (**** = large, * = small)

peptides, affibody molecules, and aptamers. Nanostructures are also being investigated as carriers of radionuclides. In their unmodified form, the targeting capabilities of nanostructures are rather nonspecific, targeting largely due to enhanced permeability of the tumor vasculature and resulting retention. They will not be further discussed.

Peptides are small amino acid sequences (typically 7–14 amino acids) that serve as opioides, hormones, sweeteners, protein substrate inhibitors, releasing factors, antibiotics, and cytoprotectors (Tesauro et al. 2011; Pedone et al. 2006). The overexpression of receptors, specific for various peptides, has lead to the development of peptide-based radiopharmaceuticals. Table 4 lists the various peptides, targets, and receptors that show promise for TRIT. Somatostatin is one of the most common peptides and is overexpressed in a multitude of malignancies including breast cancer, small-cell lung cancer, medullary thyroid cancer, and neuroendocrine tumors (NETs). Somatostatin is rapidly degraded but its derivative, octreotide, is very stable (Fig. 5). Octreoscan (^{111}In-DTPA[diethylenediaminepentaacetic acid]) has been shown to be highly diagnostic for NETs. Affibody molecules (Stahl et al. 2011; Milenic 2010) are classified as affinity ligands or scaffold proteins that are approximately 7–9 kDa. These proteins are based upon a 58 amino acid residue derived from staphylococcus protein A, which binds immunoglobulin. A wide variety of applications have been applied to affibody use, including radiolabeled targeting for therapy (Table 5). Aptamers are small (8–12 kDa; 10–100 bases) single- or double-stranded oligonucleotides that are selected in vitro from a random library termed SELEX (systemic evolution of ligands by exponential enrichment). Aptamers are an attractive alternative to larger mAbs because they are easy to produce, have a low cost of production, exhibit high affinities, have a small size, are rapidly cleared from the circulation, have an unlimited shelf life, and are of low immunogenicity. Their major detriment is a short serum half-life (measured in minutes to hours) in their unmodified form. Aptamers are

Targeted Radioimmunotherapy. Table 4 Peptides, cancer target, and receptor candidates for peptide radiation therapy in the future

Peptide	Cancer target	Receptor
Somatostatin analogs	Neuroendocrine, small cell lung, breast, monocytes, and lymphocytes	Somatostatin 1–5
VIP	Non-small cell lung, breast, colon, pancreatic, prostate, bladder, and ovarian cancer	VIP 1 and 2
Glucagon-like peptide 1	Insulinomas	Glucagon-like peptide 1 receptors
RGD analogs	Tumor-induced angiogenesis	$\alpha_v\beta_3$ integrin
Neurotensin	Exocrine pancreatic cancer, meningioma, Ewing sarcomas, prostate and pancreatic cancer	Neurotensin (NT) 1–3
Substance P	Glial tumors, astrocytomas, medullary thyroid, and breast cancer	NK1, NK2 and NK3
CCK/gastrin derivates	GI tumors, pancreatic adenoma, medullary thyroid cancer	CCK 1 CCK 2
Neuropeptide Y	Breast, ovarian, and adrenal tumors	NPY receptors
Bombesin (7–14) Bombesin antagonist Gastrin-releasing peptide	Prostate, breast, gastric, ovarian, colon, and pancreatic cancer	GRP-bombesin

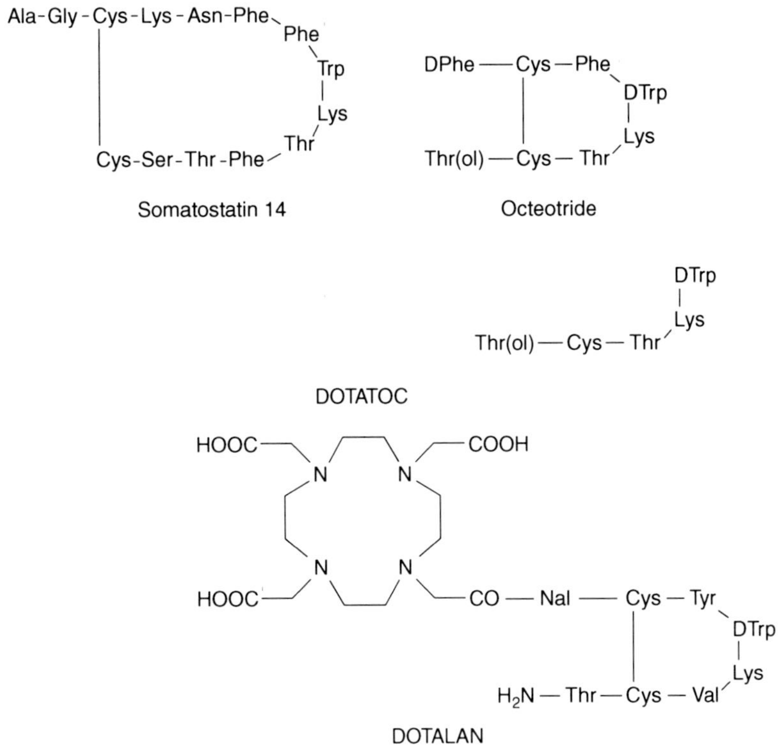

Targeted Radioimmunotherapy. Fig. 5 Somatostatin and octreotide sequences

amazingly versatile and can recognize nearly any type of target, from metal ions to whole cells and even entire organisms. A complete database (updated monthly) of known Aptamers can be found at http://aptamer.icmb.utexas.edu. The current lack of radiolabeled aptamers is simply a portrayal of a very promising technology in its infancy.

The Science of Targeted Radioimmunotherapy

TRIT delivers radiation to the target tissue in a continuous, declining, low dose-rate (LDR) fashion. Typical dose rates for TRIT are in the range of 10–20 cGy/h. The total dose delivered by TRIT is low, in the range of 1,500–2,000 cGy (Fowler 1990), with an ▶ effective half-life of 24–72 h. This can be compared to the high dose-rate

(HDR) delivery of radiation by external beam radiation therapy (EBRT). EBRT typically will deliver radiation at a dose rate of 100–500 cGy/min. It should be noted that these total dose ranges for TRIT occur in spite of overall very low percent injected doses (0.1–10.0%) that ultimately localize in target tissue (Murry and McEwan 2007); however, radiation-induced ▶ apoptosis is still induced.

The most radiosensitive component of a cell is the deoxyribonucleic acid (DNA) (Speer and Khuntia 2011). Irradiation of tissue results in DNA damage. This damage may be either repaired or results in permanent damage. Permanent damage will cause cell death. By using a target-hit model, the tissue response end point of cell death may be used to relate absorbed dose of ionizing radiation to cell death. When the log

Targeted Radioimmunotherapy. Table 5 Applications of affibody molecules

Application	Target protein	Comment
Biotechnology		
ELISA	IgA, apolipoprotein A-1	Two-site affibody/antibody ELISA to avoid false-positive signals
Protein microarray	Taq DNA polymerase, IgA, IgE, IgG, insulin, TNF-α	Capture ligands on protein microarrays
Affinity purification	Taq DNA polymerase, apolipoprotein A-1, RSV G-protein, factor VIII	Ligands in affinity chromatography for capture of recombinant proteins from cell lysates
Depletion	IgA, transferrin, Alzheimer Aβ peptide	Protein recovery by affinity chromatography from human plasma or serum
Ion exchange	Ion exchange chromatography media	Novel purification tag for general use as fusion partner to different target proteins
Biological research		
Structure determination	Alzheimer amyloid beta peptide	Stabilizing complex formation for structure determination
Inhibition of receptor interaction	CD28 TNF	Interference of CD28 and CD80 receptor interaction Blocking ligand binding to its receptor in vitro
Intracellular capture	HER2, EGFR	Reduction of cell surface level of HER2 and EGFR receptors and reduction of cell growth
Gene therapy (vector engineering)	HER2, HIV-1 gp120 HER2	Engineering of adenovirus tropism Engineering of nonviral delivery systems
Medicine		
Molecular imaging	HER2, EGFR	Radiolabeled targeting agent for cancer diagnosis Fluorescent targeting agent for superficial tumors
Radiotherapy	HER2	Radiolabeled targeting agent for cancer therapy

surviving fraction of irradiated cells is plotted on the ordinate and the dose (gray; Gy) is plotted on the abscissa, a cell survival curve is generated (Fig. 6). The "hit" that results in most lethal events is a double-strand break (DSB) of DNA. The mathematical term, α, represents the initial slope of the cell survival curve. It is a constant for a given tumor (or tissue) and can be thought of as the probability, per unit of absorbed dose, of creating a lethal DSB (Speer et al. 2011). The target is the resulting DSB and the cell

survival versus absorbed dose is a pure exponential function:

$$S = e^{-\alpha D} \tag{1}$$

where S is the surviving cell fraction and D is the mean absorbed dose. Ionizing irradiation may also cause nonlethal single-strand breaks (SSB). If these events accumulate, they may become lethal. The constant, β, is used to describe this phenomenon and it represents the more distant, "linear" portion of the cell survival curve. The

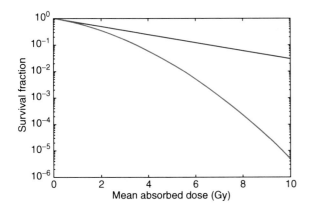

Targeted Radioimmunotherapy. Fig. 6 Cell survival curves following treatment with radiotherapy. The *blue* curve represents low dose-rate radiotherapy; the *green* curve represents high dose-rate radiotherapy

linear-quadratic (LQ) model combines the two processes into a continuously bending curve:

$$S = e^{-\alpha D - \beta D^2} \tag{2}$$

The shoulder on the cell survival curve is typically observed when high dose rates of radiation are employed (*green line*, Fig. 6). In TRIT, the dose rate is 1,000-fold lower and therefore the quadratic portion to the curve will have a much lower impact on survival as many SSBs, considered sublethal damage, will be repaired during the more lengthy delivery of low dose-rate radiation. This will result in a "small" or "no" observable shoulder. Therefore, when estimating cell survival for TRIT, α alone will define the radiosensitivity of the tumor (*blue line*, Fig. 6). Thus, considering dose rate, TRIT is approximately 20% less effective than the HDR external beam radiotherapy. TRIT, however, does appear to be relatively effective. This phenomenon can be attributed to many radiobiological processes that appear to cause greater than predicted rates of apoptosis. These processes include low dose/dose-rate apoptosis, low dose hyper-radiosensitivity-increased radioresistance, inverse dose-rate effect

(G$_2$ synchronization), radiation-induced biological bystander effect, and the crossfire effect (Murry and McEwan 2007).

Various radionuclides have been used for TRIT (Table 6) and their physical properties have been extensively reviewed in the nuclear medicine literature. They can be grouped into three basic categories depending upon the type of emitted particulate radiation. Radionuclides that emit high-energy electrons are called β-emitters. These electrons have maximum path lengths in tissue from 1.5 to 12.0 mm. This translates into a range of approximately 130–1,100 cell diameters. The most commonly used β-emitters for TRIT are ^{90}Y and [131]I. The maximum range of electrons in tissue for ^{90}Y and ^{131}I is 12 and 2 mm, respectively. It should be noted, however, that 90% of the electron energy is deposited over 5.2 mm for ^{90}Y and 0.7 mm for [131]I. This range of 90% energy deposition is termed the R_{90}. The most commonly used α-emitter for TRIT is [211]At. An α-particle is a helium nucleus and it has a maximum range in tissue of 55–100 μm (5–10 cell diameters). Although it has a short range, the α-particle is very destructive and has a high LET. Low-energy electron emitters also emit radiation that is high LET and have path lengths between 2 and 500 nm (width of a double-strand helix). Auger emitters, such as ^{111}In are most effective if delivered to the nucleus of a cell.

Because radionuclides have different energy spectra for their emitted particulate radiation, they will each interact with tissue and deposit their energy over varying distances. There is, therefore, a relation between type of radionuclide, tumor size, absorbed dose, and ultimately tumor cure probability (TCP). If it is assumed that a tumor has a spherical volume and contains a uniform and identical activity concentration of a radionuclide, then the TCP can be calculated for different radionuclides and tumor size (Bernhardt and Speer 2011; O'Donoghue 2000). Figure 7 illustrates the relation between tumor

Targeted Radioimmunotherapy. Table 6 Commonly used radionuclides for TRT

Radionuclide	Physical half-life	E max (MeV)	Maximum range in tissue	LET (keV/μm)	Approximate cell diameters
Beta emitters		**Beta-particle**		**0.2**	
^{90}Y	2.7 days	2.30	12.0 mm		400–1,100
^{131}I	8.0 days	0.81	2.0 mm		10–230
^{177}Lu	6.7 days	0.50	1.5 mm		4–180
^{186}Re	3.8 days	1.10	3.6 mm		15–360
^{188}Re	17.0 h	2.10	11.0 mm		200–1,000
^{67}Cu	2.6 days	0.60	2.8 mm		5–210
Alpha emitters		**Alpha particle**		**80**	
^{213}Bi	45.7 min	5.87	70–100 μm		7–10
^{211}At	7.2 h	5.87	55–60 μm		5–6
Low-energy electron emitters		**Low-energy electron**		**4–26**	
^{125}I	60.1 days	0.35	2–500 nm		<1
^{67}Ga	3.3 days	0.18	2–500 nm		<1
^{111}In	2.83 days	0.04–0.2	2–500 nm		<1

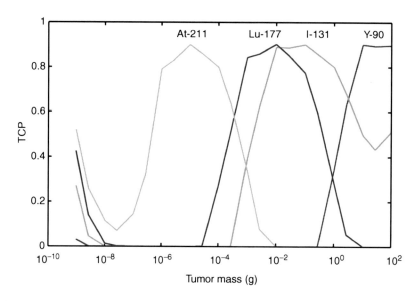

Targeted Radioimmunotherapy. Fig. 7 TCP for various radionuclides. TCP=0.9 versus tumor mass. The optimal TCP for various tumor masses when treated with ^{211}At, ^{177}Lu, ^{131}I, and ^{90}Y. This corresponds to approximately 10^{-5}, 10^{-2}, 0.1, and 10 g, respectively

mass and TCP for ^{211}At, ^{177}Lu, ^{131}I, and ^{90}Y. As can be seen, there is an optimum tumor size for the different energy spectra for each radionuclide such that the TCP is maximized. If the tumor is small relative to the emission range, then much of the energy will be lost to the surrounding tissue and the absorbed dose will be low. As the tumor size increases, more energy is absorbed until the maximum TCP is reached. As the tumor further increases in size, the absorbed energy remains high, but fewer cells are affected by the radiation and TCP begins to decrease.

Labeling the targeting construct with the appropriate radionuclide (radiochemistry) is exceedingly important and equally complex. Radionuclides are attached to targeting constructs by either using a "linker" molecule, termed a bifunctional chelating agent (BCA) or by a chemical reaction that forms a covalent bond between the radionuclide and the targeting construct. Three basic scientific fields converged to make radiochemistry a reality: coordination chemistry, directed biologic targeting, and the medical application of radiopharmaceuticals (Wilson and Brechbiel 2011). In general, metallic radionuclides will require a BCA for labeling and radiohalogens will require a chemical reaction. The most prevalent therapeutic radionuclides used in TRIT are yttrium-90 (^{90}Y; metallic radionuclide) and iodine-131 (^{131}I; radiohalogen). One of the most commonly used BCA is a polyaminopolycarboxylate straight chain ligand called diethylenetriamine pentaacetic acid (DTPA). A modified DTPA molecule, called tiuxetan, is used as a linker molecule to chelate ^{90}Y to ibritumomab (^{90}Y ibritumomab tiuxetan; Zevalin; Spectrum Pharmaceuticals, Inc., Irvine, CA). Tiuxetan forms a urea-type bond (Witzig 2010) to the antibody (ibritumomab) and its five carboxyl groups interact with and chelate ^{90}Y to form a stable coordination sphere. The halogenation reaction that bonds ^{131}I to the targeting construct (^{131}I tositumomab; Bexxar;

Glaxo-Smith Kline, Philadelphia, PA) is called iodination. Although there are many permutations of the iodination reaction, it basically inserts ^{131}I into a tyrosine group on the mAb without the need for a chelation molecule. Regardless of the required labeling technique, it is incumbent that a reasonably high labeling yield, unaltered biodistribution, stability of the radionuclide, and ▶ immunoreactivity are preserved.

To date, a single instillation, or fraction of the TRIT agent is delivered systemically (i.e., Zevalin and Bexxar). It is well known that although relatively effective for hematologic malignancies, TRIT is much less effective for treating solid tumors. Therefore, a number of strategies are being developed that will potentially increase the effectiveness of TRIT. These strategies include modulating the tumor microenvironment, using pretargeting techniques, extracorporeal delivery, combined modality therapy (CMT), fractionation, multiple radionuclides (radionuclide cocktail), increasing antibody mass (the amount of antibody delivered systemically), alteration of the physical properties (size and affinity) of the targeting construct, and employing different types of LET radiation (i.e., beta emitter versus alpha emitter). All in all, these strategies are designed to, either alone or in combination, deliver more radiation to the tumor, make the radiation more cytotoxic, or decrease the exposure of radiation to bone marrow. As a result, the tumor to blood ratio will increase and ultimately the therapeutic ratio will increase. The pretargeting strategy warrants further discussion.

Because radiolabeled mAbs take 2–3 days to localize or accrete into tumors, antibody-based TRIT results in a prolonged exposure of the bone marrow to radiation, causing hematologic toxicity and rendering the bone marrow the dose limiting normal tissue structure. Accordingly, the tumor/blood ratios of mAb will only slightly favor the tumor. This situation can seriously limit the successful prospects of antibody-based TRIT,

T

especially for treating solid tumors. Truly, smaller targeting constructs (antibody fragments) can be used for TRIT and they will exhibit pharmacokinetics that result in a more rapid blood clearance, allowing for the administration of higher activities. Unfortunately, due to the lower overall tumor accretion and retention of antibody fragments, the advantage of a more rapid blood clearance is usually offset. Therefore, the ideal targeting construct would manifest the properties of an intact monoclonal antibody, but exhibit the blood clearance pattern of a small molecular weight construct. Because no such known construct exists, pretargeting strategies have been developed. The basic premise of pretargeting is to separate the delivery of a large, macromolecule-targeting construct (prolonged circulation time) from the delivery of a much smaller cytotoxic radioconjugate (more rapid circulation time). Two main approaches have been employed: a bispecific mAb (bsmAb) system and a streptavidin-biotin system. In the bsmAb system (Fig. 8) a portion of the antibody has affinity for the tumor (anti-tumor) and another portion has affinity for the radionuclide carrier ligand or hapten-peptide (anti-hapten). Initially (step 1), a large "saturation" dose of the unlabeled bsmAb is administered and the antibody localizes in the tumor over several days. Occasionally a clearing step is used to facilitate the clearance of the bsmAb from the circulation. Subsequently (step 2), a radionuclide conjugated to a hapten-peptide is administered that has high affinity for the anti-hapten portion of the bsmAb. This step results in a rapid distribution of the radionuclide in the tumor due to the high affinity of the hapten-peptide for the bsmAb. Because the hapten-peptide has a small molecular weight, it will clear rapidly from the body and result in a low bone marrow exposure to radiation (Sharkey and Goldenberg 2011). In the streptavidin-biotin system, streptavidin is conjugated to the initial pretargeting macromolecule while biotin is conjugated to the radionuclide. Streptavidin and biotin have a very high affinity for each other (10^{15} M^{-1}). When either system is used, the tumor/blood ratios of the targeting agent are significantly increased.

FDA-Approved Therapeutic Agents

There appears to be very successful and emerging TRIT data for hematologic malignancies, but solid tumor TRIT has been less sanguine. Although there are promising phase I/II trials for solid tumor TRIT, phase III trials are lacking. For the sake of clarity and brevity, this section will only focus upon clinically relevant US FDA (or its international equivalent)–approved TRIT therapeutics.

Currently, there are two US FDA-approved TRIT agents in the United States, ^{90}Y ibritumomab tiuxetan (Zevalin 2002) and ^{131}I tositumomab (Bexxar 2003). Zevalin has FDA approval for relapsed or refractory follicular NHL and as a frontline adjuvant agent for follicular NHL achieving a complete or partial response to induction chemotherapy. Bexxar has FDA approval for the relapse or refractory setting as well as transformed NHL. Both are murine IgG mAbs that target the ▶ CD20 surface antigen on follicular NHL. A detailed comparison of both agents is shown in Table 7 (Burdick and Macklis 2011). ^{90}Y ibritumomab tiuxetan utilizes yttrium-90, a pure beta-particle emitter with a physical half-life of 2.7 days. The beta-particle has a maximum energy of 2.3 MeV and a maximum tissue penetration of approximately 12.0 mm (R_{90} = 5.2 mm). Tiuxetan is the DTPA-type chelate that attaches ^{90}Y to the mAb, ibritumomab (Fig. 9). Because there is no gamma emission in the spectrum of this isotope, it is not visualized by gamma camera scans. As a result, a biodistribution assessment cannot be performed. Therefore, a surrogate imaging radionuclide that emits gamma irradiation, indium-111 (^{111}In) is required. In contrast, ^{131}I tositumomab is a mixed

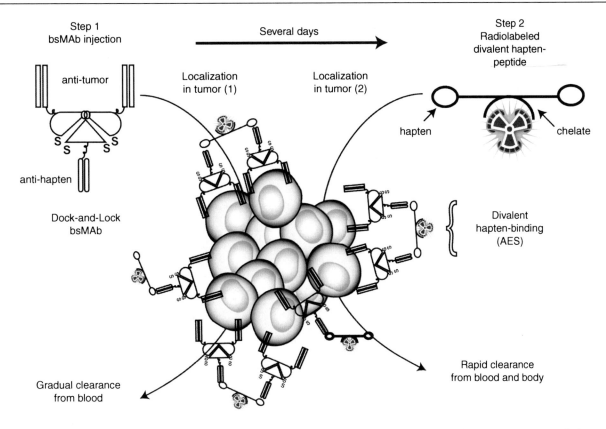

Step 1
bsMAb injection

Several days

Step 2
Radiolabeled
divalent hapten-
peptide

anti-tumor

Localization
in tumor (1)

Localization
in tumor (2)

hapten   chelate

anti-hapten

Dock-and-Lock
bsMAb

Divalent
hapten-binding
(AES)

Gradual clearance
from blood

Rapid clearance
from blood and body

Targeted Radioimmunotherapy. Fig. 8 Bispecific pretargeting procedure. The bsMAb is injected and then over several days it will localize in the tumor and clear from the blood. The bsMAb shown in this example is based on the Dock-and-Lock method for preparing recombinant bsMAb that has two binding arms for the tumor and one for the hapten. Once the molar concentration of the bsMAb is low enough, the radiolabeled hapten-peptide is given. The hapten-peptide has two haptens for more stable binding within the tumor, perhaps by cross-linking two adjacent bsMAb through a process known as the affinity-enhancement system (AES). The peptide portion usually contains 4–5 day-amino acids with a single chelator bound to one of the amino acids that is used to capture the radionuclide

beta/gamma emitter. The gamma spikes at 364 keV and the beta emission has a maximum energy of 0.6 MeV (Fig. 10). The maximum range in tissue of the beta-particle is 2.3 mm (R_{90} = 0.7 mm). This agent can be imaged on gamma camera in order to calculate total body clearance. Although theoretical arguments can be rendered as to why one or the other therapeutic agents may have an advantage based upon physical characteristics of the emission spectra, there is no convincing evidence that either Zevalin or Bexxar provides a clinical benefit for treating follicular NHL, over each other. In short, they are both mutually supportive.

For both agents, the treatment is delivered over 1–2 weeks. On day 1, both protocols deliver an infusion of nonradioactive (cold) anti-CD20 antibody (Zevalin employs rituximab; Bexxar employs tositumomab) designed to saturate CD20 antigen sink (depletion of peripheral B-cells and the binding of nonspecific sites in the liver and spleen) and improve biodistribution

Targeted Radioimmunotherapy. Table 7 Comparison of the two US FDA-approved TRIT compounds

	^{90}Y ibritumomab tiuxetan (Zevalin®)	^{131}I tositumomab (Bexxar®)
Antibody used for RIT	Ibritumomab–murine IgG1-κ	Tositumomab–murine IgG2a-λ
Specificity	CD20	CD20
Linker molecule	Tiuxetan	None (directly halogenated)
"Cold" antibody	Chimeric rituximab 250 mg/m^2	Murine tositumomab 450 mg
Pretreatment imaging agent and dose	^{111}In ibritumomab tiuxetan – 5 mCi	^{131}I tositumomab – 5 mCi
Primary intent of imaging dose	Biodistribution safety assessment	Calculation of dose based on individual clearance patterns
Number of pretreatment scans	One[a]	Three
Therapeutic isotope	Yttrium-90	Iodine-131
Major emission spectra	2.3 MeV β	0.6 MeV β and 0.36 MeV γ
Dosing parameters Platelets $\geq$ 150,000/μL Platelets 100,000–149,000/μL	0.4 mCi/kg 0.3 mCi/kg Maximum 32 mCi	75 cGy whole body dose 65 cGy whole body dose
Typical overall response rate (ORR)	60–80%	60–80%
Typical complete response rate (CR)	20–40%	20–40%

[a]Additional scans are optional

and tumor targeting. Figure 11 illustrates the benefit of "cold dosing" prior to delivering the actual therapeutic dose. For both of these radioimmunoconjugates, the treatment cycle is similar (Figs. 12 and 13). The dose for Zevalin is based on weight (0.4 mCi/kg for platelet count $\geq$ 150,000; 0.3 mCi/kg for platelet count of 100,000–149,000; maximum of 32 mCi). A single gamma scan (^{111}In ibritumomab tiuxetan) is used to confirm a normal biodistribution on day 3–4. A review of the Zevalin imaging registry reveals that only 0.6% of scans exhibited an altered biodistribution. The dose for Bexxar is based upon a calculated total body clearance (three scans over 1 week) that delivers a total body (red bone marrow) dose of 75 cGy. This calculation is reduced to a total body dose of 65 cGy for a platelet count <150,000. Eligible patients for

both Zevalin and Bexxar are also required to have an absolute neutrophil count of $\geq$1,500 and a bone marrow biopsy that reveals <25% involvement with lymphoma.

Hematologic Agents

Relapse Setting

Table 8 summarizes the most significant prospective phase II/III clinical trials providing evidence for the use of TRIT for treating relapsed or refractory follicular NHL. Together they represent greater than 200 patients treated with either Zevalin or Bexxar. Both agents appear to suggest an overall response rate (ORR) of 60–80% and a complete response rate of 20–50%. Each agent seems to have comparative response rates.

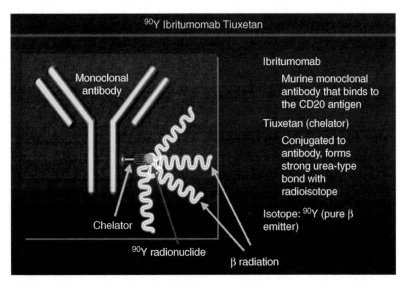

Targeted Radioimmunotherapy. Fig. 9 Summary of 90Y ibritumomab tiuxetan properties

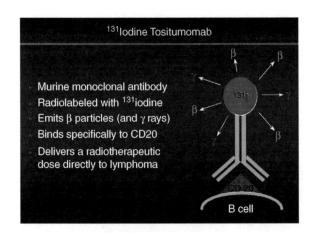

Targeted Radioimmunotherapy. Fig. 10
Summary of ^{131}I tositumomab properties

A phase III study comparing Zevalin versus rituximab for patients with relapsed or refractory low-grade follicular B-cell NHL or transformed NHL was performed (Witzig et al. 2002a). Patients were randomized to either Zevalin, 0.4 mCi/kg ($n = 73$) or rituximab, 375 mg/m^2 IV weekly for four doses ($n = 70$). The TRIT group was pretreated with two rituximab doses (250 mg/m^2) to improve biodistribution and tumor targeting. After the first rituximab dose on day 1, ^{111}In ibritumomab tiuxetan was administered in order to assess biodistribution and to aide in dosimetry. No patients received the therapeutic dose of ^{90}Y ibritumomab tiuxetan (Zevalin) if more than 20 Gy or 3 Gy was calculated to any nontumor organ or the red marrow, respectively. Zevalin was administered after the second rituximab dose, approximately 1 week (day 7–9) after the first dose of rituximab and ^{111}In ibritumomab tiuxetan. The dose of Zevalin was capped at 32 mCi. Patients in both arms of the study received two prior chemotherapy regimens. The ORR was 80% for Zevalin and 56% for rituximab ($p = 0.002$). The CR rates were 30% and 16% ($p = 0.04$), respectively, in the Zevalin and rituximab group. Durable responses of ≥6 months were 64% versus 47% ($p = 0.030$) for Zevalin versus rituximab. The conclusion of the study was that TRIT with Zevalin was well tolerated and resulted in statistically significant

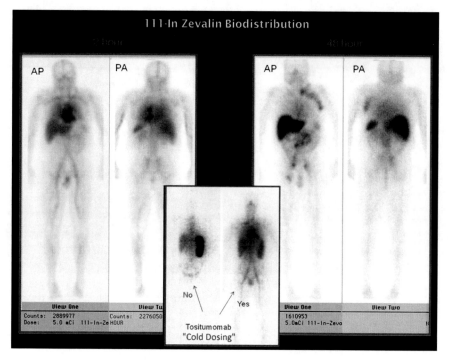

Targeted Radioimmunotherapy. Fig. 11 Biodistribution and cold dosing of TRIT. The normal 2 and 48 h biodistribution of ^{111}In ibritumomab (Zevalin). Note the lymph node targeting at 48 h. Cold antibody dosing (cold dosing), prior to imaging and therapy, will improve the biodistribution as shown in the inset (tositumomab is used prior to Bexxar; Rituxan prior to Zevalin)

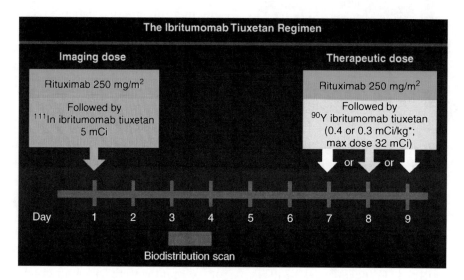

Targeted Radioimmunotherapy. Fig. 12 Treatment protocol for Zevalin. Schema for ^{90}Y ibritumomab tiuxetan treatment protocol (*0.4 mCi/kg in patients with a platelet count $\geq$ 150,000 or 0.3 mCi/kg with a platelet count of 100,000–149,000. Maximum administered activity is 32 mCi)

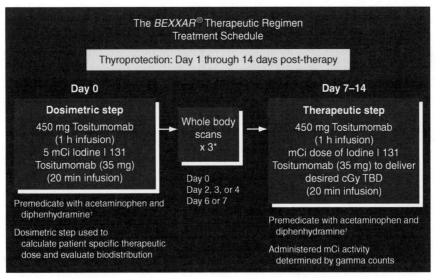

The *BEXXAR*® Therapeutic Regimen
Treatment Schedule

Thyroprotection: Day 1 through 14 days post-therapy

Day 0

Dosimetric step
450 mg Tositumomab
(1 h infusion)
5 mCi Iodine I 131
Tositumomab (35 mg)
(20 min infusion)

Premedicate with acetaminophen and
diphenhydramine†

Dosimetric step used to
calculate patient specific therapeutic
dose and evaluate biodistribution

Whole body
scans
x 3*

Day 0
Day 2, 3, or 4
Day 6 or 7

Day 7–14

Therapeutic step
450 mg Tositumomab
(1 h infusion)
mCi dose of Iodine I 131
Tositumomab (35 mg) to deliver
desired cGy TBD
(20 min infusion)

Premedicate with acetaminophen and
diphenhydramine†

Administered mCi activity
determined by gamma counts

Targeted Radioimmunotherapy. Fig. 13 Treatment protocol for Bexxar. Schema for ^{131}I tositumomab treatment protocol (*scans used to calculate bone marrow dose)

and clinically significant higher ORRs and CRs than rituxan alone.

In a pivotal, nonrandomized, phase III multicenter trial, patients with relapsed, refractory, or transformed follicular B-cell NHL were treated with Bexxar ($n = 60$) and the outcome was compared to patients' last qualifying chemotherapy (LQC) regimen ($n = 28$) (Kaminski et al. 2001). Eligible patients were required to have been treated with at least 2 prior protocol-specific chemotherapy regimens (median of 4 regimens in the study) and to either have not responded or progressed within 6 months of therapy. A partial response or CR was observed in 39 patients (65%) after Bexxar compared to 17 patients (28%) after LQC ($p < 0.001$). The median duration of response was 6.5 months for Bexxar and 3.5 months for the LQC group ($p < 0.001$). The CR rate was 20% for Bexxar and 3% for the LQC group ($p < 0.001$). The conclusion of the study was that a single dose of Bexxar was significantly more efficacious than the LQC received by heavily pretreated patients with relapse or refractory follicular B-cell NHL.

Frontline Therapy

Considering that there are concerns about TRIT for treating large bulky tumors (tumor penetration, overall required dose, nonuniform dose distributions due to antigen tissue heterogeneity), it appears that bringing TRIT into a frontline therapeutic setting after induction chemotherapy and maximum cytoreduction would be the next logical direction. A phase III trial (FIT [first-line indolent trial]) of consolidation with Zevalin compared to no additional therapy after first remission was reported for follicular B-cell NHL (Morschhauser et al. 2008). Patients with CD20+ stage III–IV follicular B-cell NHL who achieved a partial response (PR) or CR to induction chemotherapy were randomized to Zevalin ($n = 208$) or no further treatment, the control arm ($n = 206$). Prior to chemotherapy, patients had documented <25% bone marrow involvement. After induction chemotherapy, blood counts had to recover such that ANC was ≥1.5, platelets were ≥150,000, and hemoglobin was ≥9. Patients in the Zevalin arm were treated with an activity of 0.4 mCi/kg; a maximum activity of 32 mCi was

Targeted Radioimmunotherapy. Table 8 Summary of major published trials of TRIT for relapsed or refractory low-grade non-Hodgkin's lymphoma

RIT Author Date	Study design	OR (%)	CR (%)	PFS (TTP) [MDR] (months)
^{90}Y-IT Witzig et al. (1999)	Treatment failure to an anthracycline or two prior regimens or intermediate grade or mantle cell NHL in relapse	67	26	(12.9 in responders) [11.7]
^{90}Y-IT Witzig et al. (2002a)	No prior RTX. Phase III study comparing rituximab to ^{90}Y-IT	80	30	(11.2) [14.2]
^{90}Y-IT Witzig et al. (2002b)	Prior treatment with RTX and either no response to RTX or time to progression after RTX of <6 months	74	15	(6.8) [6.4]
^{90}Y-IT Wiseman et al. (2002)	RTX naïve. Platelet counts 100,000–150,000/mL	83	37	(9.4) [11.7]
^{90}Y-IT Tobinai et al. (2009)	Prior RTX eligible	83	68	9.6
^{131}I-Tos Kaminski et al. (2000)	Original report. Prior stem cell transplant allowed	71	34	12 for all responders
^{131}I-Tos Vose et al. (2000)	No prior RTX	57	32	5.3 [9.9]
^{131}I-Tos Kaminski et al. (2001)	At least two prior chemotherapy regimens with either no response or relapse within 6 months of completing their last regimen. No prior RTX	65	20	8.4 for all responders [6.5]
^{131}I-Tos Davies et al. (2004)	No prior RTX	76	49	0.8 years [1.3 years]
^{131}I-Tos Davis et al. (2004)	Trial comparing ^{131}I-Tos to unlabeled tositumomab	55	33	(6.3) [not reached]
^{131}I-Tos Horning et al. (2005)	At least one prior course of RTX	65	38	10.4 [24.5]

OR overall response, *CR* complete response, *PFS* progression-free survival, *TTP* median time to progression for all patients in study, *MDR* median duration of response in responders, ^{90}Y-IT ^{90}Y ibritumomab tiuxetan, ^{131}I-Tos ^{131}I tositumomab, *LG* low grade, *RTX* rituximab.

allowed. Although two doses of rituximab (250 mg/m^2) were used, a ^{111}In biodistribution scan was not required. The data was analyzed with a median follow-up of 3.5 years. Zevalin consolidation resulted in a median progression-free survival (PFS) advantage of 36.5 versus 13.3 months in the control arm (p <0.0001). The PFS benefit was maintained in the Zevalin arm regardless if patients achieved a PR (29.3 versus 6.2 months; p <0.0001) or CR (53.9 versus 29.5 months; p = 0.0154). The benefit of Zevalin consolidation was maintained across all Follicular Lymphoma International Prognostic Index (FLIPI) subgroups. In patients with a PR after induction chemotherapy, 77% were further converted to a CR when treated with Zevalin. This resulted in a final CR rate of

87% in the treatment arm and this result compares well with established data. In the treatment arm, 90% of patients that were bcl-2 positive converted to a negative status (90% molecular CR). Toxicity was well managed and was primarily hematologic. A total of 8% of patients experienced a grade 3–4 infection. There were no treatment-related deaths. The data from the FIT trial was recently updated at the 52nd ASH (American Society of Hematology) annual meeting in December, 2010 (http://ash.confex.com/ash/2010/webprogram/Paper28386.html). With a median follow-up of 66.2 months, the PFS advantage of Zevalin was maintained in patients undergoing a PR/CR. The overall survival was 93% and 89%, trending in favor of the Zevalin versus control arm ($p = 0.561$).

Approved Solid Tumor Therapeutics

In 2010, greater than 220,000 lung cancer cases will be diagnosed, resulting in 157,300 deaths (NCI Web page: http://www.cancer.gov/cancertopics/types/lung). Clearly new strategies are required to help improve local and systemic control. To date, most TRIT targeting constructs will bind to cell surface or extracellular matrix antigens, on or in surrounding viable malignant cells. Each antigenic target (disease site) requires a specific targeting construct (typically a mAb or antibody fragment). There is, however, emerging data to support the concept of targeting necrotic and hypoxic regions of tumors (Al-Ejeh and Brown 2011). The selective targeting of dead or dying cells will allow a cytoxic event of nearby malignant cells by the bystander and crossfire effect. Additionally, only one type of targeting construct need be manufactured to target many different types of malignancies. If the cell surface antigen does not internalize to any significant degree, then a typical targeting construct will remain on the cell surface. Because dead and dying cells (undergoing

apoptosis) exhibit disruption of their cell membrane, constructs that target intracellular products of apoptosis will then be able to gain access the cells' cytoplasm and nucleus. Although several "dead cancer cell antigens" are under investigation, tumor necrosis therapy (or treatment), designated TNT, has been investigated in human trials. TNT is an IgG_{2a} mAb that targets nuclear ▶ histones.

A pivotal trial (Chen et al. 2005) using iodine-131-chimeric tumor necrosis treatment (^{131}I-chTNT) in advanced lung cancer patients was performed. A total of 107 patients ($n = 97$, non-small cell; $n = 10$, small cell) were enrolled from 1999 to 2002. All patients had failed at least one prior therapeutic regimen (mean = 3; range = 1–5) and 86.9% of the patients had stage III–IV disease at study entry. In all cases the patients received two instillations of ^{131}I-chTNT administered over 2–4 weeks. Sixty-two patients received intravenous (IV) administrations and 45 patients received intratumoral injections of ^{131}I-chTNT. IV administrations were delivered at an activity 0.8 mCi/kg and intratumoral injections were delivered at an activity of 0.8 mCi/cm^3 of tumor size. In all patients ($n = 107$), the overall response rate (ORR) was 34.6% (3.7% CR; 30.8% PR; 55.1% no change or stable disease; 10.3% progressive disease). Of the 62 patients receiving a systemic administration of ^{131}I-chTNT, the ORR was 35.5% (3.2% CR; 32.2% PR). Of the 45 patients receiving intratumoral injection of ^{131}I-chTNT, the ORR was 33.3% (5% CR; 20.9% PR). In 58 evaluable patients, the median survival was 11.7 months and the 1-year survival rate was 41.4%. The average absorbed doses for tumor and normal lung were 8.45 Gy and 2.35 Gy for patients receiving systemic ^{131}I-chTNT and 30.0 Gy and 2.65 Gy for patients receiving intratumoral ^{131}I-chTNT. The major toxicity was hematologic and was reversible. As expected, the hematologic toxicity was lower in the intratumoral injection group. In 2003, ^{131}I-chTNT was approved by the

Chinese State Food and Drug Administration to treat refractory bronchogenic carcinoma. As a result, ^{131}I-chTNT became the first solid tumor TRIT agent in the world, approved for therapy. Recently, two studies using ^{131}I-chTNT-1/B have been completed for the treatment of CNS malignancies. The first trial was a phase I study that used ^{131}I-chTNT-1/B to treat progressive and recurrent glioblastoma multiforme (NCT00128635). The second trial was a phase II study that used ^{131}I-chTNT-1/B to treat patients with glioblastoma or anaplastic astrocytoma after conventional surgery.

Hepatocellular carcinoma (HCC), or liver carcinoma, represents a significant worldwide malignancy and has several potential etiologies: viral, metabolic (hemochromatosis, alcoholic cirrhosis), toxins (aflatoxin), hormonal, or chemical (oil industry). In addition to resection, orthotopic liver transplantation (OLT) represents the only other potential curative option. In 1989, RTOG reported a phase III study comparing EBRT+chemotherapy to the same treatment plus ^{131}I antiferritin antibody. None of the patients receiving EBRT and chemotherapy, only, were converted to a resectable state. In a separate analysis, 11 patients crossing over from the EBRT plus chemotherapy arm to further therapy with ^{131}I antiferritin antibody were converted to resection. There was, however, no significant difference in the initial "intent to treat" treatment arms based upon response rate and survival (Order 2011)

Licartin is an antibody fragment, F(ab')$_2$ that targets HAb18G/CD147, a HCC tumor-associated antigen. More recently, the safety and pharmacokinetics of Licartin (^{131}I metuximab) were investigated in phase I/II trials. The initial phase I trial evaluated 28 patients with HCC. They were treated with 0.25–1.0 mCi/kg of Licartin, via hepatic artery infusion. In a subsequent phase II trial, 106 patients with

HCC received 0.75 mCi/kg of Licartin on day 1 of a 28-day cycle. Life-threatening toxicities did not occur. In 73 patients (completing two cycles), 6 (8.22%) exhibited a partial response, 14 (19.18%) had a minor response, and 43 (58.9%) maintained stable disease. The cohort had a 21-month survival of 44.54%. It was concluded that Licartin was safe and active in patients with HCC.

Realizing that TRIT is most suited for treating microscopic disease, Licartin was tested in the adjuvant setting for patients with HCC undergoing OLT (Xu et al. 2007). A total of 60 patients with HCC, undergoing OLT, were randomized to Licartin (0.42 mCi/kg) for three fractions at 28-day intervals versus placebo. Analysis at 1 year post-therapy revealed that the recurrence rate was significantly decreased by 30.4% ($p = 0.0174$) and the survival rate was significantly increased by 20.6% ($p = 0.0289$) in the Licartin group. No significant toxicities were observed. The Chinese State Food and Drug Administration has approved Licartin as an adjuvant therapy after OLT for HCC in 2005. Currently, there are two trials using Licartin that are ongoing but not recruiting patients. The first trial (NCT00819650) randomizes patients with HCC undergoing an R0 resection to postoperative Licartin or no further treatment. Licartin is delivered in three doses (fractions) at 28 day intervals, beginning at week 4 after liver resection. In the second trial (NCT00829465), patients with unresectable HCC are randomized to transcatheter arterial chemoembolization (TACE) or Licartin combined with TACE.

Indications

Zevalin (^{90}Y Ibritumomab Tiuxetan). The Zevalin therapeutic regimen is indicated for (1) previously untreated patients with CD20 positive, follicular NHL who achieve a partial or complete response to first-line chemotherapy or (2) for patients with relapsed or refractory CD20 positive, follicular NHL.

Bexxar (^{131}I Tositumomab). The Bexxar therapeutic regimen is indicated for patients with relapse or refractory CD20 positive, follicular NHL, with or without transformation.

Licartin (^{131}I Metuximab). Licartin is approved in China as adjuvant therapy, following orthotopic liver transplant, in patients with HCC.

Tumor Necrosis Therapy (^{131}I-Chtnt). ^{131}I-chTNT is approved in China to treat refractory bronchogenic carcinoma.

Advantage

The advantage of using TRIT to treat malignancies is that various targeting constructs are used to deliver systemic radiotherapy to not only large, radiographically visible tumors, but also to distant microscopic metastatic disease. This represents the most conformal and intensity-modulated form of radiotherapy delivery to date.

Disadvantage

The disadvantage of using TRIT is that the overall low tumor penetration results in low, nonuniform doses of radiation that is delivered to malignant tissue. Due to the long required circulation time necessary for the targeting constructs to penetrate into tumors, radiation dose to bone marrow, resulting in hematologic toxicity, is a problem.

Contraindication

All known TRIT agents are contraindicated for known hypersensitivity to murine proteins and for administration during pregnancy. Their safety has not been established for >25% lymphoma bone marrow involvement, platelet count <100,000 cells/mm^3, or neutrophil count <1,500 cells/mm^3. Patients who test positive for HAMA may be at increased risk for anaphylactic reactions, reduced efficacy, and serious hypersensitivity reactions.

Cross-References

▶ Acute Radiation Toxicity
▶ Bone Marrow Toxicity in Cancer Treatment
▶ Brachytherapy
▶ Conformal Therapy: Treatment Planning, Treatment Delivery, and Clinical Results
▶ External Beam Radiation Therapy
▶ Intensity-Modulated Radiotherapy
▶ Late Radiation Toxicity
▶ Liver and Hepatobiliary Tract
▶ Lung Cancer
▶ Melanoma
▶ Non-Hodgkins Lymphoma
▶ Nuclear Medicine
▶ Radiopharmaceuticals
▶ Stage 0 Breast Cancer
▶ Thyroid Cancer

References

Abbas AK, Lichtman AH, Pillais S (eds) (2007) Cellular and molecular immunology. Saunders Elsevier, Philadelphia

Al-Ejeh F, Brown MP (2011) Combined modality therapy: relevance for targeted radionuclide therapy. In: Speer TW (ed) Targeted radionuclide therapy. Lippincott Williams & Wilkins, Philadelphia

Behr TM, Sharkey RM, Juweid ME, Dunn RM, Vagg RC, Ying ZZCH, Swayne LC, Vardi Y, Siegel JA, Goldenberg DM (1997) Phase I/II clinical radioimmunotherapy with an iodine-131-labeled anti-carcinoembryonic antigen murine monoclonal antibody IgG. J Nucl Med 38:858–870

Bernhardt P, Speer TW (2011) Modeling the systemic cure with targeted radionuclide therapy. In: Speer TW (ed) Targeted radionuclide therapy. Lippincott Williams & Wilkins, Philadelphia

Borjesson PKE, Postema EJ, Roos JC et al (2003) Phase I therapy study with Re-186-labeled humanized monoclonal antibody BIWA 4 (Bivatuzumab) in patients with head and neck squamous cell carcinoma. Clin Cancer Res 9:3961s–3972s

Breitz HB, Weiden PL, Vanderheyden J-L, Appelbaum JW, Bjorn MJ, Fer MF, Wolf SB, Ratliff BA, Seiler CA,

Foisie DC, Fisher DR, Schroff RW, Fritzberg AR, Abrams PG (1992) Clinical experience with Rhenium-186-labeled monoclonal antibodies for radioimmunotherapy: results of phase I trials. J Nucl Med 33:1099–1109

Burdick M, Macklis RM (2011) Radioimmunotherapy for non-Hodgkin lymphoma: a clinical update. In: Speer TW (ed) Targeted radionuclide therapy. Lippincott Williams & Wilkins, Philadelphia

Burvenich IJG, Scott AM (2011) The delivery construct: maximizing the therapeutic ratio of targeted radionuclide therapy. In: Speer TW (ed) Targeted radionuclide therapy. Lippincott Williams & Wilkins, Philadelphia

Campoli M, Ferrone S (2011) Cancer immune surveillance and tumor escape mechanisms. In: Speer TW (ed) Targeted radionuclide therapy. Lippincott Williams & Wilkins, Philadelphia

Chen S, Yu L, Jiang C et al (2005) Pivotal study of iodine-131-labeled chimeric tumor necrosis treatment radioimmunotherapy in patients with advanced lung cancer. J Clin Oncol 23:1538–1547

Davies AJ, Rohatiner AZ, Howell S, Britton KE, Owens SE, Micallef IN et al (2004) Tositumomab and iodine I 131 tositumomab for recurrent indolent and transformed B-cell non-Hodgkin's lymphoma. J Clin Oncol 22(8):1469–1479

Davis TA, Kaminski MS, Leonard JP, Hsu FJ, Wilkinson M, Zelenetz A et al (2004) The radioisotope contributes significantly to the activity of radioimmunotherapy. Clin Cancer Res 10(23):7792–7798

DiCara D, Nissim A (2011) Methods for development of monoclonal antibody therapeutics. In: Speer TW (ed) Targeted radionuclide therapy. Lippincott Williams & Wilkins, Philadelphia

Fowler JF (1990) Radiobiological aspects of low dose rate in radioimmunotherapy. Int J Radiat Oncol Biol Phys 18:1261–1269

Goldsmith SJ, Vallabhajosula S, Kostakoglu L, Smith-Jones P, Kotheri P, Konishi T, Ursea B, Bander NH (2002) 90Y-DOTA-huJ591: radiolabeled anti-PSMA humanized monoclonal antibody for the treatment of prostate cancer: phase I dose escalation studies. J Nucl Med 43(5):158P

Hajjar G, Sharkey RM, Burton J, Zhang C-H, Yeldell D, Matthies A, Alavi A, Losman MJ, Brenner A, Goldenberg DM (2002) Phase I radioimmunotherapy trial with iodine-131-labeled humanized MN-14 anti-carcinoembryonic antigen monoclonal antibody in patients with metastatic gastrointestinal and colorectal cancer. Clin Colorectal Cancer 2:31–42

Horning SJ, Younes A, Jain V, Kroll S, Lucas J, Podoloff D et al (2005) Efficacy and safety of tositumomab and iodine-131 tositumomab (Bexxar) in B-cell lymphoma, progressive after rituximab. J Clin Oncol 23(4):712–719

Jeoung DI (2011) Employing SEREX for identification of targets for anticancer targeted therapy. In: Speer TW (ed) Targeted radionuclide therapy. Lippincott Williams & Wilkins, Philadelphia

Juweid M, Swayne LC, Sharkey RM, Dunn R, Rubin AD, Herskovic T, Goldenberg DM (1997) Prospects of radioimmunotherapy in epithelial ovarian cancer: results with iodine-131-labeled murine and humanized MN-14 anti-carcinoembryonic antigen monoclonal antibodies. Gynecol Oncol 67:259–271

Kaminski MS, Estes J, Zasadny KR, Francis IR, Ross CW, Tuck M et al (2000) Radioimmunotherapy with iodine (131)I tositumomab for relapsed or refractory B-cell non-Hodgkin lymphoma: updated results and long-term follow-up of the University of Michigan experience. Blood 96(4):1259–1266

Kaminski MS, Zelenetz AD, Press OW, Saleh M, Leonard J, Fehrenbacher L et al (2001) Pivotal study of iodine I 131 tositumomab for chemotherapy-refractory low-grade or transformed low-grade B-cell non-Hodgkin's lymphomas. J Clin Oncol 19(19):3918–3928

Kohler G, Milstein C (1975) Continuous cultures of fused cells secreting antibody of predefined specificity. Nature 256(5517):495–497

Kramer EL, Liebes L, Wasserheit C, Noz ME, Blank EW, Zabalegui A, Melamed J, Furmanski P, Peterson JA, Ceriani RL (1998) Initial clinical evaluation of radiolabeled MX-DTPA humanized BrE-3 antibody in patients with advanced breast cancer. Clin Cancer Res 4:1679–1688

Meredith RF, Khazaeli MB, Liu T, Plott G, Wheeler RH, Russell C, Colcher D, Schlom J, Shochat D, LoBuglio AF (1992) Dose fractionation of radiolabeled antibodies in patients with metastatic colon cancer. J Nucl Med 33:1648–1653

Meredith RF, Bueschen AJ, Khazaeli MB, Plott WE, Grizzle WE, Wheeler RH, Schlom J, Russell CD, Liu T, LoBuglio AF (1994) Treatment of metastatic prostate carcinoma with radiolabeled antibody CC49. J Nucl Med 35:1017–1022

Meredith RF, Khazaeli MB, Plott WE, Spencer SA, Wheeler RH, Brady LW, Woo DV, LoBuglio AF (1995) Initial clinical evaluation of iodine-125-labeled chimeric 17-1A for metastatic colon cancer. J Nucl Med 36:2229–2233

Milenic DE (2010) Antibody engineering: optimizing the delivery vehicle. In: Reilly RM (ed) Monoclonal antibody and peptide-targeted radiotherapy of cancer. Wiley, Hoboken

Morschhauser F, Radford J, Van Hoof A et al (2008) Phase III trial of consolidation therapy with yttrium-90-ibritumomab tiuxetan compared with no additional therapy after first remission in advanced follicular lymphoma. J Clin Oncol 26:5156–5164

Mulligan T, Carrasquillo JA, Chung Y, Milenic DE, Schlom J, Feuerstein I, Paik C, Perentesis P, Reynolds J, Curt G (1995) Phase I study of intravenous Lu-labeled CC49 murine monoclonal antibody in patients with advanced adenocarcinoma. Clin Cancer Res 1: 1447–1454

Murry D, McEwan AJ (2007) Radiobiology of systemic radiation therapy. Cancer Biother Radiopharm 22:1–23

O'Donoghue JA (2000) Dosimetric principles of targeted radiotherapy. In: Abrams PG, Fritzberg AR (eds) Radioimmunotherapy of cancer. Marcel Dekker, New York

Order S (2011) Radioimmunotherapy of unresectable hepatocellular carcinoma. In: Speer TW (ed) Targeted radionuclide therapy. Lippincott Williams & Wilkins, Philadelphia

Pedone C, Morelli G, Tesauro D, Saviano M (2006) Peptide structure and analysis. In: Chinol M, Paganelli G (eds) Radionuclide peptide cancer therapy. Taylor & Francis, New York

Sharkey RM, Goldenberg DM (2011) Pretargeted radioimmunotherapy. In: Speer TW (ed) Targeted radionuclide therapy. Lippincott Williams & Wilkins, Philadelphia

Speer TW, Khuntia D (2011) Introduction to radiation oncology. In: Mehta MP (ed) Principles and practice of neuro-oncology: a multidisciplinary approach. Demos Medical Publishing, New York

Speer TW, Limmer JP, Henrich D, Buskerud J, Vogds B, Vanderkooy D, Barton D (2011) Evolution of radiotherapy toward a more targeted approach for CNS malignancies. In: Speer TW (ed) Targeted radionuclide therapy. Lippincott Williams & Wilkins, Philadelphia

Stahl S, Friedman Mikaela F, Carlsson J, Tolmachev V, Frejd F (2011) Affibody molecules for targeted radionuclide therapy. In: Speer TW (ed) Targeted radionuclide therapy. Lippincott Williams & Wilkins, Philadelphia

Tesauro D, Morelli G, Pedone C, Saviano M (2011) Radiolabeled peptides, structure and analysis. In: Speer TW (ed) Targeted radionuclide therapy. Lippincott Williams & Wilkins, Philadelphia

Tobinai K, Watanabe T, Ogura M, Morishima Y, Hotta T, Ishizawa K et al (2009) Japanese phase II study of 90Y-ibritumomab tiuxetan in patients with relapsed or refractory indolent B-cell lymphoma. Cancer Sci 100 (1):158–164

Vose JM, Wahl RL, Saleh M, Rohatiner AZ, Knox SJ, Radford JA et al (2000) Multicenter phase II study of iodine-131 tositumomab for chemotherapy-relapsed/refractory low-grade and transformed low-grade B-cell non-Hodgkin's lymphomas. J Clin Oncol 18(6):1316–1323

Weiden PL, Breitz HB, Seiler CA, Bjorn MJ, Ratliff BA, Mallett R, Beaumier PL, Appelbaum JW, Fritzberg AR, Salk D (1993) Rhenium-186-labeled chimeric antibody NR-LU-13: pharmacokinetics, biodistribution and immunogenicity relative to murine analog NR-LU-10. J Nucl Med 34:2111–2119

Welt S, Divgi CR, Kemeny N, Finn RD, Scott AM, Graham M, Germain JS, Richards EC, Larson SM, Oettgen HF et al (1994) Phase I/II study of iodine 131I-labeled monoclonal antibody A33 in patients with advanced colon cancer. J Clin Oncol 12:1561–1571

Wilson AD, Brechbiel MW (2011) Chelation chemistry. In: Speer TW (ed) Targeted radionuclide therapy. Lippincott Williams & Wilkins, Philadelphia

Wiseman GA, Gordon LI, Multani PS, Witzig TE, Spies S, Bartlett NL et al (2002) Ibritumomab tiuxetan radioimmunotherapy for patients with relapsed or refractory non-Hodgkin lymphoma and mild thrombocytopenia: a phase II multicenter trial. Blood 99 (12):4336–4342

Witzig TE (2010) Radioimmunotherapy for B-cell non-Hodgkin lymphoma. In: Reilly RM (ed) Monoclonal antibody and peptide-targeted radiotherapy of cancer. Wiley, Hoboken

Witzig TE, Gordon LI, Cabanillas F, Czuczman MS, Emmanouilides C, Joyce R et al (2002a) Randomized controlled trial of yttrium-90-labeled ibritumomab tiuxetan radioimmunotherapy versus rituximab immunotherapy for patients with relapsed or refractory low-grade, follicular, or transformed B-cell non-Hodgkin's lymphoma. J Clin Oncol 20(10):2453–2463

Witzig TE, Flinn IW, Gordon LI, Emmanouilides C, Czuczman MS, Saleh MN et al (2002b) Treatment with ibritumomab tiuxetan radioimmunotherapy in patients with rituximab-refractory follicular non-Hodgkin's lymphoma. J Clin Oncol 20(15):3262–3269

Witzig TE, White CA, Wiseman GA, Gordon LI, Emmanouilides C, Raubitschek A et al (1999) Phase I/II trial of IDEC-Y2B8 radioimmunotherapy for treatment of relapsed or refractory CD20(+) B-cell non-Hodgkin's lymphoma. J Clin Oncol 17(12): 3793–3803

Wong JYC, Chu DZ, Yamauchi DM, Odom-Maryon T, Williams LE, Liu A, Wilcyznski S, Wu AM, Shively JE, Doroshow JH, Raubitschek AA (2000) Phase I radioimmunotherapy trials evaluating Y-90 labeled anti-CEA chimeric T84.66 in patients with metastatic CEA-producing malignancies. Clin Cancer Res 6:3855–3863

Wong JYC, Williams LE, Yazaki PJ (2011) Radioimmunotherapy of colorectal cancer. In: Speer TW (ed) Targeted radionuclide therapy. Lippincott Williams & Wilkins, Philadelphia

Xu J, Shen Z-Y, Chen X-G et al (2007) A randomized controlled trial of Licartin for preventing hepatoma recurrence after liver transplantation. Hepatology 45: 269–276

Yu B, Carrasquilo J, Milenic D, Chung Y, Perentesis P, Feuerstein I, Eggensperger D, Qi C-F, Paik C, Reynolds J, Grem GC, Siler K, Schlom J, Allegra C (1996) Phase I trial of iodine 131I-labeled COL-1 in patients with gastrointestinal malignancies: influence of serum carcinoembryonic antigen and tumor bulk on pharmacokinetics. J Clin Oncol 6:1798–1809

Taxanes

RENE RUBIN
Rittenhouse Hematology/Oncology,
Philadelphia, PA, USA

Definition

These agents (paclitaxel, docetaxel, albumin bound paclitaxel, cabazitaxel: recently approved for prostate cancer) act similarly as microtubule stabilizers, halting progression through mitosis and promoting apoptosis through signaling pathways. They are used predominantly against solid tumors, primarily breast cancer, and are active against ovarian, lung, and bladder cancer. They are commonly used in combination with platinum analogs, cytotoxic agents, and monoclonal antibodies. They are also radiosensitizing agents.

Side Effects

- Neutropenia (dose-limiting toxicity)
- Acute hypersensitivity reactions
- Cardiac arrhythmias
- Cardiac heart failure (potentiates anthracycline toxicity)
- Fluid retention (taxotere)
- Neurotoxicity (sensory neuropathy/peripheral neuropathy)
- Mucositis
- Transaminitis
- Loss of nails
- Alopecia

Cross-References

▶ Principles of Chemotherapy

TBI Dosimetry

IRIS RUSU
Department of Radiation Oncology,
Loyola University Medical Center, Maywood,
IL, USA

Definition

Dosimetry of large fields at extended treatment distances.

Cross-References

▶ Total Body Irradiation (TBI)

TBI Irradiation Techniques

IRIS RUSU
Department of Radiation Oncology,
Loyola University Medical Center, Maywood,
IL, USA

Definition

Unconventional treatment geometries used to provide large fields for the effective irradiation of the whole body.

Cross-References

▶ Total Body Irradiation (TBI)

Template

Yan Yu, Laura Doyle
Department of Radiation Oncology, Thomas Jefferson University Hospital, Philadelphia, PA, USA

Definition

Grid with equally distributed holes to guide needle placement. Each hole is identified by a number and/or letter pattern. A virtual template is displayed on the TRUS images to coordinate planning and delivery of needle and seed locations.

Cross-References

▶ Brachytherapy: Low Dose Rate (LDR) Permanent Implants (Prostate)
▶ Prostate

Temporary Implant

Cheng B. Saw[1], Ning J. Yue[2]
[1]Division of Radiation Oncology, Penn State Cancer Institute, Hershey, PA, USA
[2]The Department of Radiation Oncology, The Cancer Institute of New Jersey, UMDNJ-Robert Wood Johnson Medical School, New Brunswick, NJ, USA

Definition

Temporary implant is the type of brachytherapy in which radioactive source placement is temporary and the radioactive sources are removed after treatment.

A brachytherapy implant where all radioactive sources are removed after the completion of radiation treatment.

Cross-References

▶ Brachytherapy: High Dose Rate (HDR) Implants
▶ Brachytherapy: Low Dose Rate (LDR) Temporary Implants

Testes

Johannes Classen
Department of Radiation Oncology, St. Vincentius-Kliniken Karlsruhe, Karlsruhe, Germany

Testes

Testes are the paired reproductive organs of men, located in the scrotum. They have a primary lymphatic drainage to the retroperitoneal lymph nodes. Two pituitary gland hormones control the main function of the testes: Follicle stimulating hormone (FSH) regulates growth and maturation of spermatocytes in the germinal epithelium; luteinizing hormone (LH) stimulates testosterone synthesis in the interstitial Leydig cells.

Testicular Cancer

Testicular cancer represents 1% of male malignancies but is the most frequent cancer of men in the age group 20–40 years. The incidence has doubled in all Western countries over the last 40 years and shows large geographic variations with a peak in Denmark and Switzerland (9-10/100,000/year).

Background

Ninety to ninety-five percent of testicular cancer are malignancies of the germinal epithelium; 60% of these represents seminoma, and 40% represents non-seminoma, which form a heterogeneous group. Testicular intraepithelial neoplasia is the uniform precursor lesion of all germinal testicular tumors. Leydig cell tumors, Sertoli cell tumors, non-Hodgkin's lymphomas, and metastases are among the rare testicular cancers.

Most testicular cancers are unilateral with a slight predominance of the left side. Risk factors for germinal testicular cancer are ▶ crypt-orchidism (relative risk 4–5%), a history of unilateral testicular cancer (5% lifelong risk of contralateral cancer), and a positive family history (brother: relative risk 6–10%; father: relative risk 4–6%).

Primary metastatic spread occurs by lymphatic drainage to regional retroperitoneal lymph nodes and by hematogenous spread to lung, liver, bone, brain, and other organs. Testicular cancer can be cured in all stages of the disease including visceral metastasis.

This overview entry focuses on germinal testis cancer.

Clinical Presentation

Painless swelling is the main symptom. Pain is observed in 30% of the patients. Differential diagnosis includes epididymitis, hydrocele testis, and testicular torsion. In up to 20% of the patients, clinical signs of metastasis (pain, swellings) may lead to the diagnosis.

Diagnostics

Open testicular exploration and inguinal ▶ orchiectomy is the standard procedure for local treatment of testis cancer except for symptomatic patients with advanced stage disease (e.g., brain or pulmonary metastasis) or non-testicular germinal tumors. Orchiectomy allows for definitive diagnosis based on a complete pathological workup. A contralateral testicular biopsy may be taken at the same time to rule out testicular intraepithelial neoplasia. Trans-scrotal biopsy of the tumor-bearing testis should be avoided due to the risk of aberrant lymphatic drainage ("scrotal violation").

Pathology

Pathology must specify details of rare non-germinal testis tumors, distinguish between seminomatous and non-seminomatous tumors, and provide information on tumor size, invasion of blood vessels or rete testis, proportion of embryonic cancer, or proliferation index, which are necessary for assessing clinical risk groups. For classification as seminoma, a tumor must not contain any non-seminomatous component.

Imaging

Computed tomography (CT) of abdomen and pelvis and thorax is mandatory for assessment of lymphatic (retroperitoneal and pelvic nodes) and hematogenous (liver, lung) spread. Lymph nodes with a transverse diameter of >1 cm are considered metastatic. In Stage I seminoma, chest X-ray is considered sufficient.

Positron emission tomography (PET) has a role for primary staging in higher stage, higher risk seminoma and a proven validity in assessment of vitality in residual tumor for seminoma and may guide management of residual masses in these patients.

Laboratory Studies and Tumor Markers

Lactate dehydrogenase (LDH) and tumor markers alpha-fetoprotein (AFP) and human chorionic gonadotropin (HCG) should be assessed before and after orchiectomy. They are used for assessment of prognosis and classification (seminoma versus non-seminoma) as well as monitoring of treatment and follow-up. Elevation of AFP prior to orchiectomy leads to classification of a non-seminoma cancer even in tumors that are histologically characterized as pure seminomas. HCG elevation is compatible with the diagnosis of seminoma and does not require modifications of stage- or prognosis-directed management.

Staging and Prognostic Assessment

Staging is performed according to the classification of the *Union International Contre le Cancer* (*UICC*) (Table 1). For assessment of the prognosis in metastatic disease, the classification of the *International Germ Cell Collaborative Group* (*IGCCCG*) (IGCCCG, 1997; Mead and Stenning, 1997) is used (Table 2). Patients with "good," "intermediate," or "poor" risk features have a 5-year survival of 90%, 75%, and 50%, respectively.

Therapy

Background

The aim of treatment is cure in all stages of germinal testicular cancer including distant metastases to the brain. Orchiectomy is the routine procedure for diagnosis of testicular cancer and radical local treatment. Testis-preserving surgery may be an alternative in selected cases (see below). Decisions for adjuvant or additional systemic treatment are based on the UICC stage in Stage I–IIA/B seminoma and Stage I–IIA (marker negative) non-seminoma, while risk group assessment is the basis for decision in all other patients.

Attention has to be paid to potential late effects of treatment that have gained increasing importance with long-term survivors of testicular cancer. Second cancer induction, fertility, neurotoxicity, and cardiovascular toxicity should be considered. These aspects have motivated research to establish alternative strategies in early-stage/good prognosis patients.

Testicular Intraepithelial Neoplasia (TIN – Ptis)

TIN is a precursor lesion inevitably leading to invasive cancer when left untreated. Radiotherapy with 20 Gy at 2 Gy daily fractions is the treatment of choice for this disorder in a singular testis (after contralateral orchiectomy) or for bilateral TIN, preventing invasive cancer in the vast majority of patients. In unilateral TIN (and TIN-negative contralateral biopsy), orchiectomy is appropriate. Local radiotherapy may be withheld for some time in fertile patients wishing to father a child.

TIN may persist after chemotherapy. Control biopsies are recommended 1 year after systemic treatment to guide further treatment decisions.

Seminoma Stage I

The risk of relapse without adjuvant treatment is 15–20%. Tumor size of >4 cm combined with infiltration of the rete testis indicates an increased risk of >30% (high risk) whereas a low rate of recurrence has been reported for patients without any of these factors (low risk).

The aim of adjuvant treatment is to individually control the risk of relapse at a minimal risk of late toxicity. There are three accepted alternative options (Krege et al. 2008): adjuvant radiotherapy and carboplatin single-agent chemotherapy are equally effective and reduce the risk of relapse to 5%. Watchful waiting aims at minimizing potential late toxicity by avoiding overtreatment in the majority of patients. Salvage chemotherapy in all recurring patients is highly effective, resulting in comparable rates of disease-specific survival for all three strategies (99–100%).

Radiotherapy

Adjuvant paraaortic irradiation with 20 Gy in ten fractions is the current standard of radiotherapy resulting in high cure rates (95%). Relapse is most often observed in pelvic nodes or at distant sites. Routine treatment of ipsilateral pelvic nodes is not necessary in patients without prior scrotal or inguinal surgery. Acute toxicity (mainly gastrointestinal) is moderate. There is a potential low risk of secondary cancer induction.

Testes. Table 1 Assessment of stage according to 2010 UICC classification. N: upper normal range. (**a**) UICC-stage assignment. M0: no distant metastasis, M1: distant metastasis, M1a: non-regional lymph node or pulmonary metastasis; M1b: other distant metastasis, SX: markers unknown, TX: T-category unknown. (**b**) Assessment of S-category

(a)				
Stage	**T-category**	**N-category**	**M-category**[a]	**S-category**
0	pTis	N0	M0	S0, SX
I	pT1–4	N0	M0	SX
IA	pT1	N0	M0	S0
IB	pT2	N0	M0	S0
	pT3	N0	M0	S0
	pT4	N0	M0	S0
IS	Any pT/TX	N0	M0	S1–3
II	Any pT/TX	N1–3	M0	SX
IIA	Any pT/TX	N1	M0	S0
	Any pT/TX	N1	M0	S1
IIB	Any pT/TX	N2	M0	S0
	Any pT/TX	N2	M0	S1
IIC	Any pT/TX	N3	M0	S0
	Any pT/TX	N3	M0	S1
III	Any pT/TX	Any N	M1, M1a	SX
IIIA	Any pT/TX	Any N	M1, M1a	S0
	Any pT/TX	Any N	M1, M1a	S1
IIIB	Any pT/TX	N1–3	M0	S2
	Any pT/TX	Any N	M1, M1a	S2
IIIC	Any pT/TX	N1–3	M0	S3
	Any pT/TX	Any N	M1, M1a	S3
	Any pT/TX	Any N	M1b	Any S

(b)						
Tumor markers						
S-category	**LDH**		**ß-HCG**			**AFP**
S0	N		N			N
S1	$<1.5 \times N$	and	<1,000 ng/ml (<5,000 U/l)	and		<1,000 ng/ml
S2	$1.5–10 \times N$	or	1,000–10,000 ng/ml (5,000–50,000 U/l)	or		1,000–10,000 ng/ml
S3	$>10 \times N$	or	>10,000 ng/ml (>50,000 U/l)	or		>10,000 ng/ml

Testes. Table 2 IGCCCG – classification for metastatic disease

Classification of the International Germ Cell Cancer Collaborative Group (IGCCCG) (Mead and Stenning 1997)		
Good prognosis		
Non-seminoma	Testicular/retroperitoneal tumor and "Good" markers* and No non-pulmonary visceral metastases	* "Good" markers: AFP <1,000 ng/ml and HCG <1,000 ng/mg (~5,000 IU/l) and LDH <1.5 × N
Seminoma	Any primary location and Any markers and No non-pulmonary visceral metastases	
Intermediate prognosis		
Non-seminoma	Testicular/retroperitoneal tumor and "intermediate" markers* and No non-pulmonary visceral metastases	* "Intermediate" markers: AFP 1,000–10,000 ng/ml and/or HCG 1,000–10,000 ng/mg (~5,000–50,000 IU/l) and/or LDH 1.5–10 × N
Seminoma	Any primary location and Any markers and Non-pulmonary visceral metastases	
Poor prognosis		
Non-seminoma	Primary mediastinal tumor or Testicular/retroperitoneal tumor and Non-pulmonary visceral metastases or "Poor" markers*	* "Poor" markers: AFP >10,000 ng/ml and/or HCG >10,000 ng/mg (~50,000 IU/l) and/or LDH >10 × N

N upper normal limit, *AFP* alpha-fetoprotein, *HCG* human chorionic gonadotropin, *LDH* lactate dehydrogenase

Carboplatin Single-Agent Chemotherapy

One course of carboplatin (AUC 7) is equally effective as low-dose radiotherapy and shows moderate acute toxicity (Oliver et al., 2005). Long-term experience is limited. Relapse is most often observed in paraaortic nodes. Quality of life may be less impaired by carboplatin than by adjuvant radiotherapy.

Watchful Waiting

Thorough follow-up and high patient compliance are prerequisites for this strategy. Attention should be paid to potential late relapse. Patients should be willing to accept a greater risk of relapse (15–20%) without compromise in survival. The predominant pattern of relapse is retroperitoneal nodal disease, but distant spread may occur.

Seminoma Stage IIA/B

Radiotherapy

Radiotherapy with 30 Gy in 15 fractions in Stage IIA and 36 Gy in Stage IIB given to enlarged lymph nodes and adjuvant paraaortic and ipsilateral pelvic lymphatic tissues cures 95% and 90% of the patients, respectively (Classen et al., 2003). Survival approaches 100% due to highly active salvage chemotherapy. Acute and chronic toxicity is low. ▶ Scrotal shielding is recommended to protect the contralateral testis from scattered radiation.

Chemotherapy

The role of chemotherapy in Stage IIA/B seminoma remains controversial. Three cycles of combination chemotherapy PEB (platinum, etoposide, bleomycin) or four cycles PE (▶ Principles of Chemotherapy) provide control of the disease for most patients, but acute grade III/IV toxicity is increased as compared to radiotherapy without either improving treatment outcome or reducing the hazard for ▶ secondary tumor induction. PE/PEB may serve as an alternative in advanced Stage IIB disease or in patients otherwise not suitable for radiotherapy.

Carboplatin alone yields insufficient cure rates and is not indicated in Stage II disease. Combining carboplatin and radiotherapy does not improve cure rates over radiotherapy alone, but increases the potential risk of secondary tumor induction and is therefore discouraged.

Stage I Non-seminoma

The risk of relapse without adjuvant treatment is 25–30%. Most recurrences are located in retroperitoneal lymph nodes or the lungs. Factors predicting a high risk of relapse are vascular invasion (strongest indicator), >50% embryonal carcinoma, and >70% proliferation rate (Albers et al., 2003). A combination of all three factors predicts a risk of relapse of 64%, while patients without any risk factor or without vascular invasion alone show a recurrence rate of 13% and 23%, respectively. The aims of adjuvant treatment are comparable to those in Stage I seminoma. ▶ Watchful waiting, adjuvant PEB chemotherapy, and retroperitoneal lymphadenectomy (RPLND) are three treatment options for Stage I non-seminomatous testis cancer (Krege et al. 2008). Survival approaches 99% with all three strategies.

Watchful Waiting

It is the preferred option in low-risk patients with either no vascular invasion alone or in combination with additional factors. Frequent clinical, laboratory, and imaging controls are compulsory. Relapse beyond the second year after primary diagnosis is rare, and the follow-up schedule should be tailored to this aspect. Recurring patients can be salvaged by combination chemotherapy.

Chemotherapy

Two cycles of PEB is the preferred treatment for high-risk patients or patients declining watchful waiting with low-risk disease. Disease-free survival is 97%. Overall survival reaches 99%. Current strategies focus on reduction to one cycle of PEB in order to lower acute and potential chronic toxicity.

Lymphadenectomy

Nerve-sparing retroperitoneal lymph node dissection (RPLND) is an option for patients not willing to undergo watchful waiting or adjuvant chemotherapy. The risk of relapse is reduced to 10%; most recurrences are observed outside the retroperitoneum. Overall survival is comparable to that in the other strategies.

Stage IIA Non-seminoma

The treatment strategy in Stage IIA (lymph nodes <2 cm) differs between marker positive and marker negative disease. Elevated markers are a reliable indicator of metastatic disease requiring chemotherapy for cure according to prognosis grouping (three or four cycles PEB for "good" or "intermediate" prognosis, respectively) (Krege et al. 2008). Marker negative patients may be overstaged in up to 40% by CT and require a different management. Options are primary RPLND or imaging control of nodal disease after 6 weeks and RPLND in case of progressive or stable disease. Adjuvant chemotherapy in pathologically confirmed Stage IIA is optional. Some authors advocate diagnostic RPLND for all marker negative Stage IIA patients.

Advanced Disease

Patients with seminoma >Stage IIB or non-seminoma >Stage I (except for Stage IIA marker negative, see above) are treated with primary chemotherapy according to IGCCCG risk groups. Three cycles of PEB are recommended for "good" prognosis patients. In case of contraindications to bleomycin, four cycles of PE may be applied. Four cycles of PEB are considered standard treatment for "intermediate" and "poor" risk patients.

Residual Tumor After Primary Treatment

In seminoma patients, regressing masses with a residual size of ≤3 cm do not require interventions. In non-regressing masses >3 cm, a PET scan (3–4 weeks after last course of chemotherapy) allows for differentiation between vital residual tumor which should be resected and necrosis which does not require further local treatment.

There are no parameters to reliably predict histology in residual masses in non-seminoma. Therefore, any residual mass persisting 3–4 weeks after the last cycle of chemotherapy should be resected in these patients. Necrosis can be expected in 45–50%, undifferentiated vital tumor in 15–20%, and differentiated teratoma (which bears the risk of malignant transformation if it remains in situ) in 30–40%.

Brain Metastases

Approximately 10% of testis cancer patients suffer from brain metastasis. Patients with central nervous metastasis at primary diagnosis have a 5-year survival of 30–40%, whereas patients with intracranial progressive disease under first-line treatment or concurrent with systemic relapse have a 5-year survival of 2–5%. Patients with singular brain metastasis at primary diagnosis have the best prognosis.

Curative chemotherapy is mandatory in all patients. Radiotherapy seems to improve prognosis. Whole brain irradiation with 40–45 Gy at 1.8–2 Gy fractions is common practice. A boost may be applied to metastatic sites. The optimal sequence of chemotherapy and radiotherapy is undefined. It is not clear whether radiotherapy is required in case of complete remission after chemotherapy. Surgery may be considered in case of a solitary brain metastasis.

Organ Sparing Surgery

Five percent of all testicular cancer patients develop metachronous contralateral testis cancer. For small tumors testis-preserving surgery is feasible and safe, if adjuvant radiotherapy with 20 Gy is given to the remaining testicular parenchyma in order to eliminate TIN which can be found in virtually all tumor-bearing testes. This procedure reduces the risk of lifelong androgen replacement that is necessary for standard ablative surgery in this clinical situation.

Follow-Up

Patients after primary or salvage treatment require follow-up. It is the aim of post-treatment surveillance to diagnose relapse from testis cancer, to detect and alleviate late toxicity of treatment, and to diagnose potential secondary cancers. Attention should be paid to late relapse from testicular cancer.

There is low evidence for specific follow-up schedules in any particular group of testicular cancer patients defined by stage or prognostic group. The frequency of follow-up visits as well as the use of technical investigations should be tailored to the expected risk and time course of recurrent disease. Relapse beyond the third year after primary diagnosis is rare. Imaging studies include chest X-ray, CT of abdomen and pelvis, and laboratory tests (AFP, HCG, LDH). Scrotal sonography should be performed to detect contralateral testicular cancer.

Cross-References
▶ Non-Hodgkin's Lymphoma
▶ Palliation of Bone Metastases
▶ Palliation of Brain and Spinal Cord Metastases
▶ Palliation of Metastatic Disease to the Liver
▶ Palliation of Visceral Recurrences and Metastases
▶ Pituitary
▶ Principles of Chemotherapy
▶ Principles of Surgical Oncology
▶ Statistics and Clinical Trials
▶ Stereotactic Radiosurgery: Cranial
▶ Supportive Care and Quality of Life

References

Albers P, Siener R, Kliesch S et al (2003) Risk factors for relapse in clinical stage I nonseminomatous testicular germ cell tumors: results of the German Testicular Cancer Study Group trial. J Clin Oncol 21:1505–1512

Classen J, Schmidberger H, Meisner C et al (2003) Radiotherapy for stage IIA/B testicular seminoma: final report of a prospective multicenter clinical trial. J Clin Oncol 21:1101–1106

International Germ Cell Cancer Collaborative Group (IGCCCG) (1997) The International Germ Cell Consensus Classification: a prognostic factor based staging system for metastatic germcell cancer. J Clin Oncol 15:594–603

Krege S, Beyer J, Souchon R et al (2008) European Consensus Conference on Diagnosis and Treatment of Germ Cell Cancer: a report of the second meeting of the European Germ Cell Cancer Consensus Group (EGCCCG): Part I+II. Eur Urol 53:478–513

Mead GM, Stenning SP (1997) The International Germ Cell Consensus Classification: a new prognostic factor-based staging classification for metastatic germ cell tumours. Clin Oncol (R Coll Radiol) 9:207–209.

Oliver RT, Mason MD, Mead GM et al (2005) Radiotherapy versus single-dose carboplatin in adjuvant treatment of stage I seminoma: a randomized trial. Lancet 366:293–300

Theoretical Medicine

▶ Biomedicine (also Traditional, Theoretical, Conventional, or Western Medicine)

Therapeutic Radiological Physics

▶ Radiation Oncology Physics

Therapeutic Ratio

CARSTEN NIEDER
Radiation Oncology Unit, Nordlandssykehuset HF, Bodoe, Norway

Definition
Balance between tumor control rate and treatment-related toxicity, both of which are influenced by the radiation dose administered.

Cross-References

▶ Principles of Chemotherapy
▶ Total Body Irradiation (TBI)

Therapy Physics

▶ Radiation Oncology Physics

Three-Dimensional Conformal Radiation Therapy

FENG-MING KONG, JINGBO WANG
Department of Radiation Oncology,
Veteran Administration Health Center and
University Hospital, University of Michigan,
Ann Arbor, MI, USA

Synonyms
3DCRT

Definition
Three-dimensional conformal radiation therapy is a CT-based planning technique which generates three-dimensional (3D) volumes of internal anatomy. Using multiple-shaped beams from different angles, a high-dose region is generated which encompasses the target in 3D with considerable sparing of surrounding normal tissues.

Cross-References
▶ Conformal Therapy: Treatment Planning, Treatment Delivery, and Clinical Results
▶ Lung

Thrombocytopenia

LINDSAY G. JENSEN, BRENT S. ROSE,
ARNO J. MUNDT
Center for Advanced Radiotherapy Technologies,
Department of Radiation Oncology, San Diego
Rebecca and John Moores Cancer Center,
University of California, La Jolla, CA, USA

Definition
Decreased peripheral platelet count, typically <150,000 per microliter.

Cross-References
▶ Bone Marrow Toxicity in Cancer Treatment

Thymic Neoplasms

RAMESH RENGAN[1], CHARLES R. THOMAS, JR.[2]
[1]Department of Radiation Oncology, Hospital
of the University of Pennsylvania, Philadelphia,
PA, USA
[2]Department of Radiation Medicine, Oregon
Health Sciences University, Portland, OR, USA

Synonyms
Mediastinal thymic neoplasms

Definition/Description
Tumors of the thymus account for approximately 50% of the tumors of the anterior mediastinum and most commonly arise from the epithelial cells of the thymus gland. With the exception of thymic carcinoma, these tumors are usually slow growing

with an excellent long-term prognosis for cure with surgical extirpation. Thymic tumors are associated with a variety of paraneoplastic autoimmune disorders including ▶ myasthenia gravis (35–40% of all cases), hypogammaglobulinemia (5%), and ▶ pure red cell aplasia (5–10%). Most thymomas present as an asymptomatic mass identified on routine thoracic imaging. In contrast, patients with thymic carcinoma usually present with cough, dyspnea, or even superior vena cava syndrome. The treatment of choice for thymoma is complete surgical excision. Adjuvant radiotherapy is employed in cases where there is concern for postoperative residual disease. Neoadjuvant chemotherapy may be employed to facilitate surgical resection. The treatment of choice for thymic carcinoma is usually definitive chemoradiotherapy.

Anatomy

The mediastinum occupies the central portion of the thoracic cavity. It is bounded by the lungs and parietal pleura within the pleural cavities laterally, the thoracic inlet superiorly, the diaphragm inferiorly, the sternum and attached thoracic musculature anteriorly, and by the thoracic vertebrae and associated ribs posteriorly. The mediastinum can be divided into three clinically relevant compartments: anterior, middle, and posterior. The anterior mediastinum lies posterior to the sternum and anterior to the pericardium and great vessels, extends from the thoracic inlet to the diaphragm, and contains the thymus gland, lymph nodes, and, rarely, ectopic thyroid and parathyroid glands. The middle mediastinum is defined as the space occupied by the heart, pericardium, proximal great vessels, and central airways, including both phrenic nerves and lymph nodes. The posterior mediastinum is bounded by the heart and great vessels anteriorly, the thoracic inlet superiorly, the diaphragm inferiorly, and the chest wall of the back posteriorly, and includes the paravertebral gutters, esophagus, descending aorta, sympathetic chains and vagus nerves, azygous vein, thoracic duct, and lymph nodes. Although other anatomic divisions have been proposed, these other schemes have limited clinical utility.

Epidemiology

Thymomas are a relatively rare tumor. Analysis of the Surveillance, Epidemiology and End Results (SEER) database reveals that the overall incidence of thymoma is 0.15 per 100,000 person-years and incidence increases until the eighth decade of life, with the mean age at diagnosis being between 40 and 60 years of age (Engels and Pfeiffer 2003). Males have a slightly higher risk of thymomas than females, although no clear association has been identified with sex hormones to date. Thymomas are the most common tumor of the anterior mediastinum and represent approximately 30% of all mediastinal lesions.

Clinical Presentation

Approximately 30–40% of thymomas are asymptomatic at presentation and are identified as an incidental finding on thoracic imaging. However, patients may present with chest pain, dyspnea, cough, or fatigue. In the case of thymic carcinoma, patients may present with superior vena cava syndrome. Patients with thymoma also present with associated paraneoplastic autoimmune syndromes, such as myasthenia gravis (35%–40%), ▶ hypogammaglobulinemia (5%), and pure red cell aplasia (5%). Myasthenia gravis usually presents with ocular muscle fatigue, dysphagia, and ptosis.

Differential Diagnosis

The differential diagnosis for an anterior mediastinal mass includes lymphoma, mediastinal germ cell tumors, tumors of the thyroid gland and parathyroid glands, and mesenchymal tumors such as a fibroma or leiomyosarcoma.

Imaging Studies

A contrast enhanced computed tomographic scan of the chest is the diagnostic test of choice. Magnetic resonance imaging can also be used. It has the advantage of multiplanar imaging and is superior to computed tomography in identifying vessel invasion. Additionally, MR imaging can be used with greater latitude in the setting of renal insufficiency or allergy to iodinated contrast dye. The role of FDG-PET has not yet been established in the diagnosis of thymoma; however, its role is well established in the diagnosis of lymphoma.

There is no formal AJCC staging system for thymoma. The Masaoka, although imperfect, is the most commonly used staging system and given below.

Stage	Description
I	Macroscopically completely encapsulated and microscopically no capsular invasion.
II	Macroscopic invasion into surrounding fatty tissue or mediastinal pleura; microscopic invasion into the capsule.
III	Macroscopic invasion into neighboring organs (pericardium, great vessels, lung)
IVa	Pleural or pericardial dissemination
IVb	Lymphogenous or hematogenous metastasis

Adapted from Masaoka et al. (1981).

Laboratory Studies

Complete blood count and serum chemistries should be ordered as they may be abnormal in associated syndromes. Serum tumor marker, including alpha-fetoprotein, beta human chorionic gonadotropin, and lactate dehydrogenous are secreted by many germ cell tumors. Additionally, a hormone profile including thyroid hormone and parathyroid hormone may help identify tumors of the thyroid and parathyroid glands. Adrenocorticotropic hormone may be elevated in carcinoid tumors.

Cellular Pathology

In 1999, the WHO Committee on the Classification of Thymic Tumors adopted a new classification system for thymic neoplasms (Marx and Muller-Hermelink 1999). This classification system was based in part on the previous work of Marino and Muller-Hermelink (Marino and Muller-Hermelink 1985) and classified these tumors based upon their cell of origin. Tumors arising from the epithelial cells of the cortex were classified as cortical thymomas, and those arising from the medullary spindle cells were classified as medullary thymomas, finally thymic carcinomas were categorized as a separate entity. Medullary thymomas (WHO Type A) and mixed corticomedullary thymomas (WHO Type AB) were considered benign with minimal risk of recurrence. Pure cortical tumors exhibit intermediate invasiveness and have a measurable risk of relapse after surgery (WHO Type B1-3). The final category is thymic carcinoma, which is always invasive with a high risk of relapse (WHO Type C).

Treatment

The mainstay of therapy for thymoma is complete surgical resection; however, both radiotherapy and chemotherapy may play a role in the definitive management of this disease (Moran and Suster 2008). Thymic carcinoma is often rapidly progressive requiring aggressive multimodality therapy, including cisplatin-based chemotherapy and surgery and/or definitive radiotherapy.

Surgery

Complete surgical resection results in excellent outcome in Masaoka stage I tumors with 90–100% long-term survival. The extent of surgical resection is prognostic with poorer survival (~70%). Incomplete surgical resection and biopsy alone are associated with poor survival (25–30%). In the setting of stage II and III disease adjuvant treatment may be indicated to improve outcome.

Radiation Therapy

Adjuvant radiotherapy can reduce local recurrence rates in stage II and III thymoma from 28% to 5%. (Ciernik et al. 1994) For patients with minimal capsular invasion and who successfully undergo a R0 (complete) resection for a low to intermediate-grade thymoma, adjuvant radiotherapy may not be required. The standard therapeutic approach is to include the entire surgical bed and any adjacent tissue believed to be involved. Conventionally, fractionated doses (1.8–2.0 Gy) are usually employed to a total dose of 45–54 Gy given over 4–6 weeks. Advanced treatment delivery techniques such as gated treatment delivery to minimize the impact of respiratory motion as well as and intensity-modulated radiation therapy to minimize dose to surrounding normal structures may improve the therapeutic ratio for treatment.

Chemotherapy

There has been increased use of chemotherapy in the treatment of invasive thymoma. Doxorubicin, cisplatin, ifosfamide, and cyclophosphamide have all been shown to have single agent activity in the neoadjuvant setting. Combination chemotherapeutic regimens containing cisplatin and doxorubicin have also been employed showing higher clinical response rates. Chemotherapy at the present time is used either in the setting of stage IV disease or to enhance resectability or for cytoreduction prior to radical radiotherapy as part of a multimodality approach.

Cross-References

▶ Four-Dimensional (4D) Treatment Planning/ Respiratory Gating
▶ Intensity Modulated Radiation Therapy (IMRT)
▶ Mediastinal Germ Cell Tumor

References

Ciernik IF, Meier U et al (1994) Prognostic factors and outcome of incompletely resected invasive thymoma following radiation therapy. J Clin Oncol 12(7): 1484–1490

Engels EA, Pfeiffer RM (2003) Malignant thymoma in the United States: demographic patterns in incidence and associations with subsequent malignancies. Int J Cancer 105(4):546–551

Marino M, Muller-Hermelink HK (1985) Thymoma and thymic carcinoma. Relation of thymoma epithelial cells to the cortical and medullary differentiation of thymus. Virchows Arch A Pathol Anat Histopathol 407(2):119–149

Marx A, Muller-Hermelink HK (1999) From basic immunobiology to the upcoming WHO-classification of tumors of the thymus. The second conference on biological and clinical aspects of thymic epithelial tumors and related recent developments. Pathol Res Pract 195(8):515–533

Masaoka A, Monden Y et al (1981) Follow-up study of thymomas with special reference to their clinical stages. Cancer 48(11):2485–2492

Moran CA, Suster S (2008) Thymic epithelial neoplasms: a comprehensive review of diagnosis and treatment. Preface. Hematol Oncol Clin North Am 22(3):xi–xii

Thyroid Cancer

NISHA R. PATEL, MICHAEL L. WONG
Department of Radiation Oncology, College of Medicine, Drexel University, Philadelphia, PA, USA

Synonyms

Papillary carcinoma

Definition

Thyroid cancers refer primarily to carcinomas derived from follicular epithelium or parafollicular C-cell origin. The four main histological variants include papillary, follicular, medullary, and anaplastic cancers, with various clinical and molecular features. Rare thyroid malignancies include sarcomas, hemangioendotheliomas, and lymphomas. Primary thyroid lymphomas constitute 4–8% of all thyroid neoplasms. The majority of lymphomas have been identified as diffuse, large B-cell lymphomas (DLBCLs) with the advent of immunocytochemical staining. Other types of primary thyroid lymphomas include mucosa-associated lymphoid tissue lymphomas (MALTs), mixed tumors (DLBCL+MALT), follicular lymphomas, and Hodgkin's lymphomas.

Background

The thyroid is an endocrine gland with two lateral lobes connected by an isthmus on the anterior aspect of the trachea at the level of the cricoid cartilage. The pyramidal lobe, a narrow cranial projection of tissue from the isthmus, is a remnant of the thyroglossal duct. The primary function of this endocrine gland is to produce and release tropic hormones and calcitonin in a controlled fashion. Thyroid stimulating hormone (TSH) regulates follicular cell proliferation and activity and release of T3 (triiodothyronine) and T4 (thyroxine) into systemic circulation. A negative feedback mechanism regulates hormonal levels with the hypothalamus, pituitary gland, and thyroid gland. Mutations and increased number of TSH receptors have been linked to the development of follicular thyroid cancer.

Thyroid cancer comprises 94–95% of all endocrine cancers and is considered to be the most common endocrine malignancy. According to the American Cancer Society, there has been an increasing incidence of thyroid cancer with an estimated 37,340 new cases per year in 2008 from 30,180 in 2006. Approximately three-fourth of the cases involve women illustrating a preponderance of women affected by the disease. However, thyroid cancer remains to be an uncommon cancer constituting 2% of human malignancies. The rise in incidence may be attributed to increased early detection of well-differentiated tumors.

Papillary carcinoma is the most common histological variant 76–80% followed by follicular (12–17%), medullary (1–4%), and anaplastic (2%). The majority of all thyroid cancer subtypes are sporadic, often linked to a particular molecular pathogenesis. However, factors associated with diet, ionizing radiation, and familial syndromes may impact the frequency and subtype of thyroid cancer. Endemic goiter areas tend to have a higher proportion with anaplastic and follicular variants whereas iodine-supplemented areas constitute a larger proportion of papillary thyroid cancers. Ionizing radiation is also considered to be a known risk factor for the development of papillary thyroid cancers. Most sporadic papillary cancers undergo malignant transformation through mechanistic pathways involving tyrosine kinase receptor mutations. A point mutation in the B type RAF kinase (BRAF) V600E has been associated with aggressive tumor behavior for papillary cancers. In addition, RET/PTC rearrangements have also been linked to papillary cancers developed after ionizing radiation exposure in childhood.

In the past, radiation treatments were utilized for a variety of benign conditions including ailments such as acne vulgaris, tinea capitis, thymic enlargement, and tonsillitis. Exposure to the head and neck region with radiation in this younger population accounted for an increase in frequency of papillary thyroid cancers. The atomic bomb survivors from the 1945 Hiroshima and Nagasaki attacks also have verified an increased incidence of papillary adenocarcinoma in younger women and children exposed to ionizing radiation with neutron and gamma rays, respectively. In addition, children and adolescents living in Ukraine and Belarus at the time of the 1986 Chernobyl nuclear accident were found to have a significant increase in thyroid cancer incidence.

In non-radiation associated thyroid cancers, an increased frequency of HLA-D7 positive patients has been observed particularly in follicular cancers. The majority of medullary cancers are sporadic; however 20–25% of cases arise from autosomal dominant familial syndromes such as MEN2a, MEN2b, and isolated familial MTC. Both types of the multiple endocrine neoplasias are associated with medullary adrenal tumors such as pheochromocytomas with hyperparathyroidism in type 2a and oral mucosal neuromas in type 2b. The molecular basis of these syndromes involves a point mutation in the RET proto-oncogene for a tyrosine kinase receptor. However, the molecular pathogenesis for undifferentiated aggressive, anaplastic thyroid cancers has not been completely understood. Association with a p53 tumor suppressor gene has been implicated in most anaplastic subtypes.

Initial Evaluation

The majority of well-differentiated thyroid cancers include papillary, follicular, and Hurthle cell carcinomas and tend to be asymptomatic. Palpable nodules associated with these subtypes generally are non-tender rubbery-hard in consistency. Occasionally, solitary tender nodules can be found in medullary thyroid cancers with complaints of aches around the neck. However, patients may present with more severe symptoms of airway obstruction or hemoptysis associated with anaplastic cancer and primary lymphomas. Dysphonia may represent locally progressive disease involving the recurrent laryngeal nerve to cause vocal cord dysfunction. Fatigue, weight loss, and night sweats should be concerning for possible systemic symptoms associated with lymphoma.

A palpable neck mass warrants sonographic evaluation to delineate the tumor, abnormal cervical lymph nodes, and the thyroid gland. The primary drainage of the thyroid cancer involves the central compartment with level VI lymph nodes and secondary drainage to the jugular and posterior cervical lymph nodes. Any palpable cervical lymphadenopathy or abnormal thyroid

lesion on the sonogram should have a fine needle aspiration (FNA) performed. FNA has a diagnostic sensitivity of 95–98% and specificity of 97–98%; however it may be considered inadequate in delineating follicular carcinomas from adenomas. Capsular and vascular invasion cannot be assessed on FNA to diagnose follicular or Hurthle cell carcinoma without adequate tissue from a histological surgical specimen.

Overall well-differentiated thyroid cancers have a better prognosis. Independent prognostic indicators for cause specific mortality are age and extrathyroidal invasion. The AGES, AMES, and MACIS prognostic systems have been implemented to predict cause-specific mortality for patients with papillary thyroid cancers. They all include age, tumor size, and tumor extension/invasion with variations on the inclusion of factors such as grade, complete resection, and metastases to evaluate prognosis. Papillary thyroid cancers are generally associated with regional lymph node metastasis and have an excellent prognosis. Follicular and Hurthle thyroid cell carcinomas are also considered well-differentiated, indolent tumors but have a higher likelihood to undergo hematogenous spread. Medullary thyroid cancers are the only non-follicular originated thyroid cancer and may exhibit poorly differentiated features for an aggressive type of tumor. Anaplastic thyroid cancers are considered to be highly aggressive tumors that have an increased propensity to present with distant metastases with very few long-term survivors.

Differential Diagnosis

Well-differentiated thyroid malignancies are often asymptomatic; however, they may present primarily as non-tender palpable nodules in the thyroid. Thyroid adenomas, cysts, and goiter are all benign conditions that must be excluded after sonographic evaluation and tissue diagnosis when applicable. Some patients may present with dyspnea from a locally progressive disease of undifferentiated anaplastic or progressive medullary thyroid malignancies. Possible etiologies for airway obstruction at the time of diagnosis must be excluded, such as advanced laryngeal cancers.

Imaging Studies

Standard radiographs can depict intraglandular calcifications associated with thyroid malignancies, particularly papillary cancers. However, only a limited 10% of clinical cases display such radiological features. Chest X-rays are necessary for the metastatic workup for all well-differentiated thyroid cancers with chest-computed tomography reserved for medullary and anaplastic subtypes.

Ultrasonography is the standard initial imaging evaluation for a solitary nodule in the thyroid. The sonogram should evaluate the size, characteristics of the lesion, suspicious internal microcalcifications, and central-lateral portions of the neck for abnormal cervical lymphadenopathy. Cystic lesions from solid nodules can easily be differentiated; however the presence of benign nodules may hinder early detection of thyroid cancers.

Radionuclide thyroid imaging may be used in the preoperative setting selectively to evaluate the functionality of a thyroid nodule. The TSH level at the time of initial workup may dictate the need for assessment of a "hot" or "cold" nodule in order to exclude benign conditions. The majority of radionuclide thyroid imaging is used in the postoperative setting. Radionuclide imaging primarily utilizes lower doses of Iodine-131 for identification of residual thyroid tumor or metastatic tumor after resection. The available radiopharmaceuticals are Iodine-131, Iodine-125, Iodine-123, and Technitium-99m. The preferable preoperative isotope used for scanning may be Iodine I-123 because of lower radiation doses.

Computed tomography of the neck defines the thyroid gland soft tissue to delineate anatomical extent and morphological characteristics of thyroid neoplasms. CT scans of the chest/mediastinum are used particularly for medullary and anaplastic thyroid carcinomas. Given the aggressive nature of anaplastic thyroid carcinomas, CT scans of the brain and abdomen/pelvis also are included in the initial evaluation for possible metastatic disease. An important consideration is that IV contrast contains high concentration of iodine. This may interfere with radionuclide thyroid imaging if given within 6–8 weeks of scanning, preventing adequate therapeutic uptake during radioactive ablation.

Magnetic resonance imaging has limited uses; however, it can be considered for substernal lesions, identification of recurrent sites, and medullary thyroid carcinomas. PET scans may be considered for highly aggressive lesions that have potential for distance metastasis; however they may have varied sensitivities and specificities based on multiple factors.

Laboratory Studies

The majority of the thyroid cancers are euthyroid with normal TSH levels at the time of diagnosis. However, additional laboratory markers are necessary for adequate workup of medullary subtypes. Medullary thyroid cancers secrete calcitonin, which should be evaluated for basal levels at the time of diagnosis. Carcinoembryonic antigen (CEA) levels are also primarily elevated. Additional screening for pheochromocytomas should be performed to detect metanephrines in the blood or norepinephrine metabolites in the urine for familial cases.

Postoperatively, serum thyroglobulin levels should be evaluated for all well-differentiated papillary, follicular, and HCC carcinomas for evidence of recurrence or metastasis after total thyroidectomies. Medullary thyroid cancers require calcitonin and also CEA for postoperative surveillance to ensure detection in the event that lack of differentiation prevents adequate production of calcitonin. TSH suppression is necessary after total thyroidectomy. Recommended levels postoperatively for well-differentiated resected tumors should remain from 0.1–0.5 mIU/L and <0.1 mIU/L for high-risk thyroid neoplasms.

Staging

PRIMARY TUMOR (T)

TX   Primary tumor cannot be assessed
T0   No evidence of primary tumor
T1   Tumor 2 cm or less in greatest dimension, limited to thyroid
T1a Tumor 1 cm or less, limited to the thyroid
T1b Tumor more than 1 cm but not more than 2 cm in greatest dimension, limited to the thyroid
T2   Tumor more than 2 cm but not more than 4 cm in greatest dimension, limited to the thyroid
T3   Tumor more than 4 cm in greatest dimension limited to the thyroid or any tumor with minimal extrathyroid extension (sternothyroid muscle or perithyroidal soft tissues)
T4   Moderately advanced disease
T4a Tumor extending beyond the thyroid capsule to invade subcutaneous soft tissues, larynx, trachea, esophagus, or recurrent laryngeal nerve
T4b Very advanced disease

Tumor invades prevertebral fascia or encases carotid artery or mediastinal vessels

Regional Lymph Nodes (N)

Regional lymph nodes are the central compartment, lateral cervical, and upper mediastinal lymph nodes.
NX   Regional lymph nodes cannot be assessed

N0   No regional lymph node metastasis
N1   Regional lymph node metastasis
N1a Metastasis to Level VI (pretracheal, paratracheal, and prelaryngeal/Delphian lymph nodes)
N1b Metastasis to unilateral, bilateral, or contralateral cervical (Levels I, II, III, IV, or V) or retropharyngeal or superior mediastinal lymph nodes (Level VII)

Distant Metastasis (M)

M0   No distant metastasis
M1   Distant metastasis

Staging			
Papillary or follicular (differentiated)			
UNDER 45 YEARS			
Stage I	Any T	Any N	M0
Stage II	Any T	Any N	M1
45 YEARS AND OLDER			
Stage I	T1	N0	M0
Stage II	T2	N0	M0
Stage III	T3	N0	M0
	T1	N1a	M0
	T2	N1a	M0
	T3	N1a	M0
Stage IVA	T4a	N0	M0
	T4a	N1a	M0
	T1	N1b	M0
	T2	N1b	M0
	T3	N1b	M0
	T4a	N1b	M0
Stage IVB	T4b	N1b	M0
Stage IVC	Any T	Any N	M1
Medullary carcinoma (all age groups)			
Stage I	T1	N0	M0

Stage II	T2	N0	M0
	T3	N0	M0
Stage III	T1	N1a	M0
	T2	N1a	M0
	T3	N1a	M0
Stage IVA	T4a	N0	M0
	T4a	N1a	M0
	T1	N1b	M0
	T2	N1b	M0
	T3	N1b	M0
	T4a	N1b	M0
Stage IVB	T4b	N1b	M0
Stage IVC	Any T	Any N	M1
Anaplastic carcinoma (all anaplastic considered Stage IV disease)			
Stage IVA	T4a	Any N	M0
Stage IVB	T4b	Any N	M0
Stage IVC	Any T	Any N	M1

Treatment

Surgery

The primary treatment modality for papillary, follicular, HCC, and medullary thyroid cancers is curative thyroidectomy +/− nodal neck dissections. Ten-year survival rates for papillary and follicular thyroid cancers are 93% and 85%, respectively. Total thyroidectomy remains the standard surgical option for high-risk papillary, follicular, and medullary subtypes given the greater risk of early metastatic potential. Subtotal resections such as lobectomies +/− isthmusectomies are controversial for low-risk small papillary thyroid cancers with no evidence of previous radiation, distant metastasis, cervical lymphadenopathy, aggressive histological features, and extracapsular extension within the ages of 15–45 years. According to the NCCN guidelines, <4 cm lesions with these low-risk features are candidates for thyroid preserving surgery. However, various institutions employ total thyroidectomies for all well-differentiated thyroid cancers larger >1 cm as an attempt to improve therapeutic efficacy of adjuvant radioactive ablation (RAI) and to permit thyroglobulin level surveillance for any possible recurrence postoperatively. Total thyroidectomies with adjuvant RAI and thyroid hormone suppression have been shown to have lower recurrence rates of 7.1% in comparison to 18.4% for subtotal thyroidectomies. Prognostic scoring systems such as the AGES, AMES, or MACIS may help the surgeon decipher the adequate approach in regards to papillary thyroid cancer resections. Anaplastic thyroid cancers are highly aggressive and often are not amenable to curative resection at the time of presentation. However, maximum debulking surgery should be performed prior to adjuvant chemotherapy and external beam radiation (EBRT) to improve short-term survival.

For well-differentiated thyroid cancers nodal dissections are reserved for clinically involved nodes without any prophylactic measures. However, medullary thyroid cancers with palpable primary lesions have a risk of up to 60% for nodal metastases. Selective nodal dissections for medullary lesions >1–1.5 cm are performed bilaterally for the anterior central compartment of the neck for dissection of level VI nodes. Further bilateral or unilateral modified radical nodal dissections are selected with regards to clinically or radiologically involved nodal levels from II–V. Prophylactic total thyroidectomies for hereditary conditions are recommended during infancy within the first year of life for MEN2b and prior to age 6 for patients with the 634 RET mutation. Complications from surgical interventions include recurrent laryngeal nerve injury causing vocal cord dysfunction in 1% of cases, hematomas, infections, seromas, and hypoparathyroidism.

T

Radioactive Iodine Therapy

Radioactive iodine therapy provides primary treatment for metastatic well-differentiated tumors. Adjuvant radioactive ablation is also utilized for all papillary thyroid cancers after thyroidectomy. Additional factors to employ radioactive ablation include tumor with size greater than 1 cm, capsular invasion, vascular invasion, multifocal disease, soft tissue invasion, postoperative residual disease, positive or close margins, cervical metastases, or recurrence. However, ablation is not necessary for patients with negative post-resection radionuclide scan with undetectable thyroglobulin <1 ng/mL levels after TSH stimulation and early stage I papillary neoplasm. Radionuclide iodine ablation is performed 4–12 weeks after thyroidectomy and may occur after the performance of a radionuclide scan for the detection of residual disease. About 14 days of restricted iodine intake is necessary prior to ablation treatment and a TSH level of >30uIU/mL. The potential doses of Iodine 131 range widely from 30 to 100 mCi and may require more than one treatment depending on the dose administered for ablation. Visible uptake of <0.1% on scans performed 8 months after ablation is considered to be effective therapy. Higher doses of 150–250 mCi of Iodine 131 are suggested for distant metastasis, nodal metastases, recurrent disease, and postoperative residual disease. Often posttreatment total body imaging may be performed without any further preparation in order to ensure no additional lesions were undetected with prior low dose scanning. Ablation is a relatively well-tolerated treatment modality with symptoms of nausea, emesis, parotitis, sialadenitis, and lung fibrosis for patients treated for lung metastases.

External Beam Radiation Therapy

External beam can be considered an effective modality for palliative treatment of bulky or metastatic disease such as pathological fractures from skeletal metastases, brain metastases, superior vena cava syndrome, and recurrence despite maximal radioactive iodine ablation. External beam radiation in an adjuvant setting is controversial and primarily used in cases with residual disease after incomplete resection. There is no survival benefit for adjuvant radiation in medullary thyroid neoplasm; however improved locoregional control of residual disease after resection warrants external beam therapy irrespective of the presence of metastases at the time of treatment. External beam may also be considered for carcinomas that do not avidly uptake iodine such as Hurthle cell carcinomas as well as medullary thyroid cancers. Anaplastic thyroid cancers can become lethal due to asphyxiation from airway compression caused by local progression of the disease. External beam radiation has demonstrated stabilization of tumor mass in 65% of patients with no further progression. Non-Hodgkin's lymphomas of the thyroid also have illustrated a survival advantage with combined chemotherapy and external beam radiation regimens.

Chemotherapy

Chemotherapy does not have a vital role for the primary treatment of well-differentiated thyroid malignancies. Systemic therapy is reserved primarily for thyroid malignancies that have failed curative surgical intervention. Recently, Vandetanib, an oral tyrosine kinase inhibitor, has been approved for the use of unresectable, symptomatic locally advanced medullary thyroid cancer. Given the aggressive nature of anaplastic thyroid carcinomas, these malignancies are treated with debulking surgery, adjuvant hyperfractionated radiation treatment, and sensitizing weekly doxorubicin-based chemotherapy. Overall the prognosis for anaplastic carcinomas remains dismal and accounts for over 50% of thyroid cancer deaths in the United States irrespective of the multimodality treatment.

The integral use of chemotherapy for curative treatment is employed primarily for non-Hodgkin's thyroid lymphoma. Two randomized prospective clinical trials have evaluated cyclophosphamide, hydroxydaunomycin, vincristine, prednisone (CHOP) with or without involved field irradiation for stages I and II non-Hodgkin's lymphoma with the inclusion of thyroid lymphomas. Combined cycles of CHOP with radiation treatment demonstrated an overall survival benefit. In addition, improvements in outcome have been found with the use of monoclonal antibodies such as rituximab for diffuse large B-cell lymphomas of the thyroid.

Cross-References
▶ Larynx
▶ Lymph Node Regions in Head and Neck
▶ Non-Hodgkin's Lymphoma
▶ Targeted Radioimmunotherapy

References
Edge S, Byrd D, Compton C et al (2010) AJCC cancer staging handbook, 7th edn. Springer, New York, pp 111–120

Gunderson L, Tepper J (2012) Clinical radiation oncology, 3rd edn. Elsevier, London, pp p707–p722

Hall E, Giaccia A (2012) Radiobiology for the radiologist, 7th edn. Lippincott Williams & Wilkins, Philadelphia, pp 136–156

Hoppe R, Phillips T, Roach M (2010) Leibel and Phillips textbook of radiation oncology, 3rd edn. Elsevier, Philadelphia, pp 726–736

Perez C, Halperin E, Brady L (2008) Perez and Brady's principles and practices of radiation oncology, 5th edn. Lippincott Williams & Wilkins, Philadelphia, pp 1055–1075

Tuttle M, Ball D, Byrd D et al (2011) NCCN clinical practice guidelines in oncology: thyroid cancer. National Comprehensive Cancer Network

TisN0M0

▶ Cancer of the Breast Tis

Topoisomerase Inhibitors

RENE RUBIN
Rittenhouse Hematology/Oncology, Philadelphia, PA, USA

Definition
Topoisomerase inhibitors are drugs interfering with the action of topoisomerase enzymes I and II. These enzymes control the changes in DNA structure and act cell cycle specific (S and G2 phase). Etoposide is a topoisomerase 2 inhibitor whereas irinotecan and topotecan act as topoisomerase 1 inhibitors. The drugs are used in non-Hodgkin's lymphomas, small cell lung cancer, and gastric, colon, germ cell, and ovarian cancer.

Side Effects
- Myelosuppression, pancytopenia
- Renal
- Nausea
- Radiation recall syndrome
- Leukemia
- Severe diarrhea
- Interstitial lung disease

Cross-References
▶ Principles of Chemotherapy

Torus Tubarius

BRANDON J. FISHER[1], LARRY C. DAUGHERTY[2]
[1]Department of Radiation Oncology, College of Medicine, Drexel University, Philadelphia, PA, USA
[2]Department of Radiation Oncology, College of Medicine, Drexel University, Glenside, PA, USA

Definition
A ridge in the nasopharynx that lies just posterior to the opening of the auditory tube.

The projection is caused by the cartilaginous portions of the auditory tube and is often referred to as the Eustachian cushion.

Cross-References

▶ Nasopharynx

Total Abdominal Hysterectomy

CHRISTIN A. KNOWLTON[1], MICHELLE KOLTON MACKAY[2]
[1]Department of Radiation Oncology, Drexel University, Philadelphia, PA, USA
[2]Department of Radiation Oncology, Marshfield Clinic, Marshfield, WI, USA

Synonyms

Class I hysterectomy; Extrafascial hysterectomy; TAH-BSO

Definition

A total abdominal hysterectomy (TAH) is the surgical removal of the uterus and cervix. TAH is generally performed with a vertical or horizontal incision and is advantageous because it allows the surgeon to obtain a complete unobstructed look at the uterus and surrounding area. In TAH, only a small portion of the upper vagina and small part of the connected tissues and ligaments are removed.

Cross-References

▶ Endometrium
▶ Ovary
▶ Uterine Cervix

Total Body Irradiation (TBI)

IRIS RUSU
Department of Radiation Oncology, Loyola University Medical Center, Maywood, IL, USA

Introduction

Total body irradiation (TBI) refers to a complex treatment modality that delivers a relatively uniform dose ($\pm$ 10%) of radiation to the entire patient body.

TBI is often used in the treatment of various leukemias, lymphomas, and other hematological disorders. TBI is given as part of preparatory regimens for ▶ bone marrow transplantation in both adult and pediatric patients. These regimens typically employ high dose chemotherapy administered in conjunction with radiation. The purpose of TBI is twofold: (1) to contribute to the eradication of malignant cells or cells with genetic disorders and (2) to immunosuppress the patient sufficiently to prevent rejection of the donor bone marrow.

Although the preparatory regimen can be established with chemotherapy alone, there are some advantages associated with the addition of TBI: (1) the dose delivered to the patient's body is relatively homogeneous and independent of the blood supply, (2) there is no sparing of sanctuary sites which are inaccessible to chemotherapy, and (3) the dose can be customized by shielding critical structures or by boosting areas of greater recurrence risk.

Equipment and Irradiation Techniques

Historically, TBI treatments were carried out with either specially designed machines or with modified conventional therapy equipment. To achieve the desired degree of dose uniformity ($\pm$10% is generally accepted) some of the dedicated systems employed multiple sources of irradiation; however, this method of treatment proved too expensive for most medical centers. The majority of modified conventional therapy equipment (Van Dyk et al. 1986) used either a mobile beam of radiation (e.g., Cobalt 60) that was scanned horizontally across a stationary patient (Fig. 1a) or a mobile couch that was translated through a stationary beam (Fig. 1b). Another system that used a sweeping beam of radiation over a stationary patient (Fig. 1c) was also developed.

Currently, most of the TBI procedures are performed with megavoltage photon beams from linear accelerators that are used for conventional radiation therapy treatments. Unconventional geometries are used to provide the desired large fields, typically 130 cm × 130 cm or greater.

Many different techniques have been reported for the effective irradiation of the whole body (Khan et al. 1980; Van Dyk et al. 1986). They can be divided into two groups: (1) those that utilize large field sizes that encompass the entire patient and (2) those that use multiple smaller adjacent fields to cover the patient's body.

Multiple adjacent fields are used less frequently as they present two distinct problems. First, matching adjacent fields within the accepted dose uniformity is more difficult for large fields due to large divergence of the beam edges and the large patient volumes at the junction region. Second, the cells circulating throughout the body can potentially receive a reduced dose.

The large fields that encompass the entire patient's body can be secured by positioning the patient at an extended distance, typically 3–4 m from the target. Treatments are usually delivered with a horizontal beam directed at a wall which serves as a primary barrier. These techniques are the easiest to employ and most well-established today.

The largest field size on a linear accelerator, 40 cm × 40 cm at the isocenter (1 m from the target), will project to a larger field size, e.g., 160 cm × 160 cm, using an extended source to surface distance (SSD), e.g., 4 m. Also by turning the collimator 45° the patient will lie along the square field diagonal. Positioning the patient within this field should be done carefully since the useful treatment field (90% uniformity) is substantially smaller than the projected light field. Film dosimetry at the time of TBI commissioning can be used to determine how far inside the light field the 90% decrement line lies.

Popular TBI techniques used today have the patient irradiated with parallel-opposed beam configurations: anterior-posterior (AP/PA) or left and right lateral fields (LT LAT/RT LAT).

With the AP/PA technique (Fig. 2a) the patient may be irradiated seated, standing, or lying on one side on a stretcher. This position allows the use of shielding blocks (lung, kidney, liver) when necessary.

The lateral opposed beam technique (Fig. 2b) is usually performed with the patient seated or lying down in the supine position. The ability of the patient to tolerate certain positions must be considered when choosing which technique to use. It is possible to have the patient's legs in a semi-collapsed or fetal position, to decrease the field size required to cover the whole body. Generally, bilateral irradiation requires smaller field sizes than the anterior-posterior technique. Also, careful arm positioning can be used to shield the lungs; the arms should follow the body contour anteriorly in such a way that they will shadow the lungs but not the spinal canal.

Lateral opposed beams will usually produce larger inhomogeneities in dose compared to AP/PA treatments due to larger variation in body thickness along the beam direction. The dose to the head and neck area can be 20–30% higher than that at mid-abdomen. Missing tissue

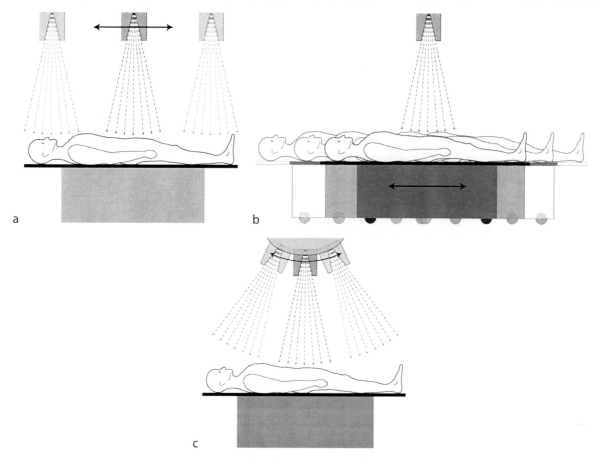

Total Body Irradiation (TBI). Fig. 1 Total body irradiation techniques using modified therapy equipment. (**a**) Mobile beam – stationary patient. (**b**) Mobile patient – stationary beam. (**c**) Sweeping beam

compensators for the head, neck, and legs can be designed to improve dose uniformity (Galvin et al. 1980; Khan et al. 1980; Van Dyk et al. 1986).

As treatment times can be long and patient weakness a common occurrence due to the combined toxicity of TBI and chemotherapy, one should also take into consideration patient comfort, stability, and reproducibility of the TBI setup.

Dose and Dose Prescription

Depending on the specific clinical situation there is a wide range in the prescribed dose-fractionation schemes in use today.

TBI was originally delivered as a single fraction treatment. The total dose was predominantly limited by fatal pulmonary toxicity from interstitial pneumonitis (IP). Since toxicity is influenced by the dose rate and total dose, fractionated and hyperfractionated TBI techniques were subsequently introduced to reduce pulmonary toxicity. High dose TBI with doses ranging from 2 to 14 Gy delivered over 1 to 9 fractions as well as low dose TBI with doses of 0.10–0.15 Gy per fraction delivered over 10–15 fractions have been used (Van Dyk et al. 1986).

The generally accepted dose prescription method for TBI, recommended by the

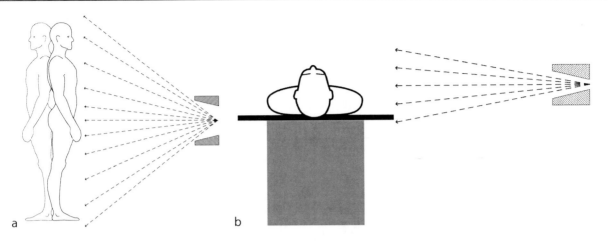

Total Body Irradiation (TBI). Fig. 2 Total body irradiation techniques commonly used today. (**a**) Anterior and posterior irradiation with a horizontal beam. (**b**) Left and right lateral irradiation with a horizontal beam

▶ American Association of Physicists in Medicine (AAPM), uses a single point specification (Van Dyk et al. 1986). The estimated uncertainties in dose delivery must be specified. The point typically used for the dose prescription is midplane at the level of the umbilicus, regardless of the delivery technique. However, many other points have been used (average midline depth of the head, neck, chest, abdomen, etc.). The manner in which the dose is prescribed must be explicitly stated in the prescription.

Dose limits to specific critical organs (e.g., lungs, kidneys) usually is included in the dose prescription. Depending on the clinical requirements the dose rate may be specified as well. Most clinical protocols require low dose rates (8–15 cGy/min) at the prescription point.

Dose Homogeneity

The International Commission of Radiation Units and Measurements (ICRU) (ICRU 1976) has suggested an overall accuracy in dose delivery of ±5%. However for large field geometries this is often difficult to achieve. If the prescribed dose is well below the onset of normal tissue toxicity, or if the dose to normal tissue can be locally limited (e.g., blocking) this accuracy level can be eased.

For TBI treatments, the AAPM suggests (Van Dyk et al. 1986) the use of APARA principle (As Precise as Readily Achievable, technical and biological factors being taken into account). In practice, the generally accepted dose inhomogeneity is ±10% relative to the prescription dose. Nevertheless, the acceptable dose uncertainty should be a clinical decision based on several variables: the available beam energy, the irradiation technique, any treatment room constraints, type of disease, prior radiation treatment history, etc.

One of the many factors that limit the dose homogeneity in TBI is related to the variations in patient thickness. Consequently, irradiation techniques that minimize these variations are more preferable (e.g., AP/PA fields instead of bilateral fields). When treatment room constraints do call for the use of bilateral fields, dose variations can be decreased with the use of compensators or bolus material. Usually, the tissue compensators are one-dimensional compensators made of lead or copper, and are placed at the head of the machine. For a head and neck compensator, the position of the absorber is crucial; an underdose of the shoulders can occur if the compensator is shifted inferiorly or an overdose to the neck can occur if the compensator is shifted superiorly. The tissue-equivalent bolus material is placed directly on the skin, thereby increasing the dose to the skin and decreasing the midplane dose.

Dose homogeneity for parallel-opposed beams can be improved by increasing the beam energy. As a result, there is increased skin sparing and the possibility of underdosing the patient surface. A large spoiler screen placed as close to the patient as possible (typically at distance of no more than 30 cm) can be used to contaminate the incident beam with secondary electrons thereby raising the surface dose to at least 90% of the prescribed dose. A ▶ beam spoiler with a low atomic number such as acrylic or Lucite and a thickness of 1–2 cm will adequately modify the buildup curve.

To further improve dose homogeneity, larger treatment distances should be used if allowed by the room geometry. Ideally distances of at least 3 m from the target to the patient midplane should be used, although techniques that use less than this have been reported (Glasgow 1982).

Shielding Critical Structures

During the course of radiation treatment some critical organs may need to be shielded to either improve dose homogeneity (reduced lung density) or reduce the dose to those particular organs (e.g., kidneys).

The lung is very sensitive to radiation and is easily affected by the therapy regimen (dose, dose rate and fractionation), so knowledge of the lung dose as well as the dose rate during treatment is critical. The lung dose can be estimated from anthropomorphic phantoms measurements or by using computational methods. Without compensating for air density, the dose inhomogeneity in the lungs can exceed the prescribed dose by 10–24% (Van Dyk et al. 1986).

Lung dose can be lowered by using shielding blocks for part of the treatment. This dose should satisfy two criteria: (1) it should be sufficiently high to suppress the immune system and (2) it should be below the dose that causes the onset of radiation pneumonitis.

The shape of the blocks can be determined from radiographic films taken in both anterior and posterior positions. The lung blocks can be placed on the treatment unit head by using a block tray, or directly on the beam spoiler using heavy duty Velcro. Port films are commonly used to check the positioning of the blocks. Since immobilization of TBI patients is not always practiced (patients need to vomit with no advanced notice), patient movement can create a significant problem.

The use of lung blocks results in an overall reduction of the lung dose but does not decrease the dose variation throughout the organ itself. A lower and uniform dose to the lungs can be achieved by using lung compensators although the production of compensators can be a time consuming process.

Depending on the treated disease, doses to other critical structures (e.g., heart, kidneys, liver, and brain) may need to be limited.

If lung blocks are used, the chest wall under the blocks may be boosted with additional electron fields to avoid a decrease in dose to the marrow in the ribs (Van Dyk et al. 1986). The dose prescribed to the inner chest wall is typically 6.0 Gy, delivered over two fractions (Shank and Simpson 1982). The energy of the electron beam is selected to position the 90% isodose line at the lung–chest wall interface.

Due to leukemic relapse in the testes, an electron boost treatment may be added for the male patients. An enface electron beam of appropriate energy, to deliver up to 4.0 Gy, in one fraction to the posterior surface of the testes can be used (Shank and Simpson 1982). Similarly, the energy of the electron beam is selected to position the 90% isodose line at the posterior aspect of the testes.

It has been shown that it is best to design kidney blocks with the patient in the treatment position (Reiff et al. 1999). When compared to the supine position, patients in the upright position show a dramatic inferior shift of the kidneys with other obvious, but less predictable, changes. For patients who must be treated lying on their side, similar shifts in the kidneys size, shape, and position occur. For TBI treatment delivered in non-supine positions, kidney blocks should not be designed on the basis of supine abdominal CT scans.

Phantom Dosimetry

The dosimetry of the large fields at extended treatment distances is significantly different than the conventional short distance treatments. TBI deviates from the standard radiation therapy techniques in multiple ways. In TBI the radiation field is larger than the irradiated volume, which is highly irregular in shape. Also, when dosimetric parameters are measured, a long length of the ionization chamber cable is irradiated in the large field geometry. Special attention should be given to ensure that the stem and cable effects are low and not impacting the measured data. The irradiated cable length should be kept as small as possible and the cable should be covered with buildup material to ensure electronic equilibrium within the cable.

Machine calibration, dosimetry, and monitor unit calculations have been extensively discussed in the literature (Van Dyk et al. 1986; Glasgow 1982; Podgorsak et al. 1985). The basic dosimetric parameters to be measured for TBI are the same as those for standard treatments, including absolute beam output calibration, percent depth dose (PDD), tissue-maximum ratio (TMR), tissue-phantom ratio (TPR), beam profiles, etc.

The minimum recommended phantom size for calibration purposes is 30 cm × 30 cm × 30 cm, although when available, larger phantoms should be used to ensure full scattering conditions (Van Dyk et al. 1986). Calibration is best to be performed under actual treatment conditions including the use of any treatment aids which will be used clinically such as shields, compensators, beam spoiler, etc.

Regardless of which dose ratio parameter will be used for TBI dosimetry, special attention should be given to its characteristics under these unusual treatment conditions. For conventional treatments, some dose ratio parameters (TMR, TPR) are considered independent of distance. The validity of this statement should be confirmed for the particular TBI geometry to be used. Also, dose ratio parameters requiring in air measurements (e.g., tissue-air ratio TAR) should not be used since they can be affected by backscatter from the treatment room wall. Furthermore, if percentage depth dose ratios are used, they should be measured for the particular treatment geometry since the use of Mayneord's factors can be erroneous at these very extended distances. The simple extrapolation of dosimetric data from conventional field sizes and treatment distances is not acceptable.

After a particular technique has been commissioned for clinical use, the calculated doses should be confirmed by performing measurements in anthropomorphic phantoms as well as in vivo verification in patients. Thermoluminescent dosimeters (TLD's) are the usual choice for monitoring the dose to the patient. Direct measurement of midline doses in patients can be performed at limited locations (mouth, between the legs or the feet, near the axilla for bilateral field irradiation). In most cases, the midline dose can be estimated from entrance and exit surface measurements. Surface measurements should be done with adequate build-up material to provide full electronic equilibrium. Corrections should be made to the exit dosimeter's reading for the lack of full scatter at this position. Accurate placement of the exit dosimeter is also very important and port films can be used to confirm it.

TBI Implementation into Clinic

Any TBI protocol should be set up as a special treatment procedure following a careful plan of implementation, with attention to the nature of the patients, the limitations of the treatment room, as well as the available equipment.

First, a medical decision must be made regarding the total dose to be prescribed, the dose-fractionation scheme, the allowable dose inhomogeneity, the dose rate at the prescription point, and the dose to the critical structures.

Second, a treatment technique should be instituted. Frequently, conventional treatment facilities do not have the optimum extended SSD to achieve the large radiation fields required for TBI treatments. Hence, the available SSD may be partially responsible for the selected TBI technique.

At extended distances, the patient is typically set up against a primary barrier wall. To deliver the desired dose at the distance of the patient, the weekly and hourly workloads at the isocenter will increase so that special consideration should be given to the existing shielding characteristics of the primary barrier. Also, the composition of the primary barrier has to be taken into account since this can influence the dose the patient receives from scattered neutrons. Steel or lead slabs present in the primary barrier will result in an increased neutron dose equivalent delivered to the patient compared to a concrete barrier.

When new rooms are designed for TBI, ideally large SSDs can be achieved and special attention can be given to the room shielding. For example, the accelerator can be offset 1 m from the room center to allow a larger SSD to one wall.

A comprehensive quality assurance program should be set up to cover performance of the equipment used for treatment planning and dose delivery. This program should be extended to treatment aids as well: positioning equipment, blocks, compensators, block cutter, etc. Furthermore an in vivo dose measurement technique should be available when setting up a new TBI program. It is a good practice to verify the patient dose on the first treatment fraction.

References

Galvin JM, D'Angio GJ, Walsh G (1980) Use of tissue compensators to improve the dose uniformity for total body irradiation. Int J Radiat Oncol Biol Phys 6:767–771

Glasgow GP (1982) The dosimetry of fixed, single source hemibody and total body irradiators. Med Phys 9:311–323

International Commission on Radiation Units and Measurements (ICRU) (1976) Determination of absorbed dose in a patient irradiated by beams of X or gamma rays in radiotherapy ICRU Report 24, 1976

Khan FM, Williamson JF, Sewchand W et al (1980) Basic data for dosage calculation and compensation. Int J Radiat Oncol Biol Phys 6:745–751

Podgorsak EB, Pla C, Evans MD et al (1985) The influence of phantom size on output, peak scatter factor, and percentage depth dose in large–field photon irradiation. Med Phys 12:639–645

Reiff JE, Werner-Wasik M, Valicenti RK et al (1999) Changes in the size and location of kidneys from the supine to standing position and the implications for block placement during total body irradiation. Int J Radiat Oncol Biol Phys 45:447–449

Shank B, Simpson L (1982) The role of total body irradiation in bone marrow transplantation for leukemia. Bull N Y Acad Sci 58:763–777

Van Dyk J, Galvin JM, Glasgow GP et al (1986) The physical aspects of total and half body photon irradiation. Task Group 29, Radiation Therapy Committee Report. American Association of Physicists in Medicine Report No. 17

Total Nodal Radiation

▶ Elective Nodal Irradiation

Total Skin Electron Beam (TSEB)

CURT HEESE
Department of Radiation Oncology, Eastern
Regional Cancer Treatment Centers of America,
Philadelphia, PA, USA

Definition

Total skin electron beam irradiation is a technique utilizing extended treatment distances and multiple patient orientations to successfully deliver electron radiation to the whole skin surface of a patient. Often, smaller fields are needed for certain surfaces not in the primary treatment fields (e.g., soles of feet).

Cross-References

▶ Cutaneous T-Cell Lymphoma

Total Skin Electron Therapy (TSET)

DAVID LIGHTFOOT
Radiation Oncology Department, Grand View
Hospital, Sellersville, PA, USA

Background

Total skin electron therapy (TSET) is used to treat a variety of shallow malignant conditions of the skin. One of the conditions in which it is considered to be a useful therapy is mycosis fungoides. Mycosis fungoides (MF) is the most common of the various classifications of cutaneous T-cell lymphoma (CTCL). CTCL is a rare disease category with an overall annual incidence of about 6.4 per million/year. The annual incidence of MF is about half of that (3–4 million/year). Due to the protracted course of the disease, the prevalence is about ten times the annual incidence. In terms of the current US population, there are about 1,600–2,000 new cases of CTCL each year with approximately half of them diagnosed as MF, resulting in an estimated prevalence of 8,000–10,000 patients. Although the term "mycosis fungoides" implies a bacterial infection that mimics a fungal infection, it is a misnomer. In MF, there is a malignant accumulation of T-helper cells (some sources specifically say CD4+ cells) within the dermis that is responsible for the symptoms of the disease. All treatments of the skin for MF are essentially palliative since they control only the T-cells that have accumulated in the skin and not the source of the T-cells which, due to their affinity for the dermis, will continue future accumulation as they are produced. TSET originally was a desperate attempt to do something to relieve suffering when all non-radiation treatments were no longer helping the patient. The results proved to be dramatic in some cases with total clearing of extensive plaques within a matter of a few weeks after a dose to the skin of 6 Gy. There was no question that even these earliest attempts at TSET relieved suffering and extended the life of the patients. The experience to date indicates the duration of remission ranges from as little as a few months to longer than a decade. With experience, it was discovered that higher doses were required to increase the probability of remission. Current prescriptions in the range of 30 to 36 Gy is associated with remission in more than 90% of the treated patients. This higher dose is also associated with a longer duration of remission. There is a growing trend to use TSET in earlier disease stages to increase its usefulness. The need for repeated treatment at the end of remission means the initial treatment dose needs to be kept low enough to allow subsequent treatment without exceeding skin tolerance. Studies are now in progress to determine the effectiveness of 12 Gy combined with systemic drugs. It may be possible to increase the permissible number of subsequent treatments with greater extension of life with such a combination.

X-Ray Contamination

X-rays are produced in some of the interactions of energetic electrons with the atoms located between the source of the electrons and the patient. The most likely types being bremsstrahlung x-rays produced by direct interaction between an electron and an atomic nucleus, and characteristic x-rays produced by the filling of inner orbit vacancies created by interaction between an energetic electron and an inner orbit electron. Such x-rays may be produced anywhere within an electron beam, including the collimating structures, the air in the beam path, shielding material placed on a patient, and the patient tissues irradiated by the beam of electrons. The dose to a patient beyond the depth of penetration of the electron beam is generally referred to as the dose due to x-ray contamination or bremsstrahlung contamination. Autopsies of seven of the first TSET patients treated in the 1950s disclosed that two of the seven had aplastic anemia that was attributed to the effects of the radiation. Hence, another requirement of TSET is to minimize the x-ray contamination of the electron beam to minimize the side effects of exposing the total body to x-rays. The recommendations of Task Group 30 of the American Association of Physicists in Medicine given in AAPM Report 23 suggest an accumulated total body x-ray dose of less than 1% of the skin dose as a desirable goal. For the various techniques of TSET described in the report, the lowest dose from x-ray contamination was associated with the Stanford technique with reported 10-cm depth x-ray contamination ranging

between 0.1% and 0.7% of the maximum electron dose for a single dual beam. Since dual beams are applied for the six patient orientations in the Stanford technique, the total dose depends on how many orientations increase skin dose and how many orientations increase the x-ray dose. All orientations increase x-ray dose but points on the skin receive significant dose from only two or three of the orientations. This results in an increase in the relative x-ray dose by a factor of about 2.0–2.4 to an overall value between 0.2% and 1.7% of the prescribed skin dose. A variety of other techniques in use at various facilities have reported acceptable whole body x-ray dose of the order of 2–3% of the prescribed skin dose. Some facilities are reportedly willing to accept x-ray doses as high as 5% of the prescribed skin dose. The AAPM report indicates that many clinicians consider values of 4% or higher clinically unacceptable. In general, higher electron energy means higher x-ray contamination. Treating a patient whose MF has reached the tumor phase of disease expression may require higher electron energy for adequate depth of treatment with a necessity to accept an increase in whole body x-ray dose. Careful attention to the atomic composition and thickness of the materials used for collimating structures, scattering foils, energy degraders, and patient shielding can reduce x-ray contamination.

Treatment Techniques and Associated Dosimetry

The use of x-rays to treat MF dates to 1903. The much higher penetrating power of x-rays places severe limits on the dose that can be administered to the skin due to the tolerance limits of underlying tissue. Recognition of the nearly absent dose beyond the extrapolated range of an electron beam sparked the interest in TSET. The earliest use of TSET in the USA dates to 1951 as a specialized application of a Van de Graaff accelerator in Boston. Scattering foils and an aluminum cone were placed in the path of a beam of

2.5 MeV electrons. The scattering foils reduced the electron energy to about 2 MeV, resulting in a beam that produced maximum dose at a depth of 4 mm with a maximum penetration (extrapolated range) of 10 mm. The end of the cone was provided with an aperture that limited the size to 1 cm in the superior/inferior dimension of the patient and 45 cm laterally at an SSD of 118 cm. With the beam aimed straight down the patient was moved feet first under the beam by a motorized couch at a rate of 6 ft/min to deliver a dose of 1 Gy to the exposed skin. The patient was initially scanned in four positions (prone, supine, right lateral, and left lateral) to treat the total skin. This was later increased to six and finally eight orientations. Shielding placed on the patient limited the lateral edges to avoid overlap of dose from adjacent scans. Under such an arrangement, there is considerable amplification of the relative total body x-ray dose. Any point on the skin surface receives electron dose only from one orientation while points deeper than the extrapolated range receive dose from each of the four, six, or eight different orientations. In addition, the defining aperture limits the size of the electron beam without necessarily limiting the amount of the x-ray contamination. An x-ray contamination beam that is five or ten times the size of the aperture in the scanning direction will amplify the relative x-ray dose by a factor of 5 or 10 as the patient is scanned. The amplification of the relative amount of x-ray dose was a definite problem in the initial stages of development that had undesirable effects on some of the initially treated patients. Appropriate modifications enabled the method to continue in use without excessive x-ray contamination.

The next significant development in TSET was the technique put into use at Stanford in 1958 to treat the total skin with electrons accelerated in an isocentrically mounted radio frequency linear accelerator (LINAC). The technique is designed to treat a patient in a standing position with a beam that provides adequate uniform coverage over an area that is approximately 200 cm in vertical dimension by 80 cm in lateral dimension. The technique is relatively easy to implement and is perhaps the most widely used TSET technique. It is designed to minimize x-ray contamination and its associated risk of harm from accumulated total body x-ray dose. The essence of the technique is to broaden a LINAC electron beam with treatment distance and scattering foils, reduce its maximum penetration to about 19 mm with energy degraders, and to minimize x-ray contamination effects by directing the maximum zone of x-ray contamination above and below the trunk of the patient. Since the beam spreads out with increasing distance, the maximum available distance between the source and the patient is usually employed. Typical facility designs usually limit the usable SSD to about 400 cm.

A typical commissioning of a Stanford TSET technique usually follows the following sequence. The LINAC is operated with the normal electron applicators removed and a special attachment to permit the extraction of the largest possible electron beam size at a high dose rate in place. Unless the LINAC is designed specifically for the beam energy and angular spread required for TSET, a beam energy in the range of 6–9 MeV is selected. With the beam aimed horizontally, the depth dose is measured in a water equivalent plastic phantom or thin-walled water phantom at the treatment distance. Based on the results, an added water equivalent thickness of material is chosen to limit the extrapolated range to 19 mm. The required thickness of polystyrene, Plexiglas, or water equivalent plastic is then added as a relatively small panel to the LINAC housing or as a large size panel placed about 20 cm in front of the plane of treatment or a combination of partial thickness in both locations. A small plastic panel added to the LINAC housing (a beam spoiler) serves as both a scattering foil that increases the size of the electron beam and an energy degrader that limits the depth of penetration. The scattering from a large plastic panel placed near the patient does not significantly increase the size of the electron beam but does aid in the uniformity of treatment.

Published results indicating that placing a small panel on the housing results in x-ray contamination exceeding 15% have not been found to be reproducible by this author. On the contrary, an initial finding of such a level on one occasion was found to be an erroneous indication due to electrons penetrating the cable attached to an ionization chamber. The correct measurement of x-ray contamination requires the proper algebraic average of results with both positive and negative collecting voltage. This is especially important in TSET measurements where significant lengths of cable may be exposed.

With the beam spoiler and/or large scattering panel in place, measurements are made at various machine angles to determine the angle above and below horizontal where the beam intensity is at half-maximum. This is then used as the starting point for producing a dual beam. If the dual-beam uniformity does not prove to be adequate (a vertical uniformity of ±8% and a horizontal uniformity of ±4% over the central 160 × 60 cm area of a 200 × 80 cm treatment plane), adjustments of angles and scattering materials are made to obtain satisfactory results (Fig. 1).

Angled beams matched at 50% of maximum yield good vertical uniformity. Gantry angles found to result in optimum uniformity vertically for the Stanford technique must produce a field size of the combined beams at the patient treatment plane approximately 200 cm in height by 80 cm in width to encompass the largest patient. Final approval of beam energy, location and thickness of beam spoiler, and angles of beams combined to form a dual beam is dependent on the acceptable uniformity of the dual beam. An evaluation of this on even a relatively coarse grid of points separated by 10 cm horizontally and

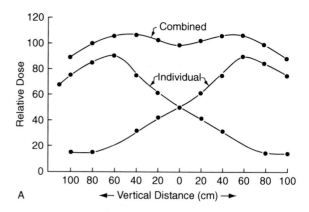

Total Skin Electron Therapy (TSET). Fig. 1

20 cm vertically as depicted on the diagram at left amounts to 77 points of measurement. This means several repeat measurements with somewhat imprecise detectors such as film, TLD, or OSL dosimeters must be performed in order to achieve adequate precision; alternatively, many exposures with a single precision detector such as an ionization chamber moved from point to point may be used (Fig. 2).

Matching the beams used in the Stanford technique will require a dual beam with a most probable energy of 3.8 MeV. The most probable energy, $E_{p,0}$ in MeV, is computed from the extrapolated range, R_p in cm, by $E_{p,0} = 1.95 R_p + 0.48$. The individual beams which are angled upward and downward to create the dual beam will each have a slightly higher most probable energy of 4.2 MeV. The difference is due to angulation of the beam through the beam spoilers. The beams can also be characterized by their average energy at surface, $\bar{E}_0$ in MeV, which is computed from the depth of 50% of the maximum dose, R_{50} in cm, by $\bar{E}_0 = 2.33 R_{50}$. The original Stanford beams individually had a 50% of maximum dose at a depth of 1.3 cm (3.03 MeV $\bar{E}_0$) and a dual beam 50% of maximum dose range of 1.13 cm (2.6 MeV $\bar{E}_0$). Since it is not highly likely that a facility can match both the most probable energy and average energy at surface of the original Stanford dual

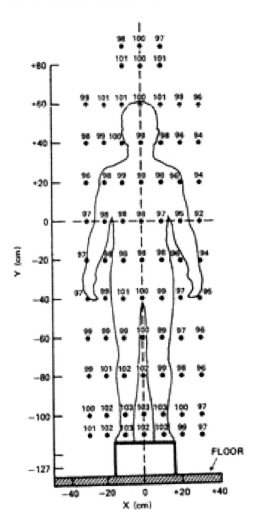

Total Skin Electron Therapy (TSET). Fig. 2

angulation between the upward and downward directed beams with a third horizontal beam to boost a central cold spot or strictly horizontal beams with different vertical positions. Another method, used at McGill University, is a strictly horizontal beam with a beam compensator placed on the LINAC housing. The compensator has a central aluminum disk mounted on a sheet of lead foil and attached to a rigid sheet of plastic with top and bottom corners removed. With the aluminum disk comprised of stepped circles of aluminum foil or a solid disk machined to create a greater reduction of the intense central portions without significantly reducing the intensity of the outer lower intensity regions, a single horizontal beam with adequate uniform size to perform TSET may be obtained. These alternatives tend to increase the x-ray contamination relative to the Stanford technique.

To lessen the risk of fall from the platform on which the patients stand, patients can simply stand on the floor and the gantry angles can be adjusted to center the dual beam at 100 cm above the floor at the treatment plane rather than at the higher isocenter height. In such a method, electrons scattered from the floor introduce some additional vertical asymmetry. For patients that are too debilitated to stand, placing them on a wheeled platform whose top surface is as close to the floor as possible allows treatment of the exposed skin surface with multiple gantry angles or an electron beam arc. Such a technique will generally have a higher dose from x-ray contamination and less than perfect uniformity than the techniques designed for a standing patient, and should therefore be reserved for appropriate clinical needs. Information about variation in beam energy as defined by depth dose characteristics at all points in the treatment plane is generally not published for any of the techniques, and an assumption of uniform energy if there is uniformity in maximum dose is implicit in technique descriptions.

beam, it is best for both measures of energy to equal or exceed the Stanford values. This frequently means a matched most probable energy and a higher than Stanford value average energy at surface. The characteristics of the dual beam should be used for calculating the descriptive beam energy terms for comparison with the characteristics of the Stanford dual beam.

In addition to variations in the beam energy chosen for TSET at various facilities, there are many facilities that do not use the dual-beam geometry. Modifications of the original dual-beam Stanford technique have included large

Electron Beam Calibration for TSET

After adjustments are completed to establish a beam of proper energy and uniformity, the final step in the commissioning process is calibration. Calibration is required of the dual beam at the depth of maximum dose, and its relationship to the surface dose for a simulated full treatment of a standardized cylindrical water or water equivalent phantom of 30 cm diameter × 30 cm height needs to be established to enable use of the calibration. The calibration is performed in a flat phantom of sufficient size to achieve full dose from electrons scattered by surrounding phantom material into the point of measurement. This may be achieved by a phantom with length, height, and width dimensions equal to twice the extrapolated range plus the dimensions of the detector. Because of the low energy of the electrons, lateral dimensions of 15 cm and thickness greater than 10 cm may be more than sufficient and convenient to used; however, larger sizes and thickness are also quite acceptable. Traceability of calibration to national standards is usually through use of ionization chambers and electrometers calibrated by an ▶ Accredited Dosimetry Calibration Laboratory (ADCL). The calibration of the TSET beam requires use of a parallel plate chamber which may not be directly calibrated by an Accredited Calibration Laboratory. The procedures recommended by the American Association of Physicists in Medicine and other recognized authoritative groups usually specify transfer of calibration from a cylindrical chamber to a parallel plate chamber by intercomparison of readings at appropriate depths for identical successive exposures of each chamber in an electron beam with the highest available energy and with full corrections applied for differences in the beam quality used for calibration of the cylindrical chamber and the quality of the beam used for intercomparison at the depth of measurement. Further correction of the parallel plate results is then based on the differences in stopping power ratio between the energy at the point used for intercomparison of the chambers and the energy at the point used for calibration of the TSET dual beam. All corrections are explained in the AAPM TG-51 protocol which is in general use at many radiation therapy facilities.

The TG-51 protocol requires a correction for the polarity of the collection voltage used by the ion chamber. This factor is a relatively minor correction factor in electron beams of limited size and there is a tendency to verify the correction less frequently than for every calibration. Because of the large size of TSET dual fields, electrons may penetrate a significant length of the cable attached to the ionization chamber, resulting in a substantial increase in the required correction, especially in lower dose regions. For TSET calibration, it is absolutely essential that measurements be made with both polarities of collection voltage with careful attention to the polarity of electrometer readings and proper algebraic averaging based on the sign of the collection voltage and not the sign of the measurement results; that is, do not average absolute numbers – subtract one result from the other and then divide by 2 to obtain a true average that does not include a contribution from direct injection of electrons into the cable that connects the ionization chamber to the electrometer.

TSET Treatment and Clinical Judgments

In the Stanford technique, the patient is placed in a standing position at the treatment distance with a varied orientation that exposes a different skin surface to the dual beam on sequential exposures. The initial use of four orientations at 90° orientation was eventually modified to the use of six orientations at 60° intervals around the circumference of the patient. A typical prescription fraction is achieved from all six orientations over two visits. At one visit, the patient has three orientations that give maximum dose to the anterior and posterior-oblique skin surfaces. On the next visit, the three different orientations give maximum dose to the posterior and anterior-oblique skin surfaces. For each orientation, the patient is positioned with feet spread and arms raised or lowered to minimize self-shielding of other skin surfaces. Since the patient does not have a perfectly cylindrical shape, there is considerable nonuniformity in dose as various body parts shield some portions of the skin. This generally requires additional radiation to the shielded areas based on the clinical judgment of the radiation oncologist of the extent of the area of the boost fields needed. These will generally not be clearly defined but will usually include the soles of the feet, the perineal area, the dorsal surface of the penis, the skin in the perianal region, and the inframammary region in females with large breasts. In some situations, boost fields have also been necessary for the top of the head and the ear canal. An indication of the size and shape of boosted regions may be gleaned from the following pictures of special shielding devices designed for such a purpose (Figs. 3, 4, 5).

Nonuniformity of TSET patient skin dose also includes areas of excessive dose, such as toes and fingers, that require added shielding during portions of the treatment. It is often customary to use either external or internal eye shields. Internal eye shields require the addition of wax, hardened tape, or aluminum casings to avoid excessive eyelid dose from back-scattered electrons. The treatment facility must also have provisions for subtotal skin electron therapy when shielding above the shoulders or below the umbilicus is medically required. Static measurements of nonuniformity may represent a worse-case assessment since variation in patient positioning during the approximately 18–20 fractions of prescribed dose tends to smooth out the

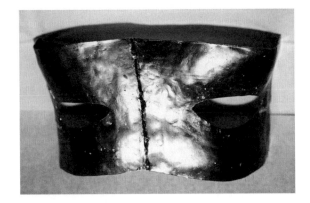

Total Skin Electron Therapy (TSET). Fig. 3 Boost for the inframammary regions

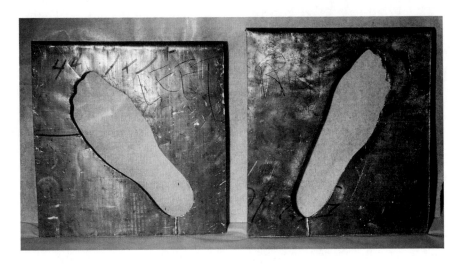

Total Skin Electron Therapy (TSET). Fig. 4 Boost for the soles of the feet

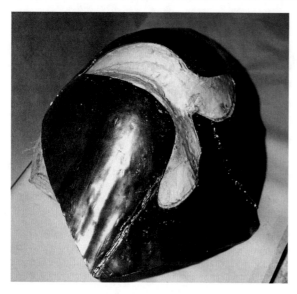

Total Skin Electron Therapy (TSET). Fig. 5 Boost for the perianal region

variations. Some facilities have developed techniques to slowly rotate the patient during TSET to reduce the nonuniformity resulting from a fixed number of orientations. The results of TSET have not been reported as significantly different between fixed patient orientations and treatments with patient rotation. A sample TSET prescription is shown in the following table.

Sample mycosis fungoides (MF) TSET treatment prescription (This example prescription is not to be construed as representative of all MF patient treatment prescriptions!!)	
1. Dose	36 Gy/9 weeks
	4 Gy/week
	4 days/week
	3 dual fields/day
2. Eyes shielded throughout	
3. Scalp shielded after 25 Gy if no involvement above neck	
4. Protect feet with 20 cm high shield after first 10 Gy when sole boost starts (Otherwise, boost blisters tops of feet)	

5. Boost soles and perineum After first 10 Gy Rate, 1 Gy/day
6. Protect fingers and other sensitive areas as needed

The Stanford technique does not result in a uniform surface dose even to a perfectly round or cylindrical shape, and does not treat with the same depth dose characteristics of the individual beams comprising the dual beam. Rather than attempting to fully account for variations due to the patient geometry, the prescription is fulfilled by considering it to represent the average surface dose on a water equivalent cylinder of 30-cm diameter and 30-cm height. For six equally spaced orientations of the cylinder, a simple consideration of geometry will reveal that a point that is centered in one of the dual beams will receive the surface dose from that beam plus the 60° oblique surface dose from two adjacent orientations. A point halfway between that point and an adjacent corresponding point will receive surface dose only from the 30° oblique surface dose of two adjacent fields. Hence, the surface dose may be expected to be on average only about 2.5 times the surface dose of a single dual field with ±20% variation around the circumference of the cylinder. Because of the diffuse cloud of electrons in the TSET dual beam, there will always be some contributions from scattered electrons to the surface dose at a point from beams that do not have a direct view of the point from a given orientation. A prime example of this is the discovery that the vertex of the scalp of a standing patient can be increased to nearly full dose by the placement of a lead sheet above the head of a patient to scatter electrons onto the vertex field.

It turns out that the maximum dose of the combined fields is at or within 1 mm of the skin surface as determined both by analysis and measurement. It also turns out that the dose decreases much more rapidly with depth than might be expected from the characteristics of a single dual beam. For example, a dual beam that has a dose equal to 80% of maximum at a depth of 8 mm will produce a combined depth-dose from all six orientations of a cylinder that delivers a dose of 80% of maximum only to a depth of 2 or 3 mm. The relationship between the calibrated maximum dose per monitor unit of the dual beam and the average surface dose for all six orientations is clearly a complex function of the dual-beam surface dose and scattering materials near the patient. The relationship is thus usually evaluated by calibrating a batch of radiographic or radiochromic film at the depth of maximum dose for a dual beam and then using other pieces of film from the same batch taped tightly to the 30 cm diameter by 30 cm height water equivalent cylindrical phantom and making a simulated treatment. The results obtained at various facilities usually show a TSET surface dose that is 2.5–3.0 times the single dual-beam maximum value. This may also be stated as 41–50% of the summated maximum dose from six dual-beam exposures. For patient rotation simulations, a value of surface dose equal to 41% of the total stationary maximum dose has been reported. Film has also been used in a horizontal orientation cut to the shape of anatomically shaped phantom material to evaluate the distribution of the summated dose.

Ozone Production

Considerable ozone is created as the large electron beam traverses the air in the treatment facility. Long-term protection of health requires a sufficiently rapid rate of exchange of room air and may require the assistance of individuals with proper expertise and equipment to assess the ozone hazard.

Quality Assurance

Quality assurance in TSEB means performing check measurements of the calibration and beam uniformity immediately before each session of patient treatments. This is necessitated by the possibility of failure to add proper beam modifiers which are usually not completely checked by the interlock circuits of the LINAC. There is also the possibility of otherwise undetectable damage to the modifiers or dose-measuring circuits. Most facilities will develop a standardized checklist and test measurements to enable a "ten-minute" QA procedure.

The development of a TSET facility should allow adequate time for its development. The required amount of time for commissioning measurements alone is expected to require several weeks and maybe even months if many adjustments are found to be necessary.

Cross-References

▶ Cutaneous T-Cell Lymphoma
▶ Electron Dosimetry and Treatment
▶ Linear Accelerators (LINAC)
▶ Mycosis Fungoides
▶ Radiation Detectors
▶ Skin Cancer

Total Vascular Exclusion

Lydia T. Komarnicky-Kocher[1], Fiori Alite[2]
[1]Department of Radiation Oncology, College of Medicine, Drexel University, Philadelphia, PA, USA
[2]College of Medicine, Drexel University, Philadelphia, PA, USA

Definition

Surgical technique for excision of hepatic tumors near the vena cava which involves cross clamping the suprahepatic and subhepatic vena cava and occluding the porta hepatis.

Cross-References

▶ Palliation of Metastatic Disease to the Liver

Traditional Medicine

▶ Biomedicine (also Traditional, Theoretical, Conventional, or Western Medicine)

Transitional Cell Carcinoma

CHRISTIAN WEISS, CLAUS ROEDEL
Department of Radiotherapy and Radiation
Oncology, University Hospital Frankfurt/Main,
Frankfurt, Germany

Definition

The predominant histology of bladder cancer in the Western countries.

Cross-References

▶ Bladder
▶ Bladder Cancer

Translational Research

▶ Clinical Research and the Practice of Evidence-Based Medicine in Radiation Oncology

Transvaginal Ultrasound Study (TVS)

PATRIZIA GUERRIERI, PAOLO MONTEMAGGI
Department of Radiation Oncology, Regional
Cancer Centre "M. Ascoli", University of Palermo
Medical School, Palermo, Italy

Definition

TVS (Transvaginal Ultrasound Study): It is an ultrasound study carried out by introducing a transducer into the vagina. It is part of the imaging studies useful for diagnosis, staging, and follow-up of female genital tract diseases.

Cross-References

▶ Endometrium
▶ Fallopian Tube
▶ Ovary
▶ Uterine Cervix

Trastuzumab (Herceptin)

TOD W. SPEER
Department of Human Oncology, University of
Wisconsin School of Medicine and Public
Health, UW Hospital and Clinics, Madison,
WI, USA

Definition

A humanized monoclonal antibody against the HER2/neu receptor. It is indicated for treatment of Her2/neu positive breast cancer.

Cross-References

▶ Her-2
▶ Targeted Radioimmunotherapy

Treatment or Management of Central Nervous System Involvement or Dissemination

▶ Palliation of Brain and Spinal Cord Metastases

Treatment or Management of Liver, Splenic, Lung, and Pelvic Metastases

▶ Palliation of Visceral Recurrences and Metastases

Trismus

LINDSAY G. JENSEN, LOREN K. MELL
Center for Advanced Radiotherapy Technologies
Department of Radiation Oncology, San Diego
Rebecca and John Moores Cancer Center,
University of California, La Jolla, CA, USA

Definition
Difficulty in opening the mouth.

Cross-References
▶ Salivary Gland Cancer

TRUS: Transrectal Ultrasound

YAN YU, LAURA DOYLE
Department of Radiation Oncology, Thomas
Jefferson University Hospital, Philadelphia,
PA, USA

Definition
Nonionizing imaging procedure involving a rectal probe with transverse and/or sagittal ultrasound crystals.

Cross-References
▶ Brachytherapy: Low Dose Rate (LDR) Permanent Implants (Prostate)
▶ Colon Cancer

Tuberous Sclerosis

STEPHAN MOSE
Department of Radiation Oncology,
Schwarzwald-Baar-Klinikum,
Villingen-Schwenningen, Germany

Definition
This is a rare disease (TSC 1, chromosome 9q34 or TSC 2 16p13) characterized by the development of benign tumors (multiple renal angiomyolipomas, renal cysts, polycystic renal disease, cardiac rhabdomyomas, angiofibromas, fibromas, nevi) in different organs (brain, kidney, lung, heart, eyes, skin) and by the rare diagnosis ($<1\%$) of a renal cell carcinoma.

Cross-References
▶ Benign Tumors
▶ Kidney

Tumor Control Probability (TCP)

BRIAN F. HASSON[1,2], DAREK MICHALSKI[3],
M. SAIFUL HUQ[4]
[1]Department of Radiation Oncology, Abington
Memorial Hospital, Abington, PA, USA
[2]Department of Radiation Oncology, College of
Medicine, Drexel University, Philadelphia,
PA, USA
[3]Division of Medical Physics, Department of
Radiation Oncology, University of Pittsburgh
Cancer Centers, Pittsburgh, PA, USA
[4]Department of Radiation Oncology, University
of Pittsburgh Medical Center Cancer Pavilion,
Pittsburgh, PA, USA

Definition
The probability that a given dose of radiation will provide tumor control or eradication considering

the specific biological cells of the tumor. The 'TCP' is used in treatment planning as a tool to differentiate among treatment plans.

Cross-References

▶ Four-Dimensional (4D) Treatment Planning/ Respiratory Gating
▶ Statistics and Clinical Trials
▶ Stereotactic Radiosurgery: Extracranial

Tumor Hypoxia

CLAUDIA E. RÜBE
Department of Radiation Oncology, Saarland University, Homburg/Saar, Germany

Definition

Situation where tumor cells have been deprived of oxygen. As a tumor grows, it rapidly outgrows its blood supply, leaving portions of the tumor with regions where the oxygen concentration is significantly lower than in healthy tissues. Hypoxic tumor cells are usually resistant to radiotherapy and Induction Chemotherapy, but they can be made more susceptible to treatment by increasing the amount of oxygen in them.

The correlation between radiosensitivity and the pressure of oxygen is generally referred to as "oxygen effect."

Eppendorf microelectrode allows the direct measurement of the oxygen tension in tumor tissue.

Hypoxia markers are surrogate endogenous or chemical markers of tumor oxygenation (e.g., hypoxia-inducible factor HIF-1α).

Cross-References

▶ Predictive In vitro Assays in Radiation Oncology

Tumor of the Adrenal Cortex

STEPHAN MOSE
Department of Radiation Oncology, Schwarzwald-Baar-Klinikum, Villingen-Schwenningen, Germany

Synonyms

ACC; Adrenal cortical carcinoma; Adrenocortical carcinoma

Definition

The adrenocortical carcinoma is a rare cancer developing within the cortex of the adrenal gland. The tumor is associated with gland-specific hormonal dysfunction.

Cross-References

▶ Carcinoma of the Adrenal Gland

Tumor Potential Doubling Time (Tpot)

CLAUDIA E. RÜBE
Department of Radiation Oncology, Saarland University, Homburg/Saar, Germany

Definition

Defined as the time within which the cell population of a tumor would double if there is no cell loss.

Cross-References

▶ Predictive In vitro Assays in Radiation Oncology

Tumor Suppressor Gene

BRADLEY J. HUTH
Department of Radiation Oncology,
Philadelphia, PA, USA

Synonyms
Anti-oncogene; Gate-keeper gene

Definition
This describes genes which downregulate genetic replication. These are often referred to as genetic gatekeepers as they often oversee key checkpoints within cellular replication. Loss of heterozygosity (LOH) in tumor suppressors may lead to malignant degeneration of a cell. This was first described by Knudson when he described the Two-Hit Hypothesis where the normal allele expression accommodates for the other mutated allele. Transmissions of these errors often occur in a recessive manner. There are exceptions, such as p53 mutation, where the mutated gene shows a dominant phenotype by impeding the normal protein function.

Cross-References
▶ Colon Cancer

Turcot Syndrome

TONY S. QUANG
Department of Radiation Oncology, VA Puget Sound Health Care System University of Washington Medical Center, Seattle, WA, USA

Definition
This is a mismatch repair syndrome having an association between familial polyposis of the colon and brain tumors such as medulloblastoma and malignant glioma.

Cross-References
▶ Primary Intracranial Neoplasms

Type I Error

EDWARD J. GRACELY
Department of Epidemiology and Biostatistics, College of Medicine, Drexel University, Philadelphia, PA, USA

Definition
Claiming that the research demonstrates a difference or effect, when in fact the observed differences or effects are due to chance.

Cross-References
▶ Statistics and Clinical Trials

Type II Error

EDWARD J. GRACELY
Department of Epidemiology and Biostatistics, College of Medicine, Drexel University, Philadelphia, PA, USA

Definition
Claiming the absence of a difference or effect, when in fact the research failed to uncover a true difference or effect due to chance.

Cross-References
▶ Statistics and Clinical Trials

Tyrer-Cuzick

▶ Breast Cancer Risk Models
▶ GAIL

U

Understanding Radiation Oncology Billing, Collections, and Insurance Issues

PAUL J. SCHILLING
Community Cancer Center of North Florida,
Gainesville, FL, USA

Understanding Medicare

For patients who have Medicare Part B as their primary insurance (these are the majority of radiation oncology patients), Medicare has a predetermined fee which is paid for each medical procedure, billed as a current procedural technology (CPT) code. Medicare pays 80% of this allowable, and the patient's secondary insurance pays the remaining 20%. Charges are electronically billed, turnaround time to receive payment can be as few as 14 days. Some secondary insurances will take between 6 and 9 months to pay the final 20%. Many secondary insurances must be billed using a paper claim sent through the mail instead of an electronic claim, thus delaying payment for up to 6 months (Schilling 2007a). Medicare Part B provides outpatient services for patients in a bundled fashion – professional and technical components of radiation treatment are paid in one lump sum.

Hospital-owned, hospital-based radiation oncology practices bill under Medicare Part A. This provides for a technical component of radiation treatment delivery for the hospital, the professional component for physician services is billed separately, also under Medicare Part A.

The basis on which the technical component is paid to the hospital is called an ambulatory payment classification (APC). APC groups have different payments based on the complexity of radiation treatment delivery. The payments under the APC classification compared to those paid to outpatient freestanding facilities vary widely. For example, radiation treatment delivery for intensity-modulated radiation treatment, code 77418, is paid to the hospital under Medicare Part A at considerably less than the rate paid to freestanding centers under Medicare Part B. Alternatively, code 77370, special medical physics consultation, is paid to the hospital at approximately twice that paid to a freestanding facility (CMS 2010a).

For a freestanding radiation oncology center, Medicare Part B is billed and a global fee is paid. This global fee combines both the professional fee to the physician and the technical fee to the equipment owner in one bundled payment. Some (CPT) codes have a professional component only, and some codes have a technical component only. Other codes have both professional and a technical component, indicating that the physician and the equipment owner split this code based on their investment of physician time or equipment ownership. Calculating the professional/technical "split" in an outpatient facility can be difficult and depends on the payer mix, as well as the complexity of patients treated. The professional/technical split is calculated using the relative value units assigned to each CPT code. The relative value units (RVUs) are units of work assigned by Medicare, with each unit of work having a standard reimbursement.

L.W. Brady, T.E. Yaeger (eds.), *Encyclopedia of Radiation Oncology*, DOI 10.1007/978-3-540-85516-3,
© Springer-Verlag Berlin Heidelberg 2013

Understanding Radiation Oncology Billing, Collections, and Insurance Issues. Table 1 Model radiation oncology treatment courses to estimate professional/technical split

IMRT prostate		
CPT Code	**Professional RVUs**	**Technical RVUs**
99245	5.89	
77263	4.40	
76370	1.18	3.09
77280	1.94	7.24
77290	4.24	13.60
77417		8.82
77300	15.48	25.20
77336		24.96
77427	36.16	
77334	23.66	47.46
77470	2.85	11.64
77301	21.46	58.34
77418		754.32
	117.26	954.67
	10.93%	89.10%
3-D conformal treatment		
99245	5.89	
77263	4.40	
76370	1.18	3.00
77280	0.97	3.60
77290	4.24	13.60
77295	6.22	29.17
77417		6.30
77300	5.16	8.40
77336		21.84
77427	31.64	6.80
77334	8.45	16.95
77414		80.52
77470	2.85	11.64

Understanding Radiation Oncology Billing, Collections, and Insurance Issues. Table 1 (continued)

77315	2.12	2.78
	73.12	197.80
	27%	73%
Palliative treatment		
99245	5.89	
77263	4.40	
76370	1.18	3.09
77290	2.12	6.80
77417		1.89
77300	7.72	2.80
77336		6.24
77427	9.04	
77334	3.38	6.78
77414		24.40
77315	2.12	2.78
	35.85	54.78
	35.30%	64.70%

The relative value units in professional/technical split are shown in Table 1 and, as can be seen, vary depending on the complexity and objective of treatment. Calculating the professional/technical split is often difficult for physicians who are in freestanding centers, and eligible to receive the professional component. In general, the professional component of global collections is approximately 11–35%, depending on the payer mix, with an average of 26%. See Table 1 for professional/technical split that varies depending on the course and complexity of treatment delivered. Patients who are hospitalized under Medicare Part A may need radiation treatment during their hospital stay. The technical component of radiation treatment is included in the diagnosis-related group payment for the patient's hospital stay. Freestanding cancer centers must collect payment from the hospital for technical component of radiation treatment and cannot bill Medicare Part B while a patient is hospitalized during radiation treatment.

Sustainable Growth Rate Versus Medical Economic Index

Medicare Part B (physician services) provides an annual update in allowable charges based on the Gross Domestic Product. From the years 2000 through 2010, this has required a reduction in Medicare payment and thus Medicare allowable. These cuts have been forestalled by congress for the past 7 years (CMS 2010b). The Medicare Economic Index (MEI) is an annual update for Medicare Part A (hospital services) that is based on the rate of medical inflation. This has resulted in a yearly increase in payments to hospitals (CMS 2010b). If physician services were paid according to the MEI, we would be reimbursed at 20% more than we are now.

Appealing Denied Medicare Claims for Radiation Oncology

In January 2006, the Centers for Medicare and Medicaid Services (CMS) reduced the maximum time for adjudicating appeals for denied claims from a maximum of 1,000 days to 300 days. Nearly 20% of processed Medicare claims are denied. However, only 5% of denied Medicare claims are appealed (Schilling 2004; Schilling 2005).

Physicians are successful in appealing payment denial in more than 60% of cases, indicating that the appeals process can be rewarding for you. If resubmitting the first rejection does not resolve the problem, the first level of appeal is called a "fair hearing," and is usually conducted by telephone. You simply need to write a letter to the Medicare carrier requesting a fair hearing. The minimum denied amount needed to appeal a denied claim is $100. Multiple denied claims on different patients can be batched together as long as the appeal is greater than $100. Include the appropriate documentation with the appeal and *Current Procedure Technology* (CPT) book definitions to describe what medical care was rendered and why you should be paid. Much to your surprise, most of the reviewers are not familiar with radiation oncology coding or the CPT coding books. Your job is to teach the reviewers to do their job and pay you.

For the carrier who habitually denies the same code, a previous favorable ruling may get the same code paid over and over again. In this situation, your goal is to use the last favorable ruling as evidence that the same denied code should be paid. This actually works, and sometimes they just pay the bill without the hearing as described above (Schilling 2005).

For all fair hearings, the Medicare carrier is required to give you a written decision within 90 days. If the fair hearing process results in additional denial, the next step is a hearing before an administrative law judge. This is much more formal, and some suggest that you should have legal representation. During the fair hearing process, the hearing officer will allow you to tell them why a patient needed the (denied) care and provide documentation that you were able to help them based on available clinical evidence. During an administrative law hearing, the judge is only interested in whether the law allows him to pay you or not. Do not be afraid to try the appeals process if you feel the denial is inappropriate, and again, most often you will win (Schilling 2004; Schilling 2005).

Medicare Medically Unlikely Edits

A Medically Unlikely Edit (MUE) is a limit on the number of units of a CPT code that would be reported for a patient on one day (Schilling 2009). Medically unlikely edits were developed based on clinical judgment, and these were reviewed by insurance medical directors of Medicare and/or

Medicare Intermediary insurance companies. MUEs are used to screen out too many units of service done in a single day. For example, an appendectomy can only be done once on a patient on one day (or ever) and reporting two appendectomies on the same day of service would be impossible. Medicine as a profession can expect Medicare to pass more medically unlikely edits in the future (Schilling 2009). These may be adopted by private insurance programs as well. MUEs apply to a number of procedures in radiation oncology including dose calculations (Code 77300), device charges (Code 77334), and IMRT plan (77301). If you find yourself the victim of not being paid due to medically unlikely edits, the first level of appeal as described above is a fair hearing, and the next level of appeal is an administrative law hearing. There is no prohibition for additional payments if clinically necessary.

Bundling Edits

Medicare and some managed care organizations "bundle procedures together" so that only one charge is paid rather than two separate services. For example, weekly physics management 77336 may not be able to be billed with dose calculation 77030, when rendered. The managed care organization may think that the dose calculation is bundled into the weekly physics management (Schilling 2006). It is essential to understand what these bundled codes are and where they conflict. Many times, this information is difficult to obtain during the contracting process. The best time to know about bundling edits is before you sign an insurance contract. It is important to have a well-trained billing staff so that they can understand when payment denials are based on bundling. Patient care decisions need to be made as to what specific service is required on a specific day.

Effective January 1, 2010, Code 77338 replaced device charge 77334 used for each multileaf pattern for Medicare patients receiving IMRT. This code is used one time per IMRT plan (77301) and replaces multiple charges for multileaf patterns. Unfortunately, the reimbursement for this code is below what would be reimbursed under the prior system. Prior to 2010, if a head and neck cancer patient receives a ten beam, ten gantry angle, IMRT treatment, code 77334 was billed for a quantity of ten separate multileaf patterns used in treatment. Currently, code 77338 replaces ALL of these charges and can only be billed with quantity of one, not ten (Schilling 2010a). Florida Medicare 2010 reimbursement for 77338 is $459 and for 77334 is $145. Thus, one charge of 77338 represents 3.2 charges of 77334, enough to pay for only 3.2 of the multileaf patterns for the above head and neck cancer patient (Schilling 2010a).

Medicare Advantage Health Maintenance Organization Insurance Plans

During 2007, Medicare Advantage Health Maintenance Insurance Programs were created. The insurance companies who administer Medicare HMOs are currently reimbursed up to 19%, more than traditional Medicare pays for each senior's care (Schilling 2007a; Schilling 2010b). The seniors who sign up for Medicare Advantage plans often receive less care, but pay higher co-pays, higher deductibles, and more than half of Medicare plans pay physicians below traditional Medicare rates. Many seniors do not realize that with a Medicare Advantage plan that they need a secondary insurance to pay for the additional costs that Medicare Advantage does not provide. More than 2,000 physicians responding to an American Medical Association survey on Medicare HMOs noted that Medicare HMOs routinely denied services typically covered by traditional Medicare plans including colonoscopies, PSA blood tests, and other cancer screenings. A survey of patients enrolled in Medicare Advantage HMOs reported that 80% of them did not understand their plans and 60% did not realize they were actually giving up traditional Medicare (Schilling 2010b). Some seniors are being sold Medicare HMO plans through abusive marketing practices. The center for Medicare and Medicaid singled out insurers including United, Humana, Coventry, and Cigna for abusive marketing techniques and these companies were advised to take steps to pay closer scrutiny to their sales personnel. Medicare Advantage plans have created an incentive for insurance companies who sponsor these plans to enroll healthy new patients. The bottom 50% of Medicare recipients spends only 3% of Medicare health dollars (Schilling 2010b). Insurance companies have found ingenious ways to enroll healthy seniors while being inconvenient to patients with many chronic diseases who might cost more. These include offering free gym memberships to those enrolled (this appeals to the healthiest, most ambulatory seniors), limiting home health-care services or requiring high co-pays, limiting chemotherapy and radiation treatment for cancer patients, holding dinner seminars for prospective enrollees in places that require a long drive at night which may be far from public transportation or which require traversing several sets of stairs. An investigation by the Medicare Payment Advisory Commission 2004 found that Medicare HMOs were designing their plans to avoid paying for kidney dialysis, chemotherapy drugs, and radiation treatment. In a New England Journal of Medicine article, currently enrolled Medicare HMO members spent only 66% of the average cost of non-Medicare HMO patients during the year prior to joining the HMO. Seniors departing from Medicare HMOs went on to spend 180% of this average, indicating that sicker patients were leaving Medicare HMOs possibly due to higher out-of-pocket costs. Cancer treatment, unfortunately, continues to be extraordinarily expensive. We must keep an eye out as to where cost shifting is going in the future and educate seniors (Schilling 2010b).

Radiation Oncology Negotiation with Managed Care Plans

In 1937, Dr. Sidney Garfield provided prepaid medical care for Henry J. Kiser's company in California, and was the beginning of managed care in the United States. Managed care proliferated with the objective to reduce health-care costs for workers covered by health-care plans paid for by their employers (Schilling 2007a; Schilling 2006).

Many physicians have experience negotiating the rate of compensation for their contracts. However, a managed care company may be reluctant to disclose their fee schedule if other physicians in the area are contracted with them. You should begin the negotiation by making an inquiry for ten codes most commonly used in radiation oncology. Oftentimes, a managed care program will send the reimbursement for ten codes total. From this it is possible to get an idea as to what their rate of payment is, and whether you wish to continue the negotiation (Schilling 2007b; Schilling 2006).

Many contracts are tied to the reimbursement rate for Medicare and pay at rates listed as a percentage of Medicare reimbursement. Some managed care plans pay you based on "100% of regional managed care company's usual and customary fees." Often, this is below Medicare rates, and it is imperative to know exactly how you are being paid (Schilling 2007a; Schilling 2006). Many managed care companies want you to take a fee reduction across the board for all radiation oncology CPT codes. Try to negotiate reduction in only a few codes (used less often), which may have a less deleterious effect on your practice. Always attach a comprehensive fee schedule to all contracts and make the insurance company signs off on this, as an exhibit, it clearly prevents confusion later. Some managed care companies will try to get you to contract for a case-rate structure. In this scenario, for any patient who requires radiation treatment, a certain dollar amount would be paid regardless of treatment complexity. Case-rate arrangements can sometimes be tiered, which allows two to three levels of complexity paid at a fixed rate. Case-rate reimbursements are difficult to manage and frequently do not increase year to year, while the complexity of treatment does increase. The physician is advised to use caution in accepting any case-rate structure (Schilling 2006).

There are a few managed care companies that reimburse based on a capitation basis. Under this scenario, a certain amount of money is paid monthly to the radiation oncology group to provide services regardless of the covered population's average age or need for radiation treatment. These contracts are extraordinarily difficult to negotiate and manage. Ultimately, to remain solvent, you would need to know the age of the population insured, as well as their cancer incidence, cancer screening availability, etc. Unfortunately, this information usually resides with the insurer, and likely they will not share this with the physician. Capitation rates can also be calculated from population-based data using the Surveillance and End Results Data (SEER data) (Schilling 2007a). Nonetheless, this data underestimates the incidence of cancer and the volume of cancer treated.

For hospital-based practices, it may be necessary for the managed care company to have a contract with the hospital for the technical component of radiation treatment and a contract with the radiation oncologist for professional services. Pitfalls to watch for include a provision that the codes with a professional/technical split must be billed on the same day by both the hospital and physician for either to obtain payment. This puts the physician in the position of auditing the hospital charge capture, a notoriously inefficient process (Schilling 2007a).

A contract with the managed care company should spell out emergency care provisions. Many

times, emergency treatment for spinal cord compression or brain metastasis, etc., will be provided, and a managed care company will later indicate that this was a noncovered service on an emergency basis. Thus, an entire course of treatment may be denied in this way (Schilling 2006).

Silent Preferred Provider Organizations

Because of the rise of managed care, a new process has been promulgated whereby a network in which a physician is contracted as a preferred provider is sold to another health plan without the physician's knowledge or consent (Schilling 2007b). This creates a "silent PPO" in which a discount is extracted from the physician's usual and customary fees without the physician's consent. The net result is a secondary discount where an insurer (often times with a low number of patients) pays only the physician's discounted fee without the physician ever receiving the benefit of any additional patient volume. In most instances, physicians become aware that they are victims of a silent PPO after providing services to a patient with indemnity insurance. When payment is made on the behalf of an insurance company, the discount is applied even though the patient is not a member of the PPO and the physician is not a contracted member of that insurance organization. Unfortunately, there is no Health Insurance Portability and Accountability Act (HIPAA) statute governing selling lists of physicians and their associated contracted discounts. The American Medical Association estimates that there are $750 million to $3 billion lost annually in the United States by physicians to silent PPOs (Schilling 2007; Tippet 2006). The American Medical Association was successful in banning silent PPOs from all federal employee health insurance benefits contracts. However, currently state insurance boards generally provide insurance regulation. A few states including North Carolina, Louisiana, Oklahoma, California, and Texas have passed legislation to combat this practice (Tippet 2006). One step to combat this practice is to carefully read all contracts. Many health insurance contracts contain provisions that allow them to enter contracts with "other payers on the physician's behalf." If this language appears in your contract, insist on striking it. Additional language to protect yourself might include the prohibition of selling, renting, or leasing networks providing any information about a fee schedule to anyone without your express permission (Schilling 2007b). Currently, the only recourse after an in-appropriate discount has been applied and you have been paid in-appropriately is to use the legal system. As always "an ounce of prevention is worth a pound of cure," so to be sure to look for the above clauses and lobby your State Medical Association to pass legislation that protects physician information and patient information.

References

CMS (2010a) Centers for medicare and medicaid services web site: sustainable growth rate 2010. www.hhs.gov.med

CMS (2010b) Centers for medicare and medicaid services web site: medical economic index 2010. www.hhs.gov.med

Schilling PJ (2004) Managing the insurance denials and appeals process. American college of radiation oncology practice management guide. American College of Radiation Oncology, Bethesda, pp 67–69

Schilling PJ (2005) Tips on how to appeal denied medicare claims for radiation oncology. American College of Radiation Oncology ACROGRAM, May 26, 2005

Schilling PJ (2006) Radiation oncology negotiation for managed care. American college of radiation oncology practice management guide. American College of Radiation Oncology, Bethesda

Schilling PJ (2007a) Economics of radiation oncology, chapter 98. In: Halperin EC, Perez CA, Brady LW (eds) Perez and Brady's principles and practice of radiation oncology, 5th edn. Philadelphia, Lippincott Williams & Wilkins, pp 2043–2049

Schilling PJ (2007b) ACRO alert: beware of the silent preferred provider organization. American College of Radiation Oncology, Bethesda, MD

Schilling PJ (2009) ACRO alert: medically unlikely edits do not mean impossible reimbursement. American College of Radiation Oncology, Bethesda, MD

Schilling PJ (2010a) ACRO alert: code 77338 replaces 77434 multiple custom multileaf device charges for medicare IMRT patients

Schilling PJ (2010b) ACRO newsletter: do medicare HMOs cherry pick healthy seniors to enroll? August 2010

Tippet TN (2006) Emergence of the silent preferred provider organization. J Fla Med Assoc 6–7

Uniform Scanning (US)

DANIEL YEUNG[1], JATINDER PALTA[2]
[1]Department of Radiation Oncology, University of Florida Proton Therapy Institute, Jacksonville, FL, USA
[2]Department of Radiation Oncology, University of Florida Health Science Center, Gainesville, FL, USA

Definition

A technique to generate a broad beam by using magnets to sweep a fairly large beam spot in both the x- and the y-direction. The beam intensity is kept constant (uniform) irrespective of the lateral position of the beam during scanning.

Cross-References

▶ Proton Therapy

Unsealed Source Brachytherapy

▶ Targeted Radioimmunotherapy

Unusual Nonepithelial Tumors of the Head and Neck

CARLOS A. PEREZ
Department of Radiation Oncology, Siteman
Cancer Center, Washington University Medical
Center, St. Louis, MO, USA

Definition
Unusual tumors and cancers of the head and
neck region are generally those presenting with
either rare incidences or with an atypical histopathology. Tumors and cancers of the head
and neck regions are frequently associated
with the development of squamous cell
or adenocarcinomas as common histopathologic
diagnoses. While more and more of these
"conventional" carcinomas are becoming associated with specific risk factors, they generally
arise from the lining membranes of the upper
aerodigestive tract. These tumors are usually
classified by the TNM staging system into distinct risk groups.

Cross-References
- ► Chloroma
- ► Chordomas
- ► Epstein-Barr Virus (EBV)
- ► Esthesioneuroblastomas
- ► Extracranial Meningioma
- ► Extramedullary Plasmacytomas
- ► Eye and Orbit
- ► Glomus Tumors
- ► Hemangiopericytomas
- ► Lethal Midline Granuloma
- ► Nasopharyngeal Angiofibroma
- ► Nasopharynx
- ► Plasma Cell Myeloma
- ► Sarcomas of the Head and Neck
- ► Soft-Tissue Sarcoma

Upper Tract Urothelial Carcinoma

- ► Renal Pelvis and Ureter

Upper Urinary Tract Carcinoma

- ► Renal Pelvis and Ureter

Ureter Cancer

- ► Renal Pelvis and Ureter

Urethral Caruncle

STEPHAN MOSE
Department of Radiation Oncology,
Schwarzwald-Baar-Klinikum,
Villingen-Schwenningen, Germany

Definition
A benign inflammatory lesion of the distal urethra that is most commonly found in elderly
women. Symptoms may be pain, dysuria, and
occasionally bleeding.

Cross-References

▶ Renal Pelvis and Ureter

Urethral Inverted Papilloma

STEPHAN MOSE
Department of Radiation Oncology,
Schwarzwald-Baar-Klinikum,
Villingen-Schwenningen, Germany

Definition

Inverted papilloma is rarely diagnosed in the male urethra. Frequent symptoms are dysuria, hematuria, and/or urethral bleeding. The diagnosis is based on ultrasound, endoscopy, and urethrocystoscopy demonstrating the filling defect. Transurethral resection is the treatment of choice.

Cross-References

▶ Human Papilloma Virus (HPV)
▶ Male Urethra

Urinary Tract

▶ Bladder
▶ Kidney

Urothelial Carcinoma

▶ Bladder
▶ Renal Pelvis and Ureter

Urothelial Carcinoma Of Upper Urinary Tract

▶ Renal Pelvis and Ureter

Uterine Cancer

▶ Endometrium

Uterine Cervix

MICHELLE KOLTON MACKAY[1], CHRISTIN A. KNOWLTON[2]
[1]Department of Radiation Oncology, Marshfield Clinic, Marshfield, WI, USA
[2]Department of Radiation Oncology, Drexel University, Philadelphia, PA, USA

Synonyms

Carcinoma of the uterine cervix; Cervical cancer; Cervical malignancy; Uterine corpus

Definition

Cervical cancer encompasses a group of malignant histologic entities that arise from diverse types of tissues contained within the uterine cervix or cervical region. This group of diseases includes squamous cell carcinoma, adenosquamous cell carcinoma, adenocarcinoma, neuroendocrine carcinoma, small cell carcinoma, glassy cell carcinoma, and sarcoma of the cervix.

Background

Cervical cancer accounted for approximately 11,000 cancer diagnoses in the United States and

4,000 cancer deaths in the year 2009 (American Cancer Society 2009). It is the third most common gynecologic malignancy after endometrial cancer and ovarian cancer. The incidence of cervical cancer has decreased in the United States; however, this disease continues to be a problem in less developed countries and is the second most common malignancy in women worldwide. Over 490,000 cases of cervical cancer are diagnosed annually worldwide and cervical cancer causes approximately 270,000 deaths worldwide. The decrease in the rates of cervical cancer in the United States can be attributed to better education and effective screening with the ▶ Papanicolaou smear (Pap smear).

A large portion of cervical cancer is caused by the human papillomavirus (▶ HPV), making exposure to HPV the greatest risk factor for cervical cancer. Because of this causative relationship, cervical cancer can be considered a sexually transmitted disease. The two types of HPV most associated with viral transmission of disease are HPV 16 and 18. HPV 16 is the most commonly associated strain and is accountable for approximately 50% of cases of cervical cancer. HPV 16 tends to be more associated with squamous cell carcinoma whereas HPV 18 is more associated with adenocarcinoma. HPV 31, 33, 45, and 59 are also known to be associated with the disease. The available vaccines for cervical cancer, Gardasil (Merck, Whitehouse Station, NJ) and Cervarix (GlaxoSmithKline, Philadelphia, PA) have been developed against the HPV 16 and 18 strains and are approved by the US Food and Drug Administration (FDA) for use in the United States.

Molecular biology studies have determined at least two pathways in which the HPV proteins interact with genetic pathways to increase cell division leading to cervical cancer. The E6 protein of HPV binds with p53, causing degradation of the p53 tumor suppression actions and leading to unrestricted cell division. The E7 protein of HPV binds to the retinoblastoma gene, causing disassociation of the retinoblastoma and the EF2 transcription factor complex. The association of this complex normally allows regulation of cell division; however, by disassociating this complex, unregulated cell proliferation occurs in excess. Other genetic abnormalities that have been associated with cervical cancer include c-*myc* overexpression and *Her*-2 neu overexpression.

Other risk factors associated with cervical cancer include smoking, chronic immunosuppression, early age of onset of coitarche, multiple sexual partners, and multiparity. HIV infection is also a risk factor and the combination of HIV and cervical cancer is an AIDS-defining illness.

The most useful screening tool for cervical cancer is the Pap smear, which has greatly reduced the incidence and mortality of cervical cancer. The Pap smear can be helpful in identifying precancerous changes. The current American Cancer Society recommendation for cervical cancer screening is to begin screening with a yearly Pap smear about 3 years after onset of vaginal intercourse or no later than 21 years of age. Beginning at 30 years of age, if a woman has had three consecutive normal Pap tests, she may transition to screening every 2–3 years (American Cancer Society 2009). Women may consider stopping cervical cancer screening after 70 years of age if they have had three or more consecutive negative Pap tests.

Cervical cancer includes a broad range of diseases from the histologic standpoint. The most common histologic subtype of cervical cancer is squamous cell carcinoma, which accounts for approximately 80% of the diagnoses. The second most common type is adenocarcinoma, accounting for 15% of cervical cancers. Adenosquamous carcinomas encompass less than 5%. Other rare pathologic types include small cell carcinoma, sarcoma, neuroendocrine carcinoma, and glassy cell carcinoma.

Staging is an important factor in determining treatment course and outcomes. Two staging systems are used in staging, the tumor-node-metastasis (TNM) classification and the Federation Internationale de Gynecologie (FIGO) classification. Table 1 details the staging for these systems. Cervical cancer is a clinically staged disease.

The TNM staging classification also categorizes patients according to anatomic stage of disease and prognostic group (detailed in Table 2).

Initial Evaluation

The first step in evaluation of cervical cancer is to perform a thorough patient history and examination including evaluation for vaginal bleeding or discharge, pelvic pain, hematuria, and rectal bleeding. An extensive examination is important in cervical cancer as it is a clinically staged disease and the stage of the disease will guide direction in treatment. Extensive gynecologic evaluation including a rectovaginal examination, preferably under anesthesia, should be performed to assess extent of tumor. During examination under anesthesia, tissue can be obtained and sent for pathologic analysis to confirm a histologic diagnosis. Cystoscopy and sigmoidoscopy should also be performed to assess whether the disease involves the bladder or rectum.

Differential Diagnosis

The differential diagnosis for cervical cancer includes cervical polyps, cervical condyloma, cervicitis, cervical pregnancy, and metastasis from other malignancies (ovarian, endometrial, gastrointestinal).

Imaging Studies

Although cervical cancer is a clinically staged disease, imaging studies are very helpful in determining treatment approach. FIGO staging allows for findings on physical exam, chest x-ray, intravenous pyelogram (IVP), cystoscopy, and proctoscopy to determine stage (National Comprehensive Cancer Network 2010).

However, after establishing the cervical cancer, diagnosis imaging studies to assess extent of disease should also be performed and include a computed tomography scan of the chest, abdomen, and pelvis, and ► positron emission tomography/computed tomography (PET/CT) scan. A barium enema may also be performed to assess disease extent involving the rectum.

PET/CT scans have been very helpful as a preoperative diagnostic tool to determine the best treatment approach. If not performed preoperatively, it should certainly be performed after surgery if risk factors for recurrence are found on pathology including lymphovascular invasion, positive margins, parametrial involvement, or positive lymph nodes.

Laboratory Studies

The Pap smear and cervical biopsy with HPV analysis should be performed and are often the first step in establishing a tissue diagnosis for cervical cancer. Other laboratory tests important in evaluation of cervical cancer include a complete blood count, metabolic panel with liver function tests, blood urea nitrogen and creatinine levels, and urinanalysis.

Treatment

Treatment options for cervical cancer depend on the stage of the disease. The stage of cervical cancer is determined clinically; therefore examination is very important. Treatment of early-stage disease generally involves surgery. In patients with stage IA1 disease, surgical options include a cone biopsy with negative margins or hysterectomy with either a ► modified radical hysterectomy or extrafascial hysterectomy. In stage IA2 disease, a ► radical hysterectomy is recommended. Some patients may wish to preserve fertility, and therefore avoiding a hysterectomy is important. ► Radical trachelectomy can be carefully considered in these patients. In patients who are not surgical candidates, radiation therapy using

Uterine Cervix. Table 1 Cervical cancer staging

Primary tumor		
TNM	**FIGO**	
TX		Primary tumor cannot be assessed
T0		No evidence of primary tumor
Tis	a	Carcinoma in situ (preinvasive carcinoma)
T1	I	Cervical carcinoma confined to uterus (extension to corpus should be disregarded)
T1a[b]	IA	Invasive carcinoma diagnosed only by microscopy. Stromal invasion with a maximum depth of 5 mm measured from the base of the epithelium and a horizontal spread of 7 mm or less. Vascular space involvement, venous or lymphatic, does not affect classification
T1a1	IA1	Measured stromal invasion 3 mm or less in depth and 7 mm or less in horizontal spread
T1a2	IA2	Measured stromal invasion more than 3 mm and not more than 5 mm with a horizontal spread 7 mm or less
T1b	IB	Clinically visible lesion confined to the cervix or microscopic lesion greater than T1a/IA2
T1b1	IB1	Clinically visible lesion 4 cm or less in greatest dimension
T1b2	IB2	Clinically visible lesion more than 4 cm in greatest dimension
T2	II	Cervical carcinoma invades beyond uterus but not to pelvic wall or to lower third of vagina
T2a	IIA	Tumor without parametrial invasion
T2a1	IIA1	Clinically visible lesion 4 cm or less in greatest dimension
T2a2	IIA2	Clinically visible lesion more than 4 cm in greatest dimension
T2b	IIB	Tumor with parametrial invasion
T3	III	Tumor extends to pelvic wall and/or involves lower third of vagina, and/or causes hydronephrosis or non-functioning kidney
T3a	IIIA	Tumor involves lower third of vagina, no extension to pelvic wall
T3b	IIIB	Tumor extends to pelvic wall and/or causes hydronephrosis or non-functioning kidney
T4	IVA	Tumor invades mucosa of bladder or rectum, and/or extends beyond true pelvis (bullous edema is not sufficient to classify a tumor as T4)
Regional lymph nodes		
TNM	**FIGO**	
NX		Regional lymph nodes cannot be assessed
N0		No regional lymph node metastasis
N1	IIIB	Regional lymph node metastasis
Distant metastasis		
TNM	**FIGO**	
M0		No distant metastasis (no pathologic M0; use clinical M to complete stage group)
M1	IVB	Distant metastasis (including peritoneal spread, involvement of supraclavicular or mediastinal lymph nodes, lung, liver, or bone)

[a]FIGO staging no longer includes Stage 0 (Tis)
[b]All macroscopically visible lesions – even with superficial invasion – are T1b/IB
Used with the permission of the American Joint Committee on Cancer (AJCC), Chicago, Illinois. The original source for this material is the AJCC Cancer Staging Manual, seventh edition (2010) published by Springer Science and Business Media LLC, www.springer.com

Uterine Cervix. Table 2 Cervical cancer anatomic stages/prognostic groups

Stage 0	Tis N0 M0
Stage I	T1N0 M0
Stage IA	T1a N0 M0
Stage IA1	T1a1 N0 M0
Stage IA2	T1a2 N0 M0
Stage IB	T1b N0 M0
Stage IB1	T1b1 N0 M0
Stage IB2	T1b2 N0 M0
Stage II	T2N0 M0
Stage IIA	T2a N0 M0
Stage IIA1	T2a1 N0 M0
Stage IIA2	T2a2 N0 M0
Stage IIB	T2b N0 M0
Stage III	T3N0 M0
Stage IIIA	T3a N0 M0
Stage IIIB	T3b any N M0
	T1–3 N1 M0
Stage IVA	T4 any N M0
Stage IVB	Any T any N M1

Used with the permission of the American Joint Committee on Cancer (AJCC), Chicago, Illinois. The original source for this material is the AJCC Cancer Staging Manual, seventh edition (2010) published by Springer Science and Business Media LLC, www.springer.com

► external beam radiation therapy with a ► brachytherapy boost can be offered.

In patients with early-stage cervical cancer demonstrating larger lesions, the decision of whether to proceed with surgery or definitive chemoradiation therapy comes into play. This decision should be made carefully after thorough evaluation and examination, because if a patient does undergo surgery and then needs postoperative radiation, she will experience side effects from both treatment modalities. Decreasing total treatment toxicity is a constant goal. If examination under anesthesia suggests that the tumor is removable by surgery, a radical hysterectomy and bilateral pelvic lymph node dissection and para-aortic lymph node sampling are performed. Alternatively, definitive chemoradiation therapy can be offered. This question of treatment course is often encountered in patients with stage IB1, IB2, and IIA disease.

In some patients with early-stage disease who undergo surgery for initial management but are found to have risk factors for recurrence including lymphovascular invasion, tumor size greater than 4 cm, and/or greater than one third stromal invasion by the tumor, postoperative radiation therapy will be offered. With factors including positive margins, positive parametrial involvement, or positive lymph node involvement, postoperative chemoradiation therapy is recommended. The general recommended chemotherapy is ► cisplatin, 40 mg/m^2 weekly, but dosing can be adjusted according to treatment scheme. External beam fields are similar to the recommendations for definitive treatment approach. This would encompass the pelvic contents in a four field approach with anterior, posterior, right lateral, and left lateral beams in 1.8 Gy fractions to a regional dose of 45 Gy. The field borders are the L4-L5 interspace or L5-S1 interspace superiorly, the bottom of the obturator foramen inferiorly, and 1.5–2 cm around the pelvic brim laterally. Postoperative brachytherapy, when utilized, would differ from definitive treatments due to difference in postoperative anatomy. Postoperative brachytherapy could be used as a boost if there are close or positive margins to the vaginal cuff and would be performed with a vaginal cylinder. An example fractionation scheme using high dose rate brachytherapy for a vaginal cylinder treatment is 6 Gy for three fractions administered over 2–3 weeks prescribed to the vaginal surface following external beam radiation therapy. A parametrial boost using external beam

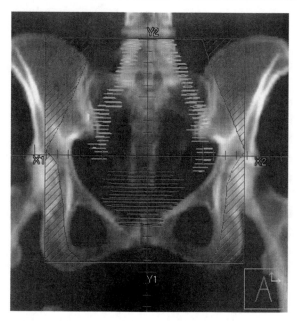

Uterine Cervix. Fig. 1 Anterior view of a 3D conformal external beam radiation pelvic field for cervical cancer

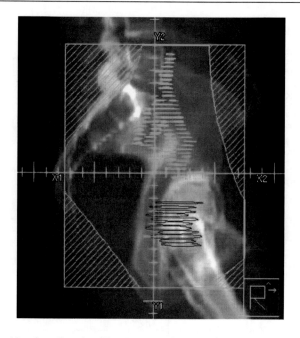

Uterine Cervix. Fig. 2 Lateral view of a 3D conformal external beam radiation pelvic field for cervical cancer

radiation therapy may be used if there is parametrial involvement. This is generally written to a dose of 54 Gy.

Generally in patients with cervical cancer stages IB2, II, III, and IVA disease, definitive chemoradiation therapy is recommended (Perez and Kavanagh 2008). Radiation therapy is administered to a pelvic treatment field with the borders being the L4-L5 interspace or L5-S1 interspace superiorly, the bottom of the obturator foramen inferiorly, and 1.5–2 cm around the pelvic brim laterally. A four-field technique is performed using an anterior, posterior, right lateral, and left lateral beam (Figs. 1 and 2). The pelvic external beam radiation treatments are administered on a daily basis for approximately 5 weeks. Standard fractionation of 1.8 Gy is used to a total dose of 45 Gy. If para-aortic lymph nodes are involved, an extended external beam radiation field treating the para-aortic lymph node region can be designed.

A boost to the intact cervical tumor is then administered with brachytherapy. Brachytherapy

can be performed with a tandem and ovoid or tandem and ring implantation (Fig. 3). The tandem is placed in the cervical os and extends into the uterine cavity. Often a cervical sleeve is inserted in the os and secured with sutures to guide insertion of the tandem throughout these treatments. Next, two ovoids or a ring are placed in the cervical fornices or around the cervix. Radioactive sources are placed into these devices for directed periods to create a desired dose distribution around the cervical tumor, sparing to a great extent the rectum and bladder. Cesium 137 and iridium 192 are the two most commonly used radioactive sources in brachytherapy for cervical cancer. Dosing of brachytherapy is administered to point A, which is located 2 cm superiorly and 2 cm laterally to the external cervical os. Total dose is 75–80 Gy.

Chemotherapy is administered intravenously and given concurrently with radiation therapy for definitive treatment of cervical cancer. Cisplatin or a cisplatin/5-fluorouracil combination is the

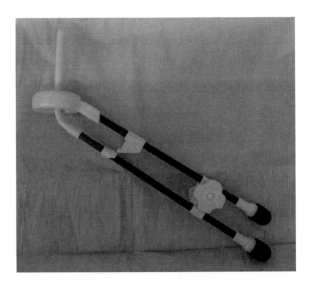

Uterine Cervix. Fig. 3 Ring and tandem implantation device for use of high-dose-rate brachytherapy for intact cervical cancer boost

current standard chemotherapy administered with radiation.

In metastatic cases of cervical cancer, chemotherapy is the standard recommended treatment. Platinum-based regimens are found to be effective, and a variety of single agents and combinations can be used including cisplatin, carboplatin, gemcitabine, docetaxel, topotecan, epirubicin, and 5-fluorouracil. Targeted therapies such as bevacizumab can be offered as well. External beam radiation therapy plays a palliative role in metastatic cervical cancer and can assist in control of pain from bone metastasis, alleviation of vaginal bleeding, and palliation of brain metastasis.

Cross-References
▶ Brachytherapy: High Dose Rate (HDR) Implants
▶ Endometrium
▶ HIV-Related Malignancies
▶ Low-Dose Rate (LDR) Brachytherapy
▶ Ovary
▶ Vagina
▶ Vulvar Carcinoma

References
American Cancer Society (2009) Cervical cancer. American Cancer Society, Atlanta

American Joint Committee on Cancer (2010) Cervix uteri. In: Edge SB, Byrd DR, Compton CC, Fritz AG, Greene FL, Trotti A (eds) AJCC cancer staging manual, 7th edn. Springer, New York

National Comprehensive Cancer Network (2010) NCCN Clinical practice guidelines in oncology: cervical cancer, V.1.2010. http://www.nccn.org/professionals/physician_gls/PDF/cervical.pdf. Accessed 31 January 31 2010

Perez C, Kavanagh BD (2008) Uterine cervix. In: Halperin EC, Perez CA, Brady LW (eds) Principles and practice of radiation oncology, 5th edn. Wolters Kluwer/Lippincott Williams & Wilkins, Philadelphia

Uterine Corpus

▶ Uterine Cervix

Uterine Lining

▶ Endometrium

Uterine Neoplasm

▶ Brachytherapy-GYN
▶ Endometrium

Uterus

▶ Brachytherapy-GYN
▶ Endometrium

V

Vagina

PATRIZIA GUERRIERI, PAOLO MONTEMAGGI
Department of Radiation Oncology, Regional
Cancer Centre "M. Ascoli", University of Palermo
Medical School, Palermo, Italy

Definition/Description

Primary cancer of the vagina is an extremely rare lesion arising in the vagina without involvement of the cervix or the vulva. It represents only 1–2% of all female genital cancer. Most of the vaginal malignancies, 80–90%, are in reality metastatic from different primary gynecologic (cervix and vulva) and non-gynecologic tumor sites, which involve the vagina either by direct extension or lymphatic or hematogenous spread. Aggressiveness of vaginal cancer is similar to that of cervix and vulva carcinomas, with a prevalent tendency to local and locoregional infiltration and relapses. However, the high complexity and richness of vascular and lymphatic networks justifies the relevant risk for distant metastasis even in a relatively early stage of the disease seen in many clinical instances.

Anatomy

The vagina is a muscular dilatable tubular structure averaging 7.5 cm in length that extends from the cervix to the vaginal introitus, marked from the vulva by the hymen. It is located dorsally to the base of the bladder and urethra and ventrally to the rectum. The upper portion of the posterior wall is separated from the rectum by a reflection of peritoneum, known the pouch of Douglas. A circular groove, called fornix, marks the separation between vagina and cervix.

The vaginal wall is composed of three layers: the mucosa, the muscularis, and the adventitia. The most inner layer, the mucosa, is composed of a thick, nonkeratinizing, stratified squamous epithelium lying over a base membrane, which contains many papillae. This epithelium does not have glands and the needed lubrification of vaginal walls originates from cervix mucinous glands. Beneath the mucosa, there is a submucosal layer of elastin and a double muscularis layer, highly vascularized and richly innervated with a complex lymphatic drainage. Skeletal muscle forms a vaginal sphincter at the introitus. The adventitia is a thin outer connective tissue, which merge with that of adjacent organs.

The proximal vagina receives blood supply by the vaginal artery branch from the uterine or cervical branch of the uterine artery. The accompanying venous plexus eventually drains into the internal iliac vein. Innervation of the vagina is provided by the lumbar and pudendal nerve, branching from sacral 2–4 roots. The lymphatic drainage of the vagina is complex and consists of an extensive and intricate network. Because of the presence of this complex network, inguinal and femoral nodes are at risk in cancer of the distal and mid-portion of the vagina, as well as the external iliac nodes, the latter even in lesions of the lower third of the vagina.

Epidemiology

Primary vaginal cancer shows a peak of incidence in the sixth and seventh decades of life

L.W. Brady, T.E. Yaeger (eds.), *Encyclopedia of Radiation Oncology*, DOI 10.1007/978-3-540-85516-3,

(Herbst et al. 1970); however, probably due to the increase of ► Human Papilloma Virus infection, it is more frequently seen in younger women. Nevertheless, the NCDB report (Creasman et al. 1998) showed only 10% of vaginal cancer patients as being younger than 40 years of age, with only 1% < 20 years, 90% of the latter presenting with in situ lesions. As the age of the patients increases, the percentage of deep infiltration of the lesions increases as well, with in situ ones accounting for no more than 11% at 80 years of age (Creasman et al. 1998; Di Domenico 1989a). The actual incidence is presently considered even lower according to more restricted diagnostic criteria, which have eliminated all primary cancer arising from adjacent organs, primarily cervix and vulva.

Potential risk factors for carcinoma of the vagina include history of HPV infection (Okagaki et al. 1983), cervical intraepithelial neoplasia (CIN) (Eversen et al. 1997), low socioeconomic status (Weitherpass et al. 2001), as well as previous pelvic irradiation, even if the latter plays a still controversial role (Boice et al. 1988; Lee et al. 1982).

A specific etiologic agent has been identified for the clear cell histology, which has been shown clearly related to the in utero exposure to diethylstilbestrol (DES) during the first weeks of pregnancy. Several reports have been published on this subject, following the increase of the incidence of this histology reported in 1971 (Herbst et al. 1971), clarifying the pathologic mechanism of the relationship between DES and vaginal cancer (Herbst et al. 1971). The relative risk for exposed women as compared to those not exposed to DES has been weighted as high as twice (Bornstein et al. 1988), even if this data has not been confirmed by others (Hatch et al. 1998).

From a pathologic point of view, squamous cell carcinoma represents the vast majority of vaginal primary cancer, accounting for 80–90%

of all cases. The pathologic aspect is similar to that of primary cervical or vulvar cancer and only those lesions showing no anatomic involvement either of cervix or vulva should be considered as primary vaginal (Zaino et al. 2002).

DES-associated clear cell adenocarcinoma (CCA) is more frequently located in the upper third of the vagina, most commonly at, or near to, the lower margin of the glandular tissue (Herbst et al. 1974). DES-associated CCA are commonly exophytic and/or superficially invasive. Size, stromal invasion, and tubulocystic growth pattern can be considered prognostic factors as well as stage in the DES-associated CCA (Herbst et al. 1974).

Up to 5% of vaginal cancer is malignant melanoma (Chung et al. 1980). They are more frequently located in the inferior third of the vagina in the anterior wall, with a strong tendency to be multifocal (Chung et al. 1980). As well as for cutaneous melanomas, thickness of the lesion can be measured through the Bresolw scale and may represent a significant prognostic factor (Breslow 1975).

A wide histological variety of sarcomas accounts for up to 3% of vaginal malignancies, with a vast majority of the cases represented by leiomyosarcomas. In young children, vaginal cancer is very rare and is typically represented by embryonal rhabdomyosarcoma and/or sarcoma botryoides. Most of the cases, up to 95%, occurs in young girls aging less than 5 years (Prempree and Amornmarn 1985). The most important prognostic factor for all non epithelial tumors of the vagina appears to be the histopathologic grade.

The natural history of vaginal cancer is dominated by the strong tendency to the local invasion and infiltration due to the absence of anatomic barriers. Even if cervix and vulva can be considered the first adjacent structures to be infiltrated, their involvement at the time of diagnosis does not permit allocation of those cases to the vagina, and they should be considered either cervical or vulvar primary cancer (Gallup et al. 1987). Following the tendency of local infiltration, lymphatic invasion is also frequent and early in the natural and clinical history of these tumors, accounting for an incidence of 6–15% in stage 1 and 25–32% in stage 2 (Al Kurdi and Monaghan 1981; Davis et al. 1991).

Metastatic lesions are frequent only in advanced cases and/or when a recurrence after primary treatment occurs, with an incidence varying from 16% in stage 1 to 62% in stage 3 (Davis et al. 1991).

Clinical Presentation

Potential risk factors are related to the presence of HPV, cervical intra epithelial neoplasia (CIN), and previous pelvic irradiation. Specifically related to HPV is the precancerous lesion normally referred to as vaginal intra epithelial neoplasia (VAIN) eventually evolving into invasive squamous cell carcinoma (SCC). While VAIN lesions are more often asymptomatic, patients with invasive disease come to the clinic with a history of irregular vaginal bleeding, often postcoital, and vaginal discharge. Dysuria may be present. Pelvic pain is normally absent until the lesion is very advanced in a late stage of the disease (Gallup et al. 1987). If the tumor arises in the posterior vaginal wall, it may resemble an ovarian mass leading to the need for a differential diagnosis (Gallup et al. 1987). Even if not frequent, asymptomatic cases cannot be considered exceptional, and account for up to 20% of the reported cases (Tjalma et al. 2001).

Imaging Studies

In the diagnostic workup of suspected vaginal cancer, clinical examination represents a cornerstone and should not be underestimated in favor of modern, even if accountable, imaging techniques. A thorough clinical examination, based on bimanual pelvic and rectal examination, along with a speculum inspection of the vagina, followed by biopsy of all the suspicious lesions, is the main, and probably the only, means to exclude those cases in which the extension to cervix or vulva, exclude them from being classified as vaginal cancer. To this effect, biopsies of cervix and vulva are mandatory to rule out primary tumor arising from these sites. Clinical examination may be completed with colposcopy, should the patient have a previous history of cervical carcinoma (Perez et al. 2008).

Lymphatic invasion is generally investigated through CT scan; CT scan of chest and abdomen are part of the imaging studies in nonepithelial tumors. MRI adds new potential efficacy to the diagnostic process of vaginal cancer, specifically T1-weighted with contrast and T2-weighted images (Hricak et al. 1988). Specificity and sensitivity of MRI in staging vaginal cancer have been reported as high as 82% and 97%, respectively. MRI also plays a role in differentiating fibrotic tissue from recurrent cancer in treated patients (Chang et al. 1988). PET scan is more and more used due to its capacity of showing at once both local and regional extension, with specific reference to the nodal extension, more efficiently than a CT scan (Grigsby et al. 2005). For the specific purpose of radiotherapy treatment planning, in order to properly cover and cure all the tumor volume, CT- and MRI-fused images will guide the planning, even if those imaging techniques are not officially allowed for staging purposes (Table 1).

Pathologic Classification and Prognostic Factors

Stage is the most significant prognostic factor (Chyle et al. 1996) accounting for a decrease of the 5-year DFS (Disease Free Survival) from 75% for stage 1 to 55% for stage 2A, 43% for stage 2B, 32% for stage 3 to 0% for stage 4 (Perez et al. 1999). Tumor size has been assigned a negative

Vagina. Table 1 Staging classification

Stage	T	N	M
1	Tumor confined to the vagina	–	–
2	A: Tumor extends to paravaginal tissues but not to the pelvic walls	–	–
	B: Tumor extends to the pelvic walls	–	–
3	As stage 2 plus	+	–
	Tumor extends beyond the true pelvis	–	–
4	A: Tumor invades mucosa of the bladder or rectum (bullous edema is not sufficient to classify tumor as a T4)	±	–
	B: any T	Any N	+

impact on survival, even though in a controversial way (Chyle et al. 1996; Perez et al. 1983). Controversial as well is considered the role of the lesion location in the vagina, with a more favorable outcome for those originating in the proximal half as opposed to those located in the distal half, or involving the entire vagina (Ali et al. 1996; Urbanski et al. 1996).

Several authors have shown the histological grade to be an independent and significant prognostic factor for survival (Urbanski et al. 1996). Similarly, histotype plays a role, having adenocarcinoma a less favorable course: with a lower incidence of local recurrence, but a higher percentage of distant metastases, and a lower 10-year survival rate (Chyle et al. 1996).

The role of age at diagnosis as an independent prognostic factor is still controversial (Perez et al. 1999; Urbanski et al. 1996).

Metastatic spread is more common in CCA, in which stage, histological tubulocystic pattern, size <3 cm and depth of invasion <3 mm, also plays a favorable role (Herbst et al. 1974).

Melanoma and nonepithelial tumors tend to behave more aggressively compared to squamous and other epithelial cancers (Reid et al. 1989; Tavassoli and Norris 1979).

Treatment

Treatment options in vaginal cancer include surgery, radiotherapy, and chemotherapy, used alone or arranged together according to the clinical stage of the disease.

In patients with VAIN, or carcinoma in situ, different approaches have been used ranging from laser (Townsend et al. 1982; Hoffman et al. 1991) to extended surgery (Robinson et al. 2000; Hoffman et al. 1992), all with encouraging even though sometimes controversial results. When surgery is used, also adverse events, mainly from a functional point of view, needs to be taken into account. Intracavitary classic low dose rate brachytherapy can be considered as an effective therapy for patients with VAIN, allowing for a control rate as high as 94% (Perez et al. 1977), with a favorable cost/benefit ratio. Doses of 50–60 Gy should be given to the entire vaginal mucosa, prescribing 70 Gy or more to the involved areas, in one or two fractions, higher doses accounting only for a higher incidence of adverse event (Perez et al. 1977). Few and sparse data are as yet available regarding the use of high dose rate brachytherapy.

When the tumor progresses into invasive lesions, even if radiation therapy remains the cornerstone of treatment, surgery can be considered a possible alternative. Patients who are surgical candidates include those with lesions arising from the upper third and from the posterior wall of the vagina, where an effective and less function impairing approach can be used (Rubin et al. 1985). Cases with positive or close margins and/or with positive nodes should be offered adjuvant radiotherapy (Perez et al. 1988; Rubin et al. 1985). However, a comparison between surgery and radiotherapy series may be inconclusive due to a possible selection bias, for patients undergoing surgery tend to be those with less-extensive lesions, in a more favorable location, younger and in better general medical conditions, all factors able to impact significantly the outcome (Tjalma et al. 2001).

In advanced stage, the role of surgery in vaginal cancer seems to be marginal, with few small series reported in the literature (Rubin et al. 1985; Stock et al. 1995), leaving radiotherapy to play a leading role in the treatment options for vaginal cancer.

In stage 1, intracavitary (ICB) and/or interstitial (ITB) brachytherapy are considered highly effective treatment modalities, local control with them ranging from 90% to 100%. A dose of 60 Gy is delivered to the entire vagina with a boost of 20–30 Gy to the tumor-involved areas. If the tumor thickness is > 0.5 cm, a combination of ICB and ITB is mandatory to adequately cover the target volume; it will allow an adequate dose both to the base as well as to the exofitic portion of the tumor (Di Domenico 1989a; Kushner et al. 2003). More controversial remains the role of external beam in stage 1.

A combination of external beam and ICB and ITB is mandatory in more advanced lesions. A clear superiority of the combination has been shown in stage 2A (Perez et al. 1999; Stock et al. 1995), as well as in stage 2B (Perez et al. 1999). The combination radiotherapy allowed for a local control ranging from 70% in stage 2A to 61% in stage 2B (Perez et al. 1999; Stock et al. 1995), with a 5-year survival respectively reported as varying from 35% to 70% in stage 2A and from 35% to 60% in stage 2B (Perez et al. 1999; Stock et al. 1995). Doses of 40–50 Gy to the entire pelvis are given, with a brachytherapy boost of 30–35 Gy. A similar, with slightly higher doses, approach of combining external radiotherapy and ICB and ITB is used in stages 3 and 4, in which, should brachytherapy not be possible, IMRT may represent a valid alternative (Mundt et al. 2002).

A more detailed discussion on radiotherapy techniques, doses distribution, and treatment modalities lies beyond the objectives of this work and we encourage those interested to refer to handbooks (Perez et al. 2008).

In patients with stages 3 and 4, the use of concomitant chemotherapy has been advocated, based on similar approaches used in other primary sites, for example, anal carcinoma. Mitomycin-C, 5-FU, and cisplatin are the more frequently used and the most effective drugs in this field (Evans et al. 1988; Roberts et al. 1991). Chemoradiation can be a valuable tool to reduce the total dose required to control the disease, improving the local control, minimizing at the same time the risk for adverse events (Dalrymple et al. 2004).

Radiotherapy remains a valid therapeutic option also in other histological types of vaginal cancer, namely, the rare melanomas and sarcomas, including malignant mixed Mullerian tumors (MMMT) (Morrow and Di Saia 1976; Chung et al. 1980; Peters et al. 1985). However, sarcomas more frequently require radical surgery. A special condition is represented by the embryonal rhabdomyosarcoma (RMS) in young girls. The latter found a significant improvement of the cure rate and an impressive decrease in the need of radical, sometimes exenterative surgery if a multimodalities approach using chemotherapy, neo adjuvant and/or adjuvant, limited surgery and radiotherapy, external and, when and if required, brachytherapy is used (Helders et al. 1972; Flamant et al. 1990).

Future Directions

Cancer of the vagina may occur in specific situation like previously irradiated patients, patients with neovagina, in which a conventional radiotherapeutic or surgical approach is not advisable or appropriate. These rare but complex clinical situations will require an innovative strategic therapeutic approach.

In these cases, strong consideration should be given to multimodalities treatment including new drugs, such as taxanes, and new radiotherapy modalities such as IMRT. This combination may help overcome drug resistance in those patients previously treated with a first-line chemotherapy as well as to allow a safe re-irradiation in pre-irradiated cases.

IMRT allows, in fact, to administer curative doses of radiotherapy even to patients who had received previous irradiation due to the possibility of varying the dose and the dose rate throughout the radiation field. In this way, it is possible to adequately spare the organ at risk from unwanted doses allowing at the same time a high dose to the target. Patients relapsing after previous primary treatment, regardless of the modality, and those who may refuse surgery to maintain organ function and integrity, can be offered a strong, valid therapeutic alternative, allowing for, at the same time, disease control probability and preservation of their quality of life.

Further improvement can be derived from image guided and adaptive radiotherapy, especially if functional imaging techniques are used to better define biological target volumes and to differentiate areas of low and high radiosensitivity, helping to better sculpt and tailor radiation doses to the actual biology of the tumor.

Cross-References

▶ Brachytherapy-GYN
▶ Brachytherapy: High Dose Rate (HDR) Implants
▶ Brachytherapy: Low Dose Rate (LDR) Temporary Implants
▶ Cervical Cancer
▶ Clinical Aspects of Brachytherapy
▶ Endometrium
▶ Female Urethra
▶ IMRT
▶ TRUS: Transrectal Ultrasound
▶ Vulvar Carcinoma

References

Al Kurdi M, Monaghan JM (1981) Thirty-two years experience in management of primary tumors of the vagina. BJOG 88:1145–1150

Ali MM, Huang DT, Goplerud DR et al (1996) Radiation alone for carcinoma of the vagina: variation in response related to the location of primary tumor. Cancer 77:1934–1939

Boice JD Jr, Engholm G, Kleinerman RA et al (1988) Radiation dose and second cancer risk in patients treated for cancer of the cervix. Radiat Res 116:3–55

Bornstein J, Adam E, Adler-Storthz K et al (1988) Development of cervical and vaginal squamous cell neoplasia as a late consequence of in utero exposure to diethylstilbestrol. Obstet Gynecol Surv 43:15–21

Breslow A (1975) Tumor thickness level of invasion and node dissection in stage 1 cutaneous melanoma. Ann Surg 182:572–575

Chang YC, Hricak H, Thurnher S et al (1988) Vagina: evaluation with MR imaging Part II. Neoplasms. Radiology 169:175–179

Chung AF, Casey MJ, Flannery JT et al (1980) Malignant melanoma of the vagina – report of 19 cases. Obstet Gynecol 55:720–727

Chyle V, Zagars GK, Wheeler JA et al (1996) Definitive radiotherapy for carcinoma of the vagina: outcome and prognostic factors. Int J Radiat Oncol Biol Phys 35:891–905

Creasman W, Phillips JL, Menck HR (1998) The National Cancer Data Base report on cancer of the vagina. Cancer 83:1033–1040

Dalrymple JL, Russel AH, Lee SW et al (2004) Chemoradiation for primary invasive squampus cell carcinoma of the vagina. Int J Gynecol Oncol 14:110–117

Davis KP, Stanhope CR, Garton GR et al (1991) Invasive vaginal carcinoma: analysis of early stage disease. Gynecol Oncol 42:131–136

Di Domenico A (1989a) Primary vaginal squamous cell carcinoma in the young patient. Gynecol Oncol 35:181–187

Di Domenico A (1989b) Primary vaginal squamous cell carcinoma in the young patient. Gynecol Oncol 58:227–231

Evans LS, Kersh CR, Constable WC et al (1988) Concomitant 5-Fluoro uracil, mitomycin C, and radiotherapy for advanced gynecologic malignancies. Int J Radiat Oncol Biol Phys 15:901–906

Eversen T, Tretli S, Jhoansen A et al (1997) Squamous cell carcinoma of the penis and of the cervix, vulva and vagina in spouses: is there any relationships? An epidemiologic study from Norway, 1960-92. Br J Cancer 76:658–660

Flamant F, Gerbaulet A, Nihoul-Fekete C et al (1990) Long term sequelae of conservative treatment by surgery, brachytherapy, and chemotherapy for vulval and vaginal rhabdomyosarcoma in children. J Clin Oncol 8:1847–1853

Gallup DG, Talledo OE, Sha KJ et al (1987) Invasive squamous cell carcinoma of the vagina: a 14-years study. Obstet Gynecol 69:782–785

Grigsby PW, Mutch DG, Rader J et al (2005) Lack of benefit of concurrent chemotherapy in patients with cervical cancer and negative lymph nodes by FDG-PET. Int J Radiat Oncol Biol Phys 61:444–449

Hatch EE, Palmer JR, Titus-Ernstoff L et al (1998) Cancer risk in women exposed to diethylstilbestrol in utero. JAMA 280:630–634

Helders R, Malkasian G, Soule E (1972) Embryional rhabdomyosarcoma of the vagina. Am J Obstet Gynecol 197:484–502

Herbst AL, Green TH Jr, Ulfelder H (1970) Primary carcinoma of the vagina. An analysis of 68 cases. Am J Obstet Gynecol 106:210–218

Herbst AL, Ulfelder H, Poskanzer DC (1971) Adenocarcinoma of the vagina. Association of maternal stilbestrol therapy with tumor appearance in young women. N Engl J Med 284:878–881

Herbst AL, Robboy SJ, Scully RE et al (1974) Clear cell adenocarcinoma of the vagina and cervix in girls: analysis of 170 registry cases. Am J Obstet Gynecol 119:713–724

Hoffman MS, Roberts WS, LaPolla JP et al (1991) Laser vaporization of grade 3 vaginal intra epithelial neoplasia. AM J Obstet Gynecol 165:1342–1344

Hoffman MS, DeCesare SL, Roberts WS et al (1992) Upper vaginectomy for in situ and occult, superficially invasive carcinoma of the vagina. Am J Obstet Gynecol 166:30–33

Hricak H, Lacey CG, Sandles LG et al (1988) Invasive cervical carcinoma: comparison of MRI imaging and surgical findings. Radiology 166:623–631

Kushner DM, Fleming PA, Kennedy AW et al (2003) High dose rate ^{192}Ir afterloading brachytherapy for cancer of the vagina. Br J Radiol 76:719–725

Lee JY, Perez CA, Ettinger N et al (1982) The risk of second primaries subsequent to irradiation for cervix cancer. Int J Radiat Oncol Biol Phys 8:207–211

Morrow CP, Di Saia PJ (1976) Malignant melanoma of the female genitalia: a clinical analysis. Obstet Gynecol Surv 31:233–271

Mundt AJ, Lujan AE, Rotmensch J et al (2002) Intensity-modulated whole pelvis radiotherapy in women with gynecologic malignancies. Int J Radiat Oncol Biol Phys 52:1330–1337

Okagaki T, Twiggs LB, Zachow KR et al (1983) Identification of human papillomavirus DNA in cervical and vaginal intra epithelial neoplasia with molecularly cloned virus specific DNA probs. Int J Gynecol Pathol 2:153–159

Perez CA, Korba A, Sharma S (1977) Dosimetric considerations in irradiation of carcinoma of the vagina. Int J Radiat Oncol Biol Phys 2:639–649

Perez CA, Bedwinek J, Breaux S et al (1983) Patterns of failures after treatment of gynecologic tumors. Cancer Treat Rep 2:217–222

Perez CA, Camel HM, Galakatos AE et al (1988) Definitive irradiation in carcinoma of the vagina: long term evaluation of results. Int J Radiat Oncol Biol Phys 15:1283–1290

Perez CA, Grigsby PW, Garipagaoplu M et al (1999) Factors affecting long term outcome of irradiation in carcinoma of the vagina. Int J Radiat Oncol Biol Phys 44:37–45

Perez CA, Brady LW, Halperin CE (2008) Principles and practice of radiation oncology, 5th edn. Lippincott Williams & Wilkins, Philadelphia, Chapter 70

Prempree T, Amornmarn R (1985) Radiation treatment of primary carcinoma of the vagina. Patterns of failures after definitive therapy. Acta Radiol Oncol 24:51–56

Peters WA 3rd, Kumar NB, Andersen WA et al (1985) Primary sarcoma of the adult vagina: a clinicopathologic study. Obstet Gynecol 65:699–704

Reid GC, Schmidt RW, Roberts JA et al (1989) Primary melanoma of the vagina: a clinicopathologic analysis. Obstet Gynecol 74:190–199

Roberts WS, Hoffman MS, Kavanagh JJ et al (1991) Further experience with radiation therapy and concomitant intra venous chemotherapy in advanced carcinoma of the lower female genital tract. Gynecol Oncol 43:233–236

Robinson JB, Sun CC, Bodurka-bevers D et al (2000) Cavitational ultrasonic surgical aspiration for the treatment of vaginal intra epithelial tumors. Gynecol Oncol 78:235–241

Rubin SC, Young J, Mikuta JJ (1985) Squamous cell carcinoma of the vagina:treatment complications and long term gollow up. Gynecol Oncol 20:346–353

Stock RG, Chen AS, Seski J (1995) A 30 year experience in the management of primary carcinoma of the vagina: analysis of prognostic factors and treatment modalities. Gynecol Oncol 56:45–52

Tavassoli FA, Norris HJ (1979) Smooth muscle tumors of the vagina. Obstet Gynecol 53:689–693

Tjalma WA, Monaghan JM, de Barros Lopes A et al (2001) The role of surgery in invasive carcinoma of the vagina. Gynecol Oncol 81:360–365

Townsend DE, Levine RU, Crum CP et al (1982) Treatment of vaginal carcinoma in situ with the carbon dioxide laser. Am J Obstet Gynecol 143:565–568

Urbanski K, Kios Z, Reinfuss M et al (1996) Primary invasive vaginal carcinoma treated with radiotherapy: analysis of prognostic factors. Gynecol Oncol 60:16–21

Weitherpass E, Ye W, Tamini R et al (2001) Alcoholism and risk for cancer of the cervix uteri, vagina, and vulva. Cancer Epidemiol Biomarkers Prev 10:899–901

Zaino R, Robboy S, Kurman R (2002) Disease of the vagina, 5th edn. Springer, New York

Various Drugs

RENE RUBIN
Rittenhouse Hematology/Oncology,
Philadelphia, PA, USA

Definition

Asparaginase is an enzyme purified from *Escherichia coli*. Tumor cells lack asparagine synthetase and need an exogenous source of l-asparagine. Without this amino acid, protein synthesis is inhibited. This drug is used in acute lymphocytic leukemia.

Side Effects

- Hypersensitivity
- Fever, chill, nausea, vomiting
- Elevation of LFT
- Bleeding and clotting abnormalities
- Pancreatitis (abnormalities in insulin and lipoproteins)
- Neurotoxicity

Sipuleucel-T is a drug used for cellular immunotherapy. It requires autologous peripheral blood mononuclear cells. They are activated with recombinant PSA linked to GM-CSF and then reinfused into the patient. It is exceedingly expensive and recommended for prostate carcinoma with rising PSA (prostate specific antigen) and no evidence of metastases.

Side Effects

- Allergic reactions
- Fever and chills

Revlimid and *thalidomide* are both are immunomodulative and acting on antiangiogenesis. They are used in myeloma and myelodysplastic syndrome. Thalidomide has been tested on primary brain cancer and melanoma.

Side Effects

- Neuropathy
- Constipation
- Fatigue
- Thrombosis (should be given with aspirin)
- Birth defects (contraindicated for pregnant women)
- Rash

Mitomycin-C, an agent with antibiotic and antitumor effectivity, is derived from *Streptomyces caespitosus* and *Streptomyces lavendulae*. It is used in head and neck cancer and esophageal, bladder, and anal carcinoma. Its combination with radiotherapy because of its radiosensitizing action (DNA break) is well known.

Side Effects

- Bone marrow depletion
- Renal damage
- Lung fibrosis

Cross-References

▶ Principles of Chemotherapy

Very Low-Dose Rate (VLDR) Brachytherapy

ERIK VAN LIMBERGEN
Department of Radiation Oncology, University
Hospital Gasthuisberg, Leuven, Belgium

Definition

The dose is delivered by low activity, low-energy seed sources (Iodine-125, Palladium-103,

Gold-198) which are implanted permanently (link) in the clinical target volume.

Cross-References
▶ Clinical Aspects of Brachytherapy (BT)
▶ High-Dose Rate (HDR) Brachytherapy
▶ Low-Dose Rate (LDR) Brachytherapy

Villous Adenoma

Filip T. Troicki[1], Jaganmohan Poli[2]
[1]College of Medicine, Drexel University, Philadelphia, PA, USA
[2]Department of Radiation Oncology, College of Medicine, Drexel University, Philadelphia, PA, USA

Definition
Polyp within the gastrointestinal tract that has the potential to become cancerous.

Cross-References
▶ Colon Cancer

Vinca Alkaloids

Rene Rubin
Rittenhouse Hematology/Oncology, Philadelphia, PA, USA

Definition
Derived from the vinca rosacea (periwinkle) plant, this class binds to beta tubulin, preventing the formation of microtubules. This, in turn, blocks cells in mitosis, and apoptosis follows. They are mainstays in therapy for Hodgkin's and non-Hodgkin's lymphoma, testicular cancer, as well as childhood malignancies (Wilm's tumor and Ewing's sarcoma). Newer derivatives (vincristin, vinorelbine) have shown activity against solid tumors such as lung and breast cancer.

Side Effects
- Myelosuppression (dose limiting toxicity)
- Neurotoxicity/peripheral neuropathy and autonomic dysfunction
- Mucositis
- Constipation
- Hypertension
- Schwartz-Bartter syndrome (SIADH): inappropriate antidiuretic hormone hypersecretion, characterized by excessive release of antidiuretic hormone
- Acute pulmonary edema

Cross-References
▶ Principles of Chemotherapy

Virchow's Node

Filip T. Troicki[1], Jaganmohan Poli[2]
[1]College of Medicine, Drexel University, Philadelphia, PA, USA
[2]Department of Radiation Oncology, College of Medicine, Drexel University, Philadelphia, PA, USA

Definition
Enlarged left supraclavicular lymph node, often associated with advanced gastric and esophagus cancer.

Cross-References
▶ Esophageal Cancer
▶ Stomach Cancer

Viscera

▶ Visceral Organs (also Viscera or Internal Organs)

Visceral Organs (also Viscera or Internal Organs)

JAMES H. BRASHEARS, III
Radiation Oncologist, Venice, FL, USA

Synonyms
Internal organs; Viscera

Definition
The organs located within the three central cavities of the body (chest, abdomen and pelvis). The main cardiovascular, pulmonary, gastrointestinal, and genitourinary organs compose the viscera, compared with splanchnic organs which are the intra-abdominal organs exclusively.

Cross-References
▶ Palliation of Visceral Recurrences and Metastases

Von Hippel-Lindau Disease

TONY S. QUANG[1], STEPHAN MOSE[2]
[1]Department of Radiation Oncology, VA Puget Sound Health Care System University of Washington Medical Center, Seattle, WA, USA
[2]Department of Radiation Oncology, Schwarzwald-Baar-Klinikum, Villingen-Schwenningen, Germany

Definition
This disease is characterized by a predisposition to bilateral and multicentric vascular tumors such as retinal angiomas, CNS hemangioblastomas, paragangliomas, cystadenomas, renal cell carcinomas, pheochromocytomas, islet cell tumors of the pancreas, endolymphatic sac tumors, and renal, pancreatic, and epididymal cysts. The Von Hippel-Lindau syndrome gene is located on chromosome 3p25-26.

Cross-References
▶ Kidney

Voxel

DAREK MICHALSKI[1], M. SAIFUL HUQ[2]
[1]Division of Medical Physics, Department of Radiation Oncology, University of Pittsburgh Cancer Centers, Pittsburgh, PA, USA
[2]Department of Radiation Oncology, University of Pittsburgh Medical Center Cancer Pavilion, Pittsburgh, PA, USA

Definition
An abbreviation for volume element.

Cross-References
▶ Four-Dimensional (4D) Treatment Planning/Respiratory Gating
▶ Imaging in Oncology

Vulvar Carcinoma

PATRIZIA GUERRIERI, PAOLO MONTEMAGGI
Department of Radiation Oncology, Regional Cancer Centre "M. Ascoli", University of Palermo Medical School, Palermo, Italy

Definition/Description
Vulvar cancer represents a rare neoplasm generally affecting elderly women, aged >70; its incidence is estimated as being 1% to 2% of all

cancers occurring in women and up to 4% of all of the cancers affecting the female genital system (Ries et al. 1983; Van der Velden et al. 1996). In recent years and decades, the incidence per annum of vulvar in-situ cancer has steeply risen, especially in the younger population, with a proportional reduction of invasive cancer cases, probably due to changes in sexual habits (Brinton et al. 1990). The occurrence of vulvar cancer is related to a higher incidence of genital and non-genital second primaries compared to the general population, even though there is no clear explanation of this phenomenon, especially for non-genital second primaries (Choo and Morley 1980; Monk et al. 1995). Immunosuppression, leukoplakia, genitourinary neoplasms, and some working conditions (cleaning industries) may predispose women to the development of a vulvar neoplasia, also a low social economic status may have an impact on the incidence of this neoplasia (Mabuchi et al. 1985).

Anatomy

The vulva is a complex anatomic structure composed of mons pubis, clitoris, majora and minora labia, vaginal vestibule, and layers of supportive connective tissues. The vulva fuses with urethral meatus anteriorly and superiorly, and with perineum and anus posteriorly. Majora and minora labia constitute the most relevant portion of the vulva; the clitoris is located 2–3 cm from the urethral meatus and is composed of erectile tissue. Its central position is crucial to understand the natural history of tumors originating from the clitoris itself. Vulva's vestibule is also centrally located, defined laterally by the labia minora and posteriorly by the perineum. Two mucous secreting glands, named Bartholin glands, lie in the subcutaneous tissue posteriorly to the labia majora; they may pose issues of differential diagnosis with vulvar carcinoma.

The lymphatic network from the vulva drains into the superficial inguinal and femoral nodes. Lymphatic vessels from clitoris can also drain into not only superficial but also deep femoral and pelvic nodes. The most important superficial inguinal and femoral nodes lie on a triangle formed by the inguinal ligament superiorly, the border of the Sartorius muscle laterally, and medially by the border of the adductor longus muscle. Three to five nodes are deeply located in it; the superior and most relevant of those is known as the Cloquet's node.

Epidemiology

As mentioned above, cancer of the vulva is a rare malignancy representing only 1–2% of all the cancers occurring in women and no more than 4% of all the gynecologic malignancies. The peak of incidence affects women 70 years of age or older, nevertheless an increasing occurrence of in situ vulvar cancer has been recently seen in the younger population, probably because of changes in sexual behavior of the new generations. This increase has occurred mainly in white women younger than 35 years old, in which the incidence rate almost tripled between 1970 and 1990 (Sturgeon et al. 1992).

Almost two-thirds of the lesions arise in the labia majora and minora, followed by those originating from the clitoris (15%), at the fourchette level and Bartholin's glands (5%); sometimes lesions are so large that may be impossible to allocate them to the precise site of origin (Plentl and Friedman 1971). Lymphatic spread tends to invade superficial inguinofemoral nodes, while direct infiltration of deep nodes, as well as contralateral inguinal, is quite unusual (Krupp and Bohm 1978). Primary tumor size and extent are crucial in determining the rate of nodal involvement (Perez et al. 1998).

Clinical Presentation

Cancer of the vulva is normally diagnosed because of symptoms such as pruritus, bleeding or spotting, discharge, and pain. However, patients often suffer symptoms for a long time before seeking medical evaluation, due to psychological discomfort and to an elderly age; as a consequence, the lesions are quite large when discovered. If not cured or if diagnosed at a more advanced stage, other symptoms as dysuria, trouble in defecation and pain or difficulties in intercourse may be present. Inguinal nodes represent a frequent event in vulvar cancer, but they are not noted until they become quite large. Nevertheless, it is uncommon to have patients presenting with a nodal disease so advanced to provoke lower extremities edema.

Imaging Studies

The staging process of vulvar cancer is mainly based on physical examination (PE) because of the location of the primary lesions and the prominent relevance and incidence of inguinal nodes. With respect to the latter a thorough evaluation of the inguinal region should be carried out according to the anatomic location of the primary. Unilateral inguinal evaluation will be sufficient in well lateralized lesions, while in those more close to or growing in the medial part of the vulva as well as in those originating from the region of either the clitoris or the fourchette, a bilateral inguinal evaluation will be necessary.

Even though the staging systems do not recommend as mandatory diagnostic imaging studies, CT and/or MRI can be used to identify the presence of nodal or potential organ involvement, determining at the same time their location so that, should it be necessary, a proper biopsy can be performed. If no biopsy is performed, both CT and MRI lack specificity with a large number of false positive findings. Location and extent of the primary lesion may indicate, as it does in other gynecologic malignancies, the need for further clinical investigations such as cystoscopy and/or proctoscopy. A precise evaluation and measurement of the infiltration depth of the primary lesion is also part of the staging procedures,

for the risk of nodal involvement directly correlates to this parameter, varying from very low when the depth is ≤3 mm, to very significant or very high in deeper infiltration (Montana and Kang 2008).

Pathologic Classification and Prognostic Factors

Epidermoid carcinoma accounts for about 90% of all vulvar cancers. It has, in the vulva, peculiar characteristics when compared to other gynecologic primary sites. It is crucial in vulvar cancer to exactly define the largest dimension in diameter as well as the depth of infiltration measured according to the specification given by the International society of Gynecological Pathologists (Creasman 1995). Size and depth of infiltration influence the new staging classification both in TNM and FIGO system as shown in Table 1.

Malignant melanoma of the vulva, characteristically seen in white women during the sixth and seventh decades of life, represents the second more common malignant condition of the vulva accounting for about 10% of all the vulvar cancers. Prognostic factors for vulvar melanoma do not differ from melanomas originating from other primary sites, level of invasion and tumor thickness dictating the prognosis (Johnson et al. 1986).

Although adenocarcinomas of the vulva are rare, they pose differential diagnostic difficulties, arising frequently from Bartholin's glands. They are frequently diagnosed at a late stage, with important nodal involvement.

Also rare is the Paget's disease of the vulva, occurring more frequently in older white women. Differential diagnosis must be made with eczema or contact dermatitis. As well as in the breast, Paget's disease of the vulva shows an invasive pattern in a quarter to a third of the patients. Up to 20% of patients with vulvar Paget's disease, also present an underlying adenocarcinoma either apocrine or of the Bartholins glands (Helwig and Graham 1963).

Vulvar Carcinoma. Table 1 Vulvar cancer staging

FIGO	Tumor characteristics included	TNM
0	Carcinoma in situ	Tis
IA	Tumor confined to vulva, including perineum involvement, ≤2 cm, depth infiltration ≤1 mm, N0	T1a
IB	Tumor confined to vulva, including perineum involvement, ≤2 cm, depth infiltration >1 mm, N0	T1b
II	Tumor confined to vulva, including perineum involvement, >2 cm, N0	T2
III	Tumor invades urethra lower tract, and/or vagina, and/or anus, unilateral inguinal nodes involvement	T3N1
1VA	Tumor extends to the upper tract of the urethra, bladder and/or rectal mucosa, and/or involves pubic bones, bilateral inguinal node involvement	T4N2
1VB	Any T, Any N, M1	T1-4N0-2,M1

Nodal involvement represents the most relevant single prognostic factor in vulvar carcinoma. Its presence dramatically cuts the long term specific survival to 50% (Farias-Eisner et al. 1994). It is of paramount importance to determine the involvement of inguinal nodes up front to avoid the severity of adverse events which may occur following radical surgery and, when necessary, adjuvant radiotherapy. Several methods are available to quite accurately forecast the risk for inguinal nodes involvement. Along with the above mentioned CT and MRI imaging studies with their lack of specificity which negatively affects their usefulness, many clinical and histologic features of the primary tumor help predict nodal metastasis and prognosis. Some of those factors have been historically known and described (Berman et al. 1989; Rutledge et al. 1991). An analysis of the GOG database done at the end of the twentieth century allowed a clearer knowledge of clinical prognostic factors in carcinoma of the vulva (Homesley et al. 1991). They were ranked as follows: clinical nodal status, GOG grade, vascular lymphatic space invasion, tumor thickness, and patient's stage. Tumor size also played a significant role.

As already said, accurately defining the risk of inguinal nodal involvement is relevant to the issue of therapeutic strategy. Recently, the sentinel node biopsy has been suggested as a final and definitive attempt to avoid inguinal radical dissection (Donaldson et al. 1981; Binder et al. 1990; Moore et al. 2003; Torne and Puig-Tintore 2004). Sentinel node dissection represent a highly accurate method of nodal involvement evaluation; it makes possible to correctly classify 97% of the cases with a 13–41% histologic finding of metastatic infiltration (Moore et al. 2003; Torne and Puig-Tintore 2004). Definitely rare is the rate of false negative sentinel nodes (Moore et al. 2003; Torne and Puig-Tintore 2004). Currently, it is assumed that only patients with a penetration depth <1 mm can safely escape a radical inguinal node dissection (Sedlis et al. 1987; Berman et al. 1989).

Even though the involvement of deep pelvic nodes is a highly negative prognostic factor, nevertheless about one third of the patients may still be curable (Boutselis 1972).

Looking at the histopathologic features of the surgical specimen, nodal extracapsular extension (Van der Velden et al. 1995) and positive or close margins (Heaps et al. 1990) correlate with the risk of loco regional and/or distant failures.

Treatment

Generally speaking, cancer of the vulva presents several challenging aspects that make it complex to determine an effective therapeutic strategy. Anatomic location with a high possibility for adjacent organs, such as bladder and rectum, involvement, age of the patients, frequent comorbidities, psychological and sexual negative impact, all these factors contribute to make it difficult to find a proper balance between tumor cure and quality of life, a satisfactory cost/benefit equilibrium.

Radical en-bloc resection of primary tumor and bilateral inguinal nodes has been the standard up front treatment for decades. More recently, looking at results obtained in other tumors like anal cancer, a multidisciplinary approach has been designed to treat vulvar carcinoma the same way. The treatment schedule proposed consists of radiotherapy, surgery, and chemotherapy assembled differently in their temporal sequence, with the intent to reduce the negative impact of radical surgery on both body-self-image and sexual function (Woodruff et al. 1973). In addition to that, important innovations have taken place in surgery and radiotherapy. Surgery has been refined in the operative procedure as well as in the postoperative care, while radiotherapy has found a way to a more clear definition and identification of the clinical target volumes thanks to the modern imaging techniques and, to the new software now available for a highly precise delivery of the dose. IMRT and, in selected cases, brachytherapy, allow the delivery of a very high dose to the tumor volume, efficiently sparing the adjacent organs at risk: primarily rectum and bladder. Even though a wide agreement on the best timing of the multidisciplinary approach is not yet on the table, a vast consensus exists about a better trend, that favors the use of concomitant chemo radiotherapy.

Early Disease

According to the recent developments in the therapeutic rationale of treating cancer of the vulva, lesions up to 2 cm in diameter and up to 5 mm depth may be treated with local excision instead of the old fashioned radical surgery, allowing highly comparable results. With both these two approaches it is possible to achieve very good results with only 6% local failure and 98% disease free survival (Hacker and Van der Velden 1993). Larger or deeper lesions require inguinal node evaluation through either mono or bilateral dissection, according to the anatomic location of the primary, bilateral dissection limited to clitoris or midline lesions (Van der Velden 2000).

In the setting of early vulvar cancer, there is a limited role for radiotherapy as adjuvant post surgery treatment. Patients suitable for radiotherapy are those showing at the pathologic exam, an invasion depth >5 mm, positive or close (<8 mm) margins, even if the results cannot be considered consolidated at the present (Faul et al. 1997). Also controversial remains the role of radiotherapy in the management of nodal disease. A GOG randomized trial conducted during the 1980s showed a definitive advantage from postoperative inguinal radiotherapy following bilateral inguinal node dissection, with 5.1% versus 23.6% groin failure rate and a 68% versus 54% survival in favor of the radiotherapy group in those patients who had more than one positive node. The number of the series was small, but nevertheless, considering the rarity of the disease, one must consider postoperative radiotherapy as positively indicated in patients with inguinal nodal involvement (Homesley et al. 1986).

Advanced Disease

Advanced vulvar cancer represents the ideal setting for the above described multimodality approach (Moore et al. 1998; Montana et al. 2000). As it has been clearly shown in other tumor locations (Gage et al. 1995; Veronesi et al. 1990; Whitney et al. 1999), concomitant chemo-radiotherapy followed by tailored surgery should be considered the standard treatment for patients with advanced vulvar cancer and/or for those with recurrent disease (Thomas et al. 1989; Koh et al. 1993; Wahlen et al. 1995; Lupi et al. 1996). This approach has been proven superior to surgery alone, allowing a significant reduction of the need for ultra-radical intervention such as pelvic exenteration.

Nonepidermoid Vulvar Cancer

Tumors of different histology, namely vulvar melanoma, and tumors arising from Bartholin's glands may present the need for a different therapeutic approach. The rationale of treatment remains based on the specific histology of the tumor; however, the role of different therapeutic tools as well as their strategic integration in multimodalities treatment schedules has to take into account the anatomy of the vulva, with special focus on its lymphatic network (Davidson et al. 1980; Copeland et al. 1986; Cardosi et al. 2001).

Role of Radiotherapy

Radiotherapy plays a relevant role in the management of vulvar cancer, either as adjuvant or exclusive treatment. Doses ranging from 60 to 70 Gy on primary and 50–60 Gy on inguinal and pelvic nodes are thought to be high enough to locally control the disease when used as exclusive treatment (Slevin and Pointon 1989; Pohar et al. 1995) for locally advanced or relapsed disease, or in patients unsuitable for curative surgery due to general medical conditions. Volumes to be treated include primary site, inguinal node, and pelvic nodes up to the origin of common iliac artery. A proper boost may be needed either with brachytherapy or electron beams to adequately cover the outer layers of the treated area. Modern technical improvements in radiotherapy have found their

place also in vulvar cancer. Specifically, IMRT has been shown coupling high efficacy with great capacity of effectively maintain organ at risk functions (Beriwal et al. 2006).

Interstitial brachytherapy also plays a relevant role especially in a conservative approach. Doses as high as 70–80 Gy can be safely used on primary tumors with a local failure rate of about 15% when brachytherapy is used as primary treatment (Pohar et al. 1995). The local control capability of brachytherapy decreases when treating relapsed tumors (Pohar et al. 1995).

During recent decades, radiotherapy efficacy has been increased thanks to a wider use of treatment schedules of concomitant chemo radiotherapy. This multimodality approach has been shown of greater advantage in patients with very large primary lesions and/or clinically macroscopically involved inguinal node, both as exclusive treatment and, even more, as neo-adjuvant treatment before a more conservative surgical intervention (Moore et al. 1998).

Treatment Sequelae

The most important chronic complication of surgery is lower extremities edema, which may be in some series as high as 69% in incidence (Gould et al. 2001). On its part, radiotherapy, alone or in combination with chemotherapy, presents two differently timed adverse events: acute and late. In an acute phase, mild to severe mucocutaneous reaction in the vulvar and perineal region, as well as in the inguinal folds area, may be seen. Intensity and duration of this inflammatory changes mainly depend on the fractionation schedule used and on the total administered dose. Some drugs, like fluoropirimidyne derivates, may also impact negatively on this adverse reaction. Late complications are more frequently seen in multimodality treatment schedules using chemotherapy, radiotherapy, and surgery, regardless of their temporal sequence. Late adverse events include skin and vaginal

V

mucosa dryness, vaginal introitus stenosis, skin and mucosa atrophy.

Besides these physical adverse events, the most relevant adverse reaction in patients with vulvar cancer remains the psychosexual impact of the treatment. This impact varies from distortion of body image self-perception, to impairment of sexual function, up to the impossibility of intercourse (Andersen et al. 1988). The severity of this psychological reaction to surgical approach, even when conservative, has been one of the powerful motives for the multimodality schedules to become a more and more widely used standard treatment method in these patients.

Future Directions

New perspectives and therapeutic gain in vulvar cancer do not differ from those expected in other gynecologic malignancies. Modern imaging techniques with special emphasis on the functional ones, such as SPECT, PET and spectroscopic MRI, should allow better volumes allowing for the identification of biological target volumes and offering treatment schedules specifically and personally tailored for every single patient. IMRT, IGRT, and adaptive technique of radiotherapy will consequently be able to sculpt the dose distribution effectively impacting on tumor control while, at the same time, sparing structures and organs at risk from adverse events.

Cross-References

▶ Brachytherapy-GYN
▶ Brachytherapy: Low Dose Rate (LDR) Temporary Implants
▶ Clinical Aspects of Brachytherapy
▶ Electron Beam Dosimetry
▶ High Dose Rate (HDR) Implants
▶ Image-Guided Radiotherapy (IGRT)
▶ IMRT
▶ Melanoma
▶ Skin Cancer
▶ Vagina

References

Andersen BL, Turquist D, LaPolla J et al (1988) Sexual functioning after treatment of in situ vulvar cancers preliminary report. Obstet Gynecol 71:15–19

Beriwal S, Heron DE, Kim H et al (2006) Intensity-modulated radiotherapy for the treatment of vulvar carcinoma: a comparative dosimetric study with early clinical outcome. Int J Radiat Oncol Biol Phys 64(5):1395–1400

Berman ML, Soper JT, Creasman WT et al (1989) Conservative surgical management of superficially invasive stage I vulvar carcinoma. Obstet Gynecol 35:352–357

Binder SW, Huang I, Fu YS et al (1990) Risk factors for the development of lymph node metastasis in vulvar squamous cell carcinoma. Obstet Gynecol 37:9–16

Boutselis JG (1972) Radical vulvectomy for invasive squamous cell carcinoma of the vulva. Obstet Gynecol 39:827–836

Brinton LA, Nasca PC, Mallin K et al (1990) Case-control study of cancer of the vulva. Obstet Gynecol 75:859–866

Cardosi RJ, Speights A, Fiorica JV et al (2001) Bartholin's gland carcinoma: a 15-year experience. Obstet Gynecol 82:247–251

Choo YC, Morley GW (1980) Double primary epidermoid carcinoma of the vulva and cervix. Obstet Gynecol 56:365–369

Copeland Lj, Sneige N, Gershenson DM et al (1986) Bartholin gland carcinoma. Obstet Gynecol 67:794–801

Creasman WT (1995) New gynecologic cancer staging. Obstet Gynecol 58:157–158

Davidson T, Kissin M, Westbury G (1980) Vulvo-vaginal melanoma – should radical surgery be abandoned? Br J Obstet Gynecol 9:63–67

Donaldson ES, Powell DE, Hanson MB et al (1981) Prognostic parameters I invasive vulvar cancer. Obstet Gynecol 11:184–190

Farias-Eisner R, Cirisano FD, Grouse D et al (1994) Conservative and individualized surgery for early squamous carcinoma of the vulva: the treatment of choice for stage I and II (T1-2, N0-1M0). Obstet Gynecol 53:55–58

Faul CM, Mirdow F, Huang Q et al (1997) Adjuvant radiation for vulvar carcinoma: improved local control. Int J Radiat Oncol Biol Phys 38:381–389

Gage I, Recht A, Gelman R et al (1995) Long term outcome following breast conservative surgery and radiation therapy. Int J Radiat Oncol Biol Phys 33:245–251

Gould N, Kamelle S, Tillmanns T et al (2001) Predictors of complications after inguinal lymphadenectomy. Obstet Gynecol 82:329–332

Hacker NF, Van der Velden J (1993) Conservative management of early vulvar cancer. Cancer 71:1673–1677

Heaps JM, Fu YS, Montz FJ et al (1990) Surgical-pathologic variables predictive of local recurrence in squamous cell carcinoma of the vulva. Obstet Gynecol 38:309–314

Helwig EB, Graham JH (1963) Anogenital (extramammary) paget's disease. Cancer 16:387–395

Homesley HD, Bundy BN, Sedlis A et al (1986) Radiation therapy versus pelvic node resection for carcinoma of the vulva with positive groin nodes. Obstet Gynecol 68:733–740

Homesley HD, Bundy BN, Sedlis A et al (1991) Assessment of current FIGO staging of vulvar carcinoma relative to prognostic factors for survival (a GOG study). Am J Obstet Gynecol 164:997–1004

Johnson TR, Kumar NB, Whitw CD et al (1986) Prognostic features of vulvar melanoma: a clinicopathologic analysis. Int J Gynecol Pathol 5:110–118

Koh WJ, Wallace HJ 3rd, Greer BE et al (1993) Combined radiotherapy and chemotherapy in the management of local-regionally advanced vulvar cancer. Int J Radiat Oncol Biol Phys 26:809–816

Krupp PJ, Bohm JW (1978) Lymph gland metastases in invasive squamous cell carcinoma of the vulva. Am J Obstet Gynecol 130:943–952

Lupi G, Raspagliesi F, Zuvali R et al (1996) Combined pre-operative chemoradiotherapy followed by radical surgery in locally advanced vulvar carcinoma. A pilot study. Cancer 77:1472–1478

Mabuchi K, Bross DS, Kessler II (1985) Epidemiology of cancer of the vulva. A case-control study. Cancer 55:1843–1848

Monk BJ, Burger RA, Lin F et al (1995) Prognostic significance of human papillomavirus DNA in vulvar carcinoma. Obstet Gynecol 85:709–715

Montana GS, Kang SK (2008) Carcinoma of the vulva. In: Perez CA, Brady LW, Halperin EC (eds) Principles and practice of radiation oncology, 5th edn. Lippincott Williams & Wilkins, Philadelphia

Montana GS, Thomas GM, Moore DH et al (2000) Preoperative chemo-radiation for carcinoma of the vulva with N2/N3 nodes: a Gynecologic Oncology Group study. Int J Radiat Oncol Biol Phys 48:1007–1013

Moore DH, Thomas GM, Montana GS et al (1998) Preoperative chemoradiation for advanced vulvar cancer: a phase II study of the Gynecologic Oncology Group. Int J Radiat Oncol Biol Phys 42:79–85

Moore RG, DePasquale SE, Steinhoff MM et al (2003) Sentinel node identification and the ability to detect metastatic tumor to inguinal lymph nodes in squamous cell carcinoma of the vulva. Obstet Gynecol 89:475–479

Perez CA, Grigsby PW, Chao C et al (1998) Irradiation in carcinoma of the vulva: factors affecting outcome. Int J Radiat Oncol Biol Phys 42:335–344

Plentl AA, Friedman EA (1971) Lymphatic system of the female genitalia. W.B. Saunders, Philadelphia

Pohar S, Foffstetter S, Peiffert D et al (1995) Effectiveness of brachytherapy in treating carcinoma of the vulva. Int J Radiat Oncol Biol Phys 32:1455–1460

Ries LG, Pollack ES, Young JL Jr (1983) Cancer patient survival: Surveillance, Epidemiology, and End Results Program, 1973-79. J Natl Cancer Inst 70:693–707

Rutledge FN, Mitchell MF, Munsell MF et al (1991) Prognostic indicators for invasive carcinoma of the vulva. Obstet Gynecol 42:239–241

Sedlis A, Homesley H, Bundy BN et al (1987) Positive groin lymph nodes in superficial squamous cell vulvar cancer. Am J Ostet Gynecol 156:1159–1164

Slevin NJ, Pointon RC (1989) Radical radiotherapy for carcinoma of the vulva. Br J Radiol 62:145–147

Sturgeon SR, Brinton LA, Devesa SS et al (1992) In situ and invasive vulvar cancer incidence trends (1973 to 1987). Am J Obstet Gynecol 166:1482–1485

Thomas GM, Dembo A, DePetrillo A et al (1989) Concurrent radiation and chemotherapy in vulvar carcinoma. Obstet Gynecol 34:263–267

Torne A, Puig-Tintore IM (2004) The use of sentinel node in gynecological malignancies. Curr Opin Obstet Gynecol 16:57–64

van der Velden J (2000) Surgery in the primary management of vulvar cancer. In: Luesley D (ed) Cancer and pre cancer of the vulva. Arnold, London, pp 106–119

van der Velden J, van Lindert AC, Lammes FB et al (1995) Extracapsular growth of lymph nodes metastases in squamous cell carcinoma of the vulva. The impact on recurrence and survival. Cancer 75:2885–2890

Van der Velden J, van Lindert AC, Gimbrere CH et al (1996) Epidemiologic data on vulvar cancer: comparison of hospital with population based data. Obstet Gynecol 62:379–383

Veronesi U, Salvadori B, Luini A et al (1990) Conservative treatment of early breast cancer. Long term results of 1232 cases treated with quadrantectomy, axillary node dissection, and radiotherapy. Ann Surg 211:250–259

Wahlen SA, Slater JD, Wagner RJ et al (1995) Concurrent radiation therapy and chemotherapy in the treatment of primary squamous cell carcinoma of the vulva. Cancer 75:2289–2294

Whitney CW, Sause W, Bundy BN et al (1999) Randomized comparison of fluorouracil plus cisplatin versus hydroxyurea as an adjunct to radiation therapy in stage IIB-IVA carcinoma of the cervix with negative para-aortic nodes: A Gynecologic Oncology Group and Southwest Oncology Group study. J Clin Oncol 17:1339–1348

Woodruff JD, Julian C, Puray T et al (1973) The contemporary challenge of carcinoma in situ of the vulva. Am J Obstet Gynecol 115:677–686

W

WAGR Syndrome

Larry C. Daugherty[1], Brandon J. Fisher[2]
[1]Department of Radiation Oncology, College of Medicine, Drexel University, Glenside, PA, USA
[2]Department of Radiation Oncology, Drexel University, College of Medicine, Philadelphia, PA, USA

Definition

Acronym for the clinical combination of *W*ilm's tumor, *a*niridia, *g*enitourinary malformations, and mental *r*etardation.

Cross-References

▶ Wilm's Tumor

Waldenstrom's Macroglobulinemia

Jo Ann Chalal
Department of Radiation Oncology, Fox Chase Cancer Center, Philadelphia, PA, USA

Definition

Also known as lymphoplasmacytic lymphoma as it is a rare type of indolent lymphoma. This is a disorder of B cells maturing to plasma cells which results in an overproduction of immunoglobulin M.

Cross-References

▶ Leukemia
▶ Multiple Myeloma

▶ Non-Hodgkins Lymphoma
▶ Plasma Cell Myeloma

Warthin's Tumor

Lindsay G. Jensen, Loren K. Mell
Center for Advanced Radiotherapy Technologies, Department of Radiation Oncology, San Diego Rebecca and John Moores Cancer Center, University of California, La Jolla, CA, USA

Definition

Benign parotid gland tumor that occurs more commonly in smokers. It is the second most common benign parotid tumor and 12% are multifocal, either bilateral or unilateral.

Cross-References

▶ Lung
▶ Salivary Gland Cancer

Watchful Waiting

Johannes Classen
Department of Radiation Oncology, St. Vincentius-Kliniken Karlsruhe, Karlsruhe, Germany

Definition

Management strategy for cancer giving active treatment only to those patients showing clinical signs of active tumor (relapse/progression).

L.W. Brady, T.E. Yaeger (eds.), *Encyclopedia of Radiation Oncology*, DOI 10.1007/978-3-540-85516-3,
© Springer-Verlag Berlin Heidelberg 2013

Cross-References

▶ Prostate

▶ Testes

Western Medicine

▶ Biomedicine (also Traditional, Theoretical, Conventional, or Western Medicine)

Whole Abdomen Irradiation (WAI)

Patrizia Guerrieri, Paolo Montemaggi
Department of Radiation Oncology, Regional Cancer Center "M. Ascoli", University of Palermo Medical School, Palermo, Italy

Synonyms

Whole abdominal radiation therapy (WART)

Definition

Irradiation through a high-voltage radiotherapy linear accelerator of the intraperitoneal space for high intraperitoneal relapse risk patients from ovary or Fallopian tube cancers.

Whole Abdominal Radiation Therapy (WART)

Christin A. Knowlton[1], Michelle Kolton Mackay[2]
[1]Department of Radiation Oncology, Drexel University, Philadelphia, PA, USA
[2]Department of Radiation Oncology, Marshfield Clinic, Marshfield, WI, USA

Synonyms

Whole abdominal irradiation (WAI)

Definition

Historically WART was used in the treatment of ovarian cancer but this method has been largely replaced with newer chemotherapy to allow for less toxicity. There has been a recent resurgence in the technique, which is used for consolidation for selected patients following maximum surgical resection and adjuvant chemotherapy at some institutions. WART is also an option for consolidative treatment for patients with minimal residual disease following surgical resection. WART is typically performed with external beam radiation therapy using anterior and posterior beams. The borders of the field include above the domes of the diaphragm superiorly, below the obturator foramen inferiorly, and covering the peritoneal reflection laterally. The dose to the field is 30 Gy in 1.2–1.5-Gy fractions to the abdominal field with a para-aortic region boost to 45 Gy and pelvis boost to 45–55 Gy.

Cross-References

▶ Carcinoma of the Fallopian Tube

▶ Ovary

Whole Breast Radiation

David E. Wazer
Radiation Oncology Department, Tufts Medical Center, Tufts University School of Medicine, Boston, MA, USA
Radiation Oncology Department, Rhode Island Hospital, Brown University School of Medicine, Providence, RI, USA

Definition

Whole breast radiation is the treatment of all ipsilateral breast tissue with external beam irradiation utilizing a conventional or hypofractionated treatment scheme.

Cross-References

Wilm's Tumor

LARRY C. DAUGHERTY[1], BRANDON J. FISHER[2]
[1]Department of Radiation Oncology, College of Medicine, Drexel University, Glenside, PA, USA
[2]Department of Radiation Oncology, College of Medicine, Drexel University, Philadelphia, PA, USA

Synonyms

Nephroblastoma

Definition/Description

Wilm's tumor (WT) is a cancerous tumor of the kidney seen in children. The term was originally coined by Dr. Ebenezer Gairdner in 1828, and the tumor was named after Max Wilms, who first described the tumor. Wilm's tumor arises from the nephroblasts.

Background

Wilm's tumor is the most common malignant renal tumor in children. The annual incidence is 7 cases per million children younger than 15 years of age, which translates to approximately 450 new cases in the USA annually. WT constitutes 6–7% of all childhood cancers in the USA. The peak incidence is between 3 and 4 years of age, with 75% of the cases occurring before the age of 5. WT affects both male and female children equally. The majority of children have a favorable histologic pattern and 4% have an unfavorable, anaplastic WT.

Wilm's tumor may arise as a sporadic or hereditary tumor (often in children with specific genetic disorders). Most WTs are solitary lesions but may also be multifocal within a single kidney in 12% and bilateral in 7%.

Genetics may also play a strong role in the development of WT. The most common genetic changes implicated in the development of WT is the *WT1* gene, which is a tumor-suppressor gene at chromosome 11p13. *WT1* is likely to play a specific role in glomerular and gonadal development; however, it can also cause abnormal cell growth. Germ-line *WT1* mutations are observed in approximately 82% of WT patients who have genitourinary anomalies or renal failure. The frequency of *WT1* mutations in sporadic and familial WT is much lower, at about 20% and 4%, respectively. ▶ Beckwith–Wiedemann syndrome maps to chromosome 11p15.5; this locus is also referred to as *WT2*. Patients with loss of heterozygosity on 16q and 1p have a worse prognosis with higher relapse and mortality rates.

Initial Evaluation

Diagnosis and evaluation of WT should begin with a thorough history and physical examination. Special attention should be paid to specific disease-related signs and symptoms. The most common presentation for WT is a healthy

W

child with abdominal swelling, discovered by the child's mother or by a physician. Physical examination typically reveals a smooth, firm mass on one side of the abdomen, which is generally nontender to palpation. Gross hematuria occurs in roughly 25% of these cases. The child may be hypertensive due to catecholamine release or have nonspecific symptoms such as malaise or fever. Symptoms of metastases are rare; however, the child can present with shortness of breath or other symptoms of more advanced disease.

Syndromes associated with WT include ▶ WAGR syndrome (WT, aniridia, genitourinary malformations, mental retardation), ▶ Denys-Drash syndrome (pseudohermaphroditism, mesangial sclerosis, renal failure, and WT), and overgrowth syndromes like Beckwith–Wiedemann syndrome (somatic gigantism, omphalocele, macroglossia, genitourinary abnormalities, ear creases, hypoglycemia, hemihypertrophy, and a predisposition to WT and other malignancies) and Simpson-Golabi-Behmel syndrome.

Surgical staging is necessary; however, a closed biopsy is not indicated unless the tumor is unresectable or bilateral. Diagnosis and staging of Wilm's tumor are based on histopathological specimens.

Wilm's Tumor. Table 1 Children's oncology group staging of Wilm's tumor, rhabdoid tumor, and clear cell sarcoma of the kidney (Brady et al. 2008)

Stage I	Tumor limited to one kidney, which was completely resected. Renal capsule is intact. No tumor rupture, and vessels of the renal sinuses are not involved. Lymph nodes examined
Stage II	The tumor is completely resected and there is no tumor at or beyond the margins. Or the tumor extends beyond the kidney with any one of the following:, as evidenced by any one of the following criteria:
	• Regional extension of the tumor (i.e., penetration of the renal capsule or extensive invasion of the soft tissue of the renal sinus, as discussed later) is present
	• Blood vessels within the nephrectomy specimen outside the renal parenchyma, including those of the renal sinus, contain tumor
Stage III	Residual nonhematogenous tumor present after surgery and confined to abdomen. Any one of the following may occur:
	• Lymph nodes within the abdomen or pelvis are involved by tumor
	• Penetrated through the peritoneal surface
	• Implants are found on the peritoneal surface
	• Gross or microscopic tumor remains postoperatively
	• The tumor is not completely resectable because of local infiltration into vital structures
	• Tumor spillage
	• The tumor was biopsied before removal
	• The tumor is removed in more than one piece
Stage IV	Hematogenous metastases (such as lung, liver, bone, brain) or lymph node metastases outside the abdominopelvic region are present. (The presence of tumor within the adrenal gland is not interpreted as metastasis, and staging depends on all other staging parameters being present.)
Stage V	Bilateral renal involvement by tumor is present at diagnosis

Wilm's Tumor. Table 2 Children's oncology group risk group classifications for favorable histology Wilm's tumors (Brady et al. 2008)

Age (years)	Tumor weight (g)	Stage	LOH (both 1p and 16q)	Risk group	COG study	Treatment
<2	<550	I	Any	Very Low	AREN0532	Surgery only
Any	≥550	I	None	Low	AREN0532	EE4A
≥2	Any	I	None	Low	AREN0532	EE4A
Any	Any	II	None	Low	AREN0532	EE4A
≥2	Any	I	Yes	Standard	AREN0532	DD4A
Any	≥550	I	Yes	Standard	AREN0532	DD4A
Any	Any	II	Yes	Standard	AREN0532	DD4A
Any	Any	III	None	Standard	AREN0532	DD4A
Any	Any	III	Yes	Higher	AREN0533	M
Any	Any	IV	Yes	Higher	AREN0533	M
Any	Any	IV	None	Standard	AREN0533	DD4A
Any	Any	IV	None	Higher	AREN0533	M

LOH loss of heterozygosity, *N/A* not applicable, AREN, DD4A (*V* vincristine, *A* dactinomycin, *D* doxorubicin); M (*VAD/Cy* cyclophosphamide, *E* etoposide), EE4A (VA)

Staging

Tumor staging is performed after examining the radiologic, surgical, and histopathologic findings. The Children's Oncology Group (COG) staging guidelines for WT are shown in Table 1. The COG risk group classification protocol for treatment assignment in the new generation of WT protocols is shown in Table 2. In addition to tumor stage, this classification also takes into consideration the patient's age, tumor weight, presence or absence of loss of heterozygosity at 1p and 16q, and response to chemotherapy in children with favorable histology tumors and lung metastases (Table 3).

Differential Diagnosis

Differential diagnoses for WT include neuroblastoma, polycystic kidney disease, rhabdomyosarcoma, hydronephrosis, mesoblastic nephroma, renal cell carcinoma, clear cell sarcoma of the kidney, rhabdoid tumor of the kidney, nonmalignant mass, multicystic kidney disease, renal cyst, renal thrombosis, dysplastic kidney, and renal hemorrhage.

Imaging Studies

Plain films of the abdomen can narrow the differential diagnosis by showing the presence or absence of calcifications. Although calcifications can be present in 5–10% of WT, the presence of calcifications is generally more diagnostic of a neuroblastoma because calcifications are present in at least 70% of those cases.

Ultrasonography is useful because it is readily available and is cost effective. A specific advantage of ultrasonography is its ability to assess vessels for flow and tumor thrombus with duplex and color Doppler.

Abdominal computed tomography (CT) imaging can demonstrate gross extrarenal spread, lymph node involvement, liver metastases, and the status of the opposite kidney. WT is generally spherical, intrarenal, and contains a small amount of fat with or without calcifications.

W

Wilm's Tumor. Table 3 Outline of Children's Oncology Group renal tumor study (Brady et al. 2008)

Tumor risk classification	Multimodality treatment
Very low-risk FH Wilm's tumor	
< 2 year, stage I tumor weight < 550 g	Nephrectomy without adjuvant therapy, if node sampling and central pathological review has been performed.
Low-risk FH Wilm's tumor	
≥2 year, stage I, tumor weight ≥ 550 g, stage II without LOH at 1p and 16q	Nephrectomy, no RT, regimen EE4A
Standard-risk FH Wilm's tumor	
Stages I and II with LOH at 1p and 16q	Nephrectomy, no RT, chemotherapy
Stage III without LOH at 1p and 16q	Nephrectomy, RT, chemotherapy
Stage IV FH: Rapid responders of lung metastases at week 6 with regimen DD4A	Nephrectomy, RT, chemotherapy; no WLI
Higher-risk FH Wilm's tumor	
Stage III with LOH at 1p and 16q	Nephrectomy, RT, chemotherapy
Stage IV slow responders (lung) and nonpulmonary metastases	Nephrectomy, RT, chemotherapy, WLI and RT to metastases
High-risk UH renal tumors	
Stages I–IV focal anaplasia	Nephrectomy, RT, regimen DD 4A
Stage I diffuse anaplasia	
Stages I–III CCSK	Nephrectomy, RT, regimen I
Stages II–IV diffuse anaplasia	Nephrectomy, RT, regimen UH1, RT
Stage IV CCSK	To all metastatic sites
Stages I–IV RTK	

FH favorable histology, *LOH* loss of heterozygosity; RT, flank or abdominal irradiation; regimen EE4A (VA); regimen DD 4A (*V* vincristine, *A* dactinomycin, *D* doxorubicin); *WLI* whole lung irradiation; regimen M (*VAD/Cy* cyclophosphamide, *E* etoposide), *UH* unfavorable histology, *CCSK* clear cell sarcoma of kidney, *RTK* rhabdoid tumor of kidney; regimen I (alternating VDCy/CyE); regimen UH1 (alternating VDCy/CyC [carboplatin] E)

Magnetic resonance imaging (MRI) scans have several advantages over CT scans, especially in identifying renal origin and vascular extension of the tumor. WT typically appears intense on T1-weighted images and hyperintense on T2-weighted images. After administration of contrast, it often appears hypointense in relation to normal renal tissue, further delineating the tumor.

Plain chest radiography and chest CT scans are also essential because asymptomatic pulmonary metastases are common.

Laboratory Studies

A complete blood cell count, including kidney function tests and routine measurements of electrolytes and calcium, and a urinalysis should be performed. Serum blood urea nitrogen and

Wilm's Tumor. Table 4 Children's Oncology Group renal tumor protocol radiation therapy guidelines (Brady et al. 2008)

Abdominal tumor stage and histological appearance	RT dose/RT field
Stages I and II FH Wilm's tumor	None
Stage III FH, stages I–III focal anaplasia, stages I–II diffuse anaplasia, stages I–III CCSK	10.8 Gy to the flank
Stage III diffuse anaplasia, stages I–III RTK	19.8 Gy (infants 10.8 Gy) to the flank, RT
Recurrent abdominal Wilm's tumor	12.6 Gy–18 Gy (< 12 months of age) or 21.6 Gy (older children) if previous radiation dose is ≤10.8 Gy. Boost dose of up to 9 Gy to gross residual tumor after surgery
Lung metastases (favorable histology)	12 Gy WLI in 8 fractions
Lung metastases (unfavorable histology)	12 Gy WLI in 8 fractions
Brain metastases	30.6 Gy whole brain in 17 fractions, or 21.6 Gy whole brain + 10.8 Gy IMRT or stereotactic boost
Liver metastases	19.8 Gy to whole liver in 11 fractions
Bone metastases	25.2 Gy to the lesion plus 3-cm margin
Unresected lymph node metastases	19.8 Gy

CCSK clear cell sarcoma of the kidney, *FH* favorable histology, *IMRT* intensity-modulated RT, *RT* radiation therapy, *RTK* rhabdoid tumor of kidney, *WLI* whole lung irradiation

creatinine levels and liver function tests are routine. If neuroblastoma is not ruled out, a test for urinary catecholamines should be performed. Coagulation studies, as well as cytogenetics studies, assessing 11p13 deletion, 11p15, and *WT1* gene, are appropriate and helpful in the workup.

Treatment

Surgery

Surgery is the treatment of choice. The contralateral kidney should be examined surgically and possibly mobilized to rule out bilateral WT before nephrectomy. The surgeon must excise the entire tumor without spillage or do what is necessary to limit as much spillage as possible. Lymph node sampling of the abdominal and pelvic, para-aortic, celiac, and iliac nodes must be performed. The use of surgical clips to identify the tumor bed, residual tumor, and

margins is typically recommended. Patients with stage I and II with favorable histology are for the most part treated with only postoperative chemotherapy. Patients with stage III disease are treated with chemoradiation. Patients with more advanced, stage IV disease require more extensive chemotherapy and radiation, with abdominal radiation and the possible addition of whole lung irradiation. Physicians are advised to follow a COG protocol for all pediatric patients with WT.

Radiation Therapy

Radiation therapy guidelines used for WT following the COG protocols are shown in Table 4.

Timing of Radiation

Radiation therapy is delivered shortly after surgery; a delay of greater than or equal to 10 days after surgery is associated with a significantly

W

higher abdominal relapse rate. All patients with WT should be scheduled to start radiation therapy no later than day 9, with the day of the surgery being day 0 (Table 4).

Dose

Typically a total of 10 Gy should be prescribed. In the COG protocols, children with stage III anaplastic tumors receive a higher dose of 19.8 Gy (Table 4).

Radiation Therapy Volume

The treatment volumes should encompass the tumor bed and the nephrectomy site with a 2- to 3-cm margin. The medial border must cross the midline to include the entire width of the vertebrae, which will decrease the likelihood of developing scoliosis and its associated morbidity. An abdominal wall shield may be used. When whole abdominal irradiation is used, special care is needed to shield and block out the femoral heads and acetabulum.

Cross-References

► Kidney
► Lung
► Neuroblastoma
► Whole Abdominal Radiation Therapy (WART)

References

Baert AL (2008) Encyclopedia of diagnostic imaging, vol 2. Springer, Berlin/Heidelberg

Brady LW, Lu JJ (eds) (2008) Radiation oncology, an evidence-based approach. Springer, Berlin

Brady LW, Perez CA, Halperin EC (eds) (2008) Principles and practice of radiation oncology, 5th edn. Philadelphia, Lippincott, Williams and Wilkins

Edge SB et al (eds) (2010) Cancer staging handbook, 7th edn. Springer, New York

Hansen EK, Roach M III (eds) (2007) Handbook of evidence-based radiation oncology. Springer, New York

WT1 Gene

LARRY C. DAUGHERTY[1], BRANDON J. FISHER[2]
[1]Department of Radiation Oncology, College of Medicine, Drexel University, Glenside, PA, USA
[2]Department of Radiation Oncology, College of Medicine, Drexel University, Philadelphia, PA, USA

Definition

A tumor suppressor gene located on chromosome 11p13. Mutation in this gene results in ► WAGR or ► Denys Drash syndromes.

Cross-References

► Wilm's Tumor

WT 2 Gene

LARRY C. DAUGHERTY[1], BRANDON J. FISHER[2]
[1]Department of Radiation Oncology, College of Medicine, Drexel University, Glenside, PA, USA
[2]Department of Radiation Oncology, College of Medicine, Drexel University, Philadelphia, PA, USA

Definition

A tumor suppressor gene located on chromosome 11p15. Mutation in this gene results in the ► Beckwith-Wiedemann syndrome.

Cross-References

► Wilm's Tumor

X

Xerostomia

LINDSAY G. JENSEN, LOREN K. MELL
Center for Advanced Radiotherapy Technologies,
Department of Radiation Oncology, San Diego
Rebecca and John Moores Cancer Center,
University of California, La Jolla, CA, USA

Definition
Decreased or absent production of saliva.

Cross-References
► Salivary Gland Cancer
► Sarcomas of the Head and Neck

X-Rays

CHERIE YAEGER
Department Radiation Oncology, Wake Forest
University School of Medicine, Winston-Salem,
NC, USA

Definition
Highly penetrating photons observed in nature and produced in medicine through the interaction of high energy electrons with matter; electromagnetic radiation, similar to gamma rays emitted from radioactive nuclei in characteristics and interaction processes; high-energy ionizing radiation produced medically for diagnostic and therapeutic purposes in medicine.

Discussion
Discovered in 1895 by William Conrad Roentgen, by observing the fluorescence produced when electrons passed through a cathode ray tube, x-rays were soon used in medical facilities to image broken bones.

All rays comprising the electromagnetic spectrum, from low quantum energy radio waves to high quantum energy gamma rays and x-rays, are characterized by wavelength, frequency, and energy as described by Max Planck in 1901. Dependent on their energy is their ability to ionize atoms, which is crucial to understanding their usefulness in medicine as well as their potential danger. Although most photons used for therapy and diagnosis are ionizing, lower-energy nonionizing radiation in the electromagnetic spectrum is also used in medicine for diagnostic and treatment purposes and includes microwaves and radiowaves, in addition to the "optical" radiations, ultraviolet, visible, and infrared.

Nonionizing radiation in the electromagnetic spectrum is produced by the release of light photons and heat (infrared) as the excited electrons in a material or tissue return to their ground state. This process also has the potential to cause cell damage. Exposure to ultraviolet (UV) rays (290–320 nm) from the sun has been linked to skin cancer. Radiofrequency waves (radiowaves), as emanating from cell phones, have been linked to cell alterations, as well as questions concerning their impact on our health from prolonged exposure. The higher quantum energy photons comprising the electromagnetic spectrum, specifically x-rays and gamma rays, are capable of ionization and excitation of the atoms

L.W. Brady, T.E. Yaeger (eds.), *Encyclopedia of Radiation Oncology*, DOI 10.1007/978-3-540-85516-3,
© Springer-Verlag Berlin Heidelberg 2013

comprising cells. The interaction processes are described in detail and include Thompson scattering, photoelectric effect, Compton scattering, and pair production processes. These higher-energy ionizing beams penetrate deep below the skin surface reaching critical organs, damaging tissues and increasing the possibility of complete cellular death as a result. Ionizing radiation is potentially harmful if not used correctly, but is used successfully in medicine to diagnose and treat life-threatening cancers, in addition to numerous other disease processes.

Specifically in medicine, these high-frequency electromagnetic rays used for diagnosis and treatment are produced by three principal interaction processes in matter. When high energy electron beams are accelerated through an electrical potential, the kinetic energy gained is converted to x-rays or electromagnetic radiation upon interaction with nuclei in the target material. If the electron is suddenly decelerated by an atomic nucleus and an x-ray is emitted, this x-ray photon is classically called Bremsstrahlung or "braking radiation." Additionally, emissions of light and heat (infrared radiation) can be produced as these high energy electrons interact with the electrons of the target material. This "excitation" occurs often and is the result of the excited electrons in the shells of the atoms in the target material returning to the ground state after the interaction. High energy electrons can also bombard a target, completely ejecting electrons (ionization) from the shells of the high atomic number nuclei in the target material. This can lead to the remaining electrons of the atom transitioning between shells. Excess energy is released from the shells as an x-ray photon in another classic conversion of kinetic energy to electromagnetic energy. Since the binding energies and, consequently, the chemical or quantum structure is unique for each element, and the electron shell binding energies are specific for particular materials, x-rays created from these electron shell transitions are referred to as characteristic x-rays and their energy is "characteristic" of the atom from which they originated.

X-ray beams produced in modern diagnostic radiology facilities typically range from energies of $35-160 \, kV_p$. These energies are used to produce images of the human body to diagnose injuries and detect physical changes such as calcifications in breast tissue and fractured bones. Observed physical variations may lead to further investigation and/or additional diagnostic or therapeutic procedures. Images obtained in radiology departments are produced by detecting x-rays that pass through the patient without interacting and, indirectly, by those x-rays whose energy is absorbed or scattered in the tissue, thus not capable of reaching the image detector. For medical purposes, high energy x-rays are produced in conventional radiography, fluoroscopy, and computed tomography (CT) imaging equipment. CT requires computer analysis of data and involves analyzing x-rays as they pass through multiple thin slices of the patient and interact with detectors. The contrast between tissues typically results from the energy of the photon produced and its primary interaction process, as well as the differential tissue densities.

Higher-energy x-ray beams produced with linear accelerators in modern radiation therapy centers to treat cancer commonly include lower-energy beams of approximately 4–6 MV and higher-energy beams of approximately 12–20 MV to treat deeper areas of the patient's body. These machines treat benign and cancerous growths, as well as tissues at risk. With sophisticated beam aperture devices and advanced computer algorithms available, users can manipulate the beam such that the radiation beam is precisely focused at the location of the tumor while sparing the adjacent normal tissue. The basis of this technology relies heavily on advanced technologies developed by radiation physicists, as well as increased knowledge of radiation effects by radiation biologists. These processes dictate complex field arrangements and treatment techniques, dose schedules, and total dose as prescribed by a radiation oncologist. The most effective treatments rely on the maturing medical expertise developed from the study of applicable radiation treatment regimens that can lead to maximum cancerous cell death. In turn, this leads to a high-yield tumor control probability (TCP) and the desired outcome for cure of the affected patient.

X-rays are often associated with gamma rays, due to their electromagnetic nature and similar interactions with matter. Gamma rays are emitted from the nucleus of radioactive atoms and their average energy is specific to the radioactive atom of origin. In general, however, comparing one "packet of energy" to another, x-rays and gamma rays differ primarily in their origin site. Gamma rays are used in nuclear medicine departments for traditional planar scans, tomographic images available from single photon emission tomography (SPECT), and positron emission tomography (PET) imaging. For most traditional nuclear medicine procedures, Technetium-99m is the radionuclide of choice and emits a gamma ray of 140 keV. It is often "tagged" chemically to particular molecules designed to reach specific target organs in the patient by injection, ingestion, and/or inhalation. Radiolabeled insoluble particles such as ^{99m}Tc sulfur colloid and ^{99m}Tc macro-aggregated albumin (MAA) (Honda et al. 1970) are frequently used, for example, to image liver and lung tissue, respectively. Technetium-99m is also tagged with molecules of certain functional ability allowing examination of physiological processes. Single photon emission computed tomography (SPECT) is widely used for this purpose as it forms three-dimensional images from gamma rays emitted from the patient. Positron emission tomography (PET) images record two annihilation photons that are emitted after electron-positron annihilation and uses fluorine-18,

a positron-emitting radionuclide. In each case, images are obtained as the gamma rays from inside the patient interact with scintillation material in the gamma camera positioned near the patient to produce light photons. The molecular information obtained from nuclear medicine studies, including single photon emission computed tomography (SPECT) and positron emission tomography (PET) images, provides valuable insights on the organ being investigated and its physiology, unavailable in other diagnostic procedures.

High energy ionizing radiation includes both particulate and electromagnetic radiation originating from radioactive atoms' nuclei and electron shells. These include beta particles, gamma rays, x-rays, neutrons, high energy electrons, high energy protons, and other particles capable of producing ions. Not having electromagnetic characteristics, particulate radiation refers to ionizing radiation with particle-like characteristics of mass and/or charge and includes, in addition to high energy electrons, alpha particles, beta particles, neutrons, and protons. The particulate radiation originating from the nucleus of radioactive atoms include alpha particles, beta particles, neutrons, and protons and are often referred to as nuclear radiation. Although gamma rays originate from the nucleus of radioactive atoms, and are often referred to as nuclear radiation, they are not particulate in nature, having no mass or charge. All types of nuclear radiation are also ionizing radiation, but the reverse is not necessarily true; for example, x-rays are a type of ionizing radiation, but they are not nuclear radiation because they do not originate from atomic nuclei. Compared to non-ionizing photons, such as radiowaves, microwaves, or visible, infrared, or ultraviolet light, x-rays and gamma rays are not only ionizing but considerably more energetic electromagnetic waves.

Particulate radiations are easily attenuated as they pass through matter compared to their high-energy electromagnetic "cousins." They interact with matter primarily through ionization and excitation, as well as through radiative losses, as described in their use to produce high-energy x-ray beams. For example, high-energy electrons can also be used to treat tumors in radiation therapy by removing the high atomic number target in the beam and flattening the beam's intensity across the field in the linear accelerator (Metcalf et al. 2004). All particulate radiations tend to lose their energy over a specified distance with electrons being no exception. Their short range in tissue limits their treatment use to relatively shallow tumors, however, close to or at the skin surface depending on their energy. Energy, mass, charge, and interaction material dictate the path length of particulate radiation in matter as all particulate radiations tend to lose their energy over a specified distance. For example, alpha particles encountered externally, with their increased mass and charge are easily absorbed by a thin piece of paper, but are very dangerous if inhaled as radon gas where the alpha particles can deposit their energy directly in adjacent lung tissue. Beta particles, originating from radioactive nuclei and with similar in characteristics to electron particles, are often used in radiation therapy as sources for brachytherapy, due to their short range and immediate deposition of energy in the tumor where the sources are placed. Varying the input energy of a proton beam, for example, allows for the treatment of a relatively deep-seated tumor where protection is needed before and after the

range of the particle is reached (Palta and Yeung in press). Theoretically, all particulate radiation exhibit Bragg peaks, the depth at which the maximum amount of energy from the particle is absorbed, but the peak for protons is unique clinically. Protons deposit very little energy as they traverse tissue until a specified depth where they release the majority of their energy. Combining different energy protons manipulates the depth to cover the tumor and spares the critical structures encountered before and after the tumor.

Cross-References

▶ Brachytherapy: High Dose Rate (HDR) Implants
▶ Bragg Peak
▶ Linear Accelerators (LINAC)
▶ Low-Dose Rate (LDR) Brachytherapy
▶ Proton Therapy
▶ Radiation Detectors
▶ Radiation Therapy Shielding
▶ Short-Term and Long-Term Health Risk of Nuclear Power Plant Accident

References

Honda T, Kazem T, Croll MN, Yaeger T, Brady LW (1970) Instant labeling of macro and microaggregated albumin with Tc99m. J Nuc Med 10:580–585
Metcalf PE, Kron T, Hoban P (eds) (2004) The physics of radiation therapy X-rays and electrons, 1st edn. Medical Physics, Madison
Palta J, Yeung D. Presicion and uncertainties in proton therapy for non-moving targets. In Pagini (ed) Proton therapy physics (in press)

Y

Yttrium-90

THEODORE E. YAEGER
Department Radiation Oncology, Wake Forest
University School of Medicine, Winston-Salem,
NC, USA

Definition

Radioactive nuclide (atomic number 39) used in
the production of glass spheres intended for transarterial injection into the liver to embolize and
deliver close-proximity, low-energy radiation to
tumors such a hepatocellular cancer or metastases.

Discussion

A low-energy beta emitter delivering 0.936 meV
mean energy and 64.1 h half-life that is currently
available in 81 to 540 mCi doses.

Cross-References

► Brachytherapy
► Liver and Hepatobiliary tract
► Targeted Radioimmunotherapy

References

TheraSphere Y-90 glass microspheres. Nordion Company

Ytterbium-169

THEODORE E. YAEGER
Department Radiation Oncology, Wake Forest
University School of Medicine, Winston-Salem,
NC, USA

Definition

Radioactive nuclide (atomic number 70) which
is an intermediate low-energy photon emitter
delivering about 100 keV energy with a 32 day
half-life. It is considered an experimental
intracavitary brachytherapy source, but an
application for high dose rate delivery is
approved.

Cross-References

► Brachytherapy
► Nuclear Medicine

References

Medich DC, Tries MA, Munro JJ (2006) Monte Carlo
    characterizations of an ytterbium-169 high dose
    rate brachytherapy source with analysis of statistical
    uncertainty. Med Phys 33(10):163–172

L.W. Brady, T.E. Yaeger (eds.), *Encyclopedia of Radiation Oncology*, DOI 10.1007/978-3-540-85516-3,
© Springer-Verlag Berlin Heidelberg 2013

Yolk Sac

THEODORE E. YAEGER
Department Radiation Oncology, Wake Forest University School of Medicine, Winston-Salem, NC, USA

Definition

A nonseminomatous testicular tumor also called an endodermal sinus tumor. It makes up less than 2% of tumors in adults but can make up about 40% of mixed germ-cell tumors. Since almost 80% of yolk-sac tumors occur in the pediatric population (aged less than 2 years) it is important to recognize that 60% of germ cell tumors contain yolk sac elements. Grossly it is a cystic tumor containing gelatinous, hemorrhagic, and necrotic materials. Elevated alpha-fetoprotein and Schiller-Duval bodies are characteristic findings. Typical presentation is a painless swelling of the scrotal sac.

Cross-References

▶ Ovary
▶ Testes

References

Morton GC, Thomas GM (2008) Testis, Chapter 64. In: Perez CA, Brady LW (eds) Principles and practice of radiation oncology, 5th edn. Lippincott Williams and Williams, Philadelphia, pp 1503–1518

Z

Zevalin

THEODORE E. YAEGER
Department Radiation Oncology, Wake Forest
University School of Medicine, Winston-Salem,
NC, USA

Definition

A radiolabeled monoclonal antibody covalently attached to the chelated tiuxetan and bound to Yttrium-90. It is designed as a targeted radio-antibody for the CD-20 receptor commonly found on normal and malignant B-cell lympho-cytes. Treating lymphoma is allowed by CD-20 receptor attachments that are expressed on 90+ % of non-Hodgkin's cells. The action is a "cross fire" effect with a range up to 5 mm that causes free-radical formation in the target population as well as neighboring cells (bystander effect) to damage essential genetic components and thus inducing cell apoptosis.

Cross-References

► Nuclear Medicine
► Targeted Radioimmunotherapy

References

Witzig TE, Gordon LI et al (2002) Randomized controlled trial of yttrium-90-labeled Ibritumomab tiuxetan radioimmunotherapy versus Rituximab immunother-apy for patients with relapsed or refractory low-grade, follicular or transformed B-cell non-Hodgkin's lym-phoma. J Clin Oncol 20:2453–2463

Zoledronic Acid

THEODORE E. YAEGER
Department Radiation Oncology, Wake Forest
University School of Medicine, Winston-Salem,
NC, USA

Definition

A bisphosphonate therapy to reduce the number and duration of skeletal events associated with metastatic disease, primarily for prostate and breast cancers. It is also used to reduce hypercal-cemia associated with malignancy.

Cross-References

► Lung Cancer
► Prostate
► Stage 0 Breast Cancer

References

Ross JR, Saunders Y et al (2004) A systemic review of the role of bisphosphonate in metastatic disease. Health Technol Assess 8:1–176

L.W. Brady, T.E. Yaeger (eds.), *Encyclopedia of Radiation Oncology*, DOI 10.1007/978-3-540-85516-3,
© Springer-Verlag Berlin Heidelberg 2013

Zycomycosis

THEODORE E. YAEGER
Department Radiation Oncology, Wake Forest
University School of Medicine, Winston-Salem,
NC, USA

Definition

A skin infection commonly appearing as a black
eschar seen on the lining of the nasal mucosa, soft
palate, or skin, such as the nasal bridge. It can
have an appearance similar to a pigmented cancer
lesion such as melanoma or basal cell carcinoma.

An opportunistic infection diagnosis should
always be considered before embarking on
empiric topical radiotherapy, especially in
patients with immunosuppression diseases.

Cross-References

▶ Principles of Chemotherapy
▶ Skin Cancer

References

Safdar N, Crnich CJ, Maki DG (2006) Infectious complications of cancer therapy. In: Chang AE (ed) Oncology,
an evidenced based approach, chapter 76. Springer,
Berlin, pp 1363–1400

List of Entries